Date Due

WOMEN'S DERMATOLOGY
From Infancy to Maturity

WOMEN'S DERMATOLOGY
From Infancy to Maturity

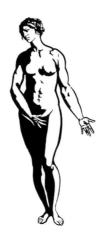

Edited by

Lawrence Charles Parish, MD

Clinical Professor of Dermatology and Cutaneous Biology, Jefferson Medical College;
and Director of the Jefferson Center for International Dermatology,
Thomas Jefferson University, Philadelphia, Pennsylvania, USA

Sarah Brenner, MD

Head, Department of Dermatology, Tel Aviv Sourasky Medical Center, Ichilov Hospital;
and Clinical Associate Professor of Dermatology, Sackler School of Medicine,
Tel Aviv University, Tel Aviv, Israel

and

Marcia Ramos-e-Silva, MD, PhD

Associate Professor of Dermatology, School of Medicine and HUCFF-UFRJ,
Federal University of Rio de Janeiro, Rio de Janeiro, Brazil

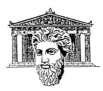

The Parthenon Publishing Group
International Publishers in Medicine, Science & Technology

NEW YORK   LONDON

Library of Congress Cataloging-in-Publication Data
Women's dermatology: from infancy to maturity/
  edited by Lawrence Charles Parish, Sarah
Brenner, and Marcia Ramos-e-Silva.
    p.; cm.
Includes bibliographical references and index.
ISBN 1-85070-086-9
1. Dermatology. 2. Women–Diseases.
3. Skin–Diseases. 4. Women–Health and hygiene.
5. Skin–Aging. I. Parish, Lawrence Charles. II.
Brenner, Sarah. III. Ramos-e-Silva, Marcia.
    [DNLM: 1. Skin Diseases. 2. Age Factors.
3. Sex Factors. 4. Skin Physiology.
5. Women's Health. WR 140 2000]
RL73.W65 W66 2000
616.5'0082–dc21
                                        00-038518

British Library Cataloguing in Publication Data
Women's dermatology: from infancy to maturity
    1. Dermatology 2. Skin - Diseases
    3. Women - Health and hygiene
    I. Parish, Lawrence Charles II. Brenner, Sarah
    III. Ramos-e-Silva, Marcia
    616.5'0082

    ISBN 1850700869

Published in the UK and Europe by
The Parthenon Publishing Group Limited
Casterton Hall, Carnforth
Lancs., LA6 2LA, UK

Published in the USA by
The Parthenon Publishing Group Inc.
One Blue Hill Plaza
PO Box 1564, Pearl River
NY 10965, USA

Copyright © 2001 The Parthenon Publishing Group

Typeset by Siva Math Setters, Chennai, India
Printed by T.G. Hostench S.A., Spain

Contents

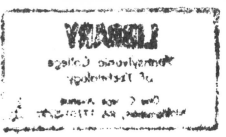

List of contributors

John Adam, MD, FRCP(C)
Professor of Medicine (Dermatology)
University of Ottawa Faculty of Medicine
Ottawa
Ontario
Canada

Sarah Bakewell, MA, MSc
Assistant Curator
Early Printed Books
Wellcome Library for the History and
    Understanding of Medicine
London
England

Robert Baran, MD
Head of the Dermatology Unit
General Hospital
Cannes
France

Anthony V. Benedetto, DO
Clinical Associate Professor of Dermatology
MCP Hahnemann University
    School of Medicine
Philadelphia
Pennsylvania
USA

Michelle L. Bennett, MD
Resident in Dermatology
Wake Forest University School of Medicine
Winston-Salem
North Carolina
USA

Wilma F. Bergfeld, MD
Senior Dermatologist and Head of the
    Section of Clinical Research
Cleveland Clinic Foundation
Cleveland
Ohio
USA

Kazal Rekha Bhowmik, MBBS
Research Associate
Paddington Testing Company Inc
Philadelphia
Pennsylvania
USA

Narayan Krishna Bhowmik, MBBS
Physician
Ibrahim Memorial Hospital
BIRDEM
Shahbagh
Dhaka
Bangladesh

Anat Bialy-Golan, MD
Dermatologist
Tel Aviv Sourasky Medical Center
Ichilov Hospital
Tel Aviv
Israel

Beatrice Bianchi, PhD
Assistant Professor of Dermatology
University of Florence
Florence
Italy

Martin M. Black, MD, FRCP, FRCPath
Honorary Consultant Dermatologist
St John's Institute of Dermatology
St Thomas' Hospital
London
England

Maria Blaszczyk, MD
Professor of Dermatology
Warsaw School of Medicine
Warsaw
Poland

Tanya O. Bleiker, MRCP
Specialist Registrar in Dermatology
The Leicester Royal Infirmary
Leicester
England

Susan Boiko, MD
Assistant Voluntary Professor of Pediatrics
University of California School of
    Medicine at San Diego
San Diego
California
USA

Sarah Brenner, MD
Head, Department of Dermatology
Tel Aviv Sourasky Medical Center
Ichilov Hospital
Clinical Associate Professor of Dermatology
Sackler School of Medicine
Tel Aviv University
Tel Aviv
Israel

Vincenzina Bruni, MD
Associate Professor of Obstetrics and
    Gynecology and Director of the Service of
    Pediatric and Adolescent Gynecology
University of Florence
Florence
Italy

Stella D. Calobrisi, MD
Assistant Professor of Dermatology
Mayo Clinic/Mayo Medical School
Rochester
Minnesota
USA

Michael Camilleri, MD, MRCP(UK)
Fellow in Dermatology
Mayo Clinic
Rochester
Minnesota
USA

Tania Ferreira Cestari, MD, PhD
Associate Professor of Dermatology
Federal University of Rio Grande do Sul
Porto Alegre
Brazil

Hyun-Joo Choi, MD
Instructor in Dermatology
Yonsei University College of Medicine
Seoul
Korea

Hae-Shin Chung, MD
Instructor in Dermatology
Yonsei University College of Medicine
Seoul
Korea

W. Patrick Coleman IV, BA
Medical Student
Tulane University School of Medicine
New Orleans
Louisiana
USA

Claudio Comacchi, MD
Assistant Professor of Dermatology
University of Florence
Florence
Italy

John A. Cotterill, MD, BSc, FRCP
Consultant Dermatologist and
    Medical Director
Lasercare Clinics
Leeds
England

Paul C. Cotterill, MD
Lecturer in Dermatology
University of Toronto Faculty of Medicine
Toronto
Ontario
Canada

J Carl Craft, MD
Head, Anti-Infective Ventures
Abbott Laboratories
Abbott Park
Illinois
USA

Mariarosaria D'Avino, MD
Dermatologist
Second University of Naples
Naples
Italy

Zoe Diana Draelos, MD
Clinical Associate Professor of
    Dermatology
Wake Forest University School of Medicine
Winston-Salem
North Carolina
USA

Nurimar Conceição Fernandes, MD, PhD
Associate Professor of Dermatology
School of Medicine and HUCFF-UFRJ
Federal University of Rio de Janeiro
Rio de Janeiro
Brazil

Timothy Corcoran Flynn, MD
Associate Professor of Dermatology &
    Otolaryngology – Head and Neck Surgery
Tulane University School of Medicine
New Orleans
Louisiana
USA

Derek Freedman, MD
Genito-Urinary Physician
St James's Hospital
Dublin
Ireland

Ilaria Ghersetich, MD
Assistant Professor of Dermatology
University of Florence
Florence
Italy

Dee Anna Glaser, MD
Professor and Acting-Chairman of
    Dermatology
St. Louis University School of Medicine
St. Louis
Missouri
USA

Robin A. C. Graham-Brown, BSc, MB, FRCP
Consultant Dermatologist
The Leicester Royal Infirmary
Leicester
England

Jean-Pierre Hachem, MD
Resident in Dermatology
Free University of Brussels (AZ-VUB)
Brussels
Belgium

Seung-Kyung Hann, MD
Clinical Professor of Dermatology
Yonsei University College of Medicine
Seoul
Korea

Doris Maria Hexsel, MD
Dermatologist
Porto Alegre
Brazil

Maria-Teresa Hojyo-Tomoka, MD
Dermatologist
Hospital General Gea González
Mexico City
Mexico

Stefania Jablonska, MD
Professor of Dermatology
Warsaw School of Medicine
Warsaw
Poland

Jivko A. Kamarashev, MD
Assistant Professor of Dermatology and
    Venereology

Medical University of Sofia
Sofia
Bulgaria

Ana Kaminsky, MD
Professor of Dermatology
University of Buenos Aires
Buenos Aires
Argentina

Paula Karam, MD
Dermatologist
St George Hospital
Beirut
Lebanon

Alexander C. Katoulis, MD
Dermatologist-Venereologist,
'A. Sygros' Hospital
Athens
Greece

Andreas D. Katsambas, MD
Associate Professor of Dermatology and
    Venereology
National University of Athens
Athens
Greece

Caroline S. Koblenzer, MD
Professor of Dermatology and
    Cutaneous Biology
Jefferson Medical College of
    Thomas Jefferson University
Philadelphia
Pennsylvania
USA

Marina Landau, MD
Dermatologist
Tel Aviv Sourasky Medical Center
Ichilov Hospital
Lecturer in Dermatology
Sackler School of Medicine
Tel Aviv University
Tel Aviv
Israel

Karolina M. Leonik, MD, MPH
Assistant Professor of Infant, Child, and
    Adolescent Psychiatry
Louisiana State University
    School of Medicine
New Orleans
Louisiana
USA

Marilyn G. Liang, MD
Resident in Dermatology
Mayo Clinic/Mayo Medical School
Rochester
Minnesota
USA

Torello M. Lotti, MD
Associate Professor of Dermatology
Director of the Dermatological
    Physiopathology Unit
University of Florence
Florence
Italy

Visiting Associate Professor of
    Dermatology and Cutaneous Biology
Jefferson Medical College of
    Thomas Jefferson University
Philadelphia
Pennsylvania
USA

Mary P. Lupo, MD
Assistant Professor of Dermatology
Tulane University School of Medicine
New Orleans
Louisiana
USA

Leonardo Magnani, MD
Specialist in Obstetrics and Gynecology
University of Florence
Florence
Italy

Amy J. McMichael, MD
Assistant Professor of Dermatology
Wake Forest University School of Medicine
Winston-Salem
North Carolina
USA

Aryeh Metzker, MD
Dermatologist
Tel Aviv Sourasky Medical Center
Ichilov Hospital

Assistant Professor of Dermatology
Sackler School of Medicine
Tel Aviv University
Tel Aviv
Israel

Barukh Mevorah, MD
Dermatologist
Tel Aviv Sourasky Medical Center
Ichilov Hospital

Assistant Professor of Dermatology
Sackler School of Medicine
Tel Aviv University
Tel Aviv
Israel

Larry E. Millikan, MD
Professor and Chairman of Dermatology
Tulane University School of Medicine
New Orleans
Louisiana
USA

Tomasz F. Mroczkowski, MD
Research Professor of Dermatology
    and Venereology
Tulane University School of Medicine

Director, Clinical Research Division
Section of Infectious Diseases
Louisiana State University School of Medicine
New Orleans
Louisiana
USA

Marianne N. O'Donoghue, MD
Associate Professor of Dermatology
Rush University College of Medicine
Chicago
Illinois
USA

Oumeish Youssef Oumeish, MD, FRCP(*Glasg*)
Consultant Dermatologist
Amman Clinic
Amman
Jordan

Visiting Professor of Dermatology
Tulane University School of Medicine
New Orleans
Louisiana
USA

Joseph L. Pace, MD, FRCP(*Edin*), FRCP(*Lond*)
Dermatologist
St Philips Hospital
Santa Venera
Malta

Visiting Professor
Dermatology and Cutaneous Biology
Jefferson Medical College of
    Thomas Jefferson University
Philadelphia
Pennsylvania
USA

Evangelia Papadavid, MD
Dermatologist
'A. Sygros' Hospital
Athens
Greece

Lawrence Charles Parish, MD
Clinical Professor of Dermatology and
    Cutaneous Biology
Jefferson Medical College
Director of the Jefferson Center for
    International Dermatology
Thomas Jefferson University
Philadelphia
Pennsylvania
USA

Neal Penneys, MD, PhD
Professor and Past-Chairman of
    Dermatology
St. Louis University School of Medicine
St. Louis
Missouri
USA

Yael Politi, MD
Dermatologist
Tel Aviv Sourasky Medical Center
Ichilov Hospital
Tel Aviv
Israel

Marcia Ramos-e-Silva, MD, PhD
Associate Professor of Dermatology
School of Medicine and HUCFF-UFRJ
Federal University of Rio de Janeiro
Rio de Janeiro
Brazil

Roy S. Rogers III, MD
Professor of Dermatology
Mayo Clinic/Mayo Medical School
Rochester
Minnesota
USA

Sarah C. F. Rogers, MSc, FRCP(*Lond*),
    FRCPI, FRCP(*Edin*)
Consultant Dermatologist and
    Clinical Lecturer
St. Vincent's University Hospital
Dublin
Ireland

Diane Roseeuw, MD, PhD
Professor of Dermatology
Free University of Brussels (AZ-VUB)
Brussels
Belgium

Hirak Behari Routh, MBBS
Senior Research Associate
Paddington Testing Company Inc
Philadelphia
Pennsylvania
USA

Eleonora Ruocco, MD
Dermatologist
Second University of Naples
Naples
Italy

Vincenzo Ruocco, MD
Professor and Chairman of Dermatology
Second University of Naples
Naples
Italy

Marcio Rutowitsch, MD, PhD
Head of Dermatology
Hospital dos Servidores do
    Estado-HSE/RJ
Rio de Janeiro
Brazil

E. Joy Schulz, MD, MMed(Derm)
Professor and Chairman of Dermatology
University of Witwatersrand
Johannesburg
South Africa

Elizabeth F. Sherertz, MD
Professor of Dermatology
Wake Forest University School of Medicine
Winston-Salem
North Carolina
USA

Rodney D. Sinclair, MBBS
Senior Lecturer in Dermatology
St. Vincent's Hospital
Melbourne
Australia

Elizabeth A. Spenceri, MD
Resident in Dermatology
St. Louis University School of Medicine
St. Louis
Missouri
USA

John D. Stratigos, MD
Emeritus Professor of Dermatology and
    Venereology
National University of Athens
Chairman of the Board of the Hellenic
    Center for the Control of AIDS and STDS
Athens
Greece

Susan Swiggum, MD, FRCP(C)
Professor of Medicine (Dermatology)
University of Ottawa Faculty of Medicine
Ottawa
Ontario
Canada

Beatriz Moritz Trope, MD, MSc
Dermatologist
University Hospital Clementino Fraga Filho
Federal University of Rio de Janeiro
Rio de Janeiro
Brazil

Rebecca C. Tung, MD
Resident in Dermatology
Cleveland Clinic Foundation
Cleveland
Ohio
USA

Ethel Tur, MD
Dermatologist
Tel Aviv Sourasky Medical Center
Ichilov Hospital
Professor of Dermatology
Sackler School of Medicine
Tel Aviv University
Tel Aviv
Israel

Walter P. Unger, MD, FRCP(C)
Assistant Professor of Dermatology
University of Toronto Faculty of Medicine
Toronto
Ontario
Canada

Snejina G. Vassileva, MD, PhD
Assistant Professor of Dermatology and
    Venereology
Medical University of Sofia
Sofia
Bulgaria

Samantha A. Vaughan Jones, MD, MRCP
Honorary Consultant Dermatologist
St John's Institute of Dermatology
St Thomas' Hospital
London
England

María-Elisa Vega-Memije, MD
Dermatologist
Hospital General Gea González
Mexico City
Mexico

Martin S. Wade, BMedSci, MBBS
Research Fellow in Dermatology
St. Vincent's Hospital
Melbourne
Australia

Daniel Wallach, MD
Dermatologist
Hôpital Tarnier
Paris
France

León M. Waxtein, MD
Dermatologist
Hospital General Gea González
Mexico City
Mexico

Joseph A. Witkowski, MD
Clinical Professor of Dermatology
University of Pennsylvania
    School of Medicine
Philadelphia
Pennsylvania
USA

Ronni Wolf, MD
Dermatologist
Tel Aviv Sourasky Medical Center
Ichilov Hospital
Assistant Professor of Dermatology
Sackler School of Medicine
Tel Aviv University
Tel Aviv
Israel

Preface

Lawrence Charles Parish, Sarah Brenner and Marcia Ramos-e-Silva

---

*Little boys are made of
snips and snails
and puppy dog tails.*

*Little girls are made of
sugar and spice
and everything nice.*

INTRODUCTION

This book has been conceived as a study of both normal and pathologic skin, as it may concern the female patient. While there has always been an undercurrent of belief in dermatology that skin diseases may vary between the sexes, to the best of our knowledge no extensive study of the gender difference exists. There have been treatises on cutaneous medicine directed towards regions and climates[1], organ systems of the body[2], or even skin manifestations of internal disease[3]. A major symposium, entitled 'Dermatologic disease and the problems of women through the life cycle'[4], edited by one of us (SB) appropriately introduces the status:

> Society has always drawn a distinction between men and women, male and female. This distinction stems as much from the biologic differences between the sexes as from their different social roles, places, and status in society. In the documentation of history, women have generally been omitted, their participation in family, work, religion, and public life made invisible as they were overshadowed by and subordinated to men. With the emergence of the women's movement, two concepts have guided the interpretation of women's place as well as the movement for social change: equality and difference[5].

THE ORIGIN OF WOMEN

Gender difference began with Creation when woman was created separate from man – first came man and from his rib came woman; and by offering the apple to man came knowledge. Since ancient times, this difference has permitted women to be treated as unequal. The most glaring example of this inequality is cloaked in biblical terms: a girl is the property of her father and at marriage this woman becomes her husband's chattel. Subsequent history has shown variations on this theme, at least until the last century with the development of the women's movement.

There can be little wonder that the social, economic and political subordination of women also found its expression in health care. Although the belief that smooth, clear skin in women is a sign of beauty, both inner and outer, the health care of such skin merited no different consideration from men by physicians.

CURRENT PROBLEMS

We can only speculate as to why more attention has not been given to the subject of gender, particularly in dermatology. At a time in the development of dermatology a century ago, etiology and morphologic descriptions were often embellished with comments about race, color, creed and social status. A possible explanation has been suggested.

> Male ideas remain present, not only in the dominant medical discourse but in society at large, which was after all organized according to an unequal sexual system. Male concerns also pervaded most source material for the study of female culture since rare glimpses into the 'private' world of women's everyday life are often only afforded the historian when contemporary male figures of authority like policemen, lawyers or journalists had scrutinized female figures in the first place. Specifically, female forms of health care were, moreover, not necessarily used to the exclusion of more conventional methods like consulting a doctor[6].

The book is meant to explore the dermatologic gender differences that entitle girls and women to gender-specific health care measures. If the skin of men and women differs in ways that impact upon how they should be treated medically, those differences demand recognition. Medical professionals have always looked at age, and sometimes even socio-economic differences, in the pursuit of better diagnostic and treatment modalities. Why not gender? The Editors of this volume hope that this book will encourage the health care community to evaluate the similarities and differences in order to bring us closer to rectifying millennia of inequity.

DEVELOPMENT OF THE TEXT

Contributors were invited from around the world to develop chapters in their areas of expertise. They were asked to examine their assignments from the point of view of gender variations. Ostensibly, the question would be whether the condition was more prevalent or different in a girl or woman. It would appear that this is easier said than done owing to the fact that the relevant data were often unavailable; there were, in addition, occasions when it became necessary to discuss skin diseases that showed no preference between the sexes, and a comparison could then be made between similar conditions affecting both men and women.

Although we attempted to be as inclusive as reasonably possible, there may be certain omissions – our intention has not been to cover every aspect of dermatology. In addition, the organization of any text of medicine, and particularly dermatology, must allow for overlap. Nomenclature and classifications create such overlaps, resulting in diseases being discussed in more than one section. Therapeutic recommendations may vary according to the authors of the various chapters.

ACKNOWLEDGEMENTS

We wish to thank Ms Carmela Ciferni, Philadelphia, for assisting in developing the project and Dr Hirak Behari Routh, Philadelphia, for reviewing the manuscripts. In particular, our deepest appreciation goes to Nat Russo, Parthenon Publishing, for seeing this project through to fruition.

REFERENCES

1. Parish LC, Millikan LE. *Global Dermatology: Diagnosis and Management According to Geography, Climate and Culture*. New York: Springer-Verlag, 1994:1–359
2. Parish LC, Kauh YC, Luscombe HA. *Color Atlas of Difficult Diagnoses in Dermatology*. New York: Igaku-Shoin, 1993:1–144
3. Braverman IM. *Skin Signs of Systemic Disease*. Philadelphia: WB Saunders, 1998:1–682
4. Brenner S. Dermatologic disease and the problems of women through the life cycle. *Clin Dermatol* 1997; 15:1–178
5. Brenner S. Commentary. *Clin Dermatol* 1997;15:1–3
6. Blécourt WE, Usborne C. Women's medicine, women's culture: abortion and fortune-telling in early twentieth-century Germany and the Netherlands. *Med Hist* 1999;43:376–92

Foreword

Ana Kaminsky

Writing the foreword of a book is not an easy task, especially when the individual chapters are written by a large number of distinguished professionals in world dermatology who, in turn, represent many countries and diverse cultures. Being acquainted with many of these individual authors and with their merits, I realize that a global understanding of the book will be required, mainly as we are in the presence of a work written with an original focus: 'Women's Dermatology'. I am not aware of the existence of any other text having undertaken a similar approach.

GENDER DIFFERENCES

Although skin diseases can be observed in both sexes, there are certain pathologies that show gender differences. The structure and function of the skin of women, the hormonal influences, socio-cultural factors, and psycho-social aspects can act as determining factors of such differences. No single detail has been neglected in the content of this book, with most dermatologic subjects being covered, including the significant topographic aspects, i.e. diseases of the breast, oral lesions, and disorders of the perineal region and vulva.

The text begins with a description of the various phases of female sexual development, from the newborn through adulthood. These include the changes that take place in the genitals during puberty and during the fertile periods. Guidelines are given for the gynecological examination, particularly of the doctor–patient relationship. Special female conditions are highlighted: menstruation, menopause, pregnancy, and the difficult and complex subject of drug selection during pregnancy, i.e. their benefits and risks, emphasizing the hard responsibility of making a selection.

HIGHLIGHTS

Several chapters are unique in their approach, particularly those related to the cultural attributes of women. The diversity of ethnic backgrounds and geographical variations add to the complexity of many cutaneous problems. Such a different and wide vision of dermatology must also encompass present world conditions and the net increase in population, particularly in the poorer countries, a situation that has given rise to a true pathology of poverty. This is not only as a result of diseases related to malnutrition, but also to those connected with the environment, as a consequence of living with promiscuity and in surroundings where primary needs and adequate hygienic conditions are lacking.

I find the reference to expatriate women especially interesting, as it discusses the problems of migrant women and their lives as part of ethnic minorities, with their traditions, language and religious beliefs, in the new countries or areas where they settle. The description of conditions which are seldom, if ever, incorporated in textbooks, such as the dermatological cultural attributes of African and African-American girls and women, their ethnic characteristics, their skin, hair and nails will be very helpful for a greater understanding of the patients, and help to establish better doctor–patient relationships which may contribute to improve compliance. The same comment is applicable to the description of beauty and culture of Arab, Korean, Caucasian, Indian, and Native American women.

The chapter discussing battered women and children stresses the importance of this real problem which does not recognize social, cultural, racial, religious or geographical boundaries. The unfortunately frequent cases of sexual abuse, rape and their psychological and medical impact and sexual abuse in children, are covered in all their facets. Other important and often neglected issues which are covered in *Women's Dermatology* include transvestism, transsexualism and gender dysphoria, a description of which may awaken the urge of dermatologists to render some form of needed assistance. Tobacco, alcohol and drug addiction and their consequences on the skin, anogenital cancer, psoriasis in the immunodeficiency syndrome, etc., are terrible problems of our time. These are also very carefully treated in this interesting book.

In the last few decades, the increasing inclusion of women in the social, political and labor environment has determined a growing demand for skin care treatments, which, after all, reflect ones' image in society. The improvement of the physical aspect, through medical or surgical methods, allows many women to strengthen their self-esteem and attain confidence in facing the challenge of entering and competing in a world previously reserved exclusively to men. These aspects are well thought-out and planned in this book which also covers the study, treatment and prevention of aging of the skin, solar damage, and the role of cosmetics in the improvement and embellishment of the skin, hair, and nails.

CONCLUSIONS

The editors have created a comprehensive text-book on the subject of women's dermatology. The contributors have followed the guidelines set forth and have carefully written their chapters, providing excellent illustrations which highlight the special characteristics of female skin physiology and pathology. This book will be of great importance not only to dermatologists but also to primary care physicians. It should provide the stimulus for the medical community to recognize and understand the differences between men and women.

Background

The skin of girls and women throughout the ages

Sarah Bakewell

INTRODUCTION

'Girls, learn from me what treatment will embellish your complexions, how beauty is best preserved'[1]. So begins the surviving fragment of Ovid's poem *On facial treatment for ladies*, composed around 15 or 20 BCE. The verses that follow reflect wryly on women's vanity and then go on to describe a number of remedies for feminine skin problems. Spots can be removed using a 'halcyon-cream' extracted from birds' nests, while any woman who uses his recommended face-pack of barley, powdered hartshorn, narcissus bulbs and honey 'will shine brighter than her own/Mirror'. The same effect can be achieved by using lupin seeds, fried beans, white lead, essence of red natron, and Illyrian iris – all 'ground/By energetic young boys'. One cannot help wondering whether it was the lotion itself or the thought of the energetic boys that made the ladies' faces shine so brightly.

ANCIENT REMEDIES

The importance of caring for the skin and treating its minor and major ailments was recognized long before Ovid's day. A healthy skin was perceived not just as a functional covering for the body, or even as an indicator of general well-being, but as the essence of beauty itself. As such, it was of particular concern to women, for whom – as a much later writer saw it – 'beauty is a duty'[2]. In the words of another nineteenth-century author, female skin 'not merely acts as an organ of sense, and a protection to the surface of the body, but it clothes it, as it were, in a garment of the most delicate texture, and of the most surpassing loveliness'. Although strong and resistant to injury, the feminine skin also 'possesses the softness of velvet, and exhibits the delicate hues of the lily, the carnation and the rose'[3]. Such a miraculous substance was surely worth preserving, and a great deal of effort was put into designing concoctions and unguents to protect it.

Medical papyri from Ancient Egypt contain numerous references to skin treatments and to ointments for cleansing or moisturizing. Both men and women used make-up, and both depilated their skin using tweezers or even bat's blood. Pimples and freckles were treated with oils, and wrinkles were kept at bay with a paste composed of wax, terebinth gum, 'behen' oil and vegetable mucilage: 'Try it and see!'[4]. A recipe for stretching and revivifying the skin involved ox bile, oil, gum and powdered ostrich egg, and a lotion for the face was made from various plant materials combined with powdered alabaster, honey and human milk. Pregnant women also used oils to smooth away stretch marks on their stomachs; they were stored in special jars shaped as a woman holding her distended belly[4].

The Greeks and Romans also took hygiene and skin care seriously. Hippocrates recommended bathing to soften the skin, although he advised caution in bathing during illness[5]. Galen discussed skin diseases and stressed the importance of good hygiene. The fanciful natural historian Pliny assembled a great deal of information about the treatments popular at the time. His favorite amongst them was 'crocodilea', a substance derived from crocodile intestines and believed to be very good for the skin of the face, clearing it of blotches, freckles and pimples. Some mixed it with cypress oil or water, while others adulterated it 'with starch or Cimolian chalk, but mostly with the dung of starlings, which they catch and feed on nothing but rice'[6]. Bovine skin treatments were also greatly approved by Pliny: cows' placenta cured skin ulcers, 'the pastern bone of a white bull-calf, boiled for forty days and nights until it melts to a jelly' was good for wrinkles, and facial lichens were treated with 'the gluey substance made from the genitals of calves, dissolved in vinegar with native sulphur, stirred up with a fig branch and applied fresh twice a day'[6]. Goose grease, mouse dung in vinegar, the ashes of hedgehogs and snails, vulture's blood and locust legs were all useful, but 'the best thing for clearing the complexion and removing wrinkles is swan's fat'[6]. 'The shell of murex or other shell-fish reduced to ash clears spots from the faces of women, remove[s] wrinkles, and fill[s] out the skin, if applied with honey for seven days … Fish-glue removes wrinkles and fills out the skin'[6].

THE EFFECT OF SMALLPOX

Traditional remedies such as these continued with undiminished popularity through to recent times and were reproduced in countless recipe books and domestic manuals aimed at women. As well as general advice on maintaining youth and beauty, such compilations included treatments for pathological conditions ranging from warts and chapped lips to eczema and leprosy. Most popular of all were techniques for preventing or disguising the signs of a disease which was as widespread as it was disfiguring: smallpox.

Many of the more successful smallpox treatments were based on sealing the skin away from the air, because they also tended to prevent scratching. Lotions and waters for bathing the pustules were composed of simple ingredients such as salt and mint water[7] or more ambitious compounds such as spermaceti, peach kernels and leek[8]. Other recipes emphasized ways of concealing the scars once they were there. In 1789, the anonymous author of *The Art of Preserving Beauty* recommended the following: 'take a piece of very lean mutton, boil it well, and dipping a sponge in the broth, gently foment the face, taking care to repeat this several times a day, till the pustules of the small-pox are quite ripe'[9]. This author also gave a very good piece of advice: don't pick off the scabs. 'The reason of this may be readily understood: when you open the pustules, and let out the matter, you let in the air at the same time, which immediately dries and hardens the cavities of the pustules, and thus prevents the flesh below from rising to fill up the hollows' (Figure 1)[9].

Queen Elizabeth I of England, who started out in life with a very fine complexion but later became a fanatical user of beauty treatments, also suffered a bout of smallpox in her youth. She treated it using an Arabic method which had been advocated by John of Gaddesden in the early fourteenth century. It involved wrapping the face in a red cloth and surrounding her bed with red things: the idea seemed to be that the red would draw out the inflammation from the skin. Pricking the spots with a needle was also recommended, but fortunately for Elizabeth this was not done in her case. She survived the disease completely unscarred[10].

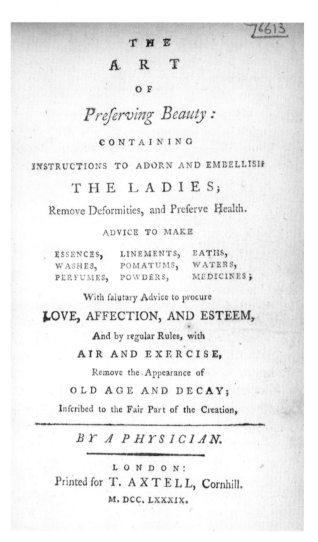

Figure 1 *The Art of Preserving Beauty* (1789). Reproduced with permission of the Wellcome Institute Library, London, England

THE PERFECT COMPLEXION

For Elizabeth, as for many of her contemporaries, the main goal of feminine beauty treatments was to keep the skin as fair as possible. So greatly was whiteness prized that thin blue lines were sometimes drawn on the bosom (which was usually bare in unmarried women) to represent veins showing through the skin[11]. This taste for pallor continued in Europe until the twentieth century, and freckles or a suntan were considered as imperfections. 'A white skin, whose surface is spread over with a colour of roses, is reckoned to be the most perfect and agreeable, as to what regards its colour', wrote the author of the *Art of Beauty* in 1760[12]. Drastic measures were employed to achieve this effect. During the sixteenth and seventeenth centuries powders were concocted from substances such as brimstone, mercury and white lead. The latter was extremely poisonous, and the brimstone and mercury tended to give the skin a mummified appearance. These effects were concealed with a glaze made from egg whites, which was supposed to make the skin look like 'polished marble'[10]. Should the woman make the mistake of smiling, the glaze would crack into a cobweb of splinters. The lead also tended to darken into a corpse-like gray after a few hours of wear, so had to be continually refreshed[11]. Other recipes for whitening the face involved powdered seashells or porcelain, or 'a powder of dried bones'[7]. Milk was much used for the same effect – presumably because of its resemblance in color. The seventeenth-century writer Hugh Platt (Figure 2) describes a trick for keeping babies' skin white while also (paradoxically one might think) protecting it against the sun: 'Wash the face and body of a sucking childe with brest milk, or cowmilk, or mixed with water, every night, and the childes skinne will wax faire and cleare, and resist sunburning'[13]. For sunburn and freckles the author of the *Art of Beauty* prescribes 'ass's milk, breast milk, almond emulsions' and so on[12]. Pierre-Joseph Buc'hoz writes of a 'Venetian water' designed to clear a sun-burnt complexion: it contains a pint of cow's milk, eight lemons, four Seville oranges, two ounces of sugar candy, half an ounce of borax, and four narcissus roots beaten to a paste[7].

If whitening with white things did not work, one could try the opposite approach. As with Elizabeth's smallpox treatment, red, fleshy or even downright bloody things applied to the skin were thought to draw out redness by sympathetic attraction. Leeches were sometimes applied to extract the blood by more direct means, too.

The creatures most favored as a source of flesh were birds. Alexis of Piedmont recommended using blood from a black hen, or compounds of chicken gall with honey and other ingredients. He also provided a recipe using a 'yonge crow even oute of the nest, yf you maye get one so: yf not take hym as yonge as you maye'[14]. The flesh should be cut into small pieces, and mixed with myrtle leaves, talcum powder, almond oil, and other materials. Pigeons were particularly popular. 'Take two young Pigeons, gut them and cut them into pieces, Crums of white Bread half a pound, peach-kernels ... the whites of twelve Eggs, and the Juice of four Limons; infuse them twelve hours in two quarts of Milk, then distil them'[15]. A Buc'hoz recipe for 'a water to preserve the Complexion' instructs: 'Take seven or eight White Pigeons, pick them, and cut off their heads and pinions, mince the rest of them small, and put them into an alembic with the other ingredients'[7].

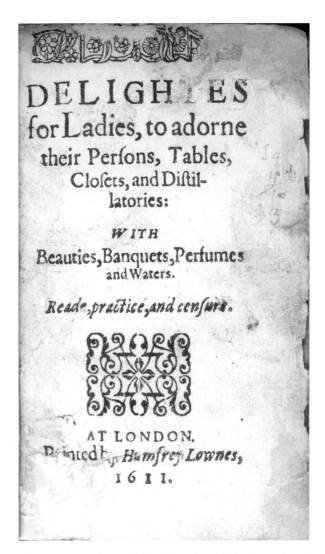

Figure 2   H. Platt, *Delightes for Ladies* (1661). Reproduced with permission of the Wellcome Institute Library, London, England

The last word in the use of gore for skin care must go to the legendary seventeenth-century 'Blood Countess', Elizabeth Bathory of Hungary. According to the story, she slapped a chambermaid so hard one day that blood spurted from the girl's nose and splashed the Countess's face. When it was washed off, her skin seemed to be whiter and softer than before (possibly because of the washing rather than the blood). She therefore took up daily bathing in virgins' blood, piercing and tearing the flesh of living victims to obtain it. Later she discovered that the blood of girls born into the nobility had a greater rejuvenating power than that of servants, and changed her sources accordingly – which was her undoing, for the missing girls were traced and she was caught. She was said to have been responsible for the deaths of 650 young women[16]. To some extent the story is a myth, but it does accord with general beliefs of the time concerning

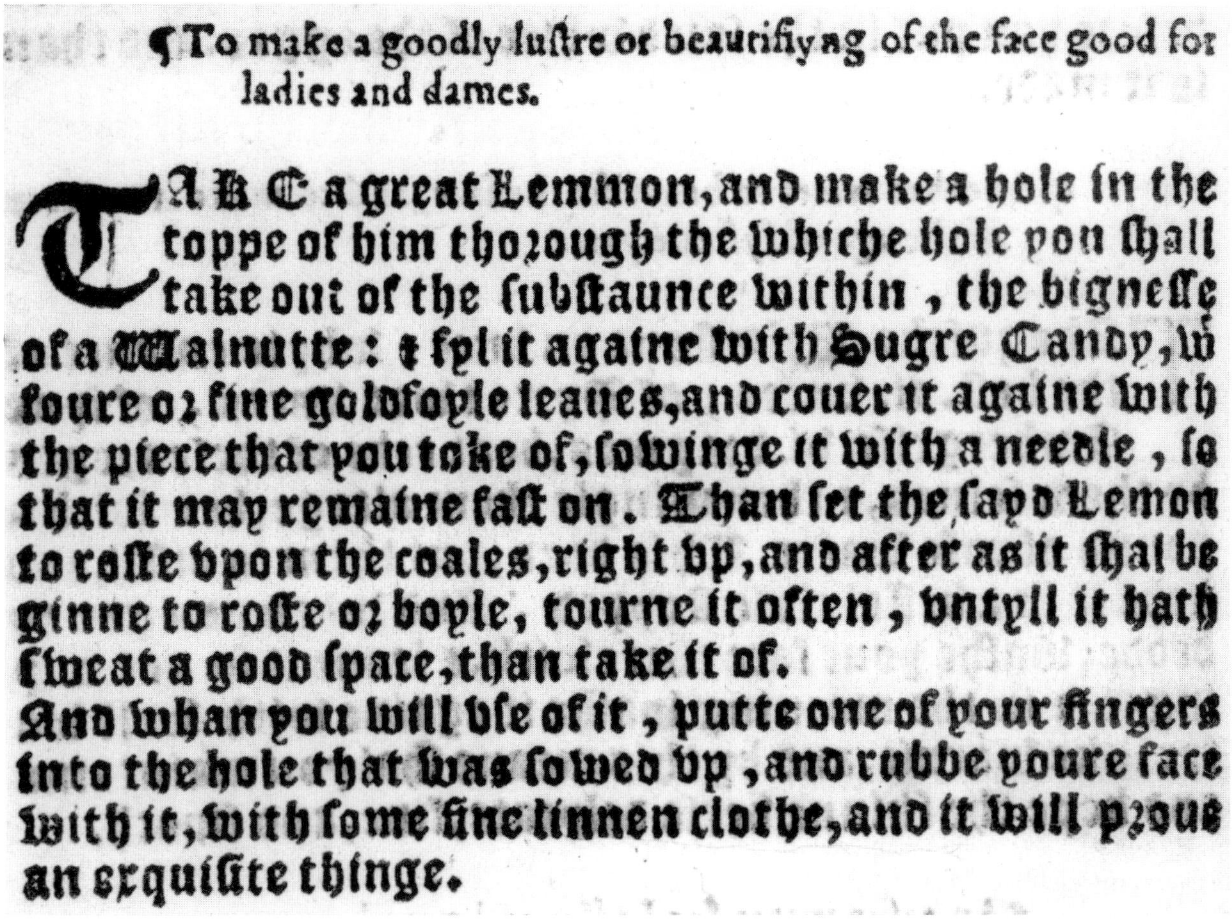

¶ To make a goodly luftre or beautifiyng of the face good for
ladies and dames.

TAK E a great Lemmon, and make a hole in the toppe of him thorough the whiche hole you shall take out of the substaunce within , the bigneſſe of a Walnutte : ¢ fpl it againe with Sugre Candy, w foure or fine goldfoyle leaues, and couer it againe with the piece that you toke of, fowinge it with a needle , fo that it may remaine faſt on . Than fet the fayd Lemon to roſte vpon the coales, right vp, and after as it ſhal be ginne to roſte or boyle, tourne it often , vntyll it hath ſweat a good fpace, than take it of. And whan you will vfe of it , putte one of your fingers into the hole that was fowed vp , and rubbe youre face with it, with fome fine linnen clothe, and it will proue an exquifite thinge.

Figure 3   Alexis of Piedmont, *The Secretes of the Reverend Maister Alexis of Piemont* (1562). Reproduced with permission of the Wellcome Institute Library, London, England

the miraculous healing and rejuvenating properties of blood and flesh. Even in modern times, similar beliefs persisted in a more innocuous form. Lola Montez in her book *The Arts of Beauty* described a tradition that thin slices of raw beef, bound over the face overnight, prevented wrinkles[17].

THE PROBLEMS OF AGING AND SPOTS

Besides achieving a whiter complexion, the great dermatological aim of women (then as now) seemed to be getting rid of wrinkles. Femininity was equated with youth, and the popular manuals are duly filled with recipes such as Alexis of Piedmont's 'verie good water to make the face appeare of the age of xxv yeares'[14]. Buc'hoz had 'a Water, christened, the Fountain of Youth' and noted that 'it is asserted also that the distilled Water of green Pine-apples takes away wrinkles, and gives the complexion an air of youth'[7]. His 'pomatum for wrinkles', a juice of white lily roots, honey and melted white wax, was to be 'applied every night, and not be wiped off until the next morning'[33] (Figure 3).

Another Hungarian aristocrat – this time the fourteenth-century Queen Elizabeth of Hungary – was credited with the invention of a successful rinse which became known as 'Hungary water'. It was said that she became so youthful and wrinkle-free from using it that the King of Poland sought her hand in marriage when she was 72 years old[9,18].

Unfortunately most of these remedies stopped considerably short of what they promised – especially the one attributed to Nostradamus which ended: 'If the work is carried out as instructed, overnight the complexion will be so changed that in the morning an old woman will look like a young girl'[19]. Serious writers later recognized that aging of the skin was essentially an incurable condition, and could be postponed but not eliminated altogether – although, of course, advertisers continued to promise the grail of eternal youth (Figure 4).

Spots were a tricky issue for the skin advisers. Some spots were considered good – those 'beauty spots' that, according to the *Art of Beauty*, 'give a certain grace to the face, set off the whiteness of the skin, and give the eye a fine amorous look. In this case one would rather consult the looking-glass

No. 6.—A wrinkled face is a starved face. Waste of tissue causes the lower skin tissue to contract and shrivel, leaving the outer covering like a loose mantle. To plump the tissues and eradicate wrinkles, apply *Oatine* with the finger tips until absorbed. Gently stroke the wrinkles crosswise with the tips of the fingers. Do this once a day for ten or fifteen minutes.

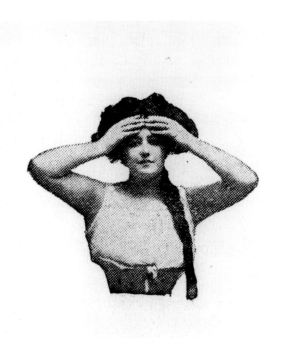

Figure 4 C. Andrews, *Beauty and Health* (1913). Reproduced with permission of the Wellcome Institute Library, London, England

than the doctor'[12]. Most spots were considered blemishes, and the recipe books abounded in instructions for removing them. Not surprisingly, early treatments involved such substances as goats' gall[14], green lizards boiled alive in oil[14], or brimstone, spermaceti and brandy[20]. The writer who records the latter treatment, Eliza Smith, also recommends an internal medicine in the form of a special diet to be eaten for 3–4 weeks: 'Take cucumbers and cut them as small as Herbs to the Pot, boil them in a small Pipkin with a piece of Mutton, and make it into Pottage with Oatmeal: So eat a Mess Morning, Noon and Night without Intermission for three Weeks or a Month'[20]. This dietary treatment points to a new recognition that spots were partly caused by physiological imbalances, and that they could be treated internally rather than simply by smearing ever more inventive substances onto the outside of the skin.

As described in the *Art of Preserving Beauty* of 1789, skin problems were caused by 'the salts being thrown off by the cutaneous glands, with ought to be washed through the kidneys'. The solution should be to promote the 'urinary discharges' as much as possible: 'any critical breakings out are by no means to be driven back, but encouraged' – '*Diuretics* are certainly the best auxiliaries to *cosmetics*'[9]. The skin was a two-way street, and so it was also very important to wash this waste matter away promptly. It was believed, for example, that if an invalid's bedlinen was not changed regularly, their foul perspirations might be sucked back in through the same pores that extruded them[21]. Constipation was a particularly dangerous condition, for if waste matter could not exit by the proper route it was likely to cause skin eruptions instead[2]. Even care of the feet was essential, wrote Susannah Cocroft, because if the sweat glands there were blocked the waste would travel around the body seeking a way out[2]. This is strangely reminiscent of 'an old Czechoslovakian remedy for clearing acne' described by C. Maxwell-Hudson in a compilation called the *Kaleidoscope of Beauty*. 'A princess who suffered from a bad complexion, on recommendation from a travelling physician, cut her little toe and left this open, not allowing it to heal. Thus all the impurities from her face were drained and excreted via the wound in her toe'[18].

A GOOD COMPLEXION

In the late eighteenth century there was already a considerable emphasis on 'natural' means to beauty, and on the importance of general health to skin tone. The *Art of Preserving Beauty* had already recommended exercise and cleanliness ('Many of the disorders among the lower classes of people are owing to a neglect in this point')[9]. By the twentieth century good skin and good health were inextricably linked: the former was a sure indicator of the latter, and the latter the *sine qua non* of the former. 'If everybody in the world had perfect health, everybody would have a good complexion', wrote Oscar Levin in 1927. Healthiness was further related to the concept of naturalness: 'A good complexion is a normal one – a natural one, intended for the individual by Nature'[22]. He regretted to note, however, that women were rarely content to leave it at that. 'There are two ways to have a satisfactory complexion – grow it, or buy it. Most women prefer the latter. Most men prefer not to bother' – 'Not one woman in ten would leave her complexion alone, if she had a naturally perfect one'.

As well as general physical well-being, mental attitude was considered a very important factor. 'Sadness, fear, too much application to study, remorse of conscience, excess of carnal pleasures' are all bad for the skin and spoil its color, wrote the author of the *Art of Beauty*[12] in 1760. H. Ellen Browning opined: 'Wrinkles are the result of pouting, frowning, making a martyr of oneself, meeting troubles half-way, and looking on the blackest side of things'[23]. And 'Myrene', author of *The Lady Beauty-Book*, advised women on how to avoid 'an anxious expression' while engaging in the otherwise commendably healthy exercise of bicycling[24]. A particularly odd manifestation of mental disturbance, widespread among young women during the eighteenth and nineteenth centuries, was chlorosis, commonly called the 'green-sickness' because of the greenish cast it gave to the skin of the face. It was believed to be caused by menstrual obstructions and sexual frustration in unmarried women, and the ideal solution was to marry the young lady off as quickly as possible. 'The health and happiness of the afflicted patient should supersede every consideration of rank or fortune in the party, where no moral causes intervene'[9]. 'If matrimony be judged improper' then alternative therapies had to be found, among them 'Russi's pills' mixed with 'salt of steel' and 'oil of savin' or 'Tincture of Hiera' with 'spirit of lavender and tincture of castor'. It was important not to go too far in seeking a cure. 'Too many of the fair sex, especially in their younger years, have frequently suffered from secret attempts to procure to themselves those delights, which Heaven has intended only as the effects of the most holy and legal union'[9]. This was equally dangerous to the complexion, making it 'pale, swarthy, and haggard'.

In the twentieth century, the care of the skin became a task of the highest importance for a woman. Susanna Cocroft (who gave her book *The Art of Keeping Young* the subtitle 'beauty a duty') wrote: 'Every woman must use her intelligence, therefore, or take up a study of this interesting subject, so that she can build up the right kind of blood and keep her skin properly nourished by forceful

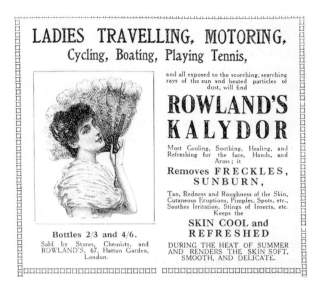

Figure 5 *The Daily Mirror Beauty Book* (early twentieth century). Reproduced with permission of the Wellcome Institute Library, London, England

circulation'[2]. 'Look in your mirror', she commanded, 'study yourself – are you satisfied? Is your complexion *clear*? Does it express the clearness of your life?'[2]. Blemishes 'symbolize imperfections within', but absence of wrinkles indicates a harmonious mind and a heart at rest, and rosy cheeks 'bespeak warm blood, circulating freely and nourishing all tissues'[2]. Beauty had increasingly become 'a science', as Browning clearly defined it in her book *Beauty Culture*[23]. It was a discipline that the advertising industry was diligent in studying. To mention mere cleaning power was not enough if you were a soap manufacturer. Other qualities had to be identified, to stake out a pitch in the market. Loveliness, delicacy, softness, femininity, attractiveness, reliability and motherliness were all co-opted to lend an extra level of appeal to skin products. 'Purity' was among the most exalted of these concepts: Woodbury's soap even founded a 'Facial Purity League', in the 1890s, issuing buttons to members proclaiming their membership of it[25].

THE FIGHT FOR BEAUTY

Early in the twentieth century there was an awareness that the slowly-won freedom for women to take part in activities such as cycling and tennis outside the home could have repercussions on the complexion (Figure 5) and a glance at a modern advertising leaflet shows skin care being promoted using an interesting new vocabulary, invoking the notion of defense against a hostile environment. The enemies of a woman's skin include stress and modernity itself, as well as the inevitable effects of time. A leaflet advertising L' Oréal Plénitude in 1993 tells us: 'Your skin is subjected to constant attack from the environment – ultra-violet rays, extremes of temperature and pollution. These factors, together with the effects of a demanding lifestyle all threaten your skin's natural vitality and contribute to the natural ageing process'[26]. The product offers to 'actively help the skin to defend itself against the signs of ageing'. Its scientific credentials are emphasized: it has been 'dermatologically and scientifically tested' by the company. Two sources of imagery, the battlefield and the laboratory, vie for dominance in this picture, and the scene is completed by evocative references to vitality and purity: 'Sometimes your skin may seem "tired" and in need of a boost. Plénitude Firming Serum Concentrate actively revitalises the skin… It improves elasticity and suppleness for a smoother more radiant complexion'.

Yet, although the language has changed, the underlying notion remains the same. The emphasis on efficacy established by experience or testing, the identification of old age as an enemy to womankind, and the notions of purity and radiance all go well back into the days of pigeon flesh and powdered porcelain.

CONCLUSIONS

Thus, from crocodile intestines to 'firming serum concentrate', the elusive double goal of youth and femininity has been pursued through treatment of the skin. To a much greater extent than men's, women's skin has been seen not just as a functional covering but as the outward manifestation of her inner self. A clear, pure skin indicates a pure soul, and a brown and roughened face betrays not only a 'lower-class' lifestyle but also the loss of a sort of spiritual virginity. It is no wonder, then, that so much has been written on the gentle art of faking this perfect, youthful state – or, at least, of preserving it long past its sell-by date.

REFERENCES

1. Ovid, 'On facial treatment for ladies' in: *The Erotic Poems*. Tr. P. Green. London: Penguin, 1982
2. Cocroft S. *The Art of Keeping Young: Beauty a Duty*. London, T. Fisher Unwin, ca. 1900
3. Cooley A J. *The Toilet in Ancient and Modern Times* (1866) reprinted New York: B. Franklin, 1970
4. *The Ebers papyrus: a new English translation, commentaries and glossaries by P. Ghalioungui*. Cairo: Academy of Scientific Research and Technology, 1987. On skin care in Egypt, see also B Watterson, *Women in Ancient Egypt*, Stroud, A. Sutton, 1994 and J Tyldesley, *Daughters of Isis*. Harmondsworth, Penguin, 1995
5. Hippocrates. Regimen in acute diseases. In *Hippocratic Writings*, ed. G E R Lloyd, tr. J Chadwick and W N Mann [et al]. London: Penguin, 1978
6. Pliny. *Natural History*, tr. W H S Jones. Cambridge, Mass.: Harvard University Press, 1963:vol 8
7. Buc'hoz P-J. *The Toilet of Flora*. New ed. London: J. Murray & W. Nicoll, 1799
8. Price E. *The New Book of Cookery*. New ed. London: The Authoress & A Hogg, [ca. 1780]
9. Anon. *The Art of Preserving Beauty*. London: T Axell, 1789
10. Hibbert C. *The Virgin Queen*, London: Viking, 1990
11. Picard L. *Restoration London*. London: Weidenfeld & Nicolson, 1997
12. *The art of beauty, or a companion for the toilet, written by a late eminent English physician at the Russian court*. London: J Williams, 1760
13. Platt H. *Delightes for Ladies*. London: H Lownes, 1611
14. Alexis of Piedmont. *The Secretes*; tr. W Warde. London: R Hall for N Englande, 1562
15. Hartman G. *The True Perserver and Restorer of Health*. London: T B for the author, 1682
16. Tannahill R. *Flesh and Blood*, Rev. ed. London: Abacus, 1996
17. Montez L. *The Arts of Beauty*. London: Blackwood, 1858
18. Maxwell-Hudson C. *Kaleidoscope of Beauty*. London: Octagon Press, 1968
19. Nostradamus. *The Elixirs*, ed. K Boeser, tr. G Slatter. London: Bloomsbury, 1995
20. Smith E. *The Compleat Housewife*. 4th ed. London: J Pemberton, 1730
21. Woolley H. *The Gentlewomans Companion*, 3rd ed. London: T J. for E Thomas, 1682
22. Levin O L. *The Care of The Face*. London: W Heinemann, 1927
23. Browning H E. *Beauty Culture*. London: Hutchinson, 1898
24. Myrene. *The Lady Beauty Book*. London: The "Lady", ca. 1900
25. Vinikas V. *Soft Soap, Hard Sell: American Hygiene in an Age of Advertisement*. Ames: Iowa State University Press, 1992
26. L' Oréal, *Plénitude: delays the signs of ageing*. London: L' Oréal, 1993

Psychodermatology of girls and women

2

Caroline S. Koblenzer

INTRODUCTION

There is no longer any doubt that psychosocial factors are able to precipitate or exacerbate physical illness in the genetically predisposed individual[1]. This is particularly true for dermatology, where numerous studies have shown that in anywhere from 30 to 70%[2,3] or more of out-patients, emotional factors play some part in the disease process. In each case, women represent a substantial portion of the population affected, a fact that the author will explore in this chapter. A working classification will also be offered, and treatment suggestions outlined, for those psychocutaneous disorders most frequently encountered in our women patients.

THE SKIN AS AN ORGAN FOR PSYCHOSOMATIC EXPRESSION

The reasons that psychophysiologic symptoms are so frequently expressed in the skin are complex. In part, the quality of the early cutaneous tactile experience and the emotional environment in which it takes place 'prime' the skin, so that it is vulnerable to the symbolic expression of psychophysiologic change[4]. This was the case, for example, for a ten-year-old girl in our practice. This little girl's mother, like the girl herself, had beautiful long dark hair, that was greatly admired in the family. When the parents divorced, to everyone's great surprise the little girl expressed little emotion; however, within a very short time, she developed extensive alopecia areata. And so, with the loss of her beautiful hair, so like her mother's, this little girl expressed symbolically the feelings of loss that she was not able to verbalize.

A second reason may have to do with the derivation of both skin and central nervous system (CNS) from the embryonic neuro-ectoderm, and the on-going communication between the two through neuro-endocrine pathways. For example, we know that one may blush from shame or embarrassment; we also know that patients with rosacea tend to blush readily; it is but a short step, then, to note that repeated vasodilatation, triggered by negative

feelings may, ultimately, be associated with the onset of rosacea[5–8]. In similar fashion, substantive links associate anxiety-driven palmar or plantar hyperhidrosis and the development of dyshidrotic eczema, in a person who is genetically so predisposed[8,9].

A third reason may be the ubiquitous presence of immunologic elements throughout the skin, and the on-going bi-directional communication between every aspect of the immune system and both axes of the stress response[10,11]. Each one of these mechanisms is characterized by the release of neuropeptides, cytokines and the various mediators of inflammation, which can be identified in the involved skin[12,13]. Whatever the mechanism, it is quite clear that biological, developmental, emotional and sociocultural factors each plays their part in determining what significance our outer covering holds over our inner lives, and whether or not it will be used to betray our inner secrets in physical symptoms.

Biological determinants

In early life the skin is a primary organ of perception, and the pathways that carry tactile perception are the very first to be fully myelinized. Already one can detect tactile perceptive function *in utero*, and by 28–32 weeks of gestation it can be demonstrated over the entire body surface[14]. Through tactile stimulation, at first by contact with the uterine wall, and later through self-exploration and the loving touch of care-takers, the physical boundaries of the self begin to be defined for the individual, and an internal picture, a body image, begins to be laid down.

Developmental and emotional determinants

The emotional environment into which the infant is born is crucial to its healthy development. This environment is important in determining the integrity and stability of the body image, and the quality of self-esteem that is engendered. It is through this medium also that emotional modulation is gradually mastered. Each of these three factors, emotional modulation, body image and self-esteem, plays a part in generating a later susceptibility to psychocutaneous disease[15].

Emotional modulation

In early infancy tension is discharged through physical pathways. Anxiety, frustration and pain are expressed in physical movement, crying and autonomic discharge. At first, this discharge is modulated by physical contact with the primary care-taker. Through this non-verbal channel, the mother establishes control of vegetative autonomic functions, through her ability to contain and modulate the infant's feelings; through it also she transmits a full range of emotional expression to her infant[15–17]. The negative feelings of the anxious, angry or hostile mother will be picked up and mirrored by her infant, while the calm, confident and loving mother will, instead, have a soothing influence, gradually helping her infant to master the modulation of anxiety, which is the infantile precursor of emotion[18,19].

It is not uncommon for a mother to feel differently towards her girl babies than towards her boys. Feelings that she has had about her own skin, or her mother's skin, may be transferred to her baby girl, without her conscious awareness, through the process of identification. The mother who is comfortable with her femininity, and knows herself to be attractive, is likely to endow her infant with those traits. But the mother who perceives her own or her mother's skin as scarred, or unattractive in some way, may in her unconscious mind 'give' those negative traits to her daughter, experiencing her baby as 'imperfect'. Alternatively, she may be disappointed that the baby is not a boy; or fear that the little girl will displace her in her husband's affections. These and other feelings that she has about her baby will be expressed in the character of the mother's touch.

The quality of this early experience has later repercussions. When the emotional environment is positive and empathic, optimal modulation of anxiety is achieved by the infant, and once speech is acquired, the girl will have words at her command through which to express emotion and discharge tension[20]. In a less empathic environment, optimal modulation may not take place, and the capacity to express feelings through words, fantasy and play may not develop. In this case, discharge of tension will continue through physiologic channels, setting the stage for later psychophysiologic disease[20].

Body image and self-esteem

The quality of the infantile tactile experience, and the emotional environment in which it takes place, affect both body image and self-esteem, two attributes that are intimately connected. As we shall see, there are a number of psychocutaneous conditions associated with a disordered body-image, just as there are with diminished self-esteem, that are integral to depression.

By body image we refer to the picture of ourselves that we carry with us, and see each time we look into the mirror[21–25]. It may not be exactly how others see us, and even for the most healthy, there may be some minor distortion. For example, in 'Look Alike Contests' some contestants will bear only the slightest resemblance to the model, and often we are surprised by the sound when we hear a recording of our own voice. A woman patient who weighed well over 200 lbs (ca. 90 kg) is a more extreme example of body image distortion. This patient reports that she does not see an obese image in the mirror, but in a photograph of herself she always wonders, 'who is that fat woman?'

Infant observation studies have shown that the greater the amount, and the more empathic the physical touching that the infant receives in the early days and weeks of life – that is to say, touching that is in tune with the specific needs of the individual infant in a warm and loving emotional environment – the more accurate and the closer to objective reality will be the body image that develops, the more stable its boundaries, and the more secure the personal and sexual identity of the individual. Studies have also shown that such a person will feel more attractive, will like herself more, and will feel closer to others. In this way, body image and self-esteem are intimately related. If a person feels secure, flexibility of character will be fostered, and the coping styles established that are essential for adaptation to the realities of changing circumstances, such as disfiguring or disabling disease and the aging process.

The concept of body image includes not only the physical image, but also the feelings, relationships and fantasies associated with the phases of its development[26]. It is not a static concept, and as the body itself changes, these changes must be accepted and integrated for emotional well-being[24,27,28]. Because his genitalia are external and visible, because touching is sanctioned during toileting, and because of the nature of the physical contact in boyish play, tactile and visual experience enable the boy to define his boundaries, and come to terms with his personal and sexual identity, as his adult persona evolves. For him, adolescence brings only enhancement and modification of organs with which he is already familiar[29].

For the little girl, life is more complicated. A large part of her genital endowment is internal, and not capable of being seen or touched. Rather than specific organs, she may experience an 'emptiness', or perhaps an excitement, that may lead to uncertainty about boundaries and personal and sexual identity[29,30]. The internal position of uterus and vagina, and their close proximity to the rectum, sometimes cause confusion about the function of these organs, leading the girl to feel dirty, or contaminated in some way, and diminishing her self-esteem[31]. This negative feeling about one's body is likely to be re-awakened and reinforced in adolescence and adult life by a concept prevalent in the media that suggests implicitly that the female genitals are inherently dirty and malodorous. Because of this, our undergarments must be protected against contamination by sweetly perfumed disposable 'panty-liners'. It is important to recognize that, male and female alike, each of us emits his or her own unique personal odor. Since perfumed boxer or jockey 'liners' are not advertised for men – whose personal hygiene, clinical observation teaches, tends to be less meticulous than our own – it can only be that our odor is experienced by men as a threat, against which they must be protected. This insight, however, does little for the self-esteem of women, who may take the implicit message at face value.

Another possible cause of confusion is the rather ubiquitous mislabeling of the external genitalia. The vulva and clitoris, the two most sensually sensitive areas of her body, are often referred to as the 'vagina', even by adult women, while the clitoris may be perceived as merely a vestigial penis, rather than an organ in its own right that the girl can enjoy and take pride in. Its very namelessness adds to her confusion, and may make her feel that the pleasurable sensations that it generates are forbidden, and 'bad', thus further diminishing her self-esteem[32,33].

The messages that the girl receives from parents and siblings too are confusing. The father takes delight in his baby daughter, making her feel very special in his eyes. But this idyll is self-limited, for as she begins to mature, threatened by sexual taboos, the father must distance himself from her. Puzzled by the change in his behavior, the little girl may feel that he is drawing away because of something that she has done, because she is unworthy, 'bad', or deficient in some way. Should the mother have body-image difficulties of her own, she may view her own body in a way that is at odds with what her daughter sees. The slender mother who does not like her body, and declares herself to be 'fat' or unattractive, may threaten the little girl's hold on reality, and cause her to wonder about her own body. Identification with her dissatisfied mother may make the girl dissatisfied with her body, also.

With the advent of adolescence, the girl must come to terms with the inevitable adolescent structural and functional bodily changes, and integrate them into the internal image that she carries of herself. Breast development alters the contours that she sees in the mirror, while the mystery, and perhaps discomfort, of menstruation focus her attention on the 'inside', and on those important organs that she cannot see. These physical ambiguities themselves may be stressful, while their portent for the future, in terms of sexuality, mature functioning and motherhood, may prove to be of even greater stress[24,30,32,33].

A mother who is comfortable with her own body, her femininity and sexuality, can be of great assistance in enabling her daughter to pass these hurdles, to identify with her mother's positive attitude, and to look forward to fulfillment as a woman. It is also possible that adolescence, pregnancy and the menopause each may be fraught with feelings of self-disgust, and with the risk of the skin problems that we associate with a disordered body image, or with depression, in those who are genetically predisposed.

Siblings, particularly boys, may add to the emotional stress for the adolescent girl, for her maturing body may be counted fair game in the arena of sibling rivalry. Cruel taunts about obesity, 'zits', or general 'ugliness' frequently compound the girl's discomfort with her changing self. If she idealizes her brother and envies the freedoms he has that are not hers, and is eager to please him, his taunts are especially damaging to her self-esteem.

The emphasis on external perfection in our culture, and the power of the media to promote that perfection, add to the girl's difficulties as she tries to adjust to her bodily changes. The influence of body image on self-concept is much greater for girls than for boys, and the girl must strive constantly to be 'as good as' the peers against whom she measures herself[34,35].

The changes of pregnancy on body image bring their own challenges, but more often we see problems later in life when the children have left home. The woman not blessed with a profession may feel that her life is now without purpose. Resentful of her husband's life outside the home, with feelings of femininity threatened by the looming menopause, the woman in middle life may become depressed, and perceive herself as ugly and undesirable. Psychocutaneous disorders are common at that time.

These, then, are some of the developmental and emotional factors that contribute to the higher incidence of depressive disorders in women, characterized by diminished self-esteem. A female to male ratio of 2–3:1 is quoted, though clinical experience would suggest that the preponderance of women is in fact much higher; psychic distress is often accepted as 'normal' in women, and goes unreported. The lifetime prevalence of major depression is believed to be 10–25% for women and 5–12% for men, but these figures do not include dysthymic disorder, a less severe depression, but one that significantly impairs the quality of life for many women[36].

Sociocultural determinants

The attitudes that we have about our skin arise in the context of relationships. These relationships include the paradigmatic ones of early childhood, those with significant others, and with the peergroup, society and the media. Acceptance or rejection of the attitudes we encounter determines our behavior, and becomes a part of our personality[14].

In the struggle to separate from the parents and establish an independent identity, the source of emotional support for the adolescent is transferred from the parents to the peer group, the adolescent girl seeking approval from peers to maintain her self-esteem. Idealization formerly bestowed on the parents is transferred onto a peer, or a media or fashion idol, with whose goals and values the adolescent identifies, and from whom she yearns for approval. Based on these models, the adolescent girl re-works her ideal image, the 'ego ideal', by which we mean the image of the person whom she would most like to become. In childhood, that image was based on an amalgam of idealized aspects of the parents, and traits and qualities the girl perceived her parents would wish in their 'ideal' daughter. Her self-esteem is now dependent on how closely, in reality, she can approximate her new ideal[37,38]. Thus it is that the adolescent will go to enormous, and sometimes dangerous, lengths to achieve the 'perfect' complexion, the 'perfect' figure and the 'perfect' tan that she sees depicted in the 'teen' magazines and on her favorite television show. Her expectations for herself may be wholly unrealistic, falling far short of the ideal and driving her to greater and greater excesses. She may subject herself to body-piercing, tattoos, too much sun,

dermatologic over-treatment, excessive camouflage and dangerous weight-loss, in her tireless attempts to enhance her shaky self-esteem, as she experiments with different personae, based on different facets of her changing idols, in quest of her evolving mature self[39].

Such is the power of our youth culture that even into and past middle life there is a push for women to maintain a youthful ego-ideal. The aged are portrayed in the media as ugly, depressive and useless, rather than the wise individuals that they may be, with an inner peace and beauty of their own. So in her quest for eternal youth, the older woman may subject herself to the quick-fixes of liposuction, laser resurfacing and other plastic procedures. All of these carry inherent procedural risks, but there are also psychological risks. If the woman's goals are unrealistic they will be unreachable, and disappointment inevitable; out of this disappointment, the surgical 'junkie' is born[40].

PSYCHOCUTANEOUS DISEASE

On the basis of the ideas discussed above, a number of different classifications of psychocutaneous diseases have been proposed, none of which is entirely satisfactory as overlap between categories is inevitable[41–43]. A classification that is useful must integrate psychopathology and pathophysiology, to formulate a rational treatment approach. Broadly, we can separate conditions that are primarily psychiatric from those that are primarily dermatologic. But difficulties arise in this latter category, because the degree of the psychiatric contribution in each case varies, and because concurrent anxiety and depression can each trigger a psychophysiologic response of its own.

Table 1 encompasses a more complete classification[18], but in Table 2 can be found a simplified, more practical version, formulated to assist in selecting effective treatment.

Descriptions of all of the listed conditions can be found in standard dermatology texts and other publications. After a brief outline of available treatment modalities, the rest of this chapter will confine itself to a discussion of those psychodermatologic conditions we are most commonly asked to treat in women and girls.

TREATMENT OF PSYCHOCUTANEOUS DISEASE
General measures

The patient with psychocutaneous disease is usually very anxious; she believes her condition to be

Table 1 Psychocutaneous diseases

Disorders in which body image is impaired
Delusions related to the skin
  parasitic infestation
  infection
  toxic damage
  disordered structure or function (dysmorphic
   delusions)
Hallucinations
  related to delusional content
   visual
   auditory
   olfactory (olfactory reference syndrome)
  arising *de novo*
   cutaneous dysesthesia
Dermatitis artefacta
Disorders in which self-esteem is impaired
Obsessive–compulsive symptoms
  obsessive worries
   parasitic infestation
   infection
   disordered structure or function (body
    dysmorphic disorder)
  compulsive behaviors
   trichotillomania
   neurotic excoriations
   lichen simplex chronicus
   onychophagia, onychotillomania
   lip-licking
   irritant dermatitis from hand washing, etc.
Dermatoses most commonly associated with
 depression
  chronic idiopathic pruritus
  chronic urticaria
  glossodynia, vulvodynia and other cutaneous
   dysesthesias
  certain inflammatory dermatoses, particularly
   psoriasis, alopecia areata
Disorders of affect regulation (psychophysiologic skin disease)
The spectrum of inflammatory dermatoses
  conditions in which the dominant affect is
   depression
    certain inflammatory dermatoses, particularly
     psoriasis, alopecia areata, etc.
  conditions in which the dominant affect is anxiety
   atopic eczema, nummular eczema, dyshidrotic
    eczema, seborrheic dermatitis, acne vulgaris,
    recurrent herpes simplex, etc.
The somatopsychic effects
The emotional cost of chronic skin disease

Reprinted with permission from Koblenzer CS. Psychodermatology of Women. *Clin Dermatol* 1997;15:129

Table 2 Psychocutaneous diseases

Psychiatric disorders with skin manifestations
Disorders of body image
  a) body dysmorphic disorder
    i) obsession
    ii) delusion
  b) dermatitis artefacta
Cutaneous delusions
    i) dysmorphic delusions (BDD)
    ii) delusions of parasitosis (DOP)
Obsessive–compulsive symptoms

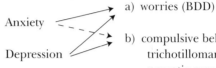
Anxiety — a) worries (BDD)
Depression — b) compulsive behavior
     trichotillomania
     neurotic excoriations, etc.

Chronic cutaneous dysesthesia syndrome

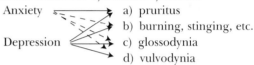
Anxiety — a) pruritus
     b) burning, stinging, etc.
Depression — c) glossodynia
     d) vulvodynia

Dermatologic conditions affected by stress
a) Primarily (but not exclusively) depression
   i) psoriasis
   ii) alopecia areata
   iii) chronic urticaria
b) Primarily (but not exclusively) anxiety
   i) atopic dermatitis
   ii) acne vulgaris
   iii) rosacea
   iv) dyshidrotic eczema
   v) recurrent herpes simplex, etc.

Somatopsychic effect
Emotional cost of chronic skin disease

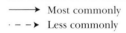
⟶ Most commonly
- - -► Less commonly

both helpless and hopeless, so it is important at the outset to let her know that you have seen conditions similar to hers before, that the condition has a name, and that treatment is available. Explanations in terms of chemical messengers, neurotransmitters or neuropeptides can help her to put her condition into a category, and therefore allay her anxiety a little. Because the skin is inherently emotionally charged, and because the patient is usually unaware, or unwilling to accept, that emotional factors contribute to the disease process, it is important to focus attention on the skin, and provide a structured regimen of topical treatment. This regimen allows the anxious patient to feel that she is doing something constructive and taking control of her disease, rather than being controlled by it.

The free use of tar or oatmeal baths, compresses, emollients, antipruritic lotions and medicated

unique, and one that no-one understands; consequently she fears that no-one can give her the answers that she is desperately seeking. She feels

shampoos is very helpful. Topical antibiotic and glucocorticoid preparations will be predicated by the clinical findings, as will the use of oral antihistamines and antibiotics. There is probably no place for oral glucocorticoids in the treatment of psychocutaneous disease, but intralesional steroids are helpful in the treatment of prurigo nodularis.

The physician must firmly and confidently set limits with regard to the laboratory studies she is willing to order, and the treatments she will prescribe, realizing that irrational anxiety cannot be allayed by rational argument. Only those studies appropriate to the specific symptom should be undertaken, and normal studies, including biopsy, should not be repeated. The physician must resist the pressure, which can be intense, to undertake ever more arcane tests and procedures.

Psychiatric referral

An inability or unwillingness to acknowledge emotional distress is common in patients who 'somatize'; were these patients able to experience and verbalize their distress, physical symptoms would not be necessary. One goal of treatment is to help the patient to become more self-aware, and more open to the possibility of psychiatric referral. Once trust has been won, the physician can begin to explore with the patient how her skin disease impairs her quality of life, and the stress it imposes; a goal of 'stress management' may then enable the patient to accept psychotropic medication, or better yet, a referral for psychiatric evaluation or counseling. The effectiveness of any psychotropic drug will be enhanced by concomitant psychotherapy, while for some patients psychotherapy alone is an effective treatment, offering the potential for long-term benefit and a better life-adjustment. Supportive, behavioral, cognitive and insight-oriented therapies all have their place in our armamentarium[26]. Psychotherapy can be of great benefit, particularly to patients with anxiety, depression and obsessive–compulsive symptoms.

Specific treatment

Specific treatment[26,42–48] is directed towards anxiety, depression, obsessive–compulsive symptoms (which include the body dysmorphic disorder), the cutaneous dysesthesias and cutaneous delusions. Table 3 shows the usual dose range for representative drugs effective in the treatment of psychocutaneous disorders.

Because few empirical data are available concerning the effect of these drugs on the developing fetus, psychotropic drugs should not be prescribed for pregnant women or nursing mothers without consulting a psychiatrist or psychopharmacologist[44]. Fluoxetine and fluvoxamine are both approved for use in children, but though risperidone and olanzepine are apparently safe and effective in the pediatric age-group, controlled studies remain to be reported.

Anxiety

Anxiety is characterized by some or all of the following: worry and apprehension, motor restlessness, physical tension, shakiness, irritability, difficulty in concentrating, inability to relax and insomnia. Physical symptoms such as anorexia or weight gain, sweating, palpitations, tachycardia, episodic shortness of breath, dry mouth, abdominal complaints, frequent urination and sudden awakening may also occur. Anxiety often accompanies depression, and these two states must be teased apart if drug treatment is to be effective. For situational anxiety, or anxiety associated with physical illness, the benzodiazepines may be prescribed on a p.r.n. basis. They are not appropriate for long-term use because they are sedating, habit-forming and subject to tachyphylaxis. Of these, alprazolam may be the most useful because, in addition to its anxiolytic properties, it has some antidepressant effect[42,45].

When a long-term anxiolytic is required, buspirone is the drug of choice. It is neither sedating nor habit-forming, but requires 2–3 weeks to take full effect, and cannot, therefore, be prescribed on a p.r.n. basis.

Depression

Depression is characterized by some or all of the following: feelings of sadness or emptiness, tearfulness, loss of interest in activities that were previously enjoyed, social withdrawal, irritability, agitation, feelings of worthlessness, hopelessness and helplessness, fatigue and inability to concentrate. There may also be insomnia or hypersomnia, anorexia or overeating, and a variety of non-specific physical complaints that cannot be explained on a physical basis. Anxiety is often a part of the picture, and one must always ensure that the patient is neither thinking of, nor planning, suicide.

The selective serotonin reuptake inhibitor (SSRI) antidepressants have largely replaced the tricyclics for treatment of depression, because of a

Table 3 Psychocutaneous drugs in dermatology

Drug	Dermatologic indications	Usual dose range in dermatology
Anxiolytics		
Alprazolam (Xanax®)	short-term situational anxiety anxiety associated with physical illness	0.25–1.0 mg at h.s., or up to q.i.d., as indicated
Buspirone (BuSpar®)	chronic anxiety pruritus aggravated by anxiety to potentiate SSRIs in BDD	5.0 mg t.i.d. gradually increasing to 10–15 mg t.i.d. as indicated
SSRI antidepressants		
Fluoxetine (Prozac®)	depression, dysesthesias, OCD (including BDD)	10–60 mg o.d. (usually 10–40 mg)
Paroxetine (Paxil®)		10–60 mg o.d. (usually 10–40 mg)
Sertraline (Zoloft®)		25–200 mg o.d. (usually 50–100 mg)
Fluvoxamine (Luvox®)		25–400 mg o.d. (usually 50–100 mg)
Antipsychotics		
Pimozide (Orap®)	delusions, hallucinations, dysesthesias, and to potentiate SSRIs in OCD and BDD	1–10 mg o.d. (usually 1–4 mg)
Risperidone (Risperdal®)		0.5–8 mg o.d. (usually 0.5–2 mg)
Olanzepine (Zyprexa®)		2.5–20 mg o.d. (usually 2.5 mg alternate days–5.0 mg o.d.)

SSRI, selective serotonin reuptake inhibitor; BDD, body dysmorphic disorder; OCD, obsessive–compulsive disorder

favorable side-effect profile and ease of dosing. They are also the drugs of choice in treatment of obsessive–compulsive disorder (OCD), and body dysmorphic disorder (BDD). Although traditionally tricyclics have been used in the treatment of the atypical pain syndromes, SSRIs are also often effective[47,48].

Potential side-effects, which usually disappear within 2–4 weeks of starting treatment, are mild nausea, heartburn or loss of appetite, headache, insomnia and restlessness, or sedation (particularly with paroxetine). Decreased libido, increased sweating, and, rarely, fluid retention, may also be troublesome. The medication is given once daily, with food, starting with a low dose and increasing gradually at weekly intervals, to minimize side-effects. Another drug in the same class may be prescribed after 3 or 4 weeks, if the desired benefit is not achieved.

Obsessive–compulsive symptoms

An obsession is an irrational thought that intrudes persistently into the mind, and a compulsion, a seemingly pointless action the patient is driven to repeat. Although she knows the thought or action to be irrational, and often self-destructive, the patient is powerless to control it, and embarrassed and ashamed by her lack of control. Obsessional concerns about the skin, and compulsive actions such as neurotic excoriations or trichotillomania respond to SSRIs, though a higher dose than that used for depression may be necessary and it may take weeks or months for significant improvement to be seen. Should the SSRIs prove partially or completely ineffective, buspirone, risperidone or olanzepine may be added to the regimen[46].

Dysesthesia

The cutaneous dysesthesias have been considered analogous to atypical pain syndromes, and traditionally have been treated with tricyclic antidepressants[47,48]. They respond equally well, however, to SSRIs. Should anxiety be prominent buspirone may be substituted or added to the regimen. Dysesthesia may sometimes be congruent with a delusional belief system; in these patients, pimozide is often effective[47].

Delusions

A delusion is a false belief that is inconsistent with the cultural or educational background of the patient, and that is held with absolute conviction in face of all reason; delusions are symptomatic of psychosis. Pimozide, risperidone and olanzepine, in low dosage, have more favorable side-effect profiles than older antipsychotics, and are effective for cutaneous delusions. In the dosage schedules used in dermatology, side-effects are minimal. Parkinsonian symptoms are rare, except with pimozide, and tardive dyskinesia does not seem to occur in dermatology patients. Rarely akathisia, or motor restlessness, is reported by patients taking pimozide; this can be relieved by diphenhydramine (Benadryl), 25–50 mg t.i.d. Though pimozide is cardiotoxic, routine electrocardiograms are not recommended if the daily dose is less than 10 mg[49].

PSYCHIATRIC DISORDERS WITH SKIN MANIFESTATIONS
Disorders of body image
Body dysmorphic disorder (cutaneous non-disease)

Clinical description

Body dysmorphic disorder[53] (BDD) refers to an incapacitating preoccupation with an imagined defect in appearance, or, if a minor abnormality is present, the preoccupation is excessive and intrusive enough to interfere in the patient's social, recreational, and academic or occupational functioning[45,50,51]. Although any body part may be involved, complaints usually center on the head and neck, or genitalia – the parts most basic to our sense of personal and sexual identity. Apart from psychiatrists, dermatologists and plastic surgeons are the specialists most frequently consulted, and it is therefore important for us to be familiar with the diagnosis and treatment of this distressing condition.

The onset of BDD most commonly occurs in adolescence – the time when, for girls especially, physical changes must be integrated into the body image, peer pressures are great, and self-esteem fragile. Feelings of shame and embarrassment often lead to secrecy and delay the diagnosis for many years. Though statistics from psychiatric studies would suggest an equal incidence in males and females, girls and women clearly predominate in our patient population.

Patients with BDD consult dermatologists about perceived abnormalities in every conceivable aspect of the structure or function of skin or its appendages. Complaints may be of disfiguring acne, abnormally large pores, changes in blood vessels, abnormalities in the texture or growth pattern of hair, excessive or malodorous sweat, or deformity or discoloration of the genitalia. Despite minimal or negative objective findings, the patient experiences her appearance as grotesque, ugly, abnormal or shameful. She thinks about it constantly, spends many hours each day scrutinizing her appearance in the mirror, and repeatedly seeks reassurance from friends and family, to an extent that strains relationships. The anxiety takes over her life, and she can think of nothing else. In 'BDD by proxy' the patient's excessive concern is about a false perception in another; usually, this is her mother, who perceives some non-existent defect in her child. For example, a mother with minimal androgenic alopecia experienced incapacitating anxiety and depression, because she had an unshakable conviction that her completely normal six-year-old daughter had inherited the trait, was losing hair, and would soon be bald. A long-recognized but only recently reported aspect of BDD is a compulsive need to pick the skin[52], a time-consuming and often ritualized activity designed to 'improve' the patient's appearance, or eradicate 'toxins', focal dysesthesia, or extraneous elements, in order to 'promote healing'. Other ritualized grooming practices and complicated camouflage regimens also occur.

Though BDD is by no means a benign condition, clinical experience would suggest that our patients are usually less severely affected, and less incapacitated, than those who consult psychiatrists; nevertheless, suicidal ideation and completed suicides do occur[53,54]. Psychiatric studies show that the majority of patients are unmarried or divorced, many are unable to work, and previous psychiatric hospitalizations are not uncommon[50].

Evidence suggests that BDD is a manifestation of obsessive–compulsive disorder (OCD), but the spectrum of severity is broad. Indeed, many 'normal' women worry about some aspect of physical appearance or functioning, and engage in mirror checking, camouflage, embarrassment and reassurance-seeking, while at the most severe end of the spectrum the symptom is truly a delusion; in that case, the anxiety it generates makes perfect sense to the patient, rather than being viewed as wholly irrational. Phenomenologically, patients with delusions of parasitosis (DOP) mirror exactly those with delusional symptoms of BDD; only the ideational content is different[55]. Cutaneous delusions will be discussed in a separate section.

Histopathology

In most cases of BDD the skin and cutaneous appendages are normal on microscopy. Should there be minor pathology, the histology will be consistent with the clinical picture. When skin-picking is present, the pathology will be that of neurotic excoriations, prurigo nodularis, or lichen simplex chronicus. Laboratory studies will depend on the specific complaints.

Differential diagnosis

The differential diagnosis falls into two parts. First, are we dealing with physical disease or with false perception? Second, how severe is the psychopathology: does the patient have an intrusive obsessional worry that does not make sense to her, or does she have a true delusion – a belief that she holds with absolute conviction; is she anxious, depressed, or suicidal?

The first question will be answered by the clinical picture. For the second question, the reader is referred to the individual sections for a summary of the clinical characteristics of obsessions, delusions, anxiety and depression. The diagnosis can only be arrived at by listening carefully to the patient.

Treatment

The physician must not dispute or make light of the patient's experience, but rather empathize with her distress. The treatment of choice for non-delusional BDD is one of the SSRI antidepressants. Reportedly, these drugs are equally as effective in delusional patients, though clinical experience would suggest that antipsychotics are significantly more, and more rapidly, effective[50]. Insight-oriented, cognitive–behavioral and supportive therapies have a place in treatment[50–52].

Prognosis

Psychiatric studies suggest that drug treatment is effective in over 80% of patients. After six months' freedom from symptoms, attempts may be made to taper off the drug, but recurrence is likely, and long-term treatment usually necessary. In less severe cases insight-oriented or psychoanalytic treatment has brought about long-term relief[55].

Dermatitis artefacta (factitious dermatitis)

Clinical description

In dermatitis artefacta (DA) the patient is driven to create lesions on her own skin, or on that of another – usually her child or ward – to satisfy a psychological need of which she is not consciously aware[26]. A wish to be taken care of, a need to define her physical and emotional boundaries through the pain and discomfort of creating lesions, an unconscious identification with an abusing childhood care-taker, or a guilty need for self-punishment are some of the unconscious reasons uncovered in working with these patients. Regardless of the reason, the activity is always carried out in secret, and strenuously denied, by the patient. Like other forms of factitious disease, DA has its onset in adolescence, and is significantly more common in girls than boys. Lack of stringency in applying diagnostic criteria makes accurate statistical analysis difficult, but the female : male incidence is variously quoted as anywhere from 3 : 1 to 20 : 1[56–60].

Lesions in DA are bizarre in appearance, often angulated or geometric, and as varied in morphology as the ingenious methods chosen to produce them. They are not in conformity with the lesions of any known dermatosis, except in 'pathomimicry', where lesions may mimic those of a dermatosis, now resolved, or of one observed in another person. Lesions may be single or multiple, unilateral, or bilateral and symmetrical, but they are always within reach of the patients' hands. A so-called 'hollow history', that makes it impossible to learn the stages in evolution of individual lesions, is characteristic, as though lesions appear mysteriously, fully formed. Characteristic also is a family dynamic in which the patient herself appears remarkably unconcerned in the face of lesions that are disfiguring, and that should be painful, while parents and family express anger and resentment, implying, overtly or covertly, that the medical community is uncaring and inept. Should one be the sixth or even the tenth physician consulted, all the wrath due to one's unsuccessful predecessors will inevitably be visited upon one's head. Equally inevitable is the thick folder of previous examinations and negative studies, and a past history of other bizarre and undiagnosed physical illnesses, that may add to the anger and frustration expressed[26,61].

The psychiatric diagnosis in the majority of patients with DA is the borderline personality disorder (BPD)[62], although occasionally an immature woman or young girl may produce lesions as a maladaptive coping mechanism in response to a psychosocial stress; more rarely, lesions may result from a dissociative phenomenon in a patient with multiple personality disorder (MPD)[63]. A co-morbid underlying depression can usually be uncovered in patients with DA, who suffer from a profound sense of isolation and emptiness, whose impulse control is poor, and whose relationships are usually dependent and manipulative[64,65]. Associated eating disorders, particularly anorexia nervosa, may co-exist in these patients. That they are able to sustain severely destructive lesions without evident distress, may be explained by an elevated level of serum metencephalin that has been detected in these patients[66], and by opioid mechanisms that may induce analgesia under stress[67]. For example, despite the depth of the ulceration, the patient in Figure 1 complained of no pain.

Histopathology

Histopathology will be determined by the particular modus operandi of the individual patient. Lyell has summarized the various methods that might be employed[62]. Laboratory studies again will be predicated by the character of the individual lesions.

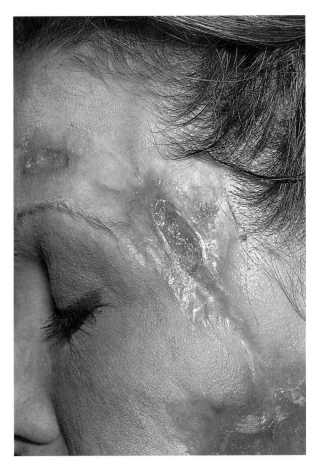

Figure 1 Dermatitis artefacta. Though initially she strenuously denied the fact, these lesions were self-induced by a patient with borderline personality disorder

Differential diagnosis

DA is to be differentiated from a primary dermatosis. It is also to be differentiated from neurotic excoriations, from other manifestations of OCD, and from malingering. Patients with DA differ from BPD patients who are wrist-cutters, since the latter openly acknowledge responsibility for the action. The hollow history, bizarre lesions, negative laboratory studies and histology will rule out a primary dermatosis. The lesions of OCD lack the secrecy of DA; they clearly bear the marks of repetitive manipulation, such as scratching, picking or rubbing, for which the patient acknowledges responsibility. In malingering, by contrast, men predominate, onset is at a later age, and the secondary gain, either financial or in terms of avoiding arduous responsibility, is quite evident.

Treatment

For a discussion of the philosophy of treatment, the reader is referred to the general section on treatment, on pp. 13–15. Patients with DA are not easy to treat, because whatever they may aver to the

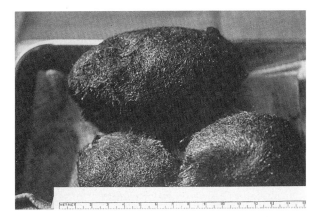

Figure 2 Trichobezoars extracted from the intestine of a patient with trichotillomania. Reprinted with permission from Navab F, Sabol J. Images in clinical medicine: trichobezoars. *N Engl J Med* 1997;336:1721

contrary, at an unconscious level they 'need' their illness, and cannot permit themselves to get well. Skin lesions are their entrée to health care, and for this reason it is important to set up regular appointments, whether or not lesions are present, so that further self-destruction in order to receive care is not necessary. Initially, visits should be frequent, though quite short, to establish rapport and provide support, but ostensibly to supervise topical therapy. One must not confront the patient about etiology, and indeed the etiology may never be spoken about by either party. In discussion, one may take an agnostic view, suggesting that although the exact cause of the problem is not known, we do know how to treat it. Alternatively, one may elect to interpret the lesions in terms of chemical neurotransmitters, or other mediators, that may be liberated in response to stress. Most patients will benefit from SSRI antidepressants, the rationale for which can be explained to the patient on the basis of chemical messengers. Antipsychotics should be added to the regimen, if the response to treatment is disappointing.

Prognosis

The prognosis depends on the severity of the psychopathology. In young adolescents, or in immature women who resort to DA as a maladaptive coping mechanism, insight-oriented or supportive therapy and increasing maturity may allow the self-destructive activity to be given up[26]. In those patients with a more severe personality disorder, long-term treatment with psychoactive agents may be necessary, and studies show that DA may continue for many years, waxing and waning in severity, in parallel with the stresses in the patient's life[68].

Cutaneous delusions

Dysmorphic delusions

Delusional beliefs about abnormal or altered structure or function of the skin have been discussed in the section on BDD.

Delusions of parasitosis

Clinical description

The clinical picture of delusions of parasitosis (DOP) is in every way similar to that of dysmorphic delusions excepting that the ideation is different. Experience would suggest that DOP is much more common than previously believed, and that although it can occur at any age, it is most common in elderly women who live alone. The majority of male patients are either on renal dialysis, or are part of a *folie à deux* (shared delusions). The clinical picture is very characteristic and has been described in detail elsewhere[26,69–71].

Differential diagnosis

Any condition that causes prolonged itching or dysesthesia may be interpreted in terms of an infestation; this then creates an overlap with the chronic cutaneous dysesthesia syndrome (vide p. 22). Hepatic or renal disease, cocaine or amphetamine intoxication, steroid psychosis, cerebral arteriosclerosis or other organic brain syndromes must be ruled out, as must a true infestation or primary dermatosis, before the diagnosis is made.

With regard to psychopathology, DOP has been regarded as a monosymptomatic hypochondriacal delusion – a term that would encompass also delusional BDD – suggesting that the patient is functioning well in other aspects of her life[72]. If one takes a little time to learn about her, invariably one finds that the patient is depressed, feels ashamed, restricts the normal activities of living, punishes herself with excessive hygiene measures, expends large sums of money in her attempts to eradicate the scourge, and isolates herself socially for fear of contaminating others[26].

Treatment

As in all psychocutaneous disorders, engagement of the patient in a treatment alliance is crucial to a successful outcome[26,73,74]. Traditionally, pimozide has been the drug of choice, perhaps because of its effect on endogenous opioid pathways, which have been associated with the transmission of itch. Both risperidone and olanzepine, however, appear to be equally as effective.

Prognosis

The patient may experience some relief within ten days to two weeks of starting medication, although it may take several months for a complete resolution of symptoms. Though anxiety, depression and cutaneous symptoms disappear, rarely does the patient gain insight, and realize that there has, in fact, been no infestation. Attempts to wean the drug gradually after six symptom-free months may result in a brief remission, but gradually symptoms will recur. Many patients are lost to follow-up, but it is doubtful whether long-term remissions really occur.

DERMATOLOGIC MANIFESTATIONS OF OCD

Obsessional worries

These have been covered in the section on BDD.

Compulsive symptoms in dermatology
Trichotillomania (hair-pulling tic)

Clinical picture

Trichotillomania (TTM) refers to a compulsive and uncontrollable urge to pull out the hair of scalp, brows, lashes or pubic area. In early childhood hair-pulling is more common in boys, and may be used temporarily as a mechanism to release tension. In adolescence, the condition is much less benign, girls predominate in a ratio of 5:1, and a disordered mother–child relationship is an almost universal finding[75].

Studies have revealed that adolescent girls with TTM are not a homogeneous group; they exhibit different triggering cues[76], favor different sites for hair-pulling, and experience differences in emotional discharge[77,78]. Psychoanalytic exploration reveals that there are also differences in the unconscious meaning of hair-pulling, in the inner life of the girl[75].

Parents are usually ashamed and depressed about an activity that does not make sense, spoils their child's looks, and cannot be controlled. It is very hard for parents to believe that the hair-loss is self-induced, and they frequently embark on an expensive peripatetic search for a physical cause before the diagnosis can be accepted. Hair-pulling is a furtive and secret activity, often ritualized and undertaken at night. Patients may carefully select specific hairs for pulling, and may be uncontrollably driven by anxiety to sniff them, stroke them across the lips or skin, or even to eat them after pulling. Intestinal obstruction from trichobezoar is reported, though usually in younger children

(Figure 2)[26,75]. The clinical picture is characteristic and has been described in detail elsewhere[26].

Histopathology

Muller, in 1990, studied biopsy material from sixty-six patients with TTM[79]. The findings included tearing of the follicles, with a hemorrhagic exudate surrounding the remnants of the bulb, trichomalacia, empty catagen follicles with torn basement membrane, and very sparse telogen hairs. He also described dilated follicular ostia, often filled with soft keratin, and large oval, comma or corkscrew-shaped pigment casts located in the isthmus, or infundibular region.

Differential diagnosis

TTM can be differentiated from alopecia areata by the ill-defined borders of the patch, and the absence of total alopecia. There are hairs of differing length within the patch, the very shortest are contiguous to long undamaged hairs at the edge of the patch, and there is a 'bristly' feeling on passing the hand gently over the surface. Scarring alopecias are excluded by the absence of inflammation, or decreased numbers of follicles, and tinea capitis by negative KOH examination and culture.

In the psychiatric literature, a question is raised as to whether TTM results from a compulsion or an impulse disorder, since the definition of compulsion requires that an intrusive obsessional thought be associated with the repetitive action. Clinical experience suggests that either may be the case, though for our purposes the distinction is irrelevant, since both respond to the same treatment.

Treatment

The treatment of TTM is the same as for OCD.

Prognosis

Without treatment TTM runs a prolonged course with remissions and exacerbations. A disease of adolescent girls *par excellence*, it should be regarded as a nonverbal communication of distress, and acted on accordingly. Once the diagnosis can be accepted by patient and parents, psychiatric referral may be possible. Psychoanalysis or psychoanalytic psychotherapy, when feasible, offers the possibility of long-term benefits, and improved functioning generally[80]; both are reported effective[81]. Behavior modification and cognitive–behavioral therapy may afford symptom relief, while the SSRIs, preferably with adjunctive cognitive–behavioral psychotherapy, address all aspects of the syndrome[42,45]. There are also early reports of a favorable response to low-dose risperidone[82], but though there may be control with these various drug regimens, it is doubtful whether permanent resolution occurs.

Neurotic excoriations

Clinical picture

The term neurotic excoriations refers to compulsive picking[26,83,85]. While there are those who have been life long 'pickers', excoriating insect bites in childhood, keratosis pilaris or acne in adolescence, and continuing into adult life, for most youngsters this is a habit, readily out-grown, and probably within the spectrum of normal behavior. The term neurotic excoriations is reserved for those who pick in a self-destructive way, who are unable to stop picking (although they know it makes no sense), who may pick in a ritualized fashion, sometimes taking hours to accomplish the task, and who experience feelings of shame and embarrassment as a result. Although neurotic excoriations occur in both genders, the condition is significantly more common in women, and particularly in those who are postmenopausal.

Significant skin-picking occurs primarily under three sets of circumstances: it may be part of the picture of BDD, as discussed previously; it may result from an obsessive–compulsive intolerance of any irregularity that is fortuitously encountered as the hands wander over the skin surface, which must then be picked off; thirdly, usually in older women, or those who are depressed, there may be a focal itch, which on rubbing develops a tiny urticarial wheal, or prurigo lesion, which in turn must be picked off.

Whatever the motivating force, once excoriations have been produced, there is an inner and uncontrollable drive to remove the resultant crusts, and a cycle of picking and crusting ensues, that may result in the development of prurigo nodularis. In some patients picking may be ritualized, occurring on a daily basis, usually in privacy, and in the evening; often the patient is driven to pick every single lesion at each sitting. For other patients, picking may be a clear expression of anger or anxiety. For example, when angered by her emotionally unresponsive husband, and unable to express her anger verbally, one patient would lock herself in the garage and remove the crust from each one of a hundred or more lesions on her legs, with the point of a kitchen knife. Unlike patients with DA or TTM, patients with neurotic excoriations usually acknowledge, if somewhat shamefacedly, that they are responsible for the lesions.

The clinical morphology and distribution have been discussed in detail elsewhere, and will not be repeated here[26,41,43,83–85].

Histology

The histology is that of a non-specific response to injury, usually with crusting, and sometimes with secondary bacterial infection. If a primary dermatosis underlies the process, the histology will reflect that.

Laboratory studies

Bacterial cultures are indicated if infection is suspected. Biopsy is necessary only if an underlying primary dermatosis is suspected, and primary lesions are not evident.

Differential diagnosis

The clinical morphology and distribution are so characteristic that other considerations are seldom entertained in the established case. Depending on the clinical picture, papular urticaria, acne vulgaris, dermatitis herpetiformis and bullous pemphigoid may need to be ruled out as underlying precipitants.

Treatment

Topical treatment is designed to make the skin as smooth as possible, thus reducing the temptation to remove irregularities. Compresses, gentle removal of crusts and topical and systemic antibiotics all have their place, as do topical and intralesional steroids. Emollients containing lactic acid, glycolic acid or urea are especially useful in helping to maintain a smooth cutaneous surface. When dermographism is present, doxepin, 10 mg at h.s., or one of the non-sedating antihistamines, may eliminate wheal formation and the need to pick. Anxiety and depression must be sought out and identified, and the psychiatric treatment is the same as for OCD.

Prognosis

Once the underlying reason for picking (BDD, OCD, anxiety, or depression), is addressed, usually the symptom will resolve, though the potential for recurrence at times of stress remains.

Chronic cutaneous dysesthesia syndrome (tactile hallucinosis; cutaneous sensory syndrome; pruritus sine materia)

Clinical picture

Chronic cutaneous dysesthesia syndrome (CCDS) refers to a condition in which altered sensations – for which no physical cause can be identified – are experienced in skin or orificial mucosae[8,42,43,47]. Occasionally the sensation is itching, but more frequently it is described as burning, stinging, crawling, pricking, shooting, 'electric' flashes, etc.; the sensation is also usually described as 'under', or 'within' the skin, rather than on the surface. Any area may be affected, and while in some it is constantly at the same site, in others it may vary, flitting from place to place. While it may be a constant unremitting presence, it may also be evanescent, coming and going in a wholly unpredictable way that makes the patient feel that she is completely out of control.

The condition is much more common in women, and though it can occur at any age patients are usually peri- or postmenopausal[43,53,86]. An underlying depression can almost always be identified. Less commonly, dysesthesia may be a primary symptom around which a delusional system, either of dysmorphic abnormality or parasitic infestation, may be woven. In these cases, BDD or DOP may evolve, or the delusion may represent a facet of a broader psychopathology such as a paranoid disorder, schizophrenia, toxic psychosis or an organic brain syndrome. Even when these latter are present, depression is usually part of the picture. Clinical experience would suggest that men who present with CCDS tend to be younger, have more severe psychopathology, and have less prominent depression.

Apart from the specific complaint, the clinical picture of CCDS is very similar to that of BDD, since the patient often interprets the cause of her discomfort as a major alteration in structure or function. Phenomenologically, dysesthetic vulvodynia[48], and glossodynia (burning mouth syndrome)[87–91] are in every way similar to cutaneous dysesthesia, and it is an artificial distinction to separate these from the condition as it occurs in skin and scalp, although of course the unconscious symbolic meaning of the symptom in the inner life of the patient is likely to be different.

As with BDD, the patient is completely absorbed by her symptom, which intrudes into every aspect of her life, and interferes in her functioning at every level. Like those with BDD, the patient often feels ashamed and embarrassed, and is frantically driven to consult numerous physicians in a variety of specialties, seeking ever more bizarre diagnoses and arcane tests, in her search for understanding and relief. Unlike the patient with DOP, who suffers alone and in isolation, the patient with CCDS often has a spouse with whom she shares a mutually dependent and often ambivalent relationship, and who colludes with her, fomenting her anxiety and perpetuating her peripatetic search for cause and cure.

Histopathology

The skin or mucous membrane is entirely normal.

Laboratory studies

These should include appropriate blood-work and CT scans to rule out a physical cause. Neurologic, dental or gynecologic consultation may be indicated, depending on the specific symptom. Biopsy is rarely helpful.

Differential diagnosis

Once physical disease has been ruled out, it is important to determine whether or not there is a delusional dysmorphic component associated with the dysesthesia.

Treatment

Tricyclic antidepressants have traditionally been prescribed for dysesthesias, in a fashion similar to post-zoster neuralgia and atypical pain syndromes[47,48,90,91]. More recently, the SSRIs have been found effective. Some slight improvement usually takes place within three or four weeks, with symptoms improving progressively over a period of months, after which most patients achieve complete relief. In some patients antipsychotics, preferably pimozide, must be added if relief is not achieved. If the dysesthesia is clearly a part of the picture of DOP it may be regarded as a tactile hallucination, and pimozide is then the first line of treatment.

Prognosis

Long-term drug therapy is usually needed, though remissions of varying length may occur.

Dermatologic conditions affected by stress

Although it is probable that any inflammatory dermatosis may be affected by stress, the major ones are listed in Table 2. Anxiety and depression are common in the elderly, and particularly so in elderly women. Many of these patients are not in touch with their feelings and present to their primary care physician only with a variety of physical complains[92,93]. This is certainly true of skin disease. The constraints of space do not permit an extensive discussion of the impact of stress on the inflammatory dermatoses, and the interested reader is referred to appropriate publications[8,10,26,41,42,94–96].

Somatopsychic effect

The somatopsychic effect refers to the emotional cost to the patient and family, when there is severe disabling or disfiguring skin disease. Much has been written about this in relation to psoriasis[97–99], acne[100,101], atopic dermatitis[102–104], hirsutism[105], port-wine stains[106], vitiligo[107] and the aging process[108–110]. Patients may experience feelings of stigmatization, shame, diminished self-esteem and guilt, because of 'imperfection', and because of the cost in terms of time, money and physical restriction incurred by the family, on account of the patient's illness. Yet we cannot fail to be impressed by the adaptability and resilience that some patients show in face of tremendous adversity[111].

Differences in the capacity of patients to adapt to adversity depend upon a number of variables. First are the inherent personality characteristics that the infant brings into the world with her. Second is the emotional environment into which the infant girl is born, and the ability of her parents to touch her lovingly without recoil, accepting her unconditionally for who she is, rather than as an idealized projection of the person they would like her to become. This unconditional acceptance enables the little girl to develop a positive sense of herself; it supports her strengths, and allows a flexibility of personality that will enable her to seek out new ways of self-expression and personal fulfillment when other avenues are closed. Thirdly the impact depends upon the age at which the condition first makes its appearance; and finally there is the impact, on the growing girl, of the societal response to her diseased skin.

The development of the body image and its importance to one's feeling of well-being has already been addressed. Integration of change into the body image is stressful at any age, and particularly stressful for those deprived of optimal nurturing in infancy. For the reasons stated, it is particularly stressful for girls and women[18,111].

A condition that is present at birth, or in early infancy, is integrated into the body image and accepted as a part of the self. The inner meaning that it has for the individual reflects the internalized attitudes of the primary care-takers during early development. Though the patient may be the butt of teasing by her peers, skin disease in childhood can be well tolerated if the parents are accepting and supportive, and help the child to lead a life that is as near to normal as possible. Support groups provide great help for parents in making them feel less isolated, and in finding ways for their daughter to adapt to her disability. Because of the stresses inherent in the girl's adolescent body-image changes, and the fragility of her self-esteem, skin disease that has its onset in adolescence is particularly stressful, and may cause the girl to exaggerate the deformity in her mind, and develop symptoms of BDD, that may continue into adult life.

The high cost of medication, treatment regimens that are arduous, the need for restriction in choice in clothing, and limited occupational and recreational activities all lead to feelings of embarrassment, guilt and shame. Patients may feel 'dirty' or 'disgusting', and may refuse to visit beauty salons or swimming pools. Feeling unattractive, the patient may withdraw, impairing intimacy and sexual activity, while negative self-worth may lead to impaired social and vocational functioning. Disease of the anogenital area is especially loaded and may lead to incapacitating feelings of shame and self-disgust. Feeling unattractive, the patient transmits a negative message socially, which, unfortunately, will generate a reciprocal response, and confirm for the patient that her self-perception is correct[112].

As dermatologists, it is important for us to be aware of these negative feelings in our patients, to accept the patient for who she is, and to make a point of showing that we find her neither dirty nor disgusting; we must show that we do not fear contamination, and that we feel free to touch. It is important for us also to support the patient's strengths and help her to accept her disease, and to find ways to adapt to it.

REFERENCES

1. Fava GA, Freyberger H, eds. *Handbook of Psychosomatic Medicine*. Madison Ct: International University Press, 1998
2. Sneddon J, Sneddon I. Acne excoriee: a protective device. *Clin Exp Dermatol* 1983;8:65–8
3. Medansky RS, Handler RM. Dermato psychosomatics: classification, physiology, and therapeutic approaches. *J Am Acad Dermatol* 1981;5:125–36
4. Spitz RA. *The First Year of Life: A Psychoanalytic Study of Normal and Deviant Development of Object Relations*. New York: International University Press, 1965: 223–42
5. Obermeyer ME. *Psychocutaneous Medicine*. Springfield IL: Charles C Thomas, 1955:280–7
6. Sneddon I. The mind and the skin. *BMJ* 1949; I/472
7. Plewig G. Rosacea. In Fitzpatrick TB, Eisen AZ, Wolff K *et al.*, eds. *Dermatology in General Medicine*, 4th edn. New York: McGraw-Hill, 1993:728
8. Panconesi E. Psychosomatic dermatology. In Panconesi E, ed. Stress and skin diseases: psychosomatic dermatology. *Clin Dermatol* 1984;2(4):94–179
9. Miller RM, Coger RW. Skin conductance conditioning with dyshidrotic eczema patients. *Br J Dermatol* 1979;101:435–7
10. Panconesi E, Hautmann G. Psychophysiology of stress in dermatology. *Dermatol Clin* 1996;14: 399–421
11. Sternberg EM. Neuroendocrine factors in susceptibility to inflammatory disease. *Horm Res* 1995;43: 159–61
12. Egan CL, Viglione Scnneck MJ, Walsh LJ, *et al.* Characterization of unmyelinated axons uniting epidermal and dermal immune cells in primate and murine skin. *J Cutan Pathol* 1998;25:20–9
13. Lotti T, Hautmann G, Panconesi E. Neuropeptides in skin. *J Am Acad Dermatol* 1995;33:482–96
14. Weiss ST. Parental touching: correlates of a child's body concept and body experience. In Barnard KE, Brazelton TB, eds. *Touch: the Foundation of Experience*. Madison: International University Press, 1990:425–59
15. Levine S, Stanton ME. The hormonal consequences of mother-infant contact in primates and rodents. In Brown CC, ed. *The Many Facets of Touch*. Johnson and Johnson Pediatric Round Table Series, 10, 1984:51–65
16. Korner AF. The many facets of touch. In Brown CC, ed. *The Many Facets of Touch*. Johnson and Johnson Pediatric Round Table Series, 10, 1984:107–13
17. Hofer MA. The mother-infant interaction as a regulator of infant physiology and behavior. In Plutchnik R, ed. *Emotion, Theory, Research and Experience*, vol II. Orlando: Academic Press, 1983:74
18. Koblenzer CS. Psychodermatology of woman. *Clin Dermatol* 1997;15:127–141
19. Koblenzer CS. A neglected but crucial aspect of skin function. *Int J Dermatol* 1990;29:185–6
20. Taylor GJ. *Psychosomatic Medicine and Contemporary Psychoanalysis*. Madison Ct: International University Press, 1987:149
21. Brown DG. The relevance of body image to neurosis. *Br J Med Psychol* 1959;32:11–38
22. Hartman H, Kris E, Lowenstein EM. Comments on the formation of psychic structure. *Psychoanalytic Study of Child* 1946;2:11–38

23. Greenspan SI. *The Development of the Ego*. Madison: International University Press, 1989:1–56

24. Pines D. *A Woman's Unconscious Use of Her Body*. New Haven: Yale University Press, 1994:42–96, 98–103

25. Anzier D. *The Skin Ego*. New Haven: Yale University Press, 1989:3–67

26. Koblenzer CS. *Psychocutaneous Disease*. Orlando: Grune and Stratton, 1987:4–5, 31–80, 85–107, 108–30, 138–68

27. Main M. Parental aversion to infant-initiated contact is correlated with parent's own rejection during childhood. In Barnard KE, Brazelton TB, eds. *Touch: the Foundation of Experience*. Madison: International University Press, 1990:461–95

28. McAnarney ER. Adolescents and touch. In Brown CC, ed. *The Many Facets of Touch*. Johnson and Johnson Pediatric Round Table Series, 10, 1984:138–45

29. Mahler MS, Pine E, Bergman A. *The Psychological Birth of the Human Infant*. New York: Basic Books, 1975:52–108

30. McDougal J. In Baruch EH, Serrano LJ, eds. *Women Analyze Women*. New York: New York University Press, 1988:63–84

31. Burton A. The meaning of perineal activity to women: an inner sphinx. *J Am Psychoanal Assoc* 1996;44(suppl):241–59

32. Lerner HE. Parental mislabeling of female genitals as a determinant of penis envy and learning inhibition in women. *J Am Psychoanal Assoc* 1976; 24(suppl):269–84

33. Renik O, Grossman L. Contemporary theories of female sexuality: clinical applications. *J Am Psychoanal Assoc* 1994;42:233–41

34. Fallon A. Culture in the mirror: sociocultural determinants of body image. In Cash TF, Pruzinsky T, eds. *Body Images: Development, Deviance, Change*. New York: Guildford Press, 1990:80–109

35. Adams GR. Attractiveness through the ages: implications of facial attractiveness over the life cycle. In Graham JL, Kligman AM, eds. *The Psychology of Cosmetic Treatments*. New York: Praeger, 1985:133–51

36. American Psychiatric Association. *Diagnostic and Statistical Manual of Mental Disorders*, 4th edn. Washington DC: American Psychiatric Press, 1994: 339–49

37. Reiser HR. Ages eleven to fourteen. In Greenspan SI, Pollock GH, eds. *The Course of Life. Adolescence*, vol IV. Madison: International University Press, 1991:99–111

38. Kaplan EH. Adolescents age fifteen to eighteen. A psychoanalytic developmental view. In Greenspan SI, Pollock GH, eds. *The Course of Life. Adolescence*. Vol IV. Madison: International University Press, 1991:201–18

39. Koblenzer CS. The psychology of sun exposure and tanning. *Clin Dermatol* 1998;16:421–8

40. Pruzinsky T, Edgerton MT. Body image change in plastic surgery. In Cash TF, Pruzinsky T, eds. *Body Images: Development, Deviance, Change*. New York: Guildford Press, 1990:217–33

41. Koblenzer CS. Psychosomatic concepts in dermatology: a dermatologist-psychoanalyst's viewpoint. *Arch Dermatol* 1983;119:501–12

42. Koo J. Psychodermatology: a practical manual for clinicians. *Curr Prob Dermatol* 1995;VII:199–234

43. Koblenzer CS. Psychiatric syndromes of interest to dermatologists. *Int J Dermatol* 1993;32:82–8

44. Kulin NA, Pastuszak A, Sage SR, *et al.* Pregnancy outcome, following maternal use of the new selective serotonin reuptake inhibitors. *JAMA* 1988;279: 609–10

45. Koblenzer CS. Pharmacology of psychotropic drugs useful in dermatologic practice. *Int J Dermatol* 1993; 32:162–8

46. Phillips KA. Pharmacologic treatment of body dysmorphic disorder. *Psychopharm Bull* 1996;32: 597–605

47. Koblenzer CS, Bostrom P. Chronic cutaneous dysesthesia syndrome. *J Am Acad Dermatol* 1994;30: 370–4

48. McKay M. Dysesthetic (essential) vulvodynia: treatment with amitriptyline. *J Reprod Med* 1993;38: 8–13

49. Schatzberg AF, Cole JO, DeBattista DMH, eds. *Manual of Clinical Psychopharmacology*, 3rd edn. Washington DC: American Psychiatric Association Press, 1997:154–5

50. Phillips KA. Body dysmorphic disorder: clinical features and drug treatment. *Pract Therapeut* 1995; 30:30–43

51. Phillips KA. Body dysmorphic disorder: diagnosis and treatment of imagined ugliness. *J Clin Psychiatry* 1996;57(suppl 8):61–65

52. Phillips KA, Taub SL. Skin picking as a symptom of body dysmorphic disorder. *Psychopharm Bull* 1995; 31:279–88

53. Cotterill JA. Dermatologic non-disease: a common and potentially fatal disturbance of cutaneous body image. *Br J Dermatol* 1981;140:611–19

54. Cotterill JA, Cunliffe WJ. Suicide in dermatological patients. *Br J Dermatol* 1997;137:246–50

55. Munro A, Chimara J. Monosymptomatic hypochondriacal psychosis: a diagnostic check-list, based on 5 cases of the disorder. *Can J Psychiatry* 1982;27: 374–6

56. Reich P, Gottfried LA. Factitious disorder in a teaching hospital. *Am J Intern Med* 1983;99:240–7

57. Gieler U. Factitious disease in the field of dermatology. *Psychother Psychosom* 1994;62:48–55

58. Fabische W. Psychiatric aspects of dermatitis artefacta. *Acad Psychiatry Scand* 1989;79:283–9

59. Sutherland AJ, Rodin GM. Factitious disorders in a general hospital setting: clinical features and a review of the literature. *Psychosom* 1990;31:392–9

60. Haenel T, Rauchfleisch U, Schuppli R, *et al*. The psychiatric significance of dermatitis artefacta. *Euro Arch Psychiatry Neurol Sci* 1984;234:38–41

61. Lyell A. Cutaneous artefactual disease: a review amplified by personal experience. *J Am Acad Dermatol* 1979;1:391–7

62. Simpson MA. Self-mutilation and the borderline syndrome. *J Am Psychiatry* 1977;42:42–8

63. Shelley WB. Dermatitis artefacta induced in a patient by one of her multiple personalities. *Br J Dermatol* 1981;105:597–89

64. Plassman R. The biography of the factitious-disorder patient. *Psychother Psychosom* 1984;62:123–8

65. Schaeffer CB, Carroll J, Abramowitz S. Self-mutilation and the borderline personality. *J Nerv Ment Dis* 1982;170:468–73

66. Coll J, Allolio B, Rees LH. Raised plasma metencephalin in patients who habitually mutilate themselves. *Lancet* 1983;2:545–6

67. Lewis JW, Cannon JT, Lieberkind JC. Opioid and non-opioid mechanisms of stress analgesia. *Science* 1980;208:623–5

68. Sneddon I, Sneddon J. Self-inflicted injury: a follow-up study of 43 patients. *Br Med J* 1975;2:527–30

69. Lyell A. Delusions of parasitosis. *Br J Dermatol* 1983;108:485–99

70. Reilly TM, Batchelor DH. The presentation and treatment of delusional parasitosis: a dermatologic perspective. *Int J Clin Psychopharm* 1986;1:340–53

71. Driscoll MS, Rothe MJ, Grant-Kels JH, *et al*. Delusional parasitosis: a dermatologic, psychiatric and psychopharmacologic approach. *J Am Acad Dermatol* 1993;29:1023–33

72. Munro A. Monosymptomatic hypochondriacal psychosis: a diagnostic entity that may respond to pimozide. *Can J Psychiatry* 1978;23:497–9

73. Gould WM, Grag TM. Delusions of parasitosis: an approach to the problem. *Arch Dermatol* 1976;112:1745–8

74. Torch EM, Bishop ER. Delusions of parasitosis. Psychotherapeutic engagement. *Am J Psychother* 1981;35:101–6

75. Koblenzer CS. Trichotillomania – psychoanalytic aspects. In Stein DJ, Hollander E, eds. *Trichotillomania*. Washington DC: American Psychiatric Association Press:in press

76. Christenson CA, Ristvedt SL, Mackenzie TB. Identification of trichotillomania cue profiles. *Behav Res Ther* 1993;31:315–20

77. Christenson CA, Mackenzie TB, Mitchell JE. Adult men and women with trichotillomania. A comparison of male and female characteristics. *Psychosom* 1994;35:142–9

78. Christenson CA, Mackenzie TB, Mitchell JE. Characteristics of 60 adult chronic hair-pullers. *Am J Psychiatry* 1991;148:365–70

79. Muller SA. Trichotillomania: a histopathologic study in sixty-six patients. *J Am Acad Dermatol* 1990;23:56–62

80. Rothstein A, ed. How does treatment help? On the modes of therapeutic action of psychoanalytic psychotherapy. *Workshop Series of the American Psychoanalytic Association*. Madison: Internatational University Press, 1988

81. Koblenzer CS. Trichotillomania – the application of a psychodynamic understanding to etiology and treatment. Presented at the *Second International Congress of Dermatology and Psychiatry*, Leeds, UK, July 9–11, 1989

82. Garnis-Jones S. Trichotillomania: an overview, and discussion of some new therapies. Presented at the *6th Annual Meeting of the Association for Psychocutaneous Medicine of North America*, Washington DC, February 9, 1996

83. Adamson HG. Acne excoriee and other forms of 'neurotic excoriations'. *Br J Dermatol* 1915;27:1–12

84. Pusey WA, Senear FE. Neurotic excoriations with report of cases. *Arch Dermatol Syphilol* 1920;1:270–8

85. Mackee GM. Neurotic excoriations. *Arch Dermatol Syphilol* 1920;1:256–69

86. Hoss D, Segal S. Scalp dysesthesia. *Arch Dermatol* 1998;134:327–30

87. Ott G, Ott C. Glossodynia – psychodynamic basis and results of psychometric investigations. *J Psychosom Res* 1992;7:677–686

88. Rojo L, Silvestre FJ, Bagan JV, DeVicente T. Psychiatric morbidity in burning mouth syndrome. *Oral Surg, Oral Med, Oral Pathol* 1993;75:308–11

89. Gorsky M, Silverman S, Chinn H. Clinical characteristics and management outcome in the burning mouth syndrome. *Oral Surg, Oral Med, Oral Pathol* 1991;72:192–5

90. Huang W, Rothe MJ, Grant-Kels JM. The burning mouth syndrome. *J Am Acad Dermatol* 1996;34:91–8

91. Grinspan D, Fernandez-Blanco C, Allevato MA, Stengel FM. Burning mouth syndrome. *Int J Dermatol* 1995;34:483–7

92. Eisenberg L. Sounding board: treating depression and anxiety in primary care. *N Engl J Med* 1992;336:1080–4

93. Rodin G, Voshard K. Depression in the medically ill. *Am J Psychiatry* 1986;143:696–705

94. Van Moffaert M. Psychodermatology. In Fava GA, Freyberger H, eds. *Handbook of Psychosomatic Medicine*. Madison: International University Press, 1998:373–92

95. Friedman S, Hatch M, Paradis C. Dermatologic Disorders. In Gatchel RJ, Blanchard EB, eds. *Psychophysiological Disorders*. Washington DC: American Psychological Association Press, 1993:205–67

96. Koo JYM, Pham CT. Psychodermatology. *Arch Dermatol* 1992;128:381–8

97. Ginsburg IH, Link BG. Feelings of stigmatization in patients with psoriasis. *J Am Acad Dermatol* 1989; 20:53–63

98. Ginsburg IH, Link BG. Psychosocial consequences of rejection and stigma feelings, in psoriatic patients. *Int J Dermatol* 1993;32:587–91

99. Fried RG. Psychosocial impact of psoriasis on the older patient. *J Geriat Dermatol* 1995;3(suppl B): 14B–16B

100. Wu SF, Kidner BN, Trunnell TN, *et al*. Role of anxiety and anger in acne patients: a relationship with the severity of the disorder. *J Am Acad Dermatol* 1988;18:325–33

101. Lim CCL, Tah-Chew T. Personality, disability and acne in college students. *Clin Exp Dermatol* 1991; 16:371–3

102. Koblenzer CS, Koblenzer PJ. Chronic intractable atopic eczema as a physical sign of impaired parent-child relationships and psychological developmental arrest. *Arch Dermatol* 1988;124:1673–8

103. Gil KM, Sampson HA. Psychological and social factors of atopic dermatitis. *Allergy* 1989;44(suppl 9): 84–9

104. David LR, Garralda MA, David TJ. Psychosocial adjustment in pre-school children with atopic eczema. *Arch Dis Child* 1993;69:670–6

105. Barth JH, Catalan J, Cherry CA, *et al*. Psychological morbidity in women referred for treatment of hirsutism. *J Psychosom Res* 1993; 37:615–19

106. Lanigan SW, Cotterill JA. Psychological disabilities among patients with port-wine stains. *Br J Dermatol* 1989;121:209–15

107. Porter JR, Hill-Beuf A. Racial variation in reaction to a physical stigma: a study of degree of disturbance by vitiligo among black and white patients. *J Health Soc Behav* 1991;32:192–204

108. Koblenzer CS. Psychological aspects of aging and the skin. *Clin Dermatol* 1996;14:171–7

109. Fried RG. Cosmetics in the older patient: why bother? *J Geriat Dermatol* 1995;3:99–102

110. Graham JA, Kligman AM. Cosmetic therapy for the elderly. *J Soc Cosmetic Chem* 1984;35:133–45

111. Koblenzer CS. The psychological and social impact of skin disease. In Pierini AM, *et al*., eds. *Pediatric Dermatology. The World's Reality in the Children's Skin*. Amsterdam: Elsevier, 1995:8–12

112. Snyder M, Tanke ED, Berscheid E. Social perception and interpersonal behavior: on the self-fulfilling nature of social psychology. *J Pers Soc Psychol* 1977;35:656–8

The examination of girls and women   3

Sarah C. F. Rogers

INTRODUCTION

One might pose the question, 'Should the examination of girls and women differ from that of boys and men?' After all, this is the age of equality of the sexes. Nevertheless, I propose that the answer is yes. Why? Simply because men and women *are* different. That's why life is so interesting – *vive la différence!* as the French exclaim. Certainly, I am not the first to address the problem[1]. Everyone of you will have a mother, a grandmother, a sister, a wife. Consider how you would like your female relative treated by a medical colleague. A greater degree of sensitivity is called for and the 'drop your pants' approach which might do for male patients simply will not do for females.

BEFORE THE CONSULTATION

If there is an opportunity to read details about the patient from a referral letter before she is introduced to you, take advantage of it. Her age, marital status and perhaps ethnic and/or religious background will help put the first brush strokes on the canvas. Observe the patient as she enters the consulting room. Is she alone or does she need her spouse or sister for moral support? Take account of her age, how she dresses and how she feels about herself. Are her eyes downcast; does she return your greeting in a whisper or does she breeze in, grasp your hand firmly and establish eye-to-eye contact? Some older women will dress accordingly, have grey hair, and look like a granny. Others of the same age may sport something trendy and have flowing, colored tresses. How these two ladies should be addressed will be quite different. And there are other guidelines.

Like the granny type, a lady 'of a certain age' who wears a hat and clutches a linen handkerchief will not appreciate your calling her by her first name. That would be too familiar. She should be addressed as Mrs, Miss or Ms. By contrast, a smart young executive will expect to be on first name terms immediately.

THE HISTORY

Before the examination comes the initial part of the consultation, the history. This is where the rapport and trust that are necessary for a good doctor–patient relationship should be established. No one wants to meet her doctor for the first time, stripped of her clothes and huddled in a crinkling and crackling paper gown. It is a basic human requirement that the patient's dignity be maintained, always. Take the history, seated at your desk, and get your patient to relax. Remember that she has a set of expectations, realistic or otherwise, about what you can do for her. Though ultimately your aim is to deliver an accurate diagnosis, prognosis and treatment, how you communicate the information to her will be your most important task. Medicine, though many of us like to think of it as an exact science, is still largely an art. The art is that which makes the patient relax, take in what you are saying, understand that theirs may be a case of palliation rather than cure, and still feel better for having consulted you.

For both men and women one must now establish a rapport with the patient by understanding their background in all spheres of their life – social, occupational, sexual orientation – in so far as this is possible without appearing intrusive. At the same time, the patient is building up a picture of you, as it were, gaining a feeling of trust and confidence in you, so essential to a satisfactory outcome of the consultation. Not every personality gels with another straight off, but you will discover common ground. You may know where your patient lives and discover landmarks and people of mutual interest. Perhaps, when asking about employment or hobbies, you will discover a mutual passion for art, or saxophone playing, which will establish a level playing field for you both. I find that having children is a unifying bond allowing one to swap experiences and anecdotes. My consulting-rooms are at home, and hearing piano practice or seeing our little dog through the waiting-room window, mooching around in the garden, helps dispel preconceived myths about doctors as untouchables.

A woman from an Islamic background, besides having an accompanying male relative with her, may be quite shy and reticent about making eye contact until you have made her feel welcome and relaxed. She may have to communicate via an interpreter which means that some of the intimacy of the doctor–patient relationship is lost. If a young woman from a Western culture sits opposite the doctor, answering in monosyllables with downcast eyes, be on guard. Such behavior indicates a severe case of shyness, a personality problem or depression, and the whole consultation may prove very difficult. One must establish the contraceptive status of a woman of childbearing age. If she is taking the contraceptive pill it may interact with medication you wish to prescribe. Alternatively, adequate contraception must be established if you are going to prescribe a teratogenic drug.

THE EXAMINATION

Most patients will gladly accept the dermatologist's offer of a full skin examination. Others may give permission for only a more limited viewing, depending, perhaps, on ethnic or religious background. To safeguard his good name a male doctor should have a female chaperone present. The examination should take place in a separate room or adjacent cubicle. Women find it embarrassing to strip off in the presence of someone who was a complete stranger until 10 minutes ago, albeit behind a curtain. Provide a blanket or gown for the patient to cover herself in until you come to examine her. She will appreciate your sensitivity and will feel less ill at ease. If a young lady has acne, you may need to ask her to remove her makeup. To minimize the embarrassment of having to come in to the consulting-room without camouflage, as it were, have a bottle of hypoallergenic makeup remover, a bag of fluffy cotton wool balls, some tissues and a mirror on hand.

At first you may be granted only a viewing of arms, ankles and head as the rest of the body remains firmly battened down under the blanket or gown. While examining the breasts make sure the patient is covered from the waist down. When examining the genital area pull the blanket from the feet to suprapubic level leaving the remaining portion of the trunk covered. This part of the examination should be carried out sympathetically and with tact, particularly if you consider there is any possibility that the patient may have at some time experienced sexual abuse. Talk to your patient while carrying out the examination, explaining what you are looking for and report what you find. Allow no one, not even a colleague, to barge in during the examination; your patient's privacy must be respected. On conclusion of the examination

withdraw to the office so that your patient may dress alone. Don't try to chat about the diagnosis and treatment there and then. You may not be fazed as she wrestles with her tights (pantyhose) but she may be mortified by the experience.

THE DIAGNOSIS AND PLAN OF MANAGEMENT

In my experience women are better informed on medical matters than men, and their questions about treatment, side-effects and expected outcome are more probing. It may be, however, that an intelligent, well-educated patient may be more nervous than you appreciate, so take care to explain everything carefully, especially the treatment. This will only work as well as the patient's compliance allows and this, in turn, will depend on both her understanding of what is to be done and her motivation. We ask a lot of our patients: 'apply the steroid cream twice a day; the emollient, three times; special oil for the bath, oh, and don't forget the dandruff shampoo'. It's enough to drive them to the healthfood shop for a packet of herbal remedies! And never assume that, if the patient is a physician herself, an abbreviated version of what you tell the lay person will do. I know this because such a consultation with a colleague led to my taking HRT in a diligent but, nevertheless, incorrect way. The result was a revving up, rather than switching off, of beacon-like flushing. While written handouts explaining both the disease in question and how to carry out treatments are helpful, they are no substitute for the doctor personally giving the information, couched in common parlance, to the patient. Elderly patients, in particular, appreciate having the written word to refer to, especially when their short-term memory is faulty.

A problem arises when there is none but a perceived pathology, as in dysmorphophobia, or where the problem is minimal but is felt to be the end of the world, such as mild androgenetic alopecia. The patient of middle years may be driven to despair by wrinkles, too little hair on top and too much on the chin. Currently, there is an unreal expectation among women of looking youthful from puberty to grave[2]. And so they come for cosmetic rather than therapeutic doctoring. This is fostered by *Hello!*, *Cosmopolitan*, and other glossy magazine images of flawless feminine faces smiling out at them month after month. In this would-be Peter Pan situation every effort must be made to ensure that the patient understands that nothing in life comes with a 'guaranteed perfect' label. The disappointment of a peel that goes wrong or a wrinkle that fails to iron out can quickly boil over into litigation.

Lastly, don't forget that we are there, not only to treat our patients' existing pathology, but to help them to prevent further insult or damage, so there must also be an educational/preventive component to the consultation.

CONCLUSIONS

We girls and women are not so different to our male relatives and colleagues. While our ability to carry out careers is the same, we have a different set of sex chromosomes, different physiology and, according to the psychologists, a different approach to problem-solving. Thus, at a consultation in the doctor's office, it is reasonable to expect that we should be treated with appropriate consideration and courtesy.

REFERENCES

1. Phillips LP, Caruso CS, Paine LL. Primary care for women. Comprehensive dermatologic assessment. *J Nurs Midwifery* 1995;40:172–86
2. Dunn LB, Damesyn M, Moore AA, *et al.* Does estrogen prevent skin aging? Results from the First National Health and Nutrition Examination Survey. *Arch Dermatol* 1997;133:339–42

Gynecologic examination 4

Vincenzina Bruni and Leonardo Magnani

INTRODUCTION

During a general examination, the dermatologist must include an evaluation of the genital area and breasts of a female patient. The female genitalia and mammary tissue undergo drastic changes over the course of a woman's life. One of the many tasks of the dermatologist is to know what is considered 'normal' during the various stages of female development. Diagnostic accuracy of trauma, inflammation, tumors or anything harmful to the patient's health can thus be improved. Furthermore, the female genitalia are extremely sensitive targets of the endocrine system. The dermatologist must therefore be well acquainted with the fundamentals of the gynecological examination. Correct evaluation of variables, choice of examination schedules and diagnostic instruments depend on the patient's age and psychological attitude.

In this chapter, normal female genitalia and, to some extent, the mammary gland, will be discussed during the various phases of sexual development. Particular emphasis has been placed on the neonatal and infantile periods. The chronological appearance and evolution of pubertal phenomena and the changes that occur once the fertile period has ended will also be described. Suggestions regarding the modalities of the gynecological examination will be put forward. Particular attention has been given to both the technical procedures and the interactive approaches involved in the examination of the child. One of the primary aims of this section is to help the physician avoid traumatizing the young subject. Not only can satisfactory compliance be obtained, but the examination can be turned into an educational experience.

The dermatologist can recognize specific gynecological pathology. In order to allow the physician to fully evaluate the gynecologist's recommendations, an overview of the diagnostic procedures in use will be described.

EVALUATION OF THE NEONATAL GENITAL APPARATUS

Anatomy of the genital apparatus

The genital apparatus of the female neonate is characterized by relevant estrogen saturation.

These estrogens are produced by the placenta and undergo a slow process of metabolization that consists of progressive increases in glucuronoconjugation. The process is completed between the second and third weeks of extrauterine life. On a clinical level, this endocrine situation determines a series of very evident – if only transitory – phenomena.

In almost all cases (more than 99%), the breasts appear congested[1]. This situation is at times associated with some nipple secretion that may persist until the second month.

The labia majora are characterized by turgor, the clitoris is prominent, and the hymen is thick. The vagina is already well developed: it is about 5 cm in length and hyperemic. It is covered by a thick epithelial layer that abounds in glycogen and is characterized by marked cellular maturation. If no premature rupture of the membranes occurs during intrauterine life, the fetal vagina does not contain any microorganisms. As the fetus descends through the birth canal, the fetal vagina is rapidly colonized. The maternal vaginal environment is the source of lactobacilli, micrococci, diphtheroids, coliforms, enterococci, streptococci, anaerobes and yeasts.

The bacillus of Doderlein is prominently present. As a consequence of good trophism of the mucosa and the high content of glycogen, the neonate vaginal pH is characterized by a value of 5–6 during the first postnatal hours, and then diminishes to a value of 4–5.

At birth, the dimensions of the uterus have increased and this organ appears to be out of proportion when compared to body weight. This is due to hypertrophy induced during intrauterine life by maternal and placental hormones. Antiversion or retroversion of the uterus initiates with puberty. At birth the length of the uterus ranges from 2.5 to 3.5 cm. The cervix : corpus ratio is 3:1. The myometrium is made up of a very thin layer. The endometrium has hardly developed. Desquamation with hemorrhage caused by the gradual loss of maternal estrogen may occur in 10% of cases. The main target organ of prenatal endocrine stimulation is the uterine cervix. During the fetal period it takes on a markedly hypertrophic appearance, with well-represented cervical glands that secrete abundant quantities of mucosa. The fallopian tubes look like slender canals about 3–4 cm long. During this period, the mucosa is not sensitive to the action of estrogen. The development of the ovaries deserves particular attention. At birth each measures about 20 mm in length, 5 mm in width and 3 mm in thickness.

Gynecological examination of the neonate

Inspection of the external genitals

Just as in every other phase of female life, careful examination of the labia majora, labia minora, clitoris, urinary meatus, vaginal aditus, hymen, perineum, anus, inguinal canal and, if required, vagina, must be carried out.

Meticulous evaluation of the fetal clitoris has special clinical importance. It is necessary to identify any increase in normal clitoral dimensions that might indicate exposure of the fetus to abnormal prenatal androgenic stimulus. Any such increase justifies a careful evaluation of the total reproductive system in order to identify possible associated abnormalities. Objective evaluation is always necessary. This is particularly useful in the premature neonate: simple subjective evaluation may lead to errors in over-evaluating the dimensions of the clitoris. This may be owing to its apparently large size in relation to the limited dimensions of the labia majora and limited body size. By holding the baby in the frog-leg position and spreading the labia minora, the skin of the prepuce is pulled back, and the clitoris can be evaluated with a caliper. A study carried out on 159 subjects, 69 premature and 90 full-term neonates, indicated that the dimensions of the clitoris at the 40th week of gestation are the same as those during the 27th week of intrauterine life. No significant differences in the size of the clitoris based on race (i.e. black vs. white) were found[2].

The transverse diameter of the clitoris normally measures between 2 and 6 mm at birth[2]. Clitoral dimensions may also be expressed using the clitoral index (CI), which is the product of the longest sagittal and transverse dimensions of the glans of the clitoris: the results are expressed in square millimeters[3]. The normal value of the clitoral index in neonates varies between 13.3 mm^2 and 15.1 mm^2 [4] (Table 1).

Virilization, which begins before the 14th week of gestation, may not only increase the dimensions of the clitoris but may also cause labioscrotal fusion. Slight forms of labioscrotal fusion may be noted by means of the anogenital ratio (AF/AC), which is defined as the ratio of the distance between the center of the anus and the posterior extremity of the fourchette (AF) to the distance between the center of the anus and the base of the clitoris (AC) (Figure 1). A study carried out on 115 newborn infants, between the ages of 25 and 40 weeks, indicated that the mean ($\pm$ SD) value of the anogenital ratio is 0.36 ± 0.07: a ratio greater than 0.50 most probably suggests labioscrotal fusion[5] (Figure 2).

The AF/AC ratio is not modified by gestational age or body size or weight of the neonate. To evaluate the AF/AC ratio, the neonate must be examined in the same position as that used for the measurement of the dimensions of the clitoris. Special attention must be paid so as not to press excessively on the abdomen: should the perineum be extended, the ratio values could be altered. The use of a caliper is indicated when evaluating the anogenital ratio. This ratio is particularly important when labioscrotal fusion is suspected. Since this condition has been described in cases of 21-hydroxylase deficiency, even in the absence of clitorimegaly, it may be the only manifestation of intrauterine exposure to androgens[6]. However, sporadic cases of families with congenital labioscrotal fusion have been reported to be the consequence of a dominant autosomic hereditary mechanism, with variable penetrance[7].

Table 1 Clitoral index (mm^2) in girls with normal and abnormal sexual development

Age (yr)	Normal (n)	Congenital adrenal hyperplasia (n)	Central precocious puberty (n)	Premature adrenarche (n)	XO/XY Karyotype (n)
0–1	15.1 ± 1.4 (16)	137.9 ± 26.9 (6)			
1–8	15.1 ± 0.9 (29)	225.0 ± 49.0 (5)	20 ± 2 (5)	26 ± 1 (4)	
8–13	16.7 ± 0.9 (18)	212.0 ± 59.0 (4)	17 ± 2 (5)	25 ± 7 (4)	242 ± 171 (2)
13–18	20.7 ± 1.6 (17)	116.0 ± 14.0 (5)			

Reproduced with permission from Sane K, Pescovitz OH. The clitoral index: a determination of clitoral size in normal girls and in girls with abnormal sexual development. *J Pediatr* 1992;120:264–6

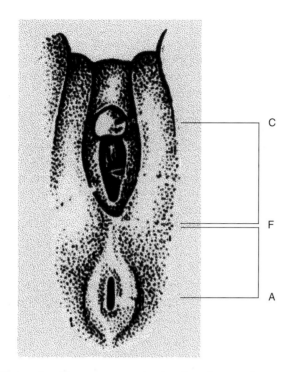

Figure 1 Measurement criteria of perineum. A, anus; C, clitoris; F, fourchette. Modified with permission from Callegari C, Everett S, Ross M, *et al.* Anogenital ratio: measure of fetal virilization in premature and full term infants. *J Pediatr* 1987;111:240–3

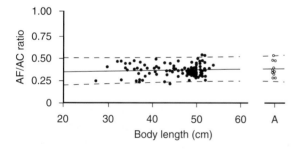

Figure 2 Correlation of AF/AC (anus to fourchette/anus to clitoris) ratio and body length. Dashed lines represent 95% confidence limits; each circle represents one subject. A, adult ratio; each open circle represents one subject. Note absence of any dispersion of data on Y axis. Reproduced with permission from Callegari C, Everett S, Ross M, *et al.* Anogenital ratio: measure of fetal virilization in premature and full term infants. *J Pediatr* 1987; 111:240–3

The use of the AF/AC ratio represents an important moment in the gynecological examination of the neonate. A pathological value may indicate exposure of the female fetus to androgenic stimulus during the first 14 weeks of intrauterine life. Even in the absence of clitorimegaly, such a value justifies an accurate morphological evaluation of the entire genital apparatus of the female neonate and an exacting endocrinological work-up

for the identification of any possible state of hyperandrogenism.

Visualization of the hymen and vaginal mucosa is obtained by dilating the labia minora and using slight traction on the fourchette. A complete description of the characteristics of the external genitalia, even those which seem normal, is important: any variation may be the expression of some important pathology. In particular, a grayish-white bump typically indicates the presence of an imperforate hymen, with a hydromucocolpos. Differential diagnosis must be established regarding hymenal cysts and paraurethral or Gartner cysts, as they can cause occlusion of the vaginal aditus. A hymen with two orifices may represent a simple malconformation, but may also be the peripheral expression of a double vaginal aditus with two hemi-vaginas, or a double uterus. A hymen with a posterior rim which covers the urinary meatus may cause the presence of vaginal urine. It can also facilitate the entry of pathogenic micro-organisms into the urethra, if present in the vaginal canal. It should be re-checked in infancy, above all in cases of recurring cystitis.

The total absence of cervical mucus at the level of the hymen or on the vaginal walls must be investigated. Verification of the possible presence of some obstructive pathology (e.g. transversal vaginal septum or vaginal atresia) is imperative, as it can prevent the outflow of physiological liquids and cause their accumulation in the genital system.

If postnatal genital blood loss continues for more than 4 days, vaginoscopy is necessary in order to exclude possible tumoral pathology of the vagina or cervix.

Examination of the internal genitalia

Today, pelvic ultrasound is the first diagnostic method used for the evaluation of the internal genitalia or of any pelvic abdominal mass. The bimanual rectoabdominal pelvic examination represents a secondary choice in either the newborn or the infant. Bimanual pelvic palpation is carried out by holding the neonate's thighs and legs flexed with the left hand. The same hand also palpates the abdomen, while the little finger of the right hand is introduced into the rectum. This procedure may provide further clinical confirmation of expansive pelvic abdominal pathology. Since the capacity of the pelvis is limited, a rapid expansion of the pelvic masses at the level of the abdominal cavity occurs. In most cases, it is sufficient only to inspect or palpate the abdomen for the identification of pelvic-abdominal tumescence.

A gynecological examination may indicate possible vulvovaginal infection. Given the age of the subject, specific procedures for laboratory confirmation of any clinical suspicion must be carried out using a vulvovaginal tampon.

Pathologies most frequently encountered

The most frequently found gynecological pathologies in the female neonate are isolated urogenital malformations (imperforation or malconformation of the hymen, hymenal and paraurethral cysts). In the neonatal period, genital infections are almost always located at the level of the vulva. Infections of the vagina, uterus, and fallopian tubes are practically non-existent during this period of life. The state of relative hyperestrogenism during the first weeks of life defends the internal genitalia against infection. Anatomical factors (e.g., vulvar, hymenal, vaginal turgor and the pluristratification of the vaginal epithelium) and some biological factors (e.g., presence of lactobacilli, acid vaginal pH of 4–4.5 two to three days after birth and desquamation of the vaginal epithelium secretions of the cervical glands) take part in this protective process. Cases of vulvovaginitis are very rare, but cases of vulvitis in newborn infants can originate from:

(1) contamination by the mother at birth (with possible infection from *Trichomonas*, *Candida*, *Gonococcus*, *Chlamydia*);
(2) infection favored by irritation from talcum or diapers;
(3) lack of hygiene; and
(4) infection contracted in the hospital nursery.

EVALUATION OF THE CHILD'S GENITAL APPARATUS

Anatomy of the genital apparatus

The clitoris of the young child who has not received any androgenic stimulus does not increase significantly in size in the first few years of life. The mean ($\pm$ SD) value of the CI is 15.1 ± 0.9 between the ages of 1 and 8 years[4] (Table 1). As a result of the continuing, gradual elimination of maternal estrogens in the newborn, owing to glucuronoconjugation, the vaginal epithelium changes. It becomes thin and lacks glycogen; the vaginal pH increases and the vaginal microclimate is modified. The bacillus of Doderlein becomes rare, but Gram-positive cocci

and both Gram-positive and Gram-negative bacilli are present. The development of anaerobes, particularly that of *Bacteroides fragilis*, is favored. After birth the uterus undergoes rapid involution. Its length is progressively reduced, and its weight decreases by 30% by the age of 6 months. The ovaries undergo a reduction in cortical thickness and in the number of primordial follicles. The increased dimensions of the organs noted during infancy can therefore be attributed to a proliferation of the stroma.

GYNECOLOGICAL EXAMINATION OF THE CHILD

The gynecological examination must be preceded by the gathering of personal and family case histories. Particular attention must be paid to the psychological make-up of the child in the school environment, at play and in sports activities. The general examination must not overlook an evaluation of the child's weight, height, growth curve, body proportions, nutritional state and possible appearance of secondary sexual characteristics. If neonatal mammary congestion lasts beyond the 6th month of age, it must be scrupulously followed up. Thus, the premature mono-bilateral appearance of the breasts may be an expression of a paraphysiological condition, such as premature thelarche. It may also, however, be the first manifestation of complete or incomplete sexual precocity, which should be investigated by means of diagnostic study and, subsequently, followed up or treated.

Inspection of the external genitalia

The co-operation of the child during the gynecological examination is of primary importance (Table 2). The carrying out of the procedure depends on patient compliance. The experience should be a positive one. In order to evaluate the anogenital area it is appropriate to invite the patient to get into one of several particular positions:

(1) frog-like position, with flexed thighs and legs splayed (this is particularly suitable for very small children);
(2) genupectoral position;
(3) lithotomic position; or
(4) on its mother's knees, if the child seems particularly anxious or frightened.

During the specific examination of the external genitalia, it is important to obtain good visualization of

Table 2 Suggestions for genital examinations of young children and adolescents

Obtain the patient's cooperation:
This is necessary for teachable moments and for adequate examinations
Get the patient to comply:
She must have control over the examination
She must be promised no physical pain
Define the information that is to be obtained
Special aspects of the prepubertal female's examination:
Inform the child that the genital examination is sanctioned
Involve the child with a hand-held mirror and magnification device
Position the child with the feet in the stirrups, with the feet on the examiner's lap, or sitting on the parent's lap drape the child's legs over the parent's thighs
Attempt both the supine and knee–chest positions
Be knowledgeable about the various spread methods to see the vestibule
There is only a limited need to use instruments
Special aspects of the peripubertal genital examination:
Understand the impact of estrogen
Use extinction of stimuli phenomenon
Choose the proper speculum width after the introitus is evaluated

Reproduced with permission from Pokorny SF, Genital examination of prepubertal and peripubertal females. In Sanfilippo JS, ed. *Pediatric and Adolescent Gynecology*, Philadelphia: WB Saunders Company, 1994:170–86

the vestibule. If the child does not want to be touched, she may be invited to visualize the vaginal entrance by laterally parting the labia majora, using her own hands. At times, correct evaluation of the anatomical structures requires the use of magnifying devices, such as lenses, lenses with aimed light sources, a vulvoscope or a vaginoscope.

The traumatized child may refuse to get undressed or be examined. This is generally owing to negative gynecological experiences at previous examination, pain, or possibly to episodes of sexual abuse. Contraction of the perineal muscles may occur in the tense child, creating inadequate visualization of the genital organs. If there are no urgent reasons for immediate examination, it is best to proceed after slight pharmacological sedation or under general anesthesia. These procedures should be used especially if other examinations such as biopsy, vaginoscopy, etc., are scheduled.

Various techniques for visualizing the hymen have been described. They have been summarized in the so-called 'multimethods approach'[8], which is characterized by separation of the labia majora in a supine position, traction of the labia majora in a supine position by exercising pressure simultaneously on the perineum, and genupectoral position. These last two positions have also been shown to be particularly efficacious in diagnosing lesions caused by sexual abuse and for evaluating both the anal region and the degree of relaxation of the sphincter. The transversal diameter of the hymenal orifice is measured in millimeters. Evaluation may be influenced by the type of anatomical configuration, the technique used for visualization, the state of contraction of the perineal muscles at the moment of observation, the degree of estrogen saturation of the tissue and by the possible presence of inflammation. Because of the multiplicity of these factors, measurement of the hymenal opening as a reliable marker of virginity has been the subject of considerable controversy. In traditional diagnostics, a horizontal diameter of less than 5 mm was considered normal. The finding had once been widely recorded in the literature. However, since smaller diameters have been reported, even in cases of sexual abuse, previous data are now considered uncertain[9].

Upon examination, the hymen may be:

(1) imperforate, and must be surgically treated. This should take place only when pubertal estrogen stimulus begins and before the first menarchal blood collection is formed. An uncommon case of non-perforation of the hymen following scarring processes that had occurred after sexual violence has been described[10];

(2) microperforated or punctiform: characterized by an orifice that is so small that at times it simulates an imperforate hymen. It should not be treated surgically if drainage of the uterovaginal secretion is assured. During the peripubertal period, the hymen may also undergo spontaneous widening with the onset of estrogen stimulation;

(3) septate: characterized by two distinct orifices, divided by a bridge of tissue which generally extends from top to bottom, but which may also be horizontal or oblique;

(4) circular: the hymenal border completely surrounds the vaginal orifice. The opening of the membrane may be centrally or anteriorly localized, below the urethra;

(5) with posterior rim: characterized by the presence of tissue that is located almost exclusively

in a posterior position. The orifice is placed so far anteriorly that the hymenal rim at the suburethral site cannot be detected at all from 10 or 11 o'clock clockwise to 1 or 2 o'clock;

(6) fimbriated: characterized by a free border which is scalloped and superabundant.

Examination of the vulva can show inflammatory processes. However, it is advisable to keep in mind the fine thinness of the vulvar mucosa and the high number of capillaries in several regions of the vulva. The sulci of the vestibule and the periurethral area may take on an erythematous appearance and be mistakenly interpreted as sites of an inflammatory process. Observation of the labia minora can frequently show anterior or posterior or, though less frequently, total synechia vulvae. Evaluation of the degree of estrogen stimulus on the external genitalia and the degree of development of secondary sexual characteristics is important. The latter may express complete or incomplete sexual precocity.

Examination of the internal genital organs

Examination of the internal genital organs of the child can begin with pelvic ultrasonography. Use of bimanual rectoabdominal pelvic examination should be limited (as it should be in the neonate). It is justified only in cases of abdominal-pelvic expansive pathology or in those cases in which phlogistic pathology of the upper genital system is suspected, though such pathology is very rare in this age group.

Vaginoscopy is not a routine examination. Its use should be limited to cases of:

(1) genital hemorrhage not associated with sexual precocity;
(2) suspected tumoral pathology;
(3) suspected congenital anomalies (partial vaginal aplasia of the uterine cervix, double genital system);
(4) traumas (accidents, sexual violence); and
(5) recurrent genital infections with suspected presence of extraneous bodies or suspicion of recurring sexual aggression.

Inspection of the vagina must be followed by a cytologic work-up of the vagina, urethra and anus to check for *Gonococcus* and *Chlamydia*. In the prepubertal child, the cells of the vaginal epithelium (mostly basal and parabasal cells), like those of the

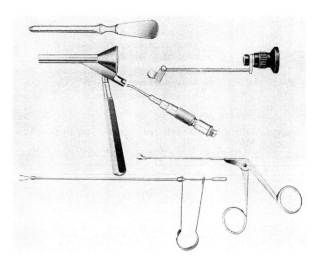

Figure 3   Huffman-Huber vaginoscope

cervix, are probable places for the development of *Chlamydia*[11].

The following is a list of the principal vaginoscopes currently in use in pediatric gynecology:

(1) Huffman-Huber vaginoscope: a rigid cylinder and variable diameter (Figure 3);
(2) Terruhn vaginoscope: a rigid cylinder with a diameter varying from 8 to 11 mm with an inflatable cuff to facilitate examination of the cervix and foreign bodies;
(3) Classical Cusco speculum, modified for pediatric use by I. Rey-Stocker; diameter is 1 cm and length is 15 cm;
(4) if a vaginoscope is not available, a Killian nasal speculum may be used for vaginal examination in the premenarcheal child. However, the blades are not long enough to expose the cervix and they can stretch the hymen and cause pain.

The most frequently encountered pathologies

Even though the genital system is relatively free of pathology in infancy, more and more case histories have been reported involving varying sites and various types of infant pathology[12]:

(1) vulvovaginitis: 60–90%;
(2) genital hemorrhage: 15–30%;
(3) traumatic lesions: 5–10%;
(4) malformations: 5%; and
(5) tumors: 1–5%.

In the child, the problems related to vulvovaginitis and traumatic lesions take on particular clinical importance. Vulvovaginal infections will be extensively treated in other chapters.

Vulvovaginal lesions in childhood

The age of the highest incidence of accidental traumas is between 4 and 12 years. The presence of an anogenital lesion may be due to:

(1) lacerations as a result of falling with splayed legs, trauma due to the splits position, those caused by gymnastic equipment or the riding of a bicycle;
(2) accidental penetration (including extraneous bodies);
(3) sexual abuse;
(4) strain at a perineal level; and
(5) laceration as a consequence of brusque abduction of the lower limbs or of pelvic fractures[13].

Falling with splayed legs is a very frequent cause of genital lesions in young girls. The lesion may be limited to a small perineal ecchymotic area, or may spread out as a rather large hematoma with relevant compression of the vulvar tissues. Furthermore, the mons pubis, clitoris, urethra, and the forward portion of the labia majora and minora may all be affected; the vaginal entrance rarely is.

Ninety per cent of perineal lesions in patients of pediatric age can be blamed on sexual abuse. Multiple tissue modifications may appear in female children who are or have been the victims of sexual violence. In addition to variations in the diameter of the hymenal orifice, other anomalous physical findings should be noted. If a physical examination is carried out shortly after an act of violence has taken place, erythemas, edemas, sub-mucosa, hemorrhages, abrasions, lacerations and hymenal breakage are the most frequently found signs[14]. At follow-up, or during an examination made long after a violent act has been committed, a series of signs can be detected. These include: pointed and jacked hymenal edges, borders with V-shaped irregularities, tightening of the hymenal rim, rolled-over borders and the presence of excrescences, intra-vaginal sulci and variations in the dimensions of the vaginal introitus. Acute tissue modifications regress rapidly (15–20 days for erythemas and edema; 30 days if sub-mucosa hemorrhage is present). Interpretation of the results of the genital examination of the child are influenced by different factors that must be taken into consideration: age, endocrine situation, individual variations, psychological condition and the interval of time between an episode of violence and the examination.

The anatomical situation can be more easily appraised by utilizing the previously-described visualization techniques. During inspection of the hymen, it might be helpful to have the child in the genupectoral position. The physician should invite her to breathe deeply and try and relax the abdominal muscles so that evagination of the hymen can be determined when the buttocks are stretched dorsally and laterally.

Sometimes, particularly if the child is in a supine position, adhesion of the thick and humid hymenal folds can prevent any visualization of the hymenal orifice. This often happens if the hymen is annular or fimbriated. If the child co-operates, the opening can be reached by utilizing a damp tampon to effect a slight shifting of the tissues. If the hymen is jagged, it may be difficult to determine whether the edges represent a particular congenital formation. If the hymen is not intact, it is necessary to note and describe the hymenal fragments, wherever visible. The anal region must also be carefully examined for the possible presence of chapping, scars, areas of hyperpigmentation, cutaneous thickenings and excrescence.

Lateral separation of the buttocks can sometimes cause a large (1–1.5 cm) widening of the anus in the child who has already undergone repeated penetration. Diameters of less than 1 cm do not necessarily signify the absence of any sexual abuse. Many girls have normal anal and rectal findings, despite a verified history of anal abuse. Cutaneous excrescence can be considered normal when localized at 12 o'clock in a supine position: if it is found in other zones, or if the growth is thick and adherent, one can probably assume that it arose from an anal trauma. If there is any doubt, a rectal examination must be carried out to determine sphincteral tone. If blood is present in the feces, or if the anamnesis contains reports of previous bleeding, a proctoscopic examination can be helpful. Diagrams of the anus and of the anal region should be made in order to gather as many data as possible regarding size and location of any possible lesions due to scars, hematomas, etc.

EVALUATION OF THE ADOLESCENT GENITAL APPARATUS

Anatomy of the genital apparatus of the adolescent

Puberty is characterized by the full expression of the estrogen stimulus. Even if the mucosa of the vulva is less responsive to estrogens (when compared to the vagina and the uterus), it becomes softer and is characteristically more turgid.

Bartholin's glands produce a clear and viscous secretion which lubricates the vaginal entrance; the labia minora develop, and become more prominent and, at times, hypertrophic. Hypertrophy can be only monolateral. During adolescence the dimensions of the clitoris increase progressively and significantly until they reach adult values. The mean value (± SD) of the CI is 16.7 ± 0.9 mm² between 8 and 13 years of age, and is 20.7 ± 1.6 mm² between 13 and 18 years of age (Table 1). A correlation between the increase in the CI and Tanner stages, as regards the breast and pubic hair, has also been suggested[4].

These CI data substantially agree with those reported by other studies[3,15] (Table 3), in which the dimensions of the clitoris were not found to be affected by height, weight, body mass index, or the use of oral contraceptives, but were correlated with parity. Moreover, all the above-mentioned authors agree that 95% of the healthy women checked had CI values of < 35 mm². If a woman has a CI value of > 35 mm², suspicion of the presence of some androgenic noxa is well founded. Therefore careful clinical and endocrinological examinations are required. The mean (± SD) value of the length of the clitoris in the healthy woman is 16.0 ± 4.3 mm: in 95% it is less than 23 mm[15] (Table 3). However the literature has been discordant regarding the usefulness of the evaluation of clitoral length in mild forms of virilization; in fact it is not always easy to identify the point of continuation of the roots in the body of the clitoris.

At puberty the hymen becomes edematous, thicker and bright pink in color; its orifice reaches a diameter of about one centimeter. However, individual differences may be noted. With the activation of ovarian function, the vaginal epithelium undergoes a maturation process characterized by an increase in its thickness owing to both the proliferation of the intermediate layer and the development of a new superficial layer.

In the period immediately preceding menarche, a series of events takes place. It is characterized by an increase in vaginal secretion, a lowering of the pH and a change in the vaginal flora. In particular, there is a reduction in staphylcocci and coliform bacteria colonization: pure cultures of lactobacilli are often found. The dimensions of the uterus increase very rapidly. Growth takes place, above all, in the upper segment, which is more responsive to hormonal stimulation than is the cervix at this time of life. Cervical volume also increases. The cervical canal, which is difficult to identify during infancy, becomes wider. The cuboidal epithelium is transformed into columnar epithelium, and secretion by the cervical glands is intensified. During the period preceding menarche, each ovary doubles its weight (to 6 g) and takes on the adult configuration, and follicular growth takes place.

The first clinical sign of the onset of puberty is the development of the breasts, which reflects the beginning of the secretory activity of the ovaries. Marshall and Tanner[16] identified and defined 5 stages of breast development (Table 4). Increases in surrenal androgens that are characteristic of adrenarche generally begin between 6 and 8 years of age. The appearance of pubic and axillary hair accompanies the development of the genitalia. The evolution of this secondary sexual characteristic has also been subdivided by Marshall and Tanner into five stages (Table 5).

The onset of menarche always takes place in subjects whose bone age is between 12.5 and 14.5 years: in the majority of cases onset is between 13 and 14 years of age. Figure 4 describes individual variations in the chronological appearance of pubertal events, according to Marshall and Tanner. Recently the age of onset of pubertal development was calculated in 8703 German girls, according to the Tanner stages[17]. Results expressed in age centiles (in years and tenths of a year) were compared to those of previous studies on the subject (Tables 6 and 7). Even though there are considerable individual variations, a continuous progression of the different pubertal phenomena represents an index of normality. This fact is almost as significant as the age at which the characteristics appear.

GYNECOLOGICAL EXAMINATION IN ADOLESCENCE

The primary objectives of a gynecological examination of an adolescent should be:

(1) evaluation of the evolutionary stage of the reproductive system and the breasts during the course of puberty and the identification of any variation from the norm;

(2) identification of organic and functional genital pathologies. Particular attention should be paid to postmenarchal oligomenorrhea, adolescent hyperandrogenism, and to pathologies related to eating disorders;

(3) education regarding knowledge of one's own body and one's own biological rhythms;

(4) prevention of sexually transmitted diseases;

Table 3 Clitoral measurements by parity

| Measurement | Mean ± SD | Confidence limits | | S-W* |
		5%	95%	
All subjects (*n* = 200)				
Total length (mm)	16.0 ± 4.3	10.1	23.0	0.97
Glans length (mm)	5.1 ± 1.4	3.0	7.0	0.94
Glans width (mm)	3.4 ± 1.0	2.0	5.0	0.90
Clitoral index (mm²)	18.5 ± 9.5	6.0	35.5	0.95
Nulliparous (*n* = 80)				
Total length (mm)	15.4 ± 4.3	9.5	23.0	0.97
Glans length (mm)	4.8 ± 1.3	2.5	7.0	0.93
Glans width (mm)	3.2 ± 1.0	1.5	5.0	0.91
Clitoral index (mm²)	16.3 ± 8.3	3.5	30.0	0.95
Parous (*n* = 120)				
Total length (mm)	16.3 ± 4.3	10	23.0	0.98
Glans length (mm)	5.3 ± 1.5	3.0	8.0	0.94
Glans width (mm)	3.6 ± 1.0	2.0	5.0	0.90
Clitoral index (mm²)	19.9 ± 10.1	7.0	38.0	0.94

*Shapiro-Wilk test for conformity to normal distribution. Reproduced from Verkauf BS, Thron J, O'Brien WF. Clitoral size in normal women. *Obstet Gynecol* 1992;80:41–4, by permission of the American College of Obstetricians and Gynecologists

Table 4 Stages of breast development in girls, according to Marshall and Tanner*

Stage	Age (years)	Characteristics
B1	9 ± 1	pre-adolescent. Elevation of papilla only
B2	11 ± 1	breast bud stage. Elevation of breast and papilla as small mound. Enlargement of areolar diameter
B3	12 ± 1	further enlargement and elevation of breast and areola with no separation of their contours
B4	13 ± 1	projection of areola and papilla to form a secondary mound above the level of the breast
B5	15 ± 1.5	mature stage. Projection of papilla only caused by recession of the areola to the general contour of the breast

*Modified from Marshall WA, Tanner JM. Variations in patterns of pubertal changes in girls. *Arch Dis Child* 1969;44:291–5, with permission

(5) counseling; and

(6) answering all questions about contraception and addressing possible requests.

For the adolescent the first step of the gynecological examination should involve the collecting of the patient's and the family's case histories. This is an excellent moment for establishing an understanding relationship by becoming aware of the subject's difficulties and questions. In the sexually active adolescent, a complete gynecological examination can be carried out in conjunction with colposcopy and cytological work-up.

In subjects who are not sexually active, pelvic ultrasonography unquestionably represents one of the first steps in gynecological evaluation. However, it must never be carried out without an examination of the external genitalia. Pelvic ultrasonography allows for an accurate evaluation of the genital organs and their evolution towards gynecological maturity. The fundamental ultrasonographic characteristics of the uterus are represented by the dimensions of the organ. The ratio between the anterior–posterior diameter of the corpus (COAP) and that of the cervix (CEAP) define its morphological state as do the ratio between the length of the corpus and that of the cervix, and the presence or absence of the endometrial rim. The uterus with infantile morphology is characterized by a COAP/CEAP ratio that is equal to or less than 0.9. In the uterus with transitional morphology the COAP/CEAP ratio is between 0.9 and 1.1, and in adult-type morphology the ratio is greater than 1.1[18] (Figure 5). The ratio of the length of the

Table 5   Stages of development in pubic hair (PH) in girls, according to Marshall and Tanner*

Stage	Age (years)	Characteristics
PH1	9 ± 1.5	pre-adolescent. The vellus over the pubes is not further developed than that over the abdominal wall; that is, no pubic hair
PH2	11.5 ± 1	sparse growth of long, slightly pigmented downy hair straight or curled, chiefly or along the labia
PH3	12.5 ± 1	considerably darker, coarser, and more curled. The hair spreads sparsely over the junction of the pubes
PH4	13 ± 1	hair now adult in type, but area covered is still considerably smaller than in the adult. No spread to the medial surface of the thighs
PH5	14 ± 1	adult in quantity and type with distribution of the horizontal (or classically 'feminine') pattern. Spread to medial surface of thighs but not up linea alba or elsewhere above the base of the inverse triangle (spread up linea alba occurs late and is Stage VI)

*Modified from Marshall WA, Tanner JM. Variations in patterns of pubertal changes in girls. *Arch Dis Child* 1969;44:291–5 with permission

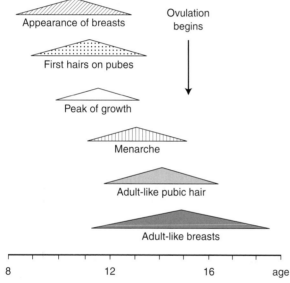

Figure 4   Chronological stages of pubertal development. Reproduced with permission from Forti G, Serio M. 'Disordini dello sviluppo puberale' In Giusti G, Serio M. *Endocrinologia: fisiopatologia e clinica*. USES, Firenze, 1988:1079–103

corpus to that of the cervix, with values of 1 to 3 in infancy, is progressively inverted up to values of 3 to 1 in the adult uterus. The finding of the endometrial rim at ultrasonography indicates that the uterus does not have infantile morphology. The endometrial rim varies a great deal during the course of puberty, as it is correlated to variations in estrogen levels. It is present in about 43% of uteri with transitional morphology and in 68% of the adult type[19]. The site, morphology and dimensions of the ovaries can also be well evaluated by using ultrasonographic examination. By using only morphological sonographic parameters, several maturational aspects of the ovaries have been defined[18]:

(1) small ovaries (volume < 2 cm^3) with homogeneous morphology;

(2) small ovaries with microfollicular (< 9 mm) morphology;

(3) relatively enlarged ovaries (volume > 2 cm^3) with homogeneous morphology;

(4) enlarged ovaries with the presence of microfollicles; and

(5) enlarged ovaries with the presence of macrofollicles (> 9 mm).

The data relative to the changes in ovarian morphology from 2 to 13 years of age are shown in Figure 6[18]. However it is more difficult to correlate sonographic morphology of the ovaries than that of the uterus with an unequivocal course of development[19]. Even if the morphology of the ovaries at ultrasound (from homogeneous to microfollicular, and then to macrofollicular) has been correlated to the production of estrogens, a constant morphological progression during the course of pubertal development cannot always be demonstrated. In particular, macrofollicular ovaries may even be present during the initial stages of development. At present, it is believed that the volume of the gonads most faithfully correlates ovarian maturation to pubertal development. The ovaries undergo continuous progressive increases in volume during puberty, and a recent study has shown that there is a significant correlation between these increases and Tanner stages[20].

Table 6 Sexual maturation centiles of healthy girls for pubertal and mature developmental stages (years)

	Stages of maturation						
	Pubertal				Mature		
Sign of maturation	3rd centile	50th centile	97th centile		3rd centile	50th centile	97th centile
Breasts (B2)	8.49	10.81	13.77	(B5)	12.30	15.74	*
Pubic hair (PH2)	9.09	11.15	13.67	(P5/6)	12.04	14.60	*
Axillary hair (AH2)	10.60	12.84	15.55	(AH3)	11.93	15.15	*
Shape of hips (SH2)	9.57	12.22	15.60	(SH3)	11.96	15.16	*
Menarche	–	–	–		11.32	13.46	16.00

*The findings of the 97th centiles could not be directly investigated, but only estimated from the probit regression line. All of these data are beyond the oldest age. Modified with permission from Engelhardt L, Willers B, Pelz L. Sexual maturation in East German girls. *Acta Pediatr* 1995;84:1362–5

Table 7 Comparison of corresponding developmental stages in sexual maturation (50th centiles) of healthy girls in selected studies (years)

Symptom and stage of maturation	Oster* 1955	This study* 1995	Roede* 1990	Dober and Kiralyfalvi* 1993	Largo and Prader[†] 1983	Buckler[†] 1990
Breasts						
B2	11.25	10.81	10.54	10.0	10.90	11.05
B5	13.62	15.74	14.21	16.4	14.00	13.90
Pubic hair						
P2	12.00	11.15	10.81	10.1	10.40	11.66
P5/6	13.46	14.60	14.00	15.5	14.00	14.02
Axillary hair						
AH2	12.95	12.84	–	–	–	–
AH3	14.46	15.15				
Menarche	13.67	13.46	13.28	12.9	13.28	13.35

*Cross-sectional study; [†]longitudinal study. Modified with permission from Engelhardt L, Willers B, Pelz L. Sexual maturation in East German girls. *Acta Pediatr* 1995;84:1362–5

The distinction between the multifollicular ovary (correlated to normal pubertal development) and the typical polycystic ovary (PCO) is unquestionably complex. Adams and colleagues[21] based their definition of the polycystic ovary on transabdominal ultrasonographic data. The PCO has 10 or more cysts that range in diameter from 2 to 8 mm. These are arranged peripherally to a dense stromal core, or are scattered throughout an increased quantity of stroma. By evaluating the same organ, but using a transvaginal probe, Fox and co-workers[22] found that the PCO can be defined by the presence of at least 15 cysts from 2 to 10 mm in diameter, arranged around prominent and highly echogenic stroma. The primary difference between the typical multifollicular ovary during puberty and the polycystic ovary is that, in the former, there are no substantial modifications in the stroma[23]. Given that the condition of the stroma can be used in the diagnostic evaluation of the ovary, it has been studied using new investigative methods. Three-dimensional ultrasonography has been shown to be more accurate than two dimensional sonography[24] and Doppler ultrasound has intimated that increased stromal blood perfusion is present in cases of PCO syndrome[25].

Ultrasonography rather than a clinical approach allows for a correlation between breast development and pubertal changes in the pelvic organs. Ultrasound evaluation also correlates well with endocrine patterns. Criteria for ultrasonographic interpretation of the breast[26] are based on progressive glandular development divided into five different stages that are easily identified (Figure 7):

Stage A: absence of glandular bud corresponding to both complete absence of clinically evident mammary growth and to adiposity of the breast region;

Stage B: first appearance of the glandular bud, which displays a linear edge, roundish shape, and

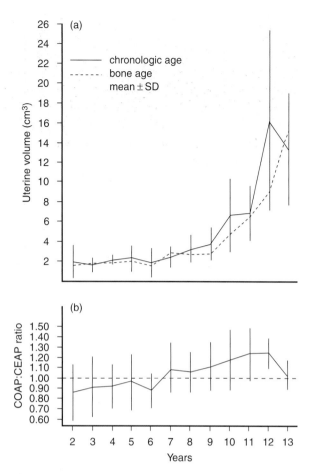

Figure 5 Uterine volume (a) and relationship between anterioposterior diameter of the corpus (COAP) and the cervix (CEAP) (b) as determined by ultrasonography from ages 2 to 13. Modified from Orsini L, Salardi S, Pilu G, *et al*. Pelvic organs in premenarchal girls: real time ultrasonography. *Radiology* 1984;153:113–16, by permission of Radiological Society of North America

appears quite distinct from the surrounding connective-adipose tissue; its maximum diameter is less than 1 cm;

Stage C: growing glandular bud with morphological features that are similar to stage B, but diameter is equal to or greater than 1 cm;

Stage D: branching glandular bud in which few ramifications appear stemming from the periphery of the bud into the stromal matrix; and

Stage E: triangular phase with glandular structure in its final phase of growth: pyramidal shape, with an upward apex, that appears triangular in sonographic scans. This situation precedes complete mammary maturation, when the glandular tissue cannot be differentiated ultrasonographically from the stroma.

The ultrasonographic approach is more accurate than the clinical one, above all during the first

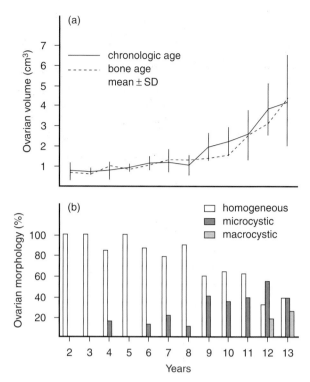

Figure 6 Ovarian volume (a) and changes in ovarian morphology (b) as determined by ultrasonography from ages 2 to 13. Modified from Orsini L, Salardi S, Pilu G, *et al*. Pelvic organs in premenarchal girls: real time ultrasonography. *Radiology* 1984;153:113–16 by permission of Radiological Society of North America

phases of puberty. A study was carried out at our clinic, on 48 healthy girls, using both Tanner staging and ultrasonography. At sonography, 6 out of 10 subjects whose clinical picture demonstrated an absence of breast development according to Tanner, showed the presence of glandular growth. On the other hand, at ultrasound the presence of adipose tissue and not that of glandular development was found in 5 out of 13 cases, defined as Tanner Stage B2[26].

EVALUATION OF THE GENITALS OF THE ADULT WOMAN

Anatomy of the genitals of the adult woman

During the phase of fertility, the adult woman's genital apparatus is not substantially different from what it was in late adolescence. It undergoes important changes only during menopause. In this period of life there is a progressive depletion of the ovarian follicular patrimony, and low estrogen levels characterize the hormonal situation. The vulva undergoes progressive atrophy. Pubic hair becomes sparser and sparser. The thickness of the

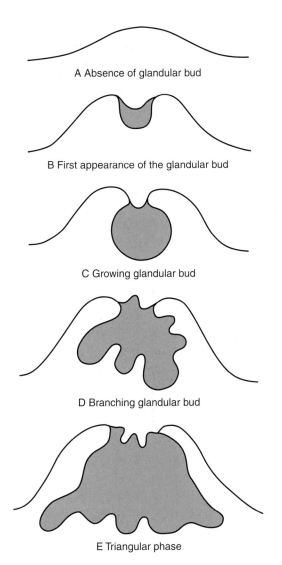

A Absence of glandular bud

B First appearance of the glandular bud

C Growing glandular bud

D Branching glandular bud

E Triangular phase

Figure 7 Schematic representation of ultrasonographic stages of the breast. Reproduced with permission of Elsevier Science from Bruni V, Dei M, Deligeoroglou E, *et al*. Breast development in adolescent girls. *Adolesc Pediatr Gynecol* 1990;3:201–5

labia majora is progressively reduced owing to atrophy of the subcutaneous tissue; the labia minora gradually become thinner, and may undergo complete regression. The vestibular mucus appears paler. Recent studies have indicated that these changes take place more markedly during the first three years of menopause[27]. The data in the literature are discordant regarding changes in the volume of the clitoris during menopause. However, the normal (threshold) value of the clitoral index, even for this phase of life, is 35 mm^2 [15]. The vagina becomes smaller and less distensible and less elastic. The folds of the mucosa tend to shrink, to the point of disappearing. The epithelial covering grows thinner and progressively lacks glycogen. Therefore the vagina becomes particularly subject to microlesions and minor episodes of bleeding

when subject to minor trauma and/or irritating stimuli. The reduced epithelial content of glycogen, due to the reduction in estrogen stimulus, determines the vaginal environment: lactobacilli can no longer proliferate and pH values increase. Vaginal atrophy accounts for the reduced secretion of fluids both at basal conditions and during sexual tension and can lead to dyspareunia.

The uterus undergoes progressive involution: the endometrial tissue becomes atrophic. The volume of the cervix is reduced and the external uterine orifice shrinks and becomes stenotic. The endometrium becomes thinner, the epithelium becomes cuboidal and the residual glands show cystic dilatations. The fallopian tubes become thinner and are reduced in diameter. The ovaries undergo a progressive loss of ovarian follicles until they are completely depleted: ovarian volume progressively decreases. The stromal cortical cells remain the last functioning structures, for a long period of time. After menopause, the breast is characterized by a reduction in adipose tissue and the glandular components; fibrous tissue is now well represented.

GYNECOLOGICAL EXAMINATIONS FOR ADULT WOMEN

The 'when' and 'how' of gynecological examinations for an adult woman are substantially no different from those carried out in late adolescence. With the onset of menopause the clinical picture takes on peculiar characteristics. The marked fragility of the capillaries of the cervix may cause the appearance of petechiae following a normal gynecological examination, or after the use of a vaginal speculum, which can provoke slight friction. Owing to diminishing estrogen stimulus, the cytological examination is characterized by the dominant presence of intermediate cells and the scarcity of superficial cells. Even during menopause an echographic examination is fundamental. At ultrasonography, the dimensions of the uterus appear smaller, having diminished progressively: a volumetric reduction becomes more evident five years after the last menstruation. The greatest decrease in dimensions can be observed in the uterine corpus: there is a reduction in the ratio between the length of the corpus and the cervix[28]. Evaluation of the thickness of the endometrium is essential for early oncological diagnosis. In premenopause, normal endometrial thickness is considered 4 mm on the 4th day of the cycle and 8 mm on the 8th. During the postmenopausal period, average endometrial thickness is 3.6 mm: it does not exceed 5 mm under normal conditions[28]. A recent meta-analysis considered a number of studies that included a total of 5892 women in menopause[29]. It revealed that the endometrium in 96% of women with endometrial carcinoma was greater than 5 mm.

During menopause, the ovaries gradually become smaller owing to the progressive reduction in the functioning tissues. Thus, they cannot always be correctly evaluated years from the onset of menopause. Ultrasonographic evaluation using a transvaginal probe allows for a more exact and objective evaluation of the condition of the organs as compared to the gynecological examination. The use of a sonographic normogram to measure ovarian dimension in menopause has been proposed[30]. The ovaries decrease progressively in volume from values of 8.6 ± 2.3 cm^3 during the first year of menopause to 2.2 ± 1.4 cm^3 fifteen years after onset. In addition to structural alterations, such as the presence of cysts or vegetation on the surface, the identification of any abnormally large ovarian mass during the menopausal period can be useful in the precocious diagnosis of tumoral conditions.

REFERENCES

1. McKiernan JF, Hull D. Breast development in the newborn. *Arch Dis Child* 1981;56:525–9
2. Riley WJ, Rosenbloom AL. Clitoral size in infancy. *J Pediatr* 1980;96:918–19
3. Tagaz GE, Kopher RA, Nagel TC, *et al*. The clitoral index: a bioassay of androgenic stimulation. *Obstet Gynecol* 1979;54:562–4
4. Sane K, Pescovitz OH. The clitoral index: a determination of clitoral size in normal girls and in girls with abnormal sexual development. *J Pediatr* 1992;120:264–6
5. Callegari C, Everett S, Ross M, *et al*. Anogenital ratio: measure of fetal virilization in premature and full term newborn infants. *J Pediatr* 1987;111:240–3
6. Marshall WN, Lightner ES. Congenital adrenal hyperplasia presenting with posterior labial fusion without clitoromegaly. *Pediatrics* 1980;66:312–14
7. Klein VR, William SP, Carr BR. Familiar posterior labial fusion. *Obstet Gynecol* 1989;73:500–3
8. McCann J, Wells R, Simon M. Genital findings in prepuberal girls selected for non abuse, a descriptive study. *Pediatrics* 1990;86:428–39
9. Heger A, Emans SJ. Introital diameter as criterion for sexual abuse. *Pediatr Comm* 1990;85:22–3
10. Berkowitz C, Elvik SL, Logan MA. A simulated 'acquired' imperforate hymen following the genital trauma of sexual abuse. *Clin Pediatr* 1987;26:307–9
11. Tipton AC. Child sexual abuse: physical examination techniques and interpretation of findings. *Adolesc Pediatr Gynecol* 1989;2:10–25
12. Bellone F, Bruni V. *Ginecologia dell'Infanzia e dell'Adolescenza*. Rome: Società Editrice Universo, 1990:100–7
13. Dudgeon D, Paidas C. Trauma of the vulva and vagina. *Pediatr Adolesc Gynecol* 1992;8:117–21
14. McCann J, Wells R, Simon M. Genital injuries resulting from sexual abuse: a longitudinal study. *Pediatrics* 1992;89:307–17
15. Verkauf BS, Thron J, O'Brien WF. Clitoral size in normal women. *Obstet Gynecol* 1992;80:41–4
16. Tanner JM, Marshall WA. Variations in patterns of pubertal changes in girls. *Arch Dis Child* 1969;44:291–5
17. Engelhardt L, Willers B, Pelz L. Sexual maturation in East German girls. *Acta Pediatr* 1995;84:1362–5
18. Orsini LF, Salardi S, Pilu G, *et al*. Pelvic organs in premenarcheal girls: real time ultrasonography. *Radiology* 1984;153:113–16
19. Bruni V, Dei M, Innocenti P, *et al*. Lo studio ecografico delle mammelle e della pelvi durante la pubertà: correlati endocrini. *Ginecologia dell'Infanzia e dell'Adolescenza* 1990;6:1–6
20. Orbak Z, Sagsoz N, Alp H, *et al*. Pelvic ultrasound measurements in normal girls: relation to puberty and sex hormone concentration. *J Pediatr Endocrinol Metab* 1998;11:525–30
21. Adams J, Polson DW, Abdulwamid N, *et al*. Multifollicular ovaries: clinical and endocrine features and response to pulsatile gonadotrophin releasing hormone. *Lancet* 1985;2:1375–8
22. Fox R, Corrigan E, Thomas P, *et al*. The diagnosis of polycystic ovaries in women with oligomenorrhoea: predictive power of endocrine tests. *Clin Endocrinol* 1991;34:127–31
23. Kyei-Mensah A, Zaidi J, Campbell S. Ultrasound diagnosis of polycystic ovary syndrome. In Jacobs HS, ed. *Polycystic Ovary Syndrome*, Bailliere's *Clin Endocr Metab* 1996;10:249–62
24. Kyei-Mensah A, Zaidi J, Pittrof R, *et al*. Transvaginal three-dimensional ultrasound: accuracy of follicular volume measurements. *Fertil Steril* 1995;65:371–6
25. Zaidi J, Campbell S, Pittrof R, *et al*. Ovarian stromal blood flow changes in women with polycystic ovaries. A possible new marker for ultrasound diagnosis? *Hum Reprod* 1995;10:1992–6
26. Bruni V, Dei M, Deligeoroglou E, *et al*. Breast development in adolescent girls. *Adolesc Pediatr Gynecol* 1990;3:201–5
27. Bianco V, Penna A, Rebora P. Correlation between trophism of the external genitalia and hormone levels during menopausal age. *Ann Obstet Gynecol Med Perinat* 1991;112:41–53
28. Merz E, Miric-Tesanic D, Bahlmann F, *et al*. Sonographic size of uterus and ovaries in pre- and

postmenopausal women. *Ultrasound Obstet Gynecol* 1996;7:38–42

29. Smith Bindman R, Kerlikowske K, Vickie A, *et al.* Endovaginal ultrasound to exclude endometrial cancer and other endometrial abnormalities. *JAMA* 1998;280:1510–17

30. Tepper R, Zalel Y, Markov S, *et al.* Ovarian volume in postmenopausal women – suggestion for an ovarian size normogram for menopausal age. *Acta Obstet Gynecol Scand* 1995;74:208–11

Basic concepts

Structure and function of the skin

5

Ilaria Ghersetich, Claudio Comacchi, Beatrice Bianchi and Torello M. Lotti

INTRODUCTION

No other organ of the body is invoked more frequently than the skin. Certainly the skin is the largest organ of the body and it is the major organ of sexual attraction. All descriptions of the skin divide it into two major layers: the inner dermis, subcutaneous tissue, and the outer epidermis[1]. The epidermis is stratified epithelium mostly composed of keratinocytes, but there are also other resident cells, such as Langerhans cells, Merkel cells and melanocytes. The epidermis has a thickness ranging from 0.04 mm on the eyelids to 1.6 mm on the palms. The dermis can be divided into two distinct compartments: a thin papillary dermis immediately beneath the epidermis and the reticular dermis that is bounded by the subcutaneous fat. The dermis comprises a supporting matrix or ground substance consisting mostly of polysaccharides (glycosaminoglycans) linked to proteins to produce macromolecules known as proteoglycans[1,2]. In this matrix is embedded a collection of collagen and elastic fibers with associated cellular elements, such as fibroblasts, the master cells of the dermis, mast cells and other cellular types constituting the nervous and the vascular networks of the skin. The thickness of the dermis varies from about 1 mm on the face to 4 mm on the back and thighs. The dermis seems to function as a mechanical support for the dynamic epidermis[1,2].

Functionally, the skin is a most extraordinary organ. First, it protects the body from injury and is responsible for preventing body fluid from escaping and external fluids from penetrating, but at the same time it is permeable to a large number of different molecules. Different body sites have different degrees of percutaneous absorption. Thus, the face is particularly permeable while the palms are relatively impermeable to many molecules. The mechanical functions of the skin and its capability to be a mobile tissue depend mainly on the dermis, in particular on the mechanical properties of the dermal fibers. The extensibility of the skin is variable, depending on body site. The skin of the abdomen has an unusual capacity for distension but if extended beyond certain limits, may become damaged, i.e. with the striae distensae of adolescence or striae gravidarum of pregnancy. These permanent marks appear on the skin of some women probably because of genetic factors. The skin has sensory functions and also produces odors[1-3]. Certain cutaneous structures, such as skin glands, and their secretions have a social or sexual significance; in fact the activity of apocrine and sebaceous glands manifests at puberty, indicating a connection with sexual development. The odors are better perceived by women than men and in particular more at the time of ovulation than during the rest of the menstrual cycle. Skin has distinctive metabolic properties, participating for example in the catabolism of steroids and in the formation of active hormones. Skin appendages respond readily to sexual steroids. Like the sebaceous glands, certain secondary sexual characteristics such as facial, axillary and pubic hair and dark, coarse body hairs are known to develop in response to androgenic stimulation[1-3].

EFFECT OF HORMONES ON HUMAN SKIN

The tissues of the skin are the targets for a wide range of chemical messengers. The effects of a number of hormones have been well documented and these hormones have been shown to be responsible for the differences between male and female skin. For example, hair follicles and sebaceous glands are the targets for androgenic steroids secreted by the gonads and the adrenal cortex, and melanocytes are directly influenced by polypeptide hormones excreted by the pituitary gland[1-3].

The effects of estrogens on the skin have not yet been fully defined, though changes following the climacteric suggest that they may stimulate epidermal mitosis[1-3]. There is good evidence that they maintain dermal as well as bone collagen, and increase the synthesis of ground substance[1-3]. There is no doubt that they may inhibit sebaceous secretion, although this effect may be preceded by some other initial stimulation[1-3].

Estradiol has been shown to bind to cytosolic receptors in homogenized mouse skin. After systemic injection of ^{3}H-labeled estradiol into mice, autoradiography revealed the label to be concentrated in the nuclei of cells of the dermis and lower epidermis[1-3]. Estrogen receptors have been identified in cytosol prepared from human skin from which the subcutaneous fat has been removed, but human receptor levels appear generally to be very low, with the highest in the face and the lowest in the breast and thigh. Receptor levels have been found to be above normal in both female and male acne patients.

Progesterone receptors have been found in cytosol fractions of whole skin, with the highest level in the breast and the lowest in the pubic region.

Androgens are known to influence strongly specific targets such as sebaceous glands, hair follicles and apocrine glands. Testosterone is metabolized to 5α-dihydrotestosterone by the enzyme 5α reductase in several tissues, including the skin. In the adult the activity of the enzyme is higher in areas that appear to be sensitive to testosterone, such as acne-bearing skin with an abnormally high level of sebaceous activity, and hairy regions of women with idiopathic hirsutism[1-3].

THE INFLUENCE OF SEX ON SKIN THICKNESS, SKIN COLLAGEN AND DENSITY

Total skin collagen content is lower in females than in males. One reason for this difference may be the effect of androgen. With aging the total collagen content decreases in both men and women, but the lower initial collagen level in women is the reason why women appear to age earlier than men. So far as their skin is concerned, women are about 15 years older than men throughout their adult life. Moreover, skin collagen is less densely packed in females than in males[3-5]. As collagen is a major component of skin thickness, the lower content and density of collagen in female skin may explain why women's skin is thinner than that of men. Measurements of skin thickness, collagen content and density have provided useful information in metabolic and endocrine diseases and may also prove useful in monitoring the effects of drugs on connective tissue and in the investigation of diseases with suspected connective tissue defects[3-5].

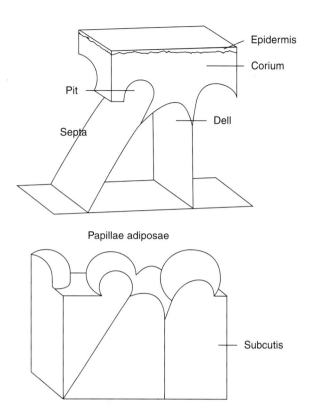

Figure 1   Reconstruction of the border zone between corium and subcutis from histologic serial sections. The plane of the subcutis with papillae adiposae rising into dells and pits on the undersurface of the corium is shown. In the upper part of the subcutis the septa are anchored in the corium

THE ANATOMIC BASIS OF SO-CALLED CELLULITE

The subcutaneous tissue of the thighs is composed of three layers of fat with two planes of connective tissue between them. On the thighs of women especially where the 'pinch test' for the 'mattress phenomenon' is elicitable, the uppermost subcutaneous layer consists of what are termed large 'standing fat cell chambers' with an average size, as seen in cross section, of 0.5×1.5 cm, and that are separated from each other by septa of connective tissue (retinacula cutis). These retinacula cutis (binders of the skin) run in a radial and arched way and anchor into the overlying corium. Papillae adiposae project from the fat cell chambers into the corium[5-10] (Figure 1). These papillae adiposae break up in the region of the stratum reticulare of the corium and surround hair bulbs, sweat glands and blood vessels, all of which are thereby protected against pressure and shearing forces. Since the fat cell units can, under pressure, change shape, but not volume, the 'mattress' phenomenon can be defined as a typical feature of the skin of women's thighs. It can be called 'status protrusus cutis' to express the fact that

(a)

(b)

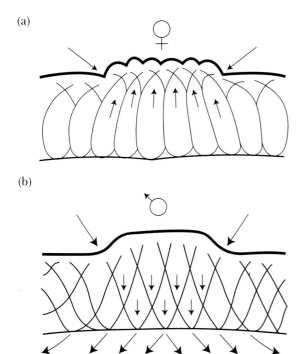

Figure 2 The pinch test on the skin of the thigh of a woman (a) and a man (b). In women, the fat cell conglomerations of the upper part of the subcutis (standing fat cell chambers, and papillae adiposae) protrude upon the overlying cutis. That produces deformation and pits, i.e., the mattress phenomenon or status protrusus cutis. In men merely folds and furrows are produced

the compression and bulging of the upper fat cell chamber system in women causes the overlying skin to protrude[5-10] (Figure 2).

In the comparable skin of men's thighs the uppermost part of the subcutaneous tissue is thinner and has a network of criss-crossing septa of connective tissue that divide the fat cell chambers into small polygonal units. Moreover, the corium is thicker in the skin of men than in women. In men, the pinch test can indeed fold or furrow the surface of the skin, but in normal men status protrusus cutis does not exist[5-10].

These characteristic structural differences of the skin of male thighs are probably due to the proliferative effect of androgens on the mesenchyme, because it has been shown that men with androgen deficiency can present the same condition of 'status protusus cutis' as women[5-10]. Thus it can be affirmed that there are, indeed, differences between male and female skin, and hormones have been shown to be responsible for these differences.

REFERENCES

1. Holbrock KA, Wolff K. The structure and development of skin. In Fitzpatrick TB, Eisen AZ, Wolff K, *et al.*, eds. *Dermatology in General Medicine*, 3rd edn. New York: McGraw Hill, 1987:93–131
2. Woodley DT, Demarcher M, Sengel P, Pruniéras M. The control of cutaneous development and behavior: the influence of extracellular and soluble factors. In Fitzpatrick TB, Eisen AZ, Wolff K, *et al.*, eds. *Dermatology in General Medicine*, 3rd edn. New York: McGraw Hill, 1987:132–45
3. Ponec M. Hormones receptors in the skin. In Fitzpatrick TB, Eisen AZ, Wolff K, *et al.*, eds. *Dermatology in General Medicine*, 3rd edn. New York: McGraw Hill, 1987:367–75
4. Shuster S, Black MM, McVitie E. The influence of age and sex on skin thickness, skin collagen and density. *Br J Dermatol* 1975;93:639–43
5. Nurnberger F. Sex differences in structure of male and female skin. *Second South African International Dermatological Congress*, Capetown, January 8–12, 1973
6. Nurnberger F, Muller G. So-called cellulite: an infective disease. *J Dermatol Surg Oncol* 1978;4:221–9
7. Scherwitz C, Braun-Falco O. So-called cellulite. *J Dermatol Surg Oncol* 1978;4:230–4
8. Lotti T, Ghersetich I, Grappone C, Dini G. Proteoglycans in so-called cellulite. *Int J Dermatol* 1990;29: 272–4
9. Braun-Falco O, Scherwitz C. Zur histopatologie der sogenannte Cellulitis. *Hautarzt* 1972;3:71–5
10. Bonnet GF. Traitment des cellulites localisées. *Rev Med Franc* 1960;5:367–9

The newborn girl

6

Daniel Wallach

INTRODUCTION

Specific cutaneous physiologic and pathologic problems are encountered in the neonatal period, i.e. the first month of life. Owing to continuous progress in neonatal medicine, *ex utero* life may start as early as 25–27 weeks after conception, and the special skin problems of the premature newborn are now a significant part of neonatal dermatology.

The differences between boys and girls are important only in a few conditions. Maternal concern about the newborn skin abnormalities is more likely to involve mothers of girls than boys: 58% of maternal questions about the skin come from mothers of girls, according to a recent survey[1]. Other sexual differences may be not only medical but cultural: girls are more likely than boys to receive applications of potentially harmful skin care products[2] or potentially sensitizing nickel jewelry. Girls and their parents may also suffer more intensely from the aesthetic consequences of all neonatal dermatoses.

THE APPEARANCE OF SKIN AT BIRTH

The appearance of neonatal skin depends on the maturity of the newborn and is one of the elements used for the assessment of gestational age. In fact, the assessment of gestational age at birth relies on history, ultrasonography, neuromuscular examination and evaluation of physical maturity[3].

The main physical criteria are:

(1) the appearance of the skin; it evolves from gelatinous and transparent with visible underlying vessels in the premature to thicker, opaque, keratinized skin with cracking and desquamation in the full-term newborn;

(2) lanugo (vellus body hair) is maximal at 27–28 weeks;

(3) creases develop from heel to toe on the plants;

(4) the ear cartilage becomes firmer;

(5) the breast areola becomes visible and the breast tissue increases in size; and

(6) the development of external genitalia is one of the most reliable indicators of gestational age; the appearance of the vulva depends on the extent of fat deposition. Labia minora are completely covered only in full-term girls. The clitoris may appear falsely hypertrophied in premature girls because of insufficient development of the labia majora (Figures 1 and 2).

The skin at birth is covered with a white, greasy coating called vernix caseosa; it is abundant mainly in infants born at full term. The vernix caseosa is mainly made of lipids deriving from the epidermis and the sebaceous secretion; it may cover the whole body or only the back and the fold areas. The vernix caseosa dries out after a few hours but is usually wiped away earlier for cosmetic purposes; in case of fetal distress, the vernix is stained yellow or brown by contact with the meconium.

PRINCIPLES OF SKIN CARE IN THE FULL-TERM NEWBORN

Curiously enough, standard guidelines for the skin care of the newborn have not been defined and as a consequence unjustified and even potentially harmful practices are still in use[4,5].

Bathing in 37°C water and gentle cleansing by clean hands using a non-medicated mild soap or syndet bar or liquid cleanser is advisable. There is no medical justification for the use of other products and parents should be advised not to use them[2]. It is probable that infant girls are at higher risk of being exposed to perfumes or other chemicals, with the possible consequence of allergic sensitization. Neither are there accepted guidelines for umbilical cord care. Many uncontrolled techniques are currently in use and the need for standardized, safe and effective antiseptic cord care is obvious. Although no standard procedure is published, chlorhexidine appears to be the best current recommendation[6].

Disposable diapers made from cellulose are used to avoid leakage of urine and feces. They are better tolerated than cloth diapers. Diapers must be changed as often as necessary, as contact of urine and feces with the skin is the main cause of diaper dermatitis. In addition to gentle cleansing, application of a protective bland ointment is useful as a barrier to protect the skin in the diaper area. In case of erythema, topical antifungals are often recommended to prevent surinfection (Figure 3).

CUTANEOUS COMPLICATIONS OF NEONATAL INTENSIVE CARE PROCEDURES

Progress in neonatal medicine has led to the successful management of ever smaller newborns. Premature babies weighing as little as 500 g at birth can now survive thanks to many sophisticated procedures. In addition to the well-known consequences of birth trauma and of antenatal investigations, cutaneous complications from the diagnostic and therapeutic procedures of the neonatal intensive care units (NICUs) have recently been recognized[7]. The number and the importance of cutaneous scars are directly correlated with the degree of prematurity and the duration of the stay in the intensive care unit[8]. Although these may appear as an unavoidable sequel of life-saving care, these complications need to be minimized. This is especially true for girls, who may be more concerned about the aesthetic appearance of neonatal scars, e.g. on the anterior chest.

Complications from antenatal procedures

Fetal scalp electrodes may hurt the scalp. This may result in a small wound and scar which must be differentiated from aplasia cutis; superinfection has been described and must be prevented. Amniocentesis occasionally induces punctiform scars in the fetus. Vacuum extractors and forceps (Figure 4) can cause skin trauma.

Complications of phototherapy

Phototherapy with visible blue light is an effective treatment of neonatal hyperbilirubinemia. This may induce non-specific transient erythematous eruptions and increased pigmentation. The bronze baby syndrome, a brown-gray discoloration, is a rare complication of phototherapy which usually reveals an underlying liver disease. It must be differentiated from cyanosis.

Acute cutaneous iatrogenic accidents in the intensive care unit

Burns

Thermal burns are usually due to transcutaneous oxygen and carbon dioxide monitoring which uses an electrode heated to 44°C in order to increase cutaneous blood flow. This induces a first-degree burn on all places where the electrode is placed (it is changed every few hours) (Figure 5). Permanent scarring is infrequent but has been reported. In addition, these burns may be involved in the so-called anetoderma of prematurity (see below). It is advisable to prevent these burns by heating the electrode as little as possible, especially when treating prematures. In girls, the anterior chest area must be avoided.

Irritant dermatitis

Irritant dermatitis is frequent in NICUs and is mainly due to two types of cutaneous agression: adhesives and surfactants.

Adhesives are numerous on the skin of infants in NICUs (Table 1) and may cover a significant part of the body surface area. The removal of adhesives is probably painful and strips the superficial stratum corneum layers. This stripping abolishes the cutaneous barrier properties. Although no satisfactory solution exists yet, the greatest attention must be focused on this problem by the medical and nursing staff. Manufacturers of adhesives should develop 'harmless adhesives for babies' (or at least as harmless as possible). Cleansing of the skin should involve the use of mild products. Antiseptics are mandatory before any invasive procedure. Care must be taken concerning not only the efficacy but also the topical and systemic safety of disinfection procedures[9]. Spontaneously or owing to these irritant factors, infant skin is often dry and cracking; emollients have proven useful to maintain it in good health and prevent additional damage[10].

Caustic dermatitis

Causticity, or chemical burns, may occur as a consequence of excessive application of irritant antiseptics. The best-documented is skin necrosis due to topical alcohol.

Table 1 Adhesive material on the skin in neonatal intensive care units

Fixation of intubation tube
Fixation of gastric tube
Cardiograph electrodes
Transcutaneous O_2/CO_2 monitoring (44°C)
Intravenous cannulae and catheters
Upper limbs contention
SaO_2 probe
Urine bag

Allergic contact dermatitis

Allergic contact dermatitis is usually said to be rare in the infant owing to immunological immaturity. In fact, allergic dermatitis on the site of ECG electrodes is sometimes observed (Figure 6). These electrodes contain an acrylic glue which may be the causative allergen. Other contact sensitizations may occur.

Others

Thrombosis in umbilical artery catheters may result in lower limb ischemia. Extravasation of intravenous fluids leads to local necrosis and permanent scars. Cutaneous or subcutaneous calcification may be a consequence of numerous heel pricks, or extravasation of calcium-containing infusions.

Long lasting scars

Long lasting, or even permanent, scars appear as an almost constant consequence of NICU stays[7]. Most of them are barely visible. The most important result from chest drain and fluid extravasations.

Anetoderma of prematurity

This is a recently described variant of anetoderma; it appears as round atrophic patches predominating at places where electrodes and other devices have been sited in prematures (Figure 7). Cutaneous irritation is believed to be the cause of this anetoderma. These long lasting or permanent sequelae of intensive care in the neonatal period may be at least partially prevented by paying special attention to the positioning of indispensable, life-saving devices in NICUs[11].

TRANSIENT NEONATAL SKIN CONDITIONS

A number of benign cutaneous conditions are frequently observed in the newborn. Although they are of no serious consequence (non-diseases of the newborn), they need to be recognized in order to avoid unnecessary concern or aggressive medical procedures. As stated earlier, parents of girls are, for cultural reasons, more prone to express concern about these conditions and to need reassurance.

Physiologic desquamation

Full-term newborns often exhibit a fine diffuse scaling, starting from the second day of life and lasting a few days; the scaling is diminished by application of emollients. When intense, physiologic desquamation may appear as ichthyosiform, but the rare neonatal ichthyoses are very different. In the peeling skin syndrome, large sheets of skin are removed and the condition is long lasting.

Milia

Milia are tiny epidermal inclusion cysts caused by retention of keratin at the extremity of hair follicles; they occur almost exclusively on the face, although at times some may be seen on the genital areas. Milia may be very numerous (Figure 8) but desquamate spontaneously, and no intervention is indicated. Widespread or lasting milia are part of rare developmental syndromes such as oro-facial-digital syndrome type I or Marie Unna hypotrichosis.

Miliaria

Miliaria is the consequence of sweat retention in immature, impermeable eccrine ducts. Sweating in newborns occurs only in term infants and must lead to a correction of excessive environmental temperature or clothing. Miliaria crystallina appears as tiny translucid vesicles; inflammation induces peripheral erythema, known as miliaria rubra; in cases of superinfection, miliaria becomes pustular.

Cutaneous consequences of hormonal transition

During the last weeks of gestation, the fetus receives important hormonal influences from her mother and the placenta. At birth, these influences cease abruptly and this cessation transiently stimulates the neonatal endocrine system. All this 'endocrine transition' has visible consequences on the skin.

Sebaceous gland hyperplasia

As a consequence of the influence of maternal androgens, the sebaceous glands on the nose and central face are often enlarged and the openings of the follicles appear as pinpoint yellowish papules. This transient hyperplasia seems to be unrelated to neonatal acne.

Neonatal acne

Neonatal acne is less frequent in girls than in boys; it predominates on the cheeks. Although papules, pustules and small nodules may be more visible, the most important lesion is the comedo, specific for acne. Except in a few instances, neonatal acne resolves in a few weeks; topical antimicrobial therapy is usually prescribed.

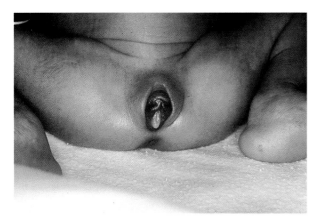

Figure 1 Normal vulva of a premature girl (31 weeks' gestation). Labia majora are not developed and the clitoris seems hypertrophied; pigmentation is ethnic

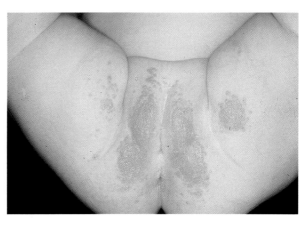

Figure 3 Diaper dermatitis (irritation dermatitis). Note that the folds are spared

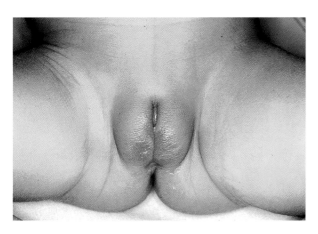

Figure 2 Normal vulva of a full-term newborn (41 weeks' gestation). The labia majora completely cover the labia minora

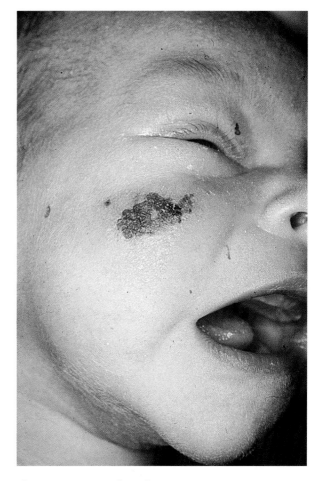

Figure 4 Trauma from forceps

The recently described facial pustulosis induced in newborns by *Malassezia furfur* is the main differential diagnosis of neonatal acne and will be discussed later.

Pseudo-puberty of the newborn

This transient consequence of stimulation by sexual hormones is seen in both sexes. In girls, it involves:

(1) hyperpigmentation of the linea alba and of external genitalia, mainly in dark-skinned newborns;

(2) edema of external genitalia;

(3) vaginal discharge, usually whitish, rarely hemorrhagic (pseudo-menses); and

(4) hypertrophy of mammary glands (Figure 9), with the possibility of a milky secretion for a few days.

Mastitis and abscess can occur, especially in cases of inadequate manipulation (Figure 10). None of these neonatal consequences of hormonal influence on the skin is related to any later cutaneous or endocrine condition.

Consequences of vascular immaturity

The change from the intra-amniotic to the aerial environment implies dramatic modifications in vasomotor tone; some instability of the cutaneous vascularization in the neonatal period may be visible.

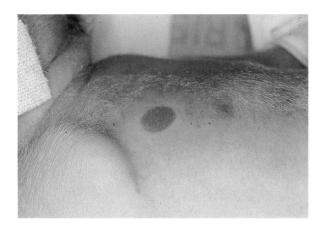

Figure 5   First-degree burn from pO_2/pCO_2 monitoring

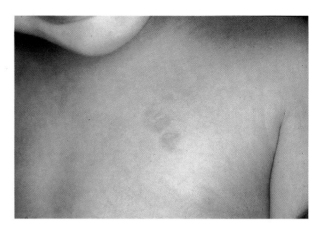

Figure 7   Anetoderma of prematurity in a three-year-old girl, prematurely born

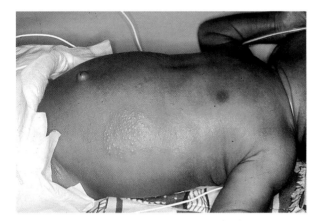

Figure 6   Acute allergic contact dermatitis from cardioscope probes

Normal skin color

Many pathological conditions may alter skin color: for example circulatory or respiratory distress, anemia, polycythemia, jaundice. In the absence of any of these conditions, normal skin color at birth associates central erythema and peripheral cyanosis. Ethnic pigmentation is usually delayed.

Cutis marmorata

Cutis marmorata (marbled skin) is a normal reaction to cold in newborns, and it disappears with warming. Physiologic neonatal cutis marmorata must be differentiated from cutis marmorata telangiectatica congenita. In this rare vascular anomaly, the mottling of the skin is more marked, permanent, and associated with areas of atrophy, ulcerations and other lesions. Systemic malformations and mental retardation may be associated.

Harlequin color change

This difference in skin coloration between the upper and lower half of the body may be seen during episodes lasting a few minutes; it is the most spectacular

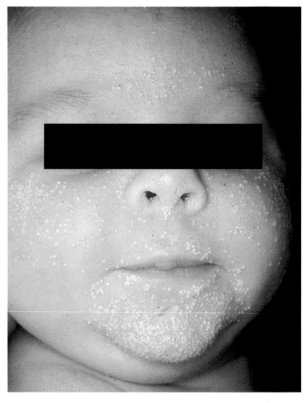

Figure 8   Numerous milia on the face of an otherwise normal newborn. Complete spontaneous healing occurred

manifestation of neonatal vascular immaturity. Its observation is limited to the first days of life.

Erythema toxicum

The condition known as erythema toxicum is the most common of all neonatal dermatoses. Its pathogenesis is unknown and the word 'toxicum' does not indicate any toxicity. Erythema toxicum occurs in about one half of term neonates and only atypical forms attract dermatological attention. It is not present at birth, begins after the first day of life and usually lasts about one week. The lesions

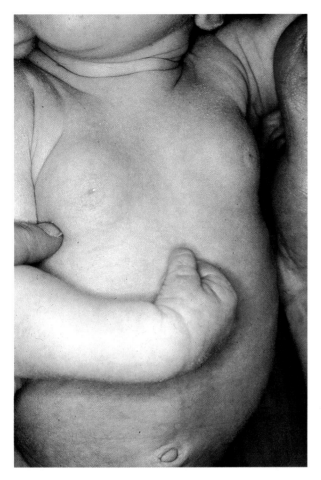

Figure 9 Pseudo-puberty of the newborn

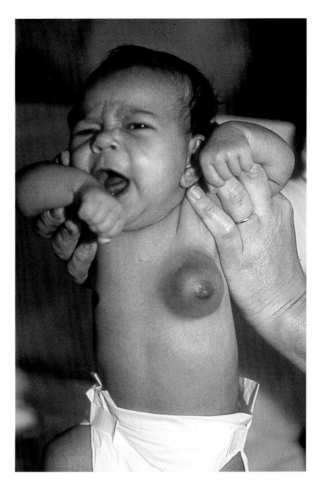

Figure 10 Acute mastitis leading to abscess formation

predominate on the trunk and proximal parts of the limbs; they consist of large (1 to 3 cm) erythematous macules and papules; the center of the lesions is more elevated than the periphery and at times may be marked by a small vesicle or even a pustule. Although vesicular or pustular erythema toxicum is usually easily differentiated from other vesicular or pustular neonatal dermatoses (see later in this chapter), one may need confirmation of the diagnosis by showing the eosinophilic content of the liquid lesions on Tzanck's smear. There is also a blood hypereosinophilia, the significance of which is unknown.

Neonatal pustular conditions

Transient neonatal pustular melanosis

This is more frequent in black newborns, and is considered as a variant of erythema toxicum with hyperpigmented sequelar macules lasting some weeks.

A benign facial neonatal pustulosis induced by Malassezia furfur

This has recently been described[12] and is probably not rare[13]. Malassezia-induced neonatal pustulosis usually starts between ages 7 and 30 days. It comprises numerous small pustules on erythematous bases, and is clinically different from other neonatal pustuloses (Figure 11). The almost unique location is the face (cheeks) but occasional lesions may be seen on the neck, nape and chest. The main differential diagnosis is neonatal acne, but in this condition comedones are always present and lesions are more long-lasting. Direct microscopic examination shows *Malassezia furfur*, and topical antifungals clear the eruption in a few days. The spontaneous course is not known but is thought to be self-limited.

Infantile acropustulosis

This is a relatively frequent disease in infancy. It may start at birth, but usually begins during the first semester of life, and lasts between one and two years. Infantile acropustulosis consists of crops of pruritic small pustules electively located on the hands and feet. The lateral sides of the hands and feet are the most common site (Figure 12), but the dorsa and the palms and plants are also involved. There may be lesions in other body areas. Lesions start as small vesicles on an erythematous macule

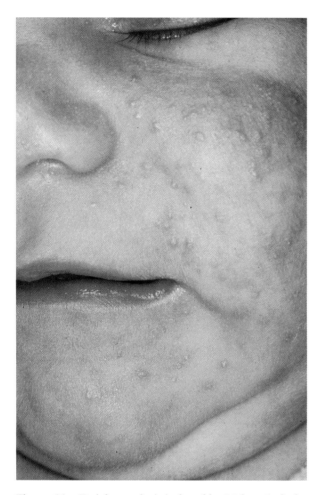

Figure 11   Facial pustulosis induced by *Malassezia furfur*

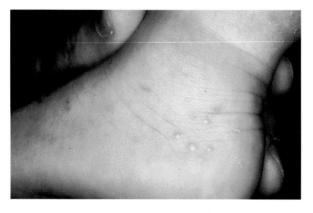

Figure 12   Typical appearance of infantile acropustulosis

and soon become pustular, before undergoing crusting and desiccation. Isolated pruritic pustules, 1–2 mm in diameter, do not tend to coalesce. A Tzanck's smear shows intact polymorphonuclear cells and a variable proportion of eosinophils. Biopsy[14] is not performed in typical cases. The main differential diagnosis is scabies. The most frequent situation is a misdiagnosis of infantile acropustulosis

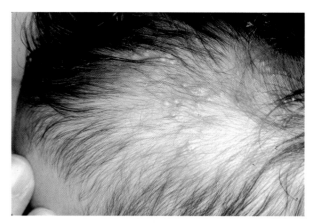

Figure 13   Eosinophilic scalp pustulosis

and useless, sometimes repeated, antiscabetic treatment. Cases of infantile acropustulosis have been reported after effective treatment of documented scabies. Great care must be taken to make a definite scabies diagnosis. Microscopic identification of sarcoptes and epidemiological data are the most reliable diagnostic clues. Infantile acropustulosis is usually responsive to topical steroids. Dapsone, with the usual caution, is advocated in resistant cases.

Eosinophilic scalp pustulosis

This is another variant of benign infantile pustulosis. The lesions are mainly located on the scalp, although other body areas may be involved as well. The pustules are usually grouped and may evoke impetigo or inflammatory tinea (Figure 13). The condition shows spontaneous remissions and bouts; Tzanck's smear, which shows eosinophils, allows diagnosis of this benign entity. Histology is not done in typical cases; these pustules may or may not be follicular, and topical steroids are effective[15].

Hair and nail conditions
Lanugo

Lanugo is a vellus, unpigmented body hair. It is usually abundant in prematures; the pattern of lanugo is not predictive of later body hair, which depends mainly on familial and ethnic factors.

Scalp hair growth

Most newborns have abundant terminal scalp hair; the normal cycle of individual growth and fall is not yet established and synchronized telogen effluvium may occur during the first months of life, followed by normal regrowth. A transient occipital alopecia is frequent; it is probably favored by repeated rubbing in bed.

Nails

The length of nails at birth is one of the indicators of the duration of gestation, and post-term babies have long nails. The nails of newborns are usually small and soft, mainly on the toes, and the surrounding skin may cover the nails' edges (pseudo-ingrown toenails). Except in cases of scratching, nails must not be cut and never cut too short.

Nodular fat necrosis

Idiopathic panniculitis, known as nodular fat necrosis of the newborn, is seen after difficult labor and delivery, especially when the baby has suffered from hypoxia and hypothermia, and also in the absence of any identifiable cause. Lesions are usually located on the upper part of the posterior trunk. The buttocks, arms and legs may also be involved. Lesions are palpable as subcutaneous indurated masses; the overlying skin is usually red. The main differential diagnosis is neonatal sclerema, a diffuse induration of the skin occurring in severely ill neonates. In contrast, babies with nodular fat necrosis remain in good health. Nodular fat necrosis heals in a few weeks; hypercalcemia has been reported and must be prevented and monitored. Infection is very rare.

REFERENCES

1. André N, Melly L, Menaud G. Tout ce que les mères ont toujours voulu savoir sur la peau de leur nouveau-né ... *Arch Pédiatr* 1988;5:578–9
2. Cetta F, Lambert GH, Ros SP. Newborn chemical exposure from over-the-counter skin care products. *Clin Pediatr* 1991;30:286–9
3. Dubowitz LMS, Dubowitz V, Goldberg C. Clinical assessment of gestational age in the newborn infant. *J Pediatr* 1970;77:1–10
4. Siegfried EC. Neonatal skin and skin care. *Dermatol Clin* 1998;16:437–46
5. Liou LW, Janniger CK. Skin care of the normal newborn. *Cutis* 1997;59:171–4
6. Verber IG, Pagan FS. What cord care – if any? *Arch Dis Child* 1993;68:594–6
7. Metzker A, Brenner S, Merlob P. Iatrogenic cutaneous injuries in the neonate. *Arch Dermatol* 1999; 135:697–703
8. Cartlidge PHT, Fox PE, Rutter N. The scars of newborn intensive care. *Early Hum Dev* 1990;21:1–10
9. Malathi I, Millar MR, Leeming JP, *et al*. Skin disinfection in preterm infants. *Arch Dis Child* 1993; 69:312–16
10. Nopper AJ, Horii KA, Sookdeo-Drost S, *et al.* Topical ointment therapy benefits premature infants. *J Pediatr* 1996;128:660–9
11. Prizant TL, Lucky AW, Frieden IJ, *et al*. Spontaneous atrophic patches in extremely premature infants. Anetoderma of prematurity. *Arch Dermatol* 1996;132:671–4
12. Aractingi S, Cadranel S, Reygagne P, Wallach D. Pustulose néo-natale induite par *Malassezia furfur*. *Ann Dermatol Vénéréol* 1991;118:856–8
13. Rapelanoro R, Mortureux P, Couprie B, *et al*. Neonatal *Malassezia furfur* pustulosis. *Arch Dermatol* 1996;132:190–3
14. Vignon-Pennamen MD, Wallach D. Infantile acropustulosis: a clinicopathologic study of six cases. *Arch Dermatol* 1986;122:1155–60
15. Taïeb A, Bassan-Andrieu L, Maleville J. Eosinophilic pustulosis of the scalp in childhood. *J Am Acad Dermatol* 1992;27:55–60

The girl and the adolescent 7

Joseph A. Witkowski and Lawrence Charles Parish

From the time a girl is no longer a toddler until she answers to being a young woman, few skin diseases are gender specific. Young people of both sexes have warts and moles, and even zits. Frogs, incantations and cucumber concoctions just will not eliminate them. Acne may occur slightly earlier in girls, owing to their more rapid maturation. Nearly all adolescents suffer from acne, but young women often aggravate the condition by excessive washing, applying occlusive cosmetics and even using moisturizing lotions, unnecessarily. Acne excoriée de jeune filles is a specific entity reflecting the patient's denial of having acne and taking measures into her hands with picking.

Stretch marks are of concern to young women who have rapid fluctuation in weight due to crash diets and even bulimia. Extensive body building can also create these elastotic problems. Similarly, folliculitis on the legs can be a nuisance, owing to improper shaving with less than adequate preshaving hydration. These problems can also occur in young men, particularly when they shave their faces in a careless fashion. Pediculosis capitis occurs more often in girls because of long hair, and more head-to-head contact. Daily or even twice daily shampooing may leave frizzled ends, but no permanent damage occurs. The concern over pantyhose causing candidosis was never borne out.

Whether there is a gender difference in atopic dermatitis or in psoriasis remains to be determined. A few diseases do have a preference for girls, and these will be discussed here.

TRICHOTILLOMANIA

This condition results in patchy non-inflammatory alopecia with broken hairs of differing lengths. The distribution appears to be artifactual with variable size and shapes of the affected areas. There is no scaling and the remaining hairs have normal resistance to epilation because telogen hairs have been pulled out. On microscopic examination the remaining anogen hairs appear twisted and broken[1]. This condition may represent a transient compulsive habit or be symptomatic of a more pervasive neurosis (Figure 1)[2]. Management includes confrontation of the patient, occlusive dressings and psychiatric referral.

TRACTION ALOPECIA

Circumscribed or linear patches of alopecia at the margins of the scalp or widening of the parts are seen. This may be accompanied by short broken hairs[1]. Follicular inflammation and later some focal scarring may be present. The causes include tight braiding, pony tails and corn rowing. The ethnic background of the patient may help to identify the cause of tension on the hair. An alternative hair style should be recommended.

ACNE EXCORIÉE

Minimal acne causes mental stress in some young women. As a result they attack the lesions with fingernails and other instruments, producing excoriations and superficial ulcerations. The forehead and cheeks are usually involved. The lesions heal slowly, leaving irregularly shaped hypopigmented atrophic scars. The condition usually represents a compulsive habit resulting from an unconscious neurosis. Treatment consists of explaining the causes, eliciting a supportive attitude on the part of the parents and management of the acne (Figure 2). Occasionally, referral for psychotherapy is necessary[2].

MELASMA

Light to dark brown patches are seen. The condition is often symmetrical, especially involving the malar eminences and the forehead. It usually becomes more prominent in the summer months and improves in the winter. Hispanics as well as inhabitants of the Middle East and Asian countries are predisposed. In this age group, oral contraceptives are the most common etiological agents. Management includes discontinuing the oral contraceptive, avoidance of sun exposure, the use of a high-potency broad-spectrum sunscreen and application of 4% hydroquinone or 20% azelaic acid[3]. Resistant lesions may require the use of a combination of hydroquinone, retinoic acid and hydrocortisone ointment or solution.

TURNER'S SYNDROME

Partial or complete absence of the short arm of one X chromosome results in Turner's syndrome[4].

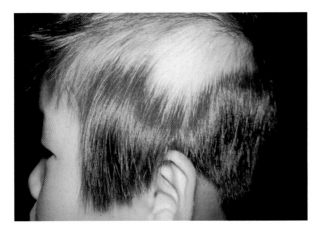

Figure 1 Trichotillomania – 4-year-old girl secretly pulled and rubbed her hair until there were bald areas

Commonly associated features are short stature, web neck and cubitus valgus. The characteristic facial features, ie. ptosis, epicanthic folds, narrow maxilla, small mandible and dysmorphic or low-set ears, and failure to develop secondary sexual changes often result in psychological problems. Patients suspected of having this condition should have a karyotypic evaluation. Those with established diagnosis should be checked periodically for diabetes mellitus and thyroid abnormalities. Counselling and psychological support are essential.

SUPERNUMERARY NIPPLES (POLYTHELIA)

The lesion resembles a normal nipple[5]. It is a brown slightly elevated papule occurring along the embryological milk line. A high incidence of associated congenital urinary tract anomalies has been reported. The renal abnormality is present on the same side as the extra nipple. Treatment of polythelia is surgical removal, usually for cosmetic reasons. Examination for urinary tract anomalies is recommended.

JOGGER'S NIPPLE

The nipples are red, swollen, eroded or hyperkeratotic[6]. Local treatment includes compresses and a steroid cream or ointment. The condition can be prevented by a properly fitted bra.

AREOLAR GLAND DISCHARGE IN GIRLS

Discharge from the areolar glands of the breast is an uncommon condition affecting adolescent women[7]. No treatment is recommended other than

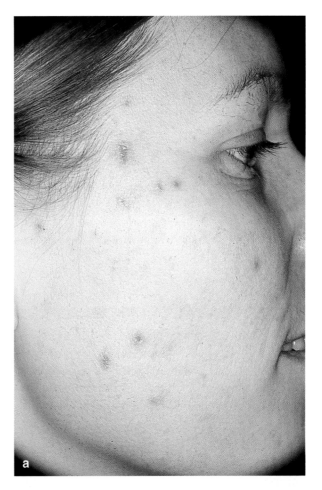

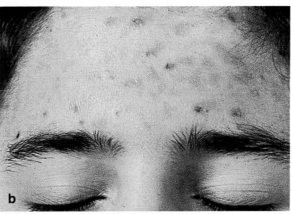

Figure 2a, b Acne excoriée de jeune fille – these teenagers constantly picked at their acne pimples, hoping to eliminate the zits

observation. The condition should be differentiated from galactorrhea. Intact pustules may resemble molluscum contagiosum (Figure 3).

NIPPLE DERMATITIS

Patchy erythema and scaling of the nipples is a minor clinical feature of atopic dermatitis[8]. The condition is associated with pruritus and other manifestations of atopy. Compresses and a steroid cream are recommended.

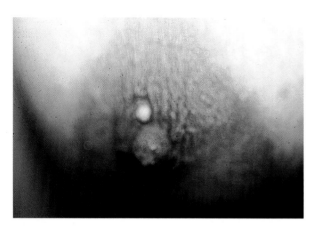

Figure 3 Molluscum contagiosum on the breast – this adolescent thought the globular lesion was a normal part of the areola

NIPPLE CONTACT DERMATITIS

Patchy erythema, scaling and occasional vesiculation of the nipples and the areolae are seen. In one study, patch tests to beeswax nipple-protective cream was positive[9]. Management includes avoidance of the substance, compresses and a steroid cream.

BODY PIERCING

While body piercing is engaged in by both sexes, adolescent women are often seen with multiple punctures on the ears. Other sites that may be pierced are the eyebrows, nose, lips, tongue, nipples, navel and areas not readily seen. Rings, studs and barbells are inserted in these man-made holes. Possible complications include nickel allergy and secondary staphylococcal and streptococcal infections. Cartilage destruction can result from pseudomonal infection of the ear. Moist areas such as the navel and genitalia are more susceptible to candidal infection, especially in hot humid climates. Broken teeth from metallic objects in the tongue often require dental consultation. There is always the risk of trauma-induced tearing, keloids and possible transmission of HIV, hepatitis, syphilis and tuberculosis. Body piercing is usually an expression of youthful rebellion.

REFERENCES

1. Olsen EA. *Disorders of Hair Growth*. New York: McGraw-Hill, 1994:79–88
2. Koblenzer CS. *Psychocutaneous Disease*. Orlando: Grune and Stratton, 1987:145–8
3. Balina L, Graupe K. The treatment of melasma with 20% azelaic acid versus 4% hydroquinone cream. *Int J Dermatol* 1991;30:893–5
4. Smith DW. XO syndrome. In Smith DW, ed. *Recognizable Patterns of Human Malformation*. Philadelphia: WB Saunders Company, 1982:72
5. Meggyessy V, Meher K. Association of supernumerary nipples with renal abnormalities. *J Pediatr* 1987;3:412
6. Levit F. Jogger's nipples. *N Engl J Med* 1977; 297:1127
7. Heyman RB, Rauh JL. Areolar gland discharge in adolescent females. *J Adolesc Health Care* 1983;4: 285–6
8. Kanwar AJ, Dhar S, Kaur S. Evaluation of minor features of atopic dermatitis. *Pediatr Dermatol* 1991;8: 114–16
9. Garcia M, del Poso MD, Diez J, *et al*. Allergic contact dermatitis from beeswax nipple protective. *Contact Dermatitis* 1995;33:440–1

The adult woman

Rebecca C. Tung and Wilma F. Bergfeld

8

INTRODUCTION

Following adolescence, a woman's skin and hair pass through many distinctive stages as she grows older. Although we can all look forward to some degree of intrinsic (chronological) aging owing to our genes, it is usually the signs of extrinsic photo-aging which prompt patients to seek our counsel. Whether the woman's initial visit occurs at age 20 or 50, we as dermatologists must be cognizant of the most commonly encountered conditions affecting each decade of life. Similarly, we should also keep gender in mind in order to select the most appropriate evaluation and treatment for a given condition.

THE TWENTIES

Acne

Whatever the age, acne can be particularly troubling psychologically. In one study, female patients with severe acne not only had a poor body image but also had a decrease in self-esteem. Both parameters improved following acne treatment[1]. Acne sufferers may even experience discrimination when trying to obtain employment[2]. Successful treatment of acne can truly give patients more than just cosmetic benefits.

Although acne vulgaris is generally considered to be a disorder of adolescence, it often continues to be a problem for many adult women. Most adult acne can be classified either as persistent acne or true late onset acne (onset after age 25)[3]. In women, it is one disorder which is particularly sensitive to hormonal changes in the monthly cycle. Up to 70% of women surveyed reported some flare acne lesions premenstrually[4]. The pathogenesis of acne is multifactorial, but androgenic stimulation of sebaceous glands plays an important role. Although sebum excretion is under genetic control, acne probably results from an exaggerated response of the pilosebaceous unit to normal levels of circulating androgens[5,6]. Other studies have actually documented increased plasma androgen levels in some female acne patients[7-9].

When acne is late-onset, has been resistant to treatment, or is accompanied by clinical signs of hyperandrogenism (hirsutism, androgenetic alopecia, or menstrual disturbances), underlying abnormalities in ovarian, adrenal, or local tissue androgens may be present[3]. Screening tests such as dehydroepiandrosterone sulfate (DHEAS) reflect adrenal androgen production, whereas testosterone and androstenedione are produced by both the ovaries and adrenals[10]. Markedly abnormal tests prompt further work-up for conditions such as polycystic ovarian syndrome, late-onset congenital adrenal hyperplasia, or virilizing malignancies[10]. When prior treatment with topical preparations, oral antibiotics, or isotretinoin have failed, addition of an anti-androgen such as spironolactone (in doses of 50 mg to 200 mg daily) and/or certain oral contraceptives, which contain non-androgenic progestins like norgestimate, desogestrel, norethindrone and ethynodiol diacetate, can benefit some patients[11,12]. See Table 1 for a list of brand names.

Smoking cessation

Young women may not at first want to hear about smoking cessation, especially from their dermatologist, but a few straight facts on the cutaneous effects of smoking may start them thinking. One study found that prominent facial wrinkling was significantly more common amongst smokers in all age, sex and sun-exposure groups[13]. Additionally, severity of wrinkling correlated with the number of 'pack-years' smoked[13,14]. Another study confirmed that women smokers had a higher relative risk of developing moderate to severe wrinkling compared to men[14,15]. The not so complimentary 'smoker's face' is defined by prominent lines or wrinkles, facial gauntness, an atrophic gray appearance of the skin, or a plethoric orange, purple, or red complexion[14,16]. Smoking-related histologic changes like fragmented thickened elastic fibers in the dermis result from chronic ischemia, increased elastase activity and decreased vitamin A levels[14].

Within all this evidence there is hope, however. Only 8% of past smokers and non-smokers clinically

Table 1 Drug names

Generic	Brand name
azelaic acid	Azelex
conjugated estrogens	Premarin
desogestrel/ethinyl estradiol	Desogen
	Orthocept
dexamethasone	Decadron
dihydroxyacetone	—
estradiol	Estraderm, Estrace, Vivelle, Climara
ethynodiol diacetate/ethinyl estradiol	Demulen
5-fluorouracil	Efudex, Fluoroplex
flutamide	Eulexin
hydroquinone USP 4% with alpha hydroxy acids	Lustra
hydroquinone USP 4% with sunscreen	Solaquin Forte
hydroquinone USP/tretinoin/dexamethasone/ascorbic acid	Kligman's bleach
isotretinoin	Accutane
medroxyprogesterone	Provera
metronidazole	Metrogel, Noritate
minoxidil	Rogaine
norethindrone/ethinyl estradiol	Orthonovum
norgestimate/ethinyl estradiol	Ortho Tri-Cyclen
	Ortho Cyclen
spironolactone	Aldactone
synthetic melanin	Melasyn™
tretinoin	Retin A, Renova

had 'smoker's face', whereas 46% of current smokers had this condition[16]. If the multiple health risks of smoking are not enough to encourage our patients to quit smoking, perhaps the threat of accelerated wrinkling may be a more powerful motivator.

Sun protection

The importance of incorporating a total sun protection regimen into a woman's everyday routine cannot be overemphasized. The sun today is not what it used to be; based on current predictions, ultraviolet B (UVB) levels are expected to peak around the millennium owing to decreases in stratospheric ozone[17]. This environmental increase in UVB coupled with underprotected exposure to the sun can translate into serious adverse effects on the skin (non-melanoma skin cancers, photoaging) and eyes (cataracts)[17,18]. Ultraviolet A (UVA), which is abundant in mid-day sunlight, can penetrate deep into the dermis, thus contributing to disproportionately more photodamage than UVB[19]. Even suberythemal doses of repetitive UVA can lead to photoaging[20]. Studies have also suggested that UVA along with UVB may also play a role in the pathogenesis of melanoma[17,18,21,22].

The cornerstone of total sun protection is a broad-spectrum (UVA and UVB) sunscreen or sunblock with a sun protection factor of at least 15[23]. Suggesting a moisturizer or foundation which has a built-in sun protection can often encourage daily compliance, but women must also be reminded that prolonged outdoor exposure necessitates more frequent sunscreen application. The benefits of regular broad spectrum sunscreen usage include a reduction in the stigmata of photoaging as well as a decrease in pre-malignant actinic keratoses and non-melanoma skin cancers[22,23]. Because complete sun avoidance is impossible, women should be encouraged to wear protective clothing, a broad brimmed hat and sunglasses when outside. Seeking shade or staying indoors at mid-day can also help minimize UV damage[24].

Not all sun damage is done outdoors. At least 18 million American women have used indoor tanning facilities one or more times[25]. While the media have done a wonderful job underscoring the evils of tanning salons, our role as physicians is to frankly explain the associated risks of accelerated photodamage and skin cancer development. Alternative topical bronzers containing dihydroxyacetone and now synthetic melanin can deliver a 'safe' tanned appearance[24,26,27].

PREGNANCY

No matter what a woman's age, pregnancy is a period of time filled with profound hormonal and physiologic changes. Pigmentary alterations are rather common during pregnancy. Hyperpigmentation occurs in 90% of pregnant women. Increasing levels of melanocyte stimulating hormone, estrogen, and possibly progesterone are causative agents[28].

Melasma is a condition of hypermelanosis affecting the face, which becomes more prominent with exposure to the sun. It generally occurs during pregnancy but can also flare premenstrually and is associated with oral contraceptive usage[28]. Although it may fade with time, treatments such as tretinoin cream applied nightly, hydroquinone preparations at a 4% concentration such as Lustra (also containing glycolic acid) and Solaquin Forte (also containing a sunscreen) applied twice daily, Kligman's bleach (hydroquinone 3–5%, 0.1% tretinoin, 0.1% dexamethasone, and ascorbic acid) applied twice daily, and azelaic acid cream applied twice daily may expedite the resolution of epidermal pigmentation[29]. Serial chemical peels with glycolic acid (30–70% increased stepwise) or trichloroacetic acid (25%) and laser treatment with the Q-switched ruby laser (694 nm) can also be utilized to treat persistent hyperpigmentation[29].

Many women may note changes in their moles during pregnancy. Previous studies have also reported darkening and enlarging nevi during pregnancy[28,30]. However, a more recent prospective study found no significant change in the size of melanocytic nevi during pregnancy[31]. Given this group's findings, any nevus which changes during pregnancy may represent atypical transformation and warrants histopathologic examination. There has also been much concern on the part of both dermatologists and patients regarding melanomas which develop during pregnancy. A recent review of controlled clinical studies found that pregnancy before, during, and after the time of diagnosis of stage I cutaneous melanoma does not appear to influence 5-year survival rates[32].

Multiple acrochordons (skin tags) may also appear in the latter trimesters of pregnancy. Because they often resolve postdelivery, it has been suggested that they are probably due to hormonal factors[33]. Stretch marks (striae gravidarum) develop in up to 90% of pregnant women[28]. Initially, they first occur on the abdominal wall and later on the breasts, buttocks and thighs. Etiologic agents include increased adrenocortical activity and physical factors resulting from increased abdominal girth. Unfortunately, treatment for striae have been disappointing. Topical tretinoin applied once or twice daily or laser therapy with the flash lamp pumped pulsed dye laser (585 nm) early on may improve cosmesis[34,35].

During pregnancy, the intravascular blood volume increases by 50%. Meanwhile, the enlarging uterus displaces and compresses the major abdominal vessels. The combined effect of these two processes is varicose veins in the legs, vulva and anus (hemorrhoids)[28,36]. While proactive steps such as leg elevation and wearing support hose can help, residual varicosities may require additional treatment like sclerotherapy, laser, or even vein stripping[37,38]. Other vascular abnormalities such as spider telangiectasias, cherry angiomas and purpura may also develop[28].

THE THIRTIES

While gazing in the mirror, women in their thirties may begin to see fine wrinkles. The frantically scheduled appointment with the dermatologist may be prompted by fears of premature aging. The majority of cosmetic problems, including fine lines, lentigines, coarseness and senile purpura may be primarily attributed to photoaging rather than the passage of time[19,39,40]. Intrinsic aging includes effects from genetics, gravity, expression, sleep and hormones[19,39]. Histologically, chronologic aging is characterized by decreased vascularity, dermal thinning, reduced cellularity of the dermis and elastic fiber loss[39]. Clinically these abnormalities are manifested as sallow color, atrophy, wrinkles and laxity[39].

Photoaging is caused by cumulative and frequent UV exposure superimposed on intrinsic aging changes. The American Academy of Dermatology consensus conference estimated that up to 80% of UV-induced photoaging occurs within the first 20 years of life, with the exception of those adults who have extensive exposure secondary to lifestyle or work[41]. Principal clinical aspects include laxity, roughness, sallowness, irregular hyperpigmentation and telangiectasia[19]. Histologically, alterations include both epidermal atrophy and acanthosis, abnormal keratinocyte progression from the basal layer, overstimulated or destroyed melanocytes, collagen loss with elastic fiber degeneration and reduction of vascular networks[19,39].

Cutaneous rejuvenation was classically initiated by women who already had significant photodamage. New research has shown that topical retinoids can actually prevent premature skin aging. Pre-treatment of the skin for 16 or more hours with retinol or tretinoin actually prevents a proto-oncogene, c-jun, from accumulating when the skin is exposed to UV light[42]. This is important because in untreated skin, sun-induced increases in c-jun can activate collagenases which degrade the dermis[42]. These findings build on previous research which demonstrated that tretinoin partially reverses the changes in photoaged skin by normalizing epidermal atypia, depositing new collagen and forming new vessels[39,43]. Therefore, adding a topical retinoid preparation to a younger woman's skin care regimen can both prevent and treat signs of photodamage.

Hirsutism

Hirsutism and androgenetic alopecia are two hormonally dependent disorders. Each condition can be emotionally disturbing for the affected individual no matter what her age. In hirsutism, there is excess terminal hair growth in a woman following the adult male pattern. Often, it is the result of androgen excess[44]. Many patients may actually recall mild hirsutism being present as early as puberty. While more specific etiologies will be discussed in a later chapter, it is important to note that up to 50% of women presenting with oligomenorrhea, hirsutism, or acne may have an ovarian source of androgen excess[45]. Sudden severe hirsutism suggests a tumor and warrants full diagnostic evaluation. Initial screening laboratory tests like DHEAS and free and total testosterone are a reasonable first step in the evaluation of the cutaneous effects of androgen excess (i.e., hirsutism, androgenetic alopecia and acne)[44]. Current therapies for hirsutism include cosmetic treatments such as bleaching, waxing, shaving, tweezing, laser hair removal and electrolysis. Severe cases may also warrant adjunctive oral medications: oral contraceptives, (as discussed in the acne section), spironolactone in doses of 50 mg to 200 mg daily, flutamide in doses of 250 mg to 750 mg daily, or corticosteroids such as dexamethasone in doses of 0.125 mg to 0.25 mg at bedtime to suppress adrenal androgen production[44].

Androgenetic alopecia

Androgenetic alopecia (AGA) is the most common type of hair loss. It represents a failure to re-initiate the anagen growth phase following shedding of telogen hairs and progressive miniaturization of the hair follicle. The result is gradual hair thinning mainly on the central scalp without an increase in the number of hairs shed. Interestingly, some cases of AGA can present as more diffuse alopecia over the entire scalp with increased telogen shedding. Other women may have a mixed type of hair loss (for example, AGA compounded by iron deficiency, telogen effluvium or thyroid disease). AGA occurs in genetically predisposed individuals whose follicles are extremely sensitive to androgen hormones. Other signs of androgen excess including hirsutism, acne and irregular menses may also be present. Many young women with AGA also have a higher incidence of polycystic ovarian syndrome and late-onset adrenal hyperplasia[44].

Initial evaluation for AGA is the same as for hirsutism; however, screening for underlying iron deficiency and thyroid disease is also of value[44]. These laboratory tests are important because studies have shown that up to 72% of women with diffuse telogen shedding are iron deficient with or without associated anemia[46]. Iron replacement in deficient individuals has resulted in cessation of shedding followed by regrowth as iron levels normalized[46]. Data suggest that ferritin levels of 40 µg/l or greater may be required for optimal hair growth[46]. In addition, diffuse hair loss may be the only symptom of new-onset hypothyroidism. Up to 50% of patients with myxedema may present with diffuse alopecia[46].

Treatment with a nutritional supplement containing biotin, topical minoxidil in concentrations of 2–5% applied twice daily, and medications also used to treat persistent acne and hirsutism including oral contraceptives, spironolactone and dexamethasone can be helpful. While finasteride has been shown to slow the progression and increase hair growth in men with AGA, it has been shown to lack efficacy in postmenopausal women with AGA[47].

Telogen effluvium

Telogen effluvium (TE) is the second most common type of hair loss; it is characterized by an alteration in the hair growth cycle[44]. Clinical features include shedding a greater than normal number of hairs accompanied by a variable amount of diffuse thinning. Hair pull tests are positive throughout the scalp. TE, which is usually self-limited, is a delayed shedding which occurs 2 to 4 months after a triggering event. Postpartum alopecia is probably the most common form of TE. During the second and third trimesters of pregnancy, women may notice that their hair seems thicker owing to a significant increase in the percentage of anagen hairs. Following delivery there is a rapid conversion of anagen to telogen hairs which can result in shedding starting 1 to 4 months postpartum. The duration of shedding is usually less than 6 months but it can persist for up to one year[46].

TE in a young woman can also occur following discontinuation of oral contraceptives, stringent dieting with or without protein malnutrition, iron deficiency, psychological stress, systemic illness, thyroid disease, certain medications, scalp inflammation and surgery[46]. Prognosis for regrowth is usually good if the cause of the alopecia is treated or eliminated[44,46].

Nevi and melanoma

Many visits to the dermatologist are scheduled for an overall skin check. In recent years, the media have raised public awareness about melanoma and changing moles. Statistics demonstrate that there is no hype – 41 600 new cases of melanoma and 7300 deaths were attributed to melanoma in the US in 1998[48]. The lifetime incidence of melanoma in Caucasian Americans is approximately 1 in 70 (1.4%)[49]. Melanoma is also more common than any non-skin cancer among individuals between 25 and 29 years old[50]. Overall, the incidence of melanoma in women is increasing more rapidly than any other malignancy except lung cancer[51]. Persons who have dysplastic nevi and a family history of melanoma can have an estimated 148-fold increased risk of developing melanoma themselves[52].

Questions may also arise regarding whether exposure to oral contraceptives or hormone replacement therapy is possibly related to an increased risk of melanoma. Epidemiological studies over the past 30 years have not shown an increased risk for cutaneous melanoma in women who ever used oral contraceptives[32]. Although fewer data are available about hormone replacement therapy, most research suggests no significant increased risk of melanoma[32].

During discussions about safe sun care, we should enlist the patient's co-operation in performing skin self-examinations on a monthly basis, minimizing sun exposure, wearing protective clothing and applying sunscreen. Surveillance of at-risk individuals should include full skin examinations at least once or twice per year[52]. Entire body examinations are essential because melanoma most often occurs on the lower limbs, followed by the trunk, in Caucasian women[53]. Serial photography and dermatoscopy are two adjunctive methods of clinical monitoring. By taking the time to educate women on the guidelines for inspection of pigmented lesions, early detection and treatment of melanoma are possible and may be life saving.

THE FORTIES AND FIFTIES
Dry skin and photodamage

As time progresses, a woman's skin has an increasing need for more moisture. Dryness (roughness) is histologically associated with thickening of the stratum corneum, which presumably results form altered keratinocyte cohesion and maturation[54,55]. Frequent application of moisturizers can help the skin maintain hydration and smoothness[54]. Although moisturizers are composed of oil and water emulsions, only a minimal amount of water is absorbed by the stratum corneum after application. It is the non-volatile oil fraction that provides lubrication by remaining on the surface[54]. Moisturizers containing alpha-hydroxy acids can additionally help skin by diminishing the thickness of the stratum corneum by decreasing corneocyte cohesion, promoting thickening of the epidermis and dermis and promoting synthesis of collagen, elastin, protein and glycosaminoglycans[39,55]. The ability of alpha-hydroxy acids such as glycolic acid to diminish corneocyte cohesion and promote normal keratinization is especially useful when treating dry or photodamaged skin which is also acne prone.

Tretinoin causes similar changes in the skin[39]. When used in conjunction with alpha-hydroxy acid products, it may provide synergistic effects for both dry skin and photodamage. Other studies have shown that tretinoin also appears to be effective in repairing chronologically aged skin unexposed to sunlight[19].

Often in the late forties and fifties, signs of photoaging become the pre-eminent cosmetic complaint. In order to restore skin that has weathered the era of baby oil and sun reflectors, a step-wise approach must be undertaken. Women should continue to use broad spectrum sunscreens on a daily basis. Topical therapies with retinoids (tretinoin and retinol), antioxidants like vitamin C and E and chemical exfoliants like the alpha- and beta-hydroxy acids can often greatly improve mild to moderate photodamage. We generally recommend that women begin with a retinoid-like tretinoin emollient cream, 0.05% formulation, which is initially applied three times weekly until nightly usage is tolerated. At the same time, we also suggest that patients use a glycolic acid cream or lotion with a concentration of 8 to 20% once or twice daily to provide needed moisture and light exfoliation. Topical preparations which contain ascorbic acid or vitamin E may also be used adjunctively. Other modalities such as serial superficial chemical peels with glycolic acid (30–70%), trichloroacetic acid (10–25%), and Jessner's solution (resorcinol, salicylic acid, lactic acid and ethanol) are most useful in improving mild to moderate photodamage. Deeper peels with trichloroacetic acid (35–50%) can be employed for more significant photoaging. Similarly, resurfacing with the erbium-YAG (2940 nm) or carbon dioxide (10 600 nm) lasers can be used effectively for moderate to severe photodamage. In some patients, medium depth chemical peels and laser resurfacing can be used on adjacent cosmetic units for uniform rejuvenation.

For localized deep furrows on the forehead and periorbital region, botulinum toxin A alone or in combination with bovine collagen injections can result in dramatic improvement. For rhytides in the nasolabial folds and perioral region, periodic collagen injections seem to be the most beneficial. Liposculpturing and plastic surgery may be needed to address more severe photoaging.

As a woman enters the perimenopausal period, the cutaneous effects of aging may become more prominent secondary to the loss of endogenous estrogen. The relationship between estrogen and the skin is complex and is influenced by a number of factors including anatomic site, dosage of estrogen, saturation of receptors and levels of other circulating hormones[51]. Research has shown that the typical reduction in levels of dermal collagen of approximately 2% per postmenopausal year for up to 15 years could be prevented by administration of oral estrogen replacement[51,56,57]. Additional studies have shown that topical estrogen compounds can also improve clinical signs of photoaging without hormonal side-effects[58,59].

Hair loss

Studies have indicated that all women have a change in scalp hair pattern following puberty[60]. The change in pattern is a gradual process but rapidly accelerates during and after menopause. During this period, women undergo a period of estrogen depletion with relative androgen excess. This hormonal shift may bring on androgenetic alopecia with or without hirsutism and acne. AGA in the perimenopausal woman initially starts as diffuse alopecia that may later develop into more advanced 'male patterns'[61]. The hair loss is gradual. There is progressive miniaturization of the hair follicles, which results in reduced hair shaft diameter[62].

Another condition presenting as diffuse hair loss may actually be chronic telogen effluvium (TE)[62]. The typical patient is 30 to 60 years old and complains of abrupt, extensive hair loss all over her scalp. Clinical examination may reveal considerable bitemporal recession with interceding new anagen hairs. Although hair pull tests are uniformly positive all over the head, there is rarely any generalized thinning of the hair. Chronic TE tends to have a fluctuating and prolonged course[62]. In either type of hair loss it is important to rule out underlying conditions such as iron deficiency, thyroid disease, or protein deficient diet. As discussed previously, work-up for AGA should include baseline hormonal parameters. Treatment for AGA in the peri-menopausal woman includes topical minoxidil, hormone replacement with conjugated estrogens or estradiol and a progestin such as medroxyprogesterone if the patient has not had a hysterectomy, and anti-androgens such as spironolactone. Supplemental vitamins containing biotin can also be helpful. Chronic TE is thought to be self-limited but does wax and wane[62]. Along with constant support and encouragement, topical minoxidil may be tried.

Acne rosacea

Rosacea frequently presents in women aged 40 to 60 as flushing erythema, telangiectasia and intermittent acneiform papulopustules on the central face. A history of severe flushing has been suggested to play a role in the pathogenesis[63]. The fact that vasomotor instability is prominent during menopause and the age group affected supports this hypothesis[64]. Patients should also be advised to avoid factors which provoke flushing such as exposure to extreme heat, cold and sunlight and consumption of spicy or hot foods and alcoholic beverages. Treatment options include topical metronidazole 0.75–1% applied once or twice daily, oral antibiotics such as tetracycline in doses of 250 mg to 1000 mg daily, oral isotretinoin in dosages of 0.1–0.5 mg/kg/day, electrosurgery and flash lamp pumped pulsed dye laser.

Lumps and bumps

Benign lesions can be a source of consternation as they seem to come up overnight and in multiple numbers. Solar lentigines are pigmented macules which predominantly occur on sun-exposed skin. Various treatments include light cryosurgery, bleaching agents like hydroquinone, tretinoin, or chemical peel and laser for more diffuse lesions. Continued sun protection is necessary to prevent further darkening of lentigines. Seborrheic keratoses are another benign lesion which frequently occur on the face and trunk. Despite being a totally pigmented benign tumor composed of epidermal keratinocytes, seborrheic keratoses are often mistaken by the patient for melanoma. Reassurance for asymptomatic keratoses usually suffices, but simple curettage or cryosurgery can remove problematic lesions.

With maturity, women may also find an increasing number of cherry angiomas, small red papules generally found on the trunk. Usually they are asymptomatic and do not require treatment. If removal is desired, shave excision, light electrocautery, cryosurgery, or flash lamp pumped pulsed dye laser can be employed.

Pre-malignant and malignant tumors

The causal relationship between ultraviolet light and the development of skin cancer is well established[19,65]. Both basal cell and squamous cell carcinoma tend to occur mainly on the skin of Caucasians that has been exposed to the sun. With increasing age, there is also an exponential rise in incidence[19,66]. Standard treatment for non-melanoma skin cancers, depending on location, includes excision, electrodessication and curettage, cryosurgery, Mohs microscopically controlled surgery and photodynamic therapy. Pre-malignant actinic keratoses also have a strong link to sun exposure. In one study, a prevalence of actinic keratosis in individuals over forty was 56%[67]. The probability of an actinic keratosis developing into a squamous cell carcinoma is estimated at 1 per 100 per year, which underscores the importance of treating visible lesions[51]. Standard therapy is cryosurgery, topical 5-fluorouracil in concentrations of 1–5% applied twice daily for a period of 3 to 6 weeks depending on location, shave excision, electrodessication and medium depth chemical peels with trichloroacetic acid (30–50%). As mentioned earlier, animal studies have shown that sunscreens can prevent the development of UV-induced non-melanoma skin cancers and also significantly suppress the development of actinic keratoses[22].

CONCLUSIONS

Each decade of a woman's life brings new changes and challenges to both the patient and her dermatologist. Environmental factors such as sun exposure, hormonal status, genetics and coexisting internal disorders are probably the most important determinants of how skin and hair will weather the passage of time. The ideal would be to cultivate a working relationship with the patient early on as a young adult, so that specific cutaneous problems of later decades may be minimized or even avoided. In addition, we must take the opportunity to emphasize the need for preventive skin care. At the minimum, women should leave our offices knowing how to launch a total sun protection regimen and perform skin self-examinations. Promoting overall good health strategies such as proper diet, exercise, stress management and sleep can only serve to additionally enhance the health of the skin.

A woman must be viewed as more than her chief complaint. We must strive to expand upon history that is offered and to draw out details which are not. In examining the skin and hair, we also get a glimpse of her body's underlying state of health or derangement. We must be willing to pursue or suggest further evaluation of possible associated conditions in order to better refine our own treatment of the dermatologic disease at hand. As specialists, it is also our responsibility not only to know the latest in standard therapy, but also to innovate when all the usual treatments have been tried. If we can work toward these goals, we will succeed in helping our patients attain and maintain healthy skin and hair at any age.

REFERENCES

1. Shuster S, Fisher GH, Harris E, *et al*. The effect of skin disease on self image. *Br J Dermatol* 1978; 99(suppl16):18–19
2. Cunliffe WJ. Acne and unemployment. *Br J Dermatol* 1986;115:386
3. Goulden V, Clark SM, Cunliffe WJ. Post-adolescent acne: review of clinical features. *Br J Dermatol* 1997;136:66–70
4. Sutherland H, Stewart I. A critical analysis of the premenstrual syndrome. *Lancet* 1965;1:1180–3
5. Walton S, Cunliffe WJ, Keczkes K, *et al*. Clinical, ultrasound, and hormonal markers of androgenicity in acne vulgaris. *Br J Dermatol* 1995;133:249–53
6. Walton S, Wyatt EH, Cunliffe WJ. Genetic control of sebum excretion and acne – a twin study. *Br J Dermatol* 1988;118:393–6
7. Lucky AW, McGuire J, Rosenfield RL, *et al*. Plasma androgens in women with acne vulgaris. *J Invest Dermatol* 1983;81:70–4
8. Lawrence D, Shaw M, Katz M. Elevated free testosterone concentration in men and women with acne vulgaris. *Clin Exp Dermatol* 1985;11:263–73
9. Schiavone F, Rietschel RL, Sgoutas D, *et al*. Elevated free testosterone levels in women with acne. *Arch Dermatol* 1983;119:799–802

10. Sperling L, Heimer W. Androgen biology as basis for the diagnosis and treatment of androgenic disorders in women. *J Am Acad Dermatol* 1993;28:669–83

11. Shaw JC. Antiandrogen and hormonal treatment of acne. *Dermatol Clin* 1996;14:803–11

12. Lucky AW, Henderson TA, Olson WH, *et al.* Effectiveness of norgestimate and ethinyl estradiol in treating moderate acne vulgaris. *J Am Acad Dermatol* 1997;37:746–54

13. Daniell HW. Smoker's wrinkles. *Ann Intern Med* 1971;75:973–80

14. Smith JB, Fenske NA. Cutaneous manifestations and consequences of smoking. *J Am Acad Dermatol* 1996;5:717–32

15. Ernster VL, Grady D, Miike R, *et al.* Facial wrinkling in men and women by smoking status. *Am J Pub Health* 1995;85:78–82

16. Model D. Smoker's face – an underrated clinical sign? *Br Med J* 1985;291:1760–2

17. Kripke M. 'Ozone, photodamage, and photoprotection'. Presentated at the *American Academy of Dermatology*, Chicago, Illinois, July 31, 1998

18. Pathak MA. UV radiation and development of non-melanoma skin cancer – clinical and experimental evidence. *Skin Pharmacol* 1991;4:85–94

19. Gilchrest BA. A review of skin ageing and its medical therapy. *Br J Dermatol* 1996;135:867–75

20. Lowe NJ, Meyers DP, Wieder JM, *et al.* Low doses of repetitive ultraviolet A induce morphologic changes in human skin. *J Invest Dermatol* 1995;105:739–43

21. Koh HK, Kligler BE, Lew RA. Sunlight and cutaneous malignant melanoma: evidence for and against causation. *Photochem Photobiol* 1990;51:765–79

22. Naylor MF, Boyd A, Smith DW, *et al.* High sun protection factor sunscreens in suppression of actinic neoplasia. *Arch Dermatol* 1995;131:170–5

23. McLean DI, Gallagher R. Sunscreens – use and misuse. *Dermatol Clin* 1998;16:219–26

24. Friedlander J, Lowe NJ. Sunscreens. In Arndt KA, Leboit PE, Robinson JK, Wintroub BE, eds. *Cutaneous Medicine and Surgery – An Integrated Program in Dermatology*. Philadelphia: WB Saunders, 1996:751–7

25. AAD 'Tanning: unsafe at any wavelength' press kit

26. Spencer JM, Amonette RA. Indoor tanning: risks, benefits, and future trends. *J Am Acad Dermatol* 1995;33:288–98

27. Pawelek JM. Melasyn™ – A new self-tanner with sun protective qualities. *Drug Cosmet Indust* 1998;163:28–33

28. Winton GB, Lewis CW. Dermatoses of pregnancy. *J Am Acad Dermatol* 1982;66:977–98

29. Torres JE, Sanchez JL. Melasma and other disorders of hyperpigmentation. In Arndt KA, Leboit PE, Robinson JK, Wintroub BE, eds. *Cutaneous Medicine and Surgery – An Integrated Program in Dermatology*. Philadelphia: WB Saunders Company, 1996:1233–41

30. Foucar E, Bentley TJ, Laube DW, *et al.* A histopathologic evaluation of nevocellular nevi in pregnancy. *Arch Dermatol* 1985;121:350–4

31. Pennoyer JW, Grin CM, Driscoll MS, *et al.* Changes in size of melanocytic nevi during pregnancy. *J Am Acad Dermatol* 1997;36:378–82

32. Grin CM, Driscoll MS, Grant-Kels JM. The relationship of pregnancy, hormones, and melanoma. *Semin Cutan Med Surg* 1998;17:167–71

33. Black MM, Mayou SC. Skin diseases in pregnancy. In de Swiet M, ed. *Medical Disorders in Obstetric Practice*, 2nd edn. Oxford: Blackwell Scientific Publications, 1989:808–29

34. Elson ML. Treatment of striae distensae with topical tretinoin. *J Dermatol Surg Oncol* 1990;16:267–70

35. Alster TS. Laser treatment of hypertrophic scars, keloids, and striae. *Dermatol Clin* 1997;15:419–29

36. Wasserstrum N. Maternal physiology. In Hacker NF, Moore G, eds. *Essentials of Obstetrics and Gynecology*, 2nd edn. Philadelphia: WB Saunders Company, 1992:61–73

37. Green D. Sclerotherapy for permanent eradication of varicose veins: theoretical and practical considerations. *J Am Acad Dermatol* 1998;38:461–75

38. Cisneros JL, Del Rio R, Palou J. Sclerosis and the Nd:YAG Q-switched laser with multiple frequency for the treatment of telangiectases, reticular veins, and residual pigmentation. *Dermatol Surg* 1998;24:1119–23

39. Lewis AB, Gendler EC. Resurfacing with topical agents. *Semin Cutan Med Surg* 1996;15:139–44

40. Taylor CR, Stern RS, Leyden JJ, *et al.* Photoaging, photodamage, and photoprotection. *J Am Acad Dermatol* 1990;22:1–15

41. Leyden JJ. Clinical features of ageing skin. *Br J Dermatol* 1990;122(suppl 35):1–3

42. Voorhees JJ. Photoaging pathophysiology. Presentated at the *American Academy of Dermatology*, Chicago, Illinois, July 31, 1998

43. Green LJ, Mc Cormick A, Weinstein G. Photoaging and the skin – the effects of tretinoin. *Dermatol Clin* 1993;11:97–105

44. Elston DM, Bergfeld WF. Disorders of hair growth. *Resident and Staff Physician* 1997;43:59–63

45. Ehrmann DA, Rosenfeld RL, Barnes RB, *et al.* Detection of functional ovarian hyperandrogenism in women with androgen excess. *N Engl J Med* 1992;327:157–62

46. Fiedler VC. Alopecia areata and other nonscarring alopecias. In Arndt KA, Leboit PE, Robinson JK, Wintroub BE, eds. *Cutaneous Medicine and Surgery – An Integrated Program in Dermatology*. Philadelphia: WB Saunders Company, 1996:1274–9

47. Kaufman KD, Olsen EA, Whiting D, *et al.* Finasteride in the treatment of men with androgenetic alopecia. *J Am Acad Dermatol* 1998;39:578–89

48. Drake L. Melanoma Monday 1998: National Skin Self-Examination Day. Presented at *Melanoma/Skin*

Cancer Detection and Prevention Campaign press conference, New York, New York, April 29, 1998

49. Atillasoy E. Direct link between UVB light and melanoma established. Presentated at *Melanoma/ Skin Cancer Detection and Prevention Campaign press conference*, New York, New York, April 29, 1998

50. American Academy of Dermatology 1998 Skin Cancer Fact Sheet

51. Bolognia JL. Dermatologic and cosmetic concerns of the older woman. *Clin Geriat Med* 1993;9:209–29

52. Koh HK. Cutaneous melanoma. *N Engl J Med* 1991;325:171–82

53. Bulliard J-L, Cox B, Elwood JM. Comparison of the site distribution of melanoma in New Zealand and Canada. *Int J Cancer* 1997;72:231–5

54. Roenigk HH. Treatment of the aging face. *Dermatol Clin* 1995;2:245–61

55. Van Scott EJ, Yu RJ. Hyperkeratinization, corneocyte cohesion, and alpha hydroxy acids. *J Am Acad Dermatol* 1984;11:867–79

56. Brincat M, Kabalan S, Studd JWW, *et al*. A study of the decrease of skin collagen content, skin thickness, and bone mass in the post menopausal woman. *Obstet Gynecol* 1987;70:840

57. Brincat M, Moniz CF, Kabalan S, *et al*. Decline in skin collagen content and metacarpal index after the menopause and its prevention with sex hormone replacement. *Br J Obstet Gynaecol* 1987;94:126

58. Schmidt JB, Binder M, Macheiner W, *et al*. Treatment of skin aging symptoms in perimenopausal females with estrogen compounds. A pilot study. *Maturitas* 1994;20:25–30

59. Creidei P, Faivre B, Agache P, *et al*. Effect of a conjugated oestrogen (Premarin) cream on aging facial skin. A comparative study with a placebo cream. *Maturitas* 1994;19:211–33

60. Venning VA, Dawber R. Patterned androgenic alopecia. *J Am Acad Dermatol* 1988;18:1073–8

61. Hordinsky MK. Androgenic disorders. In Arndt KA, Leboit PE, Robinson JK, Wintroub BE, eds. *Cutaneous Medicine and Surgery – An Integrated Program in Dermatology*. Philadelphia: WB Saunders Company, 1996:1250–7

62. Whiting DA. Chronic telogen effluvium. *Dermatol Clin* 1996;14:723–38

63. Wilkin JK. Flushing reactions – consequence and mechanisms. *Ann Intern Med* 1981;95:268–76

64. Pollack S. Rosacea. In Arndt KA, Leboit PE, Robinson JK, Wintroub BE, eds. *Cutaneous Medicine and Surgery – An Integrated Program in Dermatology*. Philadelphia: WB Saunders Company, 1996:485–96

65. 'Council on Scientific Affairs'. Harmful effects of ultraviolet radiation. *JAMA* 1989;262:380–4

66. Kripke ML. Impact of ozone depletion on skin cancers. *J Dermatol Surg Oncol* 1988;14:83–7

67. Marks R. Solar keratoses. *Br J Dermatol* 1990; 122(suppl 35):49–60

The mature adult

9

Tania Ferreira Cestari and Beatriz Moritz Trope

INTRODUCTION

The period of late adulthood, from the age of 40 plus, corresponds euphemistically to maturity and is characterized by many important changes. The psychological impact of these alterations is similar to or even stronger than the one that occurs in puberty, because visible modifications in the skin appear, providing an approximate indication of age[1]. The worship of beauty and youth has been a constant throughout history, especially for women. Occidental culture, in the very competitive recent decades, has imposed new rules regarding professional, familiar and personal aspects, always favoring a younger appearance. A longer life expectancy – of at least 30 productive years of maturity – make interest in the phenomena related to aging a matter of widespread concern[1-3].

The process of maturing is slow, with a gradual diminishing in the size and number of cells and a drop in the rate and even cessation of many organic functions associated with the systemic changes of the climacteric period, which are related to decreased hormone production by the ovaries. Most of the alterations remain hidden but the cutaneous signs of the normal degenerative process may be catastrophic in terms of social acceptance, self-esteem and even job consequences. Those disadvantages are added to the psychological impact of image alterations and changes in family life. Keeping a 'youthful' and consequently 'healthy' appearance may be fundamental for the psychological balance of middle-aged women in order to reduce the impact of climacteric adjustment.

A significant number of pathological conditions are typical of late adulthood, most of them related to the physiological process of chronological and hormonal aging[4-6]. At this point there are marked differences in the cellular structure, function and response to direct or environmental tissue injury. Studies aiming at a better knowledge of the skin physiology of the mature woman will be very rewarding, helping to replace old and out-moded concepts, changing behavior and, ultimately, improving her quality of life.

THE AGING PROCESS

Skin aging is the result of programmed senescence observed in all individuals. It is a multi-step, time-dependent continuous phenomenon manifested by clinical, histological and physiological modifications[7,8]. External damage is superimposed on the changes of intrinsic aging in an interacting process associated with a loss of maximal function and reserve capacity in human tissues. These are consequent to changes at cellular and molecular levels resulting in alterations in cell behavior, in protein production and in gene expression in response to stimuli. Practically, there is a reduction in the capacity to repair injury, predisposing the organism to disease and permanent dysfunction[3,6-10].

At the cellular level aging is a form of genetically programmed differentiation, expressed by an extension in the proportion of more differentiated cells at the expense of relatively non-differentiated ones that, perhaps, have a greater proliferative potential and/or more functional behavioral responses[8,11]. Recent studies suggest that differentiation, like age-associated changes, occurs at the mRNA level of gene expression. Therefore agents that manipulate the genetic manifestation pattern of down-regulation of proteolytic activities and up-regulation of structural protein synthesis could have marked therapeutic effects. In this respect, retinoids have shown good applicability in delaying the manifestations of skin aging since their action is connected to collagenase function and regulation of mRNA expression[12-14].

Important external influences on the normal aging process are smoking habits and life-long exposure to ultraviolet (UV) light[14-17]. In fact, many of the clinical aspects and dermatological conditions ordinarily associated with maturity are manifestations of chronic exposure to the sun, it being difficult to separate one aspect from the other[3,9,14,16,18].

The most obvious signs of progressive senile skin are distinct degrees of atrophy, laxity, wrinkling, sagging, dryness, yellowness, pigmentary alterations and hair graying[6,18]. There are quantitative differences between photoaged and chronologically aged skin (Figure 1). The main characteristic is an imbalance between atrophy and hypertrophy: intrinsic aging is manifested by a functional deterioration of the skin, while extrinsic aging involves, initially, hypertrophy as an inflammatory protective response to the damaging effects of UV radiation[10,14,17,18] (Figures 2 and 3). Moreover, many of the age-associated functional losses are accelerated in photoaged cells, including genetic mutations, a higher threshold for terminal differentiation and impaired response to acute UV radiation[3,9,17,19]. Innate aging can be characterized, clinically, by fine wrinkling, reduced elasticity and recoil, atrophy of the dermis and a decrease in subcutaneous adipose tissue, which is more visible in women's skin[18,20]. Functionally, there is a compromising of the epidermal turnover and clearance of chemical substances, alterations in the dermis, healing of wounds, mechanical protection, immune responsiveness, sensory perception, function of the glands, thermoregulation and vascular reactivity.

ANATOMICAL AND STRUCTURAL CHARACTERISTICS OF THE AGING SKIN

Normal somatic cells do not divide indefinitely and the process, in organic aging, that limits cell division is termed replicative senescence. Old cells present phenotypic changes such as growth arrest, resistance to apoptotic death and altered differentiated functions. The most affected cells in the senescence process are keratinocytes and especially fibroblasts[7,21]. These alterations, accompanied by immunological changes and tumorigenesis, make aged skin more prone to skin cancer[14,22].

The intrinsic aging process takes place in three successive stages: an early and progressive evolution at the epidermal level, a later modification of the papillary dermis at around 40 years of age and a last change, inducing subsequent effects, appearing after the age of 50[23]. Changes in the superficial cutaneous appearance are one of the first complaints of mature women, as skin roughness is significantly increased in the aged, independent of racial group or anatomic site. Studies on the evolution of physical properties of the human tegument, in individuals ranging from 8 to 89 years old, showed that the skin extendibility decreases after 35 years of age, and at a more accentuated rate after 45. Skin thickness begins to decrease at 30–40 years in both sexes but this decrease is more accentuated in women. More expressive changes occur around the age of 60 years, with alterations of the

optical characteristics of the stratum corneum, as well as in the barrier and in the dermis functions[23].

Epidermal characteristics vary according to age, gender and anatomical site but it is accepted that the whole epidermis becomes thinner and that the cells are less evenly aligned on the basement membrane and become irregular in size, shape and staining properties as the individual ages[6]. The number of cell layers remains unchanged during the aging process but the components of the superficial coating, the corneocytes, decrease in surface area; the epidermis becomes more compact; the cellular turnover rate decreases by up to 50% and the stratum corneum replacement time is nearly doubled[24]. Skin elasticity declines and the skin becomes more fragile as manifested by dry, flaky and itchy skin in old people, explaining the common superficial fissuring[6,23–25] (Figure 4). Cutaneous permeability to chemical substances also changes, and the water-binding capacity of the stratum corneum is reduced[6,23,24,26]. Transepidermal water loss is increased in postmenopausal women when compared to premenopausal ones, provoking a slower response to irritants, in a site-dependent manner[23,24,27]. Additionally, there is a significant alteration in the contents of sphingolipids of the stratum corneum after maturity, probably related to hormonal changes. These lipids are important for the cutaneous barrier, which explains the relative impairment of this function after menopause[28].

One of the most significant changes in aging skin is the flattening of the dermo-epidermal interface. The surface area decreases owing to the lack of interpenetration between the dermis and epidermis, probably causing the easy tearing and blistering in elderly skin determined by its enhanced fragility[18,25,29]. Recent ultrastructural and quantitative immunofluorescence studies in women of ages from 9 to 79 years have demonstrated that there are structural and functional changes in the components of the dermo-epidermal junction related to aging, producing a less effective epidermal anchoring system[30]. Anchoring fibrils are altered with aging and collagen VII, its main constituent, becomes less resistant to the action of proteolytic dermal enzymes, compromising the resistance of the dermal–epidermal barrier[30]. Anatomical alterations in this area lead to important changes in the physical properties of the whole skin. The process is accompanied by disruption of the capillary circulation, because of the weakness of the mechanical support of the dermis, modifications of the cutaneous micro-relief and perturbation in the synthesis of the epidermis[23].

Wrinkling is, by far, the greatest concern in maturity and is a phenomenon almost entirely dependent on dermal changes[6]. Innate and photo-damage effects lead to alterations in the relative proportion of the extracellular matrix of connective tissue, composed basically of collagen, elastic fibers and glycosaminoglycan or proteoglycan macromolecules, resulting in the clinical manifestations of cutaneous aging[31]. The reorganization of the collagen fibers that happens in this degenerative process diminishes the coefficient of deformation that permits the skin to undergo distortions without provoking stress to the dermo-epidermal junction. When this 'reservoir' decreases the injury is permanent, contributing to the older appearance[23,25]. The histology of skin sections of normal old people shows that the dermis becomes hypocellular and hypovascular, with a decrease in the content of collagen as well as in the number and size of mast cells and fibroblasts whose replicative life is limited; there is a disruption of the rhomboid network, with fragmentation and disorientation of the collagen bundles, and a progressive reduction in elastic fibers (Figures 5, 6 and 7). All these alterations are added to the ones determined by external agents such as chronic exposure to the sun[6,17,32].

The difference in skin density between women and men is an important factor in explaining why women's skin deteriorates more rapidly than men's. Skin thickness is proportional to the collagen content and is different in men and women, with age and hormones affecting both aspects. Controlled studies have shown that there is a linear decrease in skin collagen quantity of around 1% per year throughout adult life and that this is more significant in women after the age of 40[33]. It is important to note that women have a lower initial collagen concentration and that androgens exert a positive effect on its density. This can be illustrated by the increased amount of skin collagen found in women with hirsutism[34]. Considering that 90% of the body's collagen is concentrated in the bone matrix and skin and that the decline in collagen is the major causal factor in the bone loss related to menopause, skin atrophic signs could be used to predict women at risk of osteoporotic bone fracture because both are parallel manifestations of the same physiologic phenomenon[35,36].

Aged-related changes in elastic fibers are responsible for many of the features recognized as typical of aged skin such as sagging and loss of elasticity[32]. Elastic fibers suffer a gradual disintegration process with age and, by the 7th decade, most of them are abnormal[20]. It is probable that the very first event of age-related disorganization of the elastic system is represented by the loss of the perpendicular orientation and gradual change to tortuosity of thinner fibers (the oxytalan fibers) which take place in the upper papillary dermis[37]. Chronic exposure to the sun adds to this process a progressive loss of regularity in the contour of the median-diameter elastic fibers (elauninic fibers), localized in the upper mid-dermis[38]. With the advance of senescence the elastic fiber network of the reticular dermis in aged skin is irregular, with cysts and lacunae, and the anatomic damage is expressed clinically by a loss in resiliency and recoverability after stretching. The elastic content of the papillary dermis is altered as well, contributing to the superficial laxity and wrinkled surface of old skin[20].

The thickness of the whole skin is greater in men than in women, whereas the subcutaneous fat is thicker in women, owing to lipid deposits and also to collagen density[28]. With advancing age, a gradual thinning occurs in men while in women the decrease starts just after the 5th decade[28]. The subcutaneous tissue is diminished in some areas such as the face, shins, hands and feet and increased in the thighs in aging women[25].

CUTANEOUS VASCULATURE

When the normal course of aging proceeds there is a decrease of vascularity and thinning of the vascular walls. Purpura occurs easily with minimal trauma. Vascular and dermal ground alterations reduce the clearance of foreign material, prolonging cases of contact dermatitis, allowing blisters and wheals to develop and involute more slowly[18,29,39]. In aged skin there is a loss of regularly arranged capillary loops; horizontal vessels are more tortuous, elongated, disorganized and dilated, radically altering the entire vascular bed[24,39]. The reduction in surface area for nutritional exchange could have significant physiologic consequences, contributing to the degenerative changes of aging skin, including epidermal and appendageal atrophy[39]. The microcirculation is under the direct control of the autonomic nervous system which, during maturity, suffers a gradual reduction in its function. This process is expressed by a delay in blood flow, contributing to some vasoconstrictor changes detected in older individuals, especially women[24,28]. Another common complaint of perimenopausal women is hot flashes, a vasomotor symptom consequent on the instability between the autonomic nervous system and the hypothalamus. Imbalance in estrogen levels is the principal cause of this feature and appropriate hormone therapy is indicated to control it[5,40].

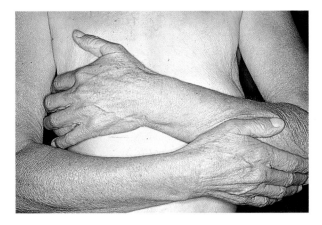

Figure 1 Sun-exposed and protected skin areas of a 53-year-old woman. The contrast is characterized by pigmentation, wrinkles and roughness of the uncovered sites, while the covered ones do not show marked alterations

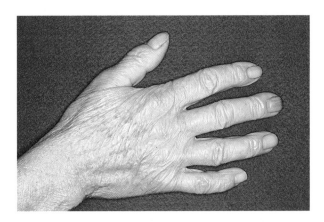

Figure 2 Extrinsic aged skin of the hand of a 42-year-old farmer. Photo-damage leads to acceleration of the degenerative process, featuring sustained wrinkles associated with laxity, atrophy and thickness of the cutaneous surface

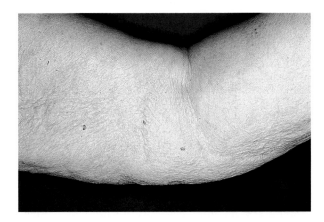

Figure 3 Intrinsically aged areas of the inner arm of a 74-year-old woman, showing slight atrophy of the epidermis, xerosis and sagging of the skin

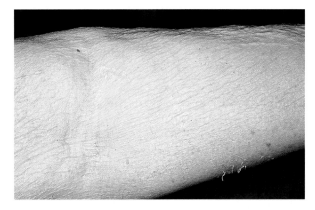

Figure 4 Intrinsically aged skin depicting a smooth skin surface, with fine wrinkles and dry scaling

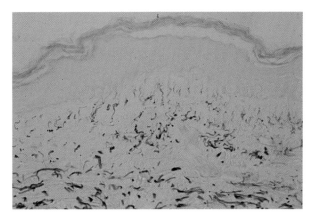

Figure 5 Light micrograph from a sun-protected skin of a mature woman. Initial intrinsic degenerative alterations of elastic fibers are represented by tortuosity of the oxitalan and elaunin fibers in the dermis, besides hyperkeratosis and epidermal flattening. Resorcin–fuchsin with previous oxidation with oxona; 100X. Courtesy of Gerson Cotta-Pereira, MD, Rio de Janeiro, Brazil

SKIN COLOR

Colorimetric measurements show that elderly skin is significantly darker than young tegument, even in areas that have not been exposed to the sun. Epidermal atrophy and increased transparency may contribute to this, leading to increased visibility of dermal components. Skin color is also influenced by the number, depth and dilatation of blood vessels, state of oxygenation of the blood and the optical properties of the entire skin structure[39]. It is well known that men's skin shows a tendency to darken with age to a greater extent than women's – a difference that most probably arises through men experiencing more exposure to the sun in their youth.

There is a decrease in and an uneven distribution of melanocytes after the age of 30, independent of phototype and sex, caused by the normal aging process. The histologic aspect is similar to a mosaic, with large and small melanocytes and modifications in the interaction of melanocytes and keratino-cytes[41]. These anatomical changes are expressed clinically by a mottled appearance of the skin with irregular pigmentation, especially in those individuals who have had extensive exposure to the sun. Additionally, the ability to tan decreases with age, making old people more vulnerable to sunburn. Melanocytic nevi are likewise affected by maturity, with a decrease in their number and a tendency of pigment cells to migrate to the dermis and become more differentiated, eventually being removed by phagocytosis or apoptosis[6,29,41].

SKIN APPENDAGES

Skin appendages decrease in number and weaken in function during the aging process[6,25,29]. Thermoregulation is decreased because eccrine sweat glands are less functional. Another consequence is the compromising of the emollient sebum film that normally covers the skin surface. Sebaceous gland secretion is hormone dependent. During a woman's forties, there is a progressive reduction in sebum production, probably as a result of decreased ovarian activity, leading to xerosis[6,16,28,29]. That is the reason why mature women and atopic individuals should be encouraged to regularly use mild soaps and emollient or moisturizing creams. Sebum becomes less dilute with maturity, increasing the possibility of developing seborrheic dermatitis in the scalp, face and chest[29]. Interestingly, the growth in size of sebaceous glands and the lack of support for the subcutaneous tissue contribute to the development of lesions such as giant comedones and sebaceous hyperplasia in seborrheic areas like the face. From the clinical point of view this can be exemplified by the Favre–Racouchaud syndrome, which is found in both sexes but is more frequent among men.

Nails usually become brittle, dull and opaque with advancing years. Nail growth is slowed and distal splitting is very easy[25,29]. White nails, similar to those seen in cirrhosis, uremia and hypoalbuminemia might be seen in healthy individuals[25,42]. Very common, as well, are longitudinal striations of the nail plate, present in some degree in most people over 50 years old (Figure 8). In spite of being a benign condition, the irregularity of the nail surface is one of the most frequent complaints of mature women and, unfortunately, it almost never regresses.

The characteristics and distribution of hair are deeply affected by the many changes that occur in the physiology of perimenopausal women. Graying of hair (canities) is one of the most outstanding markers of aging. It is due to a genetically influenced progressive reduction in melanocyte function, with decrease and eventual cessation of the activity of tyrosinase, the enzyme responsible for the first stage of melanin synthesis in the lower bulb[6]. There is a gradual dilution of pigment so that a full range of colors – from normal to white – can be seen both along individual hairs and from hair to hair[29,43]. Canities is also associated with some autoimmune conditions such as pernicious anemia, hypothyroidism and Addison's disease, including some genetic abnormalities (Rothmund–Thompson syndrome, 'cri-du-chat' syndrome, dystrophia myotonica, progeria and Werner's syndrome). In Caucasoid races, white hairs are more evident around the hairline and first appear at the age of 34.2 ± 9.6 years; by the fifth decade, almost half of the population has at least 50% of gray hairs. The onset in Africans and Japanese occurs later in life[43]. Two recent studies dealt with the association between graying of hair and osteopenia[44,45]. Reviewing normal postmenopausal populations, the authors observed that premature hair graying is inherited in an autosomal dominant pattern and is less frequent in racial groups with high bone mineral density like those with African ancestry, suggesting that genetic factors influence both trends[45].

After the menopause, thin and sparse hair is a common finding – sometimes associated with medical problems but, in the majority of women, a normal consequence of hormonal deficit[16,29]. In that period of life there is a general decrease in the density of body hair, in addition to atrophy and fibrosis of follicles[25]. The telogen phase tends to be longer and the density of hair localized in zones influenced by sex hormones, such as the axillae and pubic area, declines[6,16]. Scalp hair becomes thinner, especially in women with thyroid or estrogen deficiency. Hirsutism, however, may occur as a result of endocrine changes and androgen imbalance[6,46].

FUNCTIONAL ASPECTS

Anatomical alterations that happen after the fourth decade of life have their functional correspondence in the normal physiological processes. Women are, in general, more aware of it. With the passage of time, the immune system undergoes changes that result in decreased immunocompetence; this may account for an enhanced susceptibility to certain infections, autoimmune diseases and even malignancies[47]. Some of the available data on immunosenescence are contradictory, probably because of external influences and variability in study designs. Age-associated diseases and extrinsic factors have a known impact on the intrinsic changes of the immune system and, in some instances, cannot be separated, for example the well-known immunosuppressive effect of UV light on aged skin. Some parameters of immunosenescence are widely accepted. With advancing age T-cells are reduced in percentage and absolute number and undergo a shift from the naïve to the memory phenotype, associated with a change in cytokine profile. They also reveal a delay in the proliferative response to activation, in the diversity of the T-cell receptor antigen repertoire and in cytolytic activity[47]. Although T-cell activity is diminished, it is not completely established whether this decrease is related only to functionality. Decline in the T-type immune response can be exemplified by the reduction in sensitization to novel substances and to the so-called recall antigens[48].

B-lymphocytes of aging individuals become dysfunctional, showing a restricted diversity of their antibody repertoire owing to a decline in somatic mutations. This impairment results in a less efficient response to certain viral infections and vaccination. Whereas the total number of B-cells does not decline, the production of novel antibodies does. Clinically these abnormalities are expressed by reduced neutralization of invading microbes, increased occurrence of monoclonal gammopathies and raised levels of autoantibodies[47].

Epidermal Langerhans cells are significantly decreased in both aged skin that has been exposed to the sun and that which has not[49]. This may explain the lower rate of sensitization that occurs in normal old people since those cells are essential for the epidermal antigen presenting mechanism. Although not so evident, other components of the skin immune system such as macrophages and keratinocytes also undergo age-related changes, manifested by alterations in cytokine production, that could play a role in increased susceptibility to endotoxins in elderly individuals[47,50]. The synergistic activity of these modifications may result in an impaired cell-mediated immune response, decreased intensity of hypersensitivity reactions, increased risk of photo-carcinogenesis and greater susceptibility to chronic skin infections in old persons[49,51].

Wound healing is less efficient with aging although the mechanisms involved are not completely understood. The role of hyaluronic acid is fundamental in that process. It is a glycosaminoglycan found in the entire human body, especially in the skin, and is essential for cell proliferation and migration. The pattern of distribution of this polysaccharide in the epidermal and dermal layers changes as a function of age. It is decreased in the epidermis, at the periphery of collagen microfibrils and between collagen and elastic fibers; in contrast, the papillary dermis shows an increase in its content[52]. The extracellular matrix of the skin is composed primarily of hyaluronic acid and dermatan sulfate, with smaller amounts of chondroitin sulfate and heparan sulfate. The water-attracting property of hyaluronic acid produces a swelling pressure in the ground substance, allowing the rapid diffusion of water-soluble molecules. Decreasing levels of hyaluronic acid during maturity are manifest in shrinkage of the extracellular matrix and reduction in its viscosity, altering the rate of diffusion of ions and macromolecules from the blood to the tissues and vice-versa, probably accounting as an extra factor for the dried and wrinkled appearance of aged skin[52].

Although it may seem paradoxical, in older patients surgical incision lines are less red than in young ones, scarring is less hypertrophic and normalization of the overall appearance occurs more rapidly[53]. Wound healing stages in elderly people, though somewhat altered, are not impaired; they are delayed but still efficient. Those aspects must be remembered when dermatologists and dermatological surgeons submit their senior patients to peelings, resurfacing or other surgical procedures.

HORMONAL INFLUENCES

Hormone replacement therapy is used in a large number of perimenopausal women. It has defined indications, controlling the symptoms of the climacteric, preventing osteoporosis and reducing the risk of cardiovascular disease[54–56]. The influence of decreased ovarian hormones on the skin is catching the attention of gynecologists and dermatologists. Hormonal aging modifies the whole skin surface, exposed and non-exposed, but the main impact is in the dermis[16,57,58]. Many studies point to a relationship between dermal collagen content and cutaneous signs of menopause. The mean hydroxyproline quantity, that expresses the collagen content in the skin, was found to be 48% greater in estrogen-treated women, protecting the skin from the degenerative aging process as it protects bone from osteoporosis[58,59]. Non-invasive techniques have demonstrated that postmenopausal women on regular estrogen treatment showed a significant increase in dermal thickness, more significant in regions not exposed to the sun, and an overall younger look[58]. A double-blind placebo-controlled

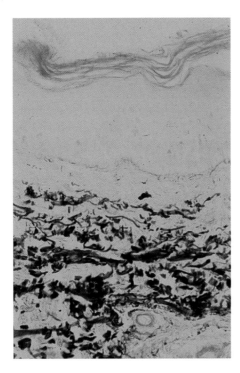

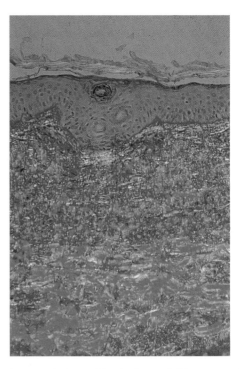

Figure 6 Sun-exposed skin biopsy of a mature woman. Light microscopy shows hyperkeratosis, epidermal atrophy, rectification of the basal layer and diminishing of oxytalan and elaunin fibers with formation of the 'Grenz zone', besides elastosis in the mid dermis. Resorcin–fuchsin with previous oxidation with oxona; 100X. Courtesy of Gerson Cotta-Pereira, MD, Rio de Janeiro, Brazil

Figure 7 Extrinsic and intrinsic aged skin. Areas of elastosis are represented by collagen III (stained in green) and sparse collagen I (stained in red). Picrocirius staining visualized by polarized light; 50X. Courtesy of Gerson Cotta-Pereira, MD, Rio de Janeiro, Brazil

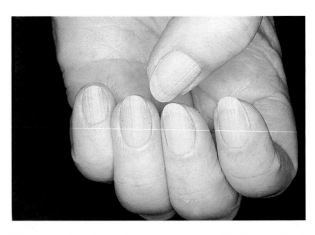

Figure 8 Brittle and opaque nails, with longitudinal striations, in spite of good cosmetic care, in a 58-year-old woman

study, assessed by ultrasonography and skin biopsies, demonstrated that treatment with conjugated estrogens significantly increases the thickness of the skin, besides impairing the progression of osteoporosis and improving the quality of life. The results demonstrated a 30% increase in dermal thickness and an 11.5% increase in skin thickness[35].

There is also a distinct effect of the hormonal imbalance on the biomechanical characteristics of the skin. A controlled investigation of the role of hormonal replacement therapy on the mechanical properties of the skin demonstrated a well-defined increase in skin laxity and a decrease in the elastic attributes of the skin, contributing to the slackness that occurs during the climacteric period. Hormonal therapy delays the process of the skin's deterioration in extendibility, slowing the progress of cutaneous slackening that follows the menopause[57,58].

The effect of estrogens on the function of the epidermis is controversial, although histopathological controlled studies indicate a consistent trend of improvement of the superficial layer of the skin in women on hormone replacement therapy, characterized by an increased number of keratinocytes layers and pronounced rete ridges after continuous treatment[35]. Oral or locally administered estrogens also improve the superficial texture of the skin, promoting an increase of up to 35% in sebum secretion and helping superficial hydration[28,58]. Large population surveys have confirmed that estrogens help to prevent tegument problems associated with aging, mainly skin dryness and wrinkling[2]. Most of the time, emphasis on women's skin care is predominantly placed on photoprotection and appropriate cosmetic measures throughout life.

Hormonal replacement therapy should always be considered when helping middle-aged women to try to preserve the best functional and aesthetic aspects of their skin.

CONCLUSIONS

Through an understanding of the molecular, structural and genetic causes of the complex phenomenon of cutaneous aging it may eventually be possible to treat, delay, or even reverse some of its features that, until now, have appeared to be inexorable.

REFERENCES

1. Koblenzer CS. Psychologic aspects of aging and the skin. *Clin Dermatol* 1996;14:171–7
2. Dunn LB, Damesyn M, Moore AA, *et al*. Does estrogen prevent skin aging: results from the First National Health and Nutrition Examination Survey (NHANES). *Arch Dermatol* 1997;133:339–42
3. Goihman-Yahr M. Skin aging and photoaging: an outlook. *Clin Dermatol* 1996;14:153–60
4. Brenner S, Politi Y. Dermatologic diseases and problems of women throughout the life cycle. *Int J Dermatol* 1995;34:369–79
5. Graham-Brown RAC. Dermatologic problems of the menopause. *Clin Dermatol* 1997;15:143–5
6. Graham-Brown RAC. The ages of man and their dermatoses. In Champion RH, Burton JL, Burns DA, Breathnach SM, eds. *Textbook of Dermatology*. Oxford, England: Blackwell Science, 1998:3259–87
7. Campisi J. The role of cellular senescence in skin aging. *J Invest Dermatol Symposium Proceedings* 1998;3:1–5
8. Gilchrest BA, Yaar M. Ageing and photoageing of the skin: observations at the cellular and molecular level. *Br J Dermatol* 1992;127(suppl 41):25–30
9. Yaar M, Gilchrest B. Aging versus photoaging: postulated mechanisms and effectors. *J Invest Dermatol Symposium Proceedings* 1998;3:47–51
10. Kligman AM, Lavker RM. Cutaneous aging: the differences between intrinsic aging and photoaging. *J Cutan Aging Cosmet Dermatol* 1988;1:5–12
11. Yaar M. Molecular mechanisms of skin aging. *Adv Dermatol* 1995;10:63–75
12. West MD. The cellular and molecular biology of skin aging. *Arch Dermatol* 1994;130:87–95
13. Gilchrest B. Retinoids and photodamage. *Br J Dermatol* 1992;127(suppl 41):14–20
14. Gilchrest B. A review of skin ageing and its medical therapy. *Br J Dermatol* 1996;135:867–75
15. Castelo-Branco C, Figueras F, Martinez de Osaba MJ, Vanrell JA. Facial wrinkling in postmenopausal women. Effects of smoking status and hormone replacement therapy. *Maturitas* 1998;29:75–86
16. Bolognia JL. Aging skin. *Am J Med* 1995;98 (suppl 1A):99S–103S
17. Fisher GJ, Wang ZQ, Datta SC, *et al*. Pathophysiology of premature skin aging induced by ultraviolet light. *N Engl J Med* 1997;337:1419–28
18. Lavker RM. Cutaneous aging: chronologic versus photoaging. In Gilchrest BA, ed. *Photodamage*. Cambridge, MA, USA: Blackwell Science, 1995: 123–35
19. Bhawan J, Andersen W, Lee J, *et al*. Photoaging versus intrinsic aging: a morphologic assessment of facial skin. *J Cutan Pathol* 1995;22:154–9
20. Uitto J, Fazio MJ, Olsen DR. Cutaneous aging: molecular alterations in elastic fibers. *J Cutan Aging Cosmet Dermatol* 1988;1:13–26
21. Stein GH, Dulic V. Molecular mechanisms for the senescent cell cycle arrest. *J Invest Dermatol Symposium Proceedings* 1998;3:14–18
22. Wei Q. Effect of aging on DNA repair and skin carcinogenesis: a minireview of population-based studies. *J Invest Dermatol Symposium Proceedings* 1998;3:19–22
23. Leveque JL, Corcuff P, de Rigal J, Agache P. *In vivo* studies of the evaluation of physical properties of the human skin with age. *Int J Dermatol* 1984; 23:322–9
24. Harvell JD, Maibach HI. Percutaneous absorption and inflammation in aged skin: a review. *J Am Acad Dermatol* 1994;31:1015–21
25. Fenske NA, Lober CW. Structural and functional changes of normal aging skin. *J Am Acad Dermatol* 1986;15:571–85
26. Manuskiatti W, Schwindt DA, Maibach HI. Influence of age, anatomic site and race on skin roughness and scaliness. *Dermatology* 1998;196:401–7
27. Elsner P, Wilhelm D, Maibach HI. Sodium lauryl sulfate-induced irritant contact dermatitis in vulvar and forearm skin of premenopausal and postmenopausal women. *J Am Acad Dermatol* 1990;23: 648–52
28. Tur E. Physiology of the skin – differences between women and men. *Clin Dermatol* 1997;15:5–16
29. O'Donoghues MN. Cosmetics for the elderly. *Dermatol Clin* 1991;9:29–34
30. Le Varlet B, Chaudagne C, Saunois A, *et al*. Age-related functional and structural changes in human dermo-epidermal junction components. *J Invest Dermatol Symposium Proceedings* 1998;3:172–9
31. Uitto J, Bernstein EF. Molecular mechanisms of cutaneous aging: connective tissue alterations in the dermis. *J Invest Dermatol Symposium Proceedings*, 1998;3:41–4
32. Dalziel KL. Aspects of cutaneous ageing. *Clin Exp Dermatol* 1991;16:315–23
33. Shuster S, Black MM, McVitie E. The influence of age and sex on skin thickness, skin collagen and density. *Br J Dermatol* 1975;93:639–43
34. Shuster S, Black MM, Bottoms E. Skin collagen and thickness in women with hirsutism. *Br Med J* 1970; 4:772

35. Maheux R, Naud F, Rioux M, *et al*. A randomized, double blind, placebo-controlled study on the effect of conjugated estrogens on skin thickness. *Am J Obstet Gynecol* 1994;170:642–9

36. Black MM, Shuster S, Bottoms E. Osteoporosis, skin collagen and androgen. *Br Med J* 1970;4:773–4

37. Bittencourt-Sampaio S, Cotta-Pereira G, Marques AS. Contribuição ao estudo da elastose actínica: alterações das fibras oxitalânicas e elaunínicas. *An Bras Dermatol* 1972;47:137

38. Cotta-Pereira G, Rodrigo FG, Bittencourt-Sampaio S. Oxytalan, elaunin and elastic fibers in the human skin. *J Invest Dermatol* 1976;66:143

39. Kelly RI, Pearse R, Bull RH, *et al*. The effect of aging on the cutaneous microvasculature. *J Am Acad Dermatol* 1995;33:749–56

40. Mishell DR. Estrogen replacement therapy: an overview. *Am J Obstet Gynecol* 1989;161:1825–7

41. Haddad MM, Xu W, Medrano EE. Aging in the epidermal melanocytes: cell cycle genes and melanins. *J Invest Dermatol Symposium Proceedings* 1998;3:36–40

42. Baran R, Dawber RPR, Tosti A, *et al*. Science of the nail apparatus and relationship to foot function. In Baran R, Dawber R, Tosti A, eds. *A Text Atlas of Nail Disorders*. London: Martin Dunitz, 1996:1–15

43. Dawber R, Van Neste D. Hair colour. In Dawber R, Van Neste D, eds. *Hair and Scalp Disorders*. London: Martin Dunitz, 1995:20–3

44. Rosen CJ, Holick MF, Millard PS. Premature graying of hair is a risk marker for osteopenia. *J Clin Endocrinol Metab* 1994;79:854–7

45. Orr-Walker B, Evans MC, Ames RW, *et al*. Premature hair graying and bone mineral density. *J Clin Endocrinol Metab* 1997;82:3580–3

46. Liang T, Hoyer S, Yu R, *et al*. Immunocytochemical localization of androgen receptors in human skin using monoclonal antibodies against the androgen receptor. *J Invest Dermatol* 1993;100:663–6

47. Sunderkötter C, Kalden H, Luger TA. Aging and the skin immune system. *Arch Dermatol* 1997;133:1256–62

48. Waldorf DS, Willkens RF, Decker JL. Impaired delayed hypersensitivity in an aging population: association with antinuclear reactivity and rheumatoid factor. *JAMA* 1968;203:111–14

49. Thiers BH, Maize JC, Spicer SS, Cantor AB. The effect of aging and chronic sun exposure on human Langerhans cell populations. *J Invest Dermatol* 1984;82:223–6

50. Gon Y, Hashimoto S, Hayashi S, *et al*. Lower serum concentrations of cytokines by peripheral blood monocytes in the elderly. *Clin Exp Immunol* 1996;106:120–6

51. Cerimele D, Celleno L, Serri F. Physiological changes in ageing skin. *Br J Dermatol* 1990;122 (suppl 35):13–20

52. Manuskiatti W, Maibach HI. Hyaluronic acid and skin: wound healing and aging. *Int J Dermatol* 1996;35:539–41

53. Cook JL, Dzubon LM. Aging of the skin: implications for cutaneous surgery. *Arch Dermatol* 1997;133:1273–7

54. Brincat M, Kabalan S, Studd JWW, *et al*. A study of the decrease of skin collagen content, skin thickness, and bone mass in the postmenopausal woman. *Obstet Gynecol* 1987;70:840–5

55. Lindsay R, Hart DM, Clark DM. The minimum effective dose of estrogen for prevention of postmenopausal bone loss. *Obstet Gynecol* 1984;63:759–63

56. Bush TL. The epidemiology of cardiovascular disease in postmenopausal women. *Ann NY Acad Sci* 1990;592:350–6

57. Piérard GE, Letawe C, Dowlati A, Piérad-Franchimont C. Effect of hormone replacement therapy for menopause on the mechanical properties of skin. *J Am Ger Soc* 1995;4:662–5

58. Callens A, Vaillant L, Lecomte P, *et al*. Does hormonal skin aging exist? A study of the influence of different hormone therapy regimens on the skin of postmenopausal women using non-invasive measurement techniques. *Dermatology* 1996;193:289–94

59. Brincat M, Moniz CF, Studd JWW, *et al*. Sex hormones and skin collagen content in postmenopausal women. *Br Med J* 1983;287:1337–8

General dermatology

Genodermatoses

10

Barukh Mevorah, Aryeh Metzker and Yael Politi

INTRODUCTION

The following genodermatoses will be discussed in this chapter: X-linked dominant chondrodysplasia punctata, congenital hemidysplasia with ichthyosiform nevus and limb defects (CHILD) syndrome, incontinentia pigmenti, focal dermal hypoplasia and oral-facial-digital syndrome type 1.

X-LINKED DOMINANT CHONDRODYSPLASIA PUNCTATA (CONRADI'S DISEASE; CONRADI–HÜNERMANN SYNDROME; X-LINKED DOMINANT ICHTHYOSIS)

Chondrodysplasia punctata (CDP) is characterized by stippled calcifications of the regions of enchondral bone formation. The epiphyseal calcifications appear *in utero*, and are usually transient. They can be visualized radiologically (Figure 1) and by ultrasound imaging. Other malformations such as eye and skin anomalies are additional findings.

History

CDP was first described by Conradi in 1914[1]. In 1931 another case was reported[2], and subsequent cases were sometimes published as Conradi's disease. In 1971 an extensive review of the literature revealed the heterogeneous nature of chondrodysplasia punctata[3]. Based on this study the authors classified CDP into two major types: an autosomal recessive rhizomelic type, usually lethal soon after birth; and the possibly autosomal dominant Conradi–Hünermann type; however, this latter type showed severe, moderate and mild clinical forms, pointing to the possibility of genetic heterogeneity. In the late seventies X-linked dominant chondrodysplasia punctata was delineated[4-7]. This type of CDP occurs almost exclusively in the female sex, and is characterized by asymmetrical limb shortening, cataracts and, in the neonatal period, patterned (mosaic) ichthyosiform skin lesions on a background of diffuse erythema. Some authors prefer the term X-linked dominant ichthyosis for this condition, because early in life the dermatosis may be even more striking than the skeletal anomalies[8].

In recent years many cases previously reported to be CDP of the autosomal dominant (Conradi–Hünermann) type have actually been shown to represent the X-linked dominant type[7,9]. The existence of an autosomal dominant type of CDP remains to be proven. Punctate calcifications as a radiologic finding can accompany diseases with various etiologies[10]. Table 1 shows a recent classification of chondrodysplasia punctata.

Clinical features

The pronounced clinical variability is characteristic in all affected systems[7-10]. In general the skeletal anomalies are asymmetrical. At birth and in early life, enchondral punctate calcifications can be observed radiologically or sonographically, and they often regress later in life. Findings include: short stature, saddle nose, frontal bossing, flat face, unilateral hypoplasia of the head, one-sided shortening of limb bones (most significant skeletal anomaly) usually of the femur and humerus (Figure 2), foot deformities, congenital hip dislocation, and flexion contractures. Scoliosis is found in most patients (Figure 3). It is the result not only of asymmetric shortening of the lower limbs but also of intrinsic anomalies of the vertebrae. Other minor skeletal malformations may also be present.

Cataracts, either congenital or appearing early in life, are the most frequent ocular finding. They occur in most patients, are often unilateral, and may be confined to only one segment of the eye (sectorial cataract). Even when bilateral, cataracts are often asymmetric in intensity. Other anomalies include epicanthus, unilateral microphthalmus with micro-cornea, nystagmus, hazy cornea, unilateral glaucoma and optic atrophy.

The cutaneous findings are the most striking feature at birth. There is a peculiar congenital ichthyosiform erythroderma. On the background of a usually generalized erythema there are thick adherent scales, arranged in a linear or blotchy pattern following the lines of Blaschko (Figure 4). These lesions clear up spontaneously within a few weeks or months. Later on, a characteristic

Table 1   Classification of chondrodysplasia punctata

Type	Characteristics
Primary chondrodysplasia	
Rhizomelic type	autosomal recessive peroxisomal disorder; high early lethality; survival possible; ichthyosiform skin lesions in 28% (not well defined)
X-linked dominant (male lethality)	asymmetric with cataracts; transient ichthyosiform skin lesions along Blaschko's lines; gene for sterol-Δ^8-isomerase (Xp11,22–11,23)
X-linked recessive	symmetric: telebrachydactyly, nasal hypoplasia; gene on Xp22.3
Sheffield mild type	symmetric. Probably heterogeneous
Tibia-metacarpal type	flat face, short limbs
Disorders with secondary punctate calcification	
Zellweger syndrome and other peroxisomal disorders	autosomal recessive; high early lethality; hypotonia, dysmorphic features
Embryopathies	fetal exposure to: warfarin, phenytoin, alcohol, rubella virus
Vit.-K-epoxide-reductase deficiency	rare autosomal recessive bleeding disorder with a warfarin embryopathy phenotype
Chromosome disorders	trisomies 18 and 21
Miscellaneous	

systematized atrophoderma involving primarily the hair follicles is observed. It most probably corresponds to the patterned hyperkeratoses of the neonatal period. The follicular atrophoderma is typically most pronounced on the dorsa of the hands and adjacent areas. In the older child and adult, ichthyotic scaling is often present and is more prominent in the atrophic areas. Its mosaic-like appearance follows the lines of Blaschko.

Pseudopelade-like areas of cicatricial alopecia are present, particularly in the older patient (Figure 5). They may be the site of hyperkeratoses. In non-alopecia areas the hair may be normal or irregularly twisted. The abnormal hair usually grows in the periphery of alopecic patches and microscopy reveals nonspecific changes. Nonalopecic areas with a mixture of normal and abnormal hair may also be observed (functional mosaicism).

The eyebrows and eyelashes are frequently involved, being sparse and disorganized. There may be minor nail anomalies such as flattening of the nail plates or onychoschisis.

A few patients will show pigmentary changes such as light and dark striated areas following the lines of Blaschko. However, these pigmentary changes, contrary to the keratotic scaly lesions, do not correspond to the patterned atrophoderma. This would indicate that the pigmentary disturbance is not a consequence of the skin lesions of the neonatal period. The striate pattern of pigmentation could

be confused with that seen in incontinentia pigmenti (Bloch–Sulzberger syndrome) which is also an X-linked dominant syndrome.

Other abnormalities

The following less characteristic anomalies have been reported: congenital heart or renal defects, pulmonary arterial stenosis, ear anomalies, increased susceptibility to infection and prematurity[7,11].

Mental development

Mental development is usually normal[7] and life expectancy is not affected provided there are no major visceral malformations or severe scoliosis.

Histology of cutaneous lesions

In the neonatal period there is hyperkeratosis with hypogranulosis or absence of the granular layer and frequent focal parakeratosis. Follicular keratotic plugging is a characteristic feature which could explain the adherence of the scales[7,12–14]. The hair follicles show signs of early or advanced atrophy depending on the patient's age[13]. The epidermis is slightly to moderately acanthotic. The changes in the superficial dermis are not significant. For some authors this histologic picture is indicative of retention hyperkeratosis[13]. Occasionally the following have been reported: calcium deposits in the epidermis, mainly in the follicular plugs[13,14], hyperpigmentation of the basal layer[13,14], marked acrosyringeal dilatation[14], and frankly psoriasiform changes of the epidermis[10-15]. A 32-year-old woman with X-linked dominant CDP was reported because of coexisting ichthyotic and psoriasiform lesions[15]. She had a 7-week history of a patterned psoriasiform eruption, in addition to streaky ichthyotic lesions involving the entire body that had been present since birth. Both types of cutaneous changes followed the lines of Blaschko. While a biopsy of the ichthyosis showed acanthosis with laminated hyperkeratosis, that of a psoriasiform lesion was compatible with pustular psoriasis. The latter was considered to be most probably part of the X-linked dominant CDP rather than a true and coincidental psoriasis 'because arrangement along Blaschko's lines has not yet been described for pustular psoriasis'[15].

The cicatricial alopecia appears histologically as pseudopelade and sometimes shows orthohyperkeratosis with a thin granular layer[7].

Electron microscopy of cutaneous lesions

The ultrastructure of the ichthyosis was first described in 1984 in a 4-week-old baby and a 14-year-old girl[13]. The epidermal changes were characterized mainly by a vacuolization of the keratinocytes of a thinned granular layer, with some of the vacuoles containing stellate or needle-like calcifications. The keratohyaline granules were reduced in number but normally structured. There was a significant reduction in the number of Langerhans cells, which showed degenerative changes[16]. The active skin lesions of a 6-month-old baby were biopsied and the ultrastructure of the epidermis supported the psoriasiform changes found with light microscopy, but there were no anomalies of subcellular structures or organelles[10]. In another case, the biopsy was taken from a region with follicular atrophoderma and there were no epidermal vacuoles with calcifications[17]. In still another patient the skin lesions were markedly improved and there was ultrastructural evidence for a self-resolving defect of multiple organelles such as lamellar bodies, peroxisomes and mitochondria[18]. Finally, a 13-year-old girl with a history of erythroderma at birth was found to have a mild patterned ichthyosis with polygonal scales adherent in the center[19]. Electron microscopy revealed thinning of the granular layer and persistence of desmosomes in the horny layer.

The ultrastructure of the lesions is striking in its variability from patient to patient, whereas the histopathologic findings are rather consistent in the majority of published cases. There is at present no satisfactory explanation for this variability.

Incomplete and atypical forms

Two mothers of affected girls were unaware that they showed minimal stigmata of the disease[9]. The women had mild cicatricial alopecia and in one of them discrete follicular atrophoderma was also present. Such minor forms of the disease are less likely to be missed 'if the clinician includes the mothers of his patients in his examination'[9]. Another report describes an affected infant girl who showed several atypical features: skeletal surveys at 6 months and one year of age did not reveal punctate calcifications; there was no cataract; there was a congenital erythroderma, but the characteristic streaky, whorled lesions appeared only after 5 months[10]. Because CDP is typically transient, it is possible that stippling was present in this child before she was six months old. That CDP is not invariably present in this syndrome is also demonstrated in another study[17]. The patient in this report had typical cutaneous and ocular manifestations, but X-ray survey of the entire skeleton at 1 week of age and of the hands and feet 9 months later did not reveal CDP. The presence of typical skeletal deformities in the absence of CDP has also been reported[20]. A 13-year-old girl was atypical only in that she had symmetrical shortening of the tubular bones[19]. A more recent report described a 7-day-old girl with unilateral distribution of the syndrome[21]. The case with ichthyotic and psoriasiform lesions along Blaschko's lines is discussed under 'Histology'[15].

Genetics and pathogenesis

X-linked dominant CDP affects almost exclusively women. Most cases are sporadic and probably represent new mutations[9,17]. In the familial instances the mothers seem to have milder symptoms than their affected daughters[9]. The following is a quotation from Happle[7], pointing out the circumstantial evidence for an X-linked dominant gene defect lethal in hemizygous males:

> X-linked dominant inheritance of this condition has been proposed to result from a connection between the mosaic phenotype and the sex ratio. The mosaic pattern of skin lesions present in a female patient, suggested functional X-chromosome mosaicism. At the time of our first report, the ratio of females to

males was 10 : 0. At present the sex ratio is 36 : 0. This mosaic pattern of skin lesions and limitation to females would be explained by an X-linked dominant gene lethal in hemizygous males. The marked asymmetry of skeletal and ocular anomalies would also be a manifestation of functional X-chromosome mosaicism. In contrast, the assumption of an autosomal dominant gene with sex-limited expression would explain the occurrence in girls, but not the mosaic pattern of defects[7].

The theory of functional X-chromosome mosaicism is based on the concept of X-inactivation (lyonization) introduced by Lyon[22]. In the early embryonal development of females one of the X chromosomes in each cell is randomly selected for inactivation[22]. This selection is retained by the progeny of that cell. The cutaneous lesions of X-linked dominant CDP are mainly distributed along the lines of Blaschko. The relationship between these lines and the phenomenon of lyonization has been thoroughly discussed[23].

Only six males have been reported with X-linked dominant chondrodysplasia punctata[24–26]. One of these had Klinefelter syndrome (XXY)[24]. This unique case lends further support to the concept of lyonization of an X-linked gene lethal in male embryos. Such rare cases are compatible with X-linked dominant inheritance and lethality in males. They could represent either a postzygotic mutation or a gametic half-chromatid mutation[24,27].

There is a murine model ('bare patches'; Bpa) for X-linked dominant CDP. In mice, 'bare patches' is transmitted in an X-linked dominant fashion lethal for male embryos[28,29]. The histologic changes of involved epidermis in affected mice have been described as psoriasiform[18], similar to two patients with the disease[10,15]. The gene for 'bare patches' has been mapped close to the murine X-linked visual pigment gene[30]. Although the mutant gene for X-linked dominant CDP is probably located within the Xq28 region, its exact mapping still defies molecular geneticists[31–33]. Recently, mutations in the gene encoding sterol-Δ^8-isomerase (Xp11, 22–11,23) have been reported[34].

Peroxisomal anomalies have been demonstrated in several patients with X-linked dominant CDP. 'Peroxisomes are subcellular organelles bounded by a single membrane; they are widely distributed in eukaryotic organisms and appear to be ubiquitous in mammalian cells'[35]. Metabolic reactions in the catabolism of substances such as amino acids and fats may produce free radicals and hydrogen peroxide, by-products which are toxic for the cell. Therefore such metabolic reactions are segregated within peroxisomes where hydrogen peroxide is degraded by catalase (abundant in these organelles)[36]. Known peroxisomal functions include: catabolism of very long chain fatty acids (> C22); biosynthesis of ether-phospholipids such as plasmalogens; biosynthesis of bile acids; catabolism of pipecolic acid; and catabolism of phytanic acid[34]. Peroxisomal disorders can be classified according to the state of peroxisomes and type of enzyme defect (Table 2)[37].

In 1987 peroxisomal enzyme deficiency was reported in a patient with 'the Conradi–Hünermann form of chondrodysplasia punctata'[38]. This was a typical example of X-linked dominant CDP. In addition to pipecolic aciduria, there was deficiency of the enzyme dihydroxyacetone phosphate acetyl transferase (DHAP-AT), which is involved in the synthesis of plasmalogens[35]. Another patient was reported with deficiency of DHAP-AT in 1989[10]. A study in 1994 investigated both an infant with X-linked dominant CDP and the homologous 'bare patches' (Bpa) mouse[18]. Samples for all tests were taken from lesional and normal-looking skin in the patient and in affected mice. Only lesional skin revealed significant ultrastructural defects of organelles such as lamellar bodies, peroxisomes and mitochondria. DHAP-AT and catalase activities were diminished in cultured fibroblasts from involved skin. In the animals these anomalies returned to normal after spontaneous resolution of the skin disorder. In 1991 the case of

Table 2   Peroxisomal disorders[*†]

Peroxisomes normal; single enzyme defects
  X-linked adrenoleukodystrophy
  Acatalasemia
  Hyperoxaluria type 1
  'Pseudo-Zellweger syndrome'
  Acyl-CoA oxidase deficiency
  Bifunctional enzyme deficiency
  Dihydroxyacetone phosphate acetyl
    transferase (DHAP-AT) deficiency
Peroxisomes present but structure abnormal;
 more than one defective enzyme
  Rhizomelic chondrodysplasia punctata
  Zellweger-like syndrome
Peroxisomes reduced or absent; multiple enzyme defects
  Zellweger syndrome
  Neonatal adrenoleukodystrophy
  Infantile Refsum disease
  Hyperpipecolic acidemia

[*]Modified with permission from reference 37. [†]Peroxisomal anomalies have recently been reported in X-linked dominant CDP and in the CHILD syndrome

a girl with normal peroxisomal function and absent skeletal manifestations was published[17]. Given that the early cutaneous changes are usually spontaneously regressive, the authors argued that the absence of peroxisomal enzyme anomaly could have been attributed to the fact that the skin lesions had already disappeared at the time of the skin biopsy. In 1998 transiently abnormal peroxisomal function tests were reported in a female infant afflicted with this disease[39]. The exact etiological role of the above-mentioned biochemical anomalies has not yet been elucidated.

Prenatal diagnosis

Prenatal diagnosis, where feasible, is mandatory both for a mother affected with X-linked dominant CDP or for an apparently healthy woman who has already had an affected child. It should be kept in mind that some patients show very few signs of the disease and may not be aware of them[9]. A primigravida with Conradi–Hünermann syndrome was reported in 1993[40]. She was 16 weeks pregnant when presenting for counseling. The karyotype of the fetal amniocytes was normal (46,XX), but sonographically there was asymmetric limb shortening. Although this finding was strongly indicative of an affected fetus the mother refused interruption of pregnancy and gave birth to a female with the clinical picture of X-linked dominant CDP. The following case does not involve the syndrome under discussion here but it does show that prenatal sonographic demonstration of premature epiphyseal calcifications is possible as early as the second trimester. A 25-year-old woman was followed during her fourth pregnancy, which had been uneventful[41]. Multiple sonographic skeletal findings of premature epiphyseal calcifications, other unusual calcifications, kyphoscoliosis and asymmetrical limb shortening led to a second-trimester prenatal diagnosis of 'non-rhizomelic chondrodysplasia punctata'. The karyotype of the amniocytes was 46,XX and pregnancy was terminated at 23 weeks. X-ray study of the abortus confirmed the suspected sonographic anomalies, but since there were no skin lesions this was probably not an example of X-linked dominant CDP.

In discussing pathogenesis we mentioned that it was recently shown that X-linked dominant CDP may well be linked to a peroxisomal disorder. Should a well-defined peroxisomal biochemical defect be established in X-linked dominant CDP, this might further enhance early prenatal diagnosis, certainly earlier than can be done with ultrasound imaging. Peroxisomal disorders can be diagnosed in the first or second trimester of pregnancy using cultures of chorionic villus cells or amniocytes[37]. Chorionic villus sampling requires facilities available in a limited number of institutions. Therefore it is important to develop diagnostic methods that require only a limited number of amniocytes[42].

CHILD SYNDROME

The acronym CHILD was coined in 1980 and stood for congenital hemidysplasia with ichthyosiform erythroderma and limb defects[43]. Recently, the unilateral skin lesions have been interpreted as a nevus, the CHILD nevus[44]. Consequently the 'i' in this acronym now stands for ichthyosiform nevus. This syndrome is a multisystem hemidysplasia, occurs almost exclusively in girls, and is transmitted as an X-linked dominant trait lethal in male embryos.

Clinical features

Skeletal anomalies are unilateral. They may involve any bone, but hypoplasia of limbs is most characteristic, and rarely, there may be aplasia of a limb. Hands or feet may be grossly deformed. Scoliosis is common and may be due to asymmetry of limbs or to genuine vertebral defects. Unilateral hypoplasia may affect the head and trunk resulting in defects of the calvarium, mandible, scapula, clavicle and ribs. Stippled calcifications of the epiphyses are quite common shortly after birth. They have also been described in the pelvis, sella-turcica, thyroid cartilage, ribs, vertebrae and larynx. Finally, contractures secondary to hypoplasia may develop[43–46].

The skin lesions, typically ipsilateral, are best described in the following quotation[46]:

> The CHILD nevus is a circumscribed inflammatory skin disorder that is usually present at birth but may also develop during the first months of life or even later. Characteristically, the disorder involves either exclusively or predominantly one side of the body, with a strict demarcation along the anterior and posterior midline. Usually the erythematous lesion is covered with waxy scales, but in some areas it may show a rather verrucous surface. As a distinguishing feature, the CHILD nevus displays a marked affinity for the body folds or ptychotropism. Sometimes parts of the nevus tend to disappear spontaneously, but even in such cases the involvement of the body folds usually persists. On the other hand, spreading of the nevus to new skin areas has been observed during infancy or later in life.

The dermatosis is either diffuse involving one half of the body or arranged in streaks along the lines of Blaschko. Often both patterns are present. Exceptionally the face and oral cavity may be affected. The opposite side of the body may also show some skin lesions.

Other abnormalities

Ipsilateral central nervous system defects may be found, such as brain hypoplasia, spinal cord and cranial nerve hypoplasia, and electroencephalogram disturbances. Ipsilateral visceral anomalies have been reported such as cardiovascular malformations, hydronephrosis, aplasia of the kidney and hypoplasia of the lung and other organs. Minor contralateral abnormalities of the skin, bones or viscera may also occur.

Incomplete and atypical forms

Exceptionally the CHILD nevus can present as an isolated dermatosis without other anomalies. A definite diagnosis can be made only if another member of the same family shows the full-blown syndrome[47,48]. Seemingly, bone anomalies may also exist in the absence of skin lesions[49]. Again, such a diagnosis requires that the complete syndrome be present in a relative of the patient.

Mental development, life expectancy

Intellectual impairment may occur and early death is usually attributed to congenital heart disease.

Histology and electron microscopy of cutaneous lesions

There are areas of parakeratosis and orthohyperkeratosis[46,50]. Also, one observes a significant acanthosis and exocytosis of neutrophils that tend to form accumulations resembling Munro abscesses. There are lymphohistiocytic infiltrates in the dermis. This histological picture is difficult to differentiate from psoriasis[45]. Verruciform xanthoma-like changes[50] may be seen mainly in biopsies taken from skin folds[45]. The enlarged papillae show histiocytes with a foamy cytoplasm[45]. Ultrastructurally the partly parakeratotic corneocytes reveal lipid vacuoles[45,49] and vesicular structures can be seen in the intercorneocyte spaces. Few vesicular structures are visible in the basal cell layer, becoming more abundant in the course of keratinization. The foamy cells of the papillary dermis show large intracytoplasmic vacuoles. Fibroblasts accumulate lamellated membranes and vacuolar structures[52]. In one study, markedly deformed keratinosomes were the most striking ultrastructural change[53]. Lipid vacuoles with occasional cholesterol crystals, in dermal cells, have also been described[54].

Genetics

The CHILD syndrome is encountered almost exclusively in women and familial cases are rare. The first instance of a mother-to-daughter transmission was reported in 1990[47]. Because the mother had minimal involvement, the authors stated: 'We conclude that the mother of a girl suffering from the CHILD syndrome cannot be considered to be unaffected unless a meticulous examination of her skin and bones has ruled out even minimal signs of involvement'. It has been proposed that this syndrome is transmitted as an X-linked dominant trait, lethal in male embryos[43,47]. This mode of inheritance is discussed in the section on X-linked dominant chondrodysplasia punctata.

Differential diagnosis

The syndrome under discussion may be confused with X-linked dominant chondrodysplasia punctata, particularly when punctate epiphyseal calcifications are present. Other common features to be kept in mind are asymmetric shortening of limbs, congenital ichthyosiform erythroderma, and limitation to the female sex. However, in contrast to the CHILD syndrome, the dermatosis of X-linked dominant chondrodysplasia punctata affects both sides of the body and the patterned hyperkeratoses always follow the lines of Blaschko; furthermore, atrophic skin lesions distributed in the same pattern are observed in the older child[43].

The CHILD nevus has often been misdiagnosed as an inflammatory linear verrucous epidermal nevus (ILVEN)[42]. 'Contrasting with ILVEN, however, the CHILD nevus is covered with large, yellow, waxy scales, shows a tendency to nonlinear arrangement and occurs almost exclusively in girls'[46]. The CHILD nevus is further characterized by ptychotropism, minimal or absent pruritus, and a histology of verruciform xanthoma, all of which are not present in ILVEN[45,46]. The CHILD nevus can be psoriasiform histologically, but the changes of verruciform xanthoma rule out psoriasis. Clinically it is easily distinguished from psoriasis. Other epidermal nevi can easily be ruled out. In addition, the histological changes of verruciform xanthoma, although nonspecific, are not encountered in other epidermal nevi. In the CHILD nevus, verruciform xanthoma is most often seen in specimens taken from the body folds[46].

Pathogenesis

Lack of expression of epidermal differentiation markers in lesional skin has recently been reported in the CHILD syndrome[55]. About the same time evidence of peroxisomal anomaly in involved skin fibroblasts was also published[52]; the number of peroxisomes was reduced and the activities of two peroxisomal enzymes, catalase and DHAP-AT, were decreased (see Table 2 and 'Pathogenesis' in the section on X-linked dominant chondrodysplasia punctata).

In another study, phenotypic dichotomy in eicosanoid metabolism and proliferative rates among cultured dermal fibroblasts were reported[55]. Dermal fibroblasts from an area of hyperkeratotic skin and from the corresponding contralateral area of 'normal' skin were maintained in culture. Compared with the 'normal' skin fibroblasts, those from lesional skin showed a slower proliferative rate, a cyclical pattern of prostaglandin E_2 (PGE$_2$) synthesis and a 20-fold greater production of PGE$_2$ in response to human purified interleukin-1 (IL-1) (the latter may be secreted by epidermal keratinocytes). PGE$_2$ is an eicosanoid with documented effects on epidermal cell and fibroblast function. The cyclical production of PGE$_2$ by the involved skin fibroblasts was responsible for their slower rate of growth compared with the uninvolved skin fibroblasts[56].

Prenatal diagnosis

Prenatal diagnosis is of the utmost importance for a mother showing only an isolated CHILD nevus because there is an increased risk of giving birth to a girl with the full-blown CHILD syndrome. The considerations here are similar to those for X-linked dominant chondrodysplasia punctata.

INCONTINENTIA PIGMENTI (BLOCH–SULZBERGER SYNDROME)
History

Incontinentia pigmenti is a rare, hereditary, multisystem disease almost exclusive to women. First reports dated from 1926[57] and 1928[58], but a previous description in 1906 relates to the same disease[59]. The name incontinentia pigmenti derives from the incontinence of melanin in the superficial dermis during the third, pigmentary stage of the disease[60].

Clinical features, cutaneous

Incontinentia pigmenti is characterized by typical skin lesions. Developmental defects, in particular of the skeleton, the eyes and the central nervous system, although not frequent, are the most serious

threats to patients' quality of life. The skin changes evolve in stages in a fixed chronological order. The first stage, present in 90% of patients at birth or within the first two weeks of life, is marked by the appearance of linear vesicular or erythematous lesions, mainly on the extremities (Figure 6)[59]. The second stage, marked by linear verrucous lesions similar to the first stage pattern (Figure 7), follows, usually between the second and sixth weeks of life. It persists for a few months and in 80% of cases fades by the age of six months[60]. The third stage, unrelated to the site(s) of the previous stages, consists of brownish linear and whorled streaks that follow the lines of Blaschko, with a wide range of involvement, mainly on the trunk (Figure 8). This stage is the hallmark of the disease and lasts from one or two years of age for a number of years, fading entirely by adolescence.

A fraction of patients exhibit a fourth stage; 14% of them show a residual hypopigmentation in the areas of the previous hyperpigmentation, and 28% show only small atrophic patches[61,62].

Clinical features, noncutaneous

About 80% of patients with incontinentia pigmenti have some systemic manifestations. About one-third have central nervous system disorders such as convulsions, mental retardation or spastic paralysis. Convulsions in infancy can result in motor and developmental delay, pointing up the importance of electroencephalographic examination in these disorders[63,64].

One-third of patients have various ocular anomalies, including strabismus, cataracts, blue sclerae, retinal detachment, microphthalmus, optic nerve atrophy or blindness[65]. Some patients have ectodermal defects such as nail dystrophy, sometimes associated with a painful subungual tumor[66], scarred alopecia[67], and dental changes like delayed dentition, peg teeth or partial anodontia[66,68].

Skeletal anomalies affect 13% of patients, and include skull deformities, dwarfism, spina bifida and cleft lip and palate[62]. Reported breast anomalies are supernumerary nipples, breast hypoplasia or aplasia, and anomalies of nipple pigmentation. The increased child mortality due to malignancies in this disease is attributed to chromosomal instability[69,70].

Histology of cutaneous lesions

The histological findings differ in the four clinical stages[71]. During the first vesicular stage there is spongiosis, and intra-epidermal vesicles are surrounded by infiltrating eosinophils which are also seen in the

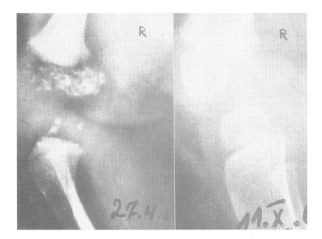

Figure 1   X-linked dominant chondrodysplasia punctata: epiphyseal stippling. Courtesy of M. Gruenbaum, MD, Petah Tiqva, Israel

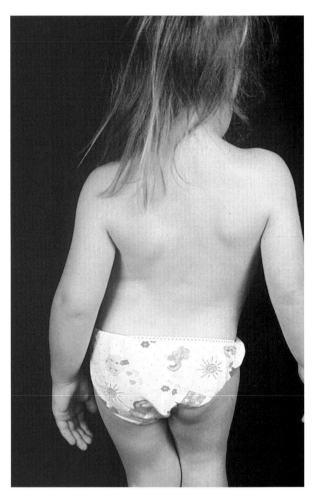

Figure 3   X-linked dominant chondrodysplasia punctata: severe scoliosis

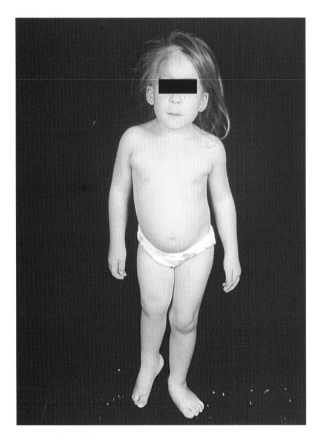

Figure 2   X-linked dominant chondrodysplasia punctata: asymmetric limb shortening

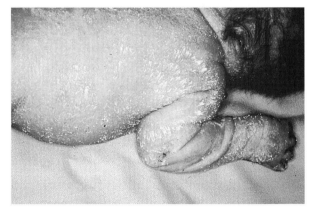

Figure 4   X-linked dominant chondrodysplasia punctata: neonate with patterned scaling along Blaschko's lines on erythematous background. Courtesy of D. Hohl, MD, Lausanne, Switzerland

dermis and within the vesicles. The peripheral blood reflects these findings, with leukocytosis (up to 40 000) and marked eosinophilia[62]. Defective neutrophil chemotaxis and altered immunologic reactivity have also been described[72,73]. The second verrucous stage is marked typically by acanthosis, irregular papillomatosis, hyperkeratosis and presence of dyskeratotic keratinocytes. The third,

whorled, pigmented stage shows, appropriately, a marked melanin deposition in the upper dermis, many melanophages and vacuolar degeneration in the basal layer. The fourth atrophic-patchy stage shows mild epidermal atrophy, lack of skin appendages, and a decreased number of small melanocytes.

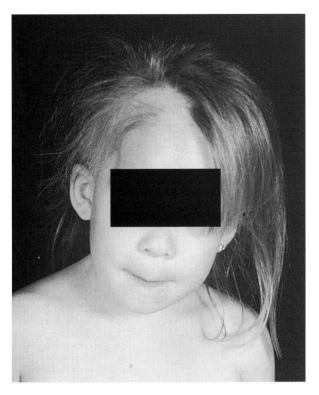

Figure 5 X-linked dominant chondrodysplasia punctata: patchy cicatricial alopecia

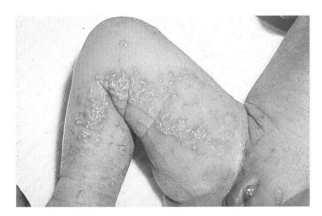

Figure 6 Incontinentia pigmenti, 1st stage: neonate with linear vesicular eruption on thigh

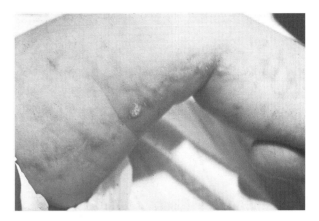

Figure 7 Incontinentia pigmenti, 2nd stage: 2-month-old female with linear verrucous lesions

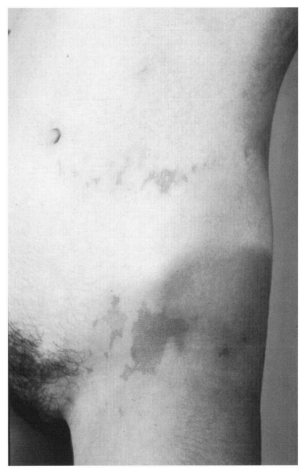

Figure 8 Incontinentia pigmenti, 3rd stage: girl with whorled pigmentation on trunk.

Genetics and pathogenesis

The inheritance is X-linked dominant, woman-to-woman transmission, with increased incidence of spontaneous abortion, usually of male fetuses[60,62,67,74]. This form of inheritance is supported by the female-to-male ratio of offspring suffering from this disease; although more than 700 cases have been documented, only 49 males are reported in the literature, and these males are more severely affected than their female counterparts. These males are grouped as incontinentia pigmenti type II with a significant occurrence of sex chromosome aneuploidy, being subjected to the

half chromatid mutation model or the postzygotic mutation, as well as mosaicism[63,75–77].

About 50% of incontinentia pigmenti cases have a positive family history, while the rest are probably due to a new mutation. The male patients have no reported family history[62]. Five infant boys with the disease also had evidence of Klinefelter's syndrome (47,XXY), which may have played a role in their survival because the second X chromosome protects them from intrauterine death[75,78–81].

The gene responsible for incontinentia pigmenti was mapped to the terminal region on the long arm of the X chromosome (Xq28) and confirmed in a large linkage study[60,82]. The location of the putative gene on chromosome Xp11.2 gained support when a number of cases with translocation between chromosomes X and 5 were described. It was suggested that two genotypes of the disease may present with the same phenotype. Sporadic cases with translocation of chromosome X were classified as incontinentia pigmenti type I[63,83]. Incontinentia pigmenti type II, on the other hand, comprises familial cases in which the gene locus is linked to Xq28[63,82]. Happle[84], an advocate of mosaicism as the explanation of the disease, points to the absence of inflammatory or bullous skin lesions and the lack of typical histological findings in incontinentia pigmenti type I. He suggests that incontinentia pigmenti type I seems to belong to hypomelanosis of Ito[84]. Genetic counseling should be offered to affected families as a preventive measure.

FOCAL DERMAL HYPOPLASIA (GOLTZ'S SYNDROME)

History

Focal dermal hypoplasia is characterized by a combination of mesodermal and ectodermal anomalies[85] involving mainly skin and skeletal changes. The first descriptions of this uncommon genodermatosis appeared under this name in 1962 and 1963[86,87], but the first known case had already been published in 1921[88]. Since that time more than 200 cases have been described[89], 90% of them in women.

Clinical features, cutaneous

The skin lesions, present at birth in all focal dermal hypoplasia patients, consist of linear or reticular atrophic and poikilodermatous streaks seen mostly on the limbs and buttocks. They resemble striae distensae, have telangiectasia adjacent to the main lesions, and sometimes follow Blaschko's lines[90]. In many cases fat tissue herniation appears in the lesion. Congenital absence of skin, similar to aplasia cutis congenita, appears as large ulcers on the scalp which heal slowly and leave an atrophic scar[91]. Small red papillomas are seen at times on mucous membranes of the mouth, larynx, esophagus, vagina and anus, or an acral locations such as palms, fingers, toes and ears.

Clinical features, noncutaneous

About 80% of affected patients display a variety of skeletal abnormalities: digital abnormalities with syndactyly, polydactyly, adactyly, or all of them in a kind of 'lobster claw' deformity; scoliosis; poor breast development; and severe spina bifida causing some neurological deficit[92]. Ocular defects are present in 40% of patients[93–95], including coloboma of the iris, microphthalmia, anophthalmia, microcornea and optic nerve hypoplasia eventually associated with diffuse cortical and cerebellar atrophy[96].

Dental changes are also frequent, presenting in about 40% of patients as hypoplastic teeth with defective enamel[97]. Patients may have sparse and brittle hair, scattered patches of alopecia on scalp and pubic areas and dystrophic nails. Occasionally there are genito-urinary defects such as bifid ureter or hypoplastic kidneys, intestinal malrotation or mediastinal dextroposition[98]. Some typical facial features are asymmetry of the face, triangular-shaped face, prominent ears or small skull. Fifteen per cent of patients have some mental retardation.

The varied features of this disease call for the differential diagnosis of Proteus syndrome, oculocerebro-cutaneous syndrome, incontinentia pigmenti, Rothmund–Thomson syndrome, nevus lipomatosus superficialis, Adams–Oliver syndrome, ectodermal dysplasia and linear scleroderma.

Histology, laboratory findings and electron microscopy

The skeletal changes present in most focal dermal hypoplasia patients appear radiologically as fine, parallel, vertical striations in the metaphysis of the long bones, the so-called osteopathia striata[99]. Histologically the dermis is hypoplastic with thin fibers of collagen that do not form bundles[91,100]. Yellow-red fat nodules are seen through a very thin hypoplastic dermis, reaching in some places into the epidermis. Electron microscopic examination of the lesion shows loose collagen bundles, collagen fibers with loss of regular bands, abnormal fibroblasts and disruption of the basement membrane zone, suggesting an abnormal function of type IV collagen[101]. The histology of the red periorificial or mucous membrane papillomas resembles that of angiofibroma[94]. An abnormal metabolism of glycosaminoglycan in the affected dermis results in a decreased amount of hyaluronic acid-derived disaccharide units, and may be a marker for defective fibroblasts in affected areas[102].

Genetics

The high predominance of women with focal dermal hypoplasia, numerous familial cases, association with a history of spontaneous abortions and stillbirth and neonatal death of males suggest an X-linked dominant trait with lethality for hemizygous males[103]. When it does occur in males it probably represents a new mutation. It has lately been interpreted as functional X-chromosome mosaicism[103] with the putative gene locus on Xp22,31. In about 20% of gene carriers, the typical osteopathia striata can be observed on radiography[94]. A multidisciplinary team including genetic counselors should follow and treat these patients as indicated.

ORAL-FACIAL-DIGITAL SYNDROME TYPE 1 (PAPILLON-LÉAGEM SYNDROME)

History

The oral-facial-digital syndrome is a genodermatosis that presents with a wide spectrum of congenital anomalies[105]. The first description dates from 1954[106], and 9 different types of the syndrome have been described since then[105,107]. The most frequent type, affecting one in 50 000 births, is the oral-facial-digital syndrome type 1 (OFD-1) seen only in females[108].

The syndrome is characterized by abnormal development of the oral cavity, digital deformities and neurological findings. Only half the OFD-1 syndrome cases exhibit oral, facial and digital abnormalities simultaneously[109,110].

Clinical features

The skin shows multiple milia and some scaly plaques. The hair is dry and coarse and at times alopecia is present. The oral and facial anomalies include cleft palate and cleft lip at the midline, cleft tongue, hematomas of the tongue, and multiple hyperplastic frenulae. One point five per cent of patients with cleft lip or cleft palate actually present the OFD-1 syndrome[111,112]. Digital anomalies are varied but are mainly syndactyly and hand deformities.

This syndrome also shows a large range of brain anomalies, including intracerebral cysts, porencephaly or arachnoid cysts and micro- or macrocephaly[107,112]. The neurologic signs include mental retardation in 50% of cases, seizures and hearing loss[109]. The presence of polycystic kidneys has been reported repeatedly, often requiring dialysis or renal transplantation[113,114].

Genetics

OFD-1 syndrome is inherited as an X-linked dominant trait with variable expression[110,115] and prenatal lethality in affected males. Nevertheless, one case of a male with OFD-1 proved to have 47,XXY karyotype[116]. The gene of the disease has been mapped to a region on the short arm of the X chromosome (Xp22,2-Xp22,3)[117]. Genetic counseling and long-term follow-up are suggested for any patient with this syndrome, both to avoid further cases and to better understand the genetics and developmental disturbances involved.

CONCLUSIONS

There are very few genodermatoses specific to females. We have reviewed those that are X-linked dominant. In such cases the disease in the male fetus leads to intrauterine death. The few cases seen in surviving boys appear to involve other mechanisms, such as new mutations and different types of mosaicism. Both genetic counseling and long-term follow-up are highly recommended in all cases. The present knowledge about the described genodermatoses, and advances in modern obstetrics, permit prenatal diagnosis in some of them.

REFERENCES

1. Conradi E. Vorzeitiges Auftreten von Knochen-und eigenartigen Verkalkungskernen bei Chondrodystrophia fötalis hypoplastica. *Z Kinderheilkd* 1914;80:86–97
2. Hünermann C. Chondrodystrophia calcificance congenita als abortive Form der Chondrodystrophie. *Z Kinderheilkd* 1931;51:1–19
3. Spranger JW, Opitz JM, Bidder U. Heterogeneity of chondrodysplasia punctata. *Hum Genet* 1971;11:190–212
4. Happle R, Matthiass HH, Macher E. Sex-linked chondrodysplasia punctata? *Clin Genet* 1977;11:73–6
5. Happle R, Kästner H. X-gecoppelt dominante Chondrodysplasia punctata. Ein osteo-kutanes Syndrome. *Hautarzt* 1979;30:590–4
6. Happle R. X-linked dominant ichthyosis. *Clin Genet* 1979;15:239–40
7. Happle R. X-linked dominant chondrodysplasia punctata. Review of literature and report of a case. *Hum Genet* 1979;53:65–73
8. Traupe H. X-linked dominant ichthyosis. In Traupe H, ed. *The Ichthyoses. A Guide to Clinical Diagnosis, Genetic Counseling, and Therapy.* Berlin, Heidelberg: Springer-Verlag, 1989:179–86
9. Manzke H, Christophers E, Wiedemann HR. Dominant sex-linked inherited chondrodysplasia

punctata: a distinct type of chondrodysplasia punctata. *Clin Genet* 1980;15:97–107

10. Kalter DC, Atherton DJ, Clayton PT. X-linked dominant Conradi–Hünermann syndrome presenting as congenital erythroderma. *J Am Acad Dermatol* 1989;21:248–56

11. Wulfsberg EA, Curtis J, Jayne CH. Chondrodysplasia punctata: a boy with X-linked recessive chondrodysplasia punctata due to an inherited X-Y translocation, with a current classification of these disorders. *Am J Med Genet* 1992;43:823–8

12. Edidin DV, Esterly NB, Bamzai AK, Fretzin DF. Chondrodysplasia punctata. Conradi–Hünermann syndrome. *Arch Dermatol* 1977;113:1431–4

·13. Kolde G, Happle R. Histologic and ultrastructural features of the ichthyotic skin in X-linked dominant chondrodysplasia punctata. *Acta Derm Venereol* (Stockh) 1984;64:389–94

14. Hamaguchi T, Bondar G, Siegried E, Penneys NS. Cutaneous histopathology of Conradi–Hünermann syndrome. *J Cutan Pathol* 1995;22:38–41

15. Bruch D, Megahed M, Majewski F, Ruzicka T. Ichthyotic and psoriasiform skin lesions along Blaschko's lines in a woman with X-linked dominant chondrodysplasia punctata. *J Am Acad Dermatol* 1995;33:356–60

16. Kolde G, Happle R. Langerhans-cell degeneration in X-linked dominant ichthyosis. A quantitative and ultrastructural study. *Arch Dermatol Res* 1985;277:245–7

17. Prendiville JS, Zaparackas ZG, Esterly NB. Normal peroxisomal function and absent skeletal manifestations in Conradi–Hünermann syndrome. *Arch Dermatol* 1991;127:539–42

18. Emami S, Hanley KP, Esterly NB, *et al.* X-linked dominant ichthyosis with peroxisomal deficiency. An ultrastructural and ultracytochemical study of Conradi–Hünermann syndrome and its murine homologue, the Bare Patches mouse. *Arch Dermatol* 1994;130:325–36

19. Gobello T, Mazzanti C, Fileccia P, *et al.* X-linked dominant chondrodysplasia punctata (Happle syndrome) with uncommon symmetrical shortening of the tubular bones. *Dermatology* 1995;191:323–7

20. Herman TE, McAlister WH, Mallory SB, *et al.* X-linked dominant chondrodysplasia punctata without stippled epiphyses. *J Perinatol* 1997;17:168–71

21. Corbi MR, Conejo-Mir JS, Linares M, *et al.* Conradi–Hünermann syndrome with unilateral distribution. *Pediatr Dermatol* 1998;15:299–303

22. Lyon MF. Gene action in the X-chromosome of the mouse (*Mus musculus* L). *Nature* 1961;190:372–3

23. Happle R. Lyonization and the lines of Blaschko. *Hum Genet* 1985;70:200–6

24. Happle R. X-linked dominant chondrodysplasia punctata/ichthyosis/cataract syndrome in males. *Am J Med Genet* 1995;57:493 (letter to the editor)

25. De Raeve L, Song M, De Dobbeleer G, *et al.* Lethal course of X-linked dominant chondrodysplasia punctata in a male. *Dermatologica* 1989;178:167–70

26. Omobono E, Goetsch W. Chondrodysplasia punctata (the Conradi–Hünermann syndrome). A clinical case report and review of the literature. *Minerva Pediatr* 1993;45:117–21

27. Lenz W. Half chromatid mutations may explain incontinentia pigmenti in males. *Am J Hum Genet* 1975;27:690

28. Phillips RJS, Hawker SH, Moseley HJ. Bare patches, a new sex-linked gene in the mouse, associated with a high production of XO females. 1. A preliminary report of breeding experiments. *Genet Res* 1973;22:91–9

29. Happle R, Phillips RJS, Roessner A, Jünemann G. Homologous genes for X-linked chondrodysplasia punctata in man and mouse. *Hum Genet* 1983;63:24–7

30. Herman GE, Walton SJ. Close linkage of the murine locus bare patches to the X-linked visual pigment gene: implications for mapping human X-linked dominant chondrodysplasia punctata. *Genomics* 1990;7:307–12

31. Traupe H, van den Ouweland AMW, van Oost BA, *et al.* Fine mapping of the human Biglycan (BGN) gene within the Xq28 region employing a hybrid cell panel. *Genomics* 1992;13:481–3

32. Traupe H, Müller D, Atherton D, *et al.* Exclusion mapping of the X-linked dominant chondrodysplasia punctata/ichthyosis/cataract/short stature (Happle) syndrome: possible involvement of an unstable premutation. *Hum Genet* 1992;89:659–65

33. Das S, Metzenberg A, Shashidar Pai G, Gitschier J. Mutational analysis of the Biglycan gene excludes it as a candidate for X-linked dominant chondrodysplasia punctata, dyskeratosis congenita and incontinentia pigmenti. *Am J Hum Genet* 1994;54:922–5

34. Braverman N, Lin P, Moebius FF, *et al.* Mutations in the gene encoding 3-beta-hydroxysteroid-delta 8, delta 7-isomerase cause linked dominant Conradi–Hünermann syndrome. *Nature Genet* 1999;22:291–4

35. Schutgens RBH, Heymans HSA, Wanders RJA, *et al.* Peroxisomal disorders: a newly recognized group of genetic diseases. *Eur J Pediatr* 1986;144:430–40

36. Lehninger AL, Nelson DL, Cox MM. *Principles of Biochemistry*, 2nd edn. New York: Worth Publishers, 1993;35

37. Moser HW. Peroxisomal disorders. In Behrman RE, Kliegman RM, Arvin AM, eds. *Nelson Textbook of Pediatrics*, 15th edn. Philadelphia: Saunders Co., 1996:363–7

38. Holmes RD, Wilson GN, Hajra AK. Peroxisomal enzyme deficiency in the Conradi–Hünermann form of chondrodysplasia punctata. *New Engl J Med* 1987;316:1608 (letter to the editor)

39. Wilson CJ, Aftimos S. X-linked dominant chondrodysplasia punctata: a peroxisomal disorder? *Am J Med Genet* 1998;78:300–2

40. Pryde PG, Bawle E, Brandt F, *et al.* Prenatal diagnosis of nonrhizomelic chondrodysplasia punctata (Conradi–Hünermann Syndrome). *Am J Med Genet* 1993;47:426–31

41. Sherer DM, Glantz JC, Allen TA, *et al.* Prenatal sonographic diagnosis of non-rhizomelic chondrodysplasia punctata. *Obstet Gynecol* 1994;83:858–60

42. Suzuki Y, Shimozawa N, Kawabata I. Prenatal diagnosis of peroxisomal disorders. Biochemical and immunocytochemical studies on peroxisomes in human amniocytes. *Brain Dev* 1994;16:27–31

43. Happle R, Koch H, Lenz W. The CHILD syndrome. Congenital hemidysplasia with ichthyosiform erythroderma and limb defects. *Eur J Pediatr* 1980;134: 27–33

44. Happle R. The lines of Blaschko: a developmental pattern visualizing functional X-chromosome mosaicism. *Curr Probl Dermatol* 1987;17:5–18

45. Happle R. Ptychotropism as a cutaneous feature of the CHILD syndrome. *J Am Acad Dermatol* 1990;23: 763–6

46. Happle R, Mittag H, Küster W. The CHILD nevus: a distinct skin disorder. *Dermatology* 1995;191:210–16

47. Happle R, Karlic D, Steijlen PM. CHILD-Syndrome bei Mutter und Tochter. *Hautarzt* 1990;41:105–8

48. Poiares Baptista A, Cortesão JM. Naevus épidermique inflammatoire variable (NEVIL atypique? entité nouvelle?) *Ann Dermatol Vénéréol* 1979;106: 443–50

49. Schlenzka K, Gehre M, Neumann HJ, Sochor H. CHILD-Syndrome-Kasuistischer Beitrag zur Kenntnis dieser seltenen Genodermatose. *Dermatol Monatsschr* 1989;175:100–6

50. Hebert AA, Esterly NB, Holbrook KA, Hall JC. The CHILD syndrome: histologic and ultrastructural studies. *Arch Dermatol* 1987;123:503–9

51. Lever WF, Schaumburg-Lever G, eds. *Histopathology of the skin*, 7th edn. Philadelphia: JB Lippincott Co., 1990;442

52. Emami S, Rizzo WB, Hanley KP, *et al.* Peroxisomal abnormality in fibroblasts from involved skin of CHILD syndrome. Case study and review of peroxisomal disorders in relation to skin disease. *Arch Dermatol* 1992;128:1213–22

53. Hashimoto K, Topper S, Sharate H, *et al.* CHILD syndrome: analysis of abnormal keratinization and ultrastructure. *Pediatr Dermatol* 1995;12:116–29

54. Hashimoto K, Prada S, Lopez AP, *et al.* CHILD syndrome with linear eruptions, hypopigmented bands, and verruciform xanthoma. *Pediatr Dermatol* 1998;15:360–6

55. Dale BA, Kimball JR, Fleckman P, *et al.* CHILD syndrome: lack of expression of epidermal differentiation markers in lesional ichthyotic skin. *J Invest Dermatol* 1992;98:442–9

56. Goldyne ME, Williams ML. CHILD syndrome. Phenotypic dichotomy in eicosanoid metabolism and proliferative rates among cultured dermal fibroblasts. *J Clin Invest* 1989;84:357–60

57. Bloch B. Eigentümliche bisher nicht beschriebene pigmentaffektion (incontinentia pigmenti). *Schweiz Med Wochenschr* 1926;7:404–5

58. Sulzberger MB. Uber eine bisher nicht beschriebene congenitale pigmentanomalie (incontinentia pigmenti). *Arch Dermatol Syph* 1928;154:19–32

59. Garrod AE. Peculiar pigmentation of the skin of an infant. *Trans Clin Soc Lond* 1906;39:216

60. Landy SJ, Donnai D. Incontinentia pigmenti (Bloch–Sulzberger syndrome). *J Med Genet* 1993;30: 53–9

61. Harre J, Millikan LE. Linear and whorled pigmentation. *Int J Dermatol* 1994;33:529–37

62. Carney RG. Incontinentia pigmenti: a world statistical analysis. *Arch Dermatol* 1976;112:535–42

63. Zvulunov A, Esterly NB. Neurocutaneous syndromes associated with pigmentary skin lesions. *J Am Acad Dermatol* 1995;32:915–35

64. O'Brian JE, Feingold M. Incontinentia pigmenti: a longitudinal study. *Am J Dis Child* 1985;139:711–12

65. Carney RG, Carney RG Jr. Incontinentia pigmenti. *Arch Dermatol* 1970;102:157–62

66. Malvehy J, Paloru J, Mascaro JM. Painful subungual tumour in incontinentia pigmenti. Response to treatment with etretinate. *Br J Dermatol* 1998;138: 554–5

67. El-Benhawi MO, George WM. Incontinentia pigmenti: a review. *Cutis* 1988;41:259–62

68. Yamashiro T, Nakagaiwa K, Takada K. Case report: orthodontic treatment of dental problems in incontinentia pigmenti. *Angle-Orthod* 1998;68:281–4

69. Canto JM, Del Castillo V, Jiminez M, *et al.* Chromosomal instability in incontinentia pigmenti. *Ann Genet* 1973;16:117–19

70. Roberts WM, Jenkins JJ, Moorhead EL, Douglas EC. Incontinentia pigmenti, a chromosomal instability syndrome, is associated with childhood malignancy. *Cancer* 1988;62:2370–2

71. Lever WF, Schaumburg-Lever G. *Histopathology of the skin*. New York: JB Lippincott, 1983:83–5

72. Mennis S, Piccino R, Bolchini A, *et al.* Immunologic investigations in eight patients with incontinentia pigmenti. *Pediatr Dermatol* 1990;7:275–7

73. Cohen PR, Kurzrock R. Genodermatoses with malignant potential. *Dermatol Clin* 1995;13:219–20

74. Wilkund DA, Weston WL. Incontinentia pigmenti: a four generation study. *Arch Dermatol* 1980;116: 701–3

75. Scheuerle AE. Male cases of incontinentia pigmenti: case report and review. *Am J Med Genet* 1998;77:201–18

76. Gartler SM, Franke U. Half chromatid mutations: transmission in humans? *Am J Hum Genet* 1975; 27:218–33

77. Lenz W. Half chromatid mutations may explain incontinentia pigmenti in males. *Am J Hum Genet* 1975;27:690–1

78. Garcia-Dorado J, De Unamuno P, Fernandez-Lopez E, *et al.* Incontinentia pigmenti: XXY male with a family history. *Clin Genet* 1990;38:128–38

79. Omerod AD, White MI, McKay E, *et al.* Incontinentia pigmenti in a boy with Klinefelter's syndrome. *J Med Genet* 1987;24:439–41

80. Kunze J, Frenzel UH, Huttig E, *et al.* Klinefelter's syndrome and incontinentia pigmenti. *Hum Genet* 1977;35:237–40

81. Prendiville JS, Gorski JL, Stein CK, *et al.* Incontinentia pigmenti in a male infant with Klinefelter syndrome. *J Am Acad Dermatol* 1989;20:937–40

82. Safiani A, M'rad R, Simard L, *et al.* Linkage relationship between incontinentia pigmenti (IP_2) and nine terminal X long arm markers. *Hum Genet* 1991;86:297–9

83. Bitoun P, Philippe C, Cherif M, *et al.* Incontinentia pigmenti (type 1) and X;5 translocation. *Ann Genet* 1992;35:51–4

84. Happle R. Mosaicism in human skin: understanding the pattern and mechanism. *Arch Dermatol* 1993;129:1460–70

85. D'Alise MD, Timmons CF, Swift DM. Focal dermal hypoplasia (Goltz syndrome) with vertebral solid aneurysmal bone cyst variant. A case report. *Pediatr Neurosurg* 1996;24:151–4

86. Goltz RW, Peterson WC, Gorlin RJ, Ravitz HG. Focal dermal hypoplasia. *Arch Dermatol* 1962;86:708–17

87. Gorlin RJ, Meskin LH, Peterson WC Jr, *et al.* Focal dermal hypoplasia syndrome. *Acta Derm Venereol* (Stockh) 1963;43:421–40

88. Jessner M. Case demonstration. Verhandlungen der Breslauer Dermatologischen Vereinigung. *Arch Dermatol Syph* 1921;133:48

89. Giam Y-C, Khoo B-P. Focal dermal hypoplasia (Goltz Syndrome). *Pediatr Dermatol* 1998;15:399–402

90. Alster TS, Wilson F. Focal dermal hypoplasia (Goltz's syndrome). *Arch Dermatol* 1995;131:143–4

91. Lever WF, Schaumburg-Lever G. *Histopathology of the Skin*, 6th edn. Philadelphia, PA: JB Lippincott Company. *Congenital diseases*, 1983:65–6

92. Mevorah B, Politi Y. Genodermatoses in women. *Clin Dermatol* 1997;15:17–29

93. Thomas JV, Yoshizumi MO, Beyer CK, *et al.* Ocular manifestations of focal dermal hypoplasia syndrome. *Arch Ophthalmol* 1977;95:1997–2001

94. Temple IK, MacDowall P, Baraitser M, *et al.* Focal dermal hypoplasia (Goltz syndrome). *J Med Genet* 1990;27:180–7

95. Gottlieb SK, Fisher BK, Violin GA. Focal dermal hypoplasia. *Arch Dermatol* 1973;108:551–3

96. Gunduz K, Gunlal I, Erden I. Focal dermal hypoplasia (Goltz's Syndrome). *Ophthalmic Genet* 1997;18:143–9

97. Valerius NH. A case of focal dermal hypoplasia syndrome (Goltz) with bilateral cheilo-gnatho-palatoschisis. *Acta Paediatr Scand* 1974;63:287–8

98. Irvine AD, Stewart FJ, Bingham EA, *et al.* Focal dermal hypoplasia (Goltz Syndrome) associated with intestinal malrotation and mediastinal dextroposition. *Am J Med Genet* 1996;62:213–215

99. Howell JB, Reynolds J. Osteopathia striata. A diagnostic osseous marker of focal dermal hypoplasia. *Trans St John's Hosp Dermatol Soc* 1974;60:178–82

100. Howell JB. Nevus angiolipomatosus versus focal dermal hypoplasia. *Arch Dermatol* 1965;92:238–48

101. Lee IJ, Cha MS, Kim SC, Bang D. Electron microscopic observation of the basement membrane zone in focal dermal hypoplasia. *Pediatr Dermatol* 1996;13:5–9

102. Sato M, Ishikawa O, Yokoyama Y, *et al.* Focal dermal hypoplasia (Goltz Syndrome): a decreased accumulation of hyaluronic acid in three-dimensional culture. *Acta Derm Venereol* 1996;76:365–7

103. Wettke-Schafer R, Kanter G. X-linked dominant diseases with lethality in hemizygous males. *Hum Genet* 1983;64:1–23

104. Van der Steen PH, Mittag H, Kuster W, Happle R. Palmar papillomatous lesions reminiscent of epidermal nevus in a case of focal dermal hypoplasia: a nosological consideration. *Dermatology* 1996;193:147–8

105. Toriello HV. Review: Oral-facial-digital syndromes, 1992. *Clin Dysmorph* 1993;2:95–105

106. Papillon-Léagem M, Psaume J. Une malformation héréditaire de la muqueuse buccale, brides et freins anormaux. *Rev Stomatol* (Paris) 1954;55:209–27

107. Leão MJ, Ribeiro-Silva ML. Orofaciodigital syndrome type I in a patient with severe CNS defects. *Pediatr Neurol* 1995;13:247–51

108. Martinot VL, Manouvrier S, Anastassov Y. Orodigitofacial syndromes types I and II: clinical and surgical studies. *Cleft Palate-Cranio-facial J* 1994;31:401–8

109. Doege TC, Thuline HC, Priest JH, *et al.* Studies of a family with the oral-facial-digital syndrome. *N Engl J Med* 1964;271:1073–80

110. Ruess AL, Pruzansky S, Lis EF, *et al.* The orofacialdigital syndrome: a multiple congenital condition of females with associated chromosomal abnormalities. *Pediatrics* 1962;29:198–9

111. Whelan DT, Feldman W, Dost I. The oro-facial-digital syndrome. *Clin Genet* 1975;89:205–12

112. Gorlin RJ, Psaume J. Orodigitofacial dysostosis: a new syndrome. A study of 22 cases. *J Pediatr* 1962;61:520–30

113. Odent S, Le-Marec B, Toutain A, *et al.* Central nervous system malformations and early end-stage renal disease in oro-facial-digital syndrome type 1: a review. *Am J Med Genet* 1998;75:389–94

114. Scolari F, Valzorio B, Carli O, *et al*. Oral-facial-digital syndrome type 1: an unusual cause of hereditary cystic kidney disease. *Nephrol Dial Transplant* 1997;12:1247–50

115. Walbaum R, Maillad E, Donazzan M, *et al*. Les syndromes orofacio digitaux: à propos de trois observations personelles. *Lille Médicales* 1970;15:917–20

116. Wahrman J, Berant M, Jacobs J, *et al*. The oral-facial-digital syndrome: a male-lethal condition in a boy with 47/XXY chromosomes. *Pediatrics* 1966;37:812–21

117. Feather SA, Woolf AS, Donnai D, *et al*. The oral-facial-digital syndrome type 1 (OFD-1), a cause of polycystic kidney disease and associated malformations, maps to Xp22.2-Xp22.3. *Hum Mol Genet* 1997;6:1163–7

Other syndromes

Marcio Rutowitsch

11

INTRODUCTION

Dermatologic syndromes might seem to be uniform between men and women, but a further inspection reveals several variations. Among the different syndromes affecting both sexes that include dermatological signs and/or symptoms some are exclusive, some predominant or with a higher incidence in girls and women. There are others with different manifestations in women when compared to men.

Several syndromes showing differences in women will be described. The ones that will be discussed are: congenital adrenal hyperplasia, Turner's syndrome, follicular degeneration syndrome, Graham–Little syndrome, Fox–Fordyce disease, hyperostosis frontalis interna, polycystic ovary syndrome, Riehl's melanosis, poikiloderma of Civatte, keratoderma climactericum and Stewart–Treves syndrome.

CONGENITAL ADRENAL HYPERPLASIA

Congenital adrenal hyperplasia increases androgen production, and its most common cause is 21-hydroxylase deficiency, an autosomal recessive disorder. Other biochemical lesions may be due to defective hydroxylation by 11β-hydroxylase, or 3β-hydroxysteroid of the steroid nucleus, but are less common[1].

Impaired 21-hydroxylase activity causes deficient production of two hormones that are essential for life: cortisol (the major glucocorticoid) and aldosterone (the major mineralocorticoid). Congenital adrenal hyperplasia or adrenal virilism syndrome presents two classic forms that manifest during the newborn period: salt losing and non-salt losing, also termed 'simple virilizing'. Patients with the salt-losing form have severe cortisol and aldosterone deficiencies, and if they remain untreated, a life-threatening adrenal crisis usually occurs between two and three weeks of age. Patients with the simple virilizing form have sufficient mineralocorticoid production to avoid such crisis and the diagnosis is made between birth and five years of age. If the virilization occurs during fetal life, pseudohermaphroditism may result. As many as 3 to 6% of women presenting with hirsutism may be affected with this form, which is an allelic variant of the classic childhood salt-wasting type; the classic form is associated with HLA-BW47 and late onset form with HLA-B14[2]. Of women with this abnormality, 75% will present with hirsutism, with or without menstrual irregularities. Deficiency of 21-hydroxylase is the commonest defect associated with late-onset congenital adrenal hyperplasia.

Hyperpigmentation of the perineum, external genitalia, axillae, aureole and nipples is present. Both types of congenital adrenal hyperplasia can result in ambiguous genitalia in girls, although the genital abnormality is usually less serious in the simple virilizing form[3]. Late onset of congenital adrenal hyperplasia due to 21-hydroxylase deficiency is one possible cause of hirsutism, acne, menstrual disorders, infertility and polycystic ovary-like symptoms[4].

Prenatal diagnosis and treatment of congenital adrenal hyperplasia have been carried out in the last 10 years. Most recently a newly developed, rapid allele-specific polymerase chain reaction has been used for DNA analysis in some cases. Steroid therapy with dexamethasone administered at or before 10 weeks' gestation is effective in reducing virilization[5].

TURNER'S SYNDROME

Turner's syndrome is the most common sex chromosome anomaly; it is due to a missing or structurally defective X chromosome (XO)[6]. The frequency of this syndrome is 1:2500 female births[7]. In around 80% of cases there are 45 chromosomes with an XO sex chromosome complement; in these cases it proved to be impossible to detect chromatin in buccal smears. It is assumed that the missing chromosome was lost before or at fertilization[8]. In some 20% of cases chromatin was detected. In these case there might be 46 chromosomes but with partial deletion of one of the X chromosomes[9]. Their phenotype may not differ from the more common XO, but they may appear more normal[10]. Also mosaicism of different types – eg XX/XO or XXX/XO – may occur[11]. The disease is a common genetic and endocrinologic disorder of women characterized by sexual infantilism, webbed neck, cubitus valgus, short stature, gonadal dysgenesis, and lymphedema[12].

The disease is also known as Ullrich–Turner syndrome or Bonnevie–Ullrich–Turner syndrome. Newborns with this syndrome exhibit small stature, webbing of the neck (Figure 1) and marked edema of the hands and feet[6]. Common skin findings include hypoplastic nails, keloids and hypertrophic scars, dry skin, low posterior hair line (Figure 2), seborrheic dermatitis, abnormal dermatoglyphics and increased number of melanocytic nevi; there is, therefore, an increased risk factor for melanoma[13]. Coarctation of the aorta may be an associated feature. Turner syndrome is associated with a variety of autoimmune disorders such as Hashimoto thyroiditis[14] and alopecia areata[15]. A linkage between Turner syndrome and vitiligo, lichen planus and neonatal lupus erythematosus has been reported[16]. Psoriasis, another possible autoimmune disorder, has also been detected in girls with this syndrome[17].

Diagnosis may be made prenatally by amniocentesis[18]. Some abnormalities may suggest the diagnosis in infancy or childhood. On the other hand it may be unsuspected until puberty, when chromosomal analysis is necessary to confirm the diagnosis of this syndrome, which is frequently associated with autoimmune diseases or with serological markers for autoimmune diseases. Estrogen replacement will allow the development of secondary sexual characteristics but does not seem to influence stature or infertility. Those individuals on growth hormone therapy should have periodic skin examinations and be advised on the use of sunscreen[13].

FOLLICULAR DEGENERATION SYNDROME

Follicular degeneration syndrome is a disorder that begins on the vertex of the scalp and expands outwards in a symmetrical fashion. Its pathophysiology is unclear and involves a premature desquamation of the inner root sheath and a marked thinning of the outer root sheath with keratinized cells. This syndrome was first described as recently as 1968[19], being called hot comb alopecia or traction alopecia, common in black women. Subsequently the hypothesis of hot comb usage was discounted as the pathogenesis of the disorder[20] and the condition was recognized as follicular degeneration syndrome, a form of scarring alopecia[21].

The first description included 51 black women with a scarring alopecia. All of them were using a hot comb to straighten their hair. Oil is applied to the hair and acts as a lubricant and conductor of heat. A metal comb, heated to 150–260°C, is applied to the hair, re-arranging the hydrogen and disulfide bonds and straightening the hair[22]. Repeated contact of the hot oil with the scalp can produce a scarring alopecia[19]. In addition to hot combs, tight hair braids, bands and rollers have been implicated. Early lesions start with erythema and follicular pustules, and atrophy and cicatricial alopecia are late sequelae. The onset can often occur between the second and fourth decades of life[19]. The affected areas vary from the crown to the temporoparietal region. Shortened hair distal to the affected area provides a useful diagnostic clue.

Recently a study was conducted in ten black women with this form of alopecia, where the condition was either unrelated to, or not primarily caused by, hot comb usage. These patients acknowledged dysesthesia of the involved area. There was no erythema, scaling, or induration, although mild perifollicular hyperpigmentation was present. The scalp did not show any signs of scarring[21]. The follicular degeneration syndrome with its clinical and histologic features was also studied in eight black men with a scarring alopecia; none of them had used any kind of procedure to straighten or style the hair[23].

Histologically, there is a premature disintegration of the inner root sheath where it desquamates and disappears at the middle portion of the follicular isthmus, without a normal lining of keratinized inner root sheath. The outer root sheath of involved follicles is markedly thinned and its cells begin to keratinize[23].

Follicular degeneration syndrome may closely resemble alopecia areata and trichotillomania. Treatment is based on prevention. Unfortunately, owing to long-standing hair care practices, the patient may dismiss the recommendations. Follicular degeneration syndrome affects both black men and black women. There are several possible explanations to account for this racial predilection. These include mechanical factors specific to the hair follicles of black people, hereditary factors, and cultural (hair grooming) factors.

GRAHAM–LITTLE SYNDROME

Graham–Little syndrome (also known as Graham–Little–Lassueur syndrome, syndrome de Lassueur–Graham–Little, syndrome de Piccardi, Graham–Little Lassueur) is a progressive disease that affects mainly women aged 20–70 years and presents, as clinical features, cicatricial alopecia, follicular keratosis and mucosal lichen planus. All three features need not be simultaneously present.

Cicatricial alopecia may result on the scalp and the axillae and pubic areas, associated with keratosis pilaris[24,25].

The symptoms may appear more or less simultaneously, but more often the alopecia precedes by months or years the sudden onset of follicular papules on the trunk and limbs. The keratosis pilaris is referred to in early case reports as lichen spinulosus, which emphasizes that the horny papules are prolonged into conspicuous spines. These papules are usually grouped in plaques but may be widely disseminated[24,25]. The end stage, of the follicular lichen planus on the scalp, may be indistinguishable from pseudopelade[24]. Whether this syndrome is or is not a form of lichen planus is still unresolved, although the immunofluorescent findings in typical cases strongly suggest lichen planus[26]. The possibility of multiple diseases as the cause of the syndrome, in particular psoriasis, has been suggested[27], though other workers feel that it is a distinct entity.

Differential diagnosis can be made with pityriasis rubra pilaris[26], and treatment of the skin lesions is by local applications of retinoic acid or surgical excision of the cicatricial alopecias.

FOX–FORDYCE DISEASE

Fox–Fordyce disease (also known as apocrine miliaria and chronic itching papular eruption of the axillae and pubes[28]) is a chronic, intensely pruritic and papular disorder with a strict localization to areas bearing apocrine glands, that usually affects women. The disease may develop in the axillae, areolae of breasts or umbilicus and pubic region, and it results from the obstruction and rupture of the intra-epidermal portion of the ducts of affected glands[28–31]. The disorder was originally described in 1902.

Clinical aspects of Fox–Fordyce disease include chronically pruritic, evenly distributed, solitary colored skin or slightly erythematous dome-shaped follicular papules (Figure 3), frequently with a central punctum[32,33]. The axillae, pubic area, labia, perineum, areola, presternal area, umbilicus and the upper medial aspect of the thighs are the sites affected, in decreasing order of frequency. Intense pruritus can be a frequent major complaint, and it is paroxysmal, especially after increased sweating. Hair growth in affected areas is often sparse possibly because of scratching[28,32]. More than 90% of cases are seen in female patients.

The cause of Fox–Fordyce disease remains unknown. Many concepts concerning its pathogenesis have been proposed, among them emotional, endocrinologic, neurologic, anatomical or chemical changes[29,33]. Genetic influence may play a role, because Fox–Fordyce disease has been reported in identical twins[34]. The cause of the disease remains elusive and it tends to be chronic, unwavering and rarely remitting.

Histopathologically, Fox–Fordyce disease is characterized by a keratotic plug in the intra-epidermal part of the apocrine duct, leading to the rupture of its spongiotic vesicle. Extravasation of sweat and inflammation could then explain the itching[29]. Important aspects of the differential diagnosis are lichen planus, syringoma, scabies and localized neurodermatitis. These can be excluded on clinical grounds or after histopathological analysis.

There is no generally accepted therapy for this disease. Fox–Fordyce has been effectively treated with a 0.1% solution of vitamin A acid[35,36]. Therapeutical trials have been reported with topical or intralesional steroids, keratolytic agents such as salicylic acid 2% with 10% urea, and oral progestational agents[37,38]. Hydrocortisone cream (1%) has been recommended to control the associated axillary discomfort[36]. Topical antibiotic preparations such as clindamycin 1% solution[39], ultraviolet light[40], surgery (eletrocoagulation[30], cold steel and laser[37]) have all been tried.

HYPEROSTOSIS FRONTALIS INTERNA

Hyperostosis frontalis interna (also known as Morgagni–Stewart–Morel syndrome) is an abnormality of the inner table of the frontal bones of the skull consisting of smooth, rounded enostosis, a bony growth within the cavity of a bone, covered by dura and projecting into the cranial cavity. These enostoses are usually smaller than 1 cm at their greatest diameter and usually do not extend posteriorly beyond the coronal suture[41]. This abnormality is almost always found in middle-aged or elderly women, with endocrine abnormalities that include obesity, hirsutism, gonadal alterations and other signs of virilization; neurologic abnormalities such as headache, epilepsy and neuropsychiatric complaints may occur[41,42]. The disorder also occurs in women with no obvious illness or associated disease. However, the presence of a skull abnormality may be a manifestation of a generalized metabolic disorder.

POLYCYSTIC OVARY SYNDROME

Polycystic ovary syndrome affects up to 10% of women of reproductive age, and in its classic form it is characterized by hyperandrogenism and anovulation[43]. The syndrome is responsible for over 70% of cases of anovulatory infertility[44], and it is the most commonly diagnosed ovarian cause of hirsutism[45]. This manifestation is also known as Stein–Leventhal syndrome.

The etiology is unclear but ovulatory and anovulatory polycystic ovary syndrome differ in their characteristics[44]. Patients with this syndrome may present with several findings including anovulation, infertility, hirsutism, obesity, bilateral polycystic ovaries[45], hyperinsulinemia and peripheral insulin resistance, both linked to dyslipidemia[46]. But this group of signs does not adequately define it. Other well defined endocrinopathies may also demonstrate the mosaic of clinical findings. They include hypothyroidism, androgen-secreting tumors, certain central nervous system tumors, congenital adrenal hyperplasia, Cushing's syndrome, acromegaly, and insulin-resistant states[45]. The circulating steroid and trophic hormone profiles can be used to differentiate these disorders[47].

In this syndrome the androgen production by the ovaries is increased and plasma testosterone levels are elevated. Polycystic ovary syndrome may be familial and, in some cases, it is difficult to separate ovarian from adrenal causes of hirsutism because the adrenal glands may also be increased in size. Acne and increased sebaceous gland activity occur in approximately 20 per cent of these patients. Some polycystic ovary syndrome family studies have found that obligate male carriers have premature male pattern baldness. This has been proposed as the putative male phenotype of the disease[48].

Antiandrogens such as spironolactone or cyproterone acetate are effective treatments. Finasteride and flutamide are effective in the treatment of hirsutism in patients with polycystic ovary syndrome[49].

RIEHL'S MELANOSIS

Riehl's melanosis, also called pigmented contact dermatitis[50] or female facial melanosis[51], is a non-pruritic pigmented dermatitis characterized by brownish-gray reticular pigmentation that rapidly develops over the greater part of the face, but is more intense on the forehead and temples; it is more frequent in women than in men. The pigmentation may extend to the chest, neck, scalp and hands. It has an unknown etiology and may be a result of contact sensitivity or photocontact dermatitis related to either a chemical – tar derivate – or compounds in cosmetics, or a particular fragrance[52].

In addition to exogenous factors, including sunlight, endogenous factors may be involved[52]. Nutrition and talcum powder also may be responsible[53].

The disease is histologically characterized by liquefactive degeneration of the basal cells accompanied by the formation of melanophages in the upper dermis with a moderate cellular infiltration of lymphoid cells and histiocytes. Ultrastructurally, there is intracellular and intercellular edema of keratinocytes, a multilayered basal lamina and many dermal melanophages[52]. The treatment is difficult, but the condition may slowly improve over many months after stopping the use of cosmetics.

POIKILODERMA OF CIVATTE

This disease is a pigmentary disorder of debated etiology. The distribution implicates exposure to light as a causative factor, and it is probable that photodynamic substances in cosmetics are an important agent. It may be caused by perfume components as it occurs mainly on the sides of the neck, especially in women. The age incidence tends to suggest that an unknown endocrine factor or age change may also play some part. Clinical features of poikiloderma of Civatte comprise a reddish-brown reticulate pigmentation with telangiectasia and atrophy. It develops in irregular, more or less symmetrical patches on the lateral cheeks and the sides of the neck but spares the areas shaded by the chin. Treatment can be successfully carried out with pulsed dye laser[54,55].

KERATODERMA CLIMACTERICUM

This disease, also known as Haxthausen disease, was first described in 1934 as keratosis of the palms and soles. The syndrome is most frequent in women aged 40–60, but it may occur in young women as a palmoplantar keratoderma. Sometimes an endocrine factor can be incriminated but not a specific one; in other cases it may follow castration[56]. Haxthausen in his report observed this condition in ten postmenopausal women in whom it was strongly associated with hypertension and obesity. The lesions were non-pruritic areas of hyperkeratosis, round or oval in shape and of different size[57].

The disease usually starts on the plantar area where the lesions first develop at the pressure point. It may be circumscribed, discrete, oval or in round patches and it slowly increases in thickness, crossed by superficial fissures, causing discomfort in walking but little if any pruritus. Hand involvement – where it may be discrete or may form an irregular band encircling the less severely involved mid

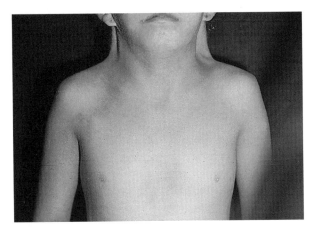

Figure 1 Turner syndrome – webbed neck. Courtesy of Joao Roberto Antonio, MD, São José do Rio Preto, Brazil

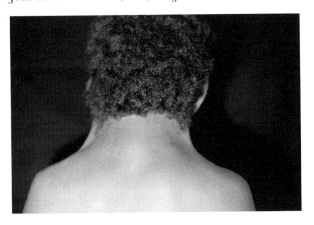

Figure 2 Turner syndrome – webbed neck and low posterior hair line. Courtesy of Joao Roberto Antonio, MD, São José do Rio Preto, Brazil

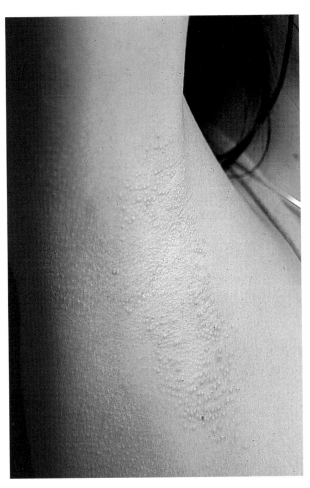

Figure 3 Fox–Fordyce disease – erythematous dome shaped follicular papules in the axillae

aspect of the palm – is not uncommon. Plantar keratoderma surrounds the margins of the heel and extends in irregular islands across the sole behind the line of the metartasal heads. During the winter symptoms may be worse. There may be some thickening over the knees, especially among obese women. In these patients the ovarian, adrenal and pituitary functions are normal[58].

Microscopic examination reveals a lichenified dermatitis with evidence of mechanical irritation. An ultrastructural study showed composite keratohyalin granules found in the granular cells of the interductal epidermis, suggesting that the intraepidermal sweat ducts may play a role in the histogenesis of palmoplantar keratoderma[59]. Keratoderma climactericum, which is usually asymptomatic, needs to be differentiated from hyperkeratotic palmar dermatitis and other forms of symptomatic keratoderma such as psoriasis, lichen planus and pityriasis rubra pilaris.

Treatment of keratoderma climactericum is notoriously difficult; weight reduction and salicylic acid ointments are helpful. Endocrine therapy might be indicated. In one report 0.05% estradiol in a water-in-oil base was successful where keratolytics and emollients had failed[60]. In one reported case of three castrated young women following bilateral oophorectomy the hyperkeratosis resolved completely with conjugated estrogens[56]. Other therapy for keratoderma climactericum includes etretinate (with partial or total remission)[58].

STEWART–TREVES SYNDROME

Stewart–Treves syndrome is a rare form of lymphangiosarcoma that arises in extremities that are chronically lymphadematous. It usually develops on the arms of women who have undergone radical mastectomy – including axillary node dissection – followed by high doses of radiation, but it also occurs in other forms of chronic lymphedema[61,62]. This disease was first reported in 1948 as lymphedema-associated angiosarcoma in the upper limb after radical mastectomy (Stewart–Treves syndrome)[63] but it is also reported in the lower limbs in association with lymphedema of many years duration[64].

The pathogenesis of the tumor cells of Stewart–Treves syndrome is unclear, as illustrated by a woman who presented with clinical signs of it on one side, and mammectomy for carcinoma on the other side, of her body. There has been controversy about whether the cells come from angiosarcoma or metastases from a mammary carcinoma[65]. Other authors think that they may originate either from endothelial cells of blood vessels[66] or from an altered immune surveillance in the lymphedematous region[67].

Although wide excision or radical amputation is recommended for early lesions, surgical treatment is disappointing in the late stage of Stewart–Treves syndrome. Immunotherapy may be a useful adjunct in the treatment[68] and anti-hormone therapy may attenuate the clinical signs in some cases of Stewart–Treves syndrome[69].

REFERENCES

1. Freinkel RK. Cutaneous manifestations of endocrine diseases. In Fitzpatrick TB, Eisen AZ, Wolf K, Freedberg IM, Austen KF, eds. *Dermatology in General Medicine*. New York: McGraw Hill, 1993:2113–31

2. Dewailly D, Vantyghen-Haudiquet MC, Saintara C, *et al*. Clinical and biological phenotypes in late onset 21 hydroxylase deficiency. *J Clin Endocrinol Metab* 1986;63:418–23

3. Merke DP, Cutler GB Jr. New approaches to the treatment of congenital adrenal hyperplasia. *JAMA* 1997;277:1073–6

4. Chryssikopoulos A, Phocas I, Sarandakou A, *et al*. New reliable biochemical marker for screening 21 alpha-hydroxylase deficiency without index person among hirsute women in agreement with HLA-haplotyping. *J Endocrinol Invest* 1995;10:754–61

5. Mercado AB, Wilson RC, Cheng KC, *et al*. Prenatal treatment and diagnosis of congenital adrenal hyperplasia owing to steroid 21 hydroxylase deficiency. *J Clin Endocrinol Metab* 1995;7:2014–20

6. Holmes LB. Congenital malformations. *N Engl J Med* 1976;295:204–9

7. Maclean N, Harnden DG, Court Brown WM. Abnormalities of sex chromosome constitution in newborn babies. *Lancet* 1961;2:406–8

8. Warburton D, Kline J, Stein Z. Monosomy X: a chromosomal anomaly associated with young maternal age. *Lancet* 1980;1:167–9

9. Bowen P. Chromosomal abnormalities. *Clin Orthoped* 1964;3:40–58

10. Grumbach MM, Conte FA. Disorders of sex differentiation. In Williams RH, ed. *Textbook of Endocrinology*. Philadelphia: WB Saunders, 1981:243–67

11. Ashby DIB. *Human Intersex*. Edinburgh: Livingstone, 1962

12. Hall J, Gilchrist D. Turner's syndrome and its variants. *Pediatr Clin North Am* 1990;37:1421–40

13. Becker B, Jospe N, Goldsmith LA. Melanocytic nevi in Turner syndrome. *Pediatr Dermatol* 1994;11:120–4

14. Kerdanet M, Lucas J, Lemee F, *et al*. Turner's syndrome with X-isochromosome and Hashimoto's thyroiditis. *Clin Endocrinol* 1994;41:673–6

15. Tebbe B, Gollnick H, Muller R, *et al*. Alopecia areata and diffuse hypertrichosis associated with Ullrich–Turner syndrome. Report on four patients. *Hautarzt* 1993;44:647–52

16. Runs E, Moreno A, Tellechea O, *et al*. Neonatal lupus erythematosus in an infant with Turner syndrome. *Pediatric Dermatol* 1996;13:298–302

17. Dacou-Voutetakis C, Kakourou T. Psoriasis and blue sclerae in girls with Turner syndrome. *J Am Acad Dermatol* 1996;35:1002–4

18. Gravholt CH, Juul S, Naeraa RW, *et al*. Prenatal and postnatal prevalence of Turner's syndrome: a registry study. *Br Med J* 1996;312:16–21

19. LoPresti P, Papa CM, Kligman AM. Hot comb alopecia. *Arch Dermatol* 1968;98:234–8

20. Price VH. Hair loss in cutaneous disease. In Baden HP, ed. *Symposium on Alopecia*. New York, NY: HP Publishing Co., 1987;6:3–11

21. Sperling LC, Sau P. The follicular degeneration syndrome in black patients. "Hot comb alopecia" revisited and revised. *Arch Dermatol* 1992;128:68–74

22. Halder RM. Hair and scalp disorders in blacks. *Cutis* 1983;32:378–80

23. Sperling LC, Skelton HG, Smith KJ, *et al*. Follicular degeneration syndrome in men. *Arch Dermatol* 1994;130:763–9

24. Bertoloino AP, Freedberg IM. Disorders of epidermal appendages and related diseases. In Fitzpatrick TB, Eisen AZ, Wolf K, Freedberg IM, Austen KF, eds. *Dermatology in General Medicine*. New York: McGraw Hill, 1993:671–96

25. Kubba R, Rook A. The Graham–Little syndrome. Follicular keratosis with cicatricial alopecia. *Br J Dermatol* 1975;93(suppl):53–5

26. Horn RT, Goette DK, Odom RB, *et al*. Immunofluorescent findings and clinical changes in two cases of follicular lichen planus. *J Am Acad Dermatol* 1982;7:203–6

27. Fernandes-Rodrigues JC, Pinto-Soares A, Garcia e Silva L. Psoriase folicular com alopecia cicatricial. Sindrome de Piccardi–Lassueur–Graham Little de natureza psoriasica. *Med Cutan Ibero Lat Am* 1983;11:1–6

28. Hurley H. Jr. Apocrine glands. In Fitzpatrick TB, Eisen AZ, Wolf K, Freedberg IM, Austen KF, eds. *Dermatology in General Medicine*. New York: McGraw Hill, 1993:753–66

29. Ranalletta M, Rositto A, Drut R. Fox–Fordyce in two prepubertal girls: histopathologic demonstration of

eccrine sweat gland involvement. *Pediatr Dermatol* 1996;13:294–7

30. Pasricha JS, Nayyar KC. Fox–Fordyce disease in the post-menopausal period treated successfully with electrocoagulation. *Dermatologica* 1973;147:271–3

31. Osment LS. Fox–Fordyce disease. Self-assessment mini-program. *Int J Dermatol* 1979;18:309–10

32. Miller ML, Harford RR, Yeager JK. Fox–Fordyce disease treated with topical clindamycin solution. *Arch Dermatol* 1995;131:1112–13

33. Effendy I, Ossowski B, Happle R. Fox–Fordyce disease in a male patient – response to oral retinoid treatment. *Clin Exp Dermatol* 1994;19:67–9

34. Graham JH, Shafer JC, Helwig EB. Fox–Fordyce disease in male identical twins. *Arch Dermatol* 1960; 82:212–21

35. Tkach JR. Tretinoin treatment of Fox–Fordyce disease. *Arch Dermatol* 1979;115:1285

36. Giacobeti R, Caro WA, Roenigk HH. Fox–Fordyce disease control with tretinoin cream. *Arch Dermatol* 1979;115:1365–6

37. Shelley WB, Levy EJ. Apocrine sweat retention in man: II. Fox–Fordyce disease (apocrine miliaria). *Arch Dermatol* 1956;73:38–49

38. Turner TW. Hormonal levels in Fox–Fordyce disease. *Br J Dermatol* 1976;94:317–18

39. Feldman R, Masouuye I, Chavaz P, et al. Fox–Fordyce disease: successful treatment with topical clindamycin in alcoholic propylene glycol solution. *Dermatology* 1992;184:310–13

40. Pinkus II. Treatment of Fox–Fordyce disease. *JAMA* 1973;223:924

41. Krane SM, Schiller AL. Disorder of bone and mineral metabolism. Hyperostosis, fibrous dysplasia and other dysplasias of bone and cartilage. In *Harrison's Principles of Internal Medicine*, vol 2 Section 3. McGraw Hill Companies Inc. International Edition, 1998;2271

42. Mallory SB, Khouri SL. Morgagni–Stewart–Morel Syndrome. In *An Illustrated Dictionary of Dermatologic Syndromes*. New York: The Parthenon Publishing Group Inc., 1994;144

43. Franks S. Polycystic ovary syndrome. *N Engl J Med* 1995;333:853–61

44. Waterworth DM, Bennett ST, Gharani N, et al. Linkage and association of insulin gene VNTR regulatory polymorphism with polycystic ovary syndrome. *Lancet* 1997;349:986–90

45. Shelley DR, Dunaif A. Polycystic ovary syndrome. *Cancer* 1990;16:26–34

46. Conway GS, Agrawal R, Betteridge DJ, et al. Risk factors for coronary artery disease in lean and obese women with polycysytic ovary syndrome. *Clin Endocrinol* 1992;37:119–25

47. Sperling LC, Heimer WL. Androgen biology as a basis for the diagnosis and treatment of androgenic disorders in women. I. *J Am Acad Dermatol* 1993;28: 669–83

48. Carey AH, Chan KL, Short F, et al. Evidence for a single gene effect causing polycystic ovaries and male pattern baldness. *Clin Endocrinol* 1993;38:653–8

49. Falsetti L, De-Fusco D, Eleftheriou G, et al. Treatment of hirsutism by finasteride and flutamide in women with polycystic ovary syndrome. *Gynecol Endocrinol* 1997;11:251–7

50. Nakayama H, Harada R, Toda M. Pigmented cosmetic dermatitis. *Int J Dermatol* 1976;15:673–7

51. Mosher DB, Fitzpatrick TB, Ortonne JP, et al. Disorders of melanocytes. In Fitzpatrick TB, Eisen AZ, Wolf K, Freedberg IM, Austen KF, eds. *Dermatology in General Medicine*. New York: McGraw Hill, 1993:903–95

52. Serrano G, Pujol C, Guadra J, et al. Riehl's melanosis: pigmented contact dermatitis caused by fragrances. *J Am Acad Dermatol* 1989;21:1057–60

53. Bose SK, Ortonne JP. Pigmentation: dyschromia. In Baran R, Maibach HI, eds. *Cosmetic Dermatology*. London: Martin Dunitz Ltd., 1994:277–98

54. Ross BS, Levine VJ, Ashinoff R. Laser treatment of acquired vascular lesions. *Dermatol Clin* 1997;15: 385–96

55. Raulin C, Schroeter C, Maushagen SE. Treatment possibilities with a high-energy pulsed light source (PhotoDerm VL). *Hautartz* 1997;48:886–93

56. Wachtel TJ. Plantar and palmar hyperkeratosis in young castrated women. *Int J Dermatol* 1981;20: 270–1

57. Haxthausen H. Keratoderma climactericum. *Br J Dermatol* 1934;6:161–4

58. Deschamps P, Leroy D, Perdailles S, et al. Keratoderma climactericum (Haxthausen disease): clinical signs, laboratory findings and etretinate treatment in 10 patients. *Dermatologica* 1986;172:258–62

59. Laurent R, Prost O, Nicolllier M, et al. Composite keratohyaline granules in palmoplantar keratoderma: an ultrastructural study. *Arch Dermatol Res* 1985;277:384–94

60. Zultak M, Bedeaux C, Blanc D. Keratodermic climactericum treatment with topical oestrogen. *Dermatologica* 1988;176:151–2

61. Woodward AH, Ivins JC, Soule EH. Lymphangiosarcoma arising in chronic lymphedematous extremities. *Cancer* 1972;30:562–72

62. Hultberg BM. Angiosarcomas in chronically lymphedematous extremities. Two cases of Stewart–Treves syndrome. *Am J Dermatopathol* 1987;9:406–12

63. Stewart FW, Treves N. Lymphangiosarcoma in postmastectomy lymphedema. *Cancer* 1948;1:64–81

64. Eby CS, Brennan MJ, Fine G. Lymphangiosarcoma: lethal complication of chronic lymphedema: report of two cases and review of the literature. *Arch Surg* 1967;94:223–30

65. Sigal M, Grossin M, Bilet S, et al. Pseudo-Syndrome de Stewart–Treves par metastases cutaneo-lymphatiques d'un carcinoma mammaire contro-lateral. *Ann Dermatol Venereol* 1987;114:677–83

66. Kanitakis J, Bendelac A, Marchand C, *et al*. Treves syndrome: a histogenetic (ultrastructural and immunohistochemical) study. *J Cutan Pathol* 1986; 13:30–9

67. Schreiber H, Barry FM, Russel WC, *et al*. Stewart–Treves syndrome: a lethal complication of postmastectomy lymphoedema and regional immune deficiency. *Arch Surg* 1979;114:82–5

68. Furue M, Yamada N, Takahashi T, *et al*. Immunotherapy for Stewart–Treves syndrome. *J Am Acad Dermatol* 1994;30:899–903

69. Fabre JF, Schneider NP, Martin PM, *et al*. Dosage et modulation des recepteurs steroidiens cutanes sous therapeutique anti-hormonale dans le cas d'un syndrome de Stewart–Treves. *Ann Dermatol Venereol* 1988;115:1035–9

Diseases of skin structure –
non-hereditary

Disorders of the sebaceous, apocrine and eccrine glands

12

Ethel Tur

INTRODUCTION

Rather than giving an instructional and detailed description of disorders of the sebaceous glands and sweat glands, this chapter will focus on several structural, anatomical, functional, biochemical and pathological aspects of the sebaceous glands and sweat glands as they relate to women. Hormonal differences, as well as genetic differences, affect skin structure and function. As a result, there are variations between women and men, and these variations change with age. In addition, exogenous factors play a role, because they may differ according to differences in lifestyle between the sexes.

STRUCTURE AND FUNCTION OF THE SEBACEOUS GLANDS: DIFFERENCES BETWEEN WOMEN AND MEN

The pilosebaceous unit is composed of the hair follicle and one or more sebaceous glands attached to it. The sebaceous glands are found in most parts of the skin, except the palms and soles. Sebaceous glands are found in greater numbers in the face, scalp and thoracic and anogenital regions. Sebaceous glands are structurally similar, but vary in size, activity and response to trophic agents according to their location in the body, as well as among individuals, ethnic groups, and according to sex and age. At puberty they also develop at the border of the lips, and are more numerous in the upper than in the lower lip. They can also differentiate in other organs, and are present between the lactiferous ducts of the tip of the nipples of both women and men, and in all ages. These are never accompanied by hair follicles. Some have referred to them as specialized sebaceous glands, but there is nothing remarkable about their structure[1]. Melanocytes are present in the sebaceous glands of all women, regardless of age and the intensity of pigmentation of the nipple and areola, but there are none in the glands of men and children. The function of these melanocytes is not known. The sides of the nipple are free of appendages. The nipples and areolae of women, men, girls and boys are qualitatively identical but quantitatively very different. In the areola there are glands of Montgomery (accessory mammary glands), clusters of large sebaceous glands, a few scattered eccrine sweat glands, some apocrine glands (particularly at the periphery), and a few vellus hairs towards the periphery.

Sebaceous glands are well developed and large over the entire surface of the skin at the end of fetal life, but after birth the size rapidly reduces. The sebaceous glands are hormone dependent, and enlarge to become functional again after puberty. The increase in their activity during puberty can be stimulated by the administration of the appropriate hormone. Androgenic steroids, of either gonadal or adrenal origin, have a direct stimulatory effect on sebaceous gland activity. Other hormones play a role too, as illustrated by the estradiol receptor-related protein that was observed in sebaceous glands of the anterior abdominal wall, whose content did not change during the normal menstrual cycle[2]. Most of the hormones – thyroid-stimulating hormone (TSH); adrenocorticotropic hormone (ACTH); follicle-stimulating hormone (FSH); luteinizing hormone (LH) – act indirectly by stimulating their respective endocrine tissues. In other cases the hormones (for instance growth hormone (GH)) act synergistically with another hormone to which the sebaceous gland is sensitive[3]. Sebaceous glands of differing activity vary in their response to hormones[4]. Similarly, the activity of hair follicles depends on the body site. High levels of testosterone inhibit the hair papilla cells and outer root sheath keratinocytes and have a lesser effect on fibroblasts and interfollicular keratinocytes, while low levels of testosterone have no effect. The opposite was found with estrogen and cyproterone[5]. Naturally, the activity of hair follicles has an influence on the sebaceous glands, as they form an integral unit. Androgens regulate sebaceous glands and hair growth by acting on both the epithelial sebocytes of sebaceous glands and the mesenchymal cells of the hair follicle dermal papilla. Androgen receptors have been identified in sebaceous glands, using mouse monoclonal antibodies against the N-terminal region of human androgen receptor[6]. Androgen receptors have also been identified in basal and differentiating sebocytes, and their concentration was found to be higher in males than in females (measured in the temple and forehead regions). They have also been found in pilosebaceous duct keratinocytes, suggesting that androgens influence pilosebaceous duct keratinization.

With aging, sebaceous glands increase in size, but their secretory output is lessened. It has been shown that the average values for sebum secretion are significantly higher in men than in women for the age range 20 to over 69 years, but not for the range 15 to 19 years[7]. This difference in sebaceous gland activity becomes more apparent in the 50 to 70 age range. In this age range the secretion in men remains unaltered, whereas in women there is a significant decrease in sebum output. This decrease is probably a result of decreased ovarian activity, as in women androgen sources for sebaceous gland stimulation are the ovary and adrenal cortex. The correlation between the decrease in sebum excretion in the aged and the decrease in the production of androgens indicates the role of androgens in sebum excretion. Blood levels of testosterone in men decline after the 6th decade but do not fall significantly until approximately the age of 70, corresponding to the drop of sebum excretion rates[8]. After the age of 50 the decrease in sebaceous gland activity occurs in women, 10 to 20 years earlier than in men. Although there is no clear evidence for a specific difference, any possible sex differences in skin function, especially as related to dryness, sensitivity and susceptibility to infection, might stem from decreased sebum. Sustainable rates of sebaceous wax ester secretion have been measured on the forehead of men and women aged 15 to 97. A decline of 23% per decade of sebum secretion in men and 32% per decade in women has been found[9]. Hormones also affect the composition of sebum: beginning in young adulthood there is an age-related decline in the secretion of wax esters. The fatty acid composition of sebum is affected by androgens in both sexes[10].

Circulating androgen levels alone could not account for the difference in the mean levels of excretion between the sexes, as there is a wide degree of overlap between men and women in their sebum excretion rate. Blood testosterone levels of women are one tenth those of men, but in a third of women sebum excretion rates are as high as the mean for men. Although androgens are essential

for providing adult levels of sebum, additional factors are operative[11].

Sebum excretion rate has been shown to be relatively constant during pregnancy. It decreases significantly postpartum, and stays low several months after delivery, indicating an increased rate during pregnancy, which is far too high to be explained by the elevation of temperature during pregnancy[12]. Sebum excretion rates were higher during pregnancy in spite of the fact that estrogens, which inhibit sebum production, are elevated during pregnancy. A sebotrophic factor might provide an explanation.

Both sebaceous glands and sweat glands have a role in the sexuality of women. Estrogens not only prime the central nervous system, acting as neurotrophic and psychotrophic factors throughout life, but they also prime the sensory organs. These include the skin with its sebaceous and sweat glands, which are the key receptors for external sexual stimuli[13].

DISORDERS OF THE SEBACEOUS GLANDS

Acne vulgaris

Acne vulgaris, a disease of the pilosebaceous unit, is the most common dermatologic condition, affecting about 85% of all adolescents. It may affect all ages but has its highest prevalence during the 2nd and 3rd decades of life. Susceptibility is influenced by genetic factors; identical twins, but not non-identical twins, had identical rates of sebum excretion but different acne severity. This indicates a genetic control of sebum excretion with modification of the development of clinical lesions by environmental factors[14]. Some epidemiological data from the seventies are given in Table 1. Since then, improved treatment has modified the clinical picture of acne and its prevalence. Table 2 shows the incidence of severe acne in school-aged boys and girls, as it changed over the years, from 1931 to 1989 (studies were done in different locations). In 1989 none had severe acne, and as few as 1.8% of boys had moderate acne whereas girls had only mild acne.

The primary lesion of acne is a microcomedo. The exact trigger for the formation of a microcomedo is unknown, but certain fractions of the sebum, such as squalene and linoleic acid, play an important role. Active sebaceous glands are needed for the development of acne. A microscopic plug forms owing to an excess of sebum production and an abnormal keratinization of the follicular lining. Accumulation of this material causes distention. In

Table 1 Incidence of acne vulgaris

Age	Reference	Affected men	Affected women	Remarks
16–19	53	35%		peak incidence and severity
14–17	53		40%	peak incidence and severity
12	54	40%	61%	
16	54	95%	83%	
40	55	3%	5%	

Table 2 Incidence of severe acne in schoolchildren

Year of study/ref.	Boys	Girls
1931[56]	57%	19%
1971[53]	30%	20%
1981[57]	35%	13%
1989[54]	none severe, 1.8% moderate	none severe, 0.3% mild

addition, the enlarged pilosebaceous structure allows the normal follicular bacterium *Propionibacterium acnes* to proliferate, releasing free fatty acids, which are inflammatory. The distended follicle may rupture, causing further inflammatory reaction, leading to the formation of papules, pustules, cysts and nodules (Figures 1 and 2). It has been shown that a high rate of sebum secretion is a decisive factor in inflammatory acne, subjects with inflammatory acne having larger secretion rates than controls[15]. Numerous compounds will induce comedones in experimental models. The vigor of the immune response directed against *Propionibacterium acnes* may be the best explanation for the variation in acne severity[16]. The antibody response and cellular response to the bacterium are proportional to the degree of inflammatory acne. Enhancement of the immune response produces an intensification of inflammation and consequently more severe acne.

Neonatal acne

This may appear in the first 6 weeks of life, resolving spontaneously within 1 to 3 months (Figure 3). It is quite common and is not associated with a later development of acne vulgaris. Stimulation of the neonatal sebaceous glands from maternal and infant androgens is believed to be the underlying cause.

Infantile acne

This has its onset at 3 to 6 months and is less common than neonatal acne (Figure 4). Male infants are more frequently affected than female. It is probably associated with a premature secretion of gonadal androgens, and these patients may develop severe acne vulgaris as teenagers.

Acne vulgaris: teenage years

Before and during puberty acne vulgaris may arise as a result of hormonal changes. Boys at this stage are more frequently affected than girls. Adrenal maturation and gonadal development cause androgen production and subsequent sebaceous gland enlargement. Both sebum production and the levels of dehydroepiandrosterone sulfate (DHEAS) increase during puberty[17]. In a study involving 871 girls aged between 10 and 15 years, the severity of acne correlated better with pubertal stage than with chronological age[18]. Testosterone and free testosterone levels had a weak correlation with the severity of acne, whereas DHEAS correlated best. In spite of the possible value of DHEAS for predicting acne severity in the general population, its levels are not predictive for individuals: only 29% of girls with severe acne had DHEAS levels of more than the 90th percentile, and, furthermore, 77% of girls with such high levels did not exhibit severe acne. An enhanced peripheral response is still the accepted explanation, and generally it is not necessary to investigate for an endocrinopathy.

Adult acne

Acne vulgaris resolves slowly after the teenage years. Most teenage boys with acne clear after the age of 20, whereas women may still carry it into adult life. Young adult acne can be a continuation of teenage acne or appear *de novo*. It may differ clinically, showing fewer comedones and more inflammation, affecting most commonly the perioral, chin, and jawline regions. The incidence of mature acne has increased in recent times. Two hundred patients with late-onset acne, with a mean age of 35.5 years (range 25–55) were evaluated[19]. Most had acne persisting from adolescence, but 18% of the women and 8% of the men had late-onset acne. The majority (76%) of patients with post-adolescent acne were women. Of these women, 37% had

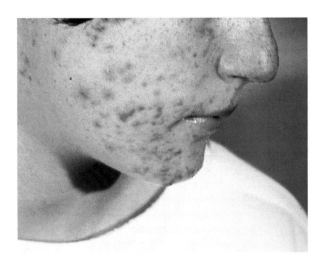

Figure 1 Acne vulgaris. Papules and pustules. Courtesy of Aryeh Metzker, MD, Tel Aviv, Israel

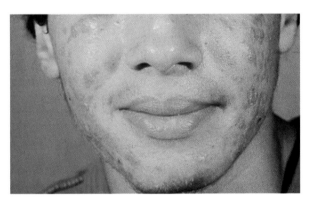

Figure 2 Acne vulgaris. Pustules and cysts. Courtesy of Aryeh Metzker, MD, Tel Aviv, Israel

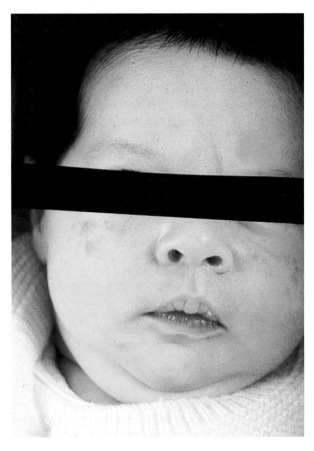

Figure 3 Neonatal acne. Courtesy of Aryeh Metzker, MD, Tel Aviv, Israel

features of hyperandrogenicity. A first degree relative with post-adolescent acne existed in 50% of the patients. External factors including cosmetics, drugs and occupation had no significant etiological role. Most of the patients (82%) failed to respond to multiple courses of antimicrobials, and 32% had relapsed after treatment with one or more courses of isotretinoin.

The majority (60–85% in various series) of women with acne experience a premenstrual flare of their acne. Surface lipid composition and sebum excretion rate show no variation throughout the menstrual cycle. Therefore, the flare is possibly related to a premenstrual change in the hydration of the pilosebaceous epithelium. In agreement with this, up to 15% of acne patients notice deterioration due to sweating, and ductal hydration may be the responsible factor. Cosmetics, drugs and occupation did not play an etiological role. A further clarification was based on measurement of the pilosebaceous duct orifices during the menstrual cycle. This was done to assess keratin hydration, on account of the dermal hydration that was known to exist premenstrually. The duct exit was significantly smaller premenstrually (between days 15 and 20), which might cause an increased resistance to sebum outflow and increased obstruction, leading to aggravation of acne[20]. It is not known why acne resolves or why it is more persistent in females. One study found significantly higher sebum excretion rates among women whose acne persisted from adolescence[21].

Acne cosmetica

Results from the use of cosmetics containing comedogenic substances. It is most commonly found in women aged 20 to 40 years, and resolves with the cessation of the use of the causative agent. Clearance is not instantaneous, but topical treatment with retinoids or benzoyl peroxide is usually successful. Lesions of cosmetic acne occur in the perioral area especially in women who have used cosmetics for a long time, and who had acne in their adolescence. Cosmetics containing lanolin, petrolatum, certain vegetable oils, butylstearate, lauryl alcohol and oleic acid are comedogenic, as shown by the rabbit-ear test.

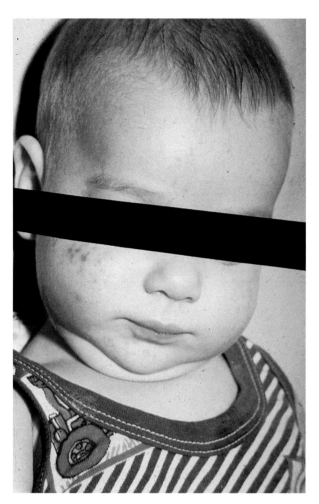

Figure 4   Infantile acne. Courtesy of Aryeh Metzker, MD, Tel Aviv, Israel

One variation of cosmetic acne is pomade acne, caused by the application of greases and oils to the scalp and face by certain ethnic groups. Lesions are non-inflamed and appear around the forehead and other areas where the greasy pomades may reach. Pomade acne occurs almost exclusively in black men.

Other forms of acne

Acne may have various psychological effects, which are an important consideration in establishing treatment even for very mild acne. Several quality of life scales have been developed for this purpose[22]. Acne induces stress, and picking of the spots will aggravate the appearance of the acne patient. This is particularly obvious in young females with acne excoriee. Acne excoriée occurs predominantly in females, and often results from personality or psychological problems. Some patients have virtually no primary acne lesions, others have some lesions.

Acne conglobata and acne fulminans are found predominantly in males.

Among drugs reported to cause acne, those relevant to the issue of women are gonadotropins and anabolic steroids. One study showed that both testosterone and anabolic steroids increased sebum excretion and the surface population of *Propionibacterium acnes* in healthy young men (power athletes)[23]. Moreover, the concentration of the various constituents of skin surface lipids changed: levels of cholesterol and free fatty acids increased. The area of sectioned sebaceous glands enlarged significantly, and the number of both differentiating and undifferentiated cell pools increased significantly after 4 weeks' use of these hormones[24]. Contraceptive pills may also aggravate acne.

Treatments

Treatments aim at controlling some of the pathologic parameters. Topical and systemic treatments are summarized in Tables 3 and 4. Surgical modalities may be employed in the treatment of the depressed scars that can result from acne. These include excision of deeply depressed scars, injections of filler substances such as collagen to depressed scars, dermabrasion, chemical peeling and carbon dioxide laser resurfacing. But the results of these therapies are limited, and they may even cause additional scarring. Pulsed dye lasers may improve both depressed and elevated scars. They may be employed in conjunction with carbon dioxide laser resurfacing, which acts well on atrophic acne scars.

Retinoids

A major breakthrough in acne treatment was achieved in 1982 with the introduction of oral isotretinoin. It battles acne on all fronts, as it reduces sebum secretion, regulates epithelial differentiation and has an anti-inflammatory effect. Teratogenicity is a well-documented systemic adverse effect of oral retinoids. Therefore, the duration of the post-therapy contraceptive period is an important safety consideration when treating women of childbearing potential with isotretinoin. Initially, the calculation of this period was based on calculating the pharmacokinetic parameters for the elimination of isotretinoin and its metabolites. Recently, knowledge about endogenous isotretinoin concentrations during early pregnancy has been used. Because isotretinoin and its metabolites are vitamin A metabolites, they are endogenous physiologic compounds. Thus, after isotretinoin therapy, the time required to reduce plasma concentrations from therapeutic levels to endogenous levels was

Table 3　Topical treatment for acne vulgaris

Treatment	Anticomedonal	Anti-inflammatory	Antimicrobial	Adverse effects: irritation
Retinoids: tretinoin, isotretinoin, microencapsulated tretinoin (less irritating), adapalene, tazarotene (higher stability)	+	+		+
Benzoyl peroxide	minimal	+	+	+
Topical antibiotics	indirect	+	+	
Benzoyl peroxide/erythromycin			+	
Erythromycin/zinc			+	
Azelaic acid (slow onset of action)	+		+	+
Salicylic acid	+			
Metronidazole		+		
Steroids in acne fulminans		+		

Table 4　Systemic treatment for acne vulgaris

Treatment	Anticomedonal	Sebum suppression	Anti-inflammatory	Antimicrobial
Retinoids	+	+	+	secondary to decrease of sebum
Estrogens		+	possible	
Antiandrogens (cyproterone acetate, spironolactone)		+		
Antimicrobials			+	+
Steroids			+	

assessed[25]. The metabolite with the longest elimination half-life (oxo-isotretinoin) reached non-teratogenic physiologic plasma concentrations after less than 2 weeks. The post-therapy contraceptive period of 1 month then proved to be adequate.

Topical all-trans retinoic acid, or tretinoin, is effective for the treatment of acne. It influences desquamation of abnormal epithelium, alters the microclimate of the microcomedo, and enhances penetration of other drugs, such as antimicrobial agents. It is widely used by young women, and therefore the question of its association with an increased risk of congenital malformations is very important. Topical tretinoin has minimal percutaneous penetration: only about 2% is absorbed both after a single dose and after 4 weeks of daily application, and absorption is even lower on long-term therapy of over 1 year[26]. Maximal concentrations of percutaneously absorbed tretinoin are approximately 100-fold lower than endogenous concentrations. The absorbed levels are so low that they do not change the endogenous concentrations of the retinoids as compared to pretreatment measurements. Hence, there is no systemic risk from commercially available topical preparations of

tretinoin. Although it is classified as pregnancy category C, the lack of effect on plasma levels indicates its safety of use during pregnancy. Topical retinoids were considered as photosensitizing agents, but the data supporting this assumption are frail. Adapalene and tazaroten are newer retinoids with higher stability, that are less irritating. But there are also differences between the irritation potential of the different topical tretinoin preparations, some of which, like a microsphere gel formulation, are only minimally irritating.

Rosacea

Rosacea is a chronic inflammatory disease of unknown etiology, usually affecting only the face (its blush areas – nose, cheeks, chin, central area of forehead) and occasionally the neck and upper trunk. It evolves through three stages: persistent flushing[27], papulopustules with telangiectasia (Figure 5), and rhinophyma (hypertrophy of sebaceous glands and soft tissue). The first stage predominantly afflicts women; the third stage is limited to men[28]. The skin lesions are notable for the absence of comedones, which distinguishes this disorder from acne vulgaris. Ultraviolet light plays a role in rosacea, as well as alcohol and extreme hot or cold temperatures. Ocular disorders, mainly conjunctivitis and rarely keratitis, occasionally accompany rosacea. The presence of pronounced sebaceous gland hypertrophy in rhinophyma has resulted in the hypothesis that rosacea is a sebaceous gland disease. However, sebaceous gland hypertrophy is not a typical feature of early rosacea lesions. On the other hand, meibomitis is a frequent accompaniment of rosacea, and a diffuse sebaceous gland abnormality has been suggested as the cause of meibomitis.

Treatment includes avoiding exposure to sunlight and extreme temperatures, topical and oral metronidazole and topical and oral antibiotics. Clonidine may also be of some value in reducing facial flushing. Telangiectasis may be treated by electrocautery or by dye laser. Rhinophyma may be treated by various laser modalities.

Sebaceous gland hyperplasia

In middle-aged or elderly people the sebaceous glands may become prominent, appearing as 1 to 3 mm papules of yellow or pink color on the forehead or temples. Sebaceous gland hyperplasia is of no clinical significance, but is associated with chronic sun damage. Its incidence is higher in heart transplant recipients receiving cyclosporine: 16% of 104 such patients had sebaceous hyperplasia in comparison with 1% of a control group[29]. It was not connected with hypertrichosis, as patients with sebaceous hyperplasia did not have a significantly higher incidence of hypertrichosis than those without sebaceous hyperplasia. In hypertrichosis it is accepted that the pilosebaceous unit is the target of the direct effect of cyclosporine, whereas the development of sebaceous hyperplasia might be related to the process of dysplastic epithelial proliferation in transplant recipients.

Ectopic sebaceous glands

Called Fordyce spots, these are present in 25% of the population over the age of 35 years. They are commonly seen in the mouth as multiple, symmetrical, slightly elevated, discrete, yellow papules (Figure 6). They may occur in the areolae and penile shaft.

SWEAT GLANDS

The eccrine sweat glands are not associated with hair follicles, whereas the apocrine glands are. There are 2 to 4 million eccrine glands over the body, with greater concentrations in the palms and soles and in the forehead. Only the glans penis, clitoris, labia minora and the inner surface of the prepuce lack eccrine glands. The eccrine sweat glands are of major importance to the body's thermal regulation through evaporation of sweat. Their function in excreting waste products is of minor significance. The sweating process is continuous, with a large output that can reach several liters per hour. In addition to induction by heat, sweating may also be induced by emotional stress, when it is confined to the palms, axillae, soles and forehead.

The apocrine glands are mainly located in the axillary and genital areas. In the embryo they are present over the entire skin surface, but most of them subsequently disappear, so that in the adult they are found in the axillae, perianal region and areolae of the breasts. Ectopic glands may appear elsewhere. The mammary glands and the glands of the external auditory meatus are modified apocrine glands. The activity of the apocrine glands is androgen dependent; they are poorly developed in childhood, and begin to enlarge before puberty. Their duct usually opens into the hair follicle above the entrance of the sebaceous glands, but some ducts open directly upon the surface of the skin. Physiologically the apocrine glands are not as important as the eccrine glands, and their secretion produces the repulsive odor that people are constantly trying to eliminate. This odorous secretion might have played a role in the chemical communication of early man, in analogy with the way animals attract or repel. There are researchers who maintain that odors are still significant for human reproduction, based on a mutual pheromonal influence between the sexes[30]. Male sweat pheromones (androstenol/androstenone) have a direct impact on female menstrual cycles and ovulation. Furthermore, female pheromones (copulins), which are present in vaginal secretions, influence male perception of females and may induce hormonal changes in men. The eccrine glands may also produce unpleasant odors owing to bacterial decomposition of the sweat, especially in the soles of the feet and intertriginous areas. Treatment consists of antiperspirants, which attempt to eliminate the cause, and fragrances, which attempt to mask the result. Antiperspirants usually contain aluminum salts, which suppress sweat production. Deodorants, which may contain mild antibacterials such as triclosan, are usually perfumed. For palmoplantar hyperhidrosis, tap water iontophoresis may be beneficial, or iontophoresis with anticholinergic drugs. Other

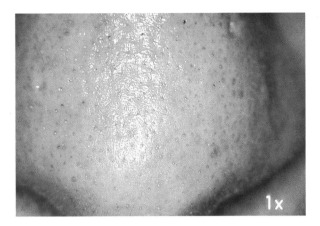

Figure 5   Rosacea, 2nd stage: papulopustules with telangiectasia

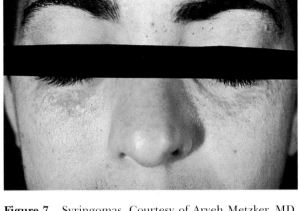

Figure 7   Syringomas. Courtesy of Aryeh Metzker, MD, Tel Aviv, Israel

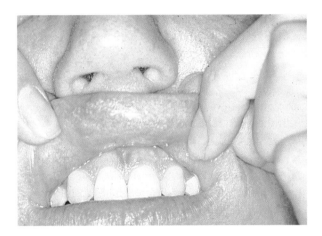

Figure 6   Fordyce spots

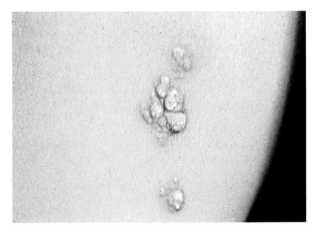

Figure 8   Syringocystadenoma papilliferum. Courtesy of Aryeh Metzker, MD, Tel Aviv, Israel

treatments, including botulinum toxin, have recently been reviewed[31]. Eccrine sweat may also gain odor owing to the excretion of certain foods and drugs, such as garlic and alcohol, and certain metabolites (like trimethylamine producing a 'fish odor') secreted in various heritable amino-acidurias.

Differences between men and women

Men have fewer eccrine and apocrine sweat glands. Pubertal sweating is more pronounced on the hands and feet of girls than boys. Eccrine secretion of men is more acid than women, with a pH about 0.5 lower. The rate of sweating in men is more than double than that in women[32]. The pilocarpine iontophoresis test showed differences between men and women[33]. Men showed higher sweat secretion rates than women, and this was true in children before and after puberty and was even more pronounced in adults. In addition, the change in sweat excretion rate from childhood to adulthood showed a gender variation. Boys (both prepubertal and pubertal) had

a lower secretion value than adult men, whereas girls showed higher secretion values than adult women. For both sexes sweat secretion rates increased significantly from prepuberty to puberty. Sweating in children was dependent on growth hormone. Similarly, sweating following pilocarpine iontophoresis measured in healthy and chronic renal-failure subjects, aged 18–75 years, revealed higher rates in men than in women in both subject groups[18].

It has been shown that women have a significantly greater sweat gland density, whereas men have a greater sweat production per gland[34]. Cholinergic-induced sweat rate was more than double in men than in women. Topical or intradermal administration of androgen did not stimulate sweat production in adult women[32]. Moreover, anti-androgens did not decrease sweat rate in men. It was concluded that the sweat rate in men is caused by androgen-induced gene expression at puberty and not by androgen modulation in adult life.

Androgen receptors were identified in luminal epithelial cells of apocrine glands in genital skin and in certain cells of the secretory coils of eccrine sweat glands in all body sites[35]. Aging causes a reduction in the number of eccrine glands, and both the eccrine and apocrine glands undergo attenuation.

A morphometric study of the distribution of hair and sweat glands of adult Koreans showed that the soles in men and palms in women were the regions of most densely distributed sweat glands, while the mammary area in both men and women was the region of lowest density[36]. Furthermore, seven regions of the body exhibited significant sexual dimorphism in terms of the density of sweat glands, and four showed dimorphism of the density of hairs.

An important consideration in women is the menstrual cycle. For example, during the luteal phase the chest sweat rate in response to heat was enhanced as related to the mean body temperature[37]. A study of perimenopausal women revealed that sweat production upon psychological stimulation decreased significantly after menopause[38]. The same study also found that after menopause the sebum content of the forehead decreased significantly, but that of the subocular region remained unchanged.

The concentration of secretory immunoglobulin A, which plays an important role in local immune defense mechanisms, was 10 times higher in men than in women. This was measured by enzyme immunoassay in the sweat glands of human axillary skin. The secretory component was localized in the terminal segment of eccrine sweat glands, and was not found in apocrine sweat glands. Hence, the IgA in sweat emerges from the eccrine sweat glands[39].

Non-neoplastic disorders of the eccrine glands

Hyperhidrosis

Hyperhidrosis represents an increased production and secretion of sweat, and most commonly affects the axillae, palms and soles. It may be primary or secondary to a number of conditions, among which is menopause, which may cause generalized hyperhidrosis. Hyperhidrosis of the feet occurs mainly in young adult men.

Syringomas

Syringoma is a quite common benign tumor of eccrine origin which derives from the eccrine ducts.

Although the variety localized on the eyelids in middle-aged women is the most frequent, many other clinical variants, differing in age of onset, location and clinical aspect, have been reported in the literature. Four principal clinical variants may be distinguished: a localized form, a familial form, a form associated with Down's syndrome, and a generalized form that encompasses multiple and eruptive syringomas[40]. Syringomas are more common in women (Figure 7). Hormonal influence is indicated by their proliferation at puberty, and by their increase in size during pregnancy and the premenstrual period. Immunohistochemical evidence supports such a hormonal control: in one study intense nuclear and cytoplasmic staining for progesterone was noted in 80% of the neoplastic cells in 8 out of 9 syringoma cases (some staining for estrogen was noted in one of the 9 cases)[41].

Non-neoplastic disorders of the apocrine glands

Hidradenitis suppurativa

Hidradenitis suppurativa is a chronic relapsing disease of apocrine gland-bearing areas, occurring in the axillary, inguinal, perianal and perineal regions, and infrequently in the breast areola. It is a disorder of the larger follicles, which include apocrine glands, and is characterized by chronic discharging abscesses and sinuses. As the disease advances, eccrine sweat glands are also involved. There is a female preponderance, the ratio between women and men being 13:5. The onset of the disease occurs after puberty, reaching a maximum during the third decade of life. All these indicate a hormonal basis. In addition, 57% of affected women experienced premenstrual flares[42]. Absence of this flare was associated with irregular menses. Patients without premenstrual flare showed a relative androgen excess and decreased progesterone levels. Enhanced peripheral androgen conversion by apocrine tissue was a possible explanation for normal serum androgen profiles in patients with a flare. Some studies have indicated an androgenic basis for the disease[43], but others found no difference between affected women and a control group: hidradenitis was not accompanied by any other signs of androgenization. The only significant differences were a shorter menstrual cycle and a longer duration of menstrual flow in the women with hidradenitis, and a higher proportion of a family history of hidradenitis[44].

Hidradenitis suppurativa is difficult to treat. Treatment includes hormonal regimens or long-term high-dose antibiotics such as minocycline. Oral isotretinoin may be tried in non-responders, but the response to isotretinoin is variable. Sometimes surgical treatment may be employed.

Multiple hidrocystomas of the face (Robinson type)

This is an uncommon variant of hidrocystoma consisting of multiple cysts of the face of middle-aged women with exacerbation in high temperatures. There is controversy about the eccrine or apocrine nature of the lesions, but recent evidence suggests that they are apocrine hidrocystomas in which characteristic 'decapitation' secretion has been effaced by the pressure of cyst contents against the lining epithelium. Serial sections have allowed identification of some areas of the cyst lining showing apocrine secretion in the luminal border of columnar cells[45].

Fox–Fordyce disease

Fox–Fordyce disease is a disorder of unknown etiology, caused by obstruction of the sweat duct of the apocrine glands (apocrine miliaria). It is predominantly observed in women, and occurs soon after puberty, but can be postmenopausal. It sometimes occurs in males and in children. It may be accompanied by intense itching in the axillae, and to a lesser extent in the anogenital region and around the breasts. The itching may be provoked by emotional stimuli which cause apocrine secretion. At first no lesions are clinically evident, but later skin colored or slightly pigmented follicular papules develop. Histologically, a small vesicle is seen in the apocrine duct, which progresses into an inflammatory lesion, followed by rupture and plugging of the duct. An accompanying involvement of eccrine sweat glands, as seen histologically, has been described[46].

Treatments include topical steroids, clindamycin or retinoic acid, ultraviolet irradiation, oral contraceptives and oral retinoids[47]. Some cases require surgical excision of the affected skin or subcutaneous removal of the apocrine glands. The response to treatment is unsatisfactory, and the disease runs a very prolonged course and may persist until menopause. Pregnancy may induce some remission.

Axillary bromhidrosis

Axillary bromhidrosis, or osmidrosis, is mainly determined by apocrine gland secretion (as discussed above), although sebaceous secretion also has some odor, as well as decomposition products of keratinization and, under certain conditions, eccrine secretion. A recent study of enzyme activity in skin appendages indicates that both apocrine and sebaceous glands are capable of sequestering dietary cholesterol and fatty acids, holding important implications for the understanding of both acne and axillary odor[48]. Axillary bromhidrosis is a distressing problem, especially in Asian societies. Surgical excision might help alleviate the problem, or the recently described superficial liposuction with subdermal scraping under local anesthesia with tumescent infiltration. Significantly more women seek surgical treatment than men, as reflected in the publication describing the latter procedure[49].

Benign tumors of sweat glands

Most adnexal tumors appear as papules on the face, scalp and neck. The most common are syringomas; others are syringocystadenoma papilliferum (Figure 8), eccrine acrospiroma, and eccrine and apocrine hidrocystomas. Apocrine hidrocystomas of the anal glands, similar to the better known cutaneous hidrocystomas of other sites that contain apocrine glands, have been described in women, in addition to the rare adenoma of the apocrine anal glands[50].

Malignant tumors of sweat glands

Eccrine porocarcinoma is a rare tumor that occurs in the elderly and affects men more frequently than women. The leg is the most common site. The tumor may develop from a pre-existing benign poroma[51]. Primary adenocarcinoma of sweat glands is a rare tumor, with no gender predilection[52].

CONCLUSIONS

A full account of sebaceous and sweat gland disorders is beyond the scope of this chapter which, however, reflects the multitude of anatomical, physiological, biochemical and clinical studies conducted in this field; many more are currently under way. It also reflects the essential symbiosis of both clinical and laboratory research. The accomplishments are enormous, both in understanding the physiological and pathological processes occurring in the sebaceous and sweat systems, and in developing appropriate treatments. This is illustrated by the discovery of retinoids, which offered a major breakthrough in this direction. But even in this context of acne treatment, the future should carry better agents. Such agents might interfere with hormone synthesis or block the active androgen metabolites that stimulate the pilosebaceous apparatus, or otherwise revolutionize our whole approach in a yet unknown manner.

REFERENCES

1. Montagna W. Histology and cytochemistry of human skin. XXXV. The nipple and areola. *Br J Dermatol* 1970;83(suppl):2–13
2. Fraser D, Padwick ML, Whitehead M, *et al*. Presence of an oestradiol receptor-related protein in the skin: changes during the normal mestrual cycle. *Br J Obstet Gynaecol* 1991;98:1277–82
3. Tur E. Physiology of the skin – differences between women and men. *Clin Dermatol* 1997;15:5–16
4. Agache P, Blanc D. Current status in sebum knowledge. *Int J Dermatol* 1982;21:304–15
5. Kiesewetter F, Arai A, Schell H. Sex hormones and antiandrogens influence *in vitro* growth of dermal papilla cells and outer root sheath keratinocytes of human hair follicles. *J Invest Dermatol* 1993;101:98S–105S
6. Choudhry R, Hodgins MB, Van der Kwast TH, *et al*. Localization of androgen receptors in human skin by immunohistochemistry: implications for the hormonal regulation of hair growth, sebaceous glands and sweat glands. *J Endocrinol* 1992;133:467–75
7. Pochi PE, Strauss JS. Endocrinologic control of the development and activity of the human sebaceous gland. *J Invest Dermatol* 1974;62:191–201
8. Pochi PE, Strauss JS, Downing DT. Age-related changes in sebaceous gland activity. *J Invest Dermatol* 1979;73:108–11
9. Jacobsen E, Billings JK, Frantz RA, *et al*. Age-related changes in sebaceous wax ester secretion rates in men and women. *J Invest Dermatol* 1985;85:483–5
10. Yamamoto A, Serizawa S, Ito M, Sato Y. Fatty acid composition of sebum wax esters and urinary androgen level in normal human individuals. *J Dermatol Sci* 1990;1:269–76
11. Downing DT, Stewart ME, Strauss JS. Changes in sebum secretion and the sebaceous gland. *Dermatol Clin* 1986;4:419–23
12. Burton JL, Cunliffe WJ, Millar DG, Shuster S. Effect of pregnancy on sebum excretion. *Br Med J* 1970;2:769–71
13. Graziottin A. The biological basis of female sexuality. *Int Clin Psychopharmacol* 1998;13(suppl 6):S15–22
14. Walton S, Wyatt EH, Cunliffe WJ. Genetic control of sebum excretion and acne – a twin study. *Br J Dermatol* 1988;118:393–6
15. Harris HH, Downing DT, Stewart ME, Strauss JS. Sustainable rates of sebum secretion in acne patients and matched normal control subjects. *J Am Acad Dermatol* 1983;8:200–3
16. Webster GF. Topical tretinoin in acne therapy. *J Am Acad Dermatol* 1998;39:S38–44
17. White GM. Recent findings in the epidemiologic evidence, classification, and subtypes of acne vulgaris. *J Am Acad Dermatol* 1998;39:S34–7
18. Lucky AW, Biro FM, Simbartl LA, *et al*. Predictors of severity of acne vulgaris in young adolescent girls: results of a five-year longitudinal study. *J Pediatr* 1997;130:30–9
19. Goulden V, Clark SM, Cunliffe WJ. Post-adolescent acne: a review of clinical features. *Br J Dermatol* 1997;136:66–70
20. Williams M, Cunliffe WJ. Explanation for premenstrual acne. *Lancet* 1973;2:1055–7
21. McGeown CH, Goulden V, Holland DB, *et al*. Sebum excretion rate in post-adolescent acne compared to controls and adolescent acne [Abstract]. *J Invest Dermatol* 1997;108:386
22. Gupta MA, Johnson AM, Gupta AK. The development of an acne quality of life scale: reliability, validity, and relation to subjective acne severity in mild to moderate acne vulgaris. *Acta Derm Venereol (Stockh)* 1998;78:451–6
23. Kiraly CL, Alen M, Korvola J, Horsmanheimo M. The effect of testosterone and anabolic steroids on the skin surface lipids and the population of *Propionibacteria acnes* in young postpubertal men. *Acta Derm Venereol (Stockh)* 1988;68:21–6
24. Kiraly CL, Collan Y, Alen M. Effect of testosterone and anabolic steroids on the size of sebaceous glands in power athletes. *Am J Dermatopathol* 1987;9:515–19
25. Wiegand UW, Chou RC. Pharmacokinetics of oral isotretinoin. *J Am Acad Dermatol* 1998;39:S8–12
26. Shapiro SS, Latriano L. Pharmacokinetics and pharmacodynamic considerations of retinoids: tretinoin. *J Am Acad Dermatol* 1998;39:S13–16
27. Tur E, Ryatt KS, Maibach HI. Idiopathic recalcitrant facial flushing syndrome. *Dermatologica* 1990;181:5–7
28. Kligman AM. Actinic rhinophyma: an old disorder with a new name. *Cutis* 1996;57:389–92
29. de Berker DAR, Taylor AE, Quinn AG, Simpson NB. Sebaceous hyperplasia in organ transplant recipients: shared aspects of hyperplastic and dysplastic processes? *J Am Acad Dermatol* 1996;35:696–9
30. Grammer K, Jutte A. Battle of odors: significance of pheromones for human reproduction. *Gynakol Geburtschilfiche Rundsch* 1997;37:150–3
31. Stolman LP. Treatment of hyperhidrosis. *Dermatol Clin* 1998;4:863–7
32. Rees J, Shuster S. Pubertal induction of sweat gland activity. *Clin Sci* 1981;60:689–92
33. Main K, Nilsson KO, Skakkebaek NE. Influence of sex and growth hormone deficiency on sweating. *Scand J Clin Lab Invest* 1991;51:475–80
34. Buono MJ, Sjoholm NT. Effect of physical training on peripheral sweat production. *J Appl Physiol* 1988;65:811–14
35. Hodgins MB, Spike RC, Mackie RM, MacLean AB. An immunohistochemical study of androgen,

oestrogen and progesterone receptors in the vulva and vagina. *Br J Obstet Gynaecol* 1998;105:216–22

36. Hwang K, Baik SH. Distribution of hairs and sweat glands on the bodies of Korean adults: a morphometric study. *Acta Anat* 1997;158:112–20

37. Hessemer V, Bruck K. Influence of menstrual cycle on shivering, skin blood flow, and sweating responses measured at night. *J Appl Physiol* 1985;59:1902–10

38. Ohta H, Makita K, Kawashima T, *et al*. Relationship between dermato-physiological changes and hormonal status in pre, peri, and postmenopausal women. *Maturitas* 1998;30:55–62

39. Okada T, Konishi H, Ito M, *et al*. Identification of secretory immunoglobulin A in human sweat and sweat glands. *J Invest Dermatol* 1988;90:648–51

40. Patrizi A, Neri I, Marzaduri S, *et al*. Syringoma: a review of twenty-nine cases. *Acta Dermatol Venereol* 1998;78:460–2

41. Wallace ML, Smoller BR. Progesterone receptor positivity supports hormonal control of syringomas. *J Cutan Pathol* 1995;22:442–5

42. Harrison BJ, Read GF, Hughes LE. Endocrine basis for the clinical presentation of hidradenitis suppurativa. *Br J Surg* 1988;75:972–5

43. Mortimer PS, Dawber RP, Gales MA, Moore RA. Mediation of hidradenitis suppurativa by androgens. *Br Med J Clin Res Ed* 1986;292:245–8

44. Jemec GB. The symptomatology of hidradenitis suppurativa in women. *Br J Dermatol* 1988;119:345–50

45. Farina MC, Pique E, Olivares M, *et al*. Multiple hidrocystoma of the face: three cases. *Clin Exp Dermatol* 1995;20:323–7

46. Ranalletta M, Rositto A, Drut R. Fox–Fordyce disease in two prepubertal girls: histopathologic demonstration of eccrine sweat gland involvement. *Pediatr Dermatol* 1996;13:294–7

47. Effendy I, Ossowski B, Happle R. Fox–Fordyce disease in a male patient – response to oral retinoid treatment. *Clin Exp Dermatol* 1994;19:67–9

48. Smythe CD, Greenall M, Kealey T. The activity of HMG-CoA reductase and acetyl-CoA carboxylase in human apocrine sweat glands, sebaceous glands, and hair follicles is regulated by phosphorylation and by endogenous cholesterol. *J Invest Dermatol* 1998;111:139–48

49. Ou LF, Yan RS, Chen IC, Tang YW. Treatment of axillary bromhidrosis with superficial liposuction. *Plast Reconstr Surg* 1998;102:1479–85

50. von Seebach HB, Stumm D, Misch P, von Seebach A. Hidrocystoma and adenoma of apocrine anal glands. *Virchows Arch Pathol Anat* 1980;386:231–7

51. Snow SN, Reizner GT. Eccrine porocarcinoma of the face. *J Am Acad Dermatol* 1992;27:306–11

52. Yugueros P, Kane WJ, Goellner JR. Sweat gland carcinoma: a clinicopathologic analysis of an expanded series in a single institution. *Plast Reconstr Surg* 1998;102:705–10

53. Burton JL, Cunliffe WJ, Stafford I, Shuster S. The prevalence of acne vulgaris in adolescence. *Br J Dermatol* 1971;85:119–26

54. Rademaker M, Garioch JJ, Simpson NB. Acne in schoolchildren: no longer a concern for dermatologists. *Br Med J* 1989;298:1217–19

55. Cunliffe WJ, Gould DJ. Prevalence of facial acne vulgaris in late adolescence and in adults. *Br Med J* 1979;1:1109–10

56. Bloch B. Metabolism, endocrine glands and skin diseases, with special reference to acne vulgaris and xanthoma. *Br J Dermatol* 1931;43:61–87

57. Fellows HM, Billewicz WZ, Thomson AM. Is acne a sign of normal puberty? A longitudinal study. *J Biosoc Sci* 1981;13:401–7

Nail disorders

13

Robert Baran

INTRODUCTION

The nail plate emerges from beneath the proximal nail fold, which adheres closely to the nail for a short distance and forms a gradually desquamating tissue, the cuticle, which seals the cul-de-sac (Figure 1). The nail plate protects the pink nail bed and the half-moon shaped white lunula which represents the distal portion of the matrix from which the nail is derived. The proximal nail fold is continuous with the similarly structured lateral nail fold on each side. The shape of the fingernail differs conspicuously between the sexes. Women's nails are more elongated than their male counterparts; men's nails tend to be broader. A British study of 9-year-old children's feet found that 25% of girls compared with 1% of boys wear unsuitable shoes; in particular the shoes are too narrow at the toes. Compared to men, women often present with the nail fragility syndrome in the fingers and with marked dystrophies related to microtrauma to the toenails. Women's nails are vulnerable to:

(1) daily chores;

(2) cosmetic procedures;

(3) repeated microtrauma;

(4) menstruation;

(5) the contraceptive pill; and

(6) pregnancy.

Finally, congenital drug-induced nail changes and congenital cutaneous candidosis can affect new borns. The terms used in this chapter are shown in Table 1.

NAIL DISORDERS RELATED TO DAILY CHORES

The nail plate takes a minimum of 5 months to regenerate; however, it is vulnerable to daily insults. The nail may be damaged by repeated trauma or by chemical agents, such as detergents, alkalis, various solvents and, especially, hot water. The housewife is very susceptible. Particularly at risk are the first three fingers of the dominant hand which may show four main types of brittle nails[1]:

(1) An isolated split at the free edge which sometimes extends proximally. This may result from onychorrhexis with shallow parallel furrows running in the superficial layer of the nail (Figure 2);

(2) Multiple, crenellated splitting which resembles the battlements of a castle. Triangular pieces may easily be torn away from the free margin (Figure 3);

(3) Lamellar splitting into fine layers of the free edge of the nail (Figure 4). This may occur alone or associated with the other types; and

(4) Transverse splitting and breaking of the lateral edge close to the distal margin.

Management of brittle nails requires preventive and protective measures to avoid quick nail plate dehydration. Affected individuals should wear cotton gloves beneath plastic gloves during household tasks, avoid repeated immersion in soap and water and keep their nails short. Frequent application of topical preparations containing hydrophilic substances may favor nail plate rehydration.

NAIL DISORDERS RELATED TO COSMETIC PROCEDURES

Cosmetic procedures may produce reactions to nail, which can be divided into two main sections[2] – reactions to cosmetics applied to the nail and nail instrument damage.

Reactions to cosmetics applied to the nail

These encompass reactions both at the site of application to the nail area and secondarily elsewhere, as the finger nails act as a reservoir for small amounts of cosmetic preparations that can be transferred

Table 1 Glossary of terms used in this chapter

Term	Meaning
Beau's line	transverse groove
Onycholysis	separation of nail from its bed
Onychorrhexis	shallow parallel longitudinal furrows
Onychoschizia	splitting of nails into layers

by the hand to other areas of skin, especially the eyelids. In addition to ectopic dermatitis, allergic airborne contact dermatitis caused by nail polish ingredients should be suspected when lesions on the face, neck and ears are symmetrical.

Fingernail coatings consist of 2 types: first, coatings that harden upon evaporation. These products include nail polishes, top coats and base coats. The possible appearance of nail plate staining (Figure 5), commonly yellow-orange in color, and superficial friability as keratin granulation should be mentioned. Second, coatings that polymerize. Nail enhancements are a special type of coating used to create artificial fingernails.

Sculptured artificial nails

Liquid and powder systems are based on the methacrylates. They consist of a liquid monomer (ethyl methacrylate) mixed with a polymer powder (polyethyl and/or polymethyl methacrylate) (Figure 6). The latter carries only the heat sensitive initiator (usually benzoyl peroxide) to the monomer. UV absorbers are polymer additives which prevent yellowing owing to exposure to sunlight. Catalysts speed up polymerization.

Light cured gels

UV or visible light-curing gels are made primarily of urethane acrylate and other acrylated oligomers. Associated with initiator, the catalyst and oligomers are combined into a single product; they come premixed and ready to use. They may be considered as a variant of sculptured artificial nails.

Preformed artificial nails

Usually made of ABS plastic, nylon or acetate these are stuck to the natural nail with cyanoacrylate monomer. Home use, retail versions of these tips may be used as temporary natural overlays, not worn for longer than 48 hours on any one occasion. They are more often used as permanent nail tip extensions. Professional nail technicians usually coat these tips with artificial nail products to create longer lasting nail extensions. Most nail technicians feel it is too time consuming to sculpt nails and these tips speed the process. The tip can be coated or overlaid with wraps (liquid and powder or gel products).

Wraps

Wraps can be used to coat the nail plate or add strength to thin, weak nails. The monomers used to create wraps are cyanoacrylates. In nail wrapping, the free edge of the nail should be long enough to be splinted by the various types of fabrics providing support and added strength to the coating. There are three fabrics in wide use – fiberglass, silk and linen.

No-light gels

These products are wrap monomers that have been thickened to have a gel-like appearance. They should be used and handled as any other wrap product.

Details of the different types of adverse reactions due to polymerized coatings are given in specialized publications[2,3]. Such reactions may occur 2–4 months, and even as long as 16 months, after the first application. The first indication is an itch in the nail bed. Paronychia, which is usually present in allergic reactions, is associated with excruciating pain in the nail area and sometimes with paresthesia. The nail bed is dry, thickened, and there is usually onycholysis. The natural nail plate becomes thinner, split and sometimes discolored. It takes several months for the nails to return to normal. Permanent nail loss is exceptional, as is intractable prolonged paraesthesia. Distant allergic contact dermatitis may affect the face and the eyelids and is probably caused by touching the face with the hands.

Instrument nail damage

The most important adverse nail and skin reactions to nail cosmetic practices are trauma and infection. Traumatic injuries from nail files, orange sticks etc. may cause not only infection, but onycholysis (Figure 7), Beau's lines and transverse white streaks may be produced by over-zealous manicuring.

NAIL DISORDERS RELATED TO REPEATED MICROTRAUMA

Improper shoe fitting started in childhood often continues into adult life. Women constantly wear shoes that are smaller than their feet. Repeated or cumulative minor injury to the toenail is a cause of onychodystrophy usually produced by shoes worn by fashion conscious women and where faulty ambulatory biomechanics plays a prominent role[4]. Poorly fitting shoes and/or abnormal biomechanics play a role in common abnormalities of the gait cycle. Hallux nail pathology appears to be the most common functional and traumatic disorder. The dystrophies encountered involve different types of alterations to the surrounding tissue of the nail.

Subungual hemorrhages, usually painless, often result from the second toe overriding the lateral aspect of the hallux. It may also produce an associated onycholysis. Hyperkeratotic changes (usually distal subungual corn or heloma, but also lateral nail fold or lateral groove onychophosis) may accompany this pathology. Ingrowing toenail has three main presentations. First, subcutaneous ingrowing toenail, which is created by impingement of the nail plate into the lateral nail fold. Second, is pincer nail with asymmetrical involvement of the halluces, the major cause being foot deformities and osteoarthritis. Third, there is hypertrophy of the lateral lip which accompanies long-standing ingrown nails. In addition, paronychia of the toes may result from rubbing against the top of the shoe.

Some other alterations of the nail itself may be observed. Worn down nails may occur in many manual occupations. We have isolated a variant of the worn-down nail syndrome, the 'bidet nail'[5]. This presents as a triangular defect with its base lying at the free edge of the nail, and affects the middle three fingers of the dominant hand. The patients are fastidious females in whom the desire for cleanliness verges on the obsessional. Multiple transverse leukonychia is a dystrophy resulting from a lack of trimming; the toenail impinges on the distal part of the shoe. The great toenail and the second toe, when longer, are usually involved. Frictional melanonychia of the toes can be initiated by repeated trauma from footwear. Alterations of the distal joint and tendon sheath may be responsible for the appearance of a myxoid pseudo-cyst in the toenail area.

NAIL DISORDERS ASSOCIATED WITH MENSTRUATION

Linear nail growth increases in the premenstrual phase[6]. Although nail disorders associated with menstruation are rarely observed, menstrual cycles may be associated with true transverse leukonychia[7]. Beau's lines have been associated with dysmenorrhea but they may also occur physiologically with each menstrual cycle[8]. The effects on artificial nails of female hormones might cause lifting; stress points start to appear between the nail plate and the artificial nail.

NAIL DISORDERS RELATED TO THE CONTRACEPTIVE PILL

Rarely, finger nails may become firm, grow faster and no longer split or chip with the use of the contraceptive pill[9]. Adverse effects have also been reported: the contraceptive pill may produce estrogen-induced porphyria cutanea tarda and variegata, and photo-onycholysis has been reported in some instances[10]. The pathogenesis of this type of porphyria is an inherited or acquired uroporphyrinogen-decarboxylase deficiency. Almost all patients with estrogen-induced porphyria cutanea tarda have the congenital type.

NAIL DISORDERS RELATED TO PREGNANCY

The increased adrenal and pituitary gland activity results in accelerated hair and nail growth during pregnancy[11], and may be as much as a third greater than normal[12]. Nail growth is, however, slowed during lactation[6].

Nail changes in pregnancy include transverse grooving, brittleness, distal subungual hyperkeratosis and distal onycholysis. The pathogenesis of these changes is not known and their relationship to pregnancy is unclear. They may not be related to hormonal factors[13]. Therefore we feel that other causes should be eliminated when these changes are observed[14]. Hyperpigmentation, which is very common in pregnancy, may rarely be associated with longitudinal melanonychia[15] while abnormal lifting of acrylic prostheses might be a possibility which could also appear in menopausal women[16].

Prevention of pregnancy has to be prolonged in female drinkers after treatment with acitretin as metabolic formation to the long-acting etretinate is enhanced by alcohol[17].

CONGENITAL DRUG-INDUCED NAIL CHANGES

Several drugs, when taken by a pregnant woman, are known to have an effect on the newborn baby. Hydantoin (phenytoin), trimethadione, paramethadione, valproic acid, carbamazepine (monotherapy) and phenobarbitone have all been observed to cause hypoplasia of nails and/or fingers in the neonate[18-23]. If the mother takes valproic acid, her child's nails can be long and hyperconvex. In one study, it was found that when carbamazepine alone was taken in late pregnancy, the hypoplastic nail changes that occurred returned to normal after some months[22]. The use of hydantoin in pregnany can, additionally, lead to hyperpigmentation of the baby's fingernails[24,25], which can be either distal with detachment of the nail plate or diffuse, or may occur as dark longitudinal streaks.

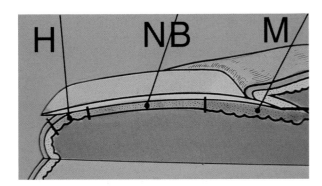

Figure 1   Nail apparatus (after E. Haneke). H, hyponychium; NB, nail bed; M, matrix

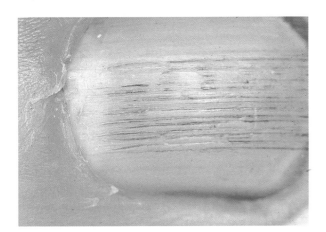

Figure 2   Onychorrhexis

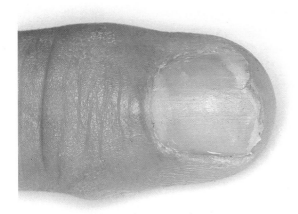

Figure 3   Multiple crenellated splitting

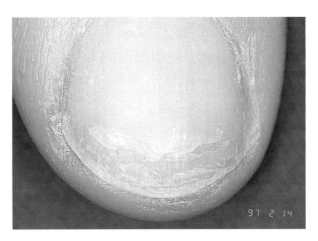

Figure 4   Onychoschizia (horizontal lamellar splitting)

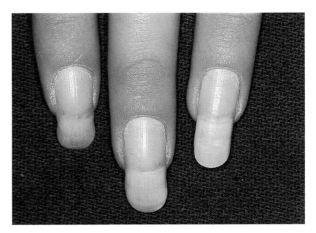

Figure 5   Nail staining due to nail polish

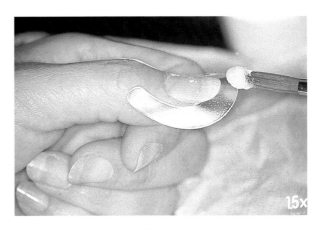

Figure 6   Sculptured artificial nail enhancement

Anticoagulant therapy with warfarin during the first trimester of pregnancy may give hypoplasia of the terminal phalanges together with stippled epiphyses: the fingernails are small and malformed[26].

Malformations in infants of chronically alcoholic women are common and may include nail hypoplasia[27]. Gladen and co-workers[28] reported koilonychia, transverse groove, hyperpigmentation and thinning of nails in children born after maternal poisoning with polychlorinated biphenyls (PCB) in rice oil. Congenital cutaneous candidosis, an uncommon condition, may be restricted to the nails[29].

CONCLUSIONS

Except for disorders related to drug intake and cosmetic procedures, most of the adverse effects

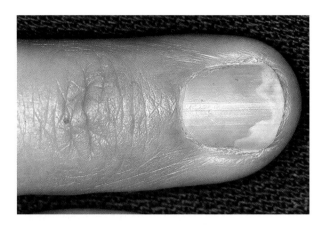

Figure 7   Onycholysis due to overzealous manicuring

observed on the nails are not specific to the female gender.

REFERENCES

1. Baran R, Schoon DD. Cosmetology for normal nails. In Baran R, Maibach HI, eds. *Textbook of Cosmetic Dermatology*. London: Martin Dunitz, 1998: 213–18

2. Brauer E, Baran R. Cosmetic: the care and adornment of the nail. In Baran R, Dawber RPR, eds. *Diseases of the Nails and their Management*. Oxford: Blackwell, 1994:285–96

3. Schoon DD. *Nail Structure and Product Industry*. Albany, New York: Milady Publishing, 1995

4. Baran R, Dawber RPR, Tosti A, Haneke E. *A Text Atlas of Nail Disorders*. London: Martin Dunitz, 1996:169–98

5. Baran R. The bidet nail: a French variant of the worn down nail syndrome. *Br J Dermatol* 1999; 140:377

6. Orentreich N, Markofsky J, Vogelman JH. The effect of aging on the rate of linear nail growth. *J Invest Dermatol* 1979;73:120–30

7. Daniel CR. Nail pigmentation abnormalities. *Dermatol Clin* 1985;3:431–43

8. Colver GB, Dawber RPR. Multiple Beau's lines due to dysmenorrhoea? *Br J Dermatol* 1984;111:111–13

9. Knight JF. Side benefits of the pill. *Med J Aust* 1974; 2:680

10. Byrne JPF, Boss JM, Dawber RPR. Contraceptive pill induced porphyria cutanea tarda presenting with onycholysis of the finger nails. *Postgrad Med J* 1976;52:535–8

11. Hellreich PD. The skin changes of pregnancy. *Cutis* 1974;13:82–6

12. Bean WB. Nail growth. Thirty-five years of observation. *Arch Intern Med* 1980;140:73–6

13. Wong RC, Ellis CN. Physiologic skin changes in pregnancy. *J Am Acad Dermatol* 1984;10:929–40

14. Demis DJ. Skin diseases during pregnancy. In Demis DJ, ed. *Clinical Dermatology*. New York: Harper and Row, 1975;2:1–9

15. Freyer JM, Werth VP. Pregnancy-associated hyperpigmentation associated with longitudinal melanonychia. *J Am Acad Dermatol* 1992;26:493–4

16. Sirdesai S. Lab reports. *Nails Magazine* 1997; July:98

17. Larsen FG, Jakobsen P, Knudsen J, *et al*. Conversion of acitretin to etretinate in psoriatic patients is influenced by ethanol. *J Invest Dermatol* 1993;100:623–7

18. Silverman AK, Fairley J, Wong RC. Cutaneous and immunologic reactions to phenytoin. *J Am Acad Dermatol* 1988;18:721–41

19. Gorlin RJ, Pindborg JJ, Cohen MM. *Syndromes of the Head and Neck*, 2nd edn. New York: McGraw Hill, 1976

20. Rosen RC, Lightner ES. Phenotypic malformations in association with maternal trimethadione therapy. *J Pediatr* 1978;92:240–4

21. Jäger-Romain E, Deichl A, Jakob S, *et al*. Fetal growth, major malformations, and minor anomalies in infants born to women receiving valproic acid. *J Paediatr* 1986;108:997–1004

22. Niesen M, Fröscher W. Finger and toenail hypoplasia after carbamazepine monotherapy in late pregnancy. *Neuropediatrics* 1985;16:167–8

23. Thakker J, Kothari SS, Desmur KL, *et al*. Hypoplasia of nails and phalanges: a teratogenic manifestation of phenobarbitone. *Indian Pediatr* 1991;28:73–5

24. Johnson RB, Goldsmith LA. Dilantin digital effects. *J Am Acad Dermatol* 1981;5:191–6

25. Verdeguer JM, Ramon D, Moragon M, *et al*. Onychopathy in a patient with fetal hydantoin syndrome. *Pediatr Dermatol* 1988;5:56–7

26. Pettifor JM, Benson R. Congenital malformations associated with the administration of oral anticoagulants during pregnancy. *J Pediatr* 1975;86:459–62

27. Crain LS, Fitsmaurice NE, Mondry C. Nail dysplasia and fetal alcohol syndrome. *Am J Dis Child* 1983;137:1069–72

28. Gladen BC, Taylor JS, Ragan NB, *et al*. Dermatological findings in children exposed transplacentally to heat-degraded polychlorinated biphenyls in Taiwan. *Br J Dermatol* 1990;122: 799–808

29. Arbegast KD, Lemberty LF, Koh JK, *et al*. Congenital candidiasis limited to the nail plates. *Pediatr Dermatol* 1990;7:310–12

Disorders of hair

Martin S. Wade and Rodney D. Sinclair

14

INTRODUCTION

In most societies, girls and boys socialize differently and segregate according to sex. Although the degree and manner of socialization varies widely in different cultures, gender differences in hair styling are almost universal. While the relative impact of nature and nurture on gender identity remain unresolved, the desire to use hair for display of sexual identity, social identity and status seems to be genetically based albeit influenced by cultural mores[1].

In Western cultures it is deemed feminine for girls to grow their hair long and to adorn it with ribbons, bows and clips. From an early age hair is emphasized as an important component of physical presentation, and its relative importance increases with age. In adult women scalp hair and its styling are commonly used for gender recognition and are important determinants of physical attractiveness. In contrast body hair, particularly when excessive, tends to be linked to masculinity and is deemed unattractive. Physical appearance has been shown to reliably influence social perceptions and reactions in various contexts, most obviously, but not exclusively, first impressions. Compared with men, women's and girls' body image perception and satisfaction are more dependent on their hair. Any loss or disturbance of their hair predisposes them to an overall negative body-image, low self-esteem and less adaptive social functioning[2].

An understanding of the social and psychological importance of hair to female patients helps to explain the considerable anxiety generated by hair loss, which occasionally seems to be out of proportion to the degree of deformity, and always out of proportion to the physiological importance of hair.

THE BIOLOGY OF HAIR

A basic knowledge of the biology of hair is required to understand the pathogenesis of hair disorders and thereby to effectively manage them. Human hair growth is cyclical with each follicle producing many distinct hairs during a lifetime. The hair follicles first form on the eyebrow, upper lip and chin at between 9 and 12 weeks' gestation. At birth the full complement of hair follicles is present. There are approximately 5 million hair follicles on the body of which on average only 100 000 are on the scalp, the number ranging from about 70 000 to 150 000.

The rate of growth of hair is relatively constant at about 1 cm per month. Hair follicle formation occurs in a frontal to occipital wave on the scalp and a cephalocaudal wave on the body, reaching the feet at about 22 weeks. The first hair grows from the follicle between weeks 16 and 22. The hair grows for about 10 to 12 weeks to a length of 2 to 3 cm and covers the entire body from head to toe. These fine and non-pigmented hairs are known as lanugo hairs. The growth then terminates in similar fronto-occipital and cephalocaudal waves, with the follicles entering telogen via the involutional catagen phase. Telogen terminates with the development of the second hair bud forming at the base of the bulb. New anagen hair growth results in shedding of the first coat of hair between weeks 32 and 36. The second hair produced by the follicle is different to the first. Site variation is introduced with the growth phase of the scalp hairs progressively elongating and the body hairs shortening to the point where most of the hairs are shorter than the first and grow for about 4 to 8 weeks, reaching a length of about 1 cm uniformly over the body. The second coat is shed during the first 3 to 4 months of life, as the second set of hairs passes through telogen and is replaced by the third set. On the body the third-growth hair is smaller than the second-growth hair and many no longer protrude from their pore, or do so only as fine light vellus hairs. In contrast, the scalp hair follicles enlarge and produce thicker and more pigmented hairs known as terminal hairs.

This site specificity also mirrors how follicles react to pubertal androgens. Scalp hairs miniaturize in response to androgens while body hairs enlarge. The degree of enlargement is highly variable, with pubic and axillary hair being most sensitive and most capable of enlarging in response to physiological levels of adrenal androgens. Facial, chest, thigh, abdominal and buttock hair require at least physiological levels of gonadal androgens but are more likely to appear with abnormally high levels of either adrenal or ovarian androgens. There is enormous person-to-person variation in the response of follicles to circulating androgens, and this is influenced by a variety of genetic and metabolic factors.

The fourth and subsequent hairs from scalp follicles continue to enlarge and elongate until a steady state is achieved. The average duration of anagen is about 3 years, producing hairs which would grow to a final length of approximately 36 cm; however, the range is large, with some women having prolonged anagen phases of up to 6 or 7 years and who are accordingly able to grow their hair twice as long. By late adolescence, the anagen duration tends to be fixed and remain constant in the absence of an acquired disorder such as androgenetic alopecia. In addition, the synchrony of neonatal hair growth is progressively lost and the wave of hair growth and shedding from the frontal to occipital scalp is disturbed. Random shedding tends to occur thereafter, so that in contrast to our mammalian counterparts who have a seasonal molt, adult humans tend to shed only a few hairs each day.

The average woman has 100 000 hairs on her scalp, a growth phase of approximately 3 years, and a resting phase of 3 months. She will shed all 100 000 hairs every 1000 or so days at a rate of 100 hairs a day. Another woman with a growth phase of 2000 days would only lose 50 a day. Most of the hair shedding goes unnoticed, particularly when they are short, and very few women are aware of losing more than 10 or 20 hairs a day. One can infer that the first 80 or so hairs go unnoticed. An increase in hair shedding of 20%, however, may double the perceived hair loss and lead the patient to seek medical advice.

DIAGNOSTIC PROCEDURES

History and clinical examination are the initial and most informative steps in forming a diagnosis. The hair pull test and trichogram are procedures that can be performed in the surgery to give further information at the time of consultation. Scrapings for fungal microscopy and culture and scalp biopsy are the definitive tests for many conditions.

Hair pull test

The clinician grasps with thumb and forefinger a clump of 50 to 100 hairs together at their base and gently pulls on the hair at the same time allowing the hair to travel through his/her fingers in a proximal to distal direction. This procedure is repeated at different locations on the scalp. Some hairs will be extracted by this test, and a total of two to five telogen hairs from six to eight pulls would be considered normal[3]. The presence of anagen hairs or hairs with abnormal bulb can be assessed for additional diagnostic information. Factors such as recent hair styling or shampooing may affect the hair pull test by reducing the number of telogen hairs *in situ* ready to be shed. Likewise, if it has been a long time since the hair has been washed, the telogen count may be higher than expected.

Hair pluck trichogram

The hair pluck involves the extraction of 15 to 20 hairs by clasping the hairs at the base with tape-coated epilating forceps and with a single, quick, forceful pull removing the hair. The original description suggested that 50 hairs be chosen[4], but this is unnecessarily painful and may distort the plucked hair fibers. If the hair is plucked too slowly, distortion of the hair bulb may also occur producing so-called dystrophic anagen bulbs[3]. For accuracy the scalp hair should not be washed for a minimum of three days prior to the pluck so as to preserve telogen hairs. The trichogram is the analysis of the hair obtained in this manner under the light microscope, which includes the telogen to anagen ratio and the examination of any abnormal hair bulbs. The normal anagen to telogen ratio in children is over 90% and in adults approximately 85%. Hairs may be extracted in this way when investigating a hair shaft disorder to diagnose fungal infections. Six to eight hairs are usually sufficient for these purposes.

Scalp biopsy

The most useful form of scalp biopsy is a 4-mm punch biopsy (Figure 1) as the normal numbers and ratios of terminal to velus and anagen to telogen hair have been defined[5]. A scalp biopsy is performed by initially anesthetizing the selected area with local anesthetic containing epinephrine, e.g. xylocaine 1% with 1 : 100 000 epinephrine. Two punch biopsies should be performed in close proximity, and the punch should be angled in the direction of hair growth and include subcutaneous fat in order to obtain anagen hair bulbs. Owing to the vascular nature of the scalp, the wound invariably requires a suture. The specimens are placed in formalin and sent for histopathology. Two specimens are required to allow for vertical and horizontal sectioning, the latter giving more detailed information on the

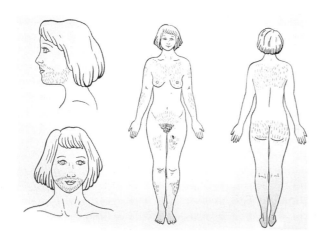

Figure 1   Tissue core from scalp punch biopsy showing sectioning for vertical and horizontal examination

Figure 2   Anatomical areas prone to the development of hirsuties in women

presence and extent of miniaturization of the hair follicles. If direct immunofluorescence is requested the punch for vertical section should be sent fresh to the laboratory where it can be divided into half. The choice of biopsy site is of the utmost importance. Where androgenetic alopecia is suspected the biopsy should be taken from the vertex, where the process is likely to be most active. To biopsy a patch of hair loss, the edge of the lesion where some hair follicles are still present is preferred. A biopsy taken from the center of the lesion may only show scarring and may not provide any information as to the cause. If folliculitis is seen clinically, then inclusion of such a pustule is helpful.

HIRSUTIES

Introduction

By convention hirsuties is a diagnosis reserved for women; men tend to be simply called hairy. Hirsuties has been defined as the growth of terminal hair on the body of a woman in the same pattern and sequence as that which develops in the

Table 1   Causes of hirsuties in adults

Ovarian	polycystic ovary syndrome
	ovarian androgen secreting tumors
	gonadal stromal tumor
	thecoma
	lipoid tumor
	postmenopausal hirsuties
Adrenal	congenital adrenal hyperplasia
	early onset 21-hydroxylase deficiency
	late onset 21-hydroxylase deficiency
	11β-hydroxylase deficiency
	3β-dehydrogenase deficiency
	Cushing's disease
	adrenal adenoma
	adrenal carcinoma
Pituitary	Cushing's syndrome
	prolactinoma
Obesity-related	HAIR-AN syndrome
Drug-related	glucocorticosteroids
	anabolic steroids
	diazoxide
	cyclosporin A
	phenytoin
	psoralens
	penicillamine
	streptomycin
Idiopathic	

post-pubertal male (Figure 2); however, as most women develop hair at puberty in an identical pattern to men that is quantitatively inferior, this definition is spurious. What differs is not that women grow hair in these sites but rather the degree and quality of the growth. At puberty every woman experiences a change in the distribution of hair on her body and scalp. Cultural norms and fashion define acceptable amounts of hair that women may accumulate on their face and body. Deviations from these norms, real or perceived, may be a source of anxiety and low self-esteem in susceptible individuals.

Hirsuties is a response of hair follicles to androgen stimulation. The progressive enlargement of the hairs seems to occur between anagen phases, with each successive anagen hair being longer and thicker than the one that went before it. Hirsuties may be caused by either an endocrine disorder associated with androgen hypersecretion (Table 1) or by a local hypersensitivity of the hair follicle to circulating androgens. This local hypersensitivity is probably mediated by quantitative differences in the amount of 5α-reductase, the enzyme that converts testosterone into dihydrotestosterone (DHT). DHT has a five-fold greater affinity than testosterone for androgen receptors.

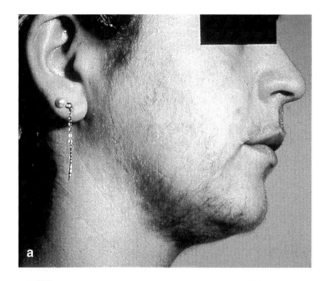

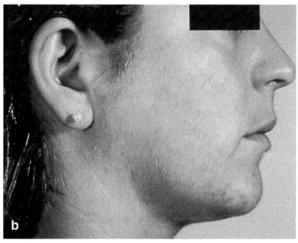

Figure 3   Facial hirsuties (a) before and (b) after treatment with cyproterone acetate

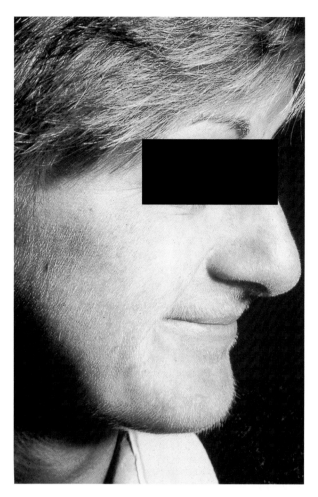

Figure 4   Facial hypertrichosis secondary to minoxidil use. Note the generalized distribution of hairs compared to hirsuties (Figure 3)

Clinical features

The physical signs of hirsuties are simply the presence of terminal hairs on certain body sites. Ferriman and Gallwey[6] have produced a grading scale that may be of use in assessing severity and monitoring progression of the hirsuties. The main differential diagnosis is hypertrichosis, which is distinguished from hirsuties by the distribution of excess hair, early onset prior to puberty and lack of response to anti-androgens (Figure 3). Other important diagnoses to consider are drug-induced hypertrichosis (Figure 4) and the paraneoplastic hypertrichosis lanuginosa.

Investigations

Whether to investigate a patient for androgen excess is determined by the age and rate of onset of the hirsutism, the degree of hirsutism and the presence of any associated features of hyperandrogenism. Such features include menstrual irregularity, acne, androgenetic alopecia, male habitus, deepening of the voice and clitoromegaly. Patients with regular menses rarely require any further investigations. An onset of hirsuties prior to puberty, rapid progression of hirsuties and clitoromegaly in particular, demand further investigation. Appropriate investigations are outlined in Table 2.

If there is a very high index of suspicion of virilism or the screening tests are abnormal, then a referral to an endocrinologist may be appropriate. If the serum testosterone or serum dehydroepiandrosterone sulfate (DHEAS) is twice the normal limit then referral is recommended. Referral may also be important for women of childbearing age seeking advice regarding their future fertility.

Treatment

Hirsutism of sufficient severity to seek medical attention has social and psychological influences on women (Figure 5). Women need reassurance that they are not becoming excessively masculine. They also need advice on cosmetic measures to remove

Table 2   Initial investigation of hirsuties

Serum testosterone (± SHBG)	uniform marked elevation in ovarian tumors
	occasional marked elevation in adrenal tumors
	small to moderate elevation with polycystic ovaries (PCO); normal in idiopathic hirsuties, congenital adrenal hyperplasia and some PCO
Serum DHEAS	uniform marked elevation in adrenal tumors
	occasional marked elevation in ovarian tumors
	usually elevated in congenital adrenal hyperplasia
	normal or small to moderate elevation in PCO

Serum 17α-hydroxyprogesterone will detect a proportion of patients with mild congenital adrenal hyperplasia otherwise missed by serum DHEAS and serum testosterone estimation alone. The low yield and relatively high expense make routine testing controversial. SHBG, sex hormone binding globulin; DHEAS, dehydroepiandrosterone sulfate

hair, particularly as many avoid cutting or shaving the excess hair owing to the baseless fear that it will worsen the problem. A minority will require pharmacological treatment of hirsutism either directed at an underlying cause or, in cases of idiopathic hirsuties, towards lowering the impact of normal levels of circulating androgens on the hair follicle. The natural history of untreated hirsuties is progression over time. Cosmetic measures do not influence the natural history, and pharmacological therapy only reverses the trend so long as it is continued.

Cosmetic measures for the removal of hair

Bleaching with hydrogen peroxide is the easiest measure but may produce an unacceptable yellow hue. Plucking and waxing stimulate reactivation of the resting telogen hairs into the anagen phase resulting in only a short delay before the new hair emerges. Waxing is painful and sometimes produces a folliculitis. In addition, the use of hot wax can burn the patient. Shaving removes all hairs, but only those that were previously in anagen regrow. Many women dislike shaving their faces, but as facial hair has a long telogen phase this is a good preliminary to plucking. Depilatory creams act by dissolving keratin and often irritate the neighbouring skin that is also made of keratin. Home epilators are in reality no more effective than plucking. Electrical epilation, which is loosely referred to as 'electrolysis', may offer a degree of permanent hair removal. It requires insertion of a fine needle through the ostium of the hair follicle (the pore) to the root, where a brief pulse of electricity is delivered with the intention of cauterizing the dermal papilla. In skilled hands it is safe but time consuming, mildly painful and expensive. Individual hairs often need multiple treatments to disappear, and up to 80% regrowth can be expected after a single treatment. In unskilled hands it can be complicated by folliculitis and scarring. Uniform training requirements for electrologists would minimize these complications.

Laser epilation

Recently, a number of lasers have been adapted to treat unwanted hair. The ruby laser shows the most promise and is designed to thermally destroy the hair bulb. The risks of scarring with these new techniques have not yet been adequately quantified, but at this stage they seem small. The main potential side-effect is hypopigmentation, which makes this laser less suitable for dark and olive skinned people. The studies on whether the hair loss is permanent are conflicting, with some showing only minimal damage to the follicle itself; nevertheless, these lasers can painlessly remove hair, without irritation of the skin or folliculitis, and the time to regrowth will be delayed by six months or more. Even if the removal is not permanent, many people would find this an acceptable alternative to waxing and electrolysis.

Pharmacological methods

Because hirsuties is a condition mediated by androgens, attempts have been made to ameliorate the growth of hair with drugs that reduce androgen bioactivity. These drugs interact at a number of sites (Table 3). It is important that hirsute women are carefully selected prior to initiating treatment and are given realistic expectations of the potential improvement. This is important because it can take six to nine months before any effect on hair growth is detectable and only partial improvement is to be expected. Additionally, because these drugs are suppressive and not curative, their effects wear off a few months after ceasing therapy. They therefore need to be taken continuously to sustain any improvement.

Table 3   Pharmacological treatment of hirsutism

Androgen receptor antagonists	spironolactone
	cyproterone acetate
	flutamide
Follicular 5α-reductase inhibitor	finasteride
Reduction in free testosterone	oral contraceptives
(increases SHBG and induces hepatic metabolism of androgens)	
Suppression of adrenal androgen production	prednisolone
(reduces pituitary ACTH secretion)	
Adrenal and gonadal steroid synthesis inhibitor	spironolactone

ACTH, adrenocorticotropic hormone; SHBG, sex hormone binding globulin

First-line therapy consists of either spironolactone or cyproterone acetate. Spironolactone is a synthetic steroid, structurally related to aldosterone, that acts as an anti-androgen by altering steroidogenesis in the adrenals and the gonads through inhibition of cytochrome p450, a coenzyme for 17α-, 11β- and 21-hydroxylases. Additionally it affects the target organ response by competitively blocking cytoplasmic receptors for DHT. The 7α-thio substituted metabolite of spironolactone is thought to be the active molecule. The dose of spironolactone is between 50 mg and 200 mg per day. Women should be advised not to fall pregnant while taking spironolactone as the pregnancy may potentially be complicated by masculinization of a female fetus. While not mandatory, many premenopausal women take it together with an oral contraceptive both to prevent a pregnancy and to correct menstrual irregularities that otherwise occur in 80% of those treated in this way. Suitable contraceptives are those with minimal androgenic effects such as those containing either desogestrel, norethindrone, or cyproterone acetate.

The main side-effects seen with spironolactone are premenstrual breast soreness and swelling, decreased libido and menstrual irregularities on stopping therapy. Hypotension does not seem to be a problem, and hyperkalemia is rarely significant in the absence of co-existing renal impairment. An appropriate starting dose is 100 mg/day and if the response at 3 months is unsatisfactory then the dose can be increased to 200 mg daily. Measurement of the baseline renal function should be considered along with annual measures of the serum potassium. It is prudent to advise patients to avoid potassium supplements.

An equally effective alternative to spironolactone is cyproterone acetate, a hydroxyprogesterone derivative. It is widely used in Europe and Australia but is not currently available in the USA. It can be used in a dose of 2 mg daily in combination with ethinyl estradiol 35 micrograms daily for 21 days in every 28 days. If the response is inadequate after 3 to 6 months then an additional 50 mg of cyproterone acetate can be taken daily for days 5 to 15 of the menstrual cycle. After a further 3 to 6 months should the response still be unsatisfactory, the dose can be further increased to 100 mg daily for days 5 to 15. This particular regimen is used in an attempt to mimic the natural hormone fluctuations of the menstrual cycle so as to prevent amenorrhea. Postmenopausal women or hysterectomized women can simply take 25–100 mg daily continuously. Side-effects are similar to those produced by aldosterone[7]. The function of the additional cyproterone acetate is to hasten the response rather than to increase the magnitude of the ultimate reduction in hair density and diameter.

Corticosteroids are first-line treatment for congenital adrenal hyperplasia and were previously used for all types of hirsuties. They have now been superseded by spironolactone and cyproterone. Flutamide, a potent anti-androgen, and finasteride, a specific 5α-reductase inhibitor, show promise in overseas clinical trials, but have significant potential side-effects and are not licensed for this indication in the USA or Australia.

Eflornithine 15% cream is a topical irreversible ornithine decarboxylase enzyme inhibitor that has recently been shown to reduce the rate of growth of unwanted facial hair in hirsute women. The mechanism of action is not completely understood but ornithine decarboxylase plays an important role in the regulation of cell growth and differentiation (unpublished data presented at the American Academy of Dermatology Meeting, San Francisco, 2000).

Conclusion

Hirsuties is a clinical diagnosis, and further investigations are rarely required. Much can be gained for the concerned patient by employing effective

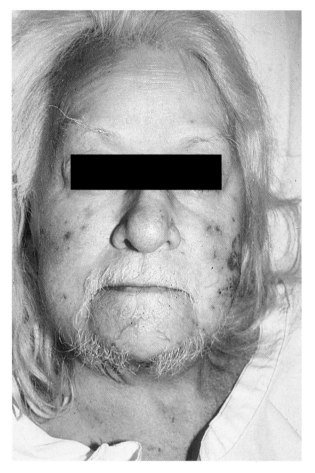

Figure 5 Long standing facial hirsuties in a post-menopausal woman

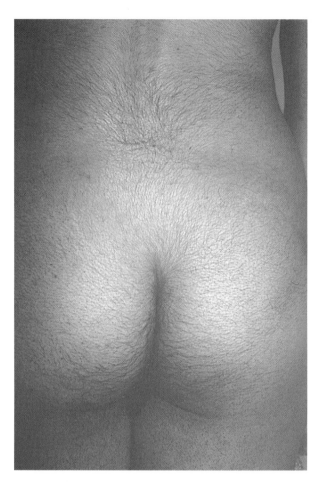

Figure 6 Generalized pattern of excessive body hair growth seen in prepubertal hypertrichosis

camouflage strategies. Medical treatment is effective but palliative. There is a new generation of drug and laser treatments on the horizon that may offer improved management.

PREPUBERTAL HYPERTRICHOSIS

Introduction

Hypertrichosis is defined as an excessive growth of hair on skin not normally hairy. The word growth is emphasized, as the number of hair follicles present is not altered. Hypertrichosis indicates a difference in the quality and length of the hair that is produced from the follicle. While the word excessive is subject to cultural and racial influences and personal preferences, most cases are self-evident. The pathogenesis of hypertrichosis predominantly involves elongation of the anagen phase. While some degree of hair follicle and hair fiber enlargement may be seen it is commonly not pronounced.

Unlike hirsuties, the hair growth in hypertrichosis is not androgen driven and the pattern does not mimic hair growth in males. The desire to distinguish hypertrichosis from hirsuties is based on

practical considerations: hypertrichosis is not androgen dependent and does not respond to anti-androgen therapy. Thus, the natural history, prognosis and response to treatment of these two conditions are different. Unfortunately, the distinction between hypertrichosis and hirsuties is not always clear clinically, and the conditions are not mutually exclusive.

Hypertrichosis can be classified as generalized or localized and can occur as an isolated phenomenon or as part of a syndrome. There are many causes including congenital, hereditary, drug-induced, or as a result of a neuroectodermal abnormality. For the purposes of this chapter the discussion will be limited to prepubertal hypertrichosis, which is an acquired form of generalized hypertrichosis.

Clinical features

The clinical presentation of prepubertal hypertrichosis is distinctive, and easily differentiated from hirsuties. The excess hair is evenly distributed along the back and limbs (Figure 6). The hair is dark and even in length (about 1–2 cm long). It is first noticed around the age of 6 and tends to remain constant until puberty. At puberty associated hirsuties commonly develops.

Investigations

The diagnosis of prepubertal hypertrichosis is a clinical one. A general assessment of the patient should be made to ensure that the hypertrichosis is not part of a syndrome. If there is a degree of suspicion then further investigations are warranted.

Treatment

The physical methods of hair removal for hirsuties are applicable to hypertrichosis, however anti-androgens have little place in the management of prepubertal hypertrichosis.

Conclusion

The clinical presentation of hypertrichosis is distinctive and easily differentiated from hirsuties, which is important as the natural history, prognosis and response to treatment of these two conditions are different; however, the pathophysiology of these two conditions is poorly understood, and it is important to acknowledge that there are areas of overlap, and dual pathology sometimes occurs. It appears that there are a number of independent and interdependent controls on hair length and hair thickness. In hypertrichosis the predominant alteration appears to be an increase in the hair length with a lesser increase in thickness, while in hirsuties there appears to be a predominant increase in hair thickness with a secondary increase in hair length.

ANDROGENETIC ALOPECIA

Introduction

Androgenetic alopecia, or common baldness, is a progressive, largely irreversible, patterned loss of an excessive amount of hair from the scalp. It occurs in both women and men as well as certain other primates, such as the macaque monkey. As the replacement of some terminal hairs by vellus hairs is a universal, physiological, secondary sexual characteristic[8] androgenetic alopecia is only abnormal when significant hair loss occurs prematurely. Pre-requisites are a genetic predisposition and the presence of sufficient circulating androgens. This is why eunuchs do not develop androgenetic alopecia. Between 95% and 100% of the population possess the polygenic inherited predisposition, but far fewer develop significant alopecia owing to variations in genetic penetrance, expression and levels of androgen production. Limited androgenetic hair loss affects all women progressively as they age. This may manifest only as diffuse thinning over the vertex of the scalp or as an alteration in the frontal hairline. Excessive or premature hair loss, which defines androgenetic alopecia, thus represents an exaggeration of a physiological event rather than a disease *per se*. The figure most often quoted is that 50% of women will have significant hair loss by the age of 60.

Clinical features

Hamilton[9] described the distinctive pattern of progression of hair loss in men and graded the severity on a scale of I to VIII (Figure 7). Alteration of the frontal hairline with bitemporal recession occurs first and is followed by balding of the vertex. Eventually a more uniform frontal recession joins the bald areas and the entire fronto-vertical region bears only an inconspicuous secondary vellus hair. The posterior and lateral scalp margins are spared even in advanced cases. Hamilton's Type I described the normal prepubertal pattern. At post-puberty this may still be seen in some women but is rare in adult men. Hamilton suggested that 79% of women develop Hamilton II alopecia after puberty, 25% of women develop Hamilton V by the age of 50, and 50% of women by the age of 60. Bitemporal recession tends to be less prominent in women than in men and is likely to go unnoticed until the late twenties[9].

Although male pattern alopecia occurs in women, more commonly women develop a hair loss over the crown with preservation of the frontal hairline. Ludwig[10] first described this pattern of alopecia and the most useful grading scale for women bears his name (Figure 8). The earliest change (Ludwig grade I) is thinning of the hair on the crown. This produces an oval area of alopecia encircled by a band of variable breadth with normal hair density. Anteriorly the fringe is narrow (1–3 cm) while at the sides the margin is 4–5 cm wide. Progression to Ludwig grade II results in further rarefaction of the crown with preservation of the fringe. Grade III is near complete baldness of the crown.

Pathogenesis

Androgenetic alopecia is the result of stepwise miniaturization of the hair follicle and alteration of the hair cycle dynamics. With each passage through the hair cycle the duration of anagen decreases while the telogen phase elongates. Because the duration of anagen is the main determinant of hair

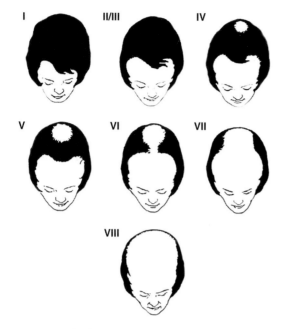

Androgenic alopecia (after Hamilton)

Figure 7   Hamilton grading for androgenetic alopecia

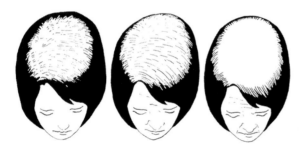

Figure 8   Ludwig pattern of hair loss

(and later modified by Norwood) and Ludwig and may reflect quantitative differences in androgen receptor numbers or 5α-reductase activity in balding and non-balding areas of the scalp.

Studies in patients with androgen insensitivity syndromes and type 2 5α-reductase deficiency[12], have suggested that the miniaturization of the follicles is due to the local effects of androgen excess and in particular dihydrotestosterone (DHT). 5α-Reductase catalyses the enzymatic conversion of testosterone to DHT, which binds to the androgen receptor five-fold more avidly than does the parent compound[13]. There are two isoenzymes of 5α-reductase, types 1 and 2, which have been defined on the basis of pH optima. While initial studies suggested that only the type 1 isoenzyme was found in the scalp in adults, with the type 2 isoenzyme being transiently expressed during infancy, this has been refuted and, using new antibodies, type 2 5α-reductase has been demonstrated in scalp hair follicles[14].

The genetics of androgenetic alopecia is complex. While it has been suggested that androgenetic alopecia is due to an autosomal dominant gene with variable penetrance[15], the prevailing view is that there is polygenic inheritance[16]. In a recent analysis of candidate genes for androgenetic alopecia by restriction fragment length polymorphism, no genetic variation in the 5α-reductase type 1 gene, the 5α-reductase type 2 gene, the aromatase gene or the 17β-hydroxysteroid dehydrogenase gene was found[17].

The miniaturization process does not occur continuously during the growing phase of the cycle. Instead it occurs in either catagen, telogen or possibly early anagen hairs, producing a stepwise reduction in size of the follicle and consequently the hair produced[18]. This is suggested by the observation that the cross-sectional area of individual hair shafts growing on the vertex of a balding scalp does not diminish over time. Thus the effect of androgens is on the early anagen hairs or, less probably, the catagen or telogen phases. This concept explains the lengthy time lag between the commencement of effective therapy and clinical response. Men have sufficient circulating androgen to maximally stimulate hair follicles such that all genetically predisposed men will develop alopecia; however, androgens in the normal female range only induce balding in premenopausal women with a strong genetic predisposition. In women with a less strong genetic predisposition, baldness only develops when androgen production is increased or drugs with androgen-like activity are taken.

length, the maximum length of the new anagen hair is less than that of its predecessor. Ultimately anagen duration is so short that the emerging hair does not reach the skin surface and the only testimony to the presence of a functioning follicle is a pore. In addition, the latency period between telogen hair shedding and anagen regrowth becomes longer, leading to a reduction in the number of hairs visible on the scalp. The follicular miniaturization that accompanies these hair cycle changes is global, affecting the papilla, the matrix and ultimately the hair shaft. The dermal papilla is fundamental to the maintenance of hair growth and is probably the target for androgen mediated changes in the hair cycle and miniaturization of the follicle (Figure 9)[11]. This combination of an altered trichogram and miniaturization of the scalp hair follicles occurs gradually over many years in reproducible patterns. As mentioned, these patterns have been described and graded by Hamilton

Investigations

The presence or absence of virilization cannot be inferred from the pattern of alopecia, be it Hamilton or Ludwig[19]. More useful is the rate of development of the alopecia, its severity and any associated evidence of androgen excess such as hirsuties, acne, menstrual irregularities and clitoromegaly. The vast majority of women do not require any investigation for virilization other than a directed history and examination. The causes and investigation of virilization have already been discussed in relation to hirsuties. It is usually more relevant to direct investigations towards excluding other causes of a diffuse alopecia, especially in patients with early androgenetic alopecia when the pattern of loss is difficult to discern (Figure 10).

The diagnosis of advanced androgenetic alopecia in a female is a clinical one based on the pattern of hair rarefaction. It is supported by a positive hair pull test restricted to the crown and a strong family history of baldness, but their absence does not exclude the diagnosis. Thyroid function tests, serum ferritin, luteinizing hormone, follicle stimulating hormone, testosterone, free androgen index and DHEAS levels should be performed to exclude potential exacerbating or reversible factors[20].

The diagnosis of early androgenetic alopecia in women is difficult. Frequently women present with diffuse hair shedding as a prodrome to the patterned hair loss from the vertex. This presentation can be clinically indistinguishable from chronic telogen effluvium. Scalp biopsy is recommended for a definitive diagnosis. Miniaturization of hair follicles on biopsy is pathognomonic.

Treatment

Camouflage

Camouflage is the simplest, easiest, cheapest and most effective way of dealing with mild androgenetic alopecia. Balding becomes most noticeable when the scalp can be seen through the hair. The easiest way to conceal the area of hair loss is to adopt a hairstyle where hair from the side is combed over the vertex. Camouflage treatments also exist that dye the scalp the same color as the hair, and give the illusion of thicker hair. Numerous brands are available in pressurized spray cans in a number of different colours and they are often combined with a holding hair spray (and sunscreen). The hair is dried and styled before the dye that matches the patient's hair color is sprayed onto the base of the hair. Although many of the newer agents are water resistant, problems may still arise in the rain if the hair gets wet and the dye runs. In addition patients should avoid touching their hair as the dye will color their hands. Towels and pillow-cases may stain, but these come out in the wash. Patients are advised to remove the dye each night by shampooing, and to reapply the dye each morning.

Minoxidil

Minoxidil is a vasodilator that was developed for the treatment of hypertension. Hypertrichosis mainly of the body and to a lesser extent of the scalp was noticed as a side-effect, and subsequently a topical preparation for use in androgenetic alopecia was developed. One milliliter of minoxidil should be applied directly to the scalp via a dropper twice daily and gently massaged in. The spray is generally unsuitable for women. The primary aim of minoxidil is to prevent further loss. It should, therefore, be applied not only to the bald areas but also to the vulnerable areas. The scalp must be dry when minoxidil is applied and the hair should not be wetted for 1 hour after the application. Once daily use is not sufficient for maintenance, and there is no extra benefit with applications more frequently than twice daily. Minoxidil is available in two concentrations, 2% and 5%. The main advantage of the 5% formulation is a more rapid onset of action. After 6 to 12 months of constant use the difference in efficacy between the two is minimal. The US Food and Drug Administration (FDA) has not yet approved the 5% solution for women as it was not convinced by the efficacy data presented.

If successful, after 2 to 4 months of continuous minoxidil 5% use, hair shedding decreases and hair regrowth may be detected at 4 to 8 months. In some patients there is an initial increase in hair shedding owing to the stimulation of hair follicles to re-enter anagen and release the old telogen hairs. If this occurs it is usually a favorable sign that the minoxidil will be effective in that patient. The hair counts usually stabilize after 12 to 18 months whereas untreated control groups continue to progressively lose hair at 5 to 10% per year.

With the 2% solution regrowth often does not begin for up to 12 months, and the treatment should not be abandoned owing to lack of efficacy before then. Most people will get a regrowth of indeterminate hairs, but for many this is not visually significant. Very occasionally there is a dramatic response with near reversion to normal, but this is unpredictable. Thus the main benefit of using minoxidil is to prevent further hair loss. Patients need to understand this before commencing the treatment so as to have realistic expectations of the probable benefits. Useful prognostic factors for regrowth are the severity and the duration of the alopecia. Good prognostic factors are a brief history of balding (fewer than 5 years), and limited alopecia on the vertex (less than 10 cm diameter). If successful, the treatment needs to be continued indefinitely because if stopped any new hair will fall out and regression to the pre-treatment state will occur within three months.

The side-effects of topical minoxidil include pruritus, a contact irritant dermatitis and occasionally contact allergic dermatitis. Hypotension does not occur with topical treatment because there is minimal systemic absorption. Oral minoxidil has also been used, however it appears to be no more effective than topical minoxidil. In addition the systemic side-effects contraindicate its routine use for androgenetic alopecia.

Oral anti-androgens

Spironolactone   The dose range required for androgenetic alopecia is 100–200 mg per day. This tends to slow the progression of balding without reversing the process. Most of the data on aldosterone relates to its use in hirsuties, and few trials have been conducted on its use in androgenetic alopecia. A contraceptive pill is not mandatory with this agent, but women of child-bearing age should be warned against becoming pregnant while on this medication owing to the risks of feminizing a male child.

Cyproterone acetate   Systemic anti-androgen therapy with cyproterone acetate decreases hair shedding but there is generally no visually significant regrowth. In premenopausal women a contraceptive pill should be used with this agent. The effects are generally not noticed for 3 to 6 months after commencing treatment and they tend to continue only for as long as the tablets are taken. About one third to one half of women taking cyproterone acetate notice a major reduction in hair fall. In premenopausal women cyproterone acetate is only given for 10 days each cycle. The reason for this is to minimize menstrual irregularities. Traditionally it is prescribed in a dose of 50–200 mg daily for days 5–15 of the cycle and used in combination with a low dose oral contraceptive or ethinyl estradiol to prevent pregnancy. In postmenopausal women the treatment may be given continuously, and the effective dose range is 25–100 mg daily. Cyproterone acetate has not been approved by the FDA for the treatment of hair loss. The combination of topical minoxidil with systemic anti-androgens could be more efficacious than either used alone; however,

properly conducted trials to verify this clinical suspicion are not available.

Hair transplantation and scalp surgery

Androgenetic alopecia in women usually presents with a thinning of hair over the vertex, and rarely produces bald patches suitable for corrective surgery. Therefore the techniques widely and successfully used for men are in general of only limited benefit to women.

Wigs

Many women with diffuse alopecia prefer wigs to medications or scalp surgery. Wigs can be either interwoven with existing hair or worn over the top of existing hair. Interwoven wigs tend to lift as the hair beneath grows and require adjustment every few weeks, which adds to their expense.

Wig hair is made from either a synthetic acrylic fiber that withstands wear and tear very well, or natural fiber (usually Asian or European human hair). Natural fiber wigs look better, are easier to style and last longer, but are considerably more expensive. Wigs can be styled and washed and modern wigs provide excellent coverage that looks natural. Wigs may become uncomfortably hot in the summer, and some patients find them difficult to wear for this reason. Unfortunately, because the only wigs people see are the bad ones they have a poor reputation. Many people require coaxing to visit a wig maker. Excellent advice on wigs is usually available from patient support groups such as the National Alopecia Areata Foundation in the USA and the Alopecia Society in Australia.

Conclusion

Common baldness already affects or will eventually affect almost all of us to some degree. Until it occurs we tend not to think much about it. How much it affects us emotionally varies enormously from person to person and is determined by our self-perception of body image. While most men cope with their hair loss, androgenetic alopecia is clearly a more distressing condition for women of any age. Compared to men, women place a greater emphasis on their appearance and are more sensitive to events that detract from their attractiveness. Hair is not only important for a woman's attractiveness but also a fundamental part of a woman's gender identity and sexuality. As hair loss in men is more visible it is regarded as an expected or normal event. In women this is not so owing to lesser public awareness. Hair loss in women engenders

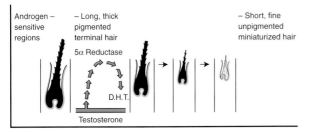

Putative effects of androgens on scalp hair
in male pattern hair loss

Figure 9   Progressive miniaturization of a scalp hair follicle due to the effect of the enzyme 5α-reductase on dihydrotestosterone (DHT) production

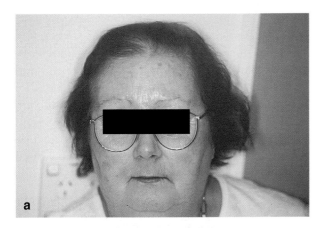

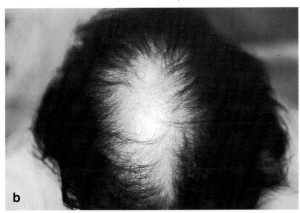

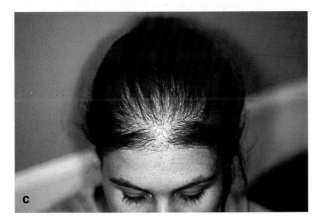

Figure 10   Ludwig stage II androgenetic alopecia (a) frontal view; (b) view of vertex; (c) young woman with Ludwig stage II androgenetic alopecia

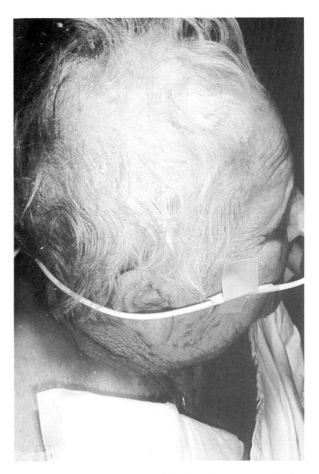

Figure 11   Acute telogen effluvium in a patient in the intensive care unit after a severe illness

considerable anxiety, helplessness and feelings of diminished attractiveness. Once balding is obvious, hair loss tends to progress at a rate of 5 to 10% per year. Pharmacological therapy can reverse the trend for as long as it continues to be taken. In all, there are a number of varied effective treatment measures available, and the appropriate implementation of these treatments relies on correct diagnosis, detailed understanding of the pathogenesis and natural history of androgenetic alopecia, and having realistic expectations of the potential benefits of these treatments.

DIFFUSE HAIR LOSS

Disease states that cause diffuse hair loss may be classified according to the type of hairs that are shed, in particular whether they are anagen or telogen hairs. As telogen hairs have a depigmented bulb, examination of the shed hairs with the naked eye will usually clarify this. The cause of the hair loss can usually be established on history together with a few simple screening blood tests, which include thyroid function tests and iron studies. In addition, serum zinc estimation, antinuclear factor antibody titer and syphilis serology may be required in some cases. Diagnostic difficulty may occur when the pattern of the loss is unclear, as occurs in early androgenetic alopecia in women. This renders it hard to distinguish it from other causes of chronic diffuse telogen hair loss such as chronic telogen effluvium. In this situation a scalp biopsy will be required to establish the diagnosis.

Acute diffuse telogen hair loss

Acute telogen effluvium and telogen gravidarum

Acute telogen effluvium is a self-limiting, non-scarring, diffuse hair loss from the scalp that occurs around 3 months after a triggering event. A wide variety of potential triggers have been implicated. Severe febrile illness, pregnancy (telogen gravidarum), chronic systemic illness, a change in medication, a large hemorrhage, a crash diet or sudden starvation, accidental trauma, surgical operations, or severe emotional stress are the most common[21]. In approximately one third of cases it is not possible to identify the precipitating event[22]. By definition, acute telogen effluvium resolves within 3 to 6 months. The hair shedding ceases and the hair density returns to normal in almost all cases. Occasionally the hair shedding continues beyond 6 months and the condition is then called chronic telogen effluvium. Telogen effluvium is the most common cause of diffuse hair loss; however, as many patients do not seek medical attention, the precise incidence is difficult to establish. Telogen gravidarum is the name given to a telogen effluvium that follows childbirth. It is estimated that significant telogen gravidarum affects one third to one half of all women following childbirth[23].

Clinical features Approximately two to three months after the triggering event there is a period of dramatic diffuse hair loss from the scalp, which may produce marked thinning of the hair (Figure 11). Patients often do not relate these events to their recent illness and become anxious that they are going to go bald. The hair pull test is strongly positive with clumps of telogen hairs being extracted with ease from both the vertex and the margins of the scalp. Beau's lines of the nails may co-exist.

Investigations A full blood count, iron studies[24] and thyroid function tests[25] should be performed to exclude other causes of diffuse telogen hair loss. Syphilis serology[26], antinuclear antibody titer[27] and serum zinc[28] tests should be performed if there are other features on history or examination to suggest these conditions. A drug history[29] should be taken and in particular a change in the oral contraceptive pill three months earlier should be inquired about, as this is a relatively common cause of a short-lived telogen effluvium and is easily overlooked.

Pathogenesis The physiological daily shedding of a few telogen club hairs from the scalp is a natural consequence of the hair cycle. Follicles normally retain telogen hairs until they have re-entered anagen[30]. Eventually the new anagen hair pushes the old telogen hair out. This shedding does not produce alopecia and does not alter the trichogram. Telogen effluvium occurs if a significant number of anagen hairs are triggered to prematurely stop growing and enter catagen and then telogen. The excessive hair shedding occurs at the end of the telogen phase some 2–3 months after the initial event. A temporary alopecia develops as the shorter new anagen hairs replace the long club hairs. Provided the insult is not repeated, the alopecia resolves as the new anagen hairs grow.

Telogen gravidarum occurs because the high circulating placental estrogens prolong anagen, leading to extra fullness of the hair during pregnancy[31]. The withdrawal of these trophic hormones at delivery causes many anagen hairs, including all the overdue anagen hairs, to simultaneously enter catagen. Telogen hairs are then shed a few months later. The trichogram from a hair pluck sample is abnormal, with more than 25% telogen hairs[21]. A biopsy is rarely required in acute cases, although it will provide reassuring prognostic information in a patient who is particularly anxious. The histology of acute telogen effluvium shows an increased number of telogen hairs without inflammation, and with no significant increase in the vellus hair count to suggest androgenetic alopecia[22].

Treatment Acute telogen effluvium and telogen gravidarum are self-limiting over 3 to 6 months. Most women get full restoration of their hair, while the hair in a small proportion of cases remains thin, possibly owing to the unmasking of underlying androgenetic alopecia. Such cases may benefit from a biopsy to further delineate the prognosis. It has been suggested that following telogen gravidarum, some hairs may not revert to the asynchrony in hair growth normally seen over the adult human scalp and cause subsequent episodic hair shedding that is either generalized or regional. Reassuring patients that they are not going bald,

Table 4 The non-scarring alopecias

Anagen hair loss		Telogen hair loss	
Diffuse	Patchy	Diffuse	Patchy
Anagen effluvium	alopecia areata	acute telogen effluvium	acute telogen effluvium
Androgenetic alopecia	loose anagen syndrome	telogen gravidarum	occipital alopecia (newborn)
Drug induced	post-op occipital alopecia	chronic telogen effluvium	alopecia areata
Radiotherapy	syphilis	early androgenetic alopecia	
Poisoning	traction alopecia	iron deficiency	
Diffuse alopecia areata	trichotillomania	malnutrition/malabsorption	
	tinea capitis	hypothyroidism	
		hyperthyroidism	
		diffuse alopecia areata	
		syphilis	
		sysytemic lupus erythematosus	
		chronic renal failure	
		hepatic failure	
		advanced malignancy	

that the telogen effluvium is temporary and that the hair will regrow is usually sufficient. Some patients require a wig while awaiting regrowth. Empirically topical minoxidil may hasten resolution by prolonging anagen and stimulating telogen hairs to re-enter anagen; however, formal studies are lacking.

Chronic diffuse telogen hair loss

Diffuse shedding of telogen hairs that persists beyond 3 months may be due to primary chronic telogen effluvium or be secondary to the causes listed in Table 4. The most common are iron deficiency, hypo- and hyperthyroidism, secondary syphilis and systemic lupus. Apart from iron deficiency these are uncommon and the other causes listed are rare. The literature to support iron deficiency as a cause of chronic diffuse hair loss is anecdotal[32], but a causative role is generally, albeit not universally, accepted.

All chronic diffuse telogen hair loss begins as acute telogen hair loss, and when patients present acutely, without an obvious explanation for their hair loss, it is appropriate to take a wait and see approach. Further investigations, in particular scalp biopsy, are indicated when the patient is very anxious or the hair loss is very severe.

Iron deficiency

Iron deficiency, with or without anemia, is an occasional finding in the investigation of diffuse alopecia. In some of these cases iron replacement therapy causes cessation of hair loss and regrowth.

In many other cases replenishment of iron stores does not stop the shedding. In these cases the iron deficiency is probably an incidental finding and an alternative cause of the hair loss, such as early androgenetic alopecia or chronic telogen effluvium, needs to be considered. Iron deficiency anemia has been reported in as many as 72% of women presenting with diffuse telogen hair loss, but this figure is an overestimate[33]. There are numerous cases in the literature where patients treated with oral iron had regrowth of their hair associated with normalization of their iron stores. On cessation of iron replacement therapy the anemia and hair loss returned, confirming that at least in some cases the iron deficiency is a causative factor in their alopecia[34].

Clinical features Patients present with diffuse telogen hair loss. Iron deficiency may also be an aggravating factor in other forms of alopecia, particularly androgenetic alopecia, and this may be missed unless specifically looked for. The patient may be pale, easily fatigued and lethargic owing to anemia. Disease states producing blood loss may be apparent or occult. Multiple vitamin deficiencies may be present in patients on poor diets or with malabsorption. A referral to a general practitioner or internal physician to establish the cause of the iron deficiency may be appropriate. In about 20% of cases the iron deficiency occurs in the absence of anemia and manifests solely with a serum ferritin below 20μg/l[34]. Therefore, iron studies should be performed in addition to a full blood examination.

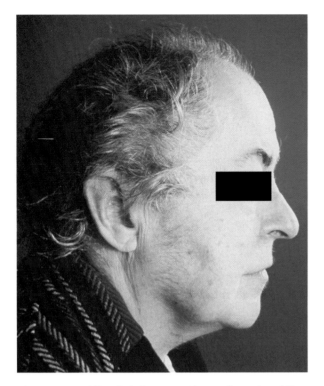

Figure 12 Diffuse hair loss secondary to hypothyroidism

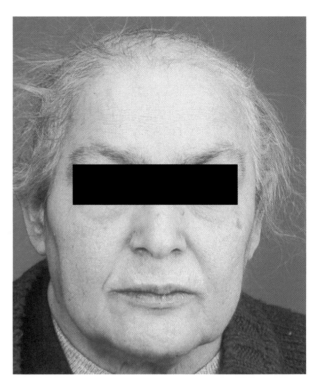

Figure 13 Drug-induced telogen hair loss. In this case the cause was acitretin

Pathogenesis As iron is an essential cofactor for ribonuclease reductase, which is involved in DNA synthesis, it has been proposed that iron deficiency reduces proliferation of matrix cells. The telogen effluvium results from the arrest of matrix proliferation. The pathology is indistinguishable from that of telogen effluvium.

Treatment Patients should be treated with oral iron supplements until their ferritin returns to normal. Some have advocated that treatment should be continued until the ferritin rises above 40µg/l[35], however the evidence for this is unconvincing. If the hair loss is due to the iron deficiency it will resolve within 3 months of correcting the iron stores. If the hair loss continues beyond this time an alternative cause for it, such as androgenetic alopecia, should be sought.

Other nutritional disorders

There are a number of other dietary causes of diffuse telogen hair loss. Sudden weight loss can precipitate a telogen effluvium[36]. Chronic starvation and in particular marasmus may result in dry, lifeless, fine, straight hair that is sparse and easily plucked[37]. Kwashiorkor results in periods of interrupted hair growth that either send the hair into telogen or, if less severe, affect the caliber of the hair more than its linear growth, hence producing multiple Pohl Pinkus lines. Changes in hair color are another prominent feature. Dark hair changes to brown or red, while brown hair becomes blond. This color change, together with the periodic constrictions, produces the so-called flag sign of kwashiorkor[37]. Essential fatty acid deficiency[38] also produces marked telogen hair loss combined with a lightening of hair colour. Zinc deficiency, both hereditary and acquired[28], leads to sparse, dry, brittle hair, and the hair loss is an important clue to the diagnosis.

Thyroid disease

Diffuse telogen hair loss may occur in association with both hypo- and hyperthyroidism[25]. Loss of the outer third of the eyebrows is seen in approximately 25% of patients with hypothyroidism, while diffuse scalp alopecia occurs in about a third of hypothyroid patients[39]. Hyperthyroidism, when severe, is said to cause a diffuse alopecia in up to 50% of cases.

Pathogenesis Hypothyroidism inhibits cell division both in the epidermis and the skin appendages. In a proportion of patients this inhibition of mitosis induces catagen and delays re-entry of telogen hairs into anagen. The mechanism of hair loss in hyperthyroidism is unknown.

Clinical features Hair loss may precede other clinical manifestations of thyroid disease by many months, and can therefore be an important clue to the diagnosis. Likewise, other stigmata of thyroid disease will help diagnose the cause for the alopecia. Drug-induced hypothyroidism also produces alopecia in a similar proportion of patients. The alopecia has a gradual onset and continues until the thyroid status is normal. Marked hair loss can occasionally occur. There appears to be no relationship between duration or severity of hypothyroidism and the degree of alopecia (Figure 12).

Investigations Serum thyroid function testing will determine the thyroid status of the patient. Both the trichogram and hair microscopy reveal an increased proportion of telogen hairs. The histopathology is that of telogen effluvium.

Treatment Referral to an endocrinologist for treatment may be appropriate. Rapid replacement therapy in a patient with long-standing hypothyroidism may precipitate myocardial infarction. The management of hyperthyroidism is complex. With thyroxine replacement the hairs rapidly re-enter anagen and the telogen count falls. Replacement therapy generally leads to regrowth of hair within a few months. An exception to this occurs when the hypothyroidism has been present for many years and the hair follicles have atrophied; nevertheless, failure of a biochemically hypothyroid patient to respond to therapy usually suggests an alternate or coincident cause of alopecia, most commonly androgenetic alopecia. Hair loss in the hyperthyroid patient usually stops within three months of becoming euthyroid.

Other metabolic disorders

Chronic renal failure and dialysis are associated with dry, brittle sparse scalp hair and loss of body hair, including pubic and axillary hair[40]. Chronic liver failure can produce a diffuse alopecia as can advanced malignancy[41]. The mechanism is unknown. Pancreatic disease and upper-gastrointestinal disorders associated with malabsorption may also be associated with diffuse alopecia[42]. Diffuse hair loss in secondary syphilis produces a classic 'moth-eaten' appearance[26]. A telogen effluvium may also follow two to three months after a primary infection or after successful treatment as a feature of the Jarisch–Herxheimer reaction. Connective tissue disorders, in particular systemic lupus erythematosus[27] and dermatomyositis[43], may also produce a non-scarring diffuse alopecia.

Drug-induced telogen hair loss

Drugs can induce alopecia through loss of either anagen or telogen hairs[29]. Anagen hair loss is usually dramatic, with the patient rapidly developing total alopecia. The long list of drugs reported to have caused hair loss is shown in Table 5. Many of these reports are not conclusive, in that other causes have not been adequately ruled out. Hair loss affects everyone who receives high-dose chemotherapy. It is very common with etretinate[44] and acitretin and is dose related. It is much less common with isotretinoin. Hair loss is frequently seen following either the cessation or commencement of oral contraceptive pills, and is more common with high-dose preparations and those that have a high progestogen to estrogen ratio. The incidence of hair loss associated with a host of other implicated drugs is unknown.

Clinical features Drug-induced telogen alopecia usually presents with diffuse hair loss leading to thinning, which may be profound. The alopecia tends to begin about 6 to 12 weeks after starting treatment and is progressive while the drug is continued (Figure 13). The diagnosis is based on demonstrating the correct chronology of relevant drug use and hair loss and the exclusion of other causes. Patients require investigation to exclude other causes of a diffuse telogen hair loss, which could be causative or exacerbating factors such as iron deficiency anemia, hypothyroidism and androgenetic alopecia. Chronic telogen effluvium may be difficult to distinguish clinically and histologically and sometimes the only way to determine whether a drug is causing the hair loss is to stop it temporarily and see if the shedding stops over the ensuing 3 months. A biopsy can exclude androgenetic alopecia.

Pathogenesis Some medications act by exacerbating androgenetic alopecia, while others produce a telogen effluvium. Most drugs that produce an anagen effluvium in high doses can also produce a telogen effluvium in low doses. Anti-thyroid drugs (including amiodarone) and anti-lipid medications most probably act by producing a deficiency state. Minoxidil has been reported to produce increased telogen shedding[22,45]; however this is due to dormant follicles re-entering anagen and pushing out the old club hair and as such is not a true alopecia.

Table 5   Drug-induced alopecia

Telogen effluvium	Heparin
	Warfarin
	Propranolol/metoprolol
	Captopril/enalopril
	Allopurinol
	Boric acid
	Phenytoin
	Glibenclamide
	Amphetamines
	Levadopa
	Bromocryptine
	Methysergide
	Interferon
	Albendazole/mebendazole
	Cimetidine
	Colchicine (low dose)
	Sulfasalazine
	Penicillamine
	Gold
Anti-thyroid action	Carbimazole
	Propylthiouracil
	Amiodarone
	Lithium
Prothyroid action	Thyroxine
Hypolipidemic agents	Clofibrate
	Triparanol
Pro-androgen action	Oral contraceptive pill
	Danazol
	Testosterone
	Anabolic steroids
Lichenoid cicatricial alopecia	Chloroquine
	Mepacrine
	Proguanil
Anagen effluvium	Radiation
	Cyclophosphamide
	Doxorubicin
	Colchicine (high dose)
	Thallium/mercury/arsenic
	Cantharadin
	Azathioprine
	Methotrexate

Almost all chemotherapeutic agents can provoke an anagen effluvium

The mechanism of hair loss with retinoids is complex. There appears to be a reduction in the duration of anagen as well as a telogen anchorage defect. There is no evidence of an anagen effluvium.

With the exception of drug-induced cicatricial alopecia, androgenetic alopecia and anagen effluvium, the histology is essentially normal, and may be indistinguishable from that of chronic telogen effluvium.

Treatment   Cessation of the drug is advised. Alopecia may also recur with other drugs that are chemically unrelated, suggesting an individual susceptibility to drug-induced hair loss rather than true cross reactivity. With the exception of drug-induced androgenetic alopecia, and cicatricial alopecias caused by drugs, regrowth of hair occurs after the medication is stopped if the drug is truly the cause of the alopecia. Reappearance of the alopecia on rechallenge helps to establish the drug, rather than the illness for which it was prescribed, as the cause of the hair loss. Occasionally patients have persisting thinning of their hair and a few notice continued shedding. This is most common after retinoid-induced hair loss, the mechanism of which is not well understood.

Chronic telogen effluvium

Chronic telogen effluvium is defined as chronic diffuse telogen hair loss that persists beyond 6 months[46]. It is much less common then acute telogen effluvium. It is a diagnosis of exclusion. Routine blood tests and a scalp biopsy are required to exclude iron deficiency, thyroid disease and early androgenetic alopecia before the diagnosis of chronic telogen effluvium can be made. In addition lupus, syphilis and drug-induced hair loss may also need to be excluded. Chronic telogen effluvium predominantly affects women. Men with short hair tend not to notice increased hair shedding, while men with long hair rarely present to doctors with this complaint for reasons that are not entirely clear. While chronic telogen effluvium may be triggered by an acute telogen effluvium, more commonly no specific trigger is evident. Stress is commonly cited as a trigger or potentiating factor for chronic diffuse hair loss; however, the evidence for this is scanty – indeed, stress may arise as a complication of the hair loss[47].

Clinical features   The presentation of chronic telogen effluvium tends to be distinctive. Affected women are between 30 and 50 and have a very full, thick head of hair. Frequently there is a history of being able to grow their hair very long in childhood, suggesting a particularly long anagen phase. They complain of an abrupt onset of hair shedding often sufficient to block the drain after a shower and with thinning of their hair (Figure 14). On examination there is prominent bitemporal recession, and a positive hair pull test equally over the vertex and occiput, but it is difficult to be convinced of any hair thinning. There is no widening of the central part as is common in androgenetic alopecia. Nevertheless, the patient is adamant that they previously had more hair and is distressed by the prospect of going bald. Usually there is no family history of early onset androgenetic alopecia and scalp biopsy shows only minimal changes.

Diagnostic difficulty occurs when the insult is prolonged or regularly repeated. Chronic telogen effluvium can be difficult to distinguish from early androgenetic alopecia, especially as periods of progression in androgenetic alopecia are preceded by increased shedding of telogen hairs. Chronic diffuse alopecia areata is very rare[48]. Acute forms are generally seen in rapidly evolving alopecia totalis and 'exclamation mark' hairs are usually present. In the absence of exclamation mark hairs the diagnosis of diffuse alopecia areata cannot be made clinically and a biopsy is required.

Investigations A scalp biopsy is required in cases of chronic telogen effluvium, mainly to exclude androgenetic alopecia[49]. Blood testing should also be performed to exclude reversible causes of diffuse hair loss.

Pathogenesis The cause of this chronic telogen effluvium is uncertain, but it may be due to shortening of the anagen phase of the cycle. It has been suggested that shedding is not noticeable until anagen is reduced by 50%, however formal studies are not available. The histology closely resembles that of the normal scalp. In particular there is no follicular miniaturization, no loss of terminal hairs and no increase in the vellus hair count. There may be a small increase of telogen hairs, but less marked than in acute telogen effluvium or androgenetic alopecia. Trichograms from the occiput and the crown show similar slight increases in the telogen count. In contrast the trichogram in early androgenetic alopecia should show an increase in telogen hairs on the vertex, but not on the occiput.

Treatment The prognosis for women with chronic telogen effluvium is less certain, but it appears that the hair shedding follows a fluctuating course, that they do not go bald and that the condition usually resolves spontaneously after 3 to 4 years. Occasionally the condition can be very persistent, lasting 10 or more years. Despite the large numbers of hairs shed over many years these women are remarkable for the amount of hair that still persists on their scalp. One treatment option is to do nothing and observe. Minoxidil, either 2 or 5%, can be used. It has been suggested that a three to six

month trial of topical minoxidil may terminate chronic telogen effluvium. Approximately half the treated women will respond, having some relapse on cessation of the minoxidil.

Diffuse androgenetic alopecia

Androgenetic alopecia is the most common cause of diffuse hair loss in women. In the early stages of androgenetic alopecia the pattern is usually not evident and patients present with diffuse hair loss. The histological hallmark of androgenetic alopecia is miniaturization of hair follicles. The ratio of big terminal hairs to small secondary vellus hairs seen on a horizontally sectioned 4 mm scalp biopsy can be used to diagnose androgenetic alopecia histologically when the clinical presentation is ambiguous. A terminal to vellus ratio of less than 4 : 1 is diagnostic of androgenetic alopecia, while a ratio greater than 7 : 1 suggests chronic telogen effluvium[5]. Between these two poles are a number of equivocal cases where the diagnosis remains unclear. Many of these equivocal cases will evolve into androgenetic alopecia with time and a proportion will respond to anti-androgen treatment.

As the natural history, prognosis and response to therapy of androgenetic alopecia and chronic telogen effluvium are considerably different, a biopsy is warranted in most women presenting with chronic diffuse telogen hair loss. The treatment of androgenetic alopecia has already been discussed.

Diffuse alopecia areata

Diffuse alopecia areata is rare. It may be seen in rapidly evolving alopecia totalis or universalis, or it may occur as a chronic state, which is particularly rare[48].

Clinical features Diffuse alopecia areata has two distinct clinical presentations. Patients may present with an acute diffuse alopecia areata or a chronic form. The acute form may occur *de novo* or in someone with established patchy disease. Patients present with a story of weeks to months of dramatic hair shedding and have a strongly positive hair pull test with hundreds of hairs extracted with light tension. Exclamation mark hairs may be seen if carefully sought. Most patients will rapidly develop alopecia totalis/universalis if left untreated (Figure 15). Chronic diffuse alopecia areata is exceptionally rare. Patients present with profound hair loss but often are not actively shedding. The hair pull test may be positive with 10 to 20 hairs released with light traction.

One or two small patches of alopecia areata may co-exist and the hair loss may have a slightly reticular pattern. Exclamation mark hairs are rarely seen and a biopsy is required to establish the diagnosis. The histology is sometimes equivocal, as a light peribulbar lymphocytic infiltrate can be a non-specific histological finding seen in normal scalps. A response to oral prednisolone with hair regrowth is sometimes required to establish the diagnosis absolutely.

Investigations   A scalp biopsy is usually performed to assist with diagnosis when there has been no history of alopecia areata, either patchy or reticular, or there are no exclamation mark hairs present.

Pathogenesis   In genetically predisposed persons, an as yet unidentified environmental trigger is thought to stimulate an autoimmune lymphocyte attack on the hair bulb. The inflammation is specific for anagen hairs and initiates anagen arrest and the onset of catagen and subsequently telogen. As the hair stem cells are unaffected, the telogen hair maintains the potential to re-enter anagen, which continues until the hair reaches anagen IV. At this stage the inflammation around the hair bulb re-ignites and stimulates anagen arrest once more. Thus the hair cycle continues, with the follicle repeatedly producing anagen hairs that are aborted before being allowed to grow long enough to reach the skin surface.

Treatment   Oral prednisolone in doses greater than 0.5 mg/kg/day for 3 to 4 weeks and then tapered will usually arrest the hair shedding and may stimulate regrowth. A more detailed description of treatment is given in the following section on alopecia areata.

Summary

Diffuse hair loss is a common clinical presentation. The diagnosis can usually be established with a history focusing particularly on the chronology of events, examination of the bulbs of the shed hairs and a few simple screening blood tests. In chronic cases a scalp biopsy may be required. Once the diagnosis has been established treatment appropriate for that diagnosis is likely to arrest the hair loss in all cases except chronic telogen effluvium. Patients with chronic telogen effluvium can, however, be consoled by the fact that their condition is non-progressive and self-limiting.

ALOPECIA AREATA
Introduction

Alopecia areata (AA) is an autoimmune, non-scarring, multifocal disorder of hair growth characterized by circular bald areas that contain pathognomonic exclamation mark hairs and which occur on any hair bearing site of the body. It occurs in approximately 0.15% of the population[50]. Most will have an occasional patch that spontaneously heals. Overall 30% will develop alopecia totalis (complete loss of hair from the scalp) or universalis (complete loss of hair from the body) during the course of their lives[51]. The chance of progressing to alopecia totalis is higher if the onset is in childhood (50%) compared to adult (25%). Once alopecia totalis has developed only 1% of children and 10% of adults will achieve complete regrowth[51]; 40 to 50% of patients develop AA before the age of 21 years and in only 20% does it begin after 40 years[52]. AA is just as common in women as in men[48].

A positive family history is present in 25–30% of patients and AA appears to have a polygenic inheritance. In addition to the genetic predisposition, a second event is required for disease expression. This event is occasionally a major life crisis, but more commonly the trigger is an unidentified event that precipitates the immunological attack on anagen hair follicles that produces alopecia. AA differs from most other known autoimmune disorders in that no permanent tissue destruction occurs. This has led some to suggest that the immunological target may be a regulatory factor or its receptor.

The incidence of alopecia areata is increased, and the prognosis for regrowth is worse, when atopy or Down's syndrome coexist. Atopy has been found in about 50% of patients with AA, compared to a general incidence of atopy of 20 to 30%. Atopics presenting with a patch of AA tend to go on to develop alopecia totalis more frequently. The incidence of AA in Down's syndrome is around 6% compared with 0.1% in mentally retarded controls. About 50% of Down's patients go on to develop alopecia totalis, and there is a higher incidence of associated autoimmune disorders, especially anti-thyroid antibodies. Prognostic indicators are listed in Table 6.

No treatment is available that modifies the natural history of alopecia areata and there is no universally successful method of producing a temporary regrowth. The best available therapies produce regrowth in more patients than does placebo, but the duration of any subsequent remission is

Table 6   Prognostic factors for alopecia areata

Childhood onset
Personal history of atopy
Down's syndrome
Co-incident endocrinopathy
Oophiasis pattern of alopecia areata
Alopecia totalis or universalis

unaltered. Partial regrowth is unlikely to be cosmetically acceptable to the patient and this should be taken into account when considering the various treatment options.

AA produces considerable distress, especially in women. Sufferers may feel embarrassed and unwelcome, and some patients alter or limit their socialization accordingly. Secondary depression and anxiety consequent to hair loss unfortunately occur commonly. Generally, children learn to cope with the alopecia quicker than their parents or adult counterparts.

Clinical features

AA appears in a variety of patterns. The most common is one or more circumscribed totally bald, smooth patches often noticed first by the hairdresser. Multiple 3 to 4 millimeter long exclamation mark hairs may be present at the margin. These exclamation mark hairs as well as normal looking hairs at the margin are easily extracted. Exclamation mark hairs are not always present, but if seen are diagnostic, and help distinguish it from secondary syphilis, a condition that can closely mimic alopecia areata. Trichotillomania may also simulate alopecia areata, and the short stubble of broken hairs can be mistaken for exclamation mark hairs. Plucking a suspected exclamation mark hair helps differentiate these two conditions. The broken hairs in trichotillomania are anagen hairs and firmly rooted to the scalp, whereas the true exclamation mark hairs are easily extracted telogen ones (Figure 16). Some patients complain of irritation, tenderness or paresthesia immediately preceding the development of a new patch, but more often they are asymptomatic. The first patch is on the scalp in over 60% of cases, although patches elsewhere are more likely to go unnoticed. The occiput and the frontovertical areas of the scalp are common sites for the initial patch. The eyebrows and eyelashes are commonly lost and may be the only site affected. Whether the first patch is on the scalp or elsewhere has no prognostic implications.

Regrowth from the first episode occurs within 6 months in about a third of cases and within a year in about two thirds. Thirty-three per cent of patients never recover from their initial patch and, some rapidly progress to alopecia totalis. Regrowth is at first fine and unpigmented, but usually the hairs resume normal colour and caliber after a short period of time. Over the ensuing years almost 100% will relapse; however this may not be for many years.

Further patches often appear after a few weeks. New patches can develop even while the initial patch is resolving. Discrete patches may coalesce with loss of the intervening hairs to produce either a reticulate pattern, alopecia totalis – with loss of all the hairs on the scalp – or alopecia universalis, with loss of all the hairs on the body.

Other patterns of hair loss occur. Patches may coalesce to form a reticular pattern (Figure 17). Alopecia oophiasis describes a band-like loss of hair around the periphery of the scalp. It has a particularly poor prognosis for regrowth. Acute diffuse alopecia areata may be the initial presentation of a rapid onset alopecia totalis, which can develop within 48 hours. As pigmented hairs are affected first, their preferential loss can produce overnight graying. Chronic diffuse loss is very rare and requires either the finding of exclamation mark hairs or supportive histology to distinguish it from telogen effluvium, androgenetic alopecia, chronic diffuse global alopecia of women or trichotillomania. Perinevoid alopecia areata is another uncommon presentation. It is characterized by the development of alopecia around nevi. The opposite of this has also been described, with the hairs within hairy nevi remaining unaffected in alopecia universalis. Nail changes occur in about 50% of children affected, but are less common in adults (around 20%). The most common finding is pitting in several fingernails. The toenails are affected much less commonly. Other potential changes include red lunulae, Beau's lines and onychomadesis, trachyonychia, onychorrhexis, thinning or thickening of nails and cross fissures. Twenty nail dystrophy, or trachyonychia of all twenty nails, may occur in children and precede the onset of the alopecia areata by a number of years. This can also be associated with the later development of psoriasis or lichen planus and as such is not specific for alopecia areata.

Investigations

The diagnosis of alopecia areata is primarily clinical. The presence of exclamation mark hairs is pathognomonic. The differential diagnosis of an

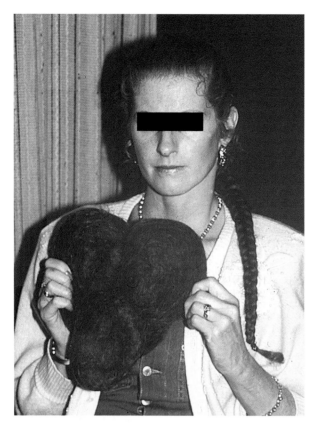

Figure 14   Chronic telogen effluvium. Despite increased hair shedding over a period of time the patient still has reasonable hair volume

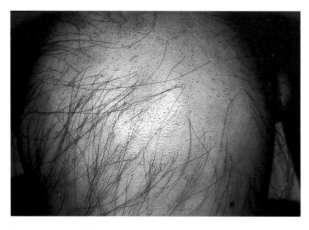

Figure 15   Diffuse alopecia areata

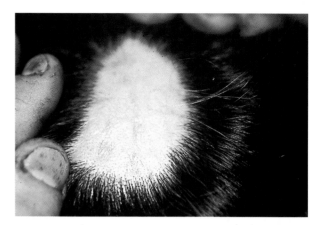

Figure 16   Patch of hair loss in alopecia areata showing pathognomonic exclamation mark hairs

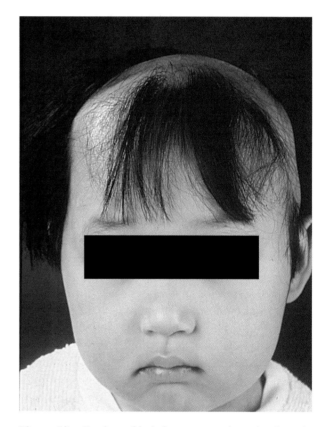

Figure 17   Patches of hair loss may coalesce in alopecia areata to form the so-called reticular pattern

atypical solitary patch of AA on the scalp includes tinea capitis, lupus erythematosus, trichotillomania, subtle scarring alopecia, or pseudopelade. (Pelade is the French term for alopecia areata.) If doubt about the diagnosis exists Wood's lamp examination, fungal culture of skin scrapings or a biopsy will enable the correct diagnosis to be made. Secondary syphilis, resembling multiple patches of AA, can be distinguished on serology. Congenital triangular alopecia and postsurgical occipital alopecia also sometimes cause difficulty with diagnosis.

Pathogenesis

There is invariably a dense peribulbar and intrafollicular lymphocytic infiltrate (predominantly CD4 positive phenotype) associated with aberrant HLA class I and class II antigen expression on the cells in the precortical matrix and presumptive cortex.

This infiltrate disappears with resolution of the alopecia (Figure 18). The perifollicular inflammation weakens anagen hairs at the keratogenous zone of the developing hair shaft and at the same time precipitates premature entry of the follicles into catagen. The weakened hairs break when the keratogenous zone reaches the surface of the skin, producing a rapid alopecia. Having entered telogen these fractured hairs are then eventually extruded as exclamation mark hairs, which are about 3 mm long. Light microscopy of exclamation mark hairs reveals a broken tip, below which the hair tapers towards a small but otherwise normal club hair. As these hairs are telogen hairs, they are easily extracted from the scalp.

Hairs in anagen III are preferentially affected and are lost first, although all anagen hairs are eventually shed in a wave running across an affected patch. Follicles continue to cycle, but as soon as a new anagen hair reaches the anagen III stage, it is damaged by the inflammatory infiltrate and sent straight back into catagen. Histology of an established lesion shows that about 70% of hairs are either in catagen or telogen (Figure 19). Anagen III is also the stage during which hair bulb melanin is transferred to cortical keratinocytes, and a number of pigmentary abnormalities occur in alopecia areata. First, the process seems to spare non-pigmented (gray) hairs in the initial phases. Second, the dystrophic anagen hairs that are also seen in this condition show variable pigmentation, and third regrowth after resolution of a patch of AA occurs initially with gray hairs.

Treatment

Many different treatments have been proposed for AA, but because of the uncertain natural history and tendency to spontaneous remission, only those agents that have an established record in studies should be considered. There is no place for the prolonged use of expensive placebos, that potentially delay the patient from coming to terms with his or her disability.

First-line pharmacological therapy

Fluorinated topical steroids applied twice daily produce regrowth in a significant proportion of patients. Alopecia of recent onset and young children below the age of 10 years appear to be the most responsive. In general a three-month trial is required before deeming the treatment unsuccessful. If hair growth occurs the treatment can be cautiously continued, observing the patient at regular intervals for early signs of scalp atrophy.

Intralesional steroids are useful for the eyebrows and for isolated small patches. It is painful and if large areas are injected there can be systemic effects. Response occurs in about two-thirds of patients as an all or nothing phenomenon. Initially the response is localized to injection sites, but a more general improvement may follow. Hairs first appear at around 2 weeks and satisfactory regrowth has usually occurred within 6 weeks. Remissions are in the order of 6 to 9 months. The injection must be delivered very superficially in the dermis as the target hair follicles lie superficially. Repeated injections eventually produce atrophy although partial recovery occurs over six to nine months. Periocular injections can induce glaucoma and cataracts. Relapse eventually occurs even with continued injections.

Second-line pharmacological therapy

For patients who fail first-line therapy, progression to second-line therapy is not automatic, and it might be better for the patient to simply change their hairstyle or to get a wig. For those patients who proceed, therapeutic options include systemic immunosuppression with either prednisolone or PUVA, contact irritants and sensitizers such as dithranol and diphencyclopropenone (DCP) or minoxidil. None is universally successful and each has its drawbacks.

Prednisolone used in a dose of 50 mg daily causes partial regrowth in three-quarters of patients treated after 3 to 6 weeks. However complete regrowth is less common and prolonged remissions are exceptional. Most patients relapse on cessation of therapy or dose reduction, while some relapse despite continued full dose therapy. Not all patients respond to steroids and even with daily intravenous pulses of methylprednisolone (500 mg) some remain refractory.

Systemic PUVA works better than topical PUVA. A minimum of 40 to 60 erythemogenic treatments are required before the treatment can be said not to have worked, and if there is a response the treatment should be continued. About 30 to 40% of AA patients will regrow hair, but relapse is common (50–90%) on discontinuation of therapy. Long-term risks include induction of skin cancer, particularly in children, and only in exceptional cases should patients receive more than 200 treatment during their life.

Dithranol has been used as a topical irritant in the treatment of AA. The mechanism of action is unknown, but two-thirds of patients treated develop some hair regrowth that in about one half is cosmetically significant. The concentration of dithranol is increased such that all patients experience irritation. Unless there is a response within six months, the treatment is abandoned. By this time there is usually significant dithranol pigmentation, but this resolves with time. The response does not correlate with the degree of pigmentation.

Diphencyclopropenone (DCP) has largely replaced dinitrochlorobenzene (DNCB) as the agent used to induce a contact allergic dermatitis on the scalp. DCP is photodegradable and so patients are told to wear a hat. The chemical is applied weekly after the patient has been sensitized. The chemical needs to be in contact with the scalp for 48 hours after application (without wetting the scalp). Many patients develop severe itching, burning, blistering or urticaria in response to treatment that makes wig wearing difficult. There is a response rate of about 50% in patients with severe alopecia areata[53]. There are no reliable predictive factors as to who will respond. Remissions are of variable duration, but are occasionally prolonged. Sometimes contact sensitivity is lost during therapy and the concentration of the DCP needs to be gradually increased. Some physicians allow the patients to apply the DCP themselves at home, while others, fearing the consequences of incautious handling, apply the DCP themselves. Sensitization of medical staff is also a hazard.

Minoxidil 5% lotion is primarily used for androgenetic alopecia, but has also been used for AA. Initial results were promising, however they were not sustained in later trials, even when the concentration was increased to 5%. Patients with alopecia totalis do not seem to respond to minoxidil and few develop cosmetically significant regrowth.

Third-line pharmacological therapy

This consists of a variety of other therapies that have at one time or another been reported as successful in small series. In general those patients with widespread AA who have not responded to any of the first- or second-line treatments are doomed to remain bald. Thrid-line treatments include cryotherapy (2 freeze–thaw cycles), azathioprine in a dose of 100 mg daily, topical nitrogen mustard 0.2 mg per ml daily over the entire scalp, oral zinc supplementation with 600 mg of zinc sulfate daily and cyclosporin A.

The natural history of AA, and in particular the tendency to spontaneous remission, should not be forgotten when evaluating treatment modalities.

Physical therapies

Some patients with extensive AA shave their head and walk about bald. Others wear a hat or a scarf. Many choose to wear a wig. Patients often have misapprehensions about wearing a wig and either speaking to another patient who has a good wig or the advice of a quality wig maker is invaluable. Patient support organizations can usually suggest a good wig maker and give useful advice on styling and wig maintenance.

Hair transplantation generally fails. The grafted hairs fall out owing to continued immunological attack. Rarely patients will be considered for hair transplantation if they have a single recalcitrant patch of AA that on biopsy shows no evidence of continuing inflammation.

Conclusions

AA is an enigmatic disorder and in no individual is a confident prognosis possible. The outcome from an episode of alopecia areata is influenced by a number of factors. Overall, about 30% of patients go on to develop alopecia totalis, and almost all patients will develop other patches of AA at some stage in their life.

Doctors need to be sensitive to the needs of their patients and allow them considerable time to voice their fears and difficulties. Patient support groups can provide a wealth of information regarding hair styling and cosmetics to minimize the impact of the hair loss. The reassurance of knowing they are not alone and others are affected too is also of considerable benefit.

CICATRICIAL ALOPECIA
Introduction

Cicatricial or scarring alopecia is a general term applied to areas of permanent hair loss evidenced histologically by destruction of the hair follicles. It can be either congenital or acquired and there are numerous possible causes. The most common causes of acquired cicatricial alopecia seen in clinical practice are lichen planus, discoid lupus erythematosus, folliculitis decalvans and pseudopelade of Brocq. Other causes include traumatic or post-infectious cicatricial alopecia, cicatricial pemphigoid and erosive pustular dermatosis of the scalp. All other causes are rare and a schematic classification is presented in Table 7. New causes continue to appear in the literature, and include frontal fibrosing alopecia, described by Kossard and colleagues in 1994. This is thought to be a variant of lichen planopilaris, is seen

Table 7   Common causes of acquired scarring alopecia

Inflammatory	Lichenoid	Lichen planus
		Pseudopelade of Brocq
	Connective tissue disease	Discoid lupus erythematosus
		Morphea
	Neutrophilic	Folliculitis decalvans
		Acne keloidalis nuchae
		Erosive pustular dermatosis
	Granulomatous	Sarcoidosis
		Temporal arteritis
Traumatic		Radiodermatitis
		Mechanical trauma
		Post surgical (flap necrosis)
		Burns
		Traction alopecia
Infectious	Bacteria	Folliculitis
	Fungal	Kerion
		Tinea capitis (rarely scarring)
	Viral	Shingles
	Protozoal	Syphilis
Neoplastic	Benign	Cylindroma (adnexal tumours)
	Malignant	Basal cell carcinoma
		Squamous cell carcinoma
		Alopecia neoplastica
		(metastatic carcinoma)

exclusively in postmenopausal women and is characterized by progressive, permanent loss of hair in a band-like pattern originating at the frontal hairline[54] (Figure 20). Tumors and in particular metastatic nodules from renal, breast and lung carcinomas should not be forgotten as a possible cause of scarring alopecia.

The natural progression of the scarring alopecias is variable, however most exhibit a progressive, patchy, permanent hair loss that can be disfiguring and upsetting to affected women and girls. Treatment at present is largely anecdotal. As the hair loss is permanent, the aim of treatment is to arrest progression.

Clinical features

Scarring in an area of alopecia is not always easy to recognize. The skin is characteristically smooth and shiny owing to atrophy, with a few single hairs emerging where isolated follicles have escaped destruction. A hand lens or a dermatoscope may allow the loss of hair follicle pores to be better seen and enable causes of non-scarring alopecia such as alopecia areata to be distinguished, while a Wood's lamp may be useful to help exclude a fungal cause. A helpful confirmatory sign is the presence of pili multigemini or tufting of hairs (multiple hairs arising from a single follicular opening) within a patch of cicatricial alopecia. This is produced by distortion of the follicles and is not seen in non-scarring alopecias.

Additional features that may be present include inflammation of the scalp, pustules, perifollicular hyperkeratosis, telangiectasia, pigmentation, perifollicular erythema and broken hairs. These signs may help determine the cause of the scarring alopecia, however no one sign in isolation is pathognomonic for a particular disease, and a correlation of clinical and histological features is usually needed to make a specific diagnosis.

When scarring is the only physical sign, examination of the entire skin surface may reveal a dermatosis, such as lichen planus, that is the cause of the scarring. Up to 70% of patients with scalp lichen planus and 30% with discoid lupus of the scalp will have specific signs of the disease elsewhere on the body.

Investigations

Scalp biopsy is required to confirm the scarring nature of the hair loss, and to help establish the etiology. Biopsies should be taken from the active

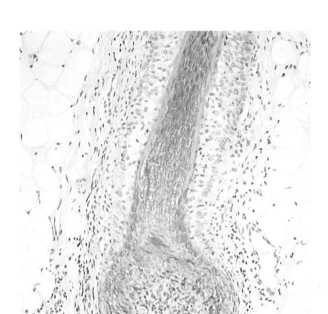

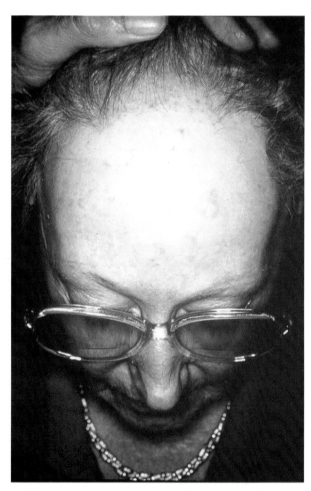

Figure 18 Perifollicular infiltrate of lymphocytes around the anagen hair bulb in alopecia areata

Figure 20 Frontal fibrosing alopecia – usually lichen planopilaris histologically. Note the difference in skin texture between the sun-exposed forehead and the shiny white skin that had previously been protected by hair

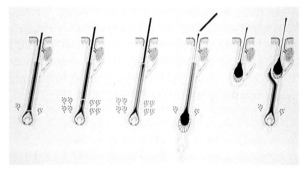

Figure 19 The hair cycle in alopecia areata. Note that only the anagen follicle is attacked by lymphocytes, preventing the growth of a hair fiber of any discernible length. The telogen follicle has no perifollicular infiltrate

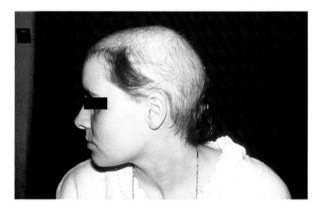

Figure 21 Trichotillomania characterized by an unusual pattern of hair loss

edge of the lesion. Examination with immuno-fluorescence will add valuable data. Even if the cicatricial alopecia seems to have burnt out, useful prognostic information may still be gained from the biopsy. If a fungal cause is suspected, hairs from the edge of the bald patch can be plucked and

sent for mycology. Any pustules should be swabbed and the fluid cultured. An antinuclear factor is suggested for suspected cases of lupus, however it should be remembered that there can be both false positive and false negative results.

Pathogenesis

Inflammation in the region of the hair bulge that leads to destruction of the hair stem cells is responsible for the permanent nature of this type of alopecia[55].

Treatment

As the hair loss is permanent the aim of treatment is to arrest progression. Any treatment is tailored to the cause. For inflammatory scarring alopecia systemic and topical steroids have been widely used, especially when a more specific diagnosis cannot be made. Antimalarials such as hydroxyquinone have a role in discoid lupus erythematosus, but may also have a role in lichen planopilaris. Oral retinoids have also been used for both lichen planopilaris and discoid lupus erythematosus. Other treatments for lichen planopilaris include minomycin and azathioprine.

If an infective agent is found then antifungals or antibiotics are indicated. Occasionally prednisolone is used in conjunction with these agents to minimize associated inflammatory damage to hair follicles.

Surgical correction of a patch of scarring alopecia can be performed once the lesion has been inactive for 12 or more months. This can be done either by hair transplantation if the area is not too large or by excision of the scar with closure using tissue expanders or a flap.

Conclusion

The scarring alopecias of inflammatory origin are at present poorly understood with regard to their natural history and response to treatment. The conditions are usually progressive and carry a high degree of morbidity owing to their deforming nature. More research is required in this field of dermatology.

TRAUMATIC ALOPECIA
Trichotillomania

Trichotillomania is twice as common in females compared to males and refers to a patient's compulsion or tic in which they twist and pluck hairs. The scalp and the eyebrows are the most common sites, but any area may be involved. The clinical findings are unusual patterns of hair loss and a stubble of short hairs of irregular length, owing to the fact that it is difficult to manually pluck hairs shorter than a few millimetres without tweezers (Figure 21). These are often better felt than seen. Fractured hair fibers and evidence of perifollicular

trauma may be seen on biopsy, but follicles devoid of their hair fiber surrounded by normal follicles may be all that is seen. Trichotillomania is mostly a non-permanent alopecia but if the same area of hair is continually plucked scarring may occur resulting in a permanent alopecia. Psychiatric referral is recommended for the treatment of recalcitrant cases.

Traction alopecia

Traction alopecia is another form of traumatic alopecia that is seen most commonly in females. It is caused by constant tension placed on the hair fiber owing to hair styling. Clinically short broken hairs, folliculitis and follicular papules may be present. It can be seen at the frontal hairline in women who constantly wear their hair in a very tight ponytail (Figure 22). Among black females, in which the condition is more common, the loss of hair may be seen anywhere on the scalp in accordance with braided hair styling. The alopecia is initially reversible, but prolonged, constant tension may induce folliculitis which may result in scarring, and thus permanent hair loss.

Hot comb alopecia

'Hot comb' alopecia is a largely historical form of permanent traumatic alopecia that was almost exclusively confined to black women. Hot combing was performed to straighten hair and consisted of applying hot oil to the hair fiber and then pulling it through a hot comb. The mode of injury was thought to be chemical and thermal follicular damage as the hot oil ran down the hair shaft and into the follicle. Scarring was the endpoint. Scalp burns from the hot comb, and traction caused by pulling the hair through the comb, may also have contributed to the hair loss.

Follicular degeneration syndrome

The follicular degeneration syndrome clinically resembles 'hot-comb' alopecia, but is seen in black women who deny ever using hot combs. Hair fiber granulomas, replacement of the follicle with fibrous tracts and follicular degeneration are seen[56]. The etiology is unknown at present.

HEREDITARY AND CONGENITAL HYPOTRICHOSIS

In hereditary hypotrichosis there is a profound reduction in the number of follicles on the scalp, usually, but not always, from birth. Congenital hypotrichosis often goes unnoticed initially, as many normal children are born without much hair and remain this way during the first year of life, making sparse hair during this period unremarkable. Hypotrichosis can occur either as an isolated defect or as part of a syndrome. Atrichia congenita, on the other hand, refers to a condition where there is total and permanent absence of scalp hair. It may begin at birth, or be delayed for up to five years. A scalp biopsy may be required to distinguish it from alopecia areata totalis. Intrafamilial variation in the degree of hair loss confirms that atrichia congenita and hypotrichosis are related, the latter being a less severe form of the former.

Atrichia congenita

Atrichia congenita is most commonly an autosomal recessive condition, usually not associated with any other anomalies. Autosomal dominant pedigrees also exist.

Clinical features

The presentation may be one of complete and permanent absence of hair from birth, or the infant may have normal hair for the first five years of life, after which there is a progressive and permanent loss of hair. Atrichia congenita usually occurs as an isolated phenomenon but may be associated with facial papular cysts, immunodeficiency, epilepsy and/or mental retardation, deafness, ocular abnormalities, ichthyosis, skeletal abnormalities, inborn errors of metabolism and premature aging syndromes, such as progeria.

Investigations

The diagnosis can be a clinical one, but a scalp biopsy is usually performed to check the histology, number of follicles, state of follicles, scarring and presence of any other cutaneous abnormalities. As already mentioned, a biopsy may be required to differentiate this condition from alopecia areata totalis.

Treatment

The only form of treatment for atrichia congenita is camouflage, in the form of a wig for example.

Hypotrichosis

As mentioned, hereditary hypotrichosis can occur either as a single abnormality or as part of a syndrome. When occurring alone, its features are similar to those of atrichia congenita, but less severe. There is a broad range of the extent of alopecia

present when associated with other abnormalities or as part of a syndrome.

Marie Unna syndrome

This is an autosomal dominant condition first described by Dr Marie Unna in 1925, and since described infrequently around the world.

Clinical features

Some variability exists, however the usual clinical picture is sparse to normal hair at birth, followed by the appearance of coarse and twisted hair on the scalp in the third year, likened to the appearance of an ill-fitting wig. At puberty there is progressive loss of scalp hair with a variable degree of scarring. Eyebrows, eyelashes and body hair, including axillary and pubic hair after puberty, are usually absent or scant. Females are usually less severely affected than their male counterparts.

Investigations

A scalp biopsy should be taken, however the histological changes seen in the scalp are not pathognomonic. There is a marked reduction in follicle number and some follicles appear to be partially destroyed with associated granulomatous reactions. Light microscopy reveals coarse, flattened hairs with shaft diameters up to 100μm. Scanning electron microscopy demonstrates hair shafts that are rigid without the usual scale pattern. Intracellular fractures of the cuticular cells are seen.

Treatment

There is no known treatment other than preserving the remaining hairs, which may be brittle and susceptible to trauma. Folliculitis can be troublesome, and is best controlled with long-term antibiotics.

STRUCTURAL ABNORMALITIES OF THE HAIR SHAFT

Numerous abnormalities of the hair shaft have been demonstrated on light microscopy, some due to an inherited disorder, but others due to the normal weathering process. This in turn can produce varied appearances of the hair including areas of alopecia, or frizzy, coarse or limp hair. Hair may be described as unruly because it is twisted, curled or irregularly shaped, all of which prevent the hair fibers from sitting together neatly. Spangled hair refers to hair which is either twisted or has alternating light and dark bands which reflect light in different directions. There are a number of recognized hair shaft disorders, each with distinctive features, the more common of which are described below.

Weathering

Weathering refers to the structural damage caused by external forces. It is caused both by environmental factors such as wetting, ultraviolet radiation and natural friction, as well as damage done by cosmetic procedures such as combing, brushing, bleaching and permanent waving. Weathering is seen more frequently and to a greater extent in females owing to the fact that women on average grow their hair longer, use more styling products and are more likely to chemically treat their hair than men.

The hair shaft consists of a hydrophobic lipid envelope which surrounds the proteinaceous cuticle, which in turn surrounds the cortex and central medulla. It is this lipid exocuticle that gives hair its luster and silky texture, and is the first to be destroyed by weathering, followed by the cuticle itself. This gives rise to limp, lusterless hair with a coarse texture. Later changes include cortical damage, terminal fraying and longitudinal fissures between exposed cortical cells, followed by transverse fissures and nodes of the type seen in trichorrhexis nodosa as the weathering becomes more severe[57]. Bleaching or perming hair may distort the shaft, which in turn increases the likelihood and extent of frictional damage. Certain hair shaft disorders will also cause hair to weather to a greater degree than normal, such as the twists in pili torti or the internodes in monilethrix.

Treatment for weathering is prevention. This includes the avoidance of all unnecessary trauma and limitation of the use of hair styling products. Washing of the hair with conditioner is advised.

Uncombable hair

This is an autosomal dominant genodermatosis characterized by triangular hair. The hair is first noted to be abnormal at about three years of age and is seen to be unruly and resistant to all forms of grooming with a brush or a comb. The pathognomonic feature on light and electron microscopy is that more than 50% of the hairs have a triangular or kidney-shaped cross-section with a longitudinal groove running along almost the entire length of the hair.

Pili torti

The hair shaft in pili torti is flattened and twisted through 180° at irregular intervals along the shaft. The hairs are fragile and snap off if subjected to moderate trauma. Not all the hairs are affected and the proportion of affected hairs varies from person to person. The twisting gives the hair a spangled appearance, and the fragility may lead to circumscribed areas of baldness at sites of friction and trauma. In severe cases there may only be a short coarse stubble over the entire scalp. In areas not subjected to trauma where the hair is allowed to grow long, the twisting renders it unruly.

Pili torti has a variable clinical presentation. Classically the hair is normal at birth and is gradually replaced by spangled, blond, abnormal hair between the third month and third year of life. The hair remains abnormal until puberty when it darkens in colour, becomes less fragile and grows to an acceptable length.

Twisting hair dystrophy

There are a number of heterogeneous disorders where half and three-quarter twists of the hair are seen at irregular intervals rather than the full 180° twists seen in pili torti. Acquired twisting is also almost invariably seen at the edge of a scarring alopecia and is due to follicular distortion as a result of the scarring process.

Woolly hair

This refers to tightly coiled hair over all or part of the scalp that resembles Negroid hair in a non-Negroid. Generalized woolly hair can be inherited in either an autosomal dominant or recessive fashion. The hairs are fine and of irregular caliber with occasional loose twists and of varying strength. Localized, nevoid woolly hair may be present at birth but appears not to be genetically determined. Acquired woolly hair also exists, but this appears to be a distinct condition that is usually a precursor of androgenetic alopecia.

Pili annulati

Patients rarely present with this autosomal dominant condition, and usually it is discovered incidentally. The patient has patches of scalp hair that have a spangled appearance. The alternating light and dark bands are well demonstrated on light microscopy, the light sections being normal hair and the dark bands areas where the medulla is expanded by air cavities which also spread into the cortex.

Monilethrix

This rare autosomal dominant condition is a type II keratin gene defect that leads to the abnormal assembly of the keratin intermediate filaments. Clinically the hair is characterized by keratosis pilaris, beaded hairs and fragile hairs. The beading may produce a slightly spangled appearance. The dominant clinical feature is hair that fails to grow long owing to fragility, and both beaded and non-beaded hairs are fragile. This condition has a high but variable penetrance giving rise to a wide spectrum of presentations, from hair that is near normal to hair that is not able to be grown more than two centimeters.

Loose anagen syndrome

Loose anagen syndrome is a newly described condition that predominantly affects girls. Here, anchorage of the growing anagen hairs to the follicle is impaired and these hairs can be easily and painlessly plucked from the follicle. As a result, most hairs do not remain *in situ* until completion of the anagen phase. This results in affected children having hair that does not grow long and that is of uneven length. The hair is unruly and has an unusual sticky feel to it. Bald patches are easily produced if a handful of hair is pulled in a childhood dispute, and is often the trigger for presentation (Figure 23).

Children between the ages of two and seven years are most commonly affected. Their hair appears normal at birth, but becomes unruly, sticky and uneven at two to three years and remains so until it spontaneously reverts to normal at five to seven years. It is inherited in an autosomal dominant fashion and it is common to find that apparently normal parents or older siblings have easily plucked hair.

The characteristic feature seen on light microscopy is an anagen hair with a misshapen bulb, and a crumpled proximal hair cuticle without an inner root sheath that has been extracted by gentle traction.

INFECTIONS AND INFESTATIONS OF THE HAIR
Tinea capitis
Introduction

Tinea capitis is the invasion of scalp hair by dermatophyte fungi which can occur in one of three ways. Anthrophilic infections are acquired from close person to person contact as well as being passed on by the shared use of hairbrushes, combs and hats. Zoophilic infections are acquired from animal contact and geophilic infections arise in children playing in infected soil. Some infections can be both zoophilic and geophilic, and *Microsporum canis*, which is classified as zoophilic, can also have limited passage from person to person.

Microsporum audouini, *Trichophyton violaceum*, and *T. schoenleinii* have a predilection for hair; however nearly all dermatophytes are able to infect hair. The predominant organism causing tinea capitis varies from country to country (Table 8) – in Europe it is *M. canis* whilst in the USA it is *T. tonsurans*.

Classification of scalp ringworm is based on the pattern of hair invasion. Endothrix (from within) infections are only due to trichophyton species. Ectothrix (from outside) infections may be divided into small spored (2–3 μm) which are only caused by *Microsporum* species, or large spored (5–10 μm) which may be caused by either *Microsporum* or *Trichophyton* species.

Clinical features

Generally anthropophilic fungi produce non-inflammatory lesions while zoophilic and geophilic fungi produce lesions with marked inflammation such as kerion and favus. Inflammatory tinea capitis tends to be self-limiting over six to ten weeks, but generally heals with scarring. Infection is far more common in children than in adults. Small-spore ectothrix infections classically produce annular lesions or gray patch ringworm. Brittle hairs break off close to the scalp surface to create circular patches of partial alopecia. The broken hairs have a dull grey appearance owing to their coating of athrospores. Inflammation of the scalp is minimal, but fine scaling is characteristic. There is usually a fairly sharp margin and there may be several such patches throughout the scalp. Each fluoresces green with Wood's lamp examination. With some infections due to *M. audouini* there may be minimal hair loss and the mild scaling may mimic seborrheic dermatitis.

Large-spored ectothrix infections may produce scalp ringworm that resembles small-spored ectothrix. Alternatively, there may be more marked inflammation of the scalp. Occasionally a folliculitis or kerion occurs, especially with zoophilic and geophilic fungi. Agminate folliculitis is a moderately severe inflammatory response and consists of well-defined dull red plaques studded with follicular pustules. A kerion is a painful, boggy, elevated, purulent inflammatory mass. Hairs fall out rather than break off and any remaining hairs can easily

Table 8   Most common cause of tinea capitis by continent

Europe	Australia	N. America	S. America	Africa	Asia
M. canis	M. canis	T. tonsurans	T. violaceum	T. violaceum	T. violaceum
	T. tonsurans	M. canis	M. canis	T. soudanense	
	(Aborigines)	M. audouini		M. audouini	
				M. canis	
				T. yaoundi	

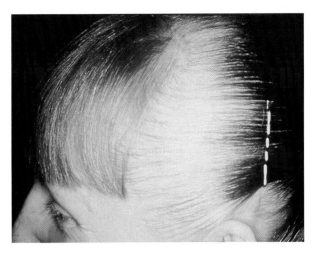

Figure 22   Traction alopecia due to repeated force placed on the hair fibers from daily hair styling into a tight pony tail

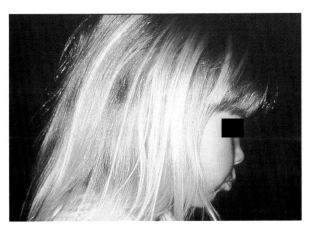

Figure 23   Loose anagen syndrome showing an inability to grow hair any longer than shoulder length

and painlessly be pulled out. Thick crusting with matting of adjacent hairs is common. The usual organisms responsible are *T. verrucosum* and *T. mentagrophytes*. Occasionally an insidious anthrophilic infection will suddenly develop into a kerion (Figure 24).

In endothrix infections the athrospores remain confined within the cuticle and affected hairs are severely damaged and break off at the scalp surface. Patients present with black dot ringworm, where

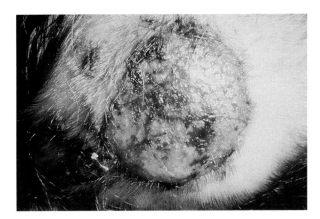

Figure 24   Kerion. Discrete, boggy, painful, purulent swelling on the scalp secondary to severe tinea capitis

broken hairs within an angular patch of alopecia appear as black dots. With the anthrophilic fungi, there is usually minimal scaling or inflammation of the scalp. Sometimes hair loss is minimal and all that can be seen is a mild folliculitis or seborrhoeic dermatitis-like scaling.

Majocchi's granuloma and tinea incognito can result from treatment of tinea capitis with potent topical steroids. Typically with tinea incognito the raised margin is lost, scaling and itch are absent and the inflammation is reduced to a few nondescript nodules. Majocchi's granuloma on the scalp are rare and present as a granulomatous folliculitis with inflammatory nodules bordering flat, scaly patches.

Yeast infection of the scalp with *Candida* is uncommon and generally occurs only in the setting of immunodeficiency.

Investigations

The Wood's lamp is an invaluable tool for diagnosing fungal conditions. Green fluorescence is seen when a fluorescent substance, possibly pteridines, is formed when hair keratin is invaded. Not all dermatophytes cause fluorescence, and scalp lotions and creams can mask fluorescence. These should be washed off before examination with the Wood's lamp. Fluorescence may confirm fungal etiology, give an indication as to the species involved and define the extent of the infection. Six to eight hairs should be plucked for fungal microscopy and culture, firstly to confirm the diagnosis and then to identify the species involved.

Treatment

The standard treatment for all ringworm of the scalp is still griseofulvin. Given late in inflammatory infections (which have a tendency to heal spontaneously), it may not alter the course of existing lesions, but it will prevent the development of new ones. Gray patch ringworm requires the full dose, which is 15 mg/kg daily of microsize griseofulvin for adults (or 10 mg/kg/day of ultramicrosize griseofulvin) and 10 mg/kg/day for children for at least six weeks. In very young children who are unable to swallow tablets, a griseofulvin suspension can be used, or, if unavailable, ketoconazole shampoo may be helpful. Cultures should be repeated after four weeks and every two weeks thereafter until mycological cure. Black dot ringworm may require slightly longer treatment, which should be continued for two weeks beyond clinical and mycological cure. Kerion generally requires six weeks of therapy.

Headache from the drug may be overcome by reducing the dose and slowly increasing it again. Griseofulvin interacts with a number of drugs such as warfarin and phenobarbitone, and dose adjustments may be required. An 'id' eruption consisting of multiple small papules on the side of the face and the trunk, or vesicles on the hands, may occur after commencing therapy with griseofulvin for tinea capitis, however a true drug hypersensitivity to griseofulvin is rare.

Secondary bacterial infection occasionally occurs and if suspected, swabs should be taken and a broad spectrum oral antibiotic such as erythromycin given.

Alternatives to griseofulvin are ketoconazole, itraconazole, fluconazole and terbinafine. Cure rates are similar, shorter treatments are required and there are fewer drug interactions. The drawbacks are that ketoconazole has problems with hepatotoxicity (1 in 10 000) and many of these newer drugs are not licensed for use in children. Few comparative studies for these newer agents in tinea capitis are available, but those to hand suggest griseofulvin is still the drug of first choice, if only on cost.

Griseofulvin treatment of kerion does not tend to prevent the development of scarring alopecia and so it is prudent to combine the griseofulvin with prednisolone 25 mg daily for the first week or two,

and this may also hasten resolution of the symptoms. Oral antibiotics are generally not required unless secondary bacterial infection is proven. Selenium sulfide or ketoconazole shampoo may also decrease the period of fungal shedding.

The source of infection should be traced. With *M. canis* cats and dogs should be examined with a Wood's lamp by a veterinary surgeon and infected animals treated with griseofulvin. Children with infection due to anthropophilic fungi and *M. canis* should be kept home from school until the infection has cleared. In school epidemics classmates should be examined with a Wood's lamp; however in new infections the fluorescent part of the hair may not yet have emerged from the follicle, and fluorescence will only be detected if the hair is plucked and the root examined.

Pediculosis and scabies

Introduction

Lice feed on the skin and deposit their eggs (nits) on the hair. Two species of louse infest man, *Pediculosis humanis* and *Pthirus pubis*. There are two subspecies of *Pediculosis humanis*; *P. humanis capitis*, the head louse, and *P. humanis corporis*, the body or clothing louse. Head lice and body lice look almost identical, and are capable of interbreeding, but on the host they tend to maintain their territorial preferences. Although the head louse occasionally wanders onto the body, the body louse rarely ventures onto the scalp.

The female head louse is 3–4 mm long. The male is slightly smaller and banded across the back. During her 40-day life span the female lays approximately 300 eggs at a rate of eight a day. The eggs are oval, white capsules with a lid (operculum) and are firmly cemented to the side of the hair shaft adjacent to the scalp. After about a week the larvae hatch close to the scalp. Larvae resemble small adults and begin feeding on the blood of the host soon after hatching. After undergoing three molts in 10 days, the louse reaches maturity and commences mating.

The life cycle of the body louse is similar to that of the head louse. Its natural habitat is clothing and it only visits its host to feed. Nits are cemented to clothing fibers, especially in the seams closest to the body. Washing in hot water and ironing kill lice, so this tends to be a disease of vagabonds and refugees.

Pthirus pubis, the pubic louse, is structurally and morphologically different to *P. humanis*. The term crab-louse is appropriate as its body is squat and the second and third pairs of legs carry heavy, pincer-like claws. In addition to pubic hair, pubic lice can colonize the axillae, eyebrows, eyelashes and also the scalp margin. Pubic lice are vessel feeders and have specially adapted mouth-parts to probe the skin and pierce blood vessels. Eggs only attach to coarse terminal hairs and so this infestation is rare prior to puberty, and can be extensive in the hirsute male. Eggs hatch in 6–8 days and the nymphs reach maturity in 15–17 days.

Clinical features

In most established infestations of head lice there are fewer than 10 adult lice and counts of more than 100 are uncommon. Most infections are acquired by direct head to head contact, but combs, brushes and hats are important in some cases. Pruritus is variable. It is often intense and only rarely absent. It is usually worst in the occipital region where the infestation is heaviest. Scratching leads to impetigenization and the hair may become matted down by exudate to produce 'plica polonica'. Nits can be seen with the naked eye and are very easily seen with a Wood's lamp. This is useful for screening in schools during epidemics. Head lice is rare in Negroids as the lice appear not to grab tightly curled hair very well.

Pubic lice are spread by sexual contact, and other sexually transmitted diseases frequently coexist. Occasionally they may be transmitted by shed hairs in clothing, towels or sleeping bags. The host immunological reaction to louse salivary antigens is variable and some subjects have intense irritation with a small louse population, while others with numerous lice are free of symptoms. The mites tend to feed at night and itching in the evening and night is the principal symptom. Blue-gray macules known as maculae ceruleae or taches bleues on the abdominal wall and thighs are characteristic, but rare. They are due to altered blood at the sites of bites. Lice and nits are visible with the naked eye on close inspection and louse feces can be seen on the skin as rust coloured speckles.

Scabies is an infestation caused by the mite *Sarcoptes scabiei var hominis*. Involvement of the scalp is rare except in infancy and in the immunocompromised. Thus when scabies is present on the scalp, immunosuppression should be suspected. Such cases tend not to be itchy and the resulting high density of mites makes this condition highly infective. Scalp lesions may occur without evidence of infestation elsewhere and simulate seborrheic dermatitis, or may be associated with crusted lesions on the trunk and limbs in the crusted scabies variant. The diagnosis requires identification of the mite.

Investigations

The diagnosis is usually a clinical one but light microscopy can be performed to identify the species involved.

Treatment

Parasitophobia is common and the diagnosis of infestation should not be accepted unless the insect or its eggs have been positively identified. Peripilar hair casts or pseudonits are a source of confusion but these can be readily slid up and down the hair shaft and are circumferential rather than eccentric. This can be visualized by light microscopy.

In the presence of severe itch, scratching may cause secondary bacterial infection, for which systemic antibiotics are usually required. Malathion and carbaryl became the mainstays of therapy for head louse infection following emergence of resistance to the organochloride antiseptics. They were required to be left in the scalp for 12 hours before being washed off. Blow drying should be avoided as heat degrades these insecticides. Both agents effectively kill lice, however they do not kill all the eggs and a second application after 7 to 10 days is usually recommended. Malathion coats the hair making it resistant to re-infection for 6 weeks. Permethrins are now the most widely used agents, and generally only require a 10 minute scalp application after shampooing. This is repeated after 7 to 10 days. Again hair dryers should be avoided.

None of these treatments removes the dead nits. Combing with a fine toothed comb is tedious and painful. Nits will eventually wear away after repeated washing but 8% formic acid in a cream rinse can be used as a nit-remover.

Head lice epidemics are common and in general malathion, carbaryl and permethrin are rotated periodically by local health authorities to prevent the build-up of resistance. Infected children should be kept home from school until the first treatment is completed.

As pubic lice may wander it is preferable to treat the whole trunk and limbs. Preparations containing gamma benzene hexachloride, malathion, carbaryl and permethrins are all effective. Eyelash infection can be treated with vaseline, 20% fluorescein drops or malathion liquid, which does not tend to irritate the eyes.

CONCLUSION

Most disease states have a similar incidence and pathological pattern with respect to gender, however hair pathology in girls and women deserves special and separate attention as there are many exceptions. Loose anagen syndrome and trichotillomania have an increased incidence in females of two to one. Hirsuties is a condition that is only described in women, and refers to excessive hair growth in the same areas as for the secondary sexual hair growth of the postpubertal male. Whether this condition is a real pathological entity or a socially unacceptable normal variant for a postpubertal female is another question. Frontal fibrosing alopecia is a true example of a pathological condition that is only described in women, and to date only postmenopausal women.

Androgenetic alopecia is a condition that occurs in both men and women by the same pathological process, yet, interestingly, has a differing clinical pattern for each sex, women following the Ludwig pattern, men the Hamilton grading. This condition carries with it a lot of social and psychological difficulties for women. In fact any hair pathology that is disfiguring has a greater morbidity in girls and women compared with their male counterparts owing to an increased sense of importance that women place on their hair for their total body image. To disguise hair loss men also have the option of shaving their heads, which is currently fashionable in Western countries for men, but not women.

Research in this area of dermatology is progressing at a fast pace, fueled by the interest generated in the community and the importance placed on maintaining a normal pattern of hair growth, and this has been reflected by recent advances in pharmacological therapies for hair loss.

REFERENCES

1. Imperato-McGinley J, Peterson R, Gautier T, et al. Androgens and the evolution of male-gender identity among male pseudohermaphrodites with 5 alpha-reductase deficiency. *N Engl J Med* 1979; 300:1233–7

2. Cash T, Price V, Savin R. Psychological effects of androgenetic alopecia on women: comparisons with balding men and female control subjects. *J Am Acad Dermatol* 1993;29:568–75

3. Olsen E. Clinical tools for assessing hair loss. In Olsen E, ed. *Disorders of Hair Growth: Diagnosis and Treatment.* New York: McGraw-Hill, 1994:59–70

4. Van Scott E, Reinerston R, Steinmuller R. The growing hair roots of the human scalp and morphologic changes therein following amethopterin therapy. *J Invest Dermatol* 1957;29:197–204

5. Whiting D. Diagnostic and predictive value of horizontal sections of scalp biopsy specimens in male pattern androgenetic alopecia. *J Am Acad Dermatol* 1993;28:755–63

6. Ferriman D, Gallwey J. Clinical assessment of body hair growth in women. *J Clin Endocrinol* 1961;21: 1440–7

7. Simpson N, Barth J. Hair patterns: hirsuties and androgenetic alopecia. In Dawber R, ed. *Diseases of the Hair and Scalp.* Oxford: Blackwell Science, 1997:71–136

8. Montagna W, Uno H. The phylogeny of baldness. In Baccareda-Boy A, Moretti G, Fray J, eds. *Biopathology of Pattern Alopecia.* Basel: Karger, 1968:9–24

9. Hamilton J. Patterned loss of hair in man: types and incidence. *Ann NY Acad Sci* 1951;53:708–28

10. Ludwig E. Classification of the types of androgenetic alopecia (common baldness) occurring in the female sex. *Br J Dermatol* 1977;97:247–54

11. Itami S, Kurata S, Takayasu S. 5α-Reductase activity in cultured human dermal papilla cells from beard compared with reticular dermal fibroblasts. *J Invest Dermatol* 1990;94:150–2

12. Harris G. Identification and selective inhibition of an isozyme of steroid 5α-reductase in human scalp. *Proc Natl Acad Sci USA* 1992;89:10787–91

13. Chen W, Zouboulis C, Orfanos C. The 5α-reductase system and its inhibitors: recent development and its perspective in treating androgen-dependent skin disorders. *Dermatology* 1996;193:177–84

14. Nakanishi J, Itami S, Adachi K, et al. Expression of androgen receptor, type I and type II 5-alpha reductase in human dermal papilla cells. In van Neste D, Randall V, eds. *Hair Research for the Next Millennium,* Brussels: *Excerpta Medica* 1996:333–7

15. Bergfeld W. Androgenetic alopecia: an autosomal dominant disorder. *Am J Med* 1995;98:95S–98S

16. Kuster W, Happle R. The inheritance of common baldness: two B or not to B? *J Am Acad Dermatol* 1984;11:921–6

17. Ellis J. Genetic analysis of male pattern baldness and the 5-alpha reductase genes. *J Invest Dermatol* 1998;110:849–53

18. Sinclair R. Male pattern androgenetic alopecia. *Br Med J* 1998;317:865–9

19. Venning V, Dawber R. Patterned androgenetic alopecia. *J Am Acad Dermatol* 1988;18:1073

20. Sinclair R. Diffuse hair loss. *Int J Dermatol* 1999;38: 8–18

21. Kligman A. Pathological dynamics of reversible hair loss in humans. I. Telogen effluvium. *Arch Dermatol* 1961;83:175–98

22. Headington J. Telogen effluvium – new concepts and review. *Arch Dermatol* 1993;129:356–63

23. Dawber R, Connor B. Pregnancy, hair loss and the pill. *Br Med J* 1971;4:234

24. Comaish J. Metabolic disorders and hair growth. *Br J Dermatol* 1971;84:83–5

25. Rook A. Endocrine influences on hair growth. *Br Med J* 1965;1:609–14

26. Kennedy C. Syphilis presenting as hair loss. *Br Med J* 1976;2:854

27. Elston D, Bergfield W. Cicatricial alopecia (and other causes of permanent hair loss). In Olsen EA, ed. *Disorders of Hair Growth – Diagnosis and Treatment.* New York: McGraw Hill, 1994:287

28. Weismann K. Zinc metabolism and the skin. In Rool ASJ, ed. *Recent Advances in Dermatology 5*, Edinburgh: Churchill Livingston, 1980:109–29

29. Feidler V, Hafeez A. Diffuse alopecia: telogen hair loss. In Olsen EA, ed. *Disorders of Hair Growth – Diagnosis and Treatment.* New York: McGraw Hill, 1994:249–52

30. Curtois M, Loussouarn G, Horseau C, *et al*. Hair cycle and alopecia. *Skin Pharmacol* 1994;7:84–9

31. Lynfield Y. The effect of pregnancy on the human hair cycle. *J Invest Dermatol* 1960;35:323–7

32. Van Neste D, Rushton D. Hair problems in women. *Clin Dermatol* 1997;15:113–25

33. Rushton D, Ramsey I, James K. Biochemical and trichological characterisation of diffuse alopecia in women. *Br J Dermatol* 1990;123:187–97

34. Hard S. Non-anaemic iron deficiency as an etiologic factor in diffuse loss of hair of the scalp in women. *Acta Derm Venereol (Stockh)* 1963;43:562–9

35. Rushton D, Ramsey I. The importance of adequate serum ferritin levels during oral cyproterone acetate and ethinyl oestradiol treatment of diffuse androgen dependent alopecia in women. *Clin Endocrinol* 1992;36:421–7

36. Kaufman J. Telogen effluvium secondary to starvation diet. *Arch Dermatol* 1976;112:731

37. Bradfield R, Bailley M. Hair root response to protein undernutrition. In Montagna W, Dobson R, eds. *Advances in Biology of Skin*. Oxford: Pergamon Press, 1968:109

38. Skolnik P, Eaglstein W, Ziboh V. Human essential fatty acid deficiency. *Arch Dermatol* 1977;113:939–41

39. Church R. Hypothyroid hair loss. *Br J Dermatol* 1965;77:661

40. Scoggins R, Harlan W. Cutaneous manifestations of hyperlipidaemia and uraemia. *Postgrad Med* 1967;41:357

41. Kelin A, Rudolf R, Leyden J. Telogen effluvium as a sign of Hodgkin's disease. *Arch Dermatol* 1973;108:702–3

42. Wells G. Skin disorders in relation to malabsorption. *Br Med J* 1962;2:937

43. Dawber R, Simpson N. Hair and scalp in systemic diseases. In Dawber R, ed. *Diseases of the Hair and Scalp*, 3rd edn. Oxford: Blackwell Science, 1997:485

44. Gupta A, Goldfarb M, Ellis C, *et al*. Side-effect profile of acitretin therapy in psoriasis. *J Am Acad Dermatol* 1989;20:1088

45. Bardelli A, Rebora A. Telogen effluvium and minoxidil. *J Am Acad Dermatol* 1989;21:572–3

46. Whiting D. Chronic telogen effluvium. *J Am Acad Dermatol* 1996;20:10

47. Eckert J. Diffuse hair loss in women. The psychopathology of those who complain. *Acta Psychiatr Scand* 1976;53:321–7

48. Messenger R, Simpson N. Alopecia areata. In Dawber R, ed. *Diseases of the Hair and Scalp.* Oxford: Blackwell Science, 1997:338–69

49. Whiting D. Chronic telogen effluvium. *Dermatol Clin* 1996;14:697–711

50. Safavi K. Prevalence of alopecia areata in the First National Health and Nutrition Examination Survey. *Arch Dermatol* 1992;128:702

51. Muller S, Winkelmann R. Alopecia areata. *Arch Dermatol* 1963;88:106–13

52. Gip L, Lodin A, Molin L. Alopecia areata: a follow-up investigation of outpatient material. *Acta Derm Venereol (Stockh)* 1969;49:180–8

53. Rokhsar C, Shupack J, Vafai J. Efficacy of topical sensitizers in the treatment of alopecia areata. *J Am Acad Dermatol* 1998;39:751–61

54. Kossard S, Lee M, Wilkininson B. Postmenopausal frontal fibrosing alopecia: a frontal variant of lichen planopilaris. *J Am Acad Dermatol* 1997;36:59–66

55. Cotsarelis G, Sun T, Lavker R. Label-retaining cells reside in the bulge area of pilosebaceous unit: implication for follicular stem cells, hair cycle, and skin carcinogenesis. *Cell* 1990;61:1329–37

56. Sperling L, Sau P. The follicular degeneration syndrome in black patients. 'Hot comb alopecia' revisited and revised. *Arch Dermatol* 1992;128:68–74

57. Jones L. Investigation of structural proteins in human hair defects using anagen follicles. *Br J Dermatol* 1996;135:80–5

Other diseases

Papulosquamous diseases including contact dermatitis

15

Michelle L. Bennett and Elizabeth F. Sherertz

INTRODUCTION

This chapter discusses the diagnosis and management of cutaneous diseases characterized by erythematous papules which have a scaly surface (Tables 1 and 2). Psoriasis is a classic example in which such scaly papules coalesce into plaques. Atopic dermatitis, seborrheic dermatitis and contact dermatitis are eczematous skin conditions with papulosquamous primary skin lesions. Some infectious conditions, such as dermatophyte infections and syphilis, often present with scaly papules and plaques. As a group, these diseases are not more common in women and girls, but there are some unique features with respect to these populations.

ATOPIC DERMATITIS

Atopic dermatitis is sometimes referred to as infantile dermatitis. Chronic pruritic inflammation of the skin occurs, often in association with a personal or family history of hay fever, allergic rhinitis, or asthma. The age of onset is within the first year of life in 60% of patients. Adult onset of symptomatic dermatitis occasionally occurs, most often in association with exogenous irritants, which may be occupational. Female patients are affected slightly less frequently than male patients. Patients tend to have dry pruritic skin leading to an itch–scratch–rash cycle that ultimately manifests as lichenification of the skin. Ichthyosis may be present as well (Figure 1). Exacerbating factors include cutaneous irritation, allergies (environmental, food and/or contact), emotional stress, infections, skin dehydration and winter weather.

Acute disease manifests as ill-defined erythematous papules, patches and plaques with a predilection for accessible sites on the face, scalp and extensor surfaces of extremities in young infants. As co-ordinated scratching develops in the third to fourth month of life, erosions and excoriations are also seen, and the distribution changes to include flexures, wrists, neck, face, hands and feet. Secondary infection often develops, and may be manifested by crusting, increased erythema, or vesicopustules. Chronic disease with prolonged scratching and rubbing results in thickening of the skin with hyperpigmentation and accentuation of skin markings known as lichenification. This is called the Dennie–Morgan sign when it involves the lower eyelids. Cataracts and retinopathy may occur in conjunction with atopic dermatitis and were found in 12 of 70 patients in a recent clinical analysis[1]. Localized atopic dermatitis with scaling on the feet, called juvenile plantar dermatosis (or sweaty sock syndrome), presents as fine peeling and fissuring and is worse with occlusive footwear like athletic shoes.

Atopic skin is reactive to multiple topical irritants, such as water (especially with intermittent dryness), soaps, detergents, fragrance and other skin product ingredients. Girls with atopic dermatitis may have a flare after frequent use of bubble bath or application of cosmetics. In atopic women, occupational (e.g. health care, hairdressing, food preparation) and domestic duties that involve hand washing and handling of irritating chemicals (e.g. soap, water, baby wipes, household cleaners, cosmetic products) can lead to localization of dermatitis to the hands (Figure 2). This hand eczema may become chronic and is usually combined with other factors, such as secondary infection. Patch testing may be helpful in identifying exacerbating allergens such as nickel, fragrance, preservatives, or rubber ingredients in sensitized patients[2].

A skin biopsy is generally not performed, as atopic dermatitis is a clinical diagnosis. Acanthosis and epidermal spongiosis are seen with a mixed inflammatory dermal infiltrate. IgE levels may be elevated in the serum. A Tokyo study revealed that serum testosterone levels are lower in men with atopic dermatitis; similar changes were not seen in female patients[3]. Some women notice a worsening of itching and dermatitis related to their menstrual cycles.

The primary consideration in differential diagnosis is contact dermatitis, since it is a common concurrent factor in atopic flares. Seborrheic dermatitis (i.e., scalp, face, intertriginous), dermatophyte

Table 1   Papulosquamous diseases commonly seen in girls and women

Disease	Distribution		Appearance	Contributing factors	Treatment
	Girls	*Women*			
Atopic dermatitis	flexures, hands, face	hands, face	erythematous papules, patches and plaques, hyperkeratosis, hyperpigmentation lichenification	irritants (water, soap, cosmetics), allergies, stress, infection, dehydration, winter	irritant avoidance, emollients, topical corticosteroids, sedating antihistamines, mild soap substitutes, antibiotics
Seborrheic dermatitis	scalp, face, 'diaper area'	scalp, face, intertriginous	erythematous patches with yellowish greasy or white dry scales	human immunodeficiency virus, Parkinson's disease, *Pityrosporum ovale*	tar, salicylic acid, selenium sulfide, topical ketoconazoles, topical corticosteroids
Psoriasis	generalized (guttate), extremities, sites of trauma, intertriginous areas, scalp, nails	extremities, sites of trauma, intertriginous areas, scalp, nails	erythematous papules and plaques with silvery-white scales	trauma, infection, stress, oral corticosteroids, lithium, antimalarials, beta blockers	emollients, topical corticosteroids, anthralins, calcipotriene, oral retinoids, methotrexate, cyclosporine, phototherapy
Contact dermatitis	face, neck	face, neck, hands	erythematous, vesicular plaques, scaling, lichenification, hyperpigmentation, fissures	exposure to irritants (water, soap, cosmetics) and allergens, (poison ivy, nickel, preservatives, fragrances, neomycin)	identification and removal of allergens and irritants, corticosteroids

infection (i.e., feet), psoriasis, or nummular dermatitis may mimic atopic dermatitis at some sites. Acrodermatitis enteropathica or immunologic disorders such as Wiskott–Aldrich syndrome or Letterer–Siwe disease are less common considerations in infants with severe atopic dermatitis. Contact dermatitis, or much less commonly early mycosis fungoides, should be considered in adult women with an acquired pattern suggestive of atopic dermatitis.

Hydration of the skin and cessation of scratching are the key goals of treatment. Frequent use of emollients is extremely important, as dry skin is more prone to pruritus. Sedating antihistamines reduce the sensation of itch and the motor activity of scratching. Topical corticosteroids also reduce itch and help heal eczematous patches. An ointment vehicle aids hydration. There are disagreements about the recommended frequency of bathing. Use of mild soaps or soap substitutes is encouraged, as is helping patients understand the important goal of 'locking in' the moisture with prompt application of emollients or topical corticosteroids while the skin is still slightly moist. Recognition and avoidance of topical irritants, such as bubble bath or fragrance, and identification and treatment of secondary factors, such as bacterial infection, are also important. *Staphylococcus aureus* and group A β-hemolytic streptococcus are the primary organisms to be covered. For limited site involvement, mupirocin ointment applied 3 times daily for 1 week is adequate. For more extensive secondary infection, a systemic antibiotic that will provide adequate coverage for staphylococcus and

Table 2 Dermatology medications, selected examples for papulosquamous disorders

Class of medication		Generic name(s)	Brand name(s)
Anthralin, topical		anthralin cream	Drithocreme, Micanol
Antibiotic, oral		azithromycin	Zithromax
		cephalexin	Keflex
		dicloxacillin	Dycill, Dynapen
		erythromycin	Ery-c, E-mycin, Ery-tabs
Antibiotic, topical		mupirocin ointment	Bactroban ointment
Antihistamine, oral, sedating		hydroxyzine HCL	Atarax
		sinequan	Doxepin
Antiviral, oral		acyclovir	Zovirax
		famciclovir	Famvir
		valaciclovir	Valtrex
Azole, cream		clotrimazole	Lotrimin
		ketoconazole	Nizoral
		miconazole	Mycatin, Mycelex
Azole, shampoo		ketoconazole	Nizoral
Corticosteroid, topical	Class I	clobetasol propionate	Temovate cream, ointment
	II	mometasone furoate	Elocon ointment
	III	triamcinolone acetonide	Aristocort A ointment
	IV	triamcinolone acetonide	Kenalog cream, ointment
	V	desonide	Desowen ointment
	VI	triamcinolone acetonide	Aristocort cream
	VII	hydrocortisone	Hytone cream, lotion, ointment, 2.5%
Cyclosporine, oral		cyclosporine	Neoral, Sandimmune
Emollient, topical		N/A (non-prescription)	Cetaphil cream, lotion, Eucerin cream Vaseline cream, lotion, petroleum jelly
Methotrexate, oral		methotrexate	Rheumatrex
Psoralen, oral		methoxsalen	Oxsoralen, Oxsoralen-Ultra, 8-MOP
Retinoid, oral		acitretin	Soriatane
		isotretinoin	Accutane
Salicylic acid, shampoo		N/A (non-prescription)	DHS Sal, Neutrogena T-Sal
Selenium sulfide, shampoo		N/A (non-prescription)	Exsel, Selsun
Soap substitute		N/A (non-prescription)	Cetaphil, Purpose cleanser
Tar, topical		coal tar ointment	MG-217
Vitamin D derivative, topical		calcipotriene	Dovonex cream, ointment, solution

streptococcus is preferable. If a patient develops an acute, febrile flare of dermatitis associated with multiple vesicles, the possibility of disseminated *Herpes simplex* superimposed on the atopic dermatitis should be considered. This so-called Kaposi's varicelliform eruption may occur with or without a history of previous *Herpes simplex*. Diagnosis is made with a Tzanck preparation, culture, or polymerase chain reaction. Treatment with a systemic antiviral agent (acyclovir, famciclovir, or valaciclovir) is essential. Individually, phototherapy, tacrolimus and cyclosporine have been used to treat severe atopic disease. It is recommended that patients with severe atopic dermatitis, in particular, be evaluated by a dermatologist before such therapy is instituted.

SEBORRHEIC DERMATITIS

Seborrheic dermatitis is a common chronic dermatosis of gradual onset characterized by scaling and erythema in areas of the head and trunk where sebaceous glands are most numerous, such as the scalp, ears, 'T-zone' of the face, the central chest, intertriginous areas and the genitalia (Figure 3). Onset may be in infancy or puberty, but most commonly is in young to middle adulthood. Rather lightly adherent yellowish greasy or white dry scales accompany ill-defined erythematous patches. Patients are asymptomatic or may experience mild pruritus. More severe involvement may be seen in patients with human immunodeficiency virus disease or Parkinson's disease or in patients under

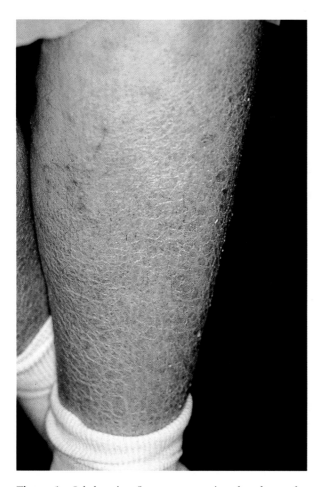

Figure 1 Ichthyosis often accompanies the dry rashy skin of atopic dermatitis

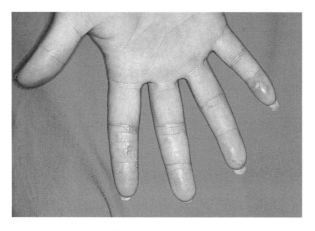

Figure 2 Distal digital involvement is shown in a patient with contact dermatitis

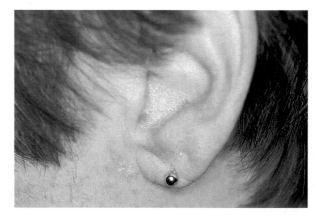

Figure 3 Seborrheic dermatitis manifests as fine white scales and erythema

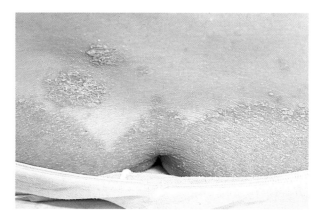

Figure 4 Typical psoriasis has well-defined erythematous plaques and silvery scale

emotional or physical stress. *Pityrosporum ovale* yeast is thought to play a role in the pathogenesis. The lower rate of sebum production and androgens in women could play a role in their having milder disease and slightly lower incidence of this condition[4]. Pomades in African-American women do not seem to aggravate this condition frequently, but more often cause folliculitis or acneiform eruptions. Less

frequent shampooing (once per 1–2 weeks) allows more scale build-up so the dermatitis seems more severe.

A skin biopsy is infrequently performed, as the diagnosis is made clinically. Focal parakeratosis, moderate acanthosis, spongiosis and neutrophils within dilated follicular ostia are observed. No laboratory studies are required. Differential diagnosis includes psoriasis, dermatophytosis and candidosis.

Tar and salicylic acid shampoos reduce scaling on the scalp. They can be alternated with selenium sulfide- or ketoconazole-containing shampoos, which have activity against pityrosporum yeasts, and also reduce scaling. These products may be used in all involved areas, including the face and chest. Used two or three times a week, they should be applied to the scalp, lathered and left on for 3–5 min before rinsing them off. Patients may use other shampoos if they desire to shampoo more frequently. For patients who routinely shampoo weekly or less often, a topical corticosteroid solution, applied sparingly daily, helps control the scaling between shampoos, and will not interfere with hair

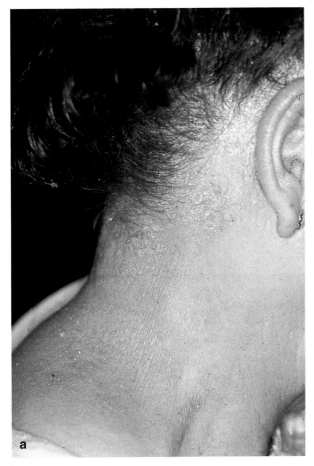
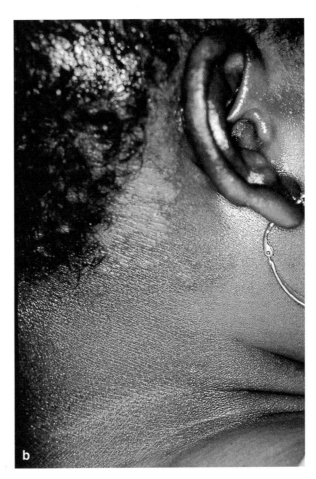

Figure 5   Erythema can be harder to detect in dark skin as evidenced by these women with scalp psoriasis. Chronic rubbing can result in thickening and accentuation of skin lines

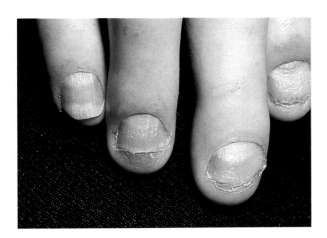

Figure 6   Nail changes in psoriasis include pitting, dystrophy and onycholysis

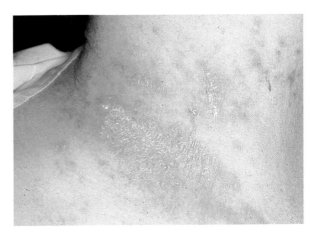

Figure 7   Contact dermatitis presents as a linear eczematous eruption on the shoulder of this woman allergic to thiuram

styling. Ketoconazole cream may be more convenient for limited involvement on the face only. Mild to moderate strength topical corticosteroids, used once a day as needed, reduce inflammation and erythema, but must be used cautiously on the face. Treatments control symptoms quite effectively, but intermittent flares of seborrheic dermatitis may occur.

PSORIASIS

Psoriasis is a hereditary disease of the skin resulting from disordered keratinocyte kinetics and differentiation. The shortened cell cycle results in a 10 to 30-fold increase in the production of epidermal cells. Gender and immunogenetics are thought to influence susceptibility to psoriasis[5], and women may be less likely to transmit the disease to their offspring than men[6].

Psoriasis is characterized by chronic scaling papules and plaques which may be pruritic and are most common in areas of minor trauma, such as the scalp, elbows, knees, lower back and buttocks. Koebnerization refers to the induction of new lesions by physical trauma including rubbing and scratching. The onset of type I (early onset) disease is on average at 16 years of age in women and 22 years of age in men; infantile onset may, however, occur. The younger the onset of plaque psoriasis, the more severe and extensive it tends to be. Type II (late onset) disease occurs in 25% of patients, on average at age 56 in both sexes[7]. There is an equal incidence of disease in men and women. Clinical expressions of the disease include psoriasis vulgaris, guttate psoriasis, psoriatic erythroderma, palmoplantar pustulosis, pustular psoriasis and psoriatic arthritis.

Sharply demarcated 'salmon pink' papules and plaques with tightly adherent silvery-white 'micaceous' scale commonly involve elbows, knees, scalp and intertriginous areas (Figures 4 and 5)[8]. Nail abnormalities, joint deformities, pustules and/or erythroderma may be present depending upon the type of psoriasis (Figure 6). Regional, generalized or universal involvement may be seen. Genital involvement may lead to vulvar itching, irritation during intercourse, and secondary loss of pubic hair due to scratching. Triggers include physical trauma, infections, psychic stress, and certain medications such as oral corticosteroids, lithium, antimalarials, and beta blockers. Guttate psoriasis, rapid appearance of multiple small scaly papules, is typically triggered by streptococcal infection in the patient or a family member, and usually remits completely between episodes. Stressful life events were significantly associated with actively spreading psoriasis in men but not in women in a study from Finland[9]. Psoriasis has been found to improve during pregnancy, but postpartum flares are experienced in 88% of patients, usually within four months of delivery[10]. Hormonal influences may play a role, as suggested by the case of a woman with breast cancer whose chronic plaque psoriasis cleared upon treatment with tamoxifen[11].

A skin biopsy is not required for diagnosis. Elongation of rete ridges, increased mitoses, parakeratotic hyperkeratosis, mononuclear cells in the dermis and neutrophils forming epidermal microabscesses of Munro are common findings.

Laboratory studies are generally not required. A complete blood count and blood cultures are indicated for generalized pustular psoriasis, looking for and treating streptococcal infection may be helpful in guttate psoriasis, and checking for HIV infection may be considered in at-risk individuals with the sudden onset of severe psoriasis.

Differential diagnosis depends upon the sites involved and may include seborrheic dermatitis (especially when site involvement is limited to the scalp and face), secondary syphilis, pityriasis rosea, dermatophytosis, candidosis, and psoriasiform drug eruptions.

Treatment also depends upon sites and extent of involvement. Relatively limited, mild disease may be treated with topical emollients and corticosteroids alone. Anthralins, vitamin D derivatives, (i.e. calcipotriene), and retinoids (i.e. tazarotene), each of which help to normalize the proliferative rate in affected skin, are useful adjunctive agents. Many patients find them irritating, but combination therapy with topical corticosteroids increases patient tolerability. More extensive disease or the presence of psoriatic arthritis calls for more aggressive therapy. Oral therapies with retinoids, cyclosporine or methotrexate are highly effective, but patients must be monitored periodically for adverse effects such as increased triglycerides, hypertension, liver and kidney damage and bone marrow suppression. Pregnancy prevention is mandatory when a female patient is to use one of these systemic treatments. Women who may become pregnant should use two forms of birth control when taking oral retinoids. Isotretinoin is preferred over acitretin in women of childbearing potential, given its significantly shorter half-life. Ultraviolet phototherapy, using ultraviolet B radiation or ultraviolet A radiation with psoralens (photosensitizers), is a relatively well tolerated means to treat extensive disease. It requires frequent office visits and carries the risk of increased incidence of skin cancer. Oral antibiotics may be helpful in the treatment of flares of psoriasis suspected to be related to streptococcal infection (so called guttate psoriasis), or for secondarily infected psoriasis plaques. Consider calcium supplementation in patients with palmoplantar pustulosis, who may have decreased bone mineral density[12]. This may be a significant problem for women, who are already at risk for osteoporosis.

CONTACT DERMATITIS

Contact dermatitis is an edematous inflammation of the skin that results from the interaction of a chemical and the skin via one of two main mechanisms.

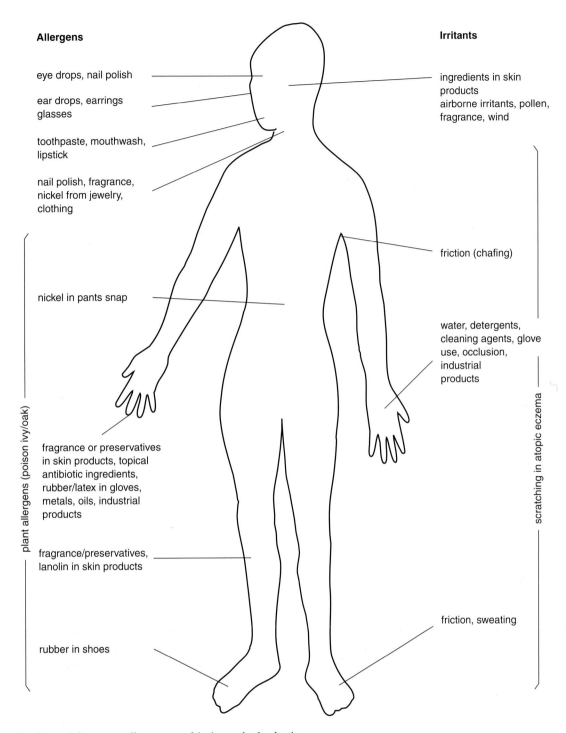

Allergens

eye drops, nail polish

ear drops, earrings glasses

toothpaste, mouthwash, lipstick

nail polish, fragrance, nickel from jewelry, clothing

nickel in pants snap

fragrance or preservatives in skin products, topical antibiotic ingredients, rubber/latex in gloves, metals, oils, industrial products

fragrance/preservatives, lanolin in skin products

rubber in shoes

plant allergens (poison ivy/oak)

Irritants

ingredients in skin products
airborne irritants, pollen, fragrance, wind

friction (chafing)

water, detergents, cleaning agents, glove use, occlusion, industrial products

friction, sweating

scratching in atopic eczema

Figure 8   Potential contact allergens and irritants by body site

Irritant contact dermatitis predominates and accounts for up to 80% of such reactions. It is a non-specific, non-immunologic process that would occur in any person given sufficient exposure to an irritant (example: hand dermatitis after dishwashing). Allergic contact dermatitis, in contrast, is immune-mediated and therefore requires pre-sensitization, the response is a delayed-type hypersensitivity, and minute cutaneous exposures may be sufficient to provoke a reaction in susceptible individuals (example: poison ivy dermatitis).

Women and men present similarly and may complain of pruritus or burning, and fissures can be especially painful. Acutely, rather well-demarcated erythematous, edematous plaques develop with superficial vesiculation (Figure 7). Superficial scaling and desquamation signify a more subacute process. Lichenification, hyperpigmentation and possibly fissures develop with longer exposures or when mechanical or frictional irritation is playing a role. The astute clinician can glean clues as to potential causative agents by observing features

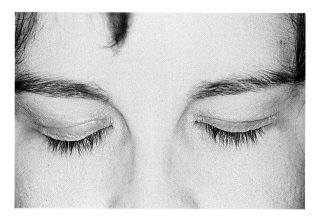

Figure 9   Eyelid dermatitis often develops in girls and women who are allergic to ingredients in skin care products and nail polish

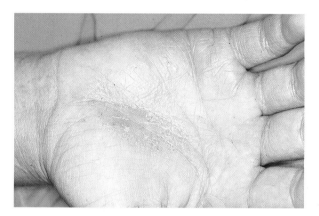

Figure 10   Allergic contact hand dermatitis is caused by acrylates in this nail technician

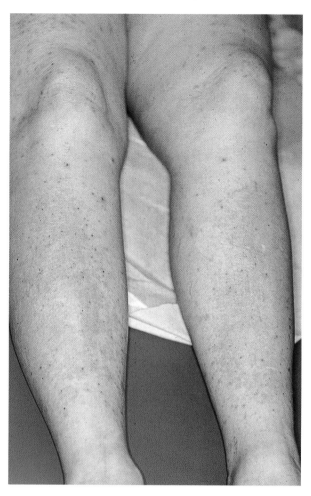

Figure 11   Contact dermatitis often develops in patients with stasis dermatitis

such as initial distribution of involvement and arrangement of lesions, with a linear pattern often on the extremities following exposure to plants such as poison ivy, or on the neck as is seen with fragrance contact dermatitis. The distribution of dermatitis and history of exposures and product use can help to narrow the likely inciting factor(s) (Figure 8).

In girls, examples of irritant contact dermatitis include diaper dermatitis, frictional chafing, chapped lips and stinging and redness after cosmetic use. The most common contact allergen in girls is nickel, found primarily in jewelry, but also in snaps on clothing, eyeglasses and metal watches. Piercing of ears and other body parts increases the likelihood of nickel allergy developing, therefore 14–18 carat gold, platinum, or stainless steel earrings are recommended. Other allergens occasionally seen in girls include nail polish (allergen is tosylamide formaldehyde resin), artificial nail adhesives (acrylates) and fragrance (Figure 9). The clinical pattern of these particular allergies is

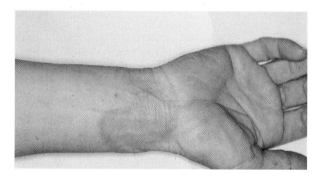

Figure 12   Patients who are latex-sensitive can develop contact urticaria from wearing latex gloves

often a subacute patchy eczema on the face and neck[13]. Similarly, irritant and allergic skin reactions in women are often localized to the face, neck and hands due to cosmetics, skin care products, and activities exposing the hands to multiple irritants and allergens (Figure 10)[14]. Contact dermatitis of the legs often develops in women with stasis dermatitis, often as a result of topical corticosteroids, antibiotic ointments, and other applied agents (Figure 11).

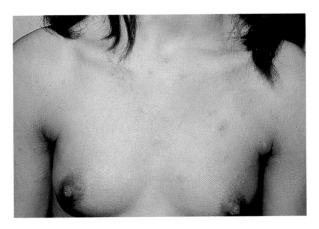

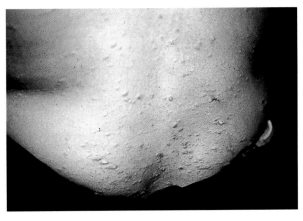

Figure 13 Pityriasis rosea presents as a scaly, sometimes pruritic eruption in a Christmas tree pattern on the trunk

Figure 15 Typical lichen planus has violaceous firm polygonal papules with lacy surface scale

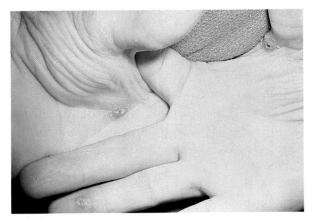

Figure 14 Secondary syphilis can present in many ways, including necrotic pustules and scaly papules on the hands

Histology is rather nonspecific and reveals spongiosis and superficial perivascular inflammatory infiltrates. Monocyte and histiocyte infiltration suggests allergic contact dermatitis, while the presence of superficial vesicles containing neutrophils suggests irritant contact dermatitis, but there is considerable overlap. More long-standing disease also exhibits hyperkeratosis, acanthosis and possibly pigment incontinence.

Closed patch testing is used to confirm a diagnosis of allergic contact dermatitis and to identify the causative agent(s). Likely substances, including some of the patient's own skin care products and agents contacted at work, are applied to the skin in appropriate concentrations in Finn chambers affixed via Scanpor tape, and are left in place for 48 hours. Contact allergy results in an erythematous papulovesicular eruption that develops within 48 to 72 hours at the site of allergen exposure. The relevance of patch test results

with respect to a patient's past and present exposures must then be determined. The most common allergens found on patch testing are nickel, preservatives, fragrances and neomycin. Balsam of Peru is a marker for commonly used fragrance, and may cross-react with flavorings such as vanilla, cinnamon, and clove; a small number of sensitized patients benefit from a low-balsam diet[15]. Poison ivy and oak are not routinely tested, since allergy to them is so common and easy to identify clinically.

Women, in general, may apply more personal care products to their skin than men, and this may result in a greater number of sensitivities to such products[16,17]. In Sweden, 90% of adverse effects reported over a 5-year period associated with cosmetics and toiletries concerned women[18]. In this study, moisturizers were the top ranking product category, followed by hair care products and nail products. Chronic vulvar irritation is a problem in women and may be a result of contact allergy or irritancy to products applied such as soaps, lubricants and feminine sprays[19]. Once begun, this process is easily sustained and exacerbated by factors such as intercourse, friction from clothing, urine and menstrual secretions[20]. Ear piercing contributes to a greater sensitivity to nickel in girls and women because of the chronic contact with the skin of earrings which contain this metal. Nickel sensitivity was seen in 30% of girls versus 3% of boys in one Finnish study[21]. Men, conversely, may have a greater number of occupational exposures leading to allergic or irritant dermatitis[22].

Contact urticaria is mentioned here because it may present as a patchy eczema, rather than an immediate urticaria at the site of contact. Fragrances and some other skin product ingredients can cause transient contact urticaria, but a latex allergy gets the most attention, because of the health care implications and potential for systemic anaphylaxis (Figure 12). Sources of contact with latex for women include gloves, diaphragms, condoms, make-up sponge applicators and balloons[23]. A serologic test known as a RAST test (radioimmunologic allergy sensitivity test) for allergen specific IgE is often performed if latex allergy is suspected[24].

Differential diagnoses of contact allergy include atopic dermatitis, nummular eczema, seborrheic dermatitis, dyshidrotic eczema and an id reaction (autosensitization phenomenon). Sometimes contact dermatitis is a factor in these other conditions.

Treatment involves identification and removal of the inciting agent and patient education about what to avoid. Patch testing is an essential diagnostic tool to confirm suspected allergens. This may involve giving the patient a list of products containing allergens to which they are sensitive, providing advice about alternative products and communication with the patient's workplace. Some patients must change job tasks or use barrier products to avoid contact with allergens at work. Topical corticosteroids are extremely useful in helping to heal dermatitic skin. For incapacitating or extensive involvement, oral corticosteroids are occasionally used.

OTHER PAPULOSQUAMOUS SKIN DISEASES

Other important papulosquamous skin diseases include pityriasis rosea, secondary syphilis, and lichen planus. A few differences are seen in these diseases in men as opposed to women, mainly with respect to incidence.

Pityriasis rosea is a self-limited acute exanthematous papulosquamous eruption, that typically begins with an erythematous scaly herald patch usually on the trunk followed over one to two weeks by multiple mildly pruritic fine scaling oval papules and plaques with marginal collarettes along skin cleavage lines on the trunk and proximal extremities (Figure 13). A viral etiology has been suspected for some time, but terbinafine and omeprazole have been reported to cause similar eruptions[25,26], and an increased incidence of *Legionella micdadei* antibodies were found in one study of 36 patients with pityriasis rosea[27]. The process generally remits in about 6 weeks without therapy.

Syphilis (both primary and secondary stages) is the second most commonly reported of the nationally notifiable diseases in the USA[28]. The greatest concentration of reported cases is in the southern states[29]. Intravenous drug abuse and prostitution are obvious risk factors. It is an acute and chronic sexually transmitted disease caused by infection with *Treponema pallidum*. It is traditionally less common in women than in men by a factor of two to four fold. Secondary syphilis begins 2 to 6 months after primary infection and may present with a scattered maculopapular, papulosquamous or pustular eruption, annular polycyclic lesions on the face, mucous patches on mucous membranes, split papules at the commissures of the lips, soft moist excrescences known as condyloma lata on genitalia, and diffuse or patchy alopecia (Figure 14). Darkfield examination or serology is positive. The disease is transmissible to an unborn baby by an infected mother; this occurs in up to 14% of cases despite appropriate treatment of syphilis in pregnancy[30]. Treatment is benzathine penicillin G. The dosage and number of treatments depends upon the stage of disease.

Lichen planus is an inflammatory dermatosis of unknown etiology that affects women more often than men, generally from 30 to 60 years of age. It is characterized by pruritic flat-topped violaceous polygonal papules with overlying Wickham's striae on the skin and lacy white hyperkeratosis in the mouth that may last months to years (Figure 15). Lichen planus can rarely involve the vaginal mucosa, and in that location is very symptomatic with vulvar burning[31]. Malignant change may occur in chronic lesions[32]. A skin biopsy confirms the diagnosis of lichen planus. Topical, intralesional or oral corticosteroids, retinoids, cyclosporine and ultraviolet A phototherapy with oral psoralens may be helpful in treatment.

REFERENCES

1. Katayama I, Taniguchi H, Matsunaga T, *et al*. Evaluation of non-steroidal ointment therapy for adult type atopic dermatitis: inquiry analysis on clinical effect. *J Dermatol Sci* 1997;14:37–44

2. Nilsson EJ, Knuttson A. Atopic dermatitis, nickel sensitivity and xerosis as risk factors for hand eczema in women. *Contact Dermatitis* 1995;33:401–6

3. Ebata T, Itamura R, Aizawa H, Niimura M. Serum sex hormone levels in adult patients with atopic dermatitis. *J Dermatol* 1996;23:603–5

4. Martignoni E, Godi L, Pacchetti C, *et al*. Is seborrhea a sign of autonomic impairment in Parkinson's disease? *J Neur Trans* 1997;104:1295–304

5. Mallon E, Bunce M, Wojnarowska F, Welsh K. HLA-CW*0602 is a susceptibility factor in type I psoriasis, and evidence Ala-73 is increased in male type I psoriatics. *J Invest Dermatol* 1997;109:183–6

6. Burden AD, Javed S, Bailey M, *et al*. Genetics of psoriasis: paternal inheritance and a locus on chromosome 6p. *J Invest Dermatol* 1998;110:958–60

7. Christophers E, Sterry W. Psoriasis. In Fitzpatrick TB, Eisen AZ, Wolff K, *et al.*, eds. *Dermatology in General Medicine*, 4th edn. New York: McGraw Hill, 1993:489–514

8. Kaur I, Handa S, Kumar B. Natural history of psoriasis: a study from the Indian subcontinent. *J Dermatol* 1997;24:230–4

9. Harvima RJ, Viinamaki H, Harvima IT, *et al.* Association of psychic stress with clinical severity and symptoms of psoriatic patients. *Acta Derm Venereol (Stockh)* 1996;76:467–71

10. Boyd AS, Morris LF, Phillips CM, Menter MA. Psoriasis and pregnancy: hormone and immune system interaction. *Int J Dermatol* 1996;35:169–72

11. Ferrari VD, Jirillo A. Psoriasis and tamoxifen therapy: a case report. *Tumori* 1996;82:262–3

12. Nymann P, Kollerup G, Jemec GB, Grossman E. Decreased bone mineral density in patients with pustulosis palmaris et plantaris. *Dermatology* 1996;192:307–11

13. Freeman S, Lee MS, Gudmundsen K. Adverse contact reactions to sculptured acrylic nails: 4 case reports and a literature review. *Contact Dermatitis* 1995;33:381–5

14. Brynzeel DP, de Boer EM. Waitresses' Itch? *Contact Dermatitis* 1997;36:308

15. Veien NK, Hattel T, Laurberg G. Can oral challenge with balsam of Peru predict possible benefit from a low-balsam diet? *Am J Contact Dermatitis* 1996;7:84–7

16. Etienne A, Piletta P, Hauser C, Pasche-Koo F. Ectopic contact dermatitis from henna. *Contact Dermatitis* 1997;37:183

17. Jagtman BA. Urticaria and contact urticaria due to basic blue 99 in a hair dye. *Contact Dermatitis* 1996;35:52

18. Berne B, Bostrom A, Grahnen AF, Tammela M. Adverse affects of cosmetics and toiletries reported to the Swedish Medical Products Agency 1989–1994. *Contact Dermatitis* 1996;34:359–62

19. Eason EL, Feldman P. Contact dermatitis associated with the use of Always sanitary napkins. *Can Med Assoc J* 1996;154:1173–6

20. Zellis S, Pincus SH. Treatment of vulvar dermatoses. *Semin Dermatol* 1996;15:71–6

21. Kerosuo H, Kullaa A, Kerosuo E, *et al.* Nickel allergy in adolescents in relation to orthodontic treatment and piercing of ears. *Am J Orthodont Dentofac Orthoped* 1996;109:148–54

22. Bangha E, Elsner P. Sensitizations to allergens of the European standard series at the department of dermatology in Zurich 1990–1994. *Dermatology* 1996;193:17–21

23. Desciak EB, Marks JG Jr. Dermatoses among housekeeping personnel. *Am J Contact Dermatitis* 1997;8:32–4

24. Miller K. Care of the latex-sensitized obstetric patient. *AWHONN Voice* 1996;4:2,13

25. Gupta AK, Lynde CW, Lauzon GJ, *et al.* Cutaneous adverse effects associated with terbinafine therapy: 10 case reports and a review of the literature. *Br J Dermatol* 1998;138:529–32

26. Buckley C. Pityriasis rosea-like eruptions in a patient receiving omeprazole. *Dermatology* 1997;194:371

27. Gjenero-Margan I, Vidovic R, Drazenovic V. Pityriasis rosea Gibert; detection of *Legionella micdadei* antibodies in patients. *Eur J Epidemiol* 1995;11:459–62

28. Niskar AS, Koo D. Differences in notifiable infectious disease morbidity among adult women – United States, 1992–1994. *J Women's Health* 1998;7:451–8

29. Anonymous. Primary and secondary syphilis – United States, 1997. *Morbid Mortal Wkly Rpt* 1998;47:493–7

30. Larkin JA, Lit L, Toney J, Haley JA. Recognizing and treating syphilis in pregnancy. *Medscape Women's Health* 1998;3:5

31. Lewis FM. Vulvar lichen planus. *Br J Dermatol* 1998;138:569–75

32. Ambros RA, Malfetano JH, Carlson JA, Mihm MC Jr. Non-neoplastic epithelial alterations of the vulva: recognition assessment and comparisons of terminologies used among the various specialties. *Mod Pathol* 1997;10:401–8

Diseases of pigment changes

16

Hyun-Joo Choi and Seung-Kyung Hann

NEVUS OF OTA

Nevus of Ota is a form of benign melanocytosis located over the ophthalmic and maxillary branches of the trigeminal nerve. It was first described by Ota and Tanino as 'naevus fuscocaeruleus ophthalmo-maxillaris' in 1939. The term 'nevus of Ota' is commonly used to refer to this anomaly.

Epidemiology

Most cases of nevus of Ota have been reported in Asia, including Japan and Korea. Nevus of Ota occurs in approximately 1 in 500 people[1], and has a prevalence in females and males in a ratio of 4.8 to 1. The general prevalence of nevus of Ota in Korea was reported as 0.03% in adolescents[2]. In dermatology clinics in Japan the prevalence was reported as 0.4–1%[1]. It also occurs in Chinese, East Indians, blacks and whites. Nevus of Ota is typically congenital but can be acquired. Inherited cases are rare and only five familial cases of nevus of Ota have been reported. There is bimodal age onset, with approximately 50% of lesions present at birth or before the age of two years[1]. The remainder arise during the first four decades of life[1].

Clinical findings

Clinically all ill-defined, brown, blue-gray or blue-black patchy hyperpigmentation intermingled with small flat brown spots is observed in the distribution of the maxillary and ophthalmic branches of the trigeminal nerve (Figure 1). In 5% of cases, the lesions are bilateral[3]. There are individuals with a unilateral nevus of Ito and a bilateral nevus of Ota. The nevus of Ito differs from the nevus of Ota only in its distribution. The nevus of Ito affects the supraclavicular, scapular and deltoid regions. It may occur alone or in association with an ipsilateral or bilateral nevus of Ota. Many patients report fluctuation of pigment intensity associated with fatigue, menstruation, insomnia and weather changes[1]. It is often associated with pregnancy or the ingestion of oral contraceptives and is aggravated by sunlight. Spontaneous regression does not occur. Hyperpigmentation may also occur on the sclera, cornea, iris, optic nerve, fundus, extraocular muscles, retrobulbar fat and periosteum[1]. Similar pigment changes can rarely be seen in the pharynx, nasal mucosa, buccal mucosa, tympanic membrane and hard palate[1].

The nevus of Ota can develop a number of complications, such as melanosis oculi, glaucoma of the involved eye, or melanoma. Abnormalities of ocular pigmentation occur in 49 to 65% of patients with nevus of Ota[1]. It is almost always unilateral. In general, nevus of Ota does not often give rise to malignant melanoma. However, malignant transformation has occurred in 4.6% of 670 cases of nevus of Ota reported. Melanoma occurs more frequently in Caucasians. The most common site for melanoma is the choroid, followed by the uveal tract. Melanoma can also arise in the skin and a few cases of intracranial melanoma have been reported.

Histopathology

An epidermal and a dermal type can be recognized, although frequently there is a combination of the two types. Light and histochemical studies reveal an increase in the number and activity of melanocytes that are engaged in increased formation, melanization and transfer of pigment granules to keratinocytes and melanophages.

Pathogenesis

Nevus of Ota is thought to represent a disorder of neural crest migration. Melanoblasts normally arise from the neural crest and migrate to the skin, leptomeninges, ocular structures and the internal ear. Deafness has been associated with nevus of Ota. In the nevus of Ota, blue nevus and Mongolian spots, melanocytes are thought to be aberrant and become arrested while remaining in the dermis. This results in a persistent discoloration and cosmetic disfigurement.

Treatment

The lesion of nevus of Ota persists throughout life and there are no reports of its spontaneous regression. If ocular pigmentation is present, patients should be followed periodically by an ophthalmologist. It is unnecessary to remove prophylactically stable cutaneous lesions.

Surgical treatment causes scarring. Cryotherapy can be effective, but success depends on the site of the lesion. Cryotherapy is not reliable and may cause atrophy or scarring if it is applied excessively.

In recent years lasers have also been used to treat successfully the nevus of Ota. The treatment of choice is laser therapy with the Q-switched ruby, Nd:YAG, or alexandrite pulsed lasers. These are helpful in reducing the intensity of pigmentation with minimal risk of scarring.

Dermabrasion can be helpful in some cases. Because most nevi are macular, many patients feel that opaque covering agents yield cosmetically acceptable results.

MELASMA

Melasma is an acquired hypermelanosis which occurs in areas of skin exposed to the sun and is exacerbated by sunlight.

Epidemiology and etiology

Melasma is common, particularly in women of child-bearing age, but up to 10% of cases have been reported in males[4]. No race is spared, but there is particular prominence among Hispanic and Asian peoples.

The cause of melasma is not known, but there are a number of factors which may be involved in causing or aggravating the condition. The majority of cases appear to be related to pregnancy or ingestion of oral contraceptives[5]. The hyperpigmentation often decreases or disappears after parturition, but may not regress in women on oral contraceptives until the medication is discontinued[5]. Both estrogen and progesterone are likely to be involved in inducing melasma, but the infrequency of melasma in postmenopausal women on estrogen replacement therapy suggests that estrogen alone is not the causative agent. The most important exacerbating factor for melasma is exposure to ultraviolet (UV) light. Melasma may be associated with endocrine dysfunction, genetic factors, cosmetics, medications, nutritional deficiency, hepatic dysfunction and other factors. Although a few familial cases have been described, melasma should not be considered a heritable disorder.

Clinical findings

Melasma is defined as a light to dark brown or slate-colored, irregular hypermelanosis of the face,

especially forehead, cheeks, temples and upper lip. It develops slowly and is usually symmetric. The onset is at puberty or later and the condition may last for many years, with relapses during summer and relative remissions during the winter.

The hyperpigmentation of melasma can be of two forms. The first is due to an increase of epidermal melanin, and the color of the affected area is brown. The second is caused by increased melanin and deposition of melanin in the dermis. The color is gray-brown or slate.

Wood's lamp examination has revealed three types of melasma: epidermal, dermal and compound. Melasma of the epidermal type is due to an increase in epidermal melanin, and the color of the affected area is brown. Wood's lamp produces an enhancement of the color contrast between affected and normal skin in the epidermal type. Melasma of the dermal type is caused by increased melanin and deposition of melanin in the dermis. The color is gray-brown or slate and there is no enhancement of color contrast under Wood's lamp. There is a mixed dermal–epidermal type, for which Wood's lamp examination shows both enhancement and no color accentuation in different areas on the same patient. Postinflammatory hyperpigmentation can usually be excluded by history. There are many different conditions that can produce increased pigmentation in skin which has been exposed to the sun, including medications such as amiodarone, phenothiazines and heavy metals.

Histopathology

In the epidermal type there is increased melanin in the basal and suprabasal layers, and in the dermal type there are melanin-laden macrophages in a perivascular array in the superficial and mid-dermis. Dihydroxyphenylalanine (DOPA) staining revealed an increase in the number and activity of melanocytes that are engaged in increased formation, melanization and transfer of pigment granules to keratinocytes and melanophages.

Treatment

Potent, broad-spectrum and high sun protection factor (SPF) sun protection is important to minimize sun-induced hyperpigmentation[6]. For patients with the epidermal type of melasma, bleaching agents are helpful when used for prolonged periods. Hydroquinone-containing agents are the most commonly used bleaching agents, but they are not always helpful because of a high incidence of contact dermatitis and postinflammatory hyperpigmentation.

The combination of hydroquinone and tretinoin has been used successfully for melasma[6]. The advised course of treatment is hydroquinone plus opaque sunscreen in the morning and hydroquinone and tretinoin at night. Jimbow has described marked to excellent improvement in epidermal melasma treated with topical 4% N-acetyl-4-S-cysteaminylphenol[7]. Kojic acid and arbutin have been described as beneficial. Treatment with physical modalities such as liquid nitrogen, cryotherapy, CO_2 laser vaporization, chemical peeling and superficial dermabrasion can be tried. Dermal melasma responds neither to hydroquinone nor to tretinoin and cannot be treated at the present. Cover up with opaque cosmetics is the only management option. Laser treatment would appear to offer some promise for the future.

ACQUIRED BILATERAL NEVUS OF OTA-LIKE MACULE (ABNOM)

Hori's nevus (acquired circumscribed dermal melanocytosis of face, acquired facial blue macules resembling a bilateral nevus of Ota, or acquired bilateral nevus of Ota-like macule) is characterized by blue-brown macules that occur bilaterally on the face (Figure 2). Blue-brown macules can be found on the sides of the forehead, temples, eyelids, malar areas and root and alae of the nose. The lesions are usually noted in women, especially in the fourth or fifth decades in Japanese women, and rarely in men[1]. These macules are clinically very similar to nevus of Ota, but do not involve the ocular and mucosal surfaces.

Histologically, bipolar or oval dermal melanocytes that are slightly DOPA positive are found scattered in the upper and middle portions of the dermis[8].

These macules can be differentiated clinically from congenital bilateral nevus of Ota. Congenital bilateral nevus of Ota is usually present at birth or soon after birth and commonly involves the conjunctivae and the mucosal membranes of the mouth and nose or tympanic membrane. Dermal melanocytes are not found in facial melanosis, Riehl's melanosis and melasma[8,9].

RIEHL'S MELANOSIS

Riehl first described several patients exhibiting a pigmented eruption of the face and neck during the First World War and attributed the problem to food substitutes or some other factors associated with war-time living conditions. This disorder is also called pigmented contact dermatitis.

Clinical findings

The patients present with rapid onset of patches of diffuse blue-gray or brown hyperpigmentation most commonly located on the face, forehead or neck. Usually there is little or no erythema and no symptoms of itch preceding the onset of pigmentation[10]. The condition persists and may become more intense if application of the offending chemicals is continued after onset[11]. It appears that darker-skinned patients or those who normally tan deeply are at greater risk for Riehl's melanosis than those who are fair skinned and tan poorly.

Histopathology

There is no epidermal acanthosis or spongiosis, but there is marked liquefaction degeneration of the basal layer along with incontinence of pigment into the dermis. A dermal lymphohistiocytic infiltrate is often present. These histological findings differ markedly from those of conventional contact dermatitis[10].

Differential diagnosis

Melasma is the disease that most closely resembles Riehl's melanosis; both conditions can coexist. A patients with melasma is likely to cover the blemishes of melasma with cosmetics containing an agent that causes Riehl's melanosis. The lateral cheeks are more commonly involved in Riehl's melanosis whereas the central face, upper lip and chin are more commonly involved in melasma. A reticulated hyperpigmentation is more typical of melasma than of Riehl's melanosis. ABNOM, photosensitivity reactions, and berloque dermatitis can resemble Riehl's melanosis. A history of the application of photosensitizers should lead one to the correct diagnosis for the latter two conditions. The histology of the former is diagnostic.

Pathogenesis

This condition represents a low-grade contact dermatitis caused by toxic agents applied to the skin. Many different chemicals have been implicated as a cause of Riehl's melanosis. It is not known how these specific agents cause basilar damage to the epidermis without signs of cutaneous injury. Brilliant Lake Red, Sudan I, hydroxycitronellal, benzyl salicylate, jasmine, canaga oil, lemon oil, or geraniol are the most common chemicals responsible for inducing Riehl's melanosis[10,12]. These chemicals are found most commonly in cosmetics. Pyrazoline derivatives in optic whiteners seem responsible for truncal pigmented contact dermatitis[12].

Treatment

Treatment consists of cessation of the causative agent, as the pigmentation changes of Riehl's melanosis will remain as long as such agents are used continuously. Most hyperpigmentation will resolve in 1 to 2 years.

PIGMENTARY DEMARCATION LINES

Matzumoto first described pigmentary demarcation lines on the upper and lower extremities of Japanese patients in 1913[13]. Later, Futcher described demarcation lines in the black population. These lines are also called Futcher's or Voigt's lines.

Epidemiology

Natural pigmentary demarcation lines of the skin have been described most frequently in dark-skinned persons, and occur most distinctly in blacks, Japanese and Hispanics. Ito reported a ratio of affected women to men of 10:1[14], but others have reported a similar incidence in both sexes[13]. Pigmentary demarcation lines have been associated with pregnancy in more recent reports[15]. In one case these lines remained unchanged eight months postpartum while other cases were reported as occurring immediately after the postpartum period. Pigmentary demarcation lines have been noted to occur in other locations and in all ethnic groups, although they are more distinct and common in blacks. Familial occurrences have been reported[13,15].

Clinical findings

Pigmentary demarcation lines correspond to a border of abrupt transition between the more deeply pigmented skin of the outer surfaces and the lighter inner surfaces. Pigmentary demarcation lines are usually bilateral and symmetrical, although unilateral variants have been described in up to 16% of cases[13]. These lines have been classified into five types (A to E) based on their location (Table 1)[13]. Types A and C are the best characterized and more common types, type A being the most common.

Histopathology

Histologic findings have been variable. Futcher did not find any significant differences between the two sides of the pigmented line. Other authors, however, reported that there were slight differences in the pigment distribution in the basal cells of the epidermis between the two halves of the demarcation line[15].

Table 1 Types of pigmentary demarcation lines

Type	Location
A	lateral aspect of upper anterior portion of arms, across pectoral area
B	posteromedial portion of lower limb
C	vertical hypopigmented line in pre- and parasternal area
D	posteromedial area of spine
E	bilateral aspect of chest, marking from mid-third of clavicle to periareolar skin

Pathogenesis

The exact mechanism underlying the phenomenon of pigmentary demarcation lines is currently unknown, but various explanations have been postulated. Some authors stated that the more pigmented dorsal skin of animals serves to protect against ultraviolet rays and to maintain thermoregulation[13]. Others considered the pigmentary demarcation lines as atavistic and indicated that they coincide with the marginal lines of cutaneous nerve distribution[13]. Also, the possibility has been raised that the demarcation lines and markings in both Japanese and black persons are dominantly inherited[14]. In cases associated with pregnancies, elevation of melanocyte-stimulating hormone, estrogen and progesterone during pregnancy probably exerts a melanocyte-stimulating effect and may cause pigmentary changes[15].

Treatment

Treatment is not necessary, since these lines are considered as normal variants and of no cosmetic concern.

RETICULATE ACROPIGMENTATION OF DOHI

Reticulate acropigmentation of Dohi (dyschromatosis symmetrica hereditaria or symmetrical dyschromatosis of the extremities) is characterized by pigmented and depigmented macules mixed in a reticulate pattern on the extremities. It was first described in 12 patients from Japan, where it appears to be a well-established condition[16].

Clinical findings

Reticulate acropigmentation of Dohi (RAD) is generally inherited as an autosomal dominant condition although sporadic cases have been reported[17].

It is characterized by pigmented and depigmented macules which merge to form a reticulate pattern on the extremities (Figure 3). The eruption starts in infancy or childhood, although it may present later, and extends slowly proximally over time, affecting the sides of the neck, the supraclavicular region and the face[16,17].

It has been suggested that RAD is an incomplete variant of xeroderma pigmentosum (XP) as the clinical appearances may show some similarities. Although decreased minimal erythema dose has been reported in some patients, others have failed to confirm this and normal DNA repair has been shown.

Histopathology

RAD demonstrates a reduced density of DOPA-positive melanocytes in the depigmented macules, and liquefaction of the basal layer has been reported[18].

Histogenesis

RAD is thought to be inherited, although the genes responsible for its expression have not been identified.

Differential diagnosis

RAD should be distinguished from the other reticulate pigmentary disorders, in particular from reticulate acropigmentation of Kitamura. Like RAD the latter is characterized by pigmented freckle-like lesions on the extremities. However, no depigmented macules are present and breaks in the epidermal ridge pattern on the palms and soles are characteristic. Other pigmentary disorders which should be considered include acromelanosis where there is diffuse hyperpigmentation over the fingers with no reticulate pattern, and pityriasis lichenoides chronica. This latter condition may cause marked pigmentary disturbances in colored skin, but a few sparse lichenoid papules can normally be found. Finally reticulate pigmented anomaly of the flexures (Dowling–Degos disease) and the generalized reticulate pigmentary disorders can be distinguished by their characteristic distribution[17].

Treatment

Treatment of RAD is difficult. Topical steroid therapy and PUVA (psoralen and ultraviolet A) have had no benefit on the depigmented component. Split-skin grafting to replace the speckled skin has been effective but would not usually be suggested. A good cosmetic result with camouflage cream may be achieved and this may be the most reasonable approach to management.

RETICULATE ACROPIGMENTATION OF KITAMURA

Reticulate acropigmentation of Kitamura (RAPK) is an autosomal dominantly inherited dermatosis reported in 1943 by Kitamura and Akamatsu[19]. Only a few cases have been reported in Western literature, whereas more than 50 cases have been reported in Japan[20].

Clinical findings

Reticulated, slightly atrophic, polygonal, hyperpigmented macules affect the extensor surfaces of the hands and feet in teenagers. There is a progression to involve the extremities, lateral neck and occasionally the trunk and face. Palmar pits and/or breaks in the epidermal ridge patterns are the other typical characteristics[19–21]. Several associations have been reported with RAPK, namely: plantar hyperkeratoderma, psoriasis, bilateral talipes, nevus spilus, nevus anemicus, acrokeratoelastoidosis and nonscarring alopecia.

Histopathology

There is hyperpigmentation of the basilar keratinocytes with either a normal or slightly increased number of melanocytes. A characteristic feature is the absence of dermal inflammation and pigment incontinence. The most prominent findings consist of club-like elongation of the rete ridges and slight atrophy on the epidermis[20]. RAPK demonstrates digitated elongation of the hyperpigmented rete ridges with a tendency to spare the suprapapillary epidermis.

Histogenesis

RAPK is thought to be inherited, although the genes responsible for its expression have not been identified.

Differential diagnosis

The differential diagnosis of RAPK includes a numbers of disorders that are thought to be genetically determined and have reticulate pigmentation as a clinical feature. The reticulate acropigmentation of Dohi differs from RAPK in that it shows a mixture of hyperpigmented and hypopigmented macules – the pigmented macules show no atrophy, and the palmar pits are absent. Franceshetti–Jadassohn syndrome includes, in addition to reticulate pigmentation keratoderma, enamel dysplasia and hypohidrosis. The presence of atrophic lesions over the knuckles, elbows and knees, as well as nail atrophy, characterizes dyskeratosis congenita and dermatopathia pigmentosa reticularis. In Dowling–Degos disease, the flexures are predominantly involved, the macules tend to be papular and the palmar pits are absent. The relation of Dowling–Degos disease to RAPK is still being debated, with some authors believing that they are one and the same disease.

IDIOPATHIC GUTTATE HYPOMELANOSIS
Epidemiology and etiology

About 50% of people in their forties and more than 70% of people in their sixties are affected by idiopathic guttate hypomelanosis[22]; exposure to the sun is assumed to play a role in this disorder, but the lack of involvement of the face has led to alternative explanations, such as somatic mutations.

Clinical findings

Idiopathic guttate hypomelanosis is a very common disorder. The lesion is probably found in all races but is simply most apparent in darker-skinned ones. Males and females are equally affected. The lesions are usually round but may be stellate and average about 5 mm in diameter. The lesions number from few to many, may increase in number and in size with age, and are most common in areas of the extremities that have been exposed to the sun, particularly the anterior lower legs, but are not observed on the face. The characteristic sharply angulated outlines are a reflection of the borders of skin lines.

Histopathology

There is a sharp demarcation in the melanin content of the basal layer between uninvolved and involved skin and there is epidermal atrophy. Melanocytes may be reduced in number but do not completely disappear, which contrasts with the absence of melanocytes seen in fully developed lesions of vitiligo[23]. Changes in collagen and elastic fibers are less common.

Differential diagnosis

Although patients and non-dermatologists sometimes confuse idiopathic guttate hypomelanosis with vitiligo, the major differential diagnosis is the confetti-like lesions of tuberous sclerosis.

Occasionally, guttate hypomelanotic lesions can be seen in patients with Darier's disease with biphasic amyloidosis, and after PUVA therapy.

Treatment

Treatment options are limited, but successful results were reported in 79 of 87 lesions of idiopathic guttate hypomelanosis in 10 patients after a light freeze with liquid nitrogen[24]. This may seem somewhat ironic, given the observation that melanocytes are more sensitive to freezing than are other cell types of the skin.

HYPOMELANOSIS DUE TO CHEMICAL, PHARMACOLOGIC AND PHYSICAL AGENTS
Etiology

Hypomelanosis may result from a multitude of types of trauma including thermal injury, hypothermia[25], X-ray, ionizing radiation, UV irradiation and chemical agents.

Clinical features

Hypomelanotic macules are milk-white and appear not only at the site of contact with the offending compound but also remotely. Remote or satellite lesions are guttate or confetti macules. A prior irritant or contact eruption is not required for the leukoderma to develop. In early stage the leukoderma may be reversible if the chemical exposure is stopped.

Histopathology

The histopathology varies according to the causative agent. When this is physical, melanocytes are present, including alterations in the length of dendrites, decreased melanosome transfer, alteration of melanin distribution in the hair and changes in the color of melanin granule[26]. However, chemical leukoderma has no typical diagnostic features to distinguish it from vitiligo: typically, melanocytes are absent, and there are no dermal or other epidermal changes in established macules.

Treatment

Established chemical leukoderma is irreversible if the offending chemical is not eliminated soon enough. Early localized cases may be reversed by topical or oral PUVA: as with vitiligo, established

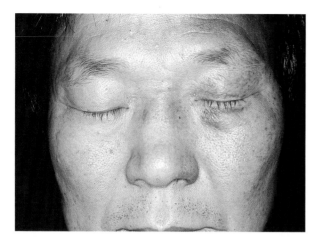

Figure 1 Nevus of Ota. Ill-defined, blue–black hyper-pigmented patch is observed in the distribution of left maxillary and ophthalmic branches of the trigeminal nerve

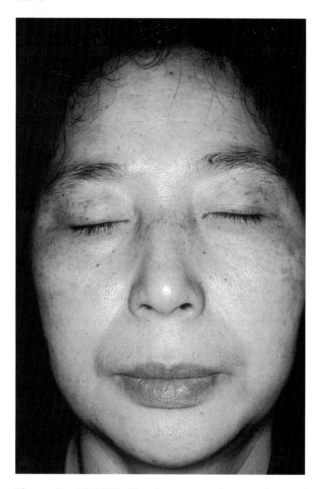

Figure 2 ABNOM. Blue–brown macules are observed on the sides of the forehead, temples and malar areas

acral and mucosal macules are usually refractory to repigmentation. Discontinuation of the exposure is mandatory; surveillance of the environment to exclude others at risk is equally prudent. Hydroquinone-induced leukoderma[27] is usually spontaneously reversible, particularly with small

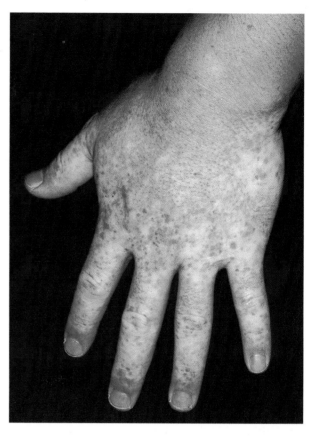

Figure 3 Reticulate acropigmentation of Dohi. Pigmented and depigmented macules form reticulate pattern on the dorsum of hand

amounts of solar irradiation. Hypomelanosis secondary to topical tretinoin is also slowly reversible upon discontinuation of the preparation. Hypopigmentation secondary to topical steroids is also usually spontaneously reversible, but that secondary to intralesional corticosteroids may be amelanotic and persistent, particularly in skin phototypes V and VI.

PROGRESSIVE MACULAR HYPOMELANOSIS

Etiology and epidemiology

Progressive macular hypomelanosis is frequently observed in the West Indies, and, occasionally, in France among persons immigrating from the Caribbean[28].

Clinical findings

The condition is characterized by a progressive and widespread hypomelanosis developing in blacks of mixed lineage living in or coming from the tropical area of the Caribbean. It occurs mainly in females from 18 to 25 years of age with extremes ranging from 13 to 35 years, with a progressive development

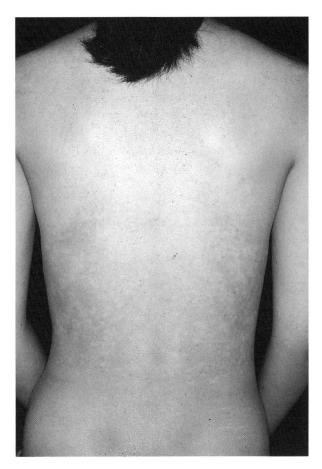

Figure 4 Progressive macular hypomelanosis. Large, hypopigmented, non-scaly patches are seen on the back

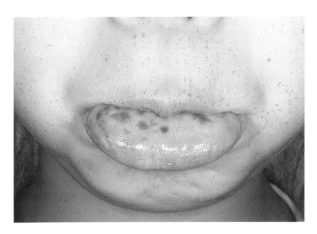

Figure 5 Peutz-Jeghers syndromr. The pigmented macules are seen on the tongue

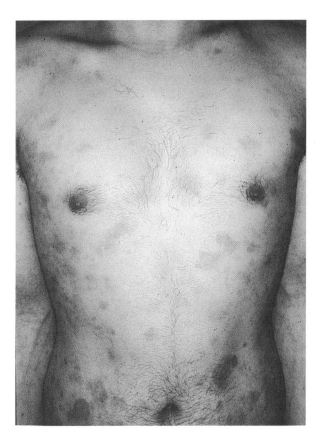

Figure 6 Erythema dyschromium perstans. The annular blue-gray macules and patches are see on the trunk

of round, pale, coalescent macules on the back and sometimes on the abdomen. They increase in number and progressively coalesce into large, hypopigmented, non-scaly patches surrounded by smaller well defined macules (Figure 4). The dyschromia is not always confined to the middle of the back; it may sometimes develop in the epigastric and/or intermammary areas, but it always spares the neck and the neckline. The resulting hypomelanosis is localized or diffuse, in a symmetrical distribution most apparent in darkest-skinned individuals[28]. The lesions are not itchy. The spots are more clearly visible under Wood's light. Because of the confluence of hypochromic macules, this disease is closer to the so-called ashy dermatosis[29,30] or erythema dyschromicum perstans than to other idiopathic diseases of pigmentation. The hypomelanosis spreads progressively over the whole trunk for about 12 months, but typically spares, at least partially, the dorso-lumbar line. Then the lesions slowly fade and disappear completely within 2 to 5 years. The lesions were found to respond to no topical treatment, including antiseptic agents, antifungal preparations and corticosteroids.

Histopathology

Both normal and hypopigmented skin revealed similar alterations in melanosome size and distribution. The surrounding normal dark skin showed that stage IV melanosomes predominated in the melanocytes, were distributed as large, single melanosomes and were regularly transferred to keratinocytes. In contrast, skin biopsy specimens from hypopigmented macules demonstrated an altered melanogenesis characterized by stages I, II and III melanosomes, predominantly in the perinucleus of melanocytes with a few stage IV melanosomes in the dendrites. These melanosomes were distributed to keratinocytes as aggregated small melanosomes[28].

LENTIGO SIMPLEX

Lentigo simplex is an acquired or congenital brown macule consisting of intradermal melanocytic hyperplasia, increased melanin formation, and a pattern of epidermal hyperplasia consisting of elongated, club shaped and often fused rete ridges.

Clinical findings

The usual finding is a sharply circumscribed, pigmented, light brown or dark brown macule, large or small. A juvenile variety of lentigo simplex appears sometimes during the first decade of life and may occur anywhere on skin or mucous membranes as a macule, usually less than 0.5 cm in diameter. There appears to be no relation between exposure to the sun and the appearance of lentigo simplex. Generalized lentigines may occur as an isolated phenomenon, without known familiar aggregation, either from birth or early infancy or appearing during adulthood[31,32].

Histopathology

Lentigo simplex consists of intra-epidermal melanocytic hyperplasia in the basal layer of elongated epidermal rete ridges, without nest formation. Melanocytes in lentigo simplex are said to be S100-negative[33]. Giant pigment granules may occur in lentigo simplex in isolation. There are varieties of lentigo simplex on cutaneous, acral and mucosal sites showing cellular atypia of melanocytes.

Differential diagnosis

Lentigo simplex must be differentiated from junctional nevomelanocytic nevus, café au lait macule, darkly pigmented varieties of solar lentigo, lentigo maligna and other varieties of freckles.

Pathogenesis

The cause of lentigo simplex is unknown. Its presence in association with somatic abnormalities in such diverse conditions suggests a developmental neural crest disorder, significantly influenced by genetic and/or racial factors. Isolated lentigo simplex on mucocutaneous sites may also be influenced by genetic and/or racial factors. The presence of melanin macroglobules in melanocytes and keratinocytes of lentigo simplex may be the result of aberrant melanogenesis and melanocyte dysfunction[31].

Treatment

There is no need to treat benign-appearing lentigo simplex. Dark or irregularly pigmented varieties of lentigo simplex should be examined histologically for cellular atypia. Atypical varieties of lentigo simplex should be completely excised with a border of at least 3 mm of normal-appearing skin. Wood's lamp examination is useful in defining the margin of lentigo simplex.

EPHELIDES

Ephelides or freckles are small, tan to dark brown macules that are promoted by exposure to the sun and fade during the winter months.

Clinical findings

Ephelides, or freckles, are small – usually less than 0.5 cm in diameter – discrete brown macules that appear on sun-exposed skin, particularly in Celts (Scottish-Irish-Welsh) with blue eyes and red or blond hair. Onset may be at any time but it often occurs early in childhood. Freckles tend to lighten in the absence of sun exposure, and are not found in unexposed areas or mucosal surfaces. Boys and girls are equally affected. Freckles are genetic in origin, following an autosomal dominant pattern. The presence of freckling in 12 members of four generations with red or red-brown hair suggests autosomal dominant inheritance[34]. Freckles exhibit immediate pigment darkening and darken more readily than does otherwise normal skin.

Histopathology

The basal layers of hyperpigmented skin show increased pigmentation without elongation of the rete ridges. The dermis is normal. In freckled skin there is no obvious increase in the concentration of melanocytes compared to nearby pale epidermis. Melanocytes are highly dendritic, are strongly DOPA-positive, and have many stage IV melanosomes, which are long and rod-shaped, analogous to darker skin photo-types[35].

Differential diagnosis

Ephelides may be found in neurofibromatosis, progeria, Moynahan's syndrome and xeroderma pigmentosum. Axillary freckling has been regarded as a marker for neurofibromatosis, though it may also be seen in progeria and Moynahan's syndrome.

Treatment

Treatment of freckles is carried out for cosmetic reasons. Application of hydroquinone or a combination of glycolic acid lotion along with maximum UVA blocking sunscreen in the morning and retinoic acid in the evening will significantly lighten freckles. Avoidance of the sun and the use of sunscreens prevent the appearance of new freckles and help prevent the darkening of existing freckles that typically accompanies exposure to the sun. Trichloroacetic acid peeling, skillful use of liquid nitrogen and dermabrasion are effective[36]. Pigment lasers, Nd: YAG, ruby, and ultrapulsed CO_2 lasers effectively remove freckles.

PEUTZ–JEGHERS SYNDROME

Peutz–Jeghers syndrome is an autosomal dominant disorder characterized by macular mucocutaneous pigmentation and hamartomatous polyps of the gastrointestinal tract.

Clinical findings

The pigmented macules are most common on the buccal mucosa and are dark brown, blue, or blue-brown in color (Figure 5). The macules, which are usually 3 to 4 mm in diameter, may resemble freckles but may be larger and resemble café au lait macules. The macules of the skin are usually found on the dorsal surfaces of the hands and feet and other common cutaneous surfaces around the mouth, eyes and umbilicus. Mucosal lesions may appear at birth or in childhood and may disappear from the skin but not from the mucosal surface. Gastrointestinal polyps are most frequent in the small bowel, particularly the jejunum. The polyps usually become symptomatic between the ages of 10 and 30 and may cause bleeding ulcers, obstruction, diarrhea and intussusception. Anemia may develop secondary to acute or chronic blood loss. Malignant changes occur, especially in the large intestine but also in the stomach and duodenum. Intestinal hemangiomas that may bleed massively have been described. Any child with recurrent, unexplained abdominal pain should be examined for the typical cutaneous, mucosal and periorificial pigmented lesion of Peutz–Jeghers syndrome.

Histopathology

Mild acanthosis and elongation of rete ridges in the pigmented macules are typical. Electron microscopy shows evidence of pigment blockade with no melanosomes in keratinocytes, but large numbers of fully melanized melanosomes in melanocytes; the dendrites are very elongated and even reach to the upper epidermal keratinocytes. Basal layer melanization is not increased, and a number of dermal melanophages have been observed in the subpapillary dermis of both the lip and finger lesions[37].

Differential diagnosis

The pigmented lesions in Peutz–Jeghers syndrome are readily distinguished from freckles, which occur in areas exposed to the sun, and from generalized lentigines, which are widely scattered. The presence of macules on the tips of the crista profunda intermedia distinguishes digital Peutz–Jeghers syndrome lesions.

Treatment

Conservative management for the bouts of abdominal pain, including bed rest, mild sedation and nasogastric suction is advisable. Spontaneous reduction of intussusception is common. However, continued bleeding or progression to obstruction of the bowel demands immediate surgical intervention[38]. Because the risk of malignancy is relatively low in the hamartomatous polyps, prophylactic resection of the bowel is not indicated. More aggressive management, consisting of endoscopic polypectomy of as many polyps as possible, and routine radiologic surveillance studies have been recommended by some authors[39].

ERYTHEMA AB IGNE
Clinical findings

Erythema ab igne is a localized dermatosis caused by repeated exposure to heat. Erythema ab igne appears as a reticulated pigmentation and telangiectasia over sites chronically exposed to heat, especially the lower legs and anterior lower legs. It is commonly seen in countries without central heating, where it tends to occur on the legs of elderly women who sit close to gas or electric heaters or in the lumbar region in patients who apply hot water bottles or electric heating pads for backache. Historically, Chinese who slept on beds of hot bricks, Kashmiris who wore pots containing hot coals next to the skin, and Japanese wearing benzene-burning flasks developed erythema ab igne in the areas that were repeatedly heated[40].

Erythema ab igne may progress to squamous cell carcinoma[41,42]. Anecdotal reports describe heat-induced carcinoma developing in the areas of erythema ab igne in individuals from northern China, India and Japan, called kanf, kangri and kairo cancers, respectively[40].

Chronic exposure to various heat sources may promote the development of cutaneous cancer.

Corson and associates have found that in individuals wearing rimless spectacles, refracted light is conducted from the upper to the lower rim of the spectacle lens and focused on the skin to produce a localized increase in temperature[43]. Fourteen cases (3 with AK, 11 with BCE) have been reported in individuals wearing such glasses[44]. Acute burns sufficient to cause ulceration may yield carcinomas in the burn scar years after the primary insult.

Histopathology

Histologic findings in early lesions include epidermal atrophy, vasodilation and a dermal mixed cell infiltrate. The pigmentary changes are due to infiltrates of melanophages, free-lying dermal melanin granules and hemosiderin. Later varying amounts of elastic fibers, similar in appearance to those seen in sun-damaged skin, and hyperkeratosis with or without dyskeratotic keratinocytes are found.

Differential diagnosis

The clinical presentation of erythema ab igne is usually diagnostic and biopsy is rarely required to confirm the diagnosis. The differential diagnosis includes livedo reticularis and cutis marmorata, each of which can be distinguished from erythema ab igne by the absence of pigmentary change.

Pathogenesis

Chronic infrared radiation produces thermal elastosis manifested by an increase in the number and thickness of elastic fibers, which form dense accretions similar to those in solar elastosis. It also may induce epidermal changes ranging from hyperkeratosis and slight keratinocytes atypia to frankly invasive squamous cell carcinoma. The changes seen in erythema ab igne are specific to repeated exposure of skin to relatively low levels of infrared radiation.

Treatment

There is no effective treatment for erythema ab igne. In patients with active disease, however, further damage can be prevented by altering the causative behavior.

ERYTHEMA DYSCHROMICUM PERSTANS

Erythema dyschromicum perstans, first described by Ramirez in 1957[45], is a cutaneous disorder of unknown etiology characterized by widespread gray-brown pigmented macules and patches that have an erythematous, raised border in the early stages.

Epidemiology and etiology

Most cases of the disease have been observed in Latin America and India. The cause of erythema dyschromicum perstans is unknown, but an immune origin is suggested by the histopathology and immunophenotypic findings. Erythema dyschromicum perstans may be a variant of lichen planus, and several cases of this latter condition have been reported preceding, following, or concominant with erythema dyschromicum perstans. The condition may be the end stage of lichen planus in darkly pigmented individuals.

Clinical findings

The disorder presents as a rare, asymptomatic, slowly progressive dermatosis characterized by annular blue-gray macules (Figure 6). The initial lesions may be erythematous patches or plaques, sometimes with an elevated border, which later in the disease become ashy gray. The macules are usually well demarcated and may coalesce to form extensive patches. The dermatosis is localized on the trunk, arms and face with sparing of palms, soles, scalp, nails and mucous membranes.

Histopathology

The histopathologic findings include vacuolar degeneration of basal layer keratinocytes and a perivascular mononuclear cell infiltrate. Civatte bodies and melanophages are often observed. Erythema dyschromicum perstans shares some histologic features with lichen planus, especially the actinic and atrophic variants[46]. Immunocytochemical analyses have revealed selective accumulation of CD-3 positive, CD8-positive and Leu-15 (CD11b)-negative T cells in the epidermis of erythema dyschromicum perstans. The dermal infiltrate in erythema dyschromicum perstans is composed of activated, CD25-expressing, CD4-positive cells and CD8-positive cells, and of macrophages, as indicated by immunoperoxidase staining[47].

Treatment

Erythema dyschromicum perstans is difficult to treat. Griseofulvin has been reported to induce complete disappearance of the disease, but the lesions recurred on discontinuation of treatment. In an open, uncontrolled study, seven of eight patients had a good to excellent response to clofazimine.

ERYTHROMELANOSIS FOLLICULARIS FACIEI ET COLLI

Erythromelanosis follicularis faciei et colli (EFFC) was first reported by Kitamura and colleagues in 1960. They reported this condition in six Japanese men, and for some time it was regarded as an entity solely confined to Japanese. However, later reports of EFFC in white men, women, and with a unilateral distribution, emphasized the ubiquity of this condition.

Epidemiology and etiology

Most patients report an onset of the condition in childhood, with a gradual extension of the lesion. To date, the majority of patients have been young and middle-aged men. The etiology of EFFC remains obscure. Mishima and Rudner have proposed the possibility of a labile autonomic nerve function in the erythromelanotic lesion[48]. A major textbook of dermatology has placed this condition under both disorders of pigmentation and disorders of keratinization. The true nature of this entity still awaits clarification.

Clinical findings

The triad that has been consistently observed in EFFC patients is hyperpigmentation, erythema and follicular plugging[49]. A typical lesion consists of a sharply demarcated reddish-brown pigmented patch with telangiectasia and many pale follicular papules. The site of predilection is the preauricular area with extension to the side of the neck. Most cases show a bilateral distribution, although, as mentioned above, unilateral distribution has been reported. Coarse beard growth and loss of vellus hair have been described in affected areas. No scarring or atrophy has ever been attributed to EFFC. Keratosis pilaris of the extremities, especially the upper arms, has frequently been associated with EFFC.

Histopathology

There is slight hyperkeratosis without parakeratosis. Hyperplasia of follicular appendages with follicular plugging and cyst formation can be observed[48]. The epidermis overlying the follicle is flattened and an increase in melanin in epidermal keratinocytes is evident. Electron microscopic examination has revealed abnormally large melanosomes, and in the dermis some of the vessels appear dilated with a mild lymphocytic infiltrate. None of the above features is diagnostic for EFFC.

Treatment

The condition appears to be persistent and only tretinoin cream, alone[50] or in combination with hydroquinone and ammonium lactate cream, have been reported as a treatment modality with some success.

REFERENCES

1. Hidano A, Kajima H, Ikeda S, et al. Natural history of nevus of Ota. Arch Dermatol 1967;95:187–95
2. Lee JH. A clinical observation about the nevi involving melanocytes in the Korean youth. Kor J Dermatol 1986;24:73–8
3. Hori Y, Kawashima M, Oohara K. Acquired, bilateral nevus of Ota-like macules. J Am Acad Dermatol 1984;10:961–4
4. Vazquez M, Maldonado H, Benmaman C, et al. Melasma in men. A clinical and histologic study. Int J Dermatol 1988;27:25–7
5. Resnick S. Melasma induced by oral contraceptive drugs. JAMA 1967;199:601–5
6. Pathak MA, Fitzpatrick TB, Kraus EW. Usefulness of retinoic acid in the treatment of melasma. J Am Acad Dermatol 1986;15:394–9
7. Jimbow K. N-acetyl-4-S cysteaminylphenol as a new type of depigmenting agent for the melanoderma of patients with melasma. Arch Dermatol 1991;127:1528–34
8. Hori Y, Kawashima M, Olhara K, et al. Acquired bilateral nevus of Ota-like macules. J Am Acad Dermatol 1984;10:961–4
9. Mizoguchi M, Murakami F, Ito M, et al. Clinical, pathological, and etiologic aspects of acquired dermal melanocytosis. Pigment Cell Res 1997;10:176–83
10. Nakayama H, Matsuo S, Hayakawa R, et al. Pigmented contact dermatitis. Int J Dermatol 1984;23:299–305
11. Osmundsen PE. Pigmented contact dermatitis. Br J Dermatol 1970;83:296–8
12. Rorsman H. Riehl's melanosis. Int J Dermatol 1982;21:75–8
13. James WJ, Carter JM. Pigmentary demarcation lines: a population survey. J Am Acad Dermatol 1987;16:584–90
14. Ito K. The peculiar demarcation of pigmentation along the so-called Voigt's line among the Japanese. Dermatol Int 1965;4:45–7
15. Vazquez M, Ibanez M, Sanchez JL. Pigmentary demarcation lines during pregnancy. Cutis 1986;38:263–6

16. Ostlere LS, Ratnavel RC, Lawlor F, *et al.* Reticulate acropigmentation of Dohi. *Clin Exp Dermatol* 1995; 20:477–9

17. Kim NI, Park SY, Youn JI, *et al.* Dyschromatosis symmetrica hereditaria affecting two families. *Kor J Dermatol* 1980;18:585–9

18. Taki T, Kuzuka S, Izawa Y, *et al.* Surgical treatment of speckled skin caused by dyschromatosis symmetrica hereditaria. *J Dermatol* 1986;13:471–3

19. Bajai AK, Gupta SC. Reticulate acropigmentation of Kitamura. *Dermatologica* 1974;168:247–9

20. Arzu E, Mehmet AG, Naci E. Reticulate acropigmentation of Kitamura. *Int J Dermatol* 1993;32:726–7

21. Arzu E, Guzin O. Reticulate acropigmentation of Kitamura. *J Dermatol* 1992;19:256–7

22. Cummings KI, Cottel WI. Idiopathic guttate hypomelanosis. *Arch Dermatol* 1966;93:184–6

23. Savall R, Ferrandiz C, Ferrer I, *et al.* Idiopathic guttate hypomelanosis. *Br J Dermatol* 1980;103:635–42

24. Ploysangam T, Dee-Ananlap S, Suvanprakorn P. Treatment of idiopathic guttate hypomelanosis with liquid nitrogen: light and electron microscopic studies. *J Am Acad Dermatol* 1990;23:681–4

25. Taylor AC. Survival of rat skin and changes in hair pigmentation following freezing. *J Exp Zool* 1949; 100:77

26. Straile WE. A study of the hair follicle and its melanocytes. *Dev Biol* 1964;10:45

27. Oettel H. Die Hydrochinonvergiftung. *Arch Exp Pathol Pharmacol* 1936;183:319

28. Guillet G, Helenon R, Gauthier Y, *et al.* Progressive macular hypomelanosis of the trunk: primary acquired hypopigmentation. *J Cut Pathol* 1988;15: 286–9

29. Ramierz CO. Dermatosis cenicienta. *Dermatología (Mex)* 1963;7:232

30. Stevenson MJR, Miura M. Erythema dyschromicum perstonis (ashy dermatosis). *Arch Dermatol* 1966;94: 196–9

31. Kaufmann J. Lentiginosis profusa. *Dermatologica* 1976;153:116–18

32. Uhle P, Norvell SS Jr. Generalized lentiginosis. *J Am Acad Dermatol* 1988;18:444–7

33. Nakajima T, Watanabe S, Sato Y, *et al.* Immunohistochemical demonstration of S-100 protein in malignant melanoma and pigmented nevus, and its diagnostic application. *Cancer* 1982;50:912–18

34. Jansson H. Problems of differentiation of ephelides and lentigines based on analysis of frequency. *Hautarzt* 1958;7:311–13

35. Ford D, Bliss JM, Swerdlow AJ, *et al.* Risk of cutaneous melanoma associated with pigmentation characteristics and freckling: systemic overview of 10 case-control studies. *Int J Cancer* 1995;62:377–81

36. Lee JB, Choi H-J. TCA chemical peeling – procedures, complications and self-evaluation of therapeutic effect in 242 patients. *Kor J Dermatol* 1993;31:1–8

37. Yamada K, Matsukawa A, Hori Y, Kukita A. Ultrastructural studies on pigmented macules of Peutz–Jeghers syndrome. *J Dermatol* 1981;8:367–7

38. McAllister AJ, Richards KF. Peutz–Jeghers syndrome: experience with twenty patients in five generations. *Am J Surg* 1977;134:717–20

39. Foley TR, McGarrity TJ, Abt AB. Peutz–Jeghers syndrome: a clinicopathologic survey of the "Harrisburg family" with 49-year follow-up. *Gastroenterology* 1988;95:1535–40

40. Kligman LH, Kligman AM. Reflections on heat. *Br J Dermatol* 1984;110:369–75

41. Arrington JH, Lockman DS. Thermal keratoses and squamous cell carcinoma *in situ* associated with erythema ab igne. *Arch Dermatol* 1979;115:1226–8

42. Peterkin GAG. Malignant change in erythema ab igne. *Br Med J* 1955;2:1599–602

43. Corson GF, Knoll GM, Luscombe HA, *et al.* Role of spectacle lenses in production of cutaneous changes especially epithelioma. *Arch Dermatol Syph* 1949;59: 435–48

44. Lawrence EA. Carcinoma arising in the scars of thermal burns. *Surg Gynecol Obstet* 1952;95:579–88

45. Ramirez CO. The ashy dermatosis (erythema dyschromicum perstans). *Cutis* 1967;3:244–7

46. Tschen JA, Tschen EA, McGavran MH. Erythema dyschromicum perstans. *J Am Acad Dermatol* 1980;2: 295–302

47. Miyagwa S, Komatsu M, Okuchi T, *et al.* Erythema dyschromicum perstans: immunopathologic studies. *J Am Acad Dermatol* 1989;20:882–6

48. Mishima YH, Rudner E. Erythromelanosis follicularis faciei et colli. *Dermatologica* 1966;132:269–87

49. Sodaify M, Baghestani S, Handjani F, *et al.* Erythromelanosis follicularis faciei et colli. *Int J Dermatol* 1994;33:643–4

50. Watt TL, Kaiser JS. Erythromelanosis follicularis faciei et colli: a case report. *J Am Acad Dermatol* 1981;5:533–4

Vesicular and bullous diseases 17

Sarah Brenner, Vincenzo Ruocco, Mariarosaria D'Avino,
Eleonora Ruocco and Anat Bialy-Golan

PEMPHIGUS
INTRODUCTION

Pemphigus (from Greek πέμφιξ = bulla) is a chronic, autoimmune, blistering disease involving the skin and Malpighian mucous membranes. There are several clinical subtypes, the major ones being pemphigus vulgaris with the pemphigus vegetans variant; pemphigus foliaceus with the two variants endemic pemphigus foliaceus (Brazilian pemphigus foliaceus, or 'fogo selvagem' meaning wild fire) and pemphigus erythematosus; and paraneoplastic pemphigus. When the outbreak of pemphigus is facilitated by one or more of the known heterogeneous triggers (such as drugs, physical agents, viruses, hormones and even diet components or emotional stress), the disease is usually labeled as induced pemphigus[1].

CLINICAL PRESENTATION

Pemphigus vulgaris, the most common type of pemphigus, presents in middle-aged and genetically predisposed individuals with oral lesions in two thirds of patients, in contrast to pemphigus foliaceus in which mucous membrane involvement is usually absent. Oral blisters are fragile and rupture readily, leaving erosions which heal with difficulty. Subsequently, flaccid bullae develop over several sites of the skin (trunk, scalp, flexures) (Figure 1). The blistering is not always obvious, and often most lesions consist of crusted erosions. Left untreated, the disease progresses with an almost always fatal outcome owing to uncontrolled fluid and protein loss or opportunistic infection. In pemphigus vegetans, pustular lesions and hypertrophic granulations or vegetations develop at the mucosal margins and on the intertriginous areas (axillae and, especially in women, inguinal regions and submammary folds).

Pemphigus foliaceus and pemphigus erythematosus are diseases of middle age, whereas the endemic form, clustered in jungle areas of Brazil, Colombia, Paraguay and Peru, and possibly precipitated by a biting black fly (*Simulium nigrimanum*), frequently affects children as well as adults[2]. However, an unusual incidence of pemphigus foliaceus has lately been reported in young Tunisian women[3]. The onset is frequently localized to the scalp and face, slowly spreading over the chest and upper back. Scattered, scaly and crusted lesions, intermingled with a few small flaccid bullae, involve the 'seborrheic' areas and only rarely extend, except in the endemic form in which the patient may become erythrodermic. Pemphigus erythematosus may show additional clinical lesions of lupus erythematosus. These diseases are usually more benign than pemphigus vulgaris, and spontaneous remissions can occur.

Paraneoplastic pemphigus is a distinctive form of pemphigus associated with lymphoproliferative disease, thymomas and sarcomas[4]. Clinical presentation is polymorphous and may mimic erythema multiforme, with 'target' oral and palmoplantar lesions, or lichen planus pemphigoides, with severe mucosal erosions and large blisters on the trunk. The prognosis is poor, being of course conditioned by the coexisting neoplastic disease.

The clinical pattern of induced pemphigus is variable[1]. Pemphigus foliaceus and pemphigus erythematosus are the most common presentations induced by drugs containing a sulfydryl group (thiol drugs), e.g. penicillamine, captopril and by some physical agents, e.g., sunburn. The vulgaris form, often heralded by a herpetiform presentation, can be induced by non-thiol drugs, e.g. pyrazolon derivatives, progesterone, and by different triggering factors, e.g. radiotherapy, thermal burns and viruses (especially herpetoviridae)[5–7]. The course is unpredictable. Many patients with the foliaceus and erythematosus forms recover spontaneously when the inducing factor is removed (induced pemphigus proper). In most patients with the vulgaris form, the disease continues its course despite removal of any inducing factor (triggered pemphigus)[1,5].

In women pemphigus may have some clinical peculiarities related to their physiology (pregnancy, menses) and to prevalently female habits (cooking, cosmetics). Pregnancy usually aggravates the course of pemphigus or even elicits relapse of a dormant

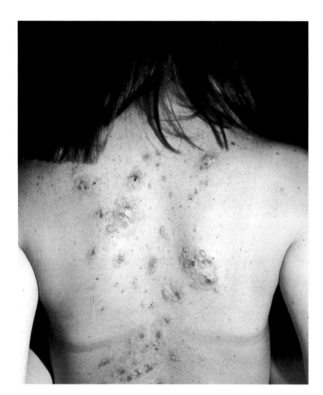

Figure 1 Pemphigus vulgaris induced by progesterone in a young woman

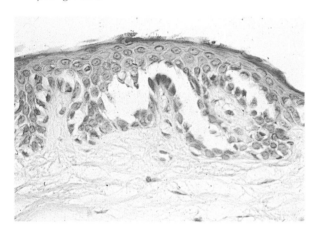

Figure 2 Standard histology showing suprabasal acantholysis in pemphigus vulgaris (HE, × 200)

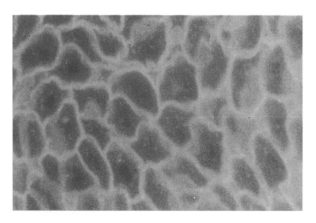

Figure 3 Pemphigus vulgaris. Direct immunofluorescence showing intercellular deposition of IgG in the perilesional epidermis (anti-IgG serum with fluorescein, × 400)

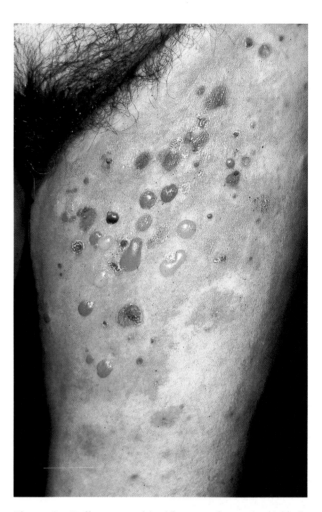

Figure 4 Bullous pemphigoid: tense, dome-shaped bullae on erythematous skin

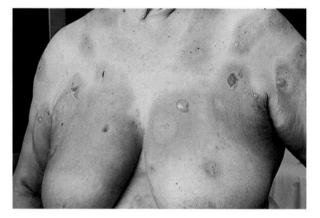

Figure 5 Bullous pemphigoid induced by a thermal burn

form. An unusual clinical presentation of pemphigus, simulating pemphigoid gestationis, was observe by one of us in a young woman during her first pregnancy. The woman gave birth to a female newborn presenting transient blisters due to transplacental transfer of maternal pemphigus antibodies[8]. Several similar cases have subsequently been reported in the literature (transient neonatal

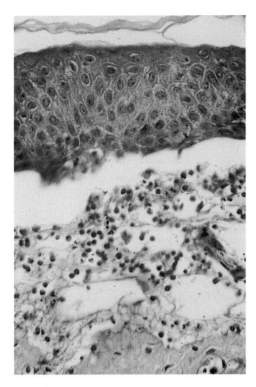

Figure 6 Bullous pemphigoid. Standard histology shows a subepidermal cavity with numerous eosinophils and neutrophils (HE, × 200)

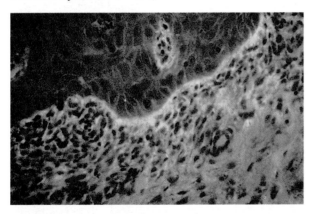

Figure 7 Bullous pemphigoid. On direct immunofluorescence of perilesional skin, a linear pattern of IgG is observed at the basement membrane zone (anti-IgG serum with fluorescein, × 200)

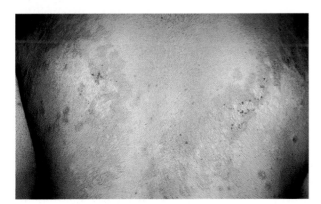

Figure 8 Dermatitis herpetiformis: a typical arrangement of the lesions on the upper back

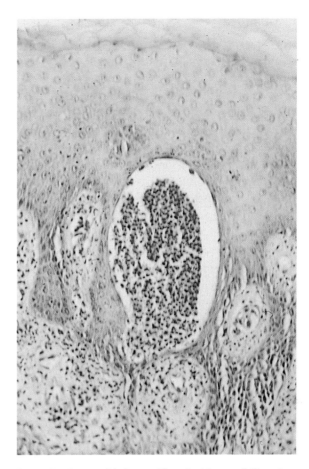

Figure 9 Dermatitis herpetiformis. Neutrophilic microabscesses within the upper papillary dermis (HE, × 100)

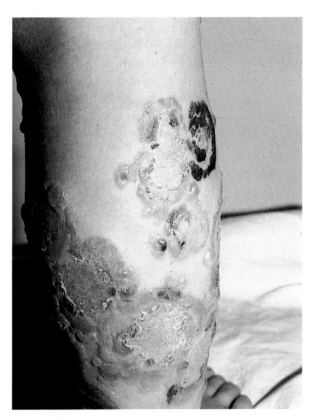

Figure 10 Linear IgA bullous dermatosis in a little girl: 'cluster of jewels' sign

pemphigus)[9]. Maternal pemphigus may be associated with fetal prematurity and death, but it is difficult to separate the effects of treatment from those of the disease. Menstruation is sometimes connected with pemphigus induction or relapse for different reasons. Women who have frequent herpes simplex recurrences in the premenstrual period may experience an exacerbation of their pemphigus because of endogenous interferon production. Irregular and painful menses are often treated with progesterone and pyrazolon derivatives, drugs capable of inducing pemphigus in genetically predisposed subjects[1,10,11] (Figure 1). Culinary activities involve an increased risk of pemphigus induction through frequent manipulation of certain spices, particularly vegetables of the *Allium* group[12], chopping poultry[13] and the possibility of minor but repeated thermal burns. Cosmetic procedures such as chemical peeling, plastic surgery[14] and the use of henna for dyeing hair[13] have also been associated with the onset of pemphigus.

Pathology

The hallmark of histologic changes in pemphigus is the intra-epithelial cleft that results from cell–cell dyshesion (acantholysis) with formation of bullae containing isolated, round-shaped, acantholytic (or Tzanck) cells. The cleft is suprabasal in pemphigus vulgaris (Figure 2) and vegetans, subcorneal in the pemphigus foliaceus subtypes. A mild to moderate inflammatory infiltrate may be seen in the upper dermis. In paraneoplastic pemphigus, dyskeratotic keratinocytes and basal cell vacuolization with interface dermatitis are additional histological findings. Eosinophils in the dermis characterize the early stages of drug-induced pemphigus.

Laboratory studies

Almost all patients with pemphigus have pathogenic circulating IgG autoantibodies, detectable in the serum at different concentrations (or titers) by indirect immunofluorescence (IIF), which bind to normal components of keratinocyte cell membrane belonging to the cadherin supergene family and involved in mediating intercellular cohesion. These components, the pemphigus antigens, have lately been identified as desmoglein 3 (130 kDa) for pemphigus vulgaris and desmoglein 1 (160 kDa) for pemphigus foliaceus. The intercellular deposition of the pathogenic autoantibodies, detectable in the perilesional epidermis (or mucosal epithelium) by direct immunofluorescence (DIF), activates the plasminogen–plasmin system. This results in loss of cell adhesion and an intra-epithelial splitting (acantholysis). Genetic factors play an essential role. There is a well-established human leukocyte antigen (HLA) association with DR4, DR14, and DQ1 genes in most forms of pemphigus, whereas an HLA-DR1 gene is linked to the endemic foliaceus form. Genetic factors may determine susceptibility to the disease but its outbreak possibly occurs when predisposed individuals are exposed to the appropriate inducing agents, which may be known (induced pemphigus) or unknown (idiopathic pemphigus).

Routine laboratory examinations for diagnostic purposes are the Tzanck test, standard histology, DIF and IIF. Smears taken by scraping the bottom of a bulla or an erosion show typical acantholytic cells (Tzanck test). Standard histology of a fresh bulla reveals suprabasilar (p. vulgaris) or subcorneal (p. foliaceus) splitting with formation of intra-epithelial cavities. Direct immunofluorescence shows the intercellular deposition of IgG and C3 in the perilesional epithelium (Figure 3). Indirect immunofluorescence (using monkey or guinea-pig esophagus) is the classic method to detect and titer pemphigus antibodies in serum. This test is also useful to monitor the course of pemphigus and to adjust the treatment since antibody titers usually parallel disease activity. In particular cases and when the diagnosis remains uncertain, more sophisticated laboratory investigations (immunoblotting, immunoprecipitation) are needed. HLA typing is useful to search for pemphigus-prone genes in the patient's genotype.

Differential diagnosis

Recurrent aphthous stomatitis (especially in women), Behçet disease, erosive lichen planus, Stevens–Johnson syndrome or cicatricial pemphigoid can simulate oral erosions of pemphigus vulgaris, but the Tzanck test is constantly negative in all these conditions. Conversely, oral surgeons and gynecologists should be alerted that a stubborn erosive stomatitis or vulvovaginitis may be common presenting signs of pemphigus vulgaris, which can easily be confirmed by a positive Tzanck test. The diagnosis is less difficult when the patient has cutaneous blisters or erosions. In pregnant women, however, pemphigus vulgaris may mimic pemphigoid gestationis with tense and hemorrhagic bullae located on the lower trunk, abdomen and thighs. The absence of acantholytic cells in Tzanck smears, the subepidermal cleavage on histology and the location of immunoreactants at the basement membrane zone on DIF and IIF, are diagnostic markers of pemphigoid. The pemphigus foliaceus subtypes may resemble seborrheic dermatitis, impetigo, discoid lupus erythematosus and even psoriasis or eruptive seborrheic keratoses[15]. Histological and immunological investigations are usually sufficient to solve all doubtful cases.

Treatment

Systemic steroid and other immunosuppressive agents are the first-line treatment of pemphigus. Prednisone or deflazacort are given initially in a high dose (100–200 mg daily), often with azathioprine (2.5 mg/kg/day) or cyclophosphamide (1–3 mg/kg/day) or cyclosporin (5 mg/kg/day). Once blistering has been controlled, the steroid dosage can gradually be lowered. Treatment usually needs to be continued for several years, which leads to the fact that nowadays mortality and morbidity are more likely to be due to side-effects of the steroid and immunosuppressive therapy than to the disease itself. In pregnant women the treatment must be restricted to steroids at moderately high dosage (60–90 mg daily deflazacort). In mild cases, and especially in pemphigus erythematosus, topical or intralesional steroid therapy alone may be attempted. Alternative treatment regimens are pulse methylprednisolone therapy, corticotropin, gold salts, antimalarials, high-dose intravenous immunoglobulin G, the association of oral tetracycline and nicotinamide, plasmapheresis and extracorporeal photophoresis.

Women with pemphigus, even in the stages of clinical remission, should be warned of the fact that pregnancy and contraceptive treatments (owing to the presence of progesterone derivatives)[10,11] are risk factors. Patients should also be discouraged from over-indulging in not absolutely necessary drugs (e.g. common analgesics for painful menses) that also carry a risk of pemphigus induction. Exposure to the sun and other UV sources requires special caution, since these physical agents may facilitate relapses of pemphigus[1,16,17]. The same can be said for intensive and prolonged emotional stress[18–20]. Finally, patients should be advised to have a balanced diet and avoid eating and even tasting or manipulating foods spiced with garlic, onion and leek, since these culinary plants (belonging to the genus *Allium*) contain allyl compounds with a proven acantholytic potential[12,21–23].

BULLOUS PEMPHIGOID

Bullous pemphigoid (or pemphigoid) is a chronic, autoimmune disease of the elderly, characterized by large, tense bullae usually developing on erythematous or urticated areas of the skin.

Clinical presentation

The disease afflicts elderly patients (rarely children), but shows no ethnic or racial predilection. With regard to sex, there are three recent reports indicating that one type, bullous pemphigoid 180, has a predilection for older men[24–26]. In particular, patients with bullous pemphigoid fail to display any increased incidence of peculiar HLA phenotypes, suggesting that genetic factors do not play a crucial role in susceptibility to the disease. In some cases a precipitating factor can be demonstrated, for example drugs (mainly furosemide, penicillin derivates, phenacetin), UV rays, thermal burns and malignancies (paraneoplastic pemphigoid)[27–32]. A nonspecific (urticaria-like or eczematous) itching rash on the limbs often precedes the onset of blistering. Weeks or months later, tense, dome-shaped bullae arise on erythematous or normal-looking skin, usually on the limbs, trunk and in flexural areas (antecubital, inguinal, popliteal folds) (Figures 4 and 5). The size of the blisters varies greatly from small vesicles to large bullae and, in contrast to pemphigus vulgaris, bullae are not fragile, so that they may last several days. By rupturing, blisters leave eroded areas which, if uncomplicated by secondary infection, heal readily without scarring. An extensive spreading of the bullous lesions with most of the body affected is possible, but despite that the patient's general condition usually remains good. Mucous membrane involvement is infrequent and in most cases confined to the mouth. The oral lesions appear as small, tense, often asymptomatic blisters that may remain intact for a couple of days before rupturing and resulting in rapidly healing erosions. The degree of pruritus varies: in the majority of patients itch is the presenting symptom and persists with fluctuations for a long time or even throughout the course of the disease; rarely it is absent or mild. The course of bullous pemphigoid is chronic, with exacerbations and remissions over months and years. Spontaneous healing can occur.

Unusual variants of the disease are the localized forms, which may be limited to the lower extremities, predominantly on the legs of women (pretibial bullous pemphigoid) or to the vulva of young girls (localized vulvar pemphigoid). The latter variant, reported in girls aged 6 months to 8 years, presents with recurrent vulvar vesicles and ulcerations that do not result in scarring[33–35]. A peculiar form of desquamative vaginitis, as a single feature of bullous pemphigoid without any scar formation, was reported in a 60-year-old-woman[36]. The clinical pattern was characterized by swelling and erosive lesions of the vaginal mucosa with contact bleeding, which made sexual intercourse very painful.

Pathology

The blister is invariably subepidermal with an intact, often flattened epidermis forming the roof. The cavity contains numerous eosinophils and neutrophils (Figure 6). Biopsy findings from non-inflammed bases or from the periphery of the blisters may be non-specific. Specimens from an erythematous base or from an early bulla show mast cells aligned along the dermo-epidermal junction and later the characteristic infiltrate, where eosinophils predominate, but lymphocytes, histiocytes and neutrophils may also be present and scattered in an edematous dermis. Ultrastructurally, the dermal–epidermal separation is located at the level of the lamina lucida.

Laboratory studies

Autoantibodies, primarily of the IgG class, directed against components of the basement membrane zone (BMZ) and aided by complement (C3) activation, are thought to be pathogenic. Their interaction with the bullous pemphigoid (BP) peculiar antigens, i.e., BP antigen-1 (230 kDa) and BP antigen-2 (180 kDa), both localized at hemidesmosomes of the basal cells, results in subepidermal splitting. Circulating anti-BMZ antibodies bind to these antigens and activate the complement cascade with the resultant production of inflammatory mediators. Mast cells that are activated by these mediators degranulate and release secondary mediators, particularly chemotactic factors, that recruit neutrophils and eosinophils. Blisters are formed by direct cytotoxic action or by proteolytic enzymes[27,29,37]. The tissue-bound antibodies and C3 are revealed by direct immunofluorescence with a linear pattern at the BMZ of perilesional skin (Figure 7). On salt-split skin technique (skin previously incubated in 1 M NaCl), immunoreactants bind to the roof alone, or to the roof and base of the split skin. Through indirect immunofluorescence (using monkey esophagus as a substrate) circulating anti-BMZ antibodies are detectable in 70% of patients. In particular cases, immunoelectron microscopy or antigen identification by immunoblotting techniques are needed to clinch the diagnosis.

Differential diagnosis

The early urticaria-like or eczematous prodromal rash is difficult to recognize as a presenting sign of bullous pemphigoid, but the possibility of this disease should always be considered in elderly patients with atypical and fixed urticarian lesions. The full-blown disease can easily be differentiated from pemphigus vulgaris on clinical grounds and through the Tzanck test (severe mucosal involvement, flaccid bullae, and acantholytic cells are characteristic of the latter). Cicatricial pemphigoid is clinically featured by a scarring and disabling nature (serious eye problems). Pemphigoid gestationis is associated with pregnancy, but it can also occur soon after delivery or even during the use of oral contraceptives. Dermatitis herpetiformis and linear IgA bullous dermatosis can be identified on the basis of immunofluorescence studies. Acquired epidermolysis bullosa can be distinguished from bullous pemphigoid on direct immunofluorescence through the aid of the salt-split skin technique, given that immunoreactants are detectable solely on the dermal side of the split.

Treatment

Bullous pemphigoid responds to a lower dose of steroids than pemphigus: 60 mg daily of oral deflazacort (or 50 mg daily of oral prednisone) is usually sufficient as attack management. A gradual reduction to 10 mg daily within one or two months is possible in the majority of patients. Stubborn cases can be treated with azathioprine, cyclophosphamide or even steroid pulse therapy and plasmapheresis, but the possibility of a coexisting malignancy (paraneoplastic pemphigoid) should always be kept in mind when the disease is refractory to conventional treatment. Localized disease, and in particular vulvar pemphigoid, may be controlled by topical steroid treatment alone[33–35].

Alternative therapies are oral erythromycin (2 g daily for four weeks), oral tetracyclines (alone or in combination with nicotinamide), sulfapyridine and dapsone (especially in patients with a neutrophil predominance in the infiltrate).

DERMATITIS HERPETIFORMIS

Dermatitis herpetiformis (DH) (or Duhring–Brocq disease) is a widespread, intensely pruritic, symmetrical papulovesicular eruption, immunologically characterized by the presence of granular deposits of IgA at the dermo-epidermal junction. Jejunal villus atrophy is an associated finding in most cases. The etiology is unknown.

Clinical presentation

DH usually occurs in the second, and especially third or fourth decades, though both the childhood and elderly may be affected. It is more common in males (3 : 2). The classical onset is with groups of small intensely itchy vesicles, intermingled with urticarial papules, on the scalp, shoulders, buttocks, knees and extensor aspects of the limbs (Figure 8). A herpetiform arrangement of the lesions is characteristic, but uncommon. Patients often complain about a painful burning sensation. In many cases scratching is severe and, therefore, excoriation and lichenification predominate over typical initial manifestations. Iodides exacerbate the eruption dramatically, so they used to be employed as a diagnostic test in the past. Oral lesions are rare and usually asymptomatic.

Although most patients have small bowel villus atrophy, symptoms of gastrointestinal disturbance and malabsorption are uncommon. A gluten-free diet may result in prolonged remission in some patients or lowering of the daily dapsone requirement in others. The disease persists for many years – usually for life. Interestingly, some female patients note exacerbations around the time of their menses[38].

Pathology

The histological hallmark of DH is the presence of neutrophilic microabscesses within the upper papillary dermis just beneath the basement membrane zone (Figure 9). These can best be seen in the vicinity of early blisters or in lesions that have not yet blistered. There are also degenerative changes of the collagen and development of edema. Multilocular vesicles may coalesce to form blisters. Typically the blister cavity contains edema fluid, a reticular network of fibrin and numerous neutrophils. A mixed inflammatory cell infiltrate, consisting of lymphocytes, histiocytes and abundant neutrophils, extends within the dermis.

Laboratory studies

DH is characterized by the finding of granular IgA at the dermal papillae on direct immunofluorescence. This is diagnostic for the disease. However, there may also be C3, IgG and rarely IgM. Immunofluorescence studies of lesions suggest that the blisters form within the lamina lucida[39]. Indirect immunofluorescence on monkey esophagus is negative for epidermal, basement membrane zone or dermal autoantibodies. IgA endomysial antibodies are frequently present, especially when jejunal villus atrophy is associated[40]. Immunoblotting studies are negative. There is a marked increase of the HLA haplotype B8-DR3 in patients with DH[41].

Differential diagnosis

Distinguishing the disease from scabies, eczema and linear IgA disease is important. Biopsy shows a subepidermal bulla, and direct immunofluorescence of normal-looking skin demonstrates granular IgA at the dermal papillae. The most difficult diagnostic problem is found in the group of patients with chronic exudative eczema, papular urticaria and chronic prurigo.

Treatment

A gluten-free diet is the treatment of choice, as this corrects both the bowel and the skin lesions. However, to control the eruption, a preliminary and often prolonged administration of dapsone is usually needed. Dapsone is started with a dose of 50 mg/day and is gradually increased to 100–200 mg/day. The dosage can be reduced and subsequently the drug can be withdrawn once the gluten-free diet proves to be beneficial and by itself sufficient to control the cutaneous lesions. Sulfamethoxypyridazine is an alternative treatment (0.5–1.5 g/day).

LINEAR IgA BULLOUS DERMATOSIS

There is considerable confusion in the literature about the terminology of linear IgA dermatosis (e.g. chronic bullous disease of childhood, juvenile pemphigoid, polymorphous pemphigoid, bullous pemphigoid with linear IgA, atypical dermatitis herpetiformis, juvenile dermatitis herpetiformis, linear dermatitis herpetiformis). The term 'linear IgA dermatosis' was suggested by Jablonska and Chorzelski[42]. Linear IgA dermatosis (LAD) is a chronic subepidermal blistering disease of children and adults, characterized by moderately pruritic vesicles and bullae, particularly about the genital and perioral regions, with a linear deposition of IgA along the basement membrane. In the majority of patients the disease is self-limiting and settles spontaneously within a few months or years.

Clinical presentation

LAD affects all ages from babies of a few months to the elderly, although the condition is rare. There is no evidence for a racial predilection, but it seems that the disease is more common in African and Asian populations[43,44]. The sex incidence is about equal or there may be slightly more female patients. Two main clinical presentations are distinguished, chronic bullous disease of childhood and adult linear IgA disease, the latter beginning any time in adult life. There is much overlap so that the immunopathology and immunogenetics are common to both disorders, but clinical differences do exist between them.

The onset of chronic bullous disease of childhood is usually abrupt with the appearance, on apparently healthy or erythematous skin, of tense bullae up to 1 cm in diameter, with clear or hemorrhagic fluid. Characteristically, the new lesions appear around those resolving, which leads to typical rosette and jewel-like patterns ('cluster of jewels' sign) (Figure 10). The lesions also comprise urticated plaques and papules, as well as annular, polycyclic erythemas. Pruritus is often present. Sites of predilection are the perioral region, the lower part of the trunk, the inner thighs and the genitalia. The mouth may be involved with ulcers and erosions, and hoarseness may indicate pharyngeal involvement. The eyes are often sore or gritty (conjunctivitis). Conjunctival scarring with subsequent blindness is a rare event[45,46]. The involvement of the perineum and vulva has been mistaken for sexual abuse in some little girls[47].

Adult linear IgA disease presents with lesions that are often clinically indistinguishable from those of dermatitis herpetiformis. Moreover, disease activity is not localized mainly in the perioral and genital regions, as with the childhood eruption. In pregnancy, there is often improvement or remission of the disease from the second trimester, so that women may be able to discontinue all drugs[48]. There is usually a relapse after delivery. The mechanism for the improvement during pregnancy is unknown, but the considerable alterations occurring in the immune system during this period seem to play an important role. In fact, increased plasma glycoprotein glycosylation during pregnancy results in an increased concentration of galactose and sialic acid in IgG[49]. Since IgA contains considerably more glycosylated side chains than IgG, the formation of the former antibody may be altered in pregnant women. Therefore, the mechanism for the clinical improvement of LAD during pregnancy (and the subsequent relapse) could be related to the modified glycosylation of IgA that may alter its ability to bind the antigen, possibly by conformational change[48].

Pathology

The histological changes are not specific. Biopsies may show features of dermatitis herpetiformis, because of the presence of neutrophilic microabscesses at the tips of dermal papillae, or of bullous pemphigoid, because of the prevalence of eosinophils. The pattern of eosinophilic spongiosis may also be detected.

Laboratory studies

Genetically, LAD is associated with HLA-B8, -Cw7, -DR3[50]. The etiology is unknown, but a number of precipitating factors (some infections and antibiotics) have been claimed. Autoimmune disorders and malignancies have been found to be associated only in the adult form[51].

Direct immunofluorescence shows deposits of linear IgA at the dermo-epidermal junction in all patients. Other immunoreactants (IgG, IgM, C3) may also be present at the same site, mostly in patients with the adult form of LAD[52]. Immunoelectron microscopy reveals that the deposits of IgA are located mainly below the lamina densa but also within the lamina lucida. The serum frequently contains a low-titer IgA anti-basement membrane antibody[52]. A broad spectrum of target antigens has been detected by immunoblotting studies.

Differential diagnosis

Conditions requiring differentiation are dermatitis herpetiformis and bullous pemphigoid. In dermatitis herpetiformis, the IgA deposition is granular and within the dermal papillae, indirect immunofluorescence is always negative; a gluten-sensitive enteropathy is constantly present. Bullous pemphigoid may be clinically and histologically similar; however, both direct and indirect immunofluorescence studies show IgG deposition at the basement membrane zone.

Treatment

Dapsone or sulfapyridine have been used successfully in the treatment of LAD. The appropriate starting dose of dapsone is 2 to 3 mg/kg/day. Dapsone is then gradually reduced to a minimum maintenance dose of 0.5 to 1 mg/kg/day. Sulfapyridine is an alternative (60 to 200 mg/kg/day with a maximum of 3 g total per day). Sulfamethoxypyridazine (adult dose 250 mg to 1.5 g daily) is often better tolerated. Dapsone and sulfonamides can be combined. Corticosteroids are added at a dose of 0.2 to 1 mg/kg/day when dapsone and sulfonamides alone fail to give good results. A few patients need azathioprine or cyclosporin. Success has been reported with tetracyclines and nicotinamide[53].

CICATRICIAL PEMPHIGOID

Cicatricial pemphigoid (CP) is a rare, autoimmune, subepidermal bullous disease that primarily affects the mucous membranes. CP is distinguished from bullous pemphigoid by the extent of the mucosal involvement and by the resultant significant scarring that often results in permanent loss of function of the structures involved.

It is widely accepted today that cicatricial pemphigoid is a heterogeneous disease with a wide spectrum of clinical presentation and clinical course. In addition, it appears that the numerous clinical subsets correlate with a variety of anti-basement membrane zone (BMZ) autoantibodies that recognize different antigens within the complex of cell surface proteins and extracellular matrix proteins in the BMZ. Although no specific subset has been found to be more frequent in women, in general there is a reported increased incidence in women. The cause of this is not known.

Clinical presentation

CP is a relatively uncommon autoimmune disease that is usually first diagnosed in the 50 to 80-year-old age group. The estimated prevalence varies depending on the different reports being considered, ranging from 1 in 15 000 to 1 in 40 000, with an average of approximately 1 in 20 000 ophthalmic patients. The disease is probably more common than recognized since diagnosis, especially in the early stages, may be difficult. The distribution of the disease seems worldwide, and there is no racial or geographical predilection. In contrast, a female dominance does exist, with reported female-to-male ratio of 1.5 : 1 to 3 : 1[54]. In literature reviews of published series[55,56], 376 of 544 cases of CP occurred in women (a ratio of 2.2 : 1). Even though CP is an autoimmune disease of the elderly, a few cases of childhood involvement have been reported, the youngest being a 4-year-old girl with vulvar lesions only[55].

The most consistent clinical feature is oral involvement, with a reported incidence ranging from 80% to almost 100% in different published series[55,58–60]. Oral lesions are believed to develop after local trauma. The primary lesion is a blister that quickly ruptures to form an erosion or an ulcer with smooth borders and distinct margins. The oral lesions may cause discomfort, heal very slowly and

have a tendency for scar formation upon healing that may lead to a white reticulated pattern resembling lichen planus. Adhesions may form as well, often between the buccal mucosa and the alveolar process. The oral lesions frequently begin as desquamative gingivitis, characterized by erythema, edema and desquamation of the gingival mucosa. In the areas of active desquamation, the gingival surface appears raw and hemorrhagic. The desquamation is aggravated by trauma.

Ocular lesions[55,59,60] are also very common, reported in up to 60–80% of patients. In contrast to the clinical presentation in the oral mucosa, erosions in the conjuctiva are a rare finding. Often the earliest manifestation is chronic, intractable conjuctival irritation. The early chronic conjuctivitis results eventually in conjuctival shrinkage, symblepharon and less often ankyloblepharon. Contraction of the conjuctiva results in eyelid inversion (entropion) and eyelash inversion (trichiasis), leading to corneal injury and terminating in blindness.

The involvement of other mucosal surfaces is a rarer event[55,59,60]. The upper aerodigestive pathway has been reported to be involved in approximately one-third of patients. Mucosal erosions manifest in symptoms of nasal discharge and epistaxis, dysphagia and phagodynia and hoarseness and dysphonia. As the lesions progress, scarring ensues that may lead to life-threatening stenosis of these organs.

Blistering cutaneous lesions affect about a quarter of CP patients, the estimated incidence ranging from 10% to 40% in the different series reported[55,59,60]. The lesions may be scarring or non-scarring, generalized with a transient nature, or localized but recurrent and chronic. The localized eruption is typically of a scarring nature, and is referred to as the Brunsting–Perry type variant when mucosal involvement is absent. Localized lesions tend to occur on the head, neck and genitalia.

Several clinical subsets have been argued for. Most authors now agree that pure ocular CP is a distinct entity in terms of disease progression, prognosis and immunopathological findings. The disease process may begin asymmetrically and be static and slowly progressive, but it results in severe scarring and crippling[60]. Mobini and colleagues[58] argued that pure oral CP (OCP) is a distinct clinical subset. Overall it has a relatively benign course compared with that in patients with CP involving the oral cavity and other mucosae and the skin. Patients with minimal disease respond favorably to topical therapy alone, while more severe involvement is adequately controlled with dapsone only.

A recently described clinical variant is anti-laminin 5 CP, with mucocutaneous lesions that are generally resistant to treatment. All patients reported suffered oral lesions. The lesions are non-inflammatory and widespread, and bear an interesting resemblance to epiligrin junctional EB. It has been shown that a common major histocompatibility complex class 2 allele HLA-DQß1*0301 is present in all clinical variants studied, as well as in bullous pemphigoid[61]. Chan and co-workers[62] argued that this allele is a marker for the ocular subset in particular.

Gender-related epidemiology
of clinical subsets

In 1971 Shklar and McCarthy[63] reported data from 85 patients with CP. The oral mucosa was involved in all the patients, and 61% had only oral involvement. The female to male ratio was as high as 6 : 1. In their published series of 87 CP patients, Chan and colleagues[64] defined three clinical subsets, with more female involvement in all of them. The female to male ratio was highest (2.9 : 1) in the subset defined by oral mucosal disease, with or without other mucosal surfaces involved. The female to male ratio of pure ocular CP was 1.6 : 1. In Mobini and colleagues' group of 29 pure oral CP patients, 83% were women, the female to male ratio being 4.9 : 1[58].

It might follow that oral involvement is a marker for female predominance. If true, the reason is not known. Person and Rogers[65] noticed a similar phenomenon; when the disease was more extensive and there was cutaneous involvement, the female predominance was less striking. The authors argued that either afflicted males got a more extensive disease, or males with minor disease were less likely than women to be seen at a referral center.

The Brunsting and Perry variant is a unique form of CP characterized by chronic, recurrent, circumscribed vesiculobullous eruption at the head and neck region, leaving atrophic scars. Mucous membranes are usually unaffected. This may be the only clinical subset of CP that is more prevalent in men[66,67].

Genital involvement

Genital involvement has been observed in about 20% of cases. The frequency of genital disease in women is reported to be even higher, with vulval involvement of about 50% described in some series. In most patients, scarring ensued that resulted in structural architectural changes of the vulva[68,69]. The lesions of the labia majora and labia minora are usually vesicular and rupture, resulting in raw, denuded areas exposed to excessive moisture, rubbing and excoriation. There is pain on urination and with intercourse. Scarring may result in loss of the labia minora and agglutination of the clitoral hood. Adhesions may form because of fibrosis and may cause narrowing of the vaginal orifice and urethral stenosis. Sexual dysfunction has been reported[59,60].

Pathology

Histologic examination reveals a subepidermal cleft with a dermal mixed inflammatory infiltrate. Ultrastructurally, the split occurs in the lamina lucida. Mapping the BMZ molecular components in the blister suggests that the site of the separation is within the lower portion of the lamina lucida, at the lamina lucida–lamina densa interface.

Laboratory studies

Direct immunofluorescent studies are estimated to be positive in about 90% of patients with CP[55,60]. C3 is the most common immunoreactant found (66% of studied specimens), followed by IgG (57%), IgA (28%) and IgM (22%). These immunoreactants are deposited in a linear fashion and have been demonstrated in lesional, perilesional and normal mucous membrane biopsy specimens. In approximately 20–30% of CP patients circulating autoantibodies may be found, often in low titers. The estimated incidence of positive indirect immunofluorescent studies is presumed to be much higher when salt-split mucosal epithelium is used as a substrate. The facts that CP is a rare disease, that the demonstration of circulating autoantibodies is an infrequent event, and that when circulating autoantibodies are present they are found in low titers, have greatly limited indirect immuno-electronmicroscopy studies. Recently, two ultrastructural binding sites of circulating autoantibodies were identified[70]. One group of patients had circulating IgG autoantibodies that bound to the dermal side of salt-split skin and were localized ultrastructurally in the lowermost aspect of the lamina lucida at its interface with the lamina densa. In contrast, another group of patients had circulating IgG that bound to the epidermal side of a salt-split preparation, and ultrastructurally were localized to hemidesmosomes and the junction between hemidesmosomes and the plasma membranes of basal keratinocytes.

IgG subclass distribution in CP also defines two groups of patients. Some CP sera reacting with BP antigens showed an IgG4/IgG1 subclass restriction, with a predominance of IgG4 in 10 of 14 sera studied, and of IgG1 in 4 of 14 sera. Sera that contained IgG4 autoantibodies alone never fixed complement, whereas all complement fixing sera had IgG1 antibodies[71]. Non-complement fixing IgG4 were also found to predominate in anti-laminin 5 CP patients. Lesion induction in such patients is believed to result by their direct, specific pathogenicity, rather than via a nonspecific inflammatory response that is dependent on complement activation, mast cell degranulation and leukocyte accumulation.

Is cicatricial pemphigoid a distinct disease entity?

Cicatricial pemphigoid is regarded nowadays as a disease phenotype rather than a disease entity. This concept is based on the fact that patients presenting with clinical and routine immunopathological findings characteristic of CP have autoantibodies directed against BP Ags, laminin and other at present unidentified BM constituents. Reclassifying patients on the basis of antigens targeted by their sera offers a new view of the disease process and will allow future studies to focus on more homogenous patient groups. Patient management may also be influenced as a consequence of defining target antigens, since BP is more responsive to treatment.

Several subsets of patients have now been identified both clinically and by immunopathological and immunochemical criteria. Chan and colleagues[64] suggested three major subsets: (1) Pure ocular cicatricial pemphigoid (POCP) characterized by ocular involvement only, by the paucity of IgG and C3 *in vivo* deposits and high frequency of fibrin deposits along the BMZ, and by the virtual absence of detectable circulating autoantibodies. The sera of patients belonging to this subgroup show no activity against bullous pemphigoid antigens by immunoblotting and immunoprecipitation methods. (2) When both mucosal and cutaneous lesions are present, the frequency of circulating and tissue bound autoantibodies is similar to that of bullous pemphigoid. As in bullous pemphigoid, these circulating autoantibodies bind to the epidermal side of a salt-split skin specimen. Furthermore, these patients demonstrate similar serologic reactivity to BP Ags by immunoblotting and immunoprecipitation as compared with classical BP patients. This group may therefore be classified as anti-BP Ag mucosal pemphigoid. (3) The nosologic status of patients with mucosal disease without skin involvement probably includes several entities. With further understanding of the disease, some could probably be regrouped with anti-BP Ag mucosal pemphigoid should antibodies to BP antigens be detected. Others could eventually be regrouped with POCP owing to the presence of severe ocular disease (together with other mucosal surfaces involved) and the absence of serologic reactivity to BP Ags. As mentioned earlier, pure oral CP has recently been justifiably argued to be a distinct entity in terms of disease course and progression[58]. Lastly, patients with prominent mucosal lesions and minor skin lesions, and with anti-laminin 5 autoantibodies, will possibly define a fourth subset[72].

Anti BP Ag cicatricial pemphigoid

The bullous pemphigoid 180 kDa antigen is a transmembrane glycoprotein with an extracellular domain that harbors an immunodominant epitope recognized by both BP and HG autoantibodies. Balding and co-workers[73] established that the BP180 epidermal antigen is also a major antigenic target of CP autoantibodies: 78% of the CP sera studied recognized this antigen. The authors have shown that these autoantibodies react with at least two different sites of the extracellular domain of BP180: one located in the non-collagenous (NC) 16A domain – at or near the previously defined site recognized by BP and HG sera – and the other in the carboxy-terminal region of this protein. Some of the CP sera in this study failed to react with either site, yet reacted with the BP180 antigen by immunoblot, suggesting the existence of additional sites that remain to be identified. The newly identified reactivity of CP autoantibodies with the C-terminal region of BP180 may account for the lower lamina lucida–upper lamina densa localization of the immunoreactants at the BMZ. Independent data suggest that the BP180 ectodomain exists in an extended conformation that traverses the lamina lucida, such that the C-terminus possibly projects into the lamina densa. Fewer patients have antibodies to the bullous pemphigoid 230 kDa antigen[73].

Anti-laminin 5 cicatricial pemphigoid

Recently a group of patients with similar clinical and histological features but with distinct immunopathological features has been identified. This group has antibodies to laminin 5 (epiligrin). It has been estimated that about 5% of well-characterized CP patients have these autoantibodies. Laminin 5 is a keratinocyte-derived protein located in the BMZ composed of three disulfide bonded glycoprotein subunits of 175, 145, and 125 kDa[72,74].

In vitro, laminin 5 serves as the major ligand for integrin α3β1 in human keratinocyte plasma membranes and focal adhesions, and co-localizes with integrin α6β4 in hemidesmosome-like structures called stable anchoring complexes. In human skin, laminin 5 is found at the lamina lucida–lamina densa interface in epidermal BMZ, where it is believed to be associated with anchoring filaments and play an important role in keratinocyte adhesion. Experimental studies have demonstrated that the antigenic epitope is most often located in the alpha subunit of laminin 5, but other subunits were also found to be rarely targeted by autoantibodies[75].

Patients with anti-laminin 5 CP have dominant mucosal involvement, especially of the oral cavity. Skin lesions are minor, and ocular involvement may be absent. Direct immunofluorescence examination of perilesional skin discloses IgG and C3 deposited at the BMZ. Some have additional reactants. The circulating immunoreactants are deposited on the dermal side of salt-split skin. Immunogold electron microscopy has localized anti-laminin antibodies to the lamina densa–lamina lucida interface. Complement activation is not assumed to play a major role in the pathophysiology of this disease subset, as noncomplement fixing IgG4 autoantibodies predominate in these patients[76,77]. The subepidermal blisters probably develop via a direct effect of anti-laminin 5 IgG itself. This notion could explain the clinical finding of minimal inflammation in the mucosal lesions, the cell-poor infiltrate observed in light microscopy and the often-disappointing response to corticoid treatment.

Differential diagnosis

Desquamative gingivitis may represent other chronic conditions such as lichen planus, pemphigus, EBA, or acute conditions like contact dermatitis. When only oral lesions are present, or when the conjunctiva solely is involved, and the process is subtle, many conditions such as herpetic infection or allergic inflammation may be suspected. When erosive lesions that result in scarring are obvious, and pathologic examination reveals a subepidermal blistering disorder, immunofluorescence procedures on salt-split preparations and antigen identification may be needed to differentiate CP from

EBA, linear IgA bullous dermatitis and, rarely, complicated bullous pemphigoid[55,59,60].

The differential diagnosis in patients with vulvar scarring and labial fusion includes lichen sclerosus, CP, possibly pemphigus, toxic epidermal necrolysis (TEN) and erosive lichen planus[78]. In pemphigus, TEN and CP, vulvar hypopigmentation, scarring and fragility are associated with vaginal, oral and cutaneous erosions and blisters. Ocular involvement may be part of the clinical set-up of these diseases, but is not found in lichen planus or LSA, and is therefore often a feature of utmost diagnostic importance. Firth and colleagues[79] reported on two patients with recurrent scarring lesions of the vulva that persisted for many years and were eventually diagnosed by silent ocular signs. Several cases were reported with vulval signs suggestive of lichen sclerosus, in which the correct diagnosis of CP was unfortunately much delayed[80,81]. Clues to the correct clinical diagnosis were a lack of fine wrinkling and purpuric features in the lesional skin. Also, the hypopigmentation was diffuse rather than sharply demarcated and careful examination revealed vaginal involvement that does not occur in LSA.

A biopsy is often necessary to confirm the diagnosis, and should be taken from the edge of a blister or an erosion, as a biopsy taken at the site of scar tissue or from the center of an erosion will often yield non-specific results.

Treatment

There is no generally accepted treatment for CP. It is also a matter of debate whether asymptomatic patients require treatment at all, because even though the natural history of untreated CP is not known, the condition may be self-limiting.

Several treatment regimens have been proposed. Patients with limited disease may be treated with topical steroids, but those with more extensive disease may warrant systemic treatment. Most authors agree that the first treatment trial should be dapsone, beginning with a dose of 25 mg/day and gradually increasing up to 100–150 mg/day. When the response is inadequate, systemic corticosteroids (1 mg/kg/day) preferably combined with immunosuppressive agents like azathioprine (1–2 mg/kg/day) or cyclophosphamide (0.5–2 mg/kg/day) are indicated[60,62].

Some authors have also reported encouraging results with topical cyclosporine for oral CP, and high-dose pulse intravenous cyclophosphamide or high-dose intravenous immunoglobulin infusion for grave, refractory disease[82–84]. Recently, tetracycline alone or combined with nicotinamide were also reported to be effective in selected patients. A satisfactory response to topical application of tetracycline was even reported[85]. Treatment of vulval involvement consists of the local application of potent topical corticosteroids and treatment of secondary infection with antibiotics if necessary. Systemic therapy as detailed above is determined by the extent of the disease and the scarring nature.

Surgical intervention should not be attempted in active disease. Scarring recurred in several reported cases of adhesiolysis, but a successful vaginoplasty for vaginal stenosis has also been reported. The conclusion may well be that selected patients can benefit from well-chosen procedures[73].

EPIDERMOLYSIS BULLOSA ACQUISITA

Epidermolysis bullosa acquisita (EBA) is a chronic, autoimmune, subepidermal blistering disease affecting the skin and mucous membranes, characterized by tissue-bound and circulating antibodies directed against the anchoring fibril type 7 collagen (C7). EBA is a clinicopathologic heterogeneous entity comprised of inflammatory and noninflammatory variants. As far as we know at present, there is no increased frequency in women, and disease phenotype seems to be the same for both sexes. However, since the disease is relatively rare and only the classical phenotype of EBA was recognized in the era when advanced diagnostic tools were not available, the true gender incidence is not known. This issue is even more emphasized in light of the increasing evidence of an association between EBA and bullous systemic lupus erythematosus (BSLE), both diseases of C7 autoimmunity sharing the same genetic susceptibility. BSLE is a disease of young women, and does not display the clinical features of classical EBA. This issue will be further discussed below.

Clinical presentation

EBA is most commonly manifested in the 4th and 5th decades, but has been reported from early childhood to late adult life[86–88]. Although the true incidence of EBA is not known, it appears to be less common than bullous pemphigoid (BP) but more common than cicatricial pemphigoid, pemphigoid gestationis, or linear IgA bullous dermatosis[87].

The reason that the full extent of the epidemiological features of EBA has not been clearly defined is the paucity of descriptions of the disease in the new era of characterization of the distinctive immunologic basis of EBA, and the ability of the disease to mimic other subepidermal bullous disorders and therefore to be underdiagnosed. It has been estimated that 5–15% of patients with circulating anti-basement membrane zone (BMZ) autoantibodies and referred to medical centers with a diagnosis of BP, actually have EBA[86].

An association between the expression of HLA DR2, more specifically DRB1*1501 (one of the DR2-split subtypes), with autoantibodies to C7 has been reported among white and black people with EBA[86].

The most commonly encountered EBA patient displays a somewhat polymorphic eruption: bullae on both erythematous and non-erythematous skin, atrophic scars and milia formation, some degree of mucosal disease and gradual loss of fingernails and hair. This disease phenotype is actually reminiscent of hereditary dystrophic epidermolysis bullosa, and therefore, before modern diagnostic tools were available, disease criteria were based on late onset and negative family history. Employing advanced immunopathological methods, patients diagnosed as suffering from other bullous disorders were actually found to manifest the 'mimicking' ability of EBA, a disease now known to be surprisingly heterogeneous.

The heterogeneity of EBA is reflected by the existence of several distinct clinical patterns: (1) the classical phenotype, distinguished by skin fragility and trauma-induced non-inflammatory blisters mainly on extensor surfaces that heal with scarring and milia. Scarring alopecia and nail dystrophy are present in some cases; (2) the bullous pemphigoid phenotype, presenting with a generalized eruption with flexural prominence of inflammatory lesions (erythematous macules, papules, plaques and blisters on erythematous base). Skin fragility is absent, and healing is usually without scarring. Mucous membranes are often involved. This phenotype is probably the most common presentation of EBA. It is noteworthy that patients may often present with features of both classic EBA and bullous pemphigoid EBA; and (3) the cicatricial pemphigoid phenotype, featuring a severe scarring mucosal disease resulting in blindness or aerodigestive stenosis, with minimal, if any, skin lesions, confined to the head, neck and genitalia[86–88].

Generally speaking, mucosal lesions are found in almost half the patients with EBA. Vulvar lesions may be severe in the cicatricial phenotype, followed by scarring that may result in structural architectural changes of the vulva. In other phenotypes, vulvar involvement may manifest as erosions that heal with or without scars or atrophy.

Disease duration varies from less than a year to more than 20 years, but the most common biologic behavior is that of a chronic disease process that usually persists for several years and impairs the patient's ability to perform tasks involving friction with the environment[86–88].

EBA may accompany diseases such as amyloidosis, ulcerative colitis, Crohn's disease, diabetes mellitus, lung carcinoma and multiple myeloma. Some claim that almost 30% of EBA cases are associated with an inflammatory bowel disease[89].

Drug-induced EBA-like eruptions have been attributed to furosemide, sulfonamides, D-penicillamine, and sulfamethoxypyridazine; however, in most of these reports definite disease diagnosis was lacking.

The female angle in EBA

Autoimmune diseases have repeatedly been conceived of as the inevitable outcome of interacting genetic and environmental factors. Environmental factors may be exogenic, like drugs, or endogenic, like cancer, systemic illness, or hormones. Sex hormones have been proposed as a causative factor for the female preponderance in many autoimmune diseases, and an increased estrogen-to-testosterone ratio is considered a risk factor in systemic lupus erythematosus (SLE). Conversely, female sex hormones have also been considered to have a suppressing effect on the immune system, as is the case in pregnancy. Thus, the immunomodulating effect of female sex hormones is manifested in both hyper- and hypo-immune states, and it is not surprising therefore that hormonal therapy and pregnancy have been reported to either exacerbate or improve autoimmune diseases.

There are only a few observations relating to the effects of female sex hormones on EBA. Kubo and colleagues[90] described an interesting case of a persuasive correlation between female hormones and EBA exacerbations. Their patient had an onset of EBA following systemic estrogen and progesterone treatment, an exacerbation in her first month of gestation necessitating abortion that was rewarded by improvement, and another outburst during the luteal phase of her menstrual cycle. Kero and co-workers[91] reported a 38-year-old woman who developed EBA in connection with her third pregnancy, with remission at menopause.

Bullous SLE (BSLE) is a relapsing blistering eruption that occurs in young adults with established SLE, and is more frequent in blacks and in women. There appears to be an interesting association between BSLE and EBA[86,87]. Both are diseases of autoimmunity to C7. The same genes were found to predispose to C7 autoimmunity in both diseases.

BSLE and EBA share so many features that it has often been argued whether BSLE is the manifestation of EBA in SLE patients, or part of the autoantibody repertoire of the autoimmune phenomena of SLE. A convincing report of C7 autoantibodies in an SLE patient without a blistering eruption argues strongly for the latter view. Yet some distinguishing features between the two diseases do exist. Not all BSLE patients have autoantibodies to C7. Patients with BSLE respond well to dapsone, whereas EBA patients generally do not. The histology of BSLE is quite distinctive, with such severe dermal inflammation as to create neutrophilic papillary microabscesses. The immunoglobulin deposits are not necessarily linear as in EBA, but may have a granular, thready or fibrillar pattern. Last but not least, BSLE is a disease of young adults in their 2nd or 3rd decade unlike the midlife-onset of EBA, and is not highlighted clinically by skin fragility, atrophic scars and milia formation.

But the most intriguing reports are those of patients with EBA who subsequently developed SLE, patients with SLE followed by EBA and concurrent SLE and EBA. Mounting evidence suggests that it may be prudent to closely follow patients with EBA for the development of SLE: Gammon and Briggaman[92] reported that of 60 patients they have seen with autoimmunity to C7, approximately 30% had, once had, or developed SLE.

Pathology

Lesional skin displays dermal–epidermal separation. In the classical phenotype, a sparse dermal infiltrate of mononuclear cells may be found. In the bullous pemphigoid phenotype, the infiltrate may be moderate or dense, of mononuclear cells and granulocytes, with the predominant granulocyte being the neutrophil rather than the eosinophil typical of BP. The electron microscope localizes the level of separation in the upper dermis, just beneath the lamina densa.

Laboratory studies

All EBA patients exhibit linear immunoglobulin deposits along the dermal–epidermal junction in perilesional skin. The tissue-bound anti-basement membrane IgG autoantibodies may be accompanied by complement components, and less often by antibodies of other classes. Circulating IgG autoantibodies can be found in less than half the patients.

The ultrastructural location of the autoantibodies may be determined in two ways: first by direct and indirect immunofluorescence analysis on the patient's skin or epithelial substrates, respectively, pretreated in 0.1 M sodium chloride solution that cleaves the BMZ at the lamina lucida level. EBA autoantibodies bind to the dermal side (bottom of the split) of such preparations[93]; and second by identifying the deposition level of the immuno-reactants by immuno-electron microscopy. The EBA autoantibodies are deposited either in the upper dermis just below the lamina densa, or on and just below the lamina densa.

The EBA antigen collagen 7 is composed of three identical alpha chains, each consisting of an amino-terminal 145-kDa noncollagenous (NC1) domain and a 145-kDa carboxyl-terminal collagenous domain. These molecules aggregate to form the anchoring fibrils that 'anchor' the lamina densa to the dermis. The NC1 domain is the region that appears to link the anchoring fibrils to the lamina densa and the dermis by interacting with matrix proteins such as type IV collagen. It has recently been shown[94] that EBA autoantibodies recognize epitopes in a fibronectin-like region of the noncollagenous (NC1) domain of C7.

The autoantibodies cause epidermal–dermal separation by at least two non-exclusive mechanisms. Antibody binding to the epitopes could disrupt the secondary structure of the fibronectin-like region, which in turn could lead to altered matrix-binding properties, or to the inability of such distorted C7 molecules to aggregate appropriately into anchoring fibrils. The other mechanism may be mediated by complement-dependent inflammation. The two mechanisms may account for the various clinico-pathologic manifestations of EBA: noninflammatory vs. inflammatory phenotypes.

Differential diagnosis

The potential for EBA to mimic other sub-epidermal blistering disorders calls for diagnostic aids. EBA can be differentiated from all bullous pemphigoid cases and from the majority of CP patients by indirect immunofluorescence on salt-split skin and by immuno-electron microscopy studies. Differential diagnosis of EBA from other diseases of the dermal side of split skin, like some of the linear IgA bullous dermatoses, a few CP cases and BSLE, is successfully achieved by antigen identification or by the occurrence of SLE criteria[86,88].

Treatment

Response to treatment is unpredictable and often disappointing. Too often patients are refractory to every treatment modality available. Patients may respond to corticosteroids alone, or in combination with either azathioprine or cyclophosphamide. Cyclosporin in doses of 3–5 mg/kg/day might be effective in some patients. Because the onset of the disease is sometimes explosive, but activity later levels off and the disease becomes milder, pulse corticosteroid therapy might be beneficial.

Interestingly, the combined use of dapsone and prednisone is considered the most effective treatment in pediatric EBA[95]. Dapsone has also been tried successfully in BSLE. In contrast, dapsone treatment in adult EBA has rarely resulted in disease control, and the few patients who did respond typically developed very inflammatory lesions that were microscopically rich with neutrophilic infiltrate. Colchicine was also reported effective in a selected patient group[96]. Recently extracorporeal photochemotherapy was reported to be a worthwhile therapeutic option in patients with refractory disease[97]. Other treatments anecdotally reported to suppress unresponsive EBA outbreaks include intravenous immunoglobulin[98] and mesalazine in a patient concomitantly suffering from inflammatory bowel disease[99].

REFERENCES

1. Ruocco V, Pisani M. Induced pemphigus. *Arch Dermatol Res* 1982;274:123–40
2. Hans-Filho G, dos Santos V, Katayama JH, *et al*. An active focus of high prevalence of fogo selvagem on an Amerindian reservation in Brasil. *J Invest Dermatol* 1996;107:68–75
3. Bastuji-Garin S, Souissi R, Blum L, *et al*. Comparative epidemiology of pemphigus in Tunisia and France: unusual incidence of pemphigus foliaceus in young Tunisian women. *J Invest Dermatol* 1995;104:302–5
4. Anhalt GJ, Kim SC, Stanley JR, *et al*. Paraneoplastic pemphigus. *N Engl J Med* 1990;323:1729–35
5. Brenner S, Wolf R, Ruocco V. Drug-induced pemphigus. I. A survey. *Clin Dermatol* 1993;11:501–5
6. Hogan P. Pemphigus vulgaris following a cutaneous thermal burn. *Int J Dermatol* 1992;31:46–9
7. Ruocco V, Wolf R, Ruocco E, Baroni A. Viruses in pemphigus: a casual or causal relationship? *Int J Dermatol* 1996;35:782–4
8. Ruocco V, Rossi A, Astarita C, *et al*. A congenital acantholytic bullous eruption in the newborn infant of a pemphigous mother. *It Gen Rev Dermatol* 1975;12:169–74
9. Chowdhury MMV, Natarajan S. Neonatal pemphigus vulgaris associated with mild oral pemphigus vulgaris in the mother during pregnancy. *Br J Dermatol* 1998;139:500–3

10. Honeyman JF, Eguiguren G, Pinto A, *et al.* Bullous dermatoses of pregnancy. *Arch Dermatol* 1981;117: 264–7

11. Lo Schiavo A, D'Avino M. Progesterone, insospettato induttore di pemfigo. *G Ital Dermatol Venereol* 1999;134:331–4

12. Brenner S, Ruocco V, Wolf R, *et al.* Pemphigus and dietary factors. *In vitro* acantholysis by allyl compounds of the genus *Allium. Dermatology* 1995; 190:197–202

13. Bastuji-Garin S, Turki H, Mokhtar I, *et al.* Facteurs de risque des pemphigus tunisiens: une étude castémoins. *Ann Dermatol Venereol* 1997;124(suppl 1):S15

14. Kaplan RP, Detwiler SP, Saperstein HW. Physically induced pemphigus after cosmetic procedures. *Int J Dermatol* 1993;32:100–3

15. Jacyk WK, Simson IW. Pemphigus erythematosus resembling multiple seborrheic keratoses. *Arch Dermatol* 1990;126:543–4

16. Muramatsu T, Iida T, Ko T, Shirai T. Pemphigus vulgaris exacerbated by exposure to sunlight. *J Dermatol* 1996;23:559–63

17. Fryer EJ, Lebwohl M. Pemphigus vulgaris after initiation of psoralen and UVA therapy for psoriasis. *J Am Acad Dermatol* 1994;30:651–3

18. Brenner S, Bar-Nathan EA. Pemphigus vulgaris triggered by emotional stress. *J Am Acad Dermatol* 1984;11:524–5

19. Tamir A, Ophir J, Brenner S. Pemphigus vulgaris triggered by emotional stress. *Dermatology* 1994; 189:210

20. Cremniter D, Baudin M, Roujeau JC, Prost C. Stressful life events as potential triggers of pemphigus. *Arch Dermatol* 1998;134:1486–7

21. Ruocco V, Brenner S, Lombardi ML. A case of diet-related pemphigus. *Dermatology* 1996;192:373–4

22. Chorzelski TP, Hashimoto T, Jablonska S, *et al.* Can pemphigus be induced by nutritional factors? *Eur J Dermatol* 1996;6:284–6

23. Tur E, Brenner S. Diet and pemphigus. In pursuit of exogenous factors in pemphigus and fogo selvagem. *Arch Dermatol* 1998;134:1406–10

24. Jiao D, Bystryn JC. Relation between antibodies to BP180 and gender in bullous pemphigoid. *J Am Acad Dermatol* 1999;41:269–70

25. Jung M, Kippes W, Messer G, *et al.* Increased risk of bullous pemphigoid in male and very old patients: a population-based study on incidence. *J Am Acad Dermatol* 1999;41:266–8

26. Banfield CC, Wojnarowska F, Allen J, *et al.* The association of HLA-DQ7 with bullous pemphigoid is restricted to men. *Br J Dermatol* 1998;138: 1085–90

27. Anhalt GJ. Pemphigoid. Bullous and cicatricial. *Dermatol Clin* 1990;8:701–16

28. Ruocco V, Sacerdoti G. Pemphigus and bullous pemphigoid due to drugs. *Int J Dermatol* 1991;30:307–12

29. Korman NJ. Bullous pemphigoid. *Dermatol Clin* 1993;11:483–98

30. Ahmed AR, Hameed A. Bullous pemphigoid and dermatitis herpetiformis. *Clin Dermatol* 1993;11: 47–52

31. Balato N, Ayala F, Patruno C, *et al.* Bullous pemphigoid induced by a thermal burn. *Int J Dermatol* 1994;33:55–6

32. Ogawa H, Sakuma M, Morioka S, *et al.* The incidence of internal malignancies in bullous pemphigoid in Japan. *J Dermatol Sci* 1995;9:136–40

33. De Castro P, Jorizzo JL, Rajaram S, *et al.* Localized vulvar pemphigoid in a child. *Pediatr Dermatol* 1985; 2:302–7

34. Guenther LC, Shum D. Localized childhood vulvar pemphigoid. *J Am Acad Dermatol* 1990;22:762–4

35. Kirtschig G, Wojnarowska F, Marsden RA, *et al.* Acquired bullous disease of childhood: re-evaluation of diagnosis by indirect immunofluorescence examination on 1 M NaCl split skin and immunoblotting. *Br J Dermatol* 1994;130:610–16

36. Haustein UF. Localized nonscarring bullous pemphigoid of the vagina. *Dermatologica* 1988;176:200–1

37. Liu Z, Giudice GJ, Swartz SJ, *et al.* The role of complement in experimental bullous pemphigoid. *J Clin Invest* 1995;95:1539–44

38. Fine JD. Immunobullous diseases. In Sams WMJ, Lynch PJ, eds. *Principles and Practice of Dermatology* 2nd edition. New York: Churchill Livingstone, 1996:455–73

39. Smith J, Taylor T, Zone J. The site of the blister formation in dermatitis herpetiformis is within the lamina lucida. *J Am Acad Dermatol* 1992;27:209–13

40. Hall RP, Waldbauer GV. Characterization of the mucosal immune response to dietary antigens in patients with dermatitis herpetiformis. *J Invest Dermatol* 1988;90:658–63

41. Szabo E, Husz S, Varkonyi T, *et al.* Dermatitis herpetiformis: relation between circulating immune complexes, small-intestinal mucosal status, and immunohistopathological findings. *Arch Dermatol Res* 1987;279:315–20

42. Jablonska S, Chorzelski TP. Dermatose a IgA lineare. *Ann Dermatol Venereol* 1979;106:651–5

43. Edwards S, Wojnarowska F. Chronic bullous disease of childhood in three patients of Polynesian extraction. *Clin Exp Dermatol* 1990;15:367–9

44. Aboobaker J, Wojnarowska F, Bhogal B, Black M. Chronic bullous disease of childhood. Clinical and immunological features seen in African patients. *Clin Exp Dermatol* 1991;16:160–4

45. Wojnarowska F, Marsden R, Bhogal B, Black M. Childhood cicatricial pemphigoid with linear IgA deposits. *Clin Exp Dermatol* 1984;9:407–15

46. Webster G, Raber I, Penne R, *et al.* Cicatrizing conjunctivitis as a predominant manifestation of linear IgA bullous dermatosis. *J Am Acad Dermatol* 1994;30: 355–7

47. Jacobson M, Krumholz B, Franks A. Desquamative inflammatory vaginitis. A case report. *J Reprod Med* 1989;34:647–50

48. Collier P, Kelley SE, Wojnarowska F. Linear IgA disease and pregnancy. *J Am Acad Dermatol* 1994;30: 407–12

49. Raynes J. Variations in the relative proportions of microheterogeneous forms of plasma glycoproteins in pregnancy and disease. *Biomed Pharmacother* 1982;36:77–86

50. Collier PM, Wojnarowska F. MHC class I and II antigens in linear IgA dermatosis. *J Invest Dermatol* 1992;98:526 (abstract)

51. Combemale P, Prost C. Maladie a IgA lineaire de l'adulte. Revue de la littérature. *Ann Dermatol Venereol* 1987;114:1605–15

52. Wojnarowska F, Marsden R, Bhogal B, Black M. Chronic bullous disease of childhood, childhood cicatricial pemphigoid and linear IgA disease of adult, a comparative study demonstrating clinical and immunopathological overlap. *J Am Acad Dermatol* 1988;19:792–805

53. Peoples D, Fivenson D. Linear IgA bullous dermatosis: successful treatment with tetracycline and nicotinamide. *J Am Acad Dermatol* 1992;26:498–9

54. Nguyen QD, Foster CS. Cicatricial pemphigoid: diagnosis and treatment. *Int Ophthalmol Clin* 1966; 36:41–60

55. Vincent SD, Lilly GE, Baker KA. Clinical, historic, and therapeutic features of cicatricial pemphigoid. A literature review and open therapeutic trial with corticosteroids. *Oral Surg Oral Med Oral Pathol* 1993; 76:453–9

56. Laskaris G, Triantafyllou A, Economopoulou P. Gingival manifestations of childhood cicatricial pemphigoid. *Oral Surg Oral Med Oral Pathol* 1988;66:349–52

57. Rogers M, Painter D. Cicatricial pemphigoid in a four-year-old child: a case report. *Aust J Dermatol* 1981;22:21–3

58. Mobini N, Nagarwalla N, Ahmed AE. Oral pemphigoid. Subset of cicatricial pemphigoid? *Oral Surg Oral Med Oral Pathol* 1998;85:37–43

59. Mutasim DF, Pelc NJ, Anhalt GJ. Cicatricial pemphigoid. *Dermatol Clin* 1993;11:499–510

60. Ahmed AR, Kurgis BS, Rogers RS. Cicatricial pemphigoid. *J Am Acad Dermatol* 1991;24:987–1001

61. Delgado JC, Turbay D, Yunis EJ, *et al*. A major histocompatibility complex class 2 allele HLA-DQβ1*0301 is present in clinical variants of pemphigoid. *Proc Natl Acad Sci USA* 1996;93: 8569–71

62. Chan LS, Hammerberg C, Cooper KD. Significantly increased occurrence of HLA-DQβ1*0301 allele in patients with ocular cicatricial pemphigoid. *J Invest Dermatol* 1997;108:129–32

63. Shklar G, McCarthy PL. Oral lesions of mucous membrane pemphigoid. *Arch Otolaryngol* 1971;93: 354–64

64. Chan LS, Yancey KB, Hammerberg C, *et al*. Immune mediated subepithelial blistering diseases of mucous membranes. Pure ocular cicatricial pemphigoid is a unique clinical and immuno-pathological entity distinct from bullous pemphigoid and other subsets identified by antigenic specificity of autoantibodies. *Arch Dermatol* 1993;129:448–55

65. Person JR, Rogers RS. Bullous and cicatricial pemphigoid. Clinical, histopathologic, and immunopathologic correlations. *Mayo Clin Proc* 1977;52: 54–66

66. Kurzhals G, Stolz W, Maciejewski W, *et al*. Localized cicatricial pemphigoid of the Brunsting–Perry type with transition into disseminated cicatricial pemphigoid. *Arch Dermatol* 1995;131:580–5

67. Joly P, Ruto F, Thomine E, *et al*. Brunsting–Perry cicatricial bullous pemphigoid: a clinical variant of localized acquired epidermolysis bullosa? *J Am Acad Dermatol* 1993;28:89–92

68. Marren P, Wojnarowska F, Venning V, *et al*. Vulvar involvement in autoimmune bullous diseases. *J Reprod Med* 1993;38:101–7

69. Venning VA, Firth PA, Bron AJ, *et al*. Mucosal involvement in bullous and cicatricial pemphigoid. *Br J Dermatol* 1987;118:7–15

70. Shimizu H, Masunaga T, Ishiko A, *et al*. Autoantibodies from patients with cicatricial pemphigoid target different sites in epidermal basement membrane. *J Invest Dermatol* 1995;104:370–3

71. Bernard P, Prost C, Aucouturier P, *et al*. The subclass distribution of IgG autoantibodies in cicatricial pemphigoid and epidermolysis bullosa acquisita. *J Invest Dermatol* 1991;97:259–63

72. Domolge-Hultsch N, Gammon WR, Briggaman RA, *et al*. Epiligrin, the major human keratinocyte integrin ligand, is a target in both an acquired autoimmune and an inherited subepidermal blistering skin disease. *J Clin Invest* 1992;90:1628–33

73. Balding SD, Prost C, Diaz LA, *et al*. Cicatricial pemphigoid autoantibodies react with multiple sites on the BP180 extracellular domain. *J Invest Dermatol* 1996;106:141–6

74. Allbritton JI, Nousari HC, Anhalt GJ. Anti-epiligrin (laminin 5) cicatricial pemphigoid. *Br J Dermatol* 1997;137:992–6

75. Lazarova Z, Hsu R, Yee C, Yancey KB. Antiepiligrin cicatricial pemphigoid represents an autoimmune response to subunits present in laminin 5 (α3β3γ2). *Br J Dermatol* 1998;139:791–7

76. Hsu R, Lazarova Z, Yee C, *et al*. Noncomplement fixing IgG4 autoantibodies predominate in patients with anti-epiligrin cicatricial pemphigoid. *J Invest Dermatol* 1997;109:557–61

77. Lazarova Z, Yee C, Darling T, *et al*. Passive transfer of anti-laminin 5 antibodies induces subepidermal blisters in neonatal mice. *J Clin Invest* 1996;98:1509–18

78. Ridley CM. General dermatological conditions and dermatoses of the vulva. In *The Vulva*. Edinburgh: Churchill Livingstone, 1988:138–211

79. Firth P, Charnock M, Wojnarowska F. Cicatricial pemphigoid diagnosed from ocular features in

recurrent severe vulval scarring. Two case reports. *Br J Obstet Gynaecol* 1991;98:482–4

80. Edwards L, Hays S. Vulvar cicatricial pemphigoid as a lichen sclerosus imitator. A case report. *J Reprod Med* 1992;37:561–4

81. Marren P, Walkden V, Mallon E, *et al*. Vulval cicatricial pemphigoid may mimic lichen sclerosus. *Br J Dermatol* 1996;134:522–4

82. Azana JM, Misa RF, Boixeda JP, *et al*. Topical cyclosporine for cicatricial pemphigoid. *J Am Acad Dermatol* 1993;28:134–5

83. Urcelay ML, McQueen A, Douglas WS. Cicatricial pemphigoid treated with intravenous immunoglobulin. *Br J Dermatol* 1997;137:477–8

84. Pandya AG, Warren KJ. Cicatricial pemphigoid successfully treated with pulse intravenous cyclophosphamide. *Arch Dermatol* 1997;133:245–7

85. Bauco van der Wal V, Jonkman MF. Topical tetracycline in cicatricial pemphigoid. *J Am Acad Dermatol* 1997;36:492–3

86. Gammon WR, Briggaman RA. Epidermolysis bullosa acquisita and bullous systemic lupus erythematosus. Diseases of autoimmunity to type 7 collagen. *Dermatol Clin* 1993;11:535–47

87. Gammon WR. Epidermolysis bullosa acquisita: a disease of autoimmunity to type 7 collagen. *J Autoimmunity* 1991;4:59–71

88. Woodely DT, Briggaman RA, Gammon WR. Acquired epidermolysis bullosa. A bullous disease associated with autoimmunity to type 7 (anchoring fibril) collagen. *Dermatol Clin* 1990;8:717–26

89. Raab B, Fretzin DF, Bronson DM, *et al*. Epidermolysis bullosa acquisita and inflammatory bowel disease. *JAMA* 1983;250:1746–8

90. Kubo A, Hashimoto K, Inoue C, *et al*. Epidermolysis bullosa acquisita exacerbated by systemic estrogen and progesterone treatment and pregnancy. *J Am Acad Dermatol* 1997;36:792–4

91. Kero M, Niemi K-M, Kanerva L. Pregnancy as a trigger of epidermolysis bullosa acquisita. *Acta Derm Venereol (Stockh)* 1983;63:353–6

92. Gammon WR, Briggaman RA. Bullous SLE: a phenotypically distinctive but immunologically heterogeneous bullous disorder. *J Invest Dermatol* 1993; 100:28S–34S

93. Medenica-Mojsilovic L, Fenske NA, Espinoza CG. Epidermolysis bullosa acquisita. Direct immunofluorescence and ultrastructural studies. *Am J Dermatol* 1987;9:324–33

94. Gammon WR, Murrell DF, Jenison MW, *et al*. Autoantibodies to type VII collagen recognize epitopes in a fibronectin-like region of the noncollagenous (NC1) domain. *J Invest Dermatol* 1993; 100:618–22

95. Callot-Mellot C, Bodemer C, Caux F, *et al*. Epidermolysis bullosa acquisita in childhood. *Arch Dermatol* 1997;133:1122–6

96. Cunningham BB, Kirchmann TTT, Woodely D. Colchicine for epidermolysis bullosa acquisita. *J Am Acad Dermatol* 1996;34:781–4

97. Gordon KB, Chan LS, Woodely DT. Treatment of refractory epidermolysis bullosa acquisita with extracorporeal photochemotherapy. *Br J Dermatol* 1997;136:415–20

98. Mohr C, Sunderkotter C, Hildebrand A, *et al*. Successful treatment of epidermolysis bullosa acquisita using intravenous immunoglobulins. *Br J Dermatol* 1995;132:824–6

99. Robinowitz BN, Towery DS, Meyers SW, *et al*. Successful treatment of epidermolysis bullosa acquisita with mesalazine. *Br J Dermatol* 1997;137: 154–5

Connective tissue diseases 18

Stefania Jablonska and Maria Blaszczyk

INTRODUCTION

Connective tissue diseases (CTD) occur preferentially in women, presumably owing to immunogenetics, sex hormones and pregnancies. The recent findings on the fetal–maternal cell transfer and mother–child relationship as a risk factor for autoimmune disease, particularly for systemic scleroderma (SSc), might at least partly explain the high prevalence of these diseases in women. Although the risk factors for women in various CTD differ considerably, in all of them women are more at risk than men.

SYSTEMIC LUPUS ERYTHEMATOSUS

The incidence of systemic lupus erythematosus (SLE) in women is much higher than in men[1]: the mean ratio is reported by several authors as 9 : 1, and in our series it was about 7 : 1 for adults (Table 1). The serological markers, present in 98% of patients, in general did not differ between women and men. The most common antibody was Ro/SS-A/ and La/SS-B/, found in 345 of 600 women and in 43 of 85 men; the most frequent other antibodies were dsDNA, U1RNP, Sm, and ribosomal antibodies. Several antibodies often coexisted both in women and in men.

The predominance of SLE in women and tendency to flare during pregnancy point to the role of sex hormones. Similarly, female mice developed SLE-like changes more frequently than males, and the disease could be ameliorated by androgens[2]. Dehydroepiandrosterone (DHEA) was reported to be beneficial for a mild to moderate SLE in females[3]. Testosterone was found to suppress *in vitro* anti-DNA antibody production in peripheral blood mononuclear cells from patients with SLE, both by inhibiting B cell hyperactivity and down-regulating IL-6 production in monocytes[4]. In contrast, estradiol stimulated production of SS-A/Ro protein[5] and enhanced response to UV-B[6]. It also increased levels of anti-dsDNA antibodies and circulating immune complexes[7]. The role of sex hormones could explain the increased incidence of SLE after puberty[8], and a preferential occurrence of SLE in women of childbearing age. The severity and course of the disease do not differ significantly between the genders[9], but in a recent study men were reported to have a poorer prognosis[10], possibly because of a frequent functional hypogonadism[11].

SLE and pregnancy

SLE is frequently exacerbated during pregnancy with possible hypertension, pre-eclampsia and increased markers of disease activity. Pregnancy is therefore regarded as a risk factor[12], although this is denied by some authors[13] who stress that exacerbations occur only in cases not controlled by therapy, especially by the active disease with renal or central nervous system involvement. A risk for fetal loss, prematurity, neonatal lupus (NLE) and perinatal mortality is increased by the presence in mothers of anticardiolipins, lupus anticoagulant and/or anti-Ro/SS-A/ antibodies.

SLE and contraceptives

The prevailing view is that oral contraceptives should be avoided in women with active disease, especially in patients with renal involvement and high-titer antiphospholipid antibodies because of the risk of flare and thrombosis[14]. Although the use of combined oral contraceptives on the activity of SLE might be deleterious, the contraceptives of newer generations are believed not to be contraindicated in patients with inactive and stable disease, in carefully selected and controlled cases[7]. Caution is needed since frequent exposure to ovulation induction agents is followed by a significant rise in levels of gonadotropins and estradiol, and may lead to development of SLE in genetically predisposed women[15].

SUBACUTE CUTANEOUS LUPUS ERYTHEMATOSUS (SCLE)

This variety of cutaneous LE differs from SLE by erythematous annular and/or papulosquamous skin lesions (Figure 1a, b), significantly less frequent kidney involvement, serositis and arthritis, rare

Table 1   Immunological markers in systemic lupus erythematosus: females vs. males

Type of ANA	Adults		Children	
	Female	Male	Female	Male
Ro/La (total 401)				
alone	272	36	5	4
with other Ab	73	7	3	1
dsDNA (total 227)				
alone	83	14	9	5
with other Ab	103	8	3	2
Sm (total 55)				
alone	7	2	—	—
with other Ab	35	6	3	2
U1RNP (total 129)				
alone	60	4	3	—
with other Ab	53	6	2	1
No markers (total 73)	61	9	2	1

The total number of patients in the study was 738, of whom 723 (98%) were ANA positive, with a female : male ratio of ~6 : 1; 685 of the ANA positive were adults, with a female : male ratio of ~7 : 1, and 38 were children with a female : male ratio of ~3 : 1. ANA, antinuclear antibodies; Ab, antibody

presence of antibodies characteristic of SLE (ds-DNA, U1-RNP, Sm), and association with Ro/SS-A and/or La/SS-B/ antibodies in over 70% of patients[16–18]. In our series of 79 patients the female: male ratio was about 4 : 1, i.e. prevalence in women was significantly lower than for SLE[18].

In our most recent study of a cohort of 112 SCLE patients (88 women and 24 men), the association with Ro/La antibodies was found in 82.1% patients (data not published).

The course of SCLE is usually milder and the prognosis better than that for SLE. In our series, 96% of patients were controlled with chloroquine combined with small doses of corticosteroids, whereas over 65% of SLE patients required higher doses of corticosteroids, and 26% were controlled only by combined therapy with corticosteroids and immunosuppressive drugs[18].

NEONATAL LUPUS ERYTHEMATOSUS (NLE)

The most important problem for women with SCLE is a possible transplacental transfer of Ro/La antibodies, which produce in infants of both genders usually transient cutaneous changes, but in some cases an irreversible congenital heart block. The lesions are commonly located on the face and neck but may appear elsewhere, develop during the first weeks or months of life, and are often exacerbated by exposure to the sun.

Systemic involvement is uncommon. NLE can also occur in infants born from mothers with inactive disease, even with no detectable Ro/La antibodies. The serologic study might be negative in immunodiffusion and ELISA techniques, and positive in immunoblotting (52-kDa, 60-kDa Ro proteins, 48-kDa La protein), and therefore all methods of detection should be employed for negative sera of mothers and neonates. More than 95% of infants with NLE are Ro-positive, but single cases may be associated with U1-RNP[19,20]. The cases of twins with identical antibodies and HLA but discordant for congenital heart block point to the role of some other factors in the development of congenital heart block, in addition to Ro antibodies and genetic set-up[21].

CHILDHOOD LUPUS ERYTHEMATOSUS

Both SLE and cutaneous LE (CLE) are rare in children (Figure 2). In our series the female : male ratio for childhood SLE was about 3 : 1 (28/10), but in CLE which developed before the age of 10 years (only 2% of cases) no female predominance was reported. There was also a low incidence of photosensitivity and very rare progression to SLE[22].

SYSTEMIC SCLEROSIS; SYSTEMIC SCLERODERMA (SSc)

The prevalence of systemic scleroderma in women is mainly related to the subtype of the disease. In our cohort of 507 patients the overall female : male ratio was 8 : 1, with a ratio of 5.7 : 1 for the diffuse variety (dSSc) and 12 : 1 for the limited subtype (lSSc) (Tables 2 and 3). In our study there was a high frequency of anti-Scl 70 (Topo I) antibody not only in diffuse scleroderma (79.5%) but also in limited variety (51%), both in women and men. The anticentromere antibodies were found in lSSc in both genders. The course of the disease was more severe in men with diffuse and limited varieties, and in rare cases of both sexes with no detectable antibodies.

The relationship of SSc to sex hormone dysfunction is not clear despite a strong female predominance. In contrast to SLE, which is prevalent in younger women, the incidence of SSc increases following childbearing years and the peak incidence of the disease is in the fifth and sixth decades[23]. The course is variable, not always progressive and tends to be more severe in younger females and in males. Life expectancy differs in various subsets of SSc depending on the severity and extent of visceral involvement.

Systemic scleroderma and pregnancy

There are only a few reports on SSc and pregnancy because over 50% of patients who have children had pregnancies before the onset of the disease, and over 30% were never pregnant. Therefore the studies, except one larger series[24], were performed on small groups of patients. Steen and colleagues[24] showed in a large cohort prematurity and abortions in about 11% and 6% respectively, with neonatal death in about 2%. A much higher incidence of complications was reported by Slate and Graham[25]. This discrepancy might arise because of more effective therapies and better condition of the patients in the study by Steen *et al*. A recent report[26] showed that the outcome of pregnancy in SSc patients may be good if the disease is stabilized. In such cases the risk of premature babies, miscarriages and baby mortality is not increased. The exception is renal crisis, which should be aggressively treated with ACE inhibitors[26]. Thus, pregnancy for patients with scleroderma does not present such a risk factor as for patients with SLE, and some even improve during the pregnancy, although with exacerbation after the delivery. The problem of SSc in pregnancy remains unclear and needs to be further investigated.

Microchimerism in systemic scleroderma

The most intriguing problem is a relationship between pregnancy and the pathogenesis of SSc. Recently it was shown that fetal hematopoietic cells may traverse placenta and persist in the mother's circulation for decades; also maternal cells found in cord blood may persist in the child. The presence of a small amount of genetically different cells, i.e., microchimerism, might be responsible for graft-versus host reaction (GVHR) and induction of SSc[27]. In women with SSc who have borne at least one male infant, male cell DNA or Y chromosome sequences were disclosed in peripheral blood mononuclear cells and in active skin lesions[28]. The children born from these women had HLA class II compatibility with the mothers and strongest association with DQA1*0501 alleles[29]. Fetal–maternal cell transfer is a frequent phenomenon which may also occur in healthy women[30]. Graft versus host disease (GVHD), as after allogenic cell transfusion, might be induced by compatible but not identical HLA in a mother and child, if the antigen is sufficiently different from self antigen to break tolerance but not different enough to induce immunity[30]. The women with SSc were found to harbor (for up to 27 years) fetal cell lines derived from their offspring that might be responsible for the disease[31]. Seventy per cent of SSc females were compatible with their children for class II alleles, compared to 21% of control individuals. Because of this, the fetal or maternal cells (present in up to 40% of pregnancies) which have crossed the placenta remain unrecognized by the host. SSc develops after their subsequent activation by yet unknown stimuli. Thus, microchimerism in pregnancy might be involved in the pathogenesis of SSc, and HLA-class II compatible mother–child relationship is a risk factor for scleroderma. Although tolerance induced by microchimerism might be a risk factor for developing other connective tissue autoimmune diseases, this has been up to now shown only for SSc. The reason for this might be immunogenetic differences, for example only 20% of patients with rheumatoid arthritis were found compatible with their children for class II alleles compared with 70% of patients with SSc[30]. Microchimerism might be responsible for a very high female prevalence of SSc, an increased incidence of the disease in women past childbearing years and for the similarity of SSc and graft versus host disease.

SYSTEMIC SCLERODERMA IN CHILDREN

SSc of childhood is a rare disease. In our recent study it was found in 18 of 525 patients (3.4%) and in our older series it constituted 1.75% of the cohort[32]. Tuffanelli and Winkelmann[33] reported the incidence as 1.5% of the Mayo Clinic series. Some

Table 2 Systemic scleroderma (SSc) in adult females vs. males

	Total	Female	Male	f : m
Total	507	451 (88.9%)	56 (11.1%)	8 : 1
Diffuse SSc (dSSc)	234 (46.1%)	199 (85%)	35 (15%)	~6 : 1
Limited SSc (lSSc)	273 (53.9%)	252 (92.3%)	21 (7.7%)	12 : 1

Table 3 Immunological markers in systemic scleroderma (SSc): females vs. males

Marker	Diffuse SSc (n = 234)			Limited SSc (n = 273)			Overall total (%)
	f (n = 199)	m (n = 35)	Total (%)	f (n = 252)	m (n = 21)	Total (%)	
Topo I	160	26	186 (79.5)	131	9	140 (51.3)	326 (64.3)
ACA	—	—	—	73	8	81 (29.7)	81 (16.0)
Fibrillarin	7	4	11 (4.7)	—	—	—	11 (2.2)
Other antibody	20	3	23 (9.8)	39	2	41 (15.0)	64 (12.6)
ANA negative	12	2	14 (6.0)	9	2	11 (4.0)	25 (4.9)

ANA, antinuclear antibodies; ACA, anticentromere antibodies; f, female; m, male

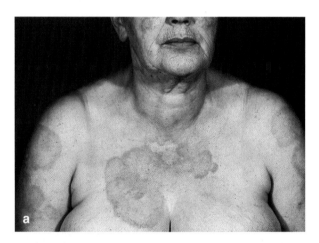

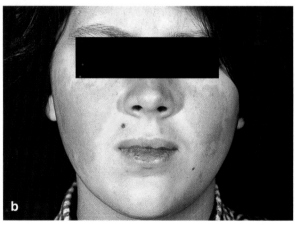

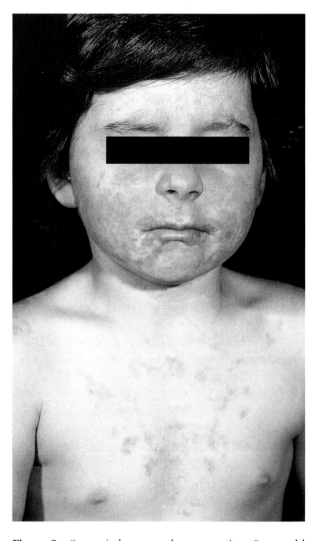

Figure 1 (a) Subacute cutaneous lupus erythematosus in a 51-year-old woman, with characteristic annular lesions on the face, thorax and forearms. There was no kidney involvement, and the course was rather mild. This case was associated with anti Ro/SS-A/ antibodies. (b) Systemic lupus erythematosus (SLE) with characteristic malar rash on the face. This case was associated with RNP, Sm and Ro/SS-A/ antibodies

Figure 2 Systemic lupus erythematosus in a 9-year-old girl, with widespread lesions on the face, trunk and limbs. This case was associated with RNP and Ro/SS-A/ antibodies

cases of overlap syndromes, mixed connective tissue disease (MCTD) and scleromyositis, which are not infrequent in children, might have been identified as juvenile SSc[34,35]. This could lead to confusion concerning the prevalence of SSc in childhood. In our series the ratio female : male in children was 3.5 : 1 (14 : 4). The association of clinical subtypes with antibodies is presented in Table 4.

A peculiarity of childhood SSc was, in our series, the association of Topo I mainly with lSSc. The diffuse subtype was found mainly in boys, and the prevailing marker was fibrillarin. In these children the course of the disease was most severe, and two of them died within several months.

Treatment depends on the severity and activity of the disease; in non-active cases aggressive therapies should be avoided.

LOCALIZED SCLERODERMA; MORPHEA

The relationship of morphea to systemic scleroderma is not clear. Although the cutaneous indurations may show similarities, localized scleroderma differs very markedly from SSc because Raynaud's phenomenon, visceral involvement and immunological abnormalities, except for antinuclear antibodies (ANA) mainly in linear scleroderma, are absent. The incidence of various subsets of localized scleroderma in both genders of adults and children in our series is presented in Table 5, which shows that the prevalence in women is less marked than in SSc: the female : male ratio in adults in our series was about 5 : 1, and in children about 3 : 1. Linear scleroderma was more frequent in children (found in over half of them), and severe generalized morphea prevailed in boys. In essence localized scleroderma, except for the linear subtype, is a self-limiting disease with a mean duration of 3.5 to 5 years. Linear scleroderma, especially in children, may lead to atrophies, contractures and severe disability. Generalized or pansclerotic morphea, occurring with the same frequency in girls and boys, may have a lethal outcome[36].

PROGRESSIVE FACIAL HEMIATROPHY (PFH)

PFH, a unilateral linear shrinkage of the skin and subcutis of the face, scalp and neck, shows similarity to band-like atrophies of involutionary linear scleroderma (Figure 3). The close relationship of PFH with scleroderma *en coup de sabre* is favored by their not uncommon co-existence, overlapping symptoms or transition of typical scleroderma *en coup de sabre*

into PFH, as well as the co-existence of localized scleroderma in other areas[37,38]. In our series of 62 children or young adults in whom the disease started before the age of 14 years, in 19 cases morphea plaques or linear scleroderma were present also on the limbs and trunk. In children the prevalence in females was less marked than in young adults in whom the changes appeared after 14 years of age, with a female : male ratio of 7 : 1 (Table 6).

The incidence in women in this group was comparable to that in morphea. Neurological complications – epilepsy and others, frequently preceded by head trauma – often occurred in younger children. In several patients abnormalities were detectable only by special techniques. In rare cases the involvement of the central nervous system could be severe, often with only slight cutaneous atrophies.

ATROPHODERMA PASINI–PIERINI

The primary cutaneous atrophies described as an idiopatic atrophoderma are regarded by some authors as an entity different from morphea in clinical presentation and course, and by others as a primarily atrophic morphea[32,39]. The coexistence with morphea, either in other localization or within the same plaques, and similarity to the atrophies after involution of morphea, favor their close relationship. The female : male ratio in cases with no coexistent morphea was similar to that in morphea both in adults (5.8) and children (2.6), as shown in Table 7. The prevalence in females was greater in cases coexisting with morphea or morphea-like changes. The pigmentation and slight atrophies usually persist for several years, and do not require any therapy.

DERMATOMYOSITIS (DM)

DM, an autoimmune inflammatory myopathy, occurs twice as often in females as in males. Two peaks of incidence were reported, one for children (juvenile dermatomyositis – JDM), and another for adults aged 40–60 years. In the USA blacks are affected more than whites by a 4 : 1 ratio, and black women have the highest incidence of all groups[40]. In our series, the female : male ratio was 3.3 : 1, while in JDM there was no female predominance, as reported also by others[41,42]. This differs from a Taiwanese study, in which the disease predominated in girls by a 6 : 3 ratio[43].

The association with specific serologic marker Mi2 antibody was found in about 12% of adults and 17% of children (Table 8). In many patients the antibodies were either absent or could not be identified (in 40% of cases). In a proportion of

Table 4   Immunological markers in 18 cases of childhood systemic scleroderma (SSc) (females/males)

SSc type	Topo I	Fibrillarin	ACA
diffuse, n = 5	2 (m)	3 (2 m)	
limited, n = 12	8 (f)	1 (f)	3 (f)*
SSc incipiens – Raynaud only (1)	1 (f)	—	—

ACA, anticentromere antibodies; *clinical type CREST

Table 5   Clinical varieties of morphea in adults and children (359 cases): females vs. males

	Adults (n = 186)		Children (n = 173)	
Variety	f (n = 154)	m (n = 32)	f (n = 131)	m (n = 42)
Morphea en plaques (101)	64	8	25	4
disseminated (66)	32	12	16	6
profound (16)	3	1	10	2
generalized (15)	8	2	1	4
abortive (24)	16	3	4	1
atypical (15)	8	2	4	1
S. linearis (122)	23	4	71	24

Table 6   Progressive facial hemiatrophy in females vs. males

Group	Female	Male	f : m
Children (up to 14 years of age) (n = 27)	15	12	~1 : 1
Adults (onset in children) (n = 35)	25	10	2.5 : 1
Young adults (onset after 14 years of age) (n = 17)	15	2	~7 : 1
Total (n = 79)	55	24	~2 : 1

Table 7   Atrophoderma Pasini–Pierini in females vs. males

	Adults (n = 91)		Children (n = 48)	
	Female	Male	Female	Male
Exclusively atrophies of atrophoderma Pasini–Pierini type (84)	41	7	26	10
Coexistence with morphea within the lesions or in other localization (55)	38	5	10	2

Table 8   Dermatomyositis/polymyositis in females vs. males; association with antibodies

	Adults (n = 101)		Children (n = 17)		Total (n = 118)	
	f (n = 78)	m (n = 23)	f (n = 9)	m (n = 8)	f (n = 87)	m (n = 31)
ANA positive, n = 69 (58.5%)						
Mi2, n = 15	9	3	1	2	10	5
Ro (SS-A), n = 13	9	3	1	—	10	3
unidentified, n = 41	28	10	2	1	30	11
Total, ANA positive	46	16	4	3	50	19
ANA negative, n = 49 (41.5%)	32	7	5	5	37	12
Total, ANA positive + negative	78	23	9	8	87	31

f, female; m, male; ANA, antinuclear antibodies

patients Ro/SS-A/ antibodies were also found. Cases associated with aminoacyl-tRNA synthetases have some clinical peculiarities, and are discussed with the synthetase syndromes (see below). However, some of them have clinical presentation of DM. The association with specific antibodies is important since cases positive for Mi2 have a more chronic course, with milder muscle and skin involvement. Rare cases associated with tRNA-synthetase antibodies are usually more severe. The course of the disease in Caucasians does not differ in women and men, while in black females the prognosis was reported as less favorable[40].

The important sequelae of DM in both genders are: fibrosis leading to muscle atrophies and indurations, contractures, calcifications and iatrogenic complications due mainly to long-term corticosteroid and immunosuppressive therapies. Survival rates were reported as about 82% at 1 year, 74% at 2, 67% at 5 and 55% at 9 years[44].

Dermatomyositis and internal malignancies

About 30% of DM cases in adults over 40 to 50 years of age are associated with internal malignancies[44]. A work-up should include mammography, pelvic ultrasonography and serologic examination for ovarian tumors with marker CA-125. The paraneoplastic symptoms include necrotic ulcerations, mostly over elbows and knees, bullous eruption and panniculitis.

DERMATOMYOSITIS SINE MYOSITIS (AMYOPATHIC DM)

In about 10% of patients the cutaneous changes characteristic of DM are not associated with clinical and laboratory signs of myositis (amyopathic DM). Muscle disease may develop within several months to 2 years (Figure 4), but we have seen cases in which the first symptoms of myositis appeared over ten years after the onset of cutaneous changes. There are also cases in which myositis failed to appear within a long follow-up. In amyopathic DM there is a greater female to male ratio (3 : 1) than seen in other DM patients (2 : 1)[45,46]. In cases with no visible muscle involvement the first signs of developing myositis are laboratory abnormalities[47].

JUVENILE DERMATOMYOSITIS (JDM)

Primary susceptibility to JDM was found to be confered by HLA-DQA1*0501[47]; children with this genetic set-up are in the risk group. JDM usually develops between 2 and 5 years of age. The cutaneous and muscle involvement is in general similar to that in adults, differing by more intensive vascular changes, frequent photosensitivity and generalized calcifications[43]. The extent of muscle involvement is often difficult to assess by physical examination, histological findings and level of muscle-related enzymes, and is best evaluated by ultrasonography and magnetic resonance imaging.

INFLAMMATORY MYOPATHIES ASSOCIATED WITH ANTI-AMINOACYL-tRNA SYNTHETASE AUTOANTIBODIES: SYNTHETASE SYNDROMES

Characteristic of synthetase syndromes is polymyositis with clinical presentation somewhat mimicking systemic scleroderma: puffy fingers with sclerodactyly, facial edema, arthritis, lung fibrosis and not infrequently Raynaud's phenomenon[48,49]. The synthetase syndromes are heterogenous, but the discovery of autoantibodies directed against cytoplasmic ribonucleoproteins involved in the process of translation enabled their classification into more clinically useful groups on the basis of clinical, immunologic and immunogenetic findings[50-52].

The most frequent is the syndrome associated with anti-histidyl synthetase antibodies (Jo1) (Table 9). The main clinical features are: polymyositis with some signs of dermatomyositis and scleroderma, interstitial lung disease (ILD), arthralgia or arthritis. In our series of 28 patients, the incidence in females was three times higher than in men. In both genders the patients were in the older age group; in both the main symptoms were myositis or myalgia, arthritis or arthralgia, fever at the onset of the disease and, in a proportion of patients, lung fibrosis. Cutaneous involvement of SSc and DM type was somewhat more frequent in males, while Raynaud's phenomenon was absent in the majority of them. The course of the disease showed great variations, both in females and males. In cases of synthetase syndromes associated with other antibodies and in cases associated with anti-SRP (signal recognition particle) antibodies, the course of the disease was usually more severe.

The recognition of polymyositis associated with anti-synthetase antibodies is important from a practical point of view, mainly because of coexisting lung disease, which often might be diagnosed only with the use of special techniques. Synthetase

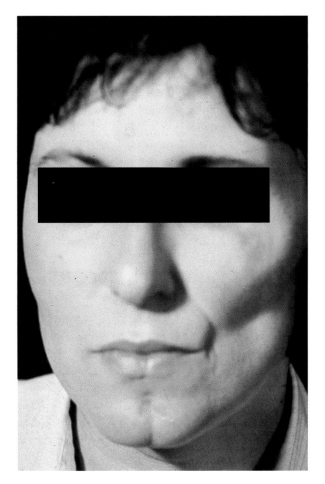

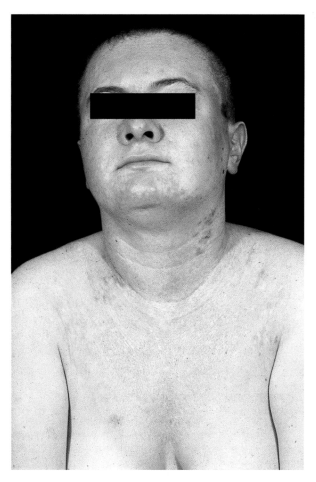

Figure 3   Progressive facial hemiatrophy. The unilateral atrophies are similar to involutionary scleroderma. In this 37-year-old woman, the first changes of morphea type were noticed in the 23rd year of life, and spread progressively

Figure 4   Dermatomyositis in a 24-year-old woman, in whom cutaneous lesions appeared 4 years previously and muscle involvement developed progressively up to full blown myositis present for about one year. Erythematous skin changes on the face, (periorbicular heliotrope sign) and neck (V sign)

syndromes with scleroderma-like cutaneous changes are not infrequently regarded as unusual scleroderma, and not treated as for polymyositis.

SCLEROMYOSITIS

This scleroderma/dermatomyositis overlap syndrome, associated with PM-Scl antibody, is still a matter of controversy owing to a variable clinical presentation mimicking SSc or DM[49,53]. The main features are: myositis or myalgia and arthralgia or non-deforming arthritis, Raynaud's phenomenon, SSc-like cutaneous changes in the hands and the face (slight thinning of the lips, radial furrowing around the mouth, mask-like facies) and DM-like changes (heliotrope rash, and Gottron's sign on the hands). ILD and esophagus hypomotility were present in one third of adult cases. Since the clinical presentation may be at one time more characteristic of SSc, and at another time more typical of DM,

Table 9   Clinical characteristics of synthetase syndrome associated with Jo 1 antibodies in females vs. males in a study involving 28 cases

Characteristic	Females (n = 21)	Males (n = 7)
Age at onset	45.5 years	46 years
Fever at onset	8 (38.1%)	2 (28.6%)
Myositis/myalgia	20 (95.2%)	7 (100%)
Arthritis/arthralgia	20 (95.2%)	5 (71.4%)
Lung fibrosis (ILD)	11 (52.3%)	5 (71.4%)
Cutaneous involvement		
type SSc	11 (52.3%)	6 (85.7%)
type DM	7 (33.3%)	4 (57.1%)
Esophageal dysmotility	6 (28.6%)	1 (14.3%)
Raynaud's phenomenon	13 (61.9%)	2 (28.6%)

ILD, interstitial lung disease; SSc, systemic scleroderma; DM, dermatomyositis

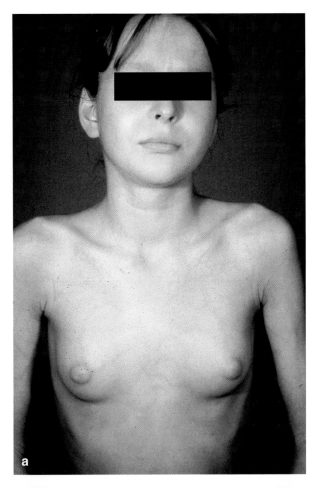

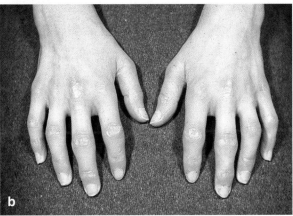

Figure 5 Scleromyositis associated with Pm-Scl antibody. In this 11-year-old girl the first symptoms appeared at the age of 10 years. (a) Cutaneous features are similar to systemic scleroderma with some symptoms of dermatomyositis (muscle involvement, periorbital edema). (b) Sclerodactyly with pronounced Raynaud's phenomenon and erythematous papules on the fingers and over intraphalangeal joints. Periungual vascular changes

the same patients are diagnosed accordingly by doctors seeing them at different times. In our cohort of 81 patients – 59 adults and 22 children – the incidence of scleromyositis was more than three

times higher in adult females than in males, and in children the ratio was about 2 : 1 (Table 10).

The clinical symptoms were in general similar in both sexes, except for Raynaud's phenomenon, absent in 30% of males, and for DM-like cutaneous involvement not present in one third of women. In children scleroderma-like changes were more pronounced than in adults (Figure 5a, b), in a majority of them with no DM-like changes[35]. In chronic cases children developed muscle atrophies, as often seen in chronic JDM. The visceral involvement differed considerably in girls and boys. In almost half of the girls functional pulmonary tests showed abnormalities, although still not of ILD type, and in about 25% of girls esophagus dysmotility was found. No visceral involvement was detected in boys. Characteristic capillaroscopy for DM (bushy capillaries, large subpapillary plexus, hemorrhages and Raynaud's loops) was found in 50% of women and in over 70% of girls, and rarely in men and boys.

All our cases were positive for PM-Scl antibody; however this antibody also appears in over 20% in other CTD, very much like U1-RNP antibody, which is present in about 70% of MCTD cases and is regarded as its marker although patients with other CTD, especially SLE and SSc, may be positive for Ul-RNP.

MIXED CONNECTIVE TISSUE DISEASE (MCTD)

This overlap syndrome, combining features of SSc and SLE with myositis, presents a heterogeneous group of cases defying classification as SSc, SLE or DM. It is still controversial whether MCTD is an entity or the co-existence of separate connective tissue diseases evolving, after a long time, into a definite CTD[54]. However most recent immunogenetic findings showed that MCTD is an independent disorder defined not only by clinical features and serology but also by immunogenetic findings[55]. In spite of three different sets of classification criteria by Alarcon-Segovia, Sharp and colleagues and Kasukawa and co-workers[56], there is no consensus concerning the recognition of cases showing overlapping CTD features, often referred to as unclassifiable.

There is a marked preponderance in women of about 8 : 1[56]. In our more recent study the incidence in females was even higher. Of 96 adult patients only 7 were men (7.3%). In children the disease, in contrast to SSc, is not uncommon. Of 28 children (about 22.5% of our cohort), 7 were boys i.e. the female : male ratio was 3 : 1. The mean age of onset in children was 10.5 (range 4–13 years). The disease

Table 10   Scleromyositis associated with PM-Scl antibody in females vs. males in a study of 81 cases

	Adults (n = 59)		Children (n = 22)	
	f (n = 46)	m (n = 13)	f (n = 15)	m (n = 7)
Gender ratio	~3.5 : 1		~2 : 1	
Age at onset (years)	41.5	52.6	9.3	9.4
Raynaud's phenomenon	41	7	13	7
Myositis/myalgia	41	8	15	7
Muscle atrophies	15	5	4	2
Skin changes				
of SSc type	31	9	13	7
of DM type	13	5	4	2
Visceral involvement				
lung	13	3	7	—
esophagus	10	2	4	—
Capillaroscopy characteristic of DM	20	—	8	2

SSc, systemic scleroderma; DM, dermatomyositis

Table 11   Heterogeneous features of mixed connective tissue disease in adult females vs. males in a study of 94 cases

	Females (n = 85)	Males (n = 9)
Cases in spectrum of SLE, n = 24	23	1
Cases in spectrum of SSc, n = 31	28	3
Cases unclassified, n = 39	34	5

SLE, systemic lupus erythematosus; SSc, systemic scleroderma

is often more severe in children than in adults, has usually more pronounced features of scleroderma and is infrequently recognized as SSc associated with U1RNP antibody.

In our study of 94 cases followed for 1 to 17 years (mean 5.9 years), 33% of patients were found to show progressively more pronounced features of SSc, the disease evolved rather in the direction of SLE in 27% of the females, but the largest subset remained unchanged (Table 11). The specific serologic markers for SSc and SLE appeared only in single cases, and U1-RNP as a marker was in most patients stable, although in some it disappeared by regression of lesions. In the majority of patients small or moderate doses of corticosteroids controlled the disease.

CONCLUSIONS

All connective tissue diseases are significantly more frequent in women. The female : male ratio varies for different CTD, and is somewhat lower in DM than in SLE and SSc. The differences in incidence and course of SLE and SSc in females vs. males appear to be related mainly to the sex hormones, and in SSc possibly also to pregnancies and induced immunotolerance. In all CTD, except JDM, girls are more commonly affected than boys, although the female : male ratio is not as high as in adults.

REFERENCES

1. Lahita RG. Sex, age, and systemic lupus erythematosus. In Lahita RG, ed. *Systemic Lupus Erythematosus*. New York: Churchill Livingstone, 1992:527–42

2. Cooper GS, Dooley MA, Treadwell EL, *et al.* Hormonal, environmental, and infectious risk factors for developing systemic lupus erythematosus. *Arthritis Rheum* 1998;41:1714–23

3. van Vollenhoven RF, Engleman EG, McGuire JL. Dehydroepiandrosterone in systemic lupus erythematosus. Results of a double-blind, placebo-controlled, randomized clinical trial. *Arthritis Rheum* 1995;38:1826–31

4. Kanda N, Tsuchida T, Tamaki K. Testosterone suppresses anti-DNA antibody production in peripheral blood mononuclear cells from patients with systemic lupus erythematosus. *Arthritis Rheum* 1997;40: 1703–11

5. Wang D, Chan EKL. 17-β-Estradiol increases expression of 52-kDa and 60-kDa SS-A/Ro autoantigens in human keratinocytes and breast cancer line MCF-7. *J Invest Dermatol* 1996;107:610–14

6. Jones SK. The effects of hormonal and other stimuli on cell-surface Ro/SSA antigen expression by human keratinocytes *in vitro*: their possible role in the induction of cutaneous lupus lesions. *Br J Dermatol* 1992;126:554–60

7. Petri M, Robinson C. Oral contraceptives and systemic lupus erythematosus. *Arthritis Rheum* 1997;40: 797–803

8. Ahmed A, Talal N. Importance of sex hormones in systemic lupus erythematosus. In Wallace DJ, Hahn BH, eds. *Dubois' Lupus Erythematosus*, 4th edn. Philadelphia: Lea & Febiger, 1993

9. Reveille JD, Bartolucci A, Alarcon GS. Prognosis in systemic lupus erythematosus. *Arthritis Rheum* 1990; 33:37–48

10. Xie SK, Feng SE, Fu H. Long term follow-up of patients with systemic lupus erythematosus. *J Dermatol* 1998;25:367–73

11. Sequeira JF, Keser G, Greenstein B, *et al*. Systemic lupus erythematosus sex hormones in male patients. *Lupus* 1993;2:315–17

12. Petri M. Systemic lupus erythematosus and pregnancy. *Rheum Dis Clin North Am* 1994;20:87–118

13. Derksen RHWM, Bruinse HW, de Groot PG, Kater L. Pregnancy in systemic lupus erythematosus: a prospective study. *Lupus* 1994;3:149–55

14. Julkunen H, Kaaja R, Jouhikainen T, *et al*. Malignant hypertension and antiphospholipid antibodies as presenting features of SLE in a young woman using oral contraceptives. *Br J Rheum* 1991; 30:471–2

15. Ben-Chetrit A, Ben-Chetrit E. Systemic lupus erythematosus induced by ovulation induction treatment. *Arthritis Rheum* 1994;37:1614–17

16. Sontheimer RD. Subacute cutaneous lupus erythematosus. *Clin Dermatol* 1985;3:58–68

17. Sontheimer RD. Subacute cutaneous lupus erythematosus: a decade's perspective. *Med Clin North Am* 1989;73:1073–90

18. Chlebus E, Wolska H, Blaszczyk M, Jablonska S. Subacute cutaneous lupus erythematosus versus systemic lupus erythematosus: diagnostic criteria and therapeutic implications. *J Am Acad Dermatol* 1998; 38:405–12

19. Crowley E, Frieden IJ. Neonatal lupus erythematosus: an unusual congenital presentation with cutaneous atrophy, erosions, alopecia and panacytopenia. *Pediatric Dermatol* 1998;15:38–42

20. Sheth AP, Esterly NB, Ratoosh SL, *et al*. U1RNP positive neonatal lupus erythematosus: association with anti-La antibodies? *Br J Dermatol* 1995;132: 520–6

21. Watson RM, Scheel JN, Petri M, *et al*. Neonatal lupus erythematosus. Report of serological and immunogenetic studies in twins discordant for congenital heart block. *Br J Dermatol* 1994;130:342–8

22. George PM, Tunnessen WW. Childhood discoid lupus erythematosus. *Arch Dermatol* 1993;129: 613–17

23. Jablonska S, Maddison PJ, Blaszczyk M. Scleroderma. In Kater L, Baart de la Faille H, eds. *Multi-systemic Autoimmune Diseases*. Amsterdam: Elsevier Science, 1995:207–25

24. Steen VD, Conte C, Day N, *et al*. Pregnancy in women with systemic sclerosis. *Arthritis Rheum* 1989; 32:151–7

25. Slate WG, Graham AR. Scleroderma and pregnancy. *Am J Obstet Gynecol* 1968;101:335–41

26. Steen VD. Scleroderma and pregnancy. *Rheum Dis Clin North Am* 1997;23:133–47

27. Nelson JL. Pregnancy, persistent microchimerism, and autoimmune disease. *J Am Med Women's Assoc* 1998;53:31–2, 47

28. Artlett CM, Smith JB, Jimenez SA. Identification of fetal DNA and cells in skin lesions from women with systemic sclerosis. *N Engl J Med* 1998;338: 1186–91

29. Artlett CM, Welsh KI, Black CM, Jimenez SA. Fetal-maternal HLA compatibility confers susceptibility to systemic sclerosis. *Immunogenetics* 1998;47:17–22

30. Tyndall A, Gratwohl A. Microchimerism: friend or foe? *Nature Med* 1998;4:386–8

31. Nelson JL, Furst DE, Maloney S, *et al*. Microchimerism and HLA-compatible relationships of pregnancy in scleroderma. *Lancet* 1997;351:559–62

32. Jablonska S. *Scleroderma and Pseudoscleroderma*. Warszawa: PZWL, 1975

33. Tuffanelli DL, Winkelmann RK. Systemic scleroderma (a clinical study of 727 cases). *Arch Dermatol* 1961;84:359

34. Blaszczyk M, Jablonska S, Szymanska-Jagiello W, *et al*. Childhood scleromyositis: an overlap syndrome associated with PM-Scl antibody. *Pediatr Dermatol* 1991;8:1–8

35. Blaszczyk M, Jablonska S, Szymanska-Jagiello W, *et al*. Immunological markers of systemic scleroderma in children. *Pediatr Dermatol* 1991;8:13–20

36. Jablonska S, Rodnan GP. Localized forms of scleroderma. *Clin Rheum Dis* 1979;5:215–41

37. Lehman TJA. The Parry–Romberg syndrome of progressive facial hemiatrophy and linear scleroderma en coup de sabre. Mistaken diagnosis of overlapping conditions. *J Rheumatol* 1992;19:844–5

38. Jablonska S, Blaszczyk M, Rosinska D. Progressive facial hemiatrophy and scleroderma en coup de sabre. Clinical presentation and course as related to the onset in early childhood and young adults. *Arch Argent Dermatol* 1998;48:125–8

39. Kencka D, Blaszczyk M, Jablonska S. Atrophoderma Pasini–Pierini is a primary atrophic abortive morphea. *Dermatology* 1995;190:203–6

40. Peake MF, Perkins P, Elston DM, *et al*. Cutaneous ulcers of refractory adult dermatomyositis responsive to intravenous immunoglobulin. *Cutis* 1998;62: 89–93

41. Pelkonen PM, Jalanko HJ, Lantto RK, *et al*. Incidence of systemic connective tissue diseases in children: a nationwide prospective study in Finland. *J Rheumatol* 1994;21:2143–6

42. Collison CH, Sinal SH, Jorizzo JL, *et al*. Juvenile dermatomyositis and polymyositis: a follow-up study of long-term sequelae. *South Med J* 1998;91:17–22

43. Chung HT, Huang JL, Wang HS, *et al*. Dermatomyositis and polymyositis in childhood.

Chung-Hua Min Kuo Hsiao Erh Ko I Hasueh Hui Tsa Chih 1994;35:407–14

44. Maugars YM, Bertelot JM, Abbas AA, *et al.* Long-term prognosis of 69 patients with dermatomyositis or polymyositis. *Clin Exp Rheumatol* 1996;14: 263–74

45. Euwer RL, Sontheimer RD. Amyopathic dermatomyositis (dermatomyositis sine myositis). Presentation of six new cases and review of the literature. *J Am Acad Dermatol* 1991;24:959–66

46. Euwer RL, Sontheimer RD. Amyopathic dermatomyositis: a review. *J Invest Dermatol* 1993;100: 124s–127s

47. Reed AM, Pachman LM, Hayford J, Ober C. Immunogenetic studies in families of children with juvenile dermatomyositis. *J Rheumatol* 1998;25: 1000–2

48. Hausmanowa-Petrsusewicz I, Kowalska-Olędzka E, Miller FW, *et al.* Clinical, serological, and immunogenetic features in Polish patients with idiopathic inflammatory myopathies. *Arthritis Rheum* 1997;40: 1257–66

49. Jablonska S, Chorzelski TP, Blaszczyk M, *et al.* Scleroderma/polymyositis overlap syndromes and their immunologic markers. *Clin Dermatol* 1993;10: 457–72

50. Love LA, Leff RL, Fraser DD, *et al.* A new approach to the classification of idiopathic inflammatory myopathy: myositis specific autoantibodies define useful homogeneous patient groups. *Medicine (Baltimore)* 1991;34:1391–6

51. Love LA, Miller FW. Noninfectious environmental agents associated with myopathies. *Curr Opin Rheumatol* 1993;5:712–18

52. Targoff IN. Autoantibodies in polymyositis. *Rheum Dis Clin North Am* 1992;18:455–82

53. Hausmanowa-Petrsusewicz I, Blaszczyk M, Kowalska E, *et al.* Neuromuscular studies in scleromyositis. *Acta Cardiomiol* 1994;6:99–110

54. Smolen JS, Steiner G. Mixed connective tissue disease. *Arthritis Rheum* 1998;41:768–77

55. Mimori T, Kuwana M. Immunogenetic factor associated with production of anti-U1RN1 antibodies and development of mixed connective tissue disease. *Arthritis Rheum* 1998;41:128

56. Maddison PJ, Jablonska S. Overlap syndromes. In Kater L, Baart de la Faille H, eds. *Multi-systemic Autoimmune Diseases.* Elsevier Science, 1995:227–40

Vasculitic disorders

19

Torello M. Lotti, Claudio Comacchi and Ilaria Ghersetich

INTRODUCTION

Vasculitic disorders refers to a group of disorders usually characterized by palpable purpura. This clinical condition of dermatologic interest is mainly related to cutaneous necrotizing vasculitis (CNV), characterized by angiocentric segmental inflammation, endothelial cell swelling and fibrinoid necrosis of blood vessel walls. Although blood vessels of any size may be affected in systemic vasculitis, CNV usually occurs in the post-capillary venules. CNV can be idiopathic or can be associated with drugs, infections, or underlying system diseases[1-4]. The disorder occurs equally in both sexes and at all ages[5,6]; approximately 10% of cases occur in children[7,8].

ETIOLOGY

No genetic factors are recognized[9,10]. Many factors (Table 1), especially drugs (insulin, penicillin, sulfonamides, etc.), chemicals (insecticides, petroleum products), food (milk proteins, etc.) and infections (viral, bacterial, fungal, protozoan, helminthic) should be considered as potential causes of CNV[1-4]. The frequency of viral or bacterial infection is probably underestimated[8]. CNV has been reported in association with coexisting diseases (collagen-vascular diseases, purpura hyperglobulinemia, cryoglobulinemia, inflammatory bowel disease, malignant neoplasm, cystic fibrosis etc.) (Table 2)[1-4]. In many cases the cause of CNV remains unknown (Table 3), for example in Henoch–Schönlein purpura and urticarial vasculitis[1-4].

CLINICAL FEATURES

Palpable purpura (Figure 1) is the major clinical presentation of CNV, while erythematous macules, wheals (Figure 2), papules, blisters, large palpable nodules, ecchymoses, pustules, hemorrhagic vesicles (Figure 3), ulcers and a mottling of the skin (livedo reticularis) are less common manifestations[1-4]. Lesions are often distributed symmetrically[11] and may occur anywhere, but are most commonly found on the lower legs (particularly in the erect patient), where elevated hydrostatic pressure and tortuosity of vessels may provoke more distorted and turbulent flow patterns and an increase

of viscosity leading to increased vasopermeability and to possible tissue deposition of circulating immune complexes[1-4]. The mucous membranes are only rarely involved (petechiae, hemorragic blisters, ulcers)[8-9]. In the skin, the lesions may be moderately itching or painful (especially in those chronic or recurrent episodes preceded by fever, myalgia, joint pain, headache and malaise)[1-4,10,11]. Usually, the lesions persist for from 1 to 4 weeks and resolve with residual scarring and hyperpigmentation[9,10]. Recently the Koebner phenomenon has been reported as an unusual cutaneous manifestation of immune complex-mediated CNV[12]. The disease is often self-limited and confined to the skin, but visceral lesions (renal, gastrointestinal, pericardial, neurologic and rheumatologic) may occur[1-6].

In about 50% of CNV cases the cause is not known (idiophatic CNV)[1-6].

TYPES OF CUTANEOUS NECROTIZING VASCULITIS

Henoch–Schönlein purpura

This disease is characterized clinically by skin lesions (present in 100% of cases), joint pains (present in 74–84%), gastrointestinal symptoms (present in 61–76%) and renal changes (present in 44–47%)[13,14]. This disorder occurs primarily in children, with a peak incidence between 4 and 8 years age and with predominance in males[14]. The syndrome often follows streptococcal or upper respiratory tract infections, with a latency period of 1 to 3 weeks[13]. In about 40% of patients the cutaneous manifestations are preceded by mild fever, headache, joint symptoms or abdominal pain for periods of up to 2 weeks[13]. The most common skin findings are represented by symmetrical petechial hemorragic or palpable purpuric lesions on the lower extremities and buttocks; the trunk is usually spared[10,13-15]. The skin lesions often regress after 10–14 days. Arthralgias and arthritis usually involve the knees and ankles. Gastrointestinal symptoms include colicky pain, vomiting, melena

Table 1 Cutaneous necrotizing vasculitis: precipitating agents

Viral infections: hepatitis A virus, hepatitis B virus, hepatitis C virus, herpes simplex, influenza virus
Bacterial infections: beta-hemolytic streptococcus group A, *Staphylococcus aureus*, *Mycobacterium leprae*
Fungal infections: *Candida albicans*
Protozoan infections: *Plasmodium malariae*
Helminthic infections: *Schistosoma haematobium*, *Schistosoma mansoni*, *Onchocerca volvulus*
Drugs: insulin, penicillin, hydantoin, streptomycin, aminosalicylic acid, sulfonamides, thiazides, phenothiazines, vitamins, phenylbutazone, quinine, streptokinase, tamoxifen, anti-influenza-vaccine, oral contraceptive, serum
Chemicals: insecticides, petroleum products
Foodstuff allergens: milk proteins, gluten

Table 2 Cutaneous necrotizing vasculitis (CNV): association with coexisting diseases

CNV associated with chronic diseases
Systemic lupus erythematous
Sjögren's syndrome
Rheumatoid arthritis
Behçet's disease
Hyperglobulinemic states
Cryoglobulinemia
Bowel bypass syndrome
Ulcerative colitis
Cystic fibrosis
Primary biliary cirrhosis
HIV seropositivity and acquired immunodeficiency syndrome
CNV associated with malignant neoplasms
a) Lymphoproliferative disorders
    Hodgkin's disease
    Mycosis fungoides
    Lymphosarcoma
    Adult T-cell leukemia
    Multiple myeloma
b) Solid tumors
    Lung cancer
    Colon carcinoma
    Renal cancer
    Prostate cancer
    Head and neck cancer
    Breast cancer

and hematemesis[10,13–15]. Acute focal or diffuse glomerulonephritis may occur and microscopic hematuria and proteinuria are a constant feature[13]. Progression to acute and chronic renal failure has

Table 3 Idiopathic cutaneous necrotizing vasculitis

Henoch–Schönlein purpura
Urticarial vasculitis
Erythema elevatum diutinum
Nodular vasculitis
Livedoid vasculitis
Atrophie blanche
Cutaneous polyarteritis nodosa

been reported[10,14]. Central nervous system involvement may occur as headaches and diplopia[14]. Direct immunofluorescence studies show deposits of immunoglobulins (IgA)[10], complement components (C3, C5) and fibrin within vessel walls[16,17].

Urticarial vasculitis

This chronic recurrent disorder is a leukocytoclastic form of CNV that usually occurs in young adult women. The clinical presentation is that of pruritic reddish wheals or elevated erythema and occasionally petechiae[18–24]. The eruption persists for 24 hours or more, in contrast with the common urticarial lesion which disappears within 24 hours[18–24]. The disease may present with atypical erythema multiforme or angioedema. This form of CNV may be associated with low grade fever, arthralgia, abdominal pain, uveitis, renal disease, polylymphadenopathy and obstructive pulmonary disease. The course of the disease is chronic[18–24]. Laboratory findings show elevated erythrocyte sedimentation rate, hypocomplementemia with depressed CH_{50}, C1q, C4 or C2, blood eosinophilia and leukocytosis. Occasional cases have antinuclear antibodies, rheumatoid factor or cryoglobulins[18–24]. This CNV may be observed in patients with infections, serum sickness, systemic lupus erythematosus and Sjögren's syndrome. Recently urticarial vasculitic has also been reported in association with monoclonal IgM gammopathy. This last association, Schnitzler's syndrome, is usually benign, even though a progression to lymphoplasmocytic maligancy has been observed[25,26]. In addition it has been reported as a variant (perhaps a new vasculitic entity) of the Muckle–Wells syndrome (recurrent urticaria, fever, deafness and renal amyloidosis) in which the histological pattern of skin lesions shows deposits of amyloid in the eccrine sweat glands and CNV[25,27].

Erythema elevatum diutinum

This is a rare disorder, more common in females. Clinically the most prominent skin lesions are nonpurpuric persistent erythematous papules localized on the extensor surface of the extremities. The lesions are often accompanied by arthralgias (in about 40% of cases) and drug intolerance. It has been suggested that the cause of this disorder might be an allergic reaction to streptococcal superantigens. The histology usually shows a pattern of leukocytoclastic vasculitis and the course is quite chronic. Sometimes lesions heal spontaneously[1–6,25,28–30].

Nodular vasculitis

Most commonly observed in females, this disorder is evident on the lower and upper extremities. The lesions, very similar to those of erythema nodosum, are nodules and plaques from 2 to 10 cm in diameter. Necrosis and ulceration may occur. The contusiform appearance of erythema nodosum is always lacking. Histopathology reveals a mixed neutrophilic and lymphocytic vasculitis. The course of the illness tends to be chronic[1–6,25].

Livedoid vasculitis

This disorder is characterized by a flat network of intersecting bluish-red lines, with a predilection for distribution on the legs, upper arms and lower trunk. Ulceration is rare. Livedoid vasculitis may be associated with cutaneous cholesterol embolism, systemic lupus erythematosus, cryoglobulinemia and cerebrovascular disease. This last association, Sneddon's syndrome, is characterized by livedoid vasculitis and hemiplegia, aphasia and hemianopsia[1–6,31,32].

Atrophie blanche

This disorder most commonly presents in adult women, occurring on the ankles and dorsa of the feet. Two phases of the disease are distinguishable: the first consists of purpuric macules and papules, the later in white atrophic areas, which develop painful ulcerations. Many patients also have livedo reticularis[1–6,33].

Cutaneous polyarteritis nodosa

The skin lesions, localized most frequently on the lower extremities, consist of a red, blanchable livedo pattern with papules or nodules. Cutaneous ulcerations are often present. In some instances arthralgia, myalgias and fever can occur. This rare disorder usually follows a long-term, benign course with frequent relapses[1–6,34].

HISTOPATHOLOGY

Two main cellular patterns of CNV are described: a leukocytoclastic form (with preponderance of neutrophils over lymphocytes) and a lymphocytic form (in which lymphocytes are predominant over neutrophils)[35].

The leukocytoclastic form is characterized by angiocentric segmental inflammation, endothelial cell swelling, fibrinoid necrosis of blood vessel walls (post-capillary venules), and cellular infiltrate around and within dermal blood vessels walls composed largely of neutrophils showing fragmentation of nuclei (karyorrhexis or leukocytoclasia) and lymphocytes. Frequently there is erythrocyte extravasation (Figure 4). Thrombosis of the affected post-capillary venules and hyalinization of blood vessel walls may be observed in the late phase of the disease[35–37].

In contrast with leukocytoclastic vasculitis, for the lymphocytic form the criteria for histopathologic diagnosis are not yet well defined. In this case, the post-capillary venules of the upper dermis show endothelial cell swelling and fibrin deposition, and a cellular infiltrate, composed largely of lymphocytes, macrophages and extravasation of red cells, is found in the vicinity both of the venules and of the capillaries[35–37].

This histopathological subdivision is not watertight. Thus, in the late phase of leukocytoclastic CNV, the number of neutrophils may be decreased and the number of lymphocytes increased with possible overlap in the histologic patterns[38–41].

PATHOGENESIS

Traditionally on the basis of the histological patterns, two major forms of CNV are recognized[7]. First is a leukocytoclastic form in which, as in the Arthus reaction, it has been suggested that the deposition of circulating immune complexes, in moderate antigen excess, initiates the vasculitic process[37,42,43]. In this case, immunofluorescence and ultrastructural studies have documented immunoglobulins (IgG, IgM, IgA), complement components (C1q, C3) and fibrin deposits within post-capillary venule walls[1–6,44,45].

The deposited immune complexes serve to activate the classic and alternative complement pathways[1–6,46,47]. The activation of the complement cascade by immune complexes results in the production of the C3a and C5a anaphylatoxins which in turn degranulate mast cells[1–6,46,47]. In addition these mediators attract polymorphonuclear leukocytes to the lesional area. During this process,

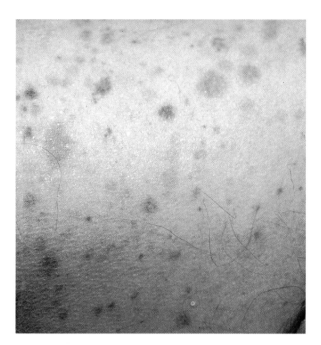

Figure 1 Cutaneous necrotizing vasculitis: palpable purpura

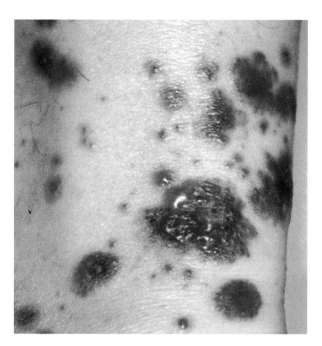

Figure 3 Cutaneous necrotizing vasculitis: hemorrhagic vesicles

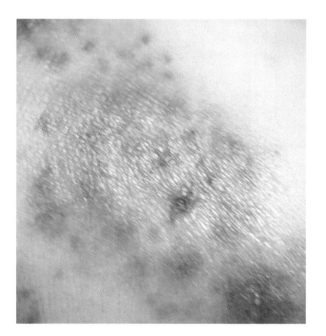

Figure 2 Cutaneous necrotizing vasculitis: wheals

circulating polymorphonuclear leukocytes become adherent to the endothelial cells and subsequently migrate into the surrounding connective tissue where they may act as phagocytes and degrade the immune complexes[1-6]. At the same time, polymorphonuclear leukocytes disintegrate and release different lysosomal enzymes (protease, collagenase, elastase, etc.) which may damage the endothelium[46]. Another way in which polymorphonuclear leukocytes damage the endothelium is

by the production of oxygen free radicals, which in presence of Fe^{2+} radicals results in especially serious consequences[1-6].

Clinical experience indicates that immunoreactants are detectable only in the early lesions (3–12 h)[1-6,44-48]. The entire chain of events from initial immune complexes and complement deposition to removal usually requires about 18–24 hours[1-6,44-48]. The synthesis and expression of a variety of surface adhesion molecules occurs on the endothelial cells, which mediate adhesion of these cells to endothelium[1-6]. Thus the 'selectins', platelet activation dependent granule external membrane protein (PADGEMP or GMP 140), endothelial leukocyte adhesion molecule-1 (ELAM-1) and the mouse lymph node homing receptor (gp90, or Mel-14 antigen), mediate the migration of neutrophils at the sites of inflammation[1-6,49-56].

The other major form of CNV is the lymphomonocytic form, in the pathogenesis of which cell-mediated immunologic mechanisms have been notoriously implicated[37], and where the cellular infiltrate consists almost entirely of T lymphocytes and dendritic cells. The majority of dermal infiltrating cells react with anti-CD4 and anti-CD1a monoclonal antibodies which stain, respectively, helper/inducer T lymphocytes and Langerhans cells/indeterminate cells (Figure 5)[57-65]. It has been suggested that the movement of lymphocytes in the vasculitic skin concentrates upon high endothelial venules, which are specialized segments of post-capillary venules, where lymphocytes selectively

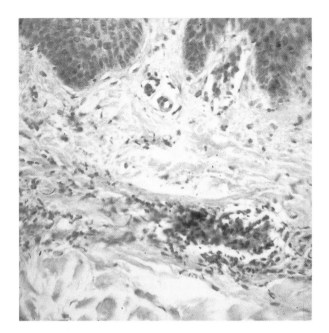

Figure 4 Histopathologic picture of leukocytoclastic vasculitis in small vessels

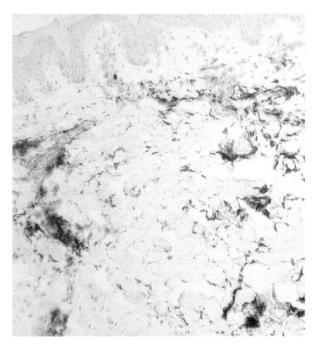

Figure 5 Lymphomonocytic form of cutaneous necrotizing vasculitis. The majority of dermal infiltrating cells react with anti-CD4 monoclonal antibodies which stain helper/inducer T lymphocytes

leave the circulation to enter perivascular tissues[49,66]. The recruitment of lymphocytes, which represents the first step in the pathogenesis of the disease, begins with their initial binding to endothelial cells[49]. Intercellular adhesion molecule (ICAM)-1 and ICAM-2 as well as leukocyte function associated antigen-1 (LFA-1) are involved in leukocyte–endothelial cell interactions[67–69]. After the induction of T-cell activation by dendritic cells, the activated T-cells release different amounts of a variety of cytokines, such as interleukin 2, interferon γ and tumor necrosis factor α, which could contribute to maintaining the vasculitic process. Immunofluorescence studies performed on lymphocytic vasculitis are generally negative. Only rarely are traces of immunoglobulin IgM present around the injured venules[37,70]. In some cases the infiltrate progressively changes from a preponderance of neutrophils to a predominance of lymphocytes, suggesting the dynamic nature of the vasculitic process and supporting the participation, also, of a secondary cell-mediated immune response in the late phase of the leukocytoclastic form, possibly owing to the expression of 'not self' antigens, consequent to the release of lysosomal proteolytic enzymes by polymorphonuclear leukocytes. On the basis of this latter hypothesis, the different histologic patterns could be mainly due to differences in the timing of the biopsies[39–41].

The fibrinolytic system is a physiologic process which effects the degradation of insoluble polymer fibrin into the soluble fibrin degradation products (FDP)[71–79]. This system is part of a complex mechanism which regulates the equilibrium between fibrinosynthesis and fibrinolysis[71–79], a balance which is a consequence of the activity of the inhibitors (plasminogen activator inhibitors (PAI)-1 and PAI-2, and antiplasmins) and activators (tissue type plasminogen activator (t-PA), M_r 74 000 and urokinase (u-PA), M_r 55 000) of fibrinolysis[71–79].

Cutaneous fibrinolytic activity is usually increased in the early form of CNV (characterized clinically by urticarial wheals), while it is reduced or absent in the late phase (clinically manifested by palpable purpura). This may lead to microvascular thrombosis, because of excessive intraperivascular deposition of fibrin, with consequent tissue hypoxia and necrosis[80]. Gamma/delta T lymphocytes and heat shock proteins have been widely represented in cases of CNV with documented infective etiology. This aspect might furnish, if supported by further studies, a clue to the infective etiology of CNV[81–92].

LABORATORY FINDINGS

In patients with CNV a laboratory screening is always required for confirmation of the diagnosis and pathogenesis and to determine the extent of systemic vasculitis involvement and/or the existence of underlying associated diseases. Laboratory evaluation includes histopathological and immunofluorescence studies and blood and urine analysis[1–6,8,10,11].

In the leukocytoclastic form, direct immunofluorescence may show immunoglobulins, complement components and fibrin deposits in and around the blood vessels; IgG rather than IgM are more likely to be present when there is an underlying collagen vascular disease, and IgA may be indicative of the Henoch–Schönlein purpura[1–6,8,10,11]. Decreased levels of complement components are often noted in leukocytoclastic CNV associated with rheumatoid arthritis (C1, C4, C2), systemic lupus erythematosus (C1q, C4, C2, C3, factor B, C9), cryoglobulinemia and Sjögren's syndrome. Circulating immune complexes, rheumatoid factor, antinuclear antibodies, antiphospholipid antibodies and cryoglobulins can be detected with antistreptolysin antibodies and hepatitis B (C and A) surface antigens. Urine analysis may reveal proteinuria, hematuria and cylindruria caused by possible renal involvement[1–6,8,10,11]. In the lymphocytic form of CNV these laboratory tests are usually normal[1–6,40,93,94].

TREATMENT

When possible, identification and removal of the causative agents (drugs, chemicals, infections, food, for example) is the etiological treatment, and this is followed by rapid clearance of the skin lesions, so that no other treatment is necessary. In other cases, local and systemic therapies are recommended[1–6,8,10,11].

Local treatments

Topical therapy (corticosteroid creams, antibiotic creams) may be helpful in some cases[1–6,95].

General treatments

These include:

(1) corticosteroids;
(2) nonsteroidal anti-inflammatory drugs;
(3) antimalarial agents;
(4) dapsone;
(5) potassium iodide;
(6) antihistamines;
(7) fibrinolytic agents;
(8) aminocaproic acid;
(9) immunosuppressive agents;
(10) monoclonal antibodies[1–6,8,10,11,96,97].

A systemic treatment with corticosteroids (prednisone 60–80 mg/day) is advised in the majority of patients for 7–15 days in the acute phase (especially in Henoch–Schönlein purpura, urticarial vasculitis and Behçet's disease)[1–6,8,10,11,96]. Nonsteroidal anti-inflammatory drugs such as acetylsalicylic acid and indomethacin have been used for vasculitis with more persistent or necrotic lesions. Some cases of urticarial vasculitis have responded to indomethacin[3,19]. Phenylbutazone, oxyphenbutazone and ibuprofen are indicated for thrombophlebitis in the course of nodular vasculitis[1–6,96,98]. Antimalarials such as oral colchicine, which inhibits neutrophil chemotaxis, in doses of 0.6 mg twice daily, may be helpful in the chronic forms of the disease[1–6]. Dapsone (50–200 mg/day) has also been used, usually in patients with skin involvement alone (especially in patients with erythema elevatum diutinum)[1–6,96,99]. Potassium iodide (0.3–1.5 g four times daily) is useful for nodular vasculitis[95]. H_1 antihistamines alone or in combination with H_2 antihistamines are used to alleviate the pruritus and to block histamine-induced endothelial gap formation with resultant trapping of immune complexes[1–6]. Fibrinolytic agents can be used in patients in whom there is a reduction of plasma and/or cutaneous fibrinolytic activity. Stanozolol (5 mg twice daily), phenformin hydrochloride (50 mg twice daily) plus ethylestrenol (2 mg four times daily) can be used for about a year. Other fibrinolytic agents such as heparin (5000 units twice daily), mesoglycans (50–100 mg/day) and defibrotide (700 mg im/day) seem beneficial in various types of hypofibrinolytic vasculitis[1–6,96,100,101]. Low molecular weight dextran is also indicated in the hypofibrinolytic phase of the disease. It seems to produce beneficial effects both in livedo reticularis and in livedoid vasculitis[1–6,96,102]. Aminocaproic acid (8–16 g/day for many months) can be used in the hyperfibrinolytic states[1–6,96,103]. Immunosuppressive agents such as cyclophosphamide (2 mg/kg/day), methotrexate (10–25 mg/week), azathioprine (150 mg/day) and cyclosporin A (3–5 mg/kg/day) are effective especially in patients with CNV (with a rapidly progressing course or with systemic involvement) which is not controlled by corticosteroids[1–6,96,97].

Recently a patient with intractable systemic vasculitis has been treated with two monoclonal antibodies, Campath-1H and rat CD4[97].

In the course of vasculitis induced by immune complexes, with concomitant arterial disease, drugs reducing platelet aggregation (dypyridamole, acetylsalicylic acid, tiklid) and plasmapheresis can be used[1–6,96]. The correction of local factors such as trauma, cold stasis and lymphedema may also be important[95].

REFERENCES

1. Lotti T, Ghersetich I, Comacchi C, Jorizzo JL. Cutaneous small-vessel vasculitis. *J Am Acad Dermatol* 1998;39:667–87

2. Lotti T, Ghersetich I, Comacchi C, Panconesi E. Purpuras and related conditions. *J Eur Acad Dermatol Venereol* 1996;7:1–25

3. Lotti T, Comacchi C, Ghersetich I. Cutaneous necrotizing vasculitis. *Int J Dermatol* 1996;35:457–74

4. Comacchi C, Ghersetich I, Lotti T. La vasculite necrotizzante cutanea. *G Ital Dermatol Venereol* 1998;133:23–49

5. Ryan TJ. Cutaneous vasculitis. In Rook A, Wilkinson DS, Ebling FJG, eds. *Textbook of Dermatology.* Oxford: Blackwell Scientific, 1992:1893–961

6. Braun-Falco O, Plewig G, Wolff HH, *et al. Dermatology.* Berlin: Springer-Verlag, 1991:620–3

7. Resnick AH, Esterly NB. Vasculitis in children. *Int J Dermatol* 1985;24:139–46

8. Lynch PJ. Vascular reactions. In Schachner LA, Hansen RC, eds. *Pediatric Dermatology.* New York: Churchill Livingstone Inc, 1988:959–1014

9. Soter NA, Wolff SM. Necrotizing vasculitis. In Fitzpatrick TB, Eisen AZ, Wolff K, *et al.*, eds. *Dermatology in General Medicine.* New York: McGraw-Hill, 1987:1300–12

10. Habif TP. *Clinical Dermatology.* St Louis: The CV Mosby Company, 1990:453–71

11. Schifferli JA, Saurat JH, Woodley DT. Cutaneous vasculitis. In Ruiz-Maldonado R, Parish LC, Beare JM, eds. *Textbook of Pediatric Dermatology.* Philadelphia: Grune & Stratton, 1989:654–61

12. Chan LS, Cooper KD, Rasmussen JE. Koebnerization as a cutaneous manifestation of immune complex-mediated vasculitis. *J Am Acad Dermatol* 1990;22:775–81

13. Saulsbury FT. Henoch–Schöenlein purpura. *Pediatr Dermatol* 1984;1:195–201

14. Paller AS. Disorders of the immune system. In Schachner LA, Hansen RC, eds. *Pediatric Dermatology.* New York: Churchill Livingstone Inc, 1988:93–137

15. Heng MCY. Henoch–Schöenlein purpura. *Br J Dermatol* 1985;112:235–40

16. VanHale HM, Gibson LE, Schroeter AL. Henoch–Schöenlein vasculitis: direct immunofluorescence study of uninvolved skin. *J Am Acad Dermatol* 1986;15:665–70

17. Stevenson JA, Leong LA, Cohen AH, *et al.* Henoch–Schönlein purpura. Simultaneous demonstration of IgA deposits in involved skin, intestine, and kidney. *Arch Pathol* 1982;106:192–5

18. Soter NA. Chronic urticaria as a manifestation of necrotizing venulitis. *N Engl J Med* 1977;296:1440–2

19. Wanderer AA, Nuss DD, Thormey AD, *et al.* Urticarial leukocytoclastic vasculitis with cold urticarial: report of a case and review of the literature. *Arch Dermatol* 1983;119:145–51

20. Monroe EF. Urticarial vasculitis: an update review. *J Am Acad Dermatol* 1981;5:88–95

21. Callen JP, Kalbfleisch S. Urticarial vasculitis: a report of nine cases and review of the literature. *Br J Dermatol* 1982;107:87–94

22. Scherer R. Urtikariavaskulitis. *Hautarzt* 1985;36(suppl VII):48–50

23. McDuffie FC, Sams WM Jr, Maldonado JE, *et al.* Hypocomplementemia with cutaneous vasculitis and arthritis: possible immune complex syndrome. *Mayo Clin Proc* 1973;48:340–8

24. Sanchez NP, Winkelmann RK, Schroeter AL, *et al.* The clinical and histopathologic spectrums of urticarial vasculitis: a study of forty cases. *J Am Acad Dermatol* 1982;7:599–605

25. Campanile G, Lotti T. Clinical aspects of cutaneous necrotizing vasculitis. *Int Angiol* 1995;14:151–61

26. Borradori L, Rybojad M, Pussant A, *et al.* Urticarial vasculitis associated with monoclonal IgM gammopathy: Schnitzler's syndrome. *Br J Dermatol* 1990;123:113–18

27. Grassegger A, Greil R, Feichtinger J, *et al.* Urticarial vasculitis as a symptom of Muckle–Wells syndrome? *Hautarzt* 1991;42:116–19

28. Cream JJ, Leven GM, Calnan CD. Erythema elevatum diutinum. *Br J Dermatol* 1971;84:393–9

29. Le Boit PE, Yen TSB, Wintroub B. The evolution of lesions in erythema elevatum diutinum. *Am J Dermatopathol* 1986;8:392–402

30. Wolff HH, Scherer R, Maciejewski W, *et al.* Erythema elevatum diutinum. II. Immunoelectromicroscopical study of leukocytoclastic vasculitis within the intracutaneous test reaction induced by streptococcal antigen. *Arch Dermatol Res* 1978;261:17–26

31. Feldacker M, Hines EA, Kierland RR. Livedo reticularis with summer ulcerations. *Arch Dermatol Syphilol* 1955;72:31–7

32. Marsch WC, Muckelmann R. Generalized racemose livedo with cerebrovascular lesions (Sneddon syndrome): an occlusive arteriolopathy due to proliferation and migration of medial smooth muscle cells. *Br J Dermatol* 1985;112:703–8

33. Braun Falco O, Plewig G, Wolff HH, *et al. Dermatology.* Berlin: Springer-Verlag, 1991:637–8

34. Diaz-Perez J, Winkelmann RK. Cutaneous periarteritis nodosa. *Arch Dermatol* 1974;110:407–12

35. Savel PH, Perroud AM, Klotz-Levy B, *et al.* Vasculite leucocytoclastique et lymphocytarie des petits vaisseaux cutanés. *Ann Dermatol Venereol (Paris)* 1982;109:503–12

36. Lever WF, Schaumburg-Lever G. *Histopathology of the Skin.* Philadelphia: JB Lippincott, 1990:188–92

37. Smoller BR, McNutt S, Contreras F. The natural history of vasculitis. *Arch Dermatol* 1990;126:84–9

38. Ghersetich I, Campanile G, Comacchi C, *et al.* The cell-mediated pathway in the pathogenesis of the leukocytoclastic form of cutaneous necrotizing

vasculitis. Presented at *Dermatology 2000*, Vienna, 18–21 May 1993;271

39. Ghersetich I, Campanile G, Comacchi C, *et al.* Cutaneous necrotizing vasculitis: are there indeed two distinct histopathological entities? Presented at the *14th Colloquium of the International Society of Dermopathology*, Siena, 26 June–1 July 1993;86

40. Zax RH, Hodge SJ, Callen JP. Cutaneous leukocytoclastic vasculitis; serial histopathologic evaluation demonstrates the dynamic nature of the infiltrate. *Arch Dermatol* 1990;126:69–72

41. Gower RG, Sams WM Jr, Thorne EG, *et al.* Leukocytoclastic vasculitis: sequential appearance of immunoreactants and cellular changes in serial biopsies. *J Invest Dermatol* 1977;69:477–84

42. Dixon FJ, Vazquez JJ, Wiegle WO, *et al.* Pathogenesis of serum sickness. *Arch Pathol Lab Med* 1958;65:18–28

43. Mackel SE, Jordon RE. Leukocytoclastic vasculitis: a cutaneous expression of immune complex disease. *Arch Dermatol* 1982;118:296–301

44. Cream JJ, Bryceson ADM, Ryder G. Disappearance of immunoglobulin and complement from the Arthus reaction and its relevance to studies of vasculitis in man. *Br J Dermatol* 1971;84:106–9

45. Braverman IM, Yen A. Demonstration of immune complexes in spontaneous and histamine-induced lesions and in normal skin of patients with leukocytoclastic vasculitis. *J Invest Dermatol* 1975;64:105–12

46. Tosca N, Stratigos JD. Possible pathogenetic mechanisms in allergic cutaneous vasculitis. *Int J Dermatol* 1988;27:291–6

47. Yancey KB, Lawley TJ. Circulating immune complexes: their immunochemistry, biology and detection in selected dermatologic and systemic diseases. *J Am Acad Dermatol* 1984;10:711

48. Cochrane GG. Mediators of the Arthus and related reactions. *Prog Allergy* 1967;11:1–35

49. Lotti T, Campanile G, Ghersetich I, *et al.* Endothelium–blood cells interactions in thrombosis. In Neri Serneri GG, eds. *Thrombosis: an Update.* Florence: Scientific Press, 1992:669–93

50. Bevilacqua MP, Stengelin S, Gimbrone MA, *et al.* ELAM-1: an inducible receptor for neutrophils related to complement regulatory proteins and lectins. *Science* 1989;243:1160–4

51. Bevilacqua MP, Pober JS, Mendrick DL, *et al.* Identification of an inducible endothelial-leukocyte adhesion molecule. *Proc Natl Acad Sci USA* 1987;84:9238–42

52. Picker LJ, Kishimoto TK, Smith CW, *et al.* ELAM-1 is an adhesion molecule for skin-homing T cells. *Nature (London)* 1991;349:737–8

53. Leeuwenberg JFM, Jeunhomme TMAA, Burman WA. Role of ELAM-1 in adhesion of monocytes to activated human endothelial cells. *Scand J Immunol* 1992;35:335–41

54. Larsen E, Celi A, Gilbert GE, *et al.* PADGEM protein: a receptor that mediates the interaction of activated platelets with neutrophils and monocytes. *Cell* 1989;59:305–12

55. Johnston GI, Cook RG, McEver RP. Cloning of GMP-140, a granule membrane protein of platelets and endothelium: sequence similarity to proteins involved in cell adhesion and inflammation. *Cell* 1989;56:1033–44

56. Jutila MA, Rott L, Berg EL, *et al.* Function and regulation of the neutrophil Mel-14 antigen *in vivo*: comparison with LFA-1 and Mac-1. *J Immunol* 1989;143:3318–24

57. Soter NA, Mihm MC Jr, Gigli I, *et al.* Two distinct cellular patterns in cutaneous necrotizing angiitis. *J Invest Dermatol* 1976;66:344–50

58. Ghersetich I, Comacchi C, Lotti T. Vasculiti necrotizzanti cutanee: caratterizzazione dell'infiltrato cellulare ed espressione di alcune molecole di adesione. Presented at *Incontri Colombiani della Riviera*, Sanremo, 24–26 April 1992;103

59. Ghersetich I, Lotti T, Campanile G, *et al.* Lymphocytes and accessory cells in the infiltrate of leukocytoclastic vasculitis. Presented at *SCUR Meet*, Lyon, 17–19 September 1992;94

60. Ghersetich I, Comacchi C, Lotti T. La vasculite cutanée nécrosante: l'infiltrat cellulaire et l'expression de quelques récepteurs de molécules d'adhesion. *Nouv Dermatol* 1992;11:852–3

61. Ghersetich I, Campanile G, Comacchi C, *et al.* Immunohistochemical and ultrastructural aspects of leukocytoclastic cutaneous necrotizing vasculitis (CNV). *J Invest Dermatol* 1993;1004:545

62. Fauci AS, Haynes BF. The spectrum of vasculitis: clinical, pathologic and therapeutic considerations. *Ann Intern Med* 1978;80:660–76

63. Tosca A, Hatzis J, Kyriakis K, *et al.* Delayed hypersensitivity and differences of histologic pattern in allergic cutaneous vasculitis. *Angiology* 1988;39:360–4

64. Lotti T, Ghersetich I, Comacchi C, *et al.* Immunophenotype and ultrastructure of infiltrate in the lymphocytic form of 'Cutaneous Necrotizing Vasculitis'. Presented at *EADV 2nd Congress*, Athens, Greece, 10–13 October 1991;204

65. Campanile G, Ghersetich I, Comacchi C, *et al.* Studio immunoistochimico e ultrastrutturale dell'infiltrato nelle vasculiti necrotizzanti cutanee linfocitarie. *G Ital Dermatol Venereol* 1992;127:337–41

66. Marchesi VT, Gowans JL. The migration of lymphocytes through the endothelium of venules in lymph node. *Proc R Soc Lond* 1964;159:283–92

67. Cagnoni ML, Ghersetich I, Lotti T. Cell adhesion molecules in inflammatory and neoplastic skin diseases. *J Eur Acad Dermatol Venereol* 1993;2:94–112

68. Makgoba MW, Sanders ME, Ginter Luce GE, *et al.* Functional evidence that intercellular adhesion

molecule-1 (ICAM-1) is a ligand for LFA-1 dependent adhesion in T cell-mediated cytotoxicity. *Eur J Immunol* 1988;18:637–40

69. Staunton DE, Dustin ML, Springer TA. Function cloning of ICAM-2, a cell adhesion ligand for LFA-1 homologous to ICAM-1. *Nature* 1989;339:61–4

70. Clayton R, Haffenden G. An immunofluorescence study of pityriasis lichenoides. *Br J Dermatol* 1978; 99:491–3

71. Lotti T, Dindelli A, Barontini A, *et al.* Fibrin deposits and fibrinolytic activity in certain dermatoses with immunological pathogenesis. *Ital Gen Rev Dermatol* 1979;2–3:189

72. Fabbri P, Lotti T, Dindelli A, *et al.* Studio della fibrinolisi tissutale e plasmatica nella vasculite necrotizzante cutanea. *Ann Ital Dermatol Clin Sper* 1981; 35:347–54

73. Bianchini G, Lotti T, Fabbri P. Fibrin deposits and fibrinolytic activity in Schönlein–Henoch syndrome. *Int J Dermatol* 1983;22:103–6

74. Ryan TJ. *Inflammation, Fibrin and Fibrinolysis in the Physiology and Pathophysiology of the Skin*, vol II. London and New York: Academic Press, 1973

75. Lotti T, Fabbri P, Panconesi E. Cutaneous fibrinolytic activity in urticaria and vasculitis. In Champion RHEA, ed. *The Urticarias.* Edinburgh: Churchill-Livingstone, 1985:161–4

76. Panconesi E, Lotti T. Fibrinolysis and fibrinolytic drugs. In Greaves MW, eds. *Handbook of Experimental Pharmacology.* Berlin: Springer-Verlag, 1989: 279–300

77. Jordan JM, Bates Allen N, Pizzo SV. Defective release of tissue plasminogen activator in systemic and cutaneous vasculitis. *Am J Med* 1987;82: 397–400

78. Lotti T, Dindelli A, Fabbri P. Cutaneous fibrinolysis: a modified method of autohistographic identification of plasminogen activators in tissue. Technical note. *Ital Gen Rev Dermatol* 1980;17:157–60

79. Lotti T, Brunetti L, Casigliani R, *et al.* A new technique for detecting inhibitors of fibrinolysis in skin section. Technical note. *Ital Gen Rev Dermatol* 1983;20:105–9

80. Teofoli P, Lotti T. Cytokines, fibrinolysis and vasculitis. *Int Angiol* 1995;14:125–9

81. Bröker B, Lydyard PM, Emmrich F. The role of gamma/delta T cells in the normal and disordered immune system. *Klin Wochenschr* 1990;68:489–94

82. Alaibac M. Gamma/delta T-lymphocytes: relevance of the current studies to dermatology. *Int J Dermatol* 1992;31:157–9

83. Comacchi C, Ghersetich I, Lotti T. Una cellula emergente in dermatologia: il linfocita T gamma/delta. *G Ital Dermatol Venereol* 1993;128: 133–40

84. Campanile G, Comacchi C. Gamma/delta TCR lymphocytes in cutaneous necrotizing vasculitis. *Int Angiol* 1995;14:119–24

85. Groh V, Porcelli S, Fabbi M, *et al.* Human lymphocytes bearing T-cell receptors gamma/delta are phenotypically diverse and evenly distributed throughout the lymphoid system. *J Exp Med* 1989; 169:1277–94

86. Janeway CA, Jones B, Hayday A. Specificity and function of T cell bearing gamma/delta receptors. *Immunol Today* 1988;9:73–5

87. Born WK, Happ MP, Dallas A, *et al.* Recognition of heat shock proteins and gamma/delta cell function. *Immunol Today* 1990;11:40–3

88. Holoshitz J, Koning F, Coligan JE, *et al.* Isolation of CD4- CD8- mycobacteria-reactive T lymphocyte clones from rheumatoid arthritis synovial fluid. *Nature* 1989;339:226–9

89. Ghersetich I, Campanile G, Comacchi C, *et al.* T lymphocytes bearing gamma/delta receptors: a clue to the etiology of cutaneous necrotizing vasculitis? Present at *XII Convegno di Immunopathologia Cutanea*, Genova, 9–10 October 1992;12

90. Ghersetich I, Campanile G, Comacchi C, *et al.* Gamma/delta TCR lymphocytes in cutaneous necrotizing vasculitis (CNV): a clue to the infective etiology. *J Invest Dermatol* 1993;100:465

91. Comacchi C, Ghersetich I, Campanile G, *et al.* Studio dei linfociti T gamma/delta nella vasculite cutanea necrotizzante leucocitoclasica. Presented at the *68th Congresso Nazionale della Società Italiana di Dermatologia e Venereologia*, Pisa, 23–26 June 1993;129

92. Ghersetich I, Campanile G, Comacchi C, *et al.* Gamma/delta TCR lymphocytes: a marker of cutaneous necrotizing venulitis with infective etiology? Presented at the *American Academy of Dermatology, 52nd Annual Meeting*, Washington DC, December 4–9, 1993

93. Alexander EL, Arnett FC, Provost TT, *et al.* Sjögren's syndrome: association of anti-Ro (SSA) antibodies with vasculitis, hematologic abnormalities, and serologic hyperreactivity. *Ann Intern Med* 1983;98:155–9

94. Molina R, Provost TT, Alexander EL. Two types of inflammatory vascular disease in Sjögren syndrome. *Arthritis Rheum* 1985;28:1251–8

95. Burge S. The management of cutaneous vasculitis. In Panconesi E, ed. *Dermatology in Europe.* Oxford: Blackwell Scientific, 1991:328–30

96. Lotti T. The management of systemic complications of vasculitis. In Panconesi E, ed. *Dermatology in Europe.* Oxford: Blackwell Scientific, 1991:330–2

97. Mathieson PW, Cobbold SP, Hale CG, *et al.* Monoclonal-antibody therapy in systemic vasculitis. *N Engl J Med* 1990;323:250–4

98. Ryan TJ. Microvascular injury. *Maj Probl Dermatol* 1976;7:373–405

99. Katz SI. Erythema elevatum diutinum. Skin and systemic manifestations, immunologic studies and successful treatment with dapsone. *Medicine* 1977;56:443–52

100. Van Vroonhoven TJMV, Van Zijl J, Muller H. Low dose subcutaneous heparin versus oral anticoagulants. *Lancet* 1974;2:375–84

101. Lotti T, Celasco G, Tsampau D, *et al*. Mesoglycan treatment restores defective fibrinolytic potential in cutaneous necrotizing venulitis. *Int J Dermatol* 1993;32:368–71

102. Isseroff SW, Whiting DA. Low molecular weight dextran in the treatment of livedo reticularis with ulceration. *Br J Dermatol* 1971;85:26–9

103. Haustein UF. Purpura hyperfibrinolytica als pathogenetisches prinzipieren hemorragieschen mikrobides miescher. *Dermatol Monatsscrift* 1969; 155:771–8

Cutaneous tumors

20

Elizabeth A. Spenceri, Dee Anna Glaser and Neal Penneys

INTRODUCTION

There are a significant number of cutaneous tumors that are of interest in the field of dermatology, including benign as well as malignant tumors. Additionally, cutaneous tumors can involve the epidermis, dermis, subcutaneous fat, vasculature, or nervous structures. It is noteworthy that these tumors can have a gender predilection or can present in a different fashion based on gender. We have reviewed many of these tumors and will discuss interesting nuances as they relate to gender differences. Although this is not an exhaustive collection, we describe many common as well as rare cutaneous tumors.

HIDRADENOMA PAPILLIFERUM

Hidradenoma papilliferum is a solitary, intradermal tumor that occurs only in postpubertal women. Although this tumor is commonly found on the vulva or in the perianal region, it can occur at other sites including the eyelid[1]. These tumors are usually asymptomatic and are frequently diagnosed during a gynecologic examination.

Histologically, hidradenoma papilliferum is located in the dermis. The cellular components of this tumor represent an adenoma with apocrine differentiation. This tumor is well circumscribed and may be surrounded by a fibrous capsule or a keratinizing epithelial wall. It consists of single or multiple cystic spaces with papilliform projections. The cystic spaces are typically lined with a double layer of cells – an inner layer of columnar cells revealing eosinophilic nuclei and decapitation secretion, and an outer layer of basophilic cuboidal, myoepithelial cells[2,3]. Occasionally, only a single row of secretory cells lines the spaces.

This tumor is benign, although one case has been reported of a metastatic squamous cell carcinoma arising within a hidradenoma papilliferum[4]. Treatment is not required unless the patient is symptomatic with local pain, bleeding, or ulceration. Surgical excision is the treatment of choice.

SYRINGOMA

Syringoma presents as discrete, flesh- or yellow-colored, one to three millimeter papules on the eyelids and upper cheeks (Figure 1a). They occur more frequently in young women[5]. There are cases of multiple, 'eruptive' syringoma occurring on the neck, chest and abdomen[6]. Other variants include vulvar syringomas, a linear unilateral variant and a familial variant[7,8].

Syringoma is a tumor differentiating toward the intra-epidermal portion of eccrine ducts[9,10]. Histochemical studies of these tumors reveal a significant amount of succinic dehydrogenase and leucine aminopeptidase, which are enzymes produced primarily in the eccrine glands and ducts as opposed to apocrine glands[11,12]. Additionally, eccrine-specific monoclonal antibody EKH6 positively stains syringoma[13]. The tumor consists of multiple small cystic ducts and solid epithelial strands in the upper and mid-dermis embedded in a fibrous stroma. The cystic ducts are typically lined with two layers of cuboidal or flat cells and show no tendencies toward secretion. Frequently, the ducts are intimately associated with comma-like tails of epithelial cells yielding a tadpole-like appearance (Figure 1b). Syringoma are sometimes connected to intra-epidermal cystic ducts, but they are never connected to the secretory portions of glands. They may contain clear cells microscopically. In this clear-cell variant, the typical syringoma cells are present along with nests of glycogen-rich clear cells[14,15].

Syringomas are benign tumors that do not require treatment. For cosmetically significant lesions, the tumor can be treated with laser ablation, cryotherapy, or electrolysis[16]. Recurrences can occur.

TRICHILEMMAL CYST

Trichilemmal cysts, also known as pilar cysts or wens, are firm, keratin-filled dermal nodules of variable size. These cysts, which occur more frequently in women, are freely mobile from the underlying tissue[17-19]. Typically, they occur on the scalp; however, other body sites may be affected. They may clinically resemble epidermoid cysts, though trichilemmal cysts are usually multiple as opposed to solitary.

The etiology is unknown; however, there is strong evidence supporting an autosomal dominant mode of inheritance[20,21].

Trichilemmal cysts form within the walls of hair follicles and differentiate towards the outer root sheath[20]. The outermost layer of epithelial cells is pallisading. The innermost layer of epithelial cells appears swollen and has pale-staining cytoplasm, and the epithelium lacks a granular layer. Occasionally the monomorphic, eosinophilic cystic material may contain nuclear material as keratinization is abrupt from the inner layer of cells. Additionally, calcification occurs in approximately 25% of trichilemmal cysts[21].

If the cyst ruptures, a granulomatous or suppurative reaction may result. A proliferating trichilemmal cyst (pilar tumor) may develop from these lesions and undergo ulceration or fungating growth[20,21].

Trichilemmal cysts typically follow a benign course. However, if the cyst undergoes rapid enlargement, it may be a sign of malignancy[22]. Generally, no treatment is required for clinically benign trichilemmal cysts. For those cysts that are painful, cosmetically significant, prone to trauma, or undergo rapid enlargement, surgical excision is curative.

DESMOPLASTIC TRICHOEPITHELIOMA

Also known as sclerosing epithelial hamartoma, desmoplastic trichoepithelioma presents as a solitary, indurated nodule measuring less than one centimeter which typically occurs on the face of young women[23,24]. Clinically, they can resemble basal cell carcinoma with their raised, annular border and central dell.

Desmoplastic trichoepitheliomas are benign tumors originating from the hair follicle[23]. The three distinguishing histologic features of a desmoplastic trichoepithelioma are anastamosing strands of small, basaloid tumor cells (one to three cells thick), sclerosing stroma and horn cysts[25]. There may be foreign body granulomas near ruptured horn cysts, and calcification within these lesions is not uncommon. Mitosis is rare in these lesions. The horn cysts tend to exclude the diagnosis of basal cell carcinoma.

These lesions typically follow a benign course and, theoretically, no treatment is necessary. However, because of the previously mentioned difficulty in making a clinical and histological distinction between a desmoplastic trichoepithelioma and morpheaform basal cell carcinoma, conservative surgical excision of such lesions is recommended[26].

DERMATOFIBROMA

Dermatofibroma is a common, benign skin lesion with several names: nodular subepidermal fibrosis, dermatofibroma lenticulare, sclerosing hemangioma, fibroma durum, and histiocytoma. The multitude of names arises from the different histologic interpretations of this lesion.

Dermatofibroma usually presents as a solitary, firm nodule which is fixed to the skin but freely mobile over the underlying subcutaneous tissue. The color is variable from pink to red or brown, and occasionally more than one color is present (Figure 2a). While most dermatofibroma have a smooth surface, some are scaly and, rarely, some ulcerate following trauma. Although they can occur at any body site, they are most frequently found on the trunk or lower extremities[27]. The size is variable, but the majority of dermatofibromas measure 4 mm to 1 cm. Dermatofibromas typically present in young adults but can occur at any age, and women are more frequently affected[27].

Diagnosis is typically based upon clinical presentation. In most cases lateral compression of the nodule produces a central indentation. The exact etiology is unknown, but dermatofibromas are believed to result from minor trauma, such as insect bites.

Histologically, dermatofibromas are collections of fibrous tissue within the dermis. Whorls of spindle-shaped cells pervade the lesion, and the borders are ill-defined as the cells intermingle with adjacent collagen bundles (Figure 2b). The lesion often extends deep to the upper aspects of the subcutaneous fat. In most cases a thin layer of unaffected papillary dermis is present above the lesion, representing the grenz zone. Mitotic figures may be seen within the lesion, but they are rarely atypical. The epidermis may show changes such as acanthosis, pseudoepitheloid hyperplasia, hyperkeratosis, or basaloid proliferation.

There are several histologic variants of dermatofibroma. Some lesions are rich in histiocytes or foamy, lipid-laden cells. Others may have prominent deposition of hemosiderin or possess a vascular component, rich in endothelial-lined spaces[28].

The majority of dermatofibromas remain stable. In some instances the lesions may involute and resolve. Basal cell carcinomas have been reported in the epidermis overlying dermatofibromas[29,30].

No treatment is required for dermatofibromas; however, surgical excision may be warranted for lesions that are prone to repeated trauma. Cryotherapy may also be beneficial[31].

DESMOID TUMOR

Desmoid tumors are benign, locally-infiltrating masses of fibrous tissue arising from the muscular aponeurosis. They are generally non-tender and slow-growing but can achieve considerable size. The most common locations are the shoulder and the anterior abdominal wall. Desmoid tumors are more common in women, where they most frequently present on the rectus abdominus following pregnancy[32,33]. In addition to pregnancy, they can result from injury, develop within surgical scars, or arise *de novo* from any skeletal muscle[34]. Although desmoid tumors tend to be solitary, multiple desmoid tumors sometimes occur. Desmoid tumors are sometimes associated with Gardner's syndrome (a syndrome with autosomal dominant inheritance consisting of adenomatous polyps with a high risk of malignancy, multiple lipomas, fibromas, facial osteomas and multiple epidermal inclusion cysts) where they can manifest as retroperitoneal masses[35].

Desmoid tumors are composed of bundles of eosinophilic spindle cells interspersed with an abundance of collagen on a background of striated muscle. They are poorly circumscribed, and mitoses are rare. They can be locally invasive and can be fatal if they encroach upon vital organs. These tumors do not metastasize. Surgery is often difficult owing to the need for wide local excision to ensure elimination. Radiation therapy has been used as adjuvant therapy and often diminishes recurrence in lesions with positive surgical margins[36-38]. Pharmacotherapy with antiestrogens (eg. tamoxifen), medroxyprogesterone, goserelin acetate and prostaglandin inhibitors such as nonsteroidal anti-inflammatory agents can be considered as well[39].

GLOMUS TUMOR

Glomus tumors present as solitary, tender, bluish-colored tumors. Although they are most commonly located in the subungual region (Figure 3a), they can occur at any anatomic site. Those lesions occurring on the digits are more frequently found in women[40,41].

Glomus tumors are composed of glomus cells, which are specialized smooth muscle cells normally found in the area bridging arterioles and venules. These cells normally function to shunt blood, bypassing the capillary system. Histologically, the tumor is well circumscribed and is classified as one of three variants: solid, glomangioma and glomangiomyoma[42]. The solid glomus tumor is composed of varying amounts of glomus cells and vessels, though glomus cells predominate. These glomus cells have eosinophilic cytoplasm and plump, ovoid nuclei and contain smooth muscle actin, muscle-specific actin and myosin[43-45]. Mitotic figures may be present, but nuclear atypia is a rarity. The stroma surrounding the tumor may be edematous with myxoid change. Glomangioma contain a large percentage of thin-walled vascular spaces that are surrounded by a thin layer of glomus cells (Figure 3b). In glomangiomyoma, the glomus cells are intermingled with spindle-shaped smooth muscle cells near the central vascular spaces. There has been a report of an infiltrative variant, which reveals subcutaneous infiltration of glomus cells; the recurrence rate for this variant is high[46].

Glomus tumors typically follow a benign course. Treatment of choice is excision of the tumor.

FAMILIAL LEIOMYOMA CUTIS ET UTERI

This variant of leiomyomas consists of multiple leiomyomas found subcutaneously as well as within the uterus. It affects women and is transmitted in an autosomal dominant pattern[47]. Pain may be the predominant symptom, and it is often difficult to manage as surgical excision of all the smooth muscle tumors may not be feasible (Figure 4).

The cutaneous lesions are simply leiomyomas. Under histologic examination, they appear as haphazardly placed bundles of smooth muscle in the dermis.

Treatment is usually focused on managing the pain. Phenoxybenzamine or calcium channel blockers (eg. nifedipine) have been used, the latter of which relaxes smooth muscle[48,49].

ANGIOLEIOMYOMA

Angioleiomyoma presents as a solitary, often painful, subcutaneous nodule measuring up to 4 cm[50]. These lesions are more frequently found on the lower extremities of middle-aged women[51].

Histologically, the lesion is composed of an encapsulated mass of vessels. There are three subtypes: capillary, venous and cavernous. The capillary type reveals numerous small vascular channels. The venous type reveals thickened muscular walls lining the lumina; the smooth muscle cells extend

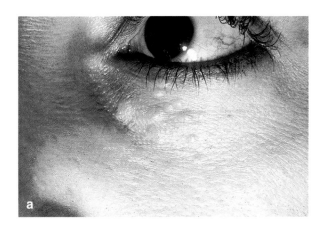

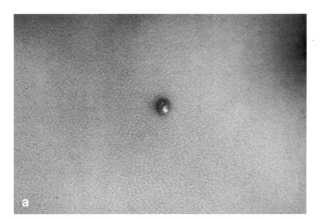

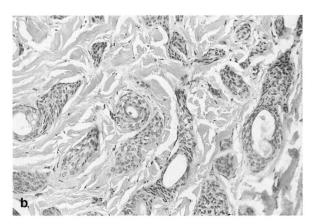

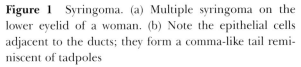

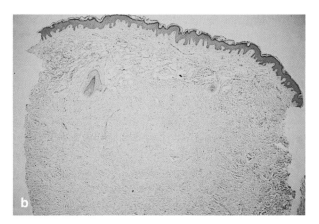

Figure 1   Syringoma. (a) Multiple syringoma on the lower eyelid of a woman. (b) Note the epithelial cells adjacent to the ducts; they form a comma-like tail reminiscent of tadpoles

Figure 2   Dermatofibroma. (a) A small, solitary, red-brown nodule on the back of a young girl. Courtesy of Elaine C. Siegfried, MD, St Louis, MO. (b) A collection of spindle cells in a whorled pattern is evident in the reticular and deep dermis. Note the grenz zone in the upper dermis

from the periphery of the veins and intermingle with the intervascular stroma. In the cavernous type, the vascular spaces are dilated with little smooth muscle.

Treatment consists of surgical excision for solitary, painful angioleiomyomas or those of cosmetic significance. Angioleiomyomas follow a benign course[51].

PYOGENIC GRANULOMA

A pyogenic granuloma (PG), also known as lobular capillary hemangioma, is a solitary, shiny red papule or nodule often with central ulceration; older lesions may be pedunculated. The moist-appearing surface resembles 'proud flesh' or exuberant granulation tissue. Initially, they undergo rapid growth over weeks to months, followed by a period of slow regression. They are commonly found on the extremities and face. They can also be found on the palms, soles, nails, or trunk. In pregnant women PGs are known as granuloma gravidarum (Figure 5a) and typically present on the gingiva[52]. PGs are seen more frequently in children than in adults.

Pyogenic granulomas were once thought to represent infection with obligatory granulomatous inflammation. Current opinion holds that PGs routinely develop at sites affected by trauma. It is believed that injury to the level of the dermis is necessary for development of this lesion; however, there have been cases of multiple PGs arising *de novo*[52]. Several variants exist including multiple PG, subcutaneous PG, and those occurring in dilated venous channels[52–56].

The lesion is characterized by an angiomatous mass that protrudes beyond the surrounding epidermis (Figure 5b). The vascular mass is typically lobulated and resembles a capillary hemangioma[57]. The overlying epidermis may be thinned and intact, or erosions and ulcerations may be present. In some histologic preparations a connection between the lesion and a neighboring vessel can be identified. Inflammatory cells may be present, particularly early in the development of the lesion, but are not essential to making the diagnosis of PG.

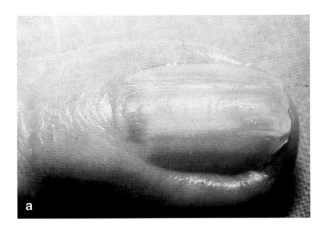

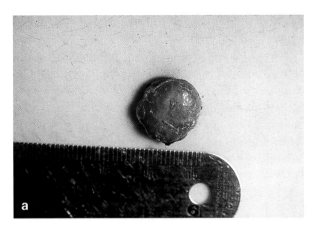

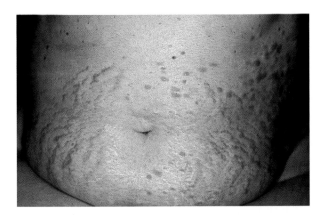

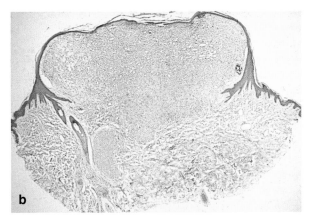

Figure 3   Glomus tumor. (a) A subungual, bluish nodule on the finger of a woman. (b) The specialized smooth muscle cells of the glomus tumor function to shunt blood. Here, a glomangioma reveals glomus cells in close association with thin-walled vascular spaces

Figure 5   Pyogenic granuloma. (a) A beefy-red, protuberant granulating papule on a pregnant woman (granuloma gravidarum). Courtesy of Elaine C. Siegfried, MD, St Louis, MO. (b) A collarette of epidermis surrounds the angiomatous mass

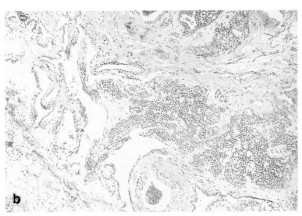

Figure 4   Multiple leiomyomata. A woman with multiple pink nodules across the abdomen in an interesting arrangement. Courtesy of Elaine C. Siegfried, MD, St Louis, MO

Pyogenic granulomas follow a benign course. Treatment generally consists of curettage or shave removal of the lesion followed by electrodesiccation of the base. Some lesions are recurrent (either as single lesions or as multiple PGs) and may require laser therapy or elliptical excision[58,59].

NEVUS ARANEUS

A nevus araneus is also referred to as spider angioma, spider nevus and vascular spider. It is essentially a solitary telangiectasia, though it often presents in multiple sites. Children, pregnant women, women on oral contraceptives and patients with hepatic disease are more frequently affected[60]. The lesion consists of a central arteriole, branching vessels and an area of surrounding erythema. It blanches under diascopy, and occasionally pulsations may be seen. Although there is no consensus, it is a common belief that these lesions are associated with a high estrogen state. Bean's early review of the relevant literature came to this conclusion[61]; however a more recent study, measuring the serum concentration of estrogens, has failed to support this[62].

Histologically, a dilated arteriole is seen in the reticular dermis. As it ascends, it branches into many dilated capillaries.

The nevus araneus of childhood may resolve with age. Those nevi associated with pregnancy also tend to gradually resolve post-partum. Nevi araneus of hepatic disease are more constant.

No treatment is required. For patients concerned about the appearance of individual lesions, electrodesiccation of the feeder arteriole or laser surgery of the lesion can be an effective treatment option[63]. Vascular lasers allow for more specific destruction of the vascular tissue compared to electrodesiccation and may result in fewer scars.

ANGIOKERATOMA OF MIBELLI

Angiokeratoma of Mibelli presents initially as individual pink papules. Progressively, the lesion takes on a dark red appearance and becomes more verrucous; the papules may even coalesce. Consequently, angiokeratoma of Mibelli has often been referred to as a 'telangiectatic wart'. Angiokeratoma of Mibelli is seen predominantly over bony prominences such as elbows, ankles, wrists, etc[64,65]. The disease is transmitted in an autosomal dominant manner and commonly presents in adolescent women[64,65].

Histologically, the lesion is characterized by acanthosis and compact hyperkeratosis; there are underlying dilated capillaries in the papillary dermis. Elongation of the rete ridges may be seen.

Angiokeratomas follow a benign course, although they may be cosmetically displeasing. Destruction via electrodesiccation, cryotherapy and laser ablation yields good results.

ANGIOMA SERPIGINOSUM

Angioma serpiginosum is a rare, asymptomatic, benign vascular lesion that can affect both sexes at any age, although up to 90% of all cases have been described in girls under the age of 16[66,67]. The lesions have a predilection for the extremities, where they present as red or violaceous punctate macules, often overlying a background of erythema or violaceous discoloration[68]. As the lesions progress, the macules develop into papules, especially at the borders. This, in addition to central involution, yields a netlike, serpiginous pattern.

The etiology is unknown, but one report noted that exposure to cold may be a precipitating cause[69]. Most cases are isolated, although familial cases of autosomal dominant inheritance have been reported[70].

Histologic examination reveals dilated capillaries in the dermal papillae and upper reticular dermis, either solitary or in a clustered configuration. The epidermis is typically unremarkable[71]. There is no associated inflammatory infiltrate or red blood cell extravasation. Neumann noted two cases where elongated epidermal rete pegs appeared to entrap dilated capillary proliferations[69].

Angioma serpiginosum can slowly progress to involve neighboring skin. It is typically a chronic condition. Spontaneous resolution of some lesions has been reported but is often incomplete[68].

BENIGN ANGIOENDOTHELIOMATOSIS

Benign (or 'reactive') angioendotheliomatosis is a rare vascular condition, sometimes associated with systemic infection like subacute bacterial endocarditis or pulmonary tuberculosis[72]. Additionally, it can be associated with paraproteinemia and cryoglobulinemia[72,73]. The individual lesions are composed of red to blue or brown, 1–5 cm, patches and plaques. Sites of predilection include the extremities, trunk, cheeks and ears, and the condition is more common in women[74].

Histologic examination reveals dilation and proliferation of vessels (particularly capillaries) in the dermis and subcutaneous tissue. The endothelial cells show marked proliferation as well and may narrow or occlude the lumina. Atypia may be present, especially within endothelial cells. In the cryoglobulin-associated lesion, refractile eosinophilic thrombi can be seen in the lumina.

Endothelial markers, including factor VIII-related antigen, blood group isoantigens, and *Ulex europaeus* I agglutinin, are reactive within these lesions[72]. However, the leukocyte common antigen marker is negative. These findings support the idea that the proliferating cells are endothelial in origin[72]. This also distinguishes the disease from the malignant angioendotheliomatosis, which represents an angiocentric lymphoma.

This benign form of angioendotheliomatosis is self-limited. The lesions usually abate within one year, although one patient has been reported as having the condition for 6 years[75].

STEWART–TREVES SYNDROME

This syndrome consists of angiosarcoma developing within a lymphedematous extremity. It occurs most often in women following mastectomy and is referred to as post-mastectomy lymphangiosarcoma (Figure 6)[76]. Radiation therapy following the mastectomy may further increase the incidence[77]. It usually appears 10 to 12 years following mastectomy and reportedly occurs in up to 0.45% of patients[78]. It consists of ecchymotic or red patches or plaques; nodules and ulceration can be found as well. Typically, the disease extends beyond the clinical boundaries.

Histologically, there can be marked variation in cellular differentiation within the tumor. In well-differentiated areas, there are irregular vascular spaces lined by large endothelial cells. These vascular channels appear to 'dissect the collagen', subdividing it into small bundles[79]. Nuclear atypia is frequent. The endothelial cells can also form papillary projections into the vascular spaces. In poorly-differentiated lesions, large pleomorphic cells are abundant and often show no luminal differentiation; it can resemble metastatic carcinoma or melanoma. The epidermis may show signs of ulceration despite the degree of differentiation. In this form of angiosarcoma secondary to chronic lymphedema, the surrounding tissue may show evidence of chronic lymphedema with dilated lymphatic channels.

Treatment consists of radical local excision; this may include amputation of the affected limb. The prognosis is poor in general, as the lesions tend to metastasize early[80].

GRANULAR CELL TUMORS

A granular cell tumor (GCT) is a benign neoplasm that typically presents as a solitary lesion on the skin, in the subcutaneous tissue, or on the oral mucosa or tongue. They can be multifocal and can also occur on internal organs such as the larynx, pituitary gland, uvea, skeletal muscle, stomach and esophagus[81,82]. Clinically, GCT appears as a well-circumscribed, firm nodule with a diameter of up to 3 cm. Sometimes the surface can have a verrucous quality. Most of the tumors occur in the head or neck region and present in the third to fifth decade[83]. Two-thirds of patients are women, and there is an increased incidence in blacks. The exact origin has been debated; most believe the Schwann cell or the 'pluripotential primitive mesenchymal cell' is the cell of origin for granular cell tumors[84].

Microscopic examination of the tumor reveals a non-encapsulated nodule of polyhedral cells in the dermis (Figure 7). These cells are arranged in nests or fascicles and contain a granular cytoplasm that is periodic acid–Schiff (PAS) positive and diastase-resistant[85]. Laminated cytoplasmic bodies with surrounding halos are also seen within the cytoplasm, and the nuclei are round and centrally located. They are typically extra-neuronal but frequently spread perineurally along peripheral nerves. Mitoses are not common, but when present do not necessarily imply malignancy. Granular cell tumors occurring on mucosa frequently have pseudo-epitheliomatous hyperplasia and can easily be mistaken for carcinoma.

Malignant granular cell tumors have frequent mitoses. There is also significant pleomorphism of the cells; giant cells and non-granular spindle cells occur commonly within malignant granular cell tumors. These malignant forms can rarely metastasize.

Excision is the treatment of choice, but incomplete excision can result in recurrence.

ADIPOSIS DOLOROSA

Adiposis dolorosa, also known as Dercum's disease, is a rare, idiopathic entity consisting of multiple lipomas. The majority of affected patients are obese, postmenopausal women who are frequently noted to have psychiatric disturbances[86,87]. The lipomas occur on the trunk, arms, or at periarticular sites and can be extremely painful.

Histologically, adiposis dolorosa consists of well-circumscribed collections of adipocytes surrounded by a thin capsule. The individual adipocytes are indistinguishable from those in the surrounding subcutaneous tissue. Occasionally, the lipomas may have an entwined mass of capillaries (angiolipoma). Other subtypes of lipomas infiltrate neighboring muscle (intramuscular lipoma) or have a substantial fibrous connective tissue component (fibrolipoma).

Surgical excision may alleviate painful lipomas. Otherwise, symptomatic relief with analgesics is the mainstay of therapy. Atkinson has successfully treated adiposis dolorosa with intravenous lidocaine[87].

ERYTHROPLASIA

Erythroplasia, or erythroplakia, presents as a solitary, velvety red plaque or smooth patch on the oral mucosa. It typically measures less than 2 cm in diameter and may have areas of leukoplakia (or white plaques) within the lesion. Erythroplasia represents either in situ or invasive squamous cell carcinoma and typically implies an unfavorable prognosis[88]. Tobacco and alcohol use are significant predisposing factors in the development of erythroplasia[89]. The exact mechanism is unclear, but the effects seem to be synergistic[88]. Erythroplasia is more predominant in men, where it is frequently located on the floor of the mouth. In contrast, erythroplasia in women occurs more frequently on the tongue or buccal mucosa[90].

In high-risk patients who have no clinical evidence of erythroplasia, one can perform a toluidine

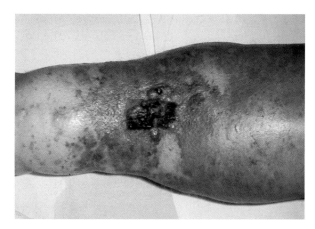

Figure 6 Lymphangiosarcoma. An ecchymotic, eroded plaque on the arm of a woman with chronic lymphedema

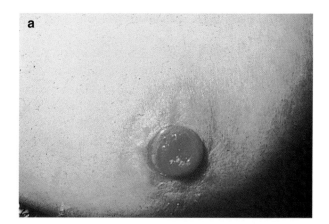

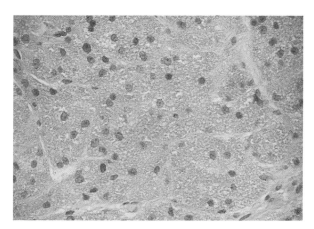

Figure 7 Granular cell tumor. Polyhedral cells with intracytoplasmic granules form a collection in the dermis

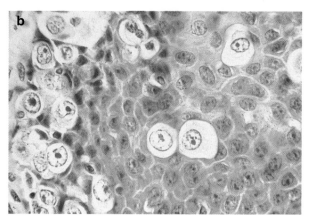

Figure 8 Paget's disease. (a) A solitary, eroded papule on the nipple of a woman. (b) In this example of extramammary Paget's disease, the Paget's cells within the epidermis are pathognomonic. These cells appear vacuolated and possess large nuclei with prominent nucleoli

blue test to aid in unmasking early disease, as indicated by Mashberg and Samit[91]. In brief, the patient rinses with water, swishes with 1% acetic acid, and dries the oral cavity with gauze prior to the application of toluidine blue. Again, the patient rinses with acetic acid followed by rinsing with water. The lesions stain blue *in vivo*.

Histologically, there is a lack of keratin on the surface of these lesions. Erythroplasia has significant nuclear atypicality throughout the epithelium, similar to Bowen's disease, though the former frequently has dermal invasion. One half of these lesions are carcinoma *in situ* and the other half are invasive carcinoma[88]. It is important to note that a random biopsy is typically not representative of the lesion as small foci of invasive carcinoma may be present throughout the lesion.

The earlier the lesion is diagnosed and treated, the better the prognosis. Surgical excision is usually curative for the *in situ* form. Invasive forms may require radiation therapy. Because many patients

with this condition have a significant tobacco and/or alcohol history, surveillance for other primary carcinomas of the digestive or respiratory tract is imperative[92,93]. The use of isotretinoin as a chemoprevention for other primary oral squamous cell carcinomas has been reportedly successful[94,95].

PAGET'S DISEASE

Paget's disease (PD) was first described by Sir James Paget in 1874[96]. He noted malignant transformation of the nipple and areola associated with underlying carcinomas of the breast (Figure 8a). In 1889, Crocker described an extramammary variant of PD (EMPD) which was histologically identical to classic PD[97]. In the years since these initial articles, many authors have provided additional case reports, reviews and histochemical and pathological studies on both classic PD and EMPD[98].

Paget's disease typically presents as a unilateral, scaly red plaque over the nipple and areola[99]. The lesion is well-circumscribed and may have areas of ulceration or retraction within the nipple[99]. Classic

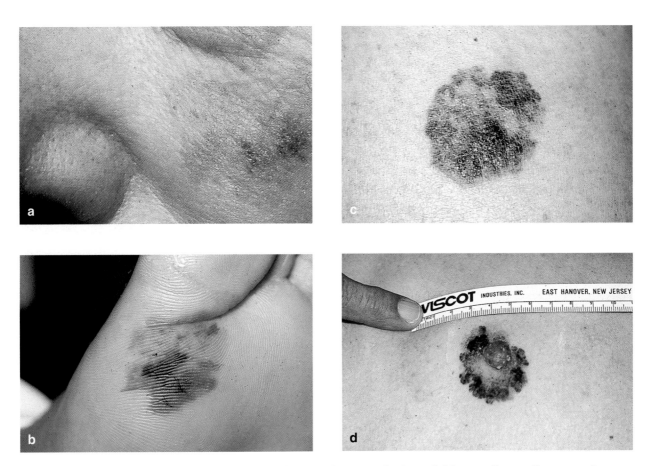

Figure 9   Malignant melanoma. (a) Lentigo maligna melanoma. (b) Superficial spreading malignant melanoma. (c) Acral lentiginous malignant melanoma. (d) Nodular malignant melanoma. Courtesy of Elaine C. Siegfried, MD, St Louis, MO

PD represents an underlying ductal carcinoma. Metastases have been reported in up to 33% of cases and typically involve the ipsilateral axillary lymph nodes[100,101].

Extramammary Paget's disease clinically resembles PD. EMPD usually measures a few centimeters in diameter, and individual lesions can be pruritic, ulcerated, eroded, or scaly. PD and EMPD both occur more frequently in women[98]. In contrast to PD, EMPD most frequently occurs on the vulva although other commonly affected sites include the perianal area and the scrotum in men. There are reports of EMPD occurring on the eyelid and within the axilla as well[102]. There may be an association between extramammary Paget's disease and an underlying visceral or adnexal carcinoma. Grow and colleagues found a concomitant carcinoma in the lower urinary tract in 78% of cases of EMPD[103], while Helwig and Graham found visceral or adnexal carcinoma within the genitourinary tract in 86% of their studied cases[104].

Histologically both types of PD contain the pathognomonic hallmark, Paget's cells within the epidermis (Figure 8b). Paget's cells appear as pale,

vacuolated cells with round or oval nuclei[105]. Nucleoli are prominent[106]. Paget's cells can also be found within appendages such as hair follicles and sweat ducts[106]. There is frequently a mixed inflammatory infiltrate in the upper dermis.

Paget's disease can be distinguished from other similar appearing entities by means of histochemical staining. Paget's cells contain cytoplasmic granules that stain positively for PAS but are diastase resistant. Other findings include positive staining for carcinogenic embryonic antigen (CEA), epithelial membrane antigen and low molecular weight keratin[107]. Because of the positive staining for CEA, PD is considered to originate from glandular components. Eccrine and apocrine sweat glands also stain positively for CEA while keratinocytes and melanocytes do not[108].

Treatment of PD is mastectomy. For EMPD, treatment consists of wide local excision, but recurrences are common[109,110]; 18–50% of vulvar EMPD and 70% of perianal EMPD[111] recurred. Mohs' micrographic surgery has proven to be successful in preventing local recurrences. Radiotherapy may have a positive role in preventing recurrences after surgery[112,113].

Lymph node dissection has not proven beneficial in the absence of palpable lymph nodes[109,114]. Chemotherapy such as 5-fluorouracil and mitomycin C has also been reported to be effective in treating EMPD[113,115].

MALIGNANT MELANOMA

Malignant melanoma (MM) results from malignant transformation of melanocytes or abnormal nevus cells. It can arise *de novo* or within a pre-existing nevus. There has been an increased incidence of MM over this century[116]. Most attribute this to a change in dress and recreational activities among Caucasians as well as changes in the histologic criteria of MM[117–120]. The reported 5-year survival rates for MM have been on the rise as well, most probably as a result of increased awareness of skin cancer signs[121–123].

Exposure to the sun is a significant risk factor in the development of the majority of MM cases. One subtype, lentigo maligna melanoma, commonly occurs on the face or other sites receiving chronic, long-term sun exposure[124–128]. Superficial spreading MM is associated with intermittent though intense sun exposure and most frequently occurs on partially protected sites[124–128]. Phenotypic characteristics such as blond hair, fair skin, blue or green eyes and a northern European ancestry are also associated with an increased risk of developing MM[124,125,129–134]. Likewise, persons with none or few of these characteristics, such as blacks and Asians, have a decreased risk of developing MM. Overall, MM has no sex predilection. However, in patients under 40 years of age, white women are more frequently affected than men[135]. Over age 45, MM is more common in white men[121].

At one time pregnancy was considered to carry an increased risk of MM but there are many reports that counter this notion[136–140]. When the depth of the melanoma is controlled, there is no worse outcome for women who are pregnant at the time of diagnosis[136,137]. A family history of MM is believed to carry an increased risk of developing the condition. Specifically, most reports note an increased risk of MM in affected first degree relatives[121]. A genetic basis for familial MM is supported by the localization of MLM2 gene on chromosome 9[141].

There are two patterns of tumor progression in MM. The first is the radial growth phase in which the neoplasm expands parallel with respect to the dermal–epidermal junction. The tumor cells lie predominantly at this junction but may invade the superficial papillary dermis. The second pattern is known as the vertical growth phase. This is characterized by nests of tumor cells extending deeper into the dermis and arranged perpendicularly to the dermal–epidermal junction. It is this vertical growth phase that indicates an increased metastatic potential.

The four most common types of MM are lentigo maligna melanoma, superficial spreading MM, acral lentiginous MM and nodular MM. The former three sub-types are frequently associated with radial growth phase while the latter one is commonly associated with the vertical growth phase.

Lentigo maligna melanoma

Lentigo maligna melanoma (LMM) (Figure 9a) occurs most frequently on the head or neck. Clinically, it presents as a brown or tan macule of variable size and border contour, but there may be multiple colors within the visible lesion. A Wood's lamp may help delineate the clinically-apparent margins[142]. Most cases of LMM occur in patients over the age of 50[143].

LMM is essentially a progression of the lentigo maligna, which possesses melanocytic atypia within the basilar layer. In contrast, LMM typically possesses an even greater degree of cytologic atypia, is invasive and has more cytologic pleomorphism. The increased number of melanocytes in the basal layer frequently outweighs the number of basal keratinocytes. In the upper and middle portions of the dermis, elastosis is prominent, consistent with a history of chronic, long-term exposure to the sun. An inflammatory infiltrate is usually commonly found in the superficial dermis, with a preponderance of melanophages or lymphocytes.

Superficial spreading malignant melanoma

Superficial spreading melanoma (SSMM) (Figure 9b) is the most common subtype of MM, occurring in about 70% of all Caucasians diagnosed with MM[144–147]. The most common sites of predilection are the back in men and the legs in women, though any body site may be affected[135]. Patients with SSMM are typically younger than those with other subtypes of MM[148,149]. SSMM is a slightly elevated papule or plaque typically less than 2–3 centimeters in diameter. The color is variable, with hues ranging from pink or tan to brown or black, and the border contour is irregular.

Histologically, SSMM shows melanocytic atypia. At low power, the epidermis may appear alternately thick and thin. There are nests of atypical melanocytes stemming from the basal layer of the epidermis. Additionally, there are single spherical melanocytes scattered throughout the middle and upper epidermis in a pagetoid pattern. The individual melanocytes reveal loss of dendritic processes but often show melanin particles scattered throughout the cytoplasm.

Acral lentiginous malignant melanoma

Acral lentiginous malignant melanoma (ALMM) (Figure 9c) is a subtype of MM that occurs on palms, soles, or ungual/periungual sites, although the sole is the most commonly affected site. ALMM is the most common type of MM in dark-skinned individuals[146,150–152]. Clinically, these lesions appear as variably colored macules or patches with irregular borders. If the neoplasm occurs at the nail matrix, the nail plate may reveal a hyperpigmented, longitudinal band; this band can extend onto the nail fold (Hutchinson's sign).

Histologically, there is 'lentiginous' proliferation of abnormal melanocytes along the dermal–epidermal junction. ALMM is distinguished from LMM because the former has a lack of elastosis, possesses irregular acanthosis, and the abnormal cells often possess dendritic features[153,154].

Nodular malignant melanoma

Nodular malignant melanoma (NMM) (Figure 9d) clinically appears as a variably pigmented papule or nodule. In fact, it may be amelanotic. Additionally, ulceration can occur. NMM is more common in men and typically is diagnosed in an older population than is SSMM[153].

Histologically, NMM is characterized by a nest of atypical melanocytes of varying size, shape and color in the dermis[155]. There is pagetoid spread of the melanoma cells into the epidermis overlying the tumor. The neighboring epidermis is typically unremarkable. An inflammatory infiltrate of varying degree is often present.

Staging

Depth of invasion is perhaps the most important aspect in determining prognosis. Two methods of measurement are commonly used. Clark's level measures the degree to which melanoma invades the dermis (Table 1)[156]. The Breslow's depth measures the tumor thickness from the granular layer to the deepest portion of the neoplasm[157–159]. This measurement is given in millimeters.

In determining prognosis several factors are reviewed, including nodal involvement and the previously mentioned Breslow's depth. Breslow's depth of less than 0.76 mm generally suggests a

Table 1 Degree of penetration of the dermis by malignant melanoma according to Clark

Clark's level	Location of tumor cells
I	Confined to the epidermis
II	Invades the papillary dermis
III	Fills the papillary dermis
IV	Invades the reticular dermis
V	Invades the subcutaneous tissue

more favorable prognosis while nodal involvement and metastases imply a poor prognosis. Vertical growth suggests greater metastatic potential[160–162]. NMM, which is characterized by vertical growth, tends to possess a greater Breslow's depth and as such carries a poorer prognosis than does SSMM. However, when controlled for thickness, the prognosis for NMM is not worse than for the other subtypes of MM[157,162].

Women with melanoma typically have longer survival rates than their male counterparts. This is attributed to women having thinner lesions and a greater frequency of anatomically-favorable extremity melanoma[135,159].

Diagnosis

The diagnosis of MM is confirmed upon histologic analysis. In addition to the previously mentioned histologic features, several immunohistochemical tests aid in the diagnosis. These include S100 and HMB 45 for which MM stains positively[163,164]. To aid in the histologic diagnosis, particularly in amelanotic variants, melanoma does not stain with leukocyte common antigen or keratin stains[165].

Treatment

Surgical excision is the mainstay of treatment for MM. The National Institutes of Health consensus conference has recommended that the lesion be excised with the following guidelines: for melanoma-in-situ, 0.5 to 1.0 cm margins beyond the clinically-apparent tumor; for lesions < 1 mm thick allow 1 cm margins; for lesions > 1 mm thick allow 2–3 cm margins[166,167].

Elective regional lymph node dissection for non-palpable lymph nodes does not increase survival in patients with MM[168,169]. However, full or modified regional lymph node dissection of palpable nodes is the standard of care in patients with MM as it affords the best control on local tumor growth and assists in tumor staging[170]. Morton and colleagues developed the concept of sentinel lymph node biopsy[171,172]. The theory behind this procedure is that the tumor will metastasize first to one of the regional lymph nodes (the sentinel node). To assess this regional lymph node metastasis, the tumor is injected with radionucleotide and dispersion of the label is localized with assistance of lymphoscintigraphy. The localization of this 'hot' node is made easier by injection of a visible dye. This technique can predict the presence of occult regional lymph node metastasis with an accuracy of greater than 96%[173]. Adjuvant therapy with chemotherapy may increase survival rates in some patients. Additionally, vaccine therapy with melanoma-assisted antigens (MAA) is a promising option for patients with advanced-stage melanoma[173].

REFERENCES

1. Santa Cruz DJ, Prioleau PG, Smith ME. Hidradenoma papilliferum of the eyelid. *Arch Dermatol* 1991;117:55–6

2. Hashimoto K. Hidradenoma papilliferum: an electron microscopic study. *Acta Derm Venereol (Stockh)* 1973;53:22–30

3. Meeker JH, Neubecker RD, Helwig EG. Hidradenoma papilliferum. *Am J Clin Pathol* 1962;37:182–95

4. Shenoy VM. Malignant perianal papillary hidradenoma. *Arch Dermatol* 1961;83:965–7

5. Wallace ML, Smoller BR. Progesterone receptor positivity supports hormonal control of syringomas. *J Cut Pathol* 1995;22:442–5

6. Hashimoto K, Dibella, Borsuk GM, *et al.* Eruptive hidradenoma and syringoma. *Arch Dermatol* 1967;96:500–19

7. Thomas J, Majmudar B, Gorelkin L. Syringoma localized to the vulva. *Arch Dermatol* 1979;115:95–6

8. Yung CW, Soltani K, Bernstein JE, *et al.* Unilateral linear nevoidal syringoma. *J Am Acad Dermatol* 1981;4:412–16

9. Asai Y, Ishii M, Hamada T. Acral syringoma: electron microscopic studies on its origin. *Acta Derm Venereol (Stockh)* 1982;62:64–8

10. Hashimoto K, Lever WF. Histogenesis of skin appendage tumors. *Arch Dermatol* 1969;100:356–69

11. Mustakallio KK. Succinic dehydrogenase activity of syringomas. *Acta Dermatol* 1964;89:827

12. Winkelmann RK, Muller SA. Sweat gland tumors. *Arch Dermatol* 1964;89:827–31

13. Hashimoto K, Blum D, Fukaya T, Eto H. Familial syringoma. Case history and application of monoclonal anti-eccrine gland antibodies. *Arch Dermatol* 1985;121:756–60

14. Headington JT, Koski J, Murphy PJ. Clear cell glycogenesis in multiple syringomas. *Arch Dermatol* 1972;106:353–6

15. Feibelman CE, Maize JC. Clear-cell syringoma. *Am J Dermatopathol* 1984;6:139–50

16. Karam P, Benedetto AV. Intralesional electrodesiccation of syringomas [published erratum appears in *Dermatol Surg* 1998;24:692]. *Dermatol Surg* 1997;23:921–4

17. Mehregan AH, Lee KC. Malignant proliferative trichilemmal tumors. *Dermatol Surg Oncol* 1987;13:1339–42

18. Lever WF, Schaumberg-Lever G. *Histopathology of the Skin*, 8th edn. Philadelphia: JB Lippincott, 1997:695–7

19. Brownstein MH, Arluk DJ. Proliferating trichilemmal cyst. *Cancer* 1981;48:1207–14

20. Weiss J, Heine M, Grimmel M, Jung EG. Malignant proliferating trichilemmal cyst. *J Am Acad Dermatol* 1995;32:870

21. Leppard BJ, Sanderson KV, Wells RS. Hereditary trichilemmal cysts. Hereditary pilar cysts. *Clin Exp Dermatol* 1977;2:23–32

22. Bulengo-Ransby SM, Johnson C, Metcalf JS. Enlarging scalp nodule. *Arch Dermatol* 1995;131:721–4

23. West AJ, Hunt SJ, Goltz R. Solitary facial plaque of long duration. *Arch Dermatol* 1995;131:213–16

24. Brownstein MH, Shapiro L. Desmoplastic trichoepithelioma. *Cancer* 1977;40:2979–86

25. Kopf AW, Shapiro PE. Familial multiple desmoplastic trichoepithelioma. *Arch Dermatol* 1991;127:83–7

26. Takei Y, Fukushiro S, Ackerman AB. Criteria for histologic differential of desmoplastic trichoepithelioma (sclerosing epithelial hamartoma) from morphea-like basal-cell carcinoma. *Am J Dermatopathol* 1985;7:207–21

27. Zelger BW, Steiner H, Kutzner H. Clear cell dermatofibroma. Case report of an unusual fibrohistiocytic lesion. *Am J Surg Pathol* 1996;20:483–91

28. Gross RE, Wolback SB. Sclerosing hemangiomas: their relationship to dermatofibroma, histiocytoma, xanthoma, and certain pigmented lesions of the skin. *Am J Pathol* 1943;19:533–51

29. Goette DK, Helwig EB. Basal cell carcinomas and basal cell carcinoma-like changes overlying dermatofibromas. *Arch Dermatol* 1975;111:589–92

30. McKenna KE, Somerville JE, Walsh MY, *et al.* Basal cell carcinoma occurring in association with dermatofibroma. *Dermatology* 1993;187:54–7

31. Spiller WF, Spiller RF. Cryosurgery in dermatologic office practice: special reference to dermatofibroma and mucous cyst of the lip. *South Med J* 1975;68:157–60

32. Das Gupta TK, Brasfield RD, O'Hara J, *et al.* Extra-abdominal desmoids: a clinicopathologic study. *Ann Surg* 1969;170:109–21

33. Lasser P, Elias D, Contesso G, *et al.* Tumeurs desmoides ou fibromatoses intra-abdominales. *Ann de Chirurgie* 1993;47:352–9

34. Gonatas NK. Extra-abdominal desmoid tumors; report of 6 cases. *Arch Pathol* 1961;71:214–21

35. Weary PE, Linthicum A, Cawley EP, *et al*. Gardner's syndrome. *Arch Dermatol* 1964;90:20–30

36. Goy BW, Lee SP, Eilber F. The role of adjuvant radiotherapy in the treatment of resectable desmoid tumors. *Int J Rad Oncol Biol Phys* 1997;39:659–65

37. Acker JC, Bossen EH, Halperin EC. The management of desmoid tumors. *Int J Rad Oncol Biol Phys* 1993;26:851–8

38. Bataini JP, Belloir C, Mazabraud A, *et al*. Desmoid tumors in adults: the role of radiotherapy in their management. *Am J Surg* 1988;155:754–60

39. Wilcken N, Tattersal MH. Endocrine therapy for desmoid tumors. *Cancer* 1991;68:1384–8

40. Tsuneyoshi M, Enjoji M. Glomus tumor: a clinicopathologic and electron microscopic study. *Cancer* 1982;50:1601–7

41. Chen WC, Lee TJ, Ku MC, Hsu KC. Glomus tumors of the upper extremity: experience with twelve cases. *Chung Hua: Tsa Chih-China Med J* 1995;55:163–7

42. Liapi-Avgeri G, Karabela-Bouropoulou V, Agnanti N. Glomus tumor: a histological, histochemical, and immunohistochemical study of the various types. *Pathol Res Pract* 1994;190:2–10

43. Masson P. Le glomus neuromyoarteriel des régions tactiles et ses tumeurs. *Lyon Chir* 1924;21:257–80

44. Porter PL, Bigler SA, McNutt M, *et al*. The immunophenotype of hemangiopericytomas and glomus tumors with special reference to muscle protein expression: an immunohistochemical study and review of the literature. *Med Pathol* 1991;4:46–52

45. Kaye VM, Dehner LP. Cutaneous glomus tumor: a comparative immuno-histochemical study with pseudoangiomatous intradermal melanocytic nevi. *Am J Dermatopathol* 1991;13:2–6

46. Gould EW, Manivel JC, Albores-Saaverda J, Monforte H. Locally infiltrative glomus tumors with glomangiosarcoma: a clinical, ultrastructural, and immuno-histochemical study. *Cancer* 1990;65:310–18

47. Thyresson HN, Su WP. Familial cutaneous leiomyomatosis. *J Am Acad Dermatol* 1981;4:430–4

48. Archer CB, Whittaker S, Greaves MW. Pharmacological modulation of cold-induced pain in cutaneous leiomyomata. *Br J Dermatol* 1988;118:255–60

49. Thompson JA Jr. Therapy for painful cutaneous leiomyomas. *J Am Acad Dermatol* 1985;13:865–7

50. Montgomery H, Winkelmann RK. Smooth-muscle tumors of the skin. *Arch Dermatol* 1959;79:32

51. Hachisuga T, Hashimoto H, Enjoji M. Angioleiomyoma. A clinicopathologic reappraisal of 562 cases. *Cancer* 1984;54:126–30

52. Warner J, Jones EW. Pyogenic granuloma recurring with multiple satellites. A report of 11 cases. *Br J Dermatol* 1968;80:218–27

53. Cooper PH, Mills SE. Subcutaneous granuloma pyogenicum: lobular capillary hemangioma. *Arch Dermatol* 1982;118:30–3

54. Saad RW, Sau P, Mulvaney MP, *et al*. Intravenous pyogenic granuloma. *Int J Dermatol* 1993;32:130–2

55. Cooper PH, McAllister HA, Helwig EB. Intravenous pyogenic granuloma: a study of 18 cases. *Am J Surg Pathol* 1979;4:221–8

56. Wilson BB, Greer KE, Cooper DH. Eruptive disseminated lobular capillary hemangioma (pyogenic granuloma). *J Am Acad Dermatol* 1989;21:391–4

57. Mills SE, Cooper PH, Fechner RE. Lobular capillary hemangioma: the underlying lesion of pyogenic granuloma. A study of 73 cases from the oral and nasal mucous membranes. *Am J Surg Pathol* 1980;4:470–9

58. Blickenstaff RD, Roeningk RK, Peters MS, Goellner JR. Recurrent pyogenic granuloma with satellitosis. *J Am Acad Dermatol* 1989;21:1241–4

59. Vincente MA, Estrach T, Zamora E, *et al*. Granuloma piogenico recidivant con lesiones satelites multiples: presentacion de dos casos. *Med Cutan Ibero Lat Am* 1990;18:331

60. Abrahamian LM, Rothe MJ, Grant-Kels JM. Primary telangiectasia of childhood. *Int J Dermatol* 1992;31:307–13

61. Bean WB. *Vascular Spiders and Related Lesions of the Skin*. Springfield, IL: Charles C. Thomas, 1958

62. Kinsell LW. Endocrinologic aspects of acute and chronic liver disease with special reference to the metabolism of endogenous androgens. *Stanford Med Bull* 1969;11:46

63. Arndt KA. Argon laser therapy of small cutaneous vascular lesions. *Arch Dermatol* 1982;118:220–4

64. Mibelli V. Di una nuova forma de cheratosis, angiocheratome. *G Ital Mal Vener* 1891;30:285

65. Haye KR, Rabello DJA. Angiokeratoma of Mibelli. *Acta Derm Venereol (Stockh)* 1961;41:56–60

66. Frain-Bell W. Angioma serpiginosum. *Br J Dermatol* 1957;69:251–5

67. Barabasch R, Baur M. [Angioma serpiginosum. A name for different dermatologic disease. Critical report of three cases.] *Hautarzt* 1971;22:436–42

68. Gautier-Smith PC, Sanders MD, Sanderson KV. Ocular and nervous system involvement in angioma serpiginosum. *Br J Ophthal* 1971;55:433–43

69. Neumann E. Some new observations on the genesis of angioma serpiginosum. *Acta Derm Venereol (Stockh)* 1971;51:194–8

70. Marriott PJ, Munro DD, Ryan T. Angioma serpiginosum—familial incidence. *Br J Dermatol* 1975;93:701–6

71. Schamberg JF. A peculiar progressive pigmentary disease of the skin. *Br J Dermatol* 1901;13:1

72. Wick MR, Rocamora A. Reactive and malignant "angioendotheliomatosis": a discriminant clinicopathological study. *J Cutan Pathol* 1988;15:260–71

73. LeBoit PE, Solomon AR, Santa Cruz DJ, *et al*. Angiomatosis with luminal cryoprotein deposition. *J Am Acad Dermatol* 1992;27:969–73

74. Berger TG, Dawson NA. Angioendotheliomatosis. *J Am Acad Dermatol* 1988;18:407–12

75. Pfleger K, Tappeiner J. Zur kenntnis der systemisierten endotheliomatose der cutanem Blutgefasse (Reticuloendotheliose?). *Hautarzt* 1959;10: 359–65

76. Brady MS, Garfein CF, Petrek JA, Brennan MF. Post-treatment sarcoma in breast cancer patients. *Ann Surg Oncol* 1994;1:66–72

77. Taghian A, deVathaire F, Terrier P, *et al*. Long term risk of sarcoma following radiation treatment for breast cancer. *Int J Rad Oncol Biol Phys* 1991;21: 361–7

78. Defraigne JO, Detroz B, Dubois J. [Lymphangiosarcoma following mastectomy: review of the literature apropos of 2 recent cases of Stewart–Treves syndrome.] *Acta Chirurgica Belgica* 1989;89: 29–33

79. Rosai J, Sumner HW, Major MC, *et al*. Angiosarcoma of the skin: a clinico-pathologic and fine structural study. *Hum Pathol* 1976;7:83–109

80. Woodward AH, Ivins JC, Soule EH. Lymphoangiosarcoma arising in chronic lymphedematous extremities. *Cancer* 1972;30:562–72

81. Moscovic EA, Azar HA. Multiple granular cell tumors (myoblastomas); case report with electron microscopic observations and review of the literature. *Cancer* 1967;20:2032–47

82. Seo IS, Azzarelli B, Warner TF, *et al*. Multiple visceral and cutaneous granular cell tumors; ultrastructural and immunocytochemical evidence of Schwann cell origin. *Cancer* 1984;53:2104–10

83. Simone J, Schneider GT, Begneaud W, Harms K. Granular cell tumor of the vulva: literature review and case report. *J LA State Med Soc* 1996;148: 539–41

84. Ulrich J, Heitz PU, Fischer T, *et al*. Granular cell tumors. Evidence for heterogeneous tumor cell differentiation: an immunocytochemical study. *Virchows Arch [B]* 1987;53:52–7

85. Reed RJ, Argenyi Z. Tumors of neural tissue. In Elder D, ed. *Lever's Histology of the Skin*, 8th edn. Philadelphia: Lippincott-Raven, 1997;994

86. Held JL, Andrew JA, Kohn SR. Surgical amelioration of Dercum's disease: a report and review. *J Dermatol Surg Oncol* 1989;15:1294–6

87. Atkinson RL. Intravenous lidocaine for the treatment of intractable pain of adiposis dolorosa. *Int J Obes* 1982;6:351–7

88. Shafer WG, Waldron CA. Erythroplakia of the oral cavity. *Cancer* 1975;36:1021–8

89. Mashberg A, Garfinkel L, Harris S. Alcohol as a primary risk factor in oral squamous carcinoma. *Ca: Cancer J Clin* 1981;31:146–55

90. Mashberg A, Samit AM. Early oral and oropharyngeal cancer. Diagnosis and management. In Schwartz RA, ed. *Skin Cancer Recognition and Management*. New York: Springer, 1988;226

91. Mashberg A, Samit A. Early diagnosis of asymptomatic oral and oropharyngeal squamous cancers. *Ca: Cancer J Clin* 1995;45:328–51

92. Kato I, Nomura AM. Alcohol in the aetiology of upper aerodigestive tract cancer. *Euro J Cancer* 1994;30B:75–81

93. Wynder EL. Tumor enhancers: underestimated factors in the epidemiology of lifestyle-associated cancers. *Environ Health Perspect* 1983;50:15–21

94. Hong WK, Endicott J, Itri LM, *et al*. 13-cis-Retinoic acid in the treatment of oral leukoplakia. *N Engl J Med* 1986;315:1501–5

95. Lippman SM, Batsakis JG, Toth BB, *et al*. Comparison of low-dose isotretinoin with beta carotene to prevent oral carcinogenesis. *N Engl J Med* 1993;328:15–20

96. Paget J. On disease of mammary areola preceeding cancer of mammary gland. *St. Bartholomew Hosp Rep* 1874;10:86

97. Crocker HR. Paget's disease affecting the scrotum and penis. *Trans Pathol Soc Lond* 1889;40:187

98. Merot Y, Mazoujian G, Pinkus G, *et al*. Extramammary Paget's disease of the perianal and perineal regions: evidence of apocrine derivation. *Arch Dermatol* 1985;121:750–2

99. Brenner S, Politi Y. Dermatologic diseases and problems of women throughout the life cycle. *Int J Dermatol* 1995;34:369–79

100. Ashikari R, Park K, Huvos HG, *et al*. Paget's disease of the breast. *Cancer* 1970;26:680–5

101. Paone JF, Baker RR. Pathogenesis and treatment of Paget's disease of the breast. *Cancer* 1981;48: 825–9

102. Kanitakis J. La maladie de Paget extramammaire. *Ann Dermatol Venereol* 1985;112:75–87

103. Grow JR, Kshirsagar V, Tolentino M. Extramammary perianal Paget's disease: report of a case. *Dis Colon Rectum* 1977;20:436–42

104. Helwig EB, Graham JH. Anogenital Paget's disease: a clinicopathological study. *Cancer* 1963;16:387–408

105. Archer CB, Louback JB, MacDonald DM. Spontaneous regression of perianal extramammary Paget's disease after partial surgical excision. *Arch Dermatol* 1987;123:379–82

106. Powell FC, Bjornsson J, Doyle JA, Cooper AJ. Genital Paget's disease and urinary tract malignancy. *J Am Acad Dermatol* 1985;13:84–90

107. Balducci L, Crawford ED, Smith GF, *et al*. Extramammary Paget's disease: an annotated review. *Cancer Invest* 1988;6:293–303

108. Nadji M, Morales AR, Girtanner RE, *et al*. Paget's disease of the skin: a unifying concept of histogenesis. *Cancer* 1982;50:2203–6

109. Mohs FE, Blanchard L. Microscopically controlled surgery for extramammary Paget's disease. *Arch Dermatol* 1979;115:706–8

110. Breen JL, Smith CI, Gregori AC. Extramammary Paget's disease. *Clin Obstet Gynecol* 1978;21:1107–15

111. Williams SL, Rogers LW, Quan SHO. Perianal Paget's disease: report of seven cases. *Dis Colon Rectum* 1976;19:30–40

112. Wada H, Urabe H. Surgical treatment of genital Paget's disease in men. *Ann Plast Surg* 1994;13:199–204

113. Dietel M, Bahnsen J, Stegner HE, Holzel F. Paget's disease of the vulva with underlying apocrine adenocarcinoma and local lymph node invasion. *Pathol Res Pract* 1981;171:353–61

114. Secco GB, Lapertosa G, Sertoli MR, *et al*. Genital Paget's disease: case report of an elderly patient treated with polychemotherapy and radiotherapy. *Tumori* 1984;70:381–3

115. Balducci L, Athar M, Smith GF, *et al*. Metastatic extramammary Paget's disease. Dramatic response to combined modality treatment. *J Surg Oncol* 1988;38:38–44

116. Boring CC, Squires TS, Tong T. Cancer statistics, 1991. *Ca: Cancer J Clin* 1991;41:19–36

117. Elwood JM, Lee JA. Recent data on epidemiology of malignant melanoma. *Semin Oncol* 1975;2:149–54

118. Lee JAH. Melanoma and exposure to sunlight. *Epidemiol Rev* 1982;4:110–36

119. Lee JAH. The melanoma epidemic thus far (editorial). *Mayo Clin Proc* 1990;6:1368–71

120. Longstreth J. Cutaneous malignant melanoma and ultraviolet radiation: a review. *Cancer Metas Rev* 1988;7:321–33

121. Ries LAG, Kosary CL, Hankey BF, *et al*., eds. SEER Cancer Statistics Review 1973–1996. Bethesda, MD: National Cancer Institute, 1999

122. Cutler SJ, Myers MH, Green SB. Trends in survival rates of patients with cancer. *N Engl J Med* 1975;293:122–4

123. Sober AJ, Day CL Jr, Koh HK, *et al*. Cutaneous melanoma in the northeastern United States: data from the Melanoma Clinical Cooperative Group. In Balch CM, Milton G, eds. *Cutaneous Melanoma: Clinical Management and Treatment Results Worldwide*. Philadelphia: Lippincott, 1985;437

124. Holman CD, Armstrong BK. Pigmentary traits, ethnic origin, benign nevi, and family history of risk factors for cutaneous malignant melanoma. *J Natl Cancer Int* 1984;72:257–66

125. Holman CD, Armstrong BK, Heenan PJ, *et al*. The causes of malignant melanoma: result from the West Australian Lions Melanoma Research project. *Recent Results Cancer Res* 1986;102:18–37

126. Holman CD, Armstrong BK. A theory of the etiology and pathogenesis of human cutaneous malignant melanoma. *J Natl Cancer Inst* 1983;71:651–6

127. Holman CD, Armstrong BK. Cutaneous malignant melanoma and indicators of total accumulating exposure to the sun. *J Natl Cancer Inst* 1984;73:75–82

128. Kopf AW, Kripke ML, Stern RS. Sun and malignant melanoma. *J Am Acad Dermatol* 1984;11:674–84

129. Elwood JM, Gallagher RP, Hill GB, Spinelli JJ. Pigmentation and skin reaction to sun as risk factors for cutaneous melanoma: Western Canada Melanoma study. *Br Med J* 1984;288:99–102

130. Dubin N, Moseson M, Pasternack BS. Epidemiology of malignant melanoma: pigmentary traits, ultraviolet radiation, and the identification of high-risk populations. *Recent Results Cancer Res* 1986;102:56–75

131. Green A, Bain C, McLennan R, Siskind V. Risk factors for cutaneous melanoma in Queensland. *Recent Results Cancer Res* 1986;102:76–97

132. Gallagher RP, Elwood JM, Hill GB. Risk factors for cutaneous malignant melanoma: the Western Canada Melanoma Study. *Recent Results Cancer Res* 1986;102:38–55

133. Evans RD, Kopf AW, Lew RA, *et al*. Risk factors for the development of malignant melanoma. I. Review of case-control studies. *J Dermatol Surg Oncol* 1988;14:393–408

134. Beitner H, Norell SE, Ringborg U, *et al*. Malignant melanoma: aetiological importance of individual pigmentation and sun-exposure. *Br J Dermatol* 1990;122:43–57

135. Streetly A, Markowe H. Changing trends in the epidemiology of malignant melanoma: gender differences and their implications for public health. *Int J Epidemiol* 1995;24:897–907

136. McManamny DS, Moss AL, Pocock PV, Briggs JC. Melanoma and pregnancy: a long-term follow-up. *Br J Obstet Gynaecol* 1989;96:1419–23

137. Slingluff CL Jr, Reintgen DS, Vollmer RT, Seigler HF. Malignant melanoma arising during pregnancy: a study of 100 patients. *Ann Surg* 1990;211:552–7

138. Reintgen DS, McCarty KS, Vollmer R, *et al*. Malignant melanoma and pregnancy. *Cancer* 1985;55:1340–4

139. Squatrito RC, Harlow SP. Melanoma complicating pregnancy. *Obstet Gynecol Clin* 1998;25:407–16

140. Wong JH, Sterns EE, Kopald KH, *et al*. Prognostic significance of pregnancy in Stage I melanoma. *Arch Surg* 1989;124:1227–30

141. Battistutta D, Palmer J, Walters M, *et al*. Incidence of familial melanoma and MLM2 gene. *Lancet* 1994;344:1607–8

142. Reyes BA, Robins P. Wood's lamp and surgical margins in malignant melanoma *in situ* [letter]. *J Dermatol Surg Oncol* 1988;14:22

143. Morris BT, Sober AJ. Cutaneous malignant melanoma in the older patient. *Dermatol Clin* 1986;4:473–80

144. Clark WH Jr. A classification of malignant melanoma in man correlated with histogenesis and biologic behavior. In Montagna W, ed. *Advances in Biology of the Skin*, vol 8. *The Pigmentary System*. New York: Pergamon, 1967;621

145. Clark WH Jr, From L, Bernardino EA, Mihm MC. The histogenesis and biologic behavior of primary

human malignant melanomas of the skin. *Cancer Res* 1969;29:705

146. Clark WH Jr, Elder DE, Van Horn M, *et al*. The biologic forms of malignant melanoma. *Hum Pathol* 1986;17:443–50

147. Milton GW, Balch CM, Shaw HM, *et al*. Clinical characteristics. In Bakh CM, Milton G, eds. *Cutaneous Melanoma: Clinical Management and Treatment Results Worldwide*. Philadelphia: Lippincott, 1985;13

148. Cox NH, Aitchison TC, Sirel JM, Mackie RM. Comparison between lentigo maligna melanoma and other histogenic types of malignant melanoma. *Br J Cancer* 1996;73:940–4

149. Garbe C, Orfanos CE. Epidemiology of malignant melanoma in central Europe: risk factors and prognostic predictors. Results of the Central Malignant Melanoma Registry of the German Dermatological Society. *Pigment Cell Research* 1992;2(suppl):285–94

150. Feibleman CE, Stoll H, Maize JC. Melanoma of the palm, sole, and nailbed: a clinicopathologic study. *Cancer* 1980;46:2492–504

151. Rippey JJ, Rippey E, Giraud RM. Pathology of malignant melanoma of the skin in black Africans. *S Afr Med J* 1975;49:789–92

152. Seiji M, Takematsu H, Hosokawa M, *et al*. Acral melanoma in Japan. *J Invest Dermatol* 1983;80(suppl):56s–60s

153. Clark WH Jr, Elder DE, Van Horn M. The biologic forms of malignant melanoma. *Hum Pathol* 1986;5:443–50

154. Paladuga RR, Winberg CD, Yonemoto RH. Acral lentiginous melanoma: a clinicopathologic study of 36 patients. *Cancer* 1983;52:161–8

155. Su WP. Malignant melanoma: basic approach to clinicopathologic correlation. *Mayo Clin Proc* 1997;72:67–72

156. Clark WH Jr, Elder DE, Guerry D IV. Model predicting survival in Stage I melanoma based on tumor progression. *J Natl Cancer Inst* 1989;81:1893–904

157. Vollmer RT. Malignant melanoma: a multivariate analysis of prognostic factors. *Pathol Ann* 1989;24:383–407

158. Breslow A. Cross-sectional areas and depth of invasion in the prognosis of cutaneous melanoma. *Ann Surg* 1970;172:902–8

159. Breslow A. Tumor thickness, level of invasion, and node dissection in Stage I cutaneous melanoma. *Ann Surg* 1975;182:572–5

160. Trozak DJ, Rowland WD, Hu F. Metastatic malignant melanoma in prepubertal children. *Pediatrics* 1975;55:191–204

161. Elder DE, Guerry D IV, Epstein MN, *et al*. Invasive malignant melanoma lacking competence for metastasis. *Am J Dermatopathol* 1984;6(suppl):55–61

162. Kopf AW, Welkovich B, Frankel RE, *et al*. Thickness of malignant melanoma: global analysis of related factors. *J Dermatol Surg Oncol* 1987;13:345–90, 401–20

163. Achilles E, Schroder S. [Positive cytokeratin results in malignant melanoma. Pitfall in differential immunohistologic diagnosis of occult neoplasm.] *Pathologe* 1994;15:235–41

164. Tousignant J, Grossin M, Toublanc M, Dauge-Geffroy MC. [Immunohistochemical characteristics of malignant melanoma. A study of 40 cases and review of the literature.] *Arch d'Anatomie Cytologie Pathologiques* 1990;38:5–10

165. Elenitsas R, Van Belle P, Elder D. Laboratory methods. In Elder D, ed. *Lever's Histology of the Skin*, 8th edn. Philadelphia: Lippincott-Raven, 1997:58–9

166. National Institutes of Health: Consensus Development Conference. Diagnosis and treatment of early melanoma. *JAMA* 1992;268:1314–19

167. Balch CM, Murad TM, Soong SJ, *et al*. Tumor thickness as a guide to surgical management of clinical stage I melanoma patients. *Cancer* 1979;43:883–8

168. Veronesi U, Adamus J, Bandiera DC, *et al*. Delayed regional lymph node dissection in Stage I melanoma of the skin of the lower extremities. *Cancer* 1982;49:2420–30

169. Sim FH, Taylor WF, Pritchard DJ, Soule EH. Lymphadenectomy in the management of stage I malignant melanoma: a prospective randomized study. *Mayo Clin Proc* 1986;61:697–705

170. Urist MM. Surgical management of primary cutaneous melanoma. *Ca: Cancer J Clin* 1996;46:217–24

171. Morton DL, Wen DR, Wong JH, *et al*. Technical details of intraoperative lymphatic mapping for early stage melanoma. *Arch Surg* 1992;127:392–9

172. Morton DL, Wen DR, Foshag LJ, *et al*. Intraoperative lymphatic mapping and selective cervical lymphadenectomy for early-stage melanomas of the head and neck. *J Clin Oncol* 1993;11:1751–6

173. Morton DL, Barth A. Vaccine therapy for malignant melanoma. *Ca: Cancer J Clin* 1996;46:225–44

Cutaneous manifestations of systemic diseases

21

Marina Landau and Barukh Mevorah

INTRODUCTION

For the most part systemic diseases affecting women are not different from those affecting men. There are several disorders, however, that occur more frequently, or manifest themselves differently, in women. The purpose of this chapter is to review these systemic disorders and to emphasize their skin manifestations. Some systemic disorders will be mentioned, not so much for their accompanying cutaneous manifestations, but because normal skin features affect their epidemiology (fair skin and gallstones) or because there is a correlation with an apparently unrelated cutaneous pathologic process (osteoporosis and skin aging). The following ailments will be discussed:

Hepatobiliary diseases, including gallstones and primary biliary cirrhosis;

Sarcoidosis;

Thyroid malfunctions;

Varicose veins and malfunction of the peripheral venous system; and

Osteoporosis and its correlation with skin aging.

Connective tissue diseases are included in a separate chapter and will not be discussed here.

HEPATOBILIARY DISORDERS IN WOMEN

Cholelithiasis

Cholelithiasis causes significant morbidity and mortality. It occurs in about 10% of the adult population in the USA, and is twice as frequent in women as in men[1], with peak incidence between 30 and 39 years of age. Gallstones are found in 20% of autopsied women and 8% of men over the age of 40.

Although usually no specific cutaneous manifestations accompany gallbladder disease, this entity is mentioned here since its occurrence correlates with the skin phenotype of the patients: 'female, fair, forty, fertile' are the classic '4 Fs' characterizing a patient with biliary disease.

Gallstones are crystalline structures formed by the concretion of abnormal bile secretion around a primary nidus. They are classified as cholesterol or pigment stones according to their major content. Cholesterol stones result from cholesterol oversaturation of the bile, while pigment stones are produced by an excess of unconjugated bilirubin. In industrialized countries 80% of gallstones consist mainly of cholesterol[2].

There are several important mechanisms involved in the formation of a lithogenic bile. The most important is an increased biliary secretion of cholesterol. Other factors are a decreased secretion of bile salts and phospholipids, and a reduced activity of hepatic cholesterol 7-hydroxylase, the rate-limiting enzyme of bile acid synthesis. It is speculated that the increased risk of gallstones in women results from a smaller total bile acid pool and an increased biliary cholesterol content of the bile. Recently chronic iron deficiency anemia has been reported to enhance the formation of cholesterol gallstones in multiparous women[3].

In 1984 a theory was suggested to explain the greater risk of gallstones in women with fair skin. The activation of the epidermal pigmentary system by UV light might increase concentrations of reactive indole metabolites both in skin and possibly in bile. In the bile these substances trigger the polymerization of the biliary nidus, thus increasing the risk of gallstone formation[4]. This holds true especially for people with light complexion, in whom storage capacity for melanin in the skin is limited, and significant quantities of reactive indole metabolites may enter the blood and bile. In a case–control study the risk of gallstones increased significantly in people with a positive attitude to sun-bathing. In people with fair skin who always burn after exposure to the sun (skin type I), the relative risk was 25 for a positive attitude compared with a negative one[5].

Primary biliary cirrhosis

Primary biliary cirrhosis (PBC) is a chronic autoimmune disease of the liver. It is seen mainly in middle-aged women, and is characterized by a progressive destruction of small intrahepatic bile ducts resulting in liver cirrhosis. PBC has been reported in all races. In England its annual incidence ranges from 5.8 to 15 cases per million population[6], and it is estimated to account for up to 2% of fatalities from liver cirrhosis[7]. More than 90% of the patients are women. The mean age of onset is 50 years. In recent years, owing to the availability and application of routine serum biochemistry tests, most patients have been diagnosed during the asymptomatic or early symptomatic stages of the disease. In symptomatic patients severe pruritus and general fatigue are the most common complaints. Other symptoms include right upper quadrant discomfort, jaundice, anorexia, diarrhea, weight loss and cutaneous manifestations, such as skin hyperpigmentation, xanthomatosis and hirsutism.

In the early stages pruritus may be the only sign of the disease, and it is not unusual for PBC patients to have first visited a dermatologist. The cause of the pruritus remains unknown. The belief that bile acids are responsible for it is supported by the observation that, in some PBC patients treated with cholestyramine, the relief in itching correlated with a fall in the serum levels of bile acids[8]. On the other hand, it is not unusual to see a patient with high serum levels of bile acids and no pruritus. Elevated levels of serum opioids have also been proposed to play a role in PBC-associated pruritus, and treatment with opioid antagonists diminished this complaint[9]. Other theories to explain pruritus in PBC patients include an imbalance of intrahepatic bile acids[10] and central nervous system receptor mediation[11]. Since pruritus is significantly less common in men with PBC, circulating sex hormones have been suggested to contribute to the itching in women[12]. Other evidence that circulating sex hormones may contribute to the higher frequency of itching in women with PBC includes clinical reports of patients in whom pruritus began during pregnancy or while taking oral contraceptives[13].

Skin pigmentation is also more frequent in women than in men[12]. This is not surprising, since pigmentation of the skin in PBC is caused by postinflammatory deposition of melanin, secondary to scratching. The interscapular area, which is difficult to reach, is usually free of the hyperpigmentation[14]. Because women scratch more, consequent to more prominent pruritus, they also have more pigmentation problems than men. Ultrastructural studies of cutaneous pigmentation in PBC show an excess of melanin, dispersed throughout the epidermis,

accumulating into giant melanosomes, and frequently spilling over into the dermis. In addition, melanosomes are packed in large membrane-bound clusters and persist in higher than usual levels of the epidermis[15].

One of the early descriptions of PBC relates to the disease as xanthomatous biliary cirrhosis, because of the frequent association with skin xanthomata[16]. The various lesions of xanthomatosis are disfiguring, and treatment is often fruitless since they tend to recur after removal. There is no correlation between these lesions and the serum level of cholesterol, and paradoxically they disappear as the disease progresses.

Other cutaneous manifestations of PBC include the nonspecific skin changes associated with liver disease. Telangiectasis on the face, the necklace area, the upper chest and palmar erythema are traditionally attributed to hyperestrogenism, since they are also found in pregnancy and during the ingestion of high estrogen content oral contraceptives. The ratio of estradiol to free testosterone was found to be highest in male cirrhosis patients with spider nevi[17]. Nevertheless, the precise pathogenesis of the vascular changes in liver cirrhosis patients is probably much more complex, since cirrhosis is associated with structural and functional defects in cutaneous capillaries, whether or not spider nevi are present[17].

Association of PBC with other autoimmune nonhepatic disorders affecting blood vessels is exceptionally high. Occurrence of PBC with scleroderma has been reported[18]. Of 83 patients with PBC, 14 had scleroderma, the calcinosis, Raynaud's phenomenon, esophageal dysmotility, sclerodactyly and telangiectasia (CREST) syndrome being identified in two of them[19]. The sicca complex occurs in about 75% of patients with PBC[20]. The association of PBC with the CREST syndrome and sicca complex has been designated by the acronym 'PACK' (primary biliary cirrhosis, anticentromere antibody, CREST, keratoconjunctivitis sicca)[21]. Cutaneous IgM and C3-mediated capillaritis, with and without renal involvement, have been reported in patients with PBC[22,23]. Circulating immune complexes of intermediate size were detected in a patient with PBC vasculitis which responded to cyclophosphamide treatment[24]. These reports and others[25,26] indicate that in PBC generalized activation of immunological mechanisms may involve the skin, clinically or subclinically.

Other skin diseases found in PBC include lichen planus, lichen sclerosus et atrophicus, cutaneous sarcoidosis and autoimmune blistering disorders. The co-existence of PBC with lichen planus was reported in five patients, suggesting that this association is more than coincidental[27]. In another study a lichen planus-like eruption was noted in PBC patients treated with D-penicillamine, and in some these skin lesions developed in the absence of the drug[28].

Serological evidence of PBC was detected in five out of 100 patients with lichen sclerosus et atrophicus (LSA)[29], and the association between these two conditions and lichen planus has also been documented clinically[30]. Since there is some evidence that LSA and lichen planus may have an autoimmune basis[31], their association with PBC is not surprising. Even less surprising are the cases of autoimmune blistering diseases, such as pemphigus or bullous pemphigoid, developing in patients with PBC, treated or not with D-penicillamine[32,33].

The co-existence of PBC and sarcoidosis has been reported. Hepatic granuloma in sarcoidosis is rarely of clinical significance, but occasionally a cholestatic picture occurs with marked similarities to PBC[34]. The majority of the reported cases describe pulmonary sarcoidosis in a patient with PBC, but a few cases of patients with cutaneous sarcoidosis and PBC have lately been published[35,36]. Until the causes of both disorders are elucidated, it is impossible to determine whether their co-existence is attributable to similar pathogenetic factors or reflects a coincidental association.

The clinical course of PBC in most cases is that of a chronic progressive disease. At the time of diagnosis most patients are found to have a liver biochemical profile of anicteric cholestasis with serum alkaline phosphatase and γ-glutamyl transpeptidase levels elevated to a greater degree than those of aminotransferases. The finding of serum antimitochondrial antibodies is extremely helpful in confirming the diagnosis of PBC, since most patients show positive results. The diagnostic histopathological pattern of PBC is that of progressive hepatic granulomatous formation with the eventual disappearance of septal and lobular bile ducts.

The course of the disease cannot be predicted in the individual patient, but the average survival time from diagnosis appears to be about 10 years. Liver transplantation in patients with PBC is associated with increased survival and a dramatic improvement in the quality of life.

SARCOIDOSIS

The first case of sarcoidosis was described by Jonathan Hutchinson more than a century ago.

Since then, cases of sarcoidosis have been reported worldwide and in all races, occurring most commonly during the winter and early spring months[37]. Estimates of prevalence of the disease are one to 40 cases per 100 000 population, with the age-adjusted annual incidence in the USA being 10.9 per 100 000 for whites and 35.5 per 100 000 for the black population[38,39]. The majority of patients in the USA are young African-American women. Moreover, there is some evidence that in blacks sarcoidosis has a more aggressive course[39].

Sarcoidosis is a multisystem granulomatous disorder of unknown cause. The majority of patients with sarcoidosis present with systemic symptoms such as fatigue, dyspnea, anorexia, weight loss and fever. However, not uncommonly asymptomatic cases are discovered when routine chest radiography is performed as part of screening programs. The lungs and intrathoracic lymph nodes are most frequently affected, but extrathoracic involvement is common. The lesions in the lungs are either nodular or disseminated with extensive parenchymal fibrosis. Peripheral lymph nodes, skin, bones and eyes are some common extrapulmonary sites of involvement. Cervical, axillary and inguinal lymph nodes are the most frequently affected. In about 25% of patients with sarcoidosis ocular involvement occurs, most commonly in a form of iridocyclitis. In 12% of patients osseous granulomata are demonstrated in X-rays of the swollen phalanges of fingers and toes or in the skull. The spleen, joints, salivary glands, upper gastrointestinal tract, heart, endocrine system and central and peripheral nervous system may all become involved in sarcoidosis.

Approximately 25% of sarcoidosis patients have skin manifestations. Most of the patients with cutaneous disease concomitant have systemic involvement, but 30% exclusively have skin lesions. When present, systemic disease is either concomitant with the appearance of skin lesions or develops during the first three years after cutaneous involvement[40]. Cutaneous lesions are classified as specific, in which typical sarcoidal granulomas are present, and nonspecific. Sarcoidal granulomas are encountered in up to 37% of patients with cutaneous involvement[40–43]. In about 70% of the cases with cutaneous findings skin lesions appear at the beginning of the disease.

Lupus pernio is rare, but considered as the most typical specific cutaneous lesion of sarcoidosis. It has a predilection for middle-aged black women with long-standing pulmonary, ophthalmic or bone disease. It presents as violaceous indurated plaques on the nose, ears, lips and other facial areas. Nasal lesions frequently involve mucosa, cartilage and bone. Lupus pernio coexists with sarcoidosis of the upper respiratory tract in about half of the cases[43]. This form of sarcoidosis usually follows a chronic course (2–25 years)[44–46].

Maculopapular eruptions are the most common type of specific cutaneous involvement in sarcoidosis. The red-brown to purple papules are usually less than 1 cm in diameter, and are primarily seen on the eyelids, around the eyes, or in the nasolabial folds (Figure 1). They are commonly associated with acute forms of sarcoidosis, such as hilar lymphadenopathy, uveitis, and parotid involvement. Such lesions are regarded as a good prognostic sign, since they are associated with mild lung involvement and usually do not persist for more than two years[46].

Infiltration of old scars and tattoos by granulomatous tissue is a characteristic finding in sarcoidosis. This is the commonest presentation of sarcoidosis in West Africa, where tribal scarification is a common practice[47]. Clinically the scars become red-purple and indurated, with histological evidence of non-caseating granuloma. The chronicity of these lesions depends on the disease activity, but they usually persist for more than 2 years[40]. Sarcoidal plaques are common. Similarly to lupus pernio they are accompanied by more severe lung involvement and have a chronic course, persisting for more than 2 years in 93% of cases[40]. The oval infiltrated purple plaques with pale atrophic centers show a symmetric distribution on the face, limbs and buttocks.

Other rare forms of cutaneous sarcoidosis include ulcerative lesions[48], hypopigmentation[49], ichthyosis-like eruption[50], erythroderma[51], lichenoid eruptions[52], and nail changes (Figure 2).

Tender subcutaneous nodules of the shins (erythema nodosum) are the most common non-specific cutaneous manifestation of sarcoidosis, affecting especially young white women (Figure 3). The association of erythema nodosum with hilar lymphadenopathy is known as Lofgren syndrome. It may be accompanied by fever, arthritis and anterior uveitis. The highest incidence of Lofgren syndrome is reported from northern Europe and Spain[53]. The prognosis of the disease is generally good, with spontaneous recovery in 2 years in most patients.

In specific skin lesions of sarcoidosis, aggregates of epithelioid cells with a few giant cells are found in the dermis (Figure 4). These granulomata are referred to as 'naked' because of the scarcity of lymphoid cells in the periphery of the epithelioid cell tubercle. The giant cells are sometimes found to contain Shaumann or asteroid bodies, which are oval, laminated and calcified intracellular particles.

The diagnosis of sarcoidosis is based on compatible history, clinical findings and histologic evidence of non-caseating granuloma. Infectious causes of granulomatous disease should be excluded by special staining of biopsy specimen and tissue cultures. An elevated serum angiotensin converting enzyme level and bronchoalveolar lavage, demonstrating an elevated CD4/CD8 ratio, can help to confirm the diagnosis of sarcoidosis. The Kveim–Siltzbach test, in which spleen or lymph node homogenate from a sarcoidosis patient is injected intradermally and subjected to biopsy, is not performed any more because of the possibility of transmitting HIV, and lack of standardization. Patients with sarcoidosis have disturbances of cell-mediated immunity. Their peripheral blood demonstrates a T-lymphopenia, yet the involved tissues, such as the lungs, are infiltrated by T-helpers.

Because of the multisystem nature of the disease, any patient found to have a cutaneous sarcoidal granuloma has to be subjected to systemic investigation. In addition to routine blood tests, the work-up should include serum calcium levels (which can be increased), chest X-rays and/or tomography, pulmonary function test, tuberculin skin test, eye examination, serum angiotensin converting enzyme level (increased in about 60% of patients with systemic sarcoidosis) and bronchoalveolar lavage.

The most effective treatment for systemic sarcoidosis is oral corticosteroids. Only severe and disfiguring forms of the cutaneous disease may require this treatment or intralesional injections of corticosteroids. Hydroxychloroquine sulfate (200–400 mg/day)[54], methotrexate (10–15 mg/week)[55] and cosmetic surgery have been shown to have a beneficial effect on the cutaneous disease. The presence of erythema nodosum usually does not require a specific treatment, except for mild anti-inflammatory drugs. The prognosis of a patient with sarcoidosis depends on the extension and severity of the systemic involvement. The presence of a specific cutaneous lesion does not affect the overall prognosis of this disease[56].

The mortality rate of sarcoidosis is about 5%. The most common cause of death is right heart insufficiency, resulting from massive parenchymal fibrosis of the lungs.

THYROID DISEASE

Thyroid disorders occur in women much more frequently than in men, probably because of the autoimmune nature of many of these disorders.

The discrepancy in the incidence of autoimmune disorders between the genders is presumably related to the effect of sex hormones on the immune system.

Thyroid hormones exert their diverse effects by binding to specific nuclear receptors, thus regulating gene expression and protein synthesis. Thyroid hormones seem to play an important role in the maintenance of normal mammalian skin function, such as oxygen consumption[57], mitotic activity and protein synthesis[58], hair growth[59], sebum secretion[60], and collagen and mucopolysaccharide production by dermal fibroblasts. The maintenance of appropriate levels of thyroid hormones requires the integration of the hypothalamic–pituitary–thyroid axis.

Thyrotropin-releasing hormone (TRH) is secreted by hypothalamic neurons and stimulates the secretion of thyroid-stimulating hormone (TSH) from the anterior pituitary. TSH stimulates the thyroid gland to produce thyroxine (T4) and triiodothyronine (T3). This system is controlled by negative-feedback interactions between circulating thyroid hormones, TSH and TRH. T3 is more potent than T4 in peripheral tissues. Both are bound to plasma proteins, and only small fractions of free hormones are active.

Hypothyroidism

Hypothyroidism is the most common abnormality of thyroid function. The prevalence rates in women are between 0.6% and 5.9%, depending on the population surveyed and the diagnostic criteria used[61–63]. The main causes of thyroid insufficiency are: chronic autoimmune disease of the gland, transient thyroiditis, iatrogenic thyroid dysfunction (post-surgical or post-irradiation) or pituitary/hypothalamic hormone deficiency. In primary thyroid failure the free T4 levels are depressed and TSH levels are elevated. Occult hypothyroidism may be expressed by elevated TSH levels exclusively. In central hypothyroidism TSH levels are low or inappropriately normal for low free T4 levels. The diagnosis of autoimmune thyroid failure is confirmed by the presence of various antithyroid antibodies, such as antithyroid peroxidase and antithyroglobulin.

The clinical syndrome is called myxedema, deriving its name from the most prominent cutaneous manifestation. Hypothyroidism is characterized clinically by symptoms of fatigue, weakness, depression, cold intolerance, constipation and disturbances in the menstrual cycle. The skin in hypothyroidism is cold and pale, because of the reduced core temperature and cutaneous vasoconstriction caused by a hypometabolic state[64]. In myxedema the entire skin is edematous, dry, pale and waxy. In spite of the edematous appearance the skin is firm and does not pit on pressure. This appearance is caused by dermal deposition of acid mucopolysaccharides, such as hyaluronic acid and chondroitin sulfate. The facial look is characterized by a broad nose, puffy eyelids and macroglossia. Drooping of the upper eyelid, even in the absence of edema, is attributed to decreased sympathetic stimulation of the superior palpebral muscle. The scalp and body hair is dry, brittle and sparse. Massive telogen effluvium may appear if the onset of hypothyroidism is abrupt. This has been attributed to premature anagen arrest and failure in initiation of anagen[65]. Loss of the lateral third of the eyebrows is a characteristic feature. Decreased sebum secretion contributes to the skin xerosis and coarse appearance of the hair. In addition there is evidence from mammalian studies that decreased epidermal sterol synthesis may contribute to the extreme skin dryness[66]. Both the hair and the nails grow slowly[67]. Yellowish discoloration of the skin, accentuated in the palms and soles, is due to carotenemia. Acquired keratoderma has been reported in association with hypothyroidism[68]. Impaired wound healing may accompany thyroid insufficiency states.

The mechanism of mucin deposition in myxedema is not clear. There is experimental evidence that thyrotropic hormone may stimulate dermal accumulation of mucopolysaccharides in mice[69]. Nevertheless, myxedematous features are less prominent in hypothyroidism secondary to pituitary failure than in primary hypothyroidism.

The histological picture of myxedematous skin, routinely stained with hematoxylin–eosin, usually does not show any abnormality. However, in severe cases swelling of the collagen bundles with splitting into their individual fibers may be observed[70]. Stains with colloidal iron or alcian blue demonstrate small amounts of mucin in the vicinity of blood vessels. All the changes are reversible on thyroid hormone replacement therapy, but may recur on its discontinuation[71].

Hyperthyroidism

Hyperthyroidism affects women 10 times as frequently as men[63,72]. Approximately 0.54% to 2.0% of women suffer from this disease[73]. Hyperthyroidism may occur in several conditions: Graves' disease, thyroiditis, multinodular goiter, single toxic nodule, excessive thyroxine intake, or TSH-secreting adenoma. The skin in hyperthyroidism

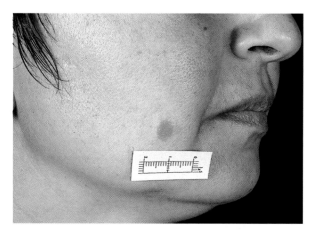

Figure 1   Red–brown papule of sarcoidosis on a face

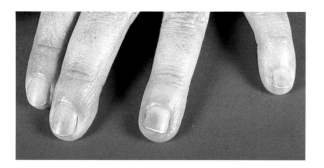

Figure 2   Nail changes in a patient with sarcoidosis

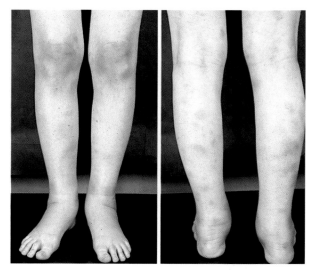

Figure 3   Erythema nodosum in a patient with Löfgren syndrome

is warm, moist and smooth. Persistent redness of the face, transient flushing and palmar erythema may occur. The warmth of the skin is caused by increased cutaneous blood flow accompanied by peripheral vasodilatation. Hyperhidrosis and thinning of the scalp hair is noticed. The change in hair quality or quantity may be a reason for the first encounter of a hyperthyroid woman with a dermatologist. Although not pathognomonic, Plummer's nails are present in about 5% of patients with hyperthyroidism. These nails are characterized by a concave contour with distal onycholysis. Hyperpigmentation, in a distribution reminiscent of Addison's disease, may appear. This is believed to result from the increased secretion of adrenocorticotropic hormone (ACTH), compensating for the accelerated degradation of cortisol[71]. Pruritus, alopecia areata, urticaria and vitiligo may be associated with hyperthyroidism.

Graves' disease

Graves' disease is the most common cause of hyperthyroidism. In this disorder autoimmune stimulation of thyrotropin receptors occurs. An association of autoimmune thyroid disease, especially Graves' disease in women, with polymorphism at the first position of codon 52 (C52–>A52) of the human thyrotropin receptor gene has been reported. This association is even more prominent in patients with skin changes[74].

Graves' disease comprises goiter, thyrotoxicosis, ophthalmopathy and skin and nail changes. The thyroid gland is diffusely enlarged. The skin changes, called pretibial myxedema, occur in 0.5–4% of patients, usually in the presence of ophthalmopathy[75]. Correction of the thyrotoxicosis does not necessarily improve the skin changes, but additional progression may occur following the treatment of thyroid dysfunction. Pretibial myxedema lesions appear on the anterior aspects of the legs and dorsa of the feet as firm pink to purple plaques or nodules (Figure 5). They are usually bilateral, but not symmetric. Sometimes they have a 'peau d'orange' appearance and woody consistence. Overlying verrucosities with hypertrichosis or hyperhidrosis may be present[76,77]. The clinical variants of thyroid dermopathy are non-pitting edema, nodular, plaque, polypoid, and elephantiasic forms. Although pretibial location is the most typical, mucin deposits in other sites may appear[78]. There is conflicting evidence that patients with this disorder may have similar abnormalities in the preradial skin[79].

On histological sections large amounts of glycosaminoglycans, especially hyaluronic acid, are found in the middle and lower thirds of the dermis, and there is damage to collagen and elastic fibers (Figure 6). During the process of fixation the deposited material may be washed out of the tissue. As a result, empty spaces are frequently seen within the mucin deposits.

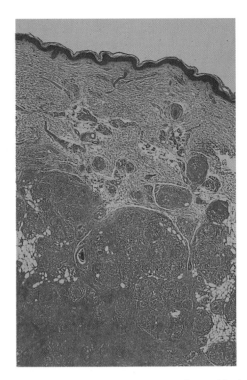

Figure 4 Typical 'naked' granuloma of sarcoidosis

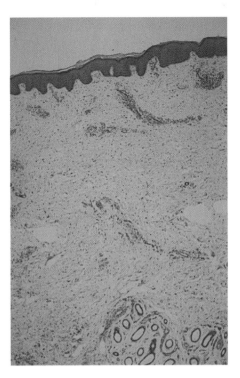

Figure 6 Mucin deposits in pretibial myxedema

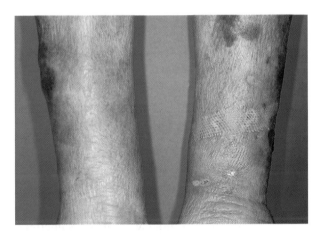

Figure 5 Pretibial myxedema in a patient with Graves' disease

The mechanism of pretibial myxedema formation is unknown. Dermal fibroblasts appear to share antigenic similarity with TSH receptors, which is a primary autoantigen in Graves' disease[80]. As a result the fibroblasts are stimulated to produce abnormally large amounts of glycosaminoglycans. The restriction of the myxedema to the pretibial area may be explained by the fact that fibroblasts from this area synthesize 2–3 times more hyaluronic acid than fibroblasts from other areas, when incubated with serum from patients with pretibial myxedema[81]. Humoral factors, such as insulin-like growth factor-I, have been suggested to be of etiological significance in the mechanism of mucin deposition in Graves' disease[82].

The development of pretibial myxedema in Graves' disease is not related to the thyroid function status. Patients may be hyperthyroid, euthyroid, or hypothyroid when lesions develop[71]. The condition may persist for years. Spontaneous regressions are accompanied by a parallel decline or disappearance of serum anti-TSH receptor antibody level. The treatment of pretibial myxedema is primarily medical, consisting of oral and topical corticosteroids. Topically applied corticosteroid therapy may induce sustained long-term partial remission in a substantial number of patients[83]. Clobetasol propionate under occlusive dressing was found to be efficient in pretibial myxedema unresponsive to other therapy[84]. Surgical excision was beneficial in a case of pseudotumorous pretibial myxedema recalcitrant to multimodal therapy[85], but this approach has failed when skin grafting of involved sites was tried[86]. Moreover, localized myxedema may appear at the donor site of a skin graft as the initial presentation of Graves' disease[87]. Recently clinical and pathological improvement of pretibial myxedema with parallel reduction in circulating autoantibodies has been observed in Graves' patients treated by high-dose intravenous immunoglobulins[88].

Thyroid acropachy is a rare manifestation of thyroid disorder, consisting of clubbing, digital soft tissue swelling and periosteal new bone formation. Although the vast majority of cases are associated with Graves' disease, it may occur in association with other thyroid dysfunction[89,90]. Most of the patients with Graves' disease develop acropachy after the diagnosis of thyrotoxicosis[91], male and female patients being equally affected[92]. Pathognomonic radiographic changes consist of a lamellar type periosteal reaction usually confined to diaphyses of the hands and wrists[93]. These radiographic changes reflect an increase in osteoblastic activity, and bone scanning of the extremities provides a sensitive test for diagnosing thyroid acropachy[94]. The natural course of thyroid acropachy is extremely variable, and spontaneous remissions have been reported[95]. Specific treatment is usually not required, since most patients are asymptomatic. When necessary, topical potent steroids under occlusion may improve clinical manifestations[95].

VENOUS DISEASE

Disease of the peripheral venous system is a public health problem affecting industrialized as well as developing countries. The cost of treatment of chronic venous disease was found to be 2–2.5% of the total 1995 health care budget in Belgium[96] and around 400 million pounds per year in the UK[97]. The prevalence of venous disease of the lower limb in the adult population ranges between 5% and 55% depending on study design and location[96,98–100]. The prevalence of varicose veins was found to be about two times higher in women than in men in Italy and the UK[98,101], four times higher in Finnish women[102] and ten times higher in French women than in men[103]. Analysis of steroid receptors, performed on stripping-removed varicose saphenous veins, showed an expression of progesterone receptors in the tunica media and the subendothelial layer of the vein, in both sexes[104]. There is at least one study demonstrating the presence of estrogen receptors in the walls of peripheral veins[105]. These observations suggest that the intergender differences in peripheral venous disease may occur owing to the direct action of sex hormones on the veins in women.

In addition to gender, advanced age, low education and ethnicity are also risk factors for varicose veins[98,101], though there is no clear relationship between varicose veins and excess weight in normal or pregnant women[99,101,106]. Up to 30% of women develop venous insufficiency during their first pregnancy, and with each pregnancy its prevalence increases. The risk of developing venous disease during pregnancy increases significantly with age[104]. Mechanical compression of an enlarged uterus on pelvic veins, hormonal changes reducing venous tonicity and other factors are considered to

be the major reasons for the increased risk for varicose disease during pregnancy[107].

Varicose veins may be either a constitutional phenomenon or develop secondary to thrombophlebitis (postphlebitic syndrome). Many patients with varicosities have no symptoms, but seek medical advice because of the cosmetic appearance. Others complain of heaviness, tension, swelling, aching, cramps and itching of the lower limbs[108]. They may report exacerbation of these symptoms by dependency and relief by elevation of the limb.

On physical examination varicose veins are seen as dilated and tortuous superficial vessels anywhere on the legs or feet, following the anatomical course of the veins. Leg edema, stasis eczema (with or without secondary infection), hyperpigmentation and ulceration may develop. Lipodermatosclerosis refers to fibrosis with induration of the dermis and subcutis secondary to venous insufficiency. Venous ulcers occur in chronic cases and are usually located on the medial aspect of the ankle. These manifestations may occur soon after an episode of deep venous thrombosis or up to twenty years later[109,110]. The majority of patients with post-phlebitic syndrome do not give a history of thrombophlebitis, and are therefore believed to have had silent thrombosis.

The diagnosis of varicose veins rests primarily on the history and physical examination of the patient. The incompetent valves of varicose veins can be demonstrated by emptying the peripheral venous system by limb elevation and subsequent application of a tourniquet at the level of the saphenofemoral junction. When the tourniquet is released, while the patient is in an erect position, rapid filling of the veins indicates the saphenofemoral valve incompetence. Duplex scanning can visualize the patency of the deep venous system and localize obstruction sites.

Patients with venous insufficiency have incompetent valves in the deep or perforating veins. As a result, increased venous pressure occurs distally to a malfunctioning valve. Moreover, pressure remains high during exertion[111]. High venous pressure is associated with capillary proliferation and increased permeability of the capillaries to large molecules, such as fibrinogen, and cells into the skin[110,112]. Stasis pigmentation is the result of the escape of red blood cells into the tissues, resulting in inflammatory reaction to the deposited hemoglobin. Fibrinogen molecules form a pericapillary barrier to the diffusion of oxygen and other nutrients, essential for the vitality of the skin[111].

The treatment of varicose veins aims at preventing venous stasis and alleviating the discomfort accompanying this disorder. Cosmetic concerns as an indication for treatment are more common in women than in men[113]. Medical compression stockings, although not curing the varicosities, prevent further progression of the disease and relieve the subjective symptoms. Usually stockings providing high compressive values of 30–40 mmHg are recommended. Recently it has been shown that even stockings with weaker compression may be useful for venous insufficiency[114]. The use of hosiery with a lower compression is cosmetically more acceptable and enhances compliance. Elastic bandages may be an alternative to stockings, and have the advantage of adapting the degree of pressure to the individual case. However, because of the cosmetic appearance, this modality of treatment has a lower compliance. Elastic bandages or stockings should be worn throughout the day and removed before retiring to bed. Elevation of the lower part of the bed to a position in which the legs are somewhat higher than the heart level helps to decrease the edema. Elastic compression stockings are particularly indicated in pregnancy[115]. Sclerotherapy is used for the treatment of varicose veins alone or in combination with surgery. The mechanism of action of sclerosants is that they cause endothelial damage with subsequent thrombus formation and fibrosis of the vessel. A wide variety of sclerosing agents is available. They produce their effect by interference with cell surface lipids (polidocanol, sodium tetradecyl sulfate), by dehydration of endothelial cells through osmosis (hypertonic saline or glucose), or by direct destruction of the endothelium (chromated glycerin).

Ligation and stripping of veins are reserved for patients with large and symptomatic varicosities. Segmental avulsion has been used to remove clusters of varicose veins. Prior to extensive sclerosing or surgical treatment, investigation should demonstrate a patent and functioning deep venous system. The treatment of varicose veins should not be postponed in young women, because of the potential for pregnancy, that worsens the condition. Early treatment prevents the further development of varicosities during the pregnancy and ensures greater comfort. Any recurrences can be treated by sclerosing or segmental avulsions after the delivery[116].

OSTEOPOROSIS AND SKIN

Osteoporosis is a skeletal disorder characterized by a structural deterioration and decrease of bone mass, resulting in increased bone fragility and fractures. About 30% of postmenopausal white women in the USA are affected by this devastating disorder.

Multiple risk factors are associated with the pathogenesis of osteoporosis. These include age, sex, low body mass index, low calcium diet, sedentary life style, prolonged corticosteroid therapy, thyroid replacement therapy, smoking and alcohol and caffeine ingestion habits.

A correlation between skin features and bone density has been suggested in various studies. In the USA the prevalence of osteoporosis is higher in white than in black women[117]. It is not clear, however, whether this difference is related to a lower bone mass observed among whites, different diet and physical activity habits or to a genetic trait. To clarify this, Nelson and colleagues compared skin color, body mass and bone mineral density in black and white normal and osteoporotic women. No significant correlation was found between skin color measured by reflectometry and bone mineral density in this work[118]. When the relationship between self-reported skin complexion and bone mineral density was evaluated in a population of Caucasian women, individuals with fairer skin were found to have lower bone mineral density[119]. It was suggested in this study that a fair skin color reflects decreased exposure to the sun. Sunlight is required for vitamin D synthesis in skin, and a positive correlation between serum 25-hydroxyvitamin D levels and bone mineral density has been previously found[120]. Therefore fair-skinned aging women, who normally reduce their sun-exposure habits, may become vitamin D depleted[121], which will contribute to the decrease in their bone mineral density. In addition to defective mineralization, evidence regarding collagen alterations within the osteoporotic bone has recently been accumulating[122]. Like bone, more than 70% of human dermis is composed of type I collagen. Thus, a possible correlation between an age-associated decrease in bone density and skin thickness, both related to matrix collagen depletion, has been extensively investigated[123]. In the early nineteen-forties patients with postmenopausal osteoporosis were described as having a wrinkled, thin, atrophic skin[124]. Later on the prevalence of osteoporosis in women with thin transparent skin, as shown by infrared photography, was reported to be higher than in women with thicker skin[125]. In a recent study by Chappard and colleagues a significant correlation between skin thickness and femoral bone mineral density was found among 133 women[126]. But when measured by A mode ultrasound scanning no difference in skin thickness was found between 20 osteoporotic females and 20 age-matched non-osteoporotic women by Pederson and co-workers[127].

Castelo-Branco and colleagues found that changes in bone mass are closely related to a decline in collagen content of the sun-protected skin during the aging process[128]. These findings are in agreement with an earlier report regarding the effect of anorexia nervosa on skin collagen and bone density[129]. Thus these studies support the hypothesis that age-related bone and skin changes are caused by a generalized loss of collagen accompanying senescence.

In a cross-sectional study performed by Whitmore and Levine, an attempt was made to predict bone density by skin thickness and to determine risk factors affecting bone density and skin thickness[130]. These authors found that skin thickness was a statistically significant independent predictor of bone density only for the femoral neck in postmenopausal women. Previously identified risk factors for osteoporosis – such as age, years past menopause, hours of exercise per week, caffeine ingestion, years of thyroid hormonal replacement and cumulative prednisone dose – were found to affect not only bone density, but also skin thickness. Although common pathogenetic mechanisms for a decrease in bone density and skin thickness are not always clear, some hypotheses have been proposed.

Prolonged thyroid replacement therapy in postmenopausal women has been found to be associated with a significant reduction in bone mass[131]. This is owing to stimulation of osteoclasts, directly or through overproduction of interleukin (IL)-1 and IL-6[132]. IL-1 may also stimulate collagenase synthesis and degradation of cutaneous collagen with consequent skin atrophy[133].

An inverse correlation between caffeine ingestion and bone mineral density in postmenopausal women[134] could be explained by an increase of urinary calcium excretion[135] and the subsequent elevation in parathyroid hormone levels. In dermal fibroblasts caffeine decreases type I procollagen mRNA levels[136], inhibits elastin gene expression[137] by enhancing 1,25-dihydroxyvitamin D3 synthesis secondary to caffeine-induced calciuria[138], and stimulates collagenase activity by increasing IL-1 production[139]. There is a direct relationship between hours of weekly exercise and bone mineral density[140]. Enhanced growth hormone secretion due to strenuous physical activity may explain the increased skin thickness, as found in patients with acromegaly. Postmenopausal hormone replacement therapy has a beneficial effect on bone density. A similar positive effect of estrogen replacement on skin thickness has also been demonstrated[141].

As life expectancy increases, so does concern about the prolonged preservation of skeletal function and unwrinkled skin. Appropriate public education regarding the prevention of risk factors and therapeutic measures for both problems, based on controlled population studies, are necessary.

REFERENCES

1. Hoover EL, Jaffe BM, Webb H, England DW. Effects of female sex hormones and pregnancy on gallbladder prostaglandin synthesis. *Arch Surg* 1988; 123:705–8
2. Baumgartner G, Sauerbruch T. Gallstones: pathogenesis. *Lancet* 1992;338:1117–21
3. Johnston SM, Murray KP, Martin SA, *et al.* Iron deficiency enhances cholesterol gallstone formation. *Surgery* 1997;122:354–61
4. Pavel S. A new possible pathogenesis of some gallstones. *Med Hypoth* 1984;14:285–92
5. Pavel S, Thijs CT, Potocky V, Knipschild PG. Fair, and still a sun lover: risk of gallstone formation. *J Epidemiol Commun Health* 1992;46:425–7
6. Triger DR. Primary biliary cirrhosis: an epidemiological study. *Br Med J* 1980;281:772–5
7. Hamlyn AN, Sherlock S. The epidemiology of primary biliary cirrhosis: a survey of mortality in England and Wales. *Gut* 1974;15:473–9
8. Datta DV, Sherlock S. Treatment of pruritus of obstructive jaundice with cholestyramine. *Br Med J* 1963;5325:216–19
9. Thornton JR, Losowsky MS. Opioid peptides and primary biliary cirrhosis. *Br Med J* 1988;297:1501–4
10. Ghent CN. Pruritus of cholestasis is related to effects of bile salts on the liver, not the skin. *Am J Gastroenterol* 1987;82:117–19
11. Bergasa NV, Thomas DA, Vergalla J, *et al.* Plasma from patients with pruritus of cholestasis induces opioid receptor-mediated scratching in monkeys. *Life Sci* 1993;53:1253–7
12. Lucey MR, Neuberger JM, Williams R. Primary biliary cirrhosis in men. *Gut* 1986;27:1373–6
13. Sherlock S. Primary biliary cirrhosis. In Schiff L, Schiff ER, eds. *Diseases of the Liver*. Philadelphia: JB Lippincott, 1982:979–1002
14. Reynolds TB. The butterfly sign in patients with chronic jaundice and pruritus. *Ann Intern Med* 1973;78:545–6
15. Mills PR, Skerrow CJ, MacKie RM. Melanin pigmentation of the skin in primary biliary cirrhosis. *J Cutan Pathol* 1981;8:404–10
16. McMahon HE, Thannhauser SJ. Xanthomatous biliary cirrhosis (a clinical syndrome). *Ann Intern Med* 1949;30:121–78
17. Pirovino M, Linder R, Boss C, *et al.* Cutaneous spider nevi in liver cirrhosis: capillary, microscopic and hormonal investigations. *Klin Wochenschr* 1988;66:289–302

18. Reynolds TB, Denison EK, Frankl HD, *et al.* Primary biliary cirrhosis with scleroderma, Raynaud's phenomenon and telangiectasia. *Am J Med* 1971;50: 302–12

19. Clarke AK, Galbraith RM, Hamilton EB, Williams R. Rheumatic disorders in primary biliary cirrhosis. *Ann Rheum Dis* 1978;37:42–7

20. Golding PL, Brown R, Mason AMS, Taylor E. 'Sicca complex' in liver disease. *Br Med J* 1987;4: 340–2

21. Powell F, Schroeter AL, Dickson ER. Primary biliary cirrhosis and the CREST syndrome: a report of 22 cases. *Q J Med* 1987;62:75–82

22. Diederrichsen H, Sorensen PG, Mickley H, *et al.* Petechiae and vasculitis in asymptomatic primary biliary cirrhosis. *Acta Derm Venereol (Stockh)* 1985;65:263–6

23. Rai GS, Hamlyn AN, Dahl MG, *et al.* Primary biliary cirrhosis, cutaneous capillaritis, and IgM-associated membranous glomerulonephritis. *Br Med J* 1977;1:817

24. Terkeltaub R, Esdaile JM, Bruneau C, *et al.* Vasculitis as a presenting manifestation of primary biliary cirrhosis: a case report. *Clin Exp Rheumatol* 1984; 2:67–73

25. Randle HW, Millins JL, Schroeterc AL, Winkelmann RK. Cutaneous immunofluorescence in primary biliary cirrhosis. *JAMA* 1981;246:1679–81

26. Hendricks AA, Hutcheon DF, Maddrey WC, *et al.* Cutaneous immunoglobulin deposition in primary biliary cirrhosis. *Arch Dermatol* 1982;118:634–7

27. Graham-Brown RA, Sarkany I, Sherlock S. Lichen planus and primary biliary cirrhosis. *Br J Dermatol* 1982;106:699–703

28. Seehafer JR, Rogers RS III, Fleming CR, Dickson ER. Lichen planus-like lesions caused by penicillamine in primary biliary cirrhosis. *Arch Dermatol* 1981;117:140–2

29. Lavery HA, Pinkerton JH, Callender M. The association of lichen sclerosis et atrophicus and primary biliary cirrhosis. *Br J Dermatol* 1985;112:729–30

30. Graham-Brown RA, Sarkany I. Lichen sclerosus et atrophicus with primary biliary cirrhosis and lichen planus. *Int J Dermatol* 1986;25:317

31. Harrington CI, Dunsmore IR. An investigation into the incidence of autoimmune disorders in patients with lichen sclerosus and atrophicus. *Br J Dermatol* 1981;104:563–6

32. Gibson LE, Dicken CH. Pemphigus erythematosus, primary biliary cirrhosis, and D-penicillamine: report of a case. *J Am Acad Dermatol* 1985;12:883–5

33. Singhal PC, Scharschmidt LA. Membranous nephropathy associated with primary biliary cirrhosis and bullous pemphigoid. *Ann Allergy* 1985;55: 484–5

34. Maddrey WC, Johns CJ, Boitnott JK, Iber FL. Sarcoidosis and chronic hepatic disease. *Medicine* 1970;49:375–95

35. Harrington AC, Gitzpatrick JE. Cutaneous sarcoidal granulomas in a patient with primary biliary cirrhosis. *Cutis* 1992;49:271–4

36. Hughes P, McGavin CR. Sarcoidosis and primary biliary cirrhosis with co-existing myositis. *Thorax* 1997;52:201–2

37. Bardinas F, Morera J, Fite E, Plasencia A. Seasonal clustering of sarcoidosis. *Lancet* 1989;2:455–6

38. Bresnitz EA, Strom BI. Epidemiology of sarcoidosis. *Epidemiol Rev* 1983;5:124–56

39. Rybicki BA, Major M, Popovich J Jr, *et al.* Racial differences in sarcoidosis incidence: a 5-year study in health maintenance organization. *Am J Epidemiol* 1997;145:234–41

40. Mana J, Marcoval J, Graells J, *et al.* Cutaneous involvement in sarcoidosis: relationship to systemic disease. *Arch Dermatol* 1997;132:882–8

41. Longcope WT, Freiman DG. A study of sarcoidosis. *Medicine* 1952;31:1–132

42. Mayock RL, Bertrand P, Morrison CE, Scott JH. Manifestations of sarcoidosis: analysis of 145 patients, with a review of nine series selected from the literature. *Am J Med* 1963;35:67–89

43. Spiteri MA, Matthey F, Gordon T, *et al.* Lupus pernio: a cliniço-radiological study of thirty-five cases. *Br J Dermatol* 1985;112:315–22

44. James DG. Dermatological aspects of sarcoidosis. *Q J Med* 1959;28:109–24

45. Sharma OM. Cutaneous sarcoidosis: clinical features and management. *Chest* 1972;61:302–5

46. Veien NK, Stahl D, Brodthagen H. Cutaneous sarcoidosis in Caucasians. *J Am Acad Dermatol* 1987;16:534–40

47. Alabi GO, George AO. Cutaneous sarcoidosis and tribal scarification in West Africa. *Int J Dermatol* 1989;28:29–31

48. Verdegem TD, Sharma OMP. Cutaneous ulcers in sarcoidosis. *Arch Dermatol* 1987;123:1531–4

49. Clayton R, Breathnach M, Martin B, Feiwel M. Hypopigmented sarcoidosis in a negro. *Br J Dermatol* 1977;96:119–25

50. Banse-Kupin L, Pelachyk JM. Ichthyosiform sarcoidosis: report of two cases and a review of the literature. *J Am Acad Dermatol* 1987;17:616–20

51. Morrison JGL. Sarcoidosis in a child presenting as an erythroderma with keratotic pines and palmar pits. *Arch Dermatol* 1973;107:758–60

52. Gange RW, Smith NP, Fox ED. Eruptive cutaneous sarcoidosis of unusual type. *Clin Exp Dermatol* 1978;3:299–306

53. Mana J, Badrinas F, Morera J, *et al.* Sarcoidosis in Spain. *Sarcoidosis* 1992;9:118–22

54. Jones E, Callen JP. Hydroxychloroquine is effective therapy for control of cutaneous sarcoidosis. *J Am Acad Dermatol* 1990;23:487–9

55. Webster GF, Razsi LK, Sanchez M, Shupack JL. Weekly low-dose methotrexate therapy for cutaneous sarcoidosis. *J Am Acad Dermatol* 1991;24:451–4

56. Mana J, Salazar J, Manresa F. Clinical factors predicting persistence of activity in sarcoidosis: a multivariate analysis of 193 cases. *Respiration* 1994;61:219–25

57. Freinkel RK. Effect of thyroxine administration on the metabolism of guinea pig skin. *J Invest Dermatol* 1962;38:31

58. Holt PJA, Marks R. The epidermis response to change in thyroid status. *J Invest Dermatol* 1977;68:299–301

59. Ebling FJ. Hormonal control and methods of measuring sebaceous gland activity. *J Invest Dermatol* 1974;62:161–71

60. Goolamali SK, Evered D, Shuster S. Thyroid disease and sebaceous gland function. *Br Med J* 1976;1: 432–3

61. dos Remedios LV, Weber PM, Feldman R, *et al.* Detecting unsuspected thyroid dysfunction by the free thyroxine index. *Arch Intern Med* 1980;140: 1045–9

62. Sawin ST, Castelli WP, Hershman JM, *et al.* The aging thyroid: thyroid deficiency in the Framingham study. *Arch Intern Med* 1985;145:1386–8

63. Tunbridge WM, Evered DC, Hall R, *et al.* The spectrum of thyroid disease in a community: the Whickham survey. *Clin Endocrinol (Oxf)* 1977;7: 481–93

64. Mullin GE, Eastern JS. Cutaneous signs of thyroid disease. *Am Fam Physician* 1986;34:93–8

65. Frienkel RK, Frienkel N. Hair growth and alopecia in hypothyroidism. *Arch Dermatol* 1972;106:349

66. Rosenberg RM, Isseroff RR, Ziboh VA, Huntley AC. Abnormal lipogenesis in thyroid hormone-deficient epidermis. *J Invest Dermatol* 1986;86:244–8

67. Feingold KR, Elias PM. Endocrine-skin interaction. *J Am Acad Dermatol* 1987;17:921–40

68. Hodak E, David M, Feurman EJ. Palmoplantar keratoderma in association with myxedema. *Acta Derm Venereol (Stockh)* 1986;66:354–7

69. Dyrbye MO, Ahlquist Y, Wegelius O, *et al.* Effect of thyroxine, thyrotropic and somatotropic hormones on skin of dwarf mice. *Proc Soc Exp Biol Med* 1959;102:417

70. Reuter MJ. Histopathology of the skin in myxedema. *Arch Dermatol Syph* 1931;24:55–71

71. Diven DG, Gwinup G, Newton RC. The thyroid. *Dermatol Clin* 1989;7:547–57

72. Sugrue D, McEvoy M, Feely J, Drury MI. Hyperthyroidism in the land of Graves: results of treatment by surgery, radio-iodine and carbimazole in 837 cases. *Q J Med* 1980;49:51–61

73. dos Remedios LV, Weber PM, Feldman R, *et al.* Detecting unsuspected thyroid dysfunction by the free thyroxin index. *Arch Intern Med* 1980;140: 1045–9

74. Cuddihy RM, Dutton CM, Bahn RS. A polymorphism in the extracellular domain of the thyrotropin receptor is highly associated with autoimmune thyroid disease in females. *Thyroid* 1995;5:89–95

75. McDougall IR. Graves' disease: current concepts. *Med Clin North Am* 1991;75:79–95

76. Mullin GE, Eastern JS. Cutaneous consequences of accelerated thyroid function. *Cutis* 1986;37:109–14

77. Gitter DG, Sato K. Localized hyperhydrosis in pretibial myxedema. *J Am Acad Dermatol* 1990;23:250–4

78. Wortsman J, Dietrich J, Traycoff RB, Stone S. Preradial myxedema in thyroid disease. *Arch Dermatol* 1981;117:635–8

79. Peacy SR, Flemming L, Messenger A, Weetman AP. Is Graves' dermopathy a generalized disorder? *Thyroid* 1996;6:41–5

80. Heufelder AE, Wenzel BE, Scriba PC. Antigen receptor variable region repertoires expressed by T cells infiltrating thyroid, retroorbital and pretibial tissue in Graves' disease. *J Clin Endocrinol Metab* 1996;81:3733–9

81. Cheung HS, Nicoloff JT, Kamiel MB, *et al.* Stimulation of fibroblast biosynthetic activity by serum of patients with pretibial myxedema. *J Invest Dermatol* 1978;71:12–17

82. Kriss JP. Pathogenesis and treatment of pretibial myxedema. *Endocrinol Metab Clin North Am* 1987;16:409–15

83. Fatourechi V, Pajouhi M, Fransway AF. Dermopathy of Graves' disease (pretibial myxedema). Review of 150 cases. *Medicine (Baltimore)* 1994;73:1–7

84. Volden G. Successful treatment of chronic skin diseases with clobetasol propionate and hydrocolloid occlusive dressing. *Acta Derm Venereol (Stockh)* 1992; 72:69–71

85. Pingsmann A, Ockenfels HM, Patsalis T. Surgical excision of pseudotumorous pretibial myxedema. *Foot Ankle Int* 1996;17:107–10

86. Kucer KA, Luscombe HA, Kauh YC. Pretibial myxedema: recurrence after skin grafting. *Arch Dermatol* 1980;116:1076–7

87. Missner SC, Ramsay EW, Houck HE, Kauffman CL. Graves' disease presenting as localized myxedema in a thigh donor graft site. *J Am Acad Dermatol* 1998;39:846–9

88. Antonelli A, Navarrane A, Palla R, *et al.* Pretibial myxedema and high-dose immunoglobulin treatment. *Thyroid* 1994;4:399–408

89. Abu Haydar N. Exophthalmus, digital clubbing and pretibial myxedema in thyroiditis. *J Clin Endocrinol* 1963;23:215–17

90. Basadjieva E, Georgieva S, Altunkov P, *et al.* Localized pretibial myxedema and thyroid acropachy in a case of Hurthle cell adenocarcinoma. *Int J Dermatol* 1971;10:170–4

91. Shaheen JS, Ellis FG, Marvasti A. Thyrotoxicosis: gross acropachy and pretibial myxedema. *J Soc Med* 1986;79:170–1

92. Sreenivasamoorthy S, Shenov BV, Krishnamurthy K. Thyroid acropachy. *Indian J Med Sci* 1969;23:492–5

93. Siegel RS, Thrall JH, Ssson JC. ^{99}Tc-pyrophosphate scan and radiographic correlation in thyroid acropachy: case report. *J Nucl Med* 1976;17:791–3

94. Parker LN, Wu SY, Lai MK, *et al.* The early diagnosis of atypical thyroid acropachy. *Arch Intern Med* 1982;142:1749–51

95. Solanski SV, Shah SS, Kothari UR. Thyroid acropachy. *Indian J Med Sci* 1973;27:708–10

96. Van den Oever R, Hepp B, Debbaut B, Simon I. Socio-economic impact of chronic venous insufficiency. An underestimated public health problem. *Int Angiol* 1998;17:161–7

97. Ruckley CV. Socioeconomic impact of chronic venous insufficiency and leg ulcers. *Angiology* 1997;48:67–9

98. Schmeiser-Reider A, Kunze U, Mitsche N, *et al.* Self-reported prevalence of venous diseases in the general population of Austria – results of the SERMO study. *Acta Med Austriaca* 1998;25:65–8

99. Canonico S, Gallo C, Paolisso G, *et al.* Prevalence of varicose veins in Italian elderly population. *Angiology* 1998;49:129–35

100. Maffei FH, Magaldi C, Pinho SZ, *et al.* Varicose veins and chronic venous insufficiency in Brazil: prevalence among 1755 inhabitants of a country town. *Int J Epidemiol* 1986;15:210–17

101. Callam MJ. Epidemiology of varicose veins. *Br J Surg* 1994;81:167–73

102. Sisto T, Reunanen A, Laurikka J, *et al.* Prevalence and risk factors of varicose veins in lower extremities: mini-Finland health study. *Eur J Surg* 1995; 1161:405–14

103. Boccalon H, Janbon C, Saumet JL, *et al.* Characteristics of chronic venous insufficiency in 895 patients followed in general practice. *Int Angiol* 1997;16:226–34

104. Perrot-Applant M, Cohen-Solal K, Milgrom E, Finet M. Progesterone receptor expression in human saphenous veins. *Circulation* 1995;92:2975–83

105. Krasinski Z, Kotwicka M, Oszkinis G, *et al.* Investigations on the pathogenesis of primary varicose veins. *Wiad Lek* 1997;50:275–80

106. Dindelli M, Parazzini F, Basellini A, *et al.* Risk factors for varicose disease before and during pregnancy. *Angiology* 1993;44:361–7

107. Krajcar J, Raadakovic B, Stefanic L. Pathophysiology of venous insufficiency during pregnancy. *Acta Med Croatica* 1998;52:65–9

108. Bradbury A, Evans C, Allan P, *et al.* What are the symptoms of varicose veins? Edinburgh vein study cross sectional population survey. *Br Med J* 1999; 318:353–6

109. Jacobs P. Pathogenesis of the postphlebitic syndrome. *Annu Rev Med* 1983;34:91–105

110. McEnroe CS, O'Donnel TF Jr, Mackey WC. Correlation of clinical findings with venous hemodynamics in 386 patients with chronic venous insufficiency. *Am J Surg* 1988;156:148–52

111. Burnand RG, Whimster IW, Clemenson G. The relationship between the number of capillaries in the skin of the venous ulcer bearing area of the lower leg and the fall in foot vein pressure during exercise. *Br J Surg* 1981;68:297–300

112. Burnand RG, Clemenson G, Whimster IW, *et al.* The effect of sustained venous hypertension in the skin capillaries of the canine hind limb. *Br J Surg* 1981;69:41–4

113. O'Leary DP, Chester JF, Jones SM. Management of varicose veins according to reason for presentation. *Ann Roy Coll Surg Engl* 1996;78:214–16

114. Gniadecka M, Karlsmark T, Bertman A. Removal of dermal edema with class I and II compression stockings in patients with lipodermatosclerosis. *J Am Acad Dermatol* 1998;39:966–70

115. Norgren L, Austrell C, Nilsson L. The effect of graduated elastic compression stockings on femoral blood flow velocity during pregnancy. *Vasa* 1995;24: 282–5

116. van der Stricht J, van Oppens C. Should varices be treated before or after pregnancy? *Phlebologie* 1991;44:321–6

117. Farmer ME, White LR, Brody JA. Race and sex differences in hip fracture incidence. *Am J Pub Health* 1984;44:1374–80

118. Nelson DA, Kleerekoper M, Peterson E, Parfitt AM. Skin color and body size as risk factors for osteoporosis. *Osteoporosis Int* 1993;3:18–23

119. May H, Murphy S, Khaw K-T. Bone mineral density and its relationship to skin color in Caucasian females. *Eur J Clin Invest* 1995;25:85–9

120. Khaw K-T, Sneyd MJ, Compston J. Bone mineral density and parathyroid hormone and 25-hydroxyvitamin D concentrations in middle-aged women. *Br Med J* 1992;305:273–7

121. McKenna M. Differences in vitamin D status between countries in young adults and the elderly. *Am J Med* 1992;93:69–77

122. Bailey AJ, Wotton SF, Sims TJ, Thompson PJ. Post-translational modifications in the collagen of human osteoporotic femoral head. *Biochem Biophys Res Commun* 1992;185:801–5

123. Uitto J. Connective tissue biochemistry of the aging dermis: age related alterations in collagen and elastin. *Dermatol Clin* 1986;4:433–46

124. Albright F, Smith P, Richardson A. Postmenopausal osteoporosis – its clinical features. *JAMA* 1941;116: 2465–74

125. McConkey B, Fraser GM, Blight AS, Whitley H. Transparent skin and osteoporosis. *Lancet* 1963; 30:693–5

126. Chappard D, Alexandre CH, Robert J-M, Riffat G. Relationships between bone and skin atrophies during aging. *Acta Anat* 1991;141:239–44

127. Pederson H, Agner T, Storm T. Skin thickness in patients with osteoporosis and controls quantified by ultrasound A scan. *Skin Pharmacol* 1995;8:207–10

128. Castelo-Branco C, Pons F, Gratuos E, *et al.* Relationship between skin collagen and bone changes during aging. *Maturitas* 1994;88:199–206

129. Savvas M, Treasure J, Studd J, *et al.* The effect of anorexia nervosa on skin thickness, skin collagen and bone density. *Br J Obstet Gynaecol* 1989;96: 1392–4

130. Whitmore SE, Levine MA. Risk factors for reduced skin thickness and bone density: possible clues regarding pathophysiology, prevention, and treatment. *J Am Acad Dermatol* 1998;38:248–55

131. Faber J, Galloe AM. Changes in bone mass during prolonged subclinical hyperthyroidism due to L-thyroxine treatment: a meta-analysis. *Eur J Endocrinol* 1994;130:350–6

132. Manolagas SC, Jilka RL. Bone marrow, cytokines, and bone remodeling. *N Engl J Med* 1995;332: 305–11

133. Boxman I, Lowik C, Aarden L, Ponec M. Modulation of IL-6 production and IL-1 activity by keratinocyte–fibroblast interaction. *J Invest Dermatol* 1993;101:316–24

134. Kiel DP, Felson DT, Hannan MT, *et al.* Caffeine and the risk of hip fracture: the Framingham study. *Am J Epidemiol* 1990;132:675–84

135. Massey LK, Whiting SJ. Caffeine, urinary calcium, calcium metabolism and bone. *J Nutr* 1993;123: 1611–14

136. Duncan MR, Hasan A, Berman B. Pentoxifylline, pentifylline, and interferons decrease type I and III procollagen mRNA levels in dermal fibroblasts: evidence for mediation by nuclear factor 1 down-regulation. *J Invest Dermatol* 1995;104:282–6

137. Parks WC. Down regulation of elastin expression in fibroblasts by 1, 25-dihydroxycholecalciferol vitamin D3 [abstract]. *J Invest Dermatol* 1989; 92:497A

138. Eli C, Liberman UA, Rosen JF, Marx SJ. A cellular defect in herditary vitamin D dependent rickets type II: defective nuclear uptake of 1, 25-dihydroxyvitamin D3 in cultured skin fibroblasts. *N Engl J Med* 1981;304:1588–91

139. Dayer J-M, de Rochemonteix B, Burrus B, *et al.* Human recombinant interleukin 1 stimulates collagenase and prostaglandin E2 production by human synovial cells. *J Clin Invest* 1986;77:645–8

140. Huddelston AL, Rockwell D, Kulund DN, Harrison RB. Bone mass in lifetime tennis athletes. *JAMA* 1980;244:1107–9

141. Maheux R, Naud F, Rioux M, *et al.* A randomized double-blind, placebo-controlled study on the effect of conjugated estrogens on skin thickness. *Am J Obstet Gynecol* 1994;170:642–9

Drug eruptions

Larry E. Millikan

22

Is this a significant issue – the gender differences in drug eruptions? Until recently, this would not have been possible to answer. At least in the USA, the process of drug evaluation and testing, until about a decade ago, was strictly limited to adult men or to a few women who no longer had child-bearing potential. This was a usual exclusion in virtually every study, to avoid potential problems such as those seen with thalidomide: the phocomelia resulting from drug usage during pregnancy. The slow process of drug approval in the USA allowed these problems from thalidomide to be identified in Europe, and vindicated the agency's usual slow *modus operandi*. This resulted in a major change in the approach of the United States Food and Drug Administration (FDA) to drug approval for the next several decades.

Such drug studies for evaluation of safety and efficacy have little bearing on practice, because there are such rigid inclusion/exclusion criteria and monotherapy is almost essential. This flies in the face of usual clinical practice, and therefore phase IV studies are perhaps more indicative of the drug's potential to create unwanted reactions and side-effects in the general population – men and women. This is now an increasing process, allowing careful follow-up and early drug withdrawal or modified usage from these findings. Usual data on incidence have been centered around hospitalization[1] and/or the elderly, which have a reported incidence of 10–17%[2].

The interesting dilemma at present is the fact that, according to some sources:

(1) Women reportedly have a higher incidence of drug eruptions[3];

(2) Women often receive more medications than men, particularly the newer psychotropic medications that can cause problems[4], hence enhancing their risk further.

Drugs are used liberally in women by clinicians, in spite of the fact that the original data for most of the older medications were not generated using a patient population including women of childbearing age. Present concerns include teratogenicity (Table 1) and proper classification of pregnancy risk (Table 2).

Perhaps a good recent historical example of gender difference relates to the hepatic problems associated with ketoconazole. While the drug passed with flying colors through initial studies, subsequent release and widespread use brought forth a 1 : 12 000–15 000 incidence of hepatic reactions, ranging from mere enzyme elevation to severe hepatotoxicity, and a few deaths. Ultimately, the usual profile began to emerge that the most common patient with this problem was an older woman, over 50 years of age, who was using ketoconazole for the treatment of onychomycosis. The idiosyncratic reaction usually occurred after 30 days on therapy, ranging from 30 to 90 days into therapy. Clinical experience from adverse reporting led clinicians to monitor patients with this profile very carefully, because they were at significant risk. The reason for female preponderance is still unclear. Again, this finding was late in appearance because of the usual rules for drug testing in the population at the phase III level. Currently, phase IV testing is allowing a greater insight into such a reaction.

DRUG REACTIONS OF PARTICULAR CONCERN IN WOMEN

A major reason for the lack of data on drug interactions and eruptions in women has been the problem of pregnancy. This came to a crisis with the thalidomide problem, and has not until recently been seriously addressed. A great deal of information has been accumulated in this particular situation, and as a baseline the US government has established a classification of drugs for pregnancy precautions: ABCD and X (Table 2). Female dermatology patients requiring systemic medication with a potential for teratogenicity are those with such diseases as acne, atopic dermatitis and asthma, and on occasion urticaria and the cutaneous eruptions of pregnancy. Additionally, many of the potent systemic treatments for psoriasis carry risks for fetal malformations. The risk of teratogenicity can be increased in patients with cutaneous malignancies and cutaneous T-cell lymphoma, and also those on systemic therapy. As a result of this, the dermatologist must use care in selection of systemic medications for the female patient of childbearing

Table 1   Known teratogenic drugs

Angiotensin converting enzyme (ACE) inhibitors
Angiotensin II blockers
Androgens
Anticonvulsants
Diethylstilbestrol
Iodides
Isotretinoin
Lithium
Live vaccines
Tetracycline
Warfarin

Table 2   Pregnancy risk category

A	No risk
B	No evidence of risk in humans
C	Cannot rule out risk
D	Positive risk
X	Contraindicated

age who is not practicing active contraception. Further, even simple therapies for acne may alter contraception, which confounds the situation further. Therefore, one can easily understand the preference of conservative dermatologists for using topical therapy only. In this area, however, there are authorities in both pediatrics and obstetrics and gynecology who consider such medications as topical retinoids to pose a risk for the fetus, and that these should therefore be avoided if at all possible during pregnancy. The new therapies for androgenetic alopecia with the 5α-reductase inhibitors have the significant potential, presumably with even very casual contact with the medications, of inducing abnormalities of the genitalia of the fetus, simulating the congenital 5α-reductase deficiency clinical picture. This is an area that is addressed in great detail by the manufacturer in the packaging of the medication for the patients' use, but is important to be considered with regards to casual prescriptions for finasteride.

SPECIAL CONSIDERATIONS IN GIRLS

The situation of drug reactions in children is similar to that with women, in that the number of subjects tested has only recently increased significantly. Additionally, the rapid appearance of many cutaneous eruptions and exanthems provides a great deal of confusion as to the role of the drugs in the evolution of certain papulosquamous and

vasculitis-like cutaneous reactions. Of significant concern with the breast-feeding mother is the transposition of drugs taken by the mother to the nursing child, and this has to be anticipated on a case-by-case basis with the drugs being extremely variable in their potential for direct passage through the milk to the child. Extreme examples are some of the H2 blockers, cimetidine or ranitidine, and erythromycin rapidly being present in large amounts in breast milk, and other drugs, such as heparin, digoxin and metoclopramide not having significant levels in mother's milk at all. With newer drugs, it is important to anticipate problems for the infant when treating the nursing mother. In reality, perhaps the most difficult area for drug reactions in children is the differential of childhood exanthems with the classical types of exanthems (Table 3), and in each case with these exanthems one has to consider the differential diagnosis, which includes various infections, including the classical five exanthems as well as drug eruptions, occasionally the TORCH syndrome and certain viral infections such as those seen with coxsackievirus, enteroviruses, echovirus and others.

MECHANISMS

The concepts of drug reactions are changing with a better understanding of the multiple mechanisms. Several major pathways occur in humans, resulting in adverse drug events. A drug can manifest untoward side-effects on several bases, including:

(1) Known side-effects, which can vary in different populations with different gene pools;

(2) Problems of drug interactions;

(3) Direct toxicity when increasing the dose, or when the amount of free drug is increased by drug interactions;

(4) Allergic reactions;

(5) Physiological effects perceived as a reaction.

Side-effects

This is an important area in therapeutic planning for the patient. Virtually every drug does not have a single target action, and multiple actions can create problems or symptoms for the patient. Sometimes these actions are perceived as a reaction to the drug that the patient subsequently lists as a drug allergy. One of the best examples is the problem with opiates inducing urticaria and pruritus. The problem of drug interactions in patients with incipient

Table 3 Exanthems and drug reactions: differential diagnosis

Infection
Bacterial
   scarlatina
   rickettsial (Rocky Mountain spotted fever, etc.)
   Gram (−) (sepsis)
   toxic shock syndrome
   staphylococcal scarlatina
Viral
   rubella
   rubeola
   roseola
   fifth disease (erythema infectiosum)
   infectious mononucleosis
Common drugs
Antibiotics – penicillin, ampicillin, sulfa drugs
Non-steroidal anti-inflammatory drugs
Phenytoins
Barbiturates

Table 4 Drug–drug interaction (abbreviated list). Check drug information for newer cautions and interactions

Cytochrome CyP450 3A
   Astemizole
   Imidizoles
   Triazoles
   Macrolides
   Statin drugs
   HIV drugs
      Amprenarivir
      Retinavir
   Viagra (sildenafil)
   Rifampin
   Amiodarone

glaucoma is another very serious potential side-effect, and involves many drugs, making it essential that the clinician evaluate the patient ahead of time and be certain that any new drug initiated is not going to increase intraocular pressure and precipitate acute problems with glaucoma.

Interactions

This is an area that has become extremely critical in the past 5 years, as we have achieved better understanding of drug metabolism and interactions. Drug interactions can include competition for a carrier site in the blood, resulting in higher levels of free drug in the blood, and possible toxicity. More important are the areas in which one drug can interfere with the normal drug metabolism of another, resulting in elevated drug levels; or the converse, where the one drug can stimulate the enzymes used in drug metabolism for a second drug, thereby diminishing the effective drug levels. This is critical in patients who are on anticoagulants. Furthermore, most recently in dermatology, the interactions of imidazole and triazole antifungals with certain antihistamines such as terfenadine and astemizole have been a serious problem, with deaths reported from cardiotoxicity, causing arrhythmias. Table 4 shows some of the interactions that face dermatologists treating patients of either gender. This is particularly important in consultation on patients who are immunosuppressed from viral HIV infection or from therapeutic immunosuppression because of organ transplantation. In these patients, the serious problem of superficial and deep fungi, and other infections, prompts use of antifungal or antimicrobial therapy that must be very carefully selected to avoid such potential interactions.

Toxicity

One of the classical examples of toxicity is the local reaction after extravasation of intravenous medication, causing local tissue necrosis. This is often a function of the pH of the infusion, causing severe local changes and cell death. Toxicity can also result in the release of various cytokines, including tumor necrosis factor, which may be one of the best candidates for the often difficult problem of drug fever.

Allergic reactions

The Coombs–Gell classification includes:

(1)   I. IgE-mediated reactions;

(2)   II. Cytotoxic reactions (IgG, IgM);

(3)   III. Immune complex reactions;

(4)   IV. Cell-mediated immunity.

A major concern in the problem of drug eruptions is the allergic type of reaction, which can be IgE-mediated or anaphylactic, and the more common reaction related to vasculitis secondary to immune complex formation. Of particular interest in this process is the role of estrogens and their effect on modulating the immune response, which can be seen so clearly in the autoimmune disorders in the New Zealand Black and New Zealand White mice. In these laboratory animals one sees the impressive role hormones and gender play, with estrogen aggravating the immunological disease and androgens moderating it. This is nearly a pure example

Table 5   Drugs generally considered safe in pregnancy

Acne
Topicals
    erythromycin, clindamycin, benzoyl peroxide
Alternatives
    oral erythromycin
Asthma
    theophylline, corticosteroids orally, inhaled
        β-agonists, steroids, cromolyn
Cough
    diphenhydramine, lozenges
Diabetes
    insulin
Headache
    acetaminophen
Hyperthyroidism
    thyroxin
Antibiotics
    penicillins, cephalosporins, cotrimoxazol,
        erythromycin
Nausea, vomiting, morning sickness
    doxylamine plus pyridoxine

of the effect of estrogens on modulation of the immune response. It points to the possibility in other animal systems as well as humans that the hormone oscillation in females can confound the predictability of drug reactions. This is especially a concern in those studies that eliminate women of childbearing age (and hence those with significant estrogen production) and may mask the possibility for additional reactions/interactions. In spite of this, there are some drugs that, through long experience, have come to be generally considered safe in pregnancy (Table 5).

Of greatest significance is the IgE-mediated reaction to certain drugs, because of its lethal (anaphylactic) potential. Penicillin deaths are perhaps the best prototype for IgE-mediated disease, but similar reactions with potential fatal complications occur with many other drugs, and this is an important aspect of testing, using skin tests, history and the radioallergosorbent test (RAST) in drug allergy. Tests in the past have included lymphocyte blast transformation, for potential detection of allergies to certain drugs, as well as modifications of the RAST test which is used for environmental allergies. Specific RAST tests for many individual drugs are unfortunately largely lacking, so this creates the major problem in confirming the diagnosis. The reaction after initiation of the production of IgE antibodies results in a drug antigen–IgE complex, with subsequent release of histamine and other vasoactive amines, and the cascade leading to urticarial and anaphylactic sequelae. For this reason, it is important, when a suspected reaction to a drug is possibly IgE mediated, that appropriate state-of-the-art testing be done by all means available, including intradermal skin testing (Figure 1), serological testing and other *in vitro* analyses that are used variably in different laboratories across the USA.

Type III reactions

Type III reactions to drugs result clinically in various vasculitis types of reaction (type III) that are microscopically associated with immune complex formation. This is usually IgM or IgG mediated, and the size of the complexes and location of their deposition determines the usual clinical picture. Serious sequelae can result from the classical immune complex reaction and its associated renal disease, arthritis and serum sickness-like phenomenon. At the present time, the most common manifestation of drug reactions is the maculopapular reaction associated with immune complex formation, so frequent in allergic reactions to antibiotics.

In women, the role of estrogen in enhancing immune reactions is an area of concern because of our awareness of the extreme in this situation: the problem of serum sickness, where immune complexes affect the cutaneous vasculature, as well as affecting other vital organs – the liver, kidney, etc.

The development of these reactions is often delayed, and this may be a point of confusion. Even after discontinuation of the offending medication, as is often seen in penicillin reactions, the extent of the maculopapular eruption progresses for as long as 2 weeks after discontinuation of the medication.

The deposition of these immune complexes in the skin as well as other organs is then followed by a cascade of reactions – cytokine release, complement activation and urticaria-like changes in the skin. In very severe reactions, the end result can be necrosis. These are usually small, punctate, sharply demarcated areas of skin necrosis.

Physiological effects

Although one can consider adverse drug interactions during pregnancy as a probable physiological situation, there are other activities that can occur that relate to the normal metabolism of a drug that causes sequelae in a fashion that varies from patient to patient. Because of this, and because of the previously mentioned occasional role of estrogenic substances on the alteration of a drug effect, women represent an unusual target and a greater potential risk. The many effects of some of the newer drugs, such as the β-blocker category of cardiovascular medications, gives the patient a significant potential for annoying and sometimes serious side-effects. The list includes such cutaneous reactions as lichenoid and papulosquamous eruptions and, as one might expect, the β-blocker interaction has been reported to cause an associated Raynaud's phenomenon. Urticaria and pruritus are not unexpected, inasmuch as these drugs will interfere with the histamine pathways in mast cells. Some of the gastrointestinal side-effects (diarrhea, etc.) can also be looked on as a direct physiological result of drugs interfering with the β-adrenergic effects in the normal physiology of the gastrointestinal tract. The sympathomimetic blockade can result in a relative overaction on the cholinergic side, and this explains many of the side-effects seen with the β-blockers that is purely physiological and not toxic or allergic. Similarly, other drugs affect cytochrome P450 and especially the 3A subset, because of their metabolism (see Table 4). This creates a competitive interaction that is physiological, and can lead to high doses of the medication and toxicity.

Additionally, as an example of physiological effects, sulfa drugs – dapsone and others that have a significant oxidizing potential – can, as the dose is increased, result in significant side-effects: methemoglobinemia, anemia, cytopenia, and even precipitation of cardiovascular sequelae because of the lowered oxygen-carrying capacity of the blood. All of these are physiological effects (and thus dose related) that can be anticipated with the understanding of the mechanisms of the drug's action. Thereby, with dosage alteration, one can avoid significant side-effects.

Hair loss with hormones and other drugs (Table 6) are another example that should be anticipated, and is of particular concern in the female patient, especially with androgenic and antiandrogenic hormones and drugs.

DIAGNOSIS

The primary problem with the establishment of the diagnosis is lack of appropriate confirmation. In a careful review of the history, timing is of the essence for the consideration of a definite drug or an alternative possibility. Therefore, one needs to review and re-review the history of the patient and the landmarks with regard to the general state of health, appearance of the rash, specific characteristics of the rash and the timing after the drug

Table 6 Drugs that can cause alopecia

β-Blockers
Antimitotics
  busulfan
  bleomycin
  cytarabine
  doxorubicin
  etoposide
Antifungals
  itraconazole
  ketoconazole
  fluconazole
Oral contraceptives, testosterone
Anticholesterol statins
  pravastatin
  simvastatin
Warfarin
Spironolactone
Stanozolol

exposure (Figure 2). Additionally, it is very important that the history reviews previous exposures to drugs, to pick up the possibility of an accelerated or anamnestic response. At the same time alternative causes need to be considered (see Table 8). The best examples of this, to rule in and rule out drug eruptions, are seen in the two cases described below.

Case 1

This was a 12-year-old girl who initially presented with low-grade fever, cervical adenopathy, a few palpable petechiae and very exudative tonsils and throat. The patient felt malaise and weakness, but was otherwise normal. There was no sign of otitis and the lungs were clear. The low-grade temperature continued, and at the first visit the patient was started on cloxacillin 500 mg daily. By day 7, at nearly the completion of the course of medication, the patient developed a widespread morbilliform eruption, the low-grade temperature continued and the initial impression was that this was the first manifestation of penicillin allergy.

Case 2

This 26-year-old woman was hospitalized in Steamboat Springs, Colorado, after fracture of her leg while skiing. As part of the general postoperative course, the patient was put on prophylactic antibiotics, namely ampicillin 250 mg four times a day.

The patient was discharged home without any obvious sequelae. She was referred to the local

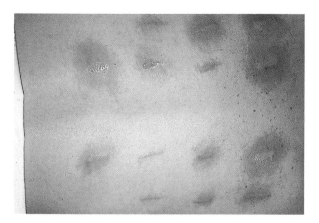

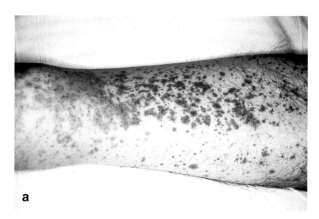

a

Figure 1 Typical example of an IgE type I reaction: scratch test in the skin

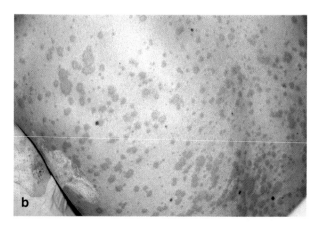

b

Figure 3 (a) Hemorrhagic residue of an ampicillin reaction that had been urticarial initially. (b) An acute morbilliform urticarial eruption occurred in this other patient receiving an ampicillin-type agent. The redness is much brighter in the acute stage

Table 7 Drugs rarely causing a reaction

Diphenhydramine
Digoxin
Potassium chloride
Aspirin
Acetaminophen
Erythromycin

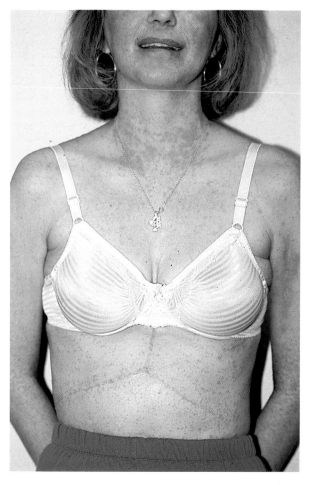

Figure 2 A morbilliform eruption developed in this woman who was taking sulfamethoxazole/trimethoprim for a urinary tract infection

dermatologist on day 5 of ampicillin therapy because of a maculopapular eruption. On her history, the patient revealed previous exposure to penicillins without any history of previous allergy, most recently treated in the past year. The maculopapular, almost urticarial reaction was considered classic for ampicillin, and the diagnosis of ampicillin drug allergy was made. The patient returned home, was treated symptomatically and the drug was discontinued. The orthopedic surgeon re-referred the patient 5 days later as the eruption continued to increase. The diagnosis of ampicillin allergy was sustained.

Comments

In case 1, this was an example of the misdiagnosis or overdiagnosis of drug allergy. This is most frequent in younger patients who are susceptible to the various exanthems (see Table 3), and the prodrome for the viral exanthem has enough suggestive signs and symptoms to mandate initial

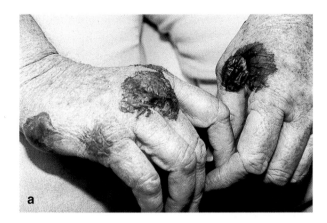

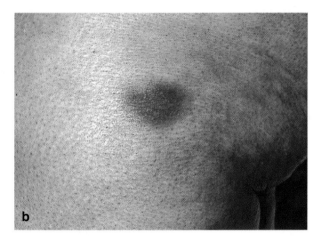

Figure 4   (a) Extensive bullae in a bullous drug eruption due to thiazides. An older woman, residing in a nursing home, received thiazides as part of her antihypertensive regimen. She developed purpuric bullae. This should not be confused with (b) a fixed drug eruption that resulted from this woman's taking a phenolphthalein laxative

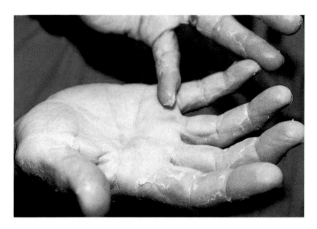

Figure 5   Extensive peeling of the skin of the hands occurred in this patient who had a toxic epidermal necrosis (TEN) type of drug eruption

Table 8   Common causes of drug reactions

Antibiotics
   penicillins
   semisynthetic penicillin
   sulfa drugs
Antiseizure medications
   phenytoin
   phenobarbital
   carbamazepine
Allopurinol

treatment with antibiotics, and quite often penicillin antibiotics. The general course of the condition and lack of any defervescence with the institution of antibiotics suggest that the infectious etiology for which the penicillin was being used was not sustainable. In fact, as so often happens with many pediatric and preadolescent patients, the diagnosis of penicillin allergy was made falsely on the basis of a viral exanthem being confused with the usual drug reaction to penicillin (Figure 3).

In contrast, in case 2, the classical ampicillin reaction – on the palms and generalized on the body; maculopapular, morbilliform or urticarial; with appropriate timing after 5 to 10 days – made a strong case for acquired ampicillin allergy. As occasionally happens, the referring physician was confused by the fact that the drug reaction could continue. It often worsens after discontinuation of the antibiotic because of the simple immunologic facts of a type III reaction, that is the development

of more antibodies with greater affinity and the resultant increase in immune complex size, causing continued or increased cutaneous reactions. The referring physician was reassured, and the reaction slowly subsided.

These are good examples of appropriate review of the patients' history and timing of drug exposure resulting in sustainable diagnoses of drug reaction in one and viral exanthem in the other. In all of these instances the differential diagnosis in Table 3 is essential to clear up any questions and to be certain not to rule out alternative diagnoses.

Match technique

The next step with several possible suspect drugs (especially in the polypharmacy scene with many older patients) involves picking the most likely. Timing here, as above in the simpler cases where a single drug was involved, is the first step: finding the appropriate 5–12-day interval for activation of the immunological reaction. On the other hand, timing can be altered by the other types of drug reactions, some of which relate to a concentration of the drug and may appear very rapidly. The knowledgeable physician has always available several alternative sources for reference to back up the diagnosis. In addition, in the match technique, one can easily dismiss several medications that fit the list of infrequent causes of reaction (Table 7). Contrast this with a knowledge of those that frequently cause eruptions (Table 8). Jerome Litt's DERM (*Drug Eruptions Reference Manual*)[5] is perhaps one of the most valuable, and is available in both a hard and soft cover, and as a CD ROM. Here one can match the reaction, lichenoid, exanthematous, etc., with long lists of drugs and pick the one most likely. More detail may be found in textbooks[6,7].

Additional tests

Some laboratory tests have been proposed, and may be of use, but many of the more sophisticated ones vary in their availability.

(1) *Complete blood count and differential*   This may be useful on the basis of a significant eosinophilia, which, if present, is a strong support for the diagnosis of drug allergy[8].

(2) *IgE*   In the atopic patient on some occasions with anaphylactoid or urticarial reactions, there may be a corresponding rise in IgE, but this is not always reliable. Elevated IgE may also suggest that a patient is at greater risk for such types of allergy.

(3) *Lymphocytoblast transformation and migration inhibition factor (MIF) assays*[9]   This test is rarely performed, but is still available in some areas, and does provide a fairly good insight into drug associations and the subsequent activation and blast formation of reactive cells of the small lymphocyte category. Certain laboratories have this available and therefore it may be useful regionally when carried out easily.

(4) *Basophil degranulation*   This test was promoted by Shelley[10] many years ago, but is rarely available currently.

(5) *Skin biopsy*   This is often a very valuable test to rule in or rule out drug eruptions, especially when one is dealing with the bullous eruptions, toxic epidermal necrosis (TEN), or Stevens–Johnson syndrome. This may be essential, and the use of cutaneous epidermal immunofluorescence is an essential part of the testing.

(6) *RAST*   The radioallergosorbent test has been used in some cases. It may be helpful when there is a crossover of *Penicillium* mold and penicillin allergy, but it also may be useful in ascertaining a definitive cause from the environment or foods other than medications. Other newer tests are regionally available in the USA and in Europe that are primarily of a research nature, looking at various cytokines and other changes, and looking at the type of cellular infiltrate in the epidermis in the patient with a drug eruption. Subsets of T cells in this infiltrate, if available, may also be a helpful guideline for the diagnosis.

Other tests in the future, such as reactive drug metabolites and other *in vitro* tests, may be of great value also[11].

TREATMENT

Obviously, the primary treatment remains discontinuation of the drug after establishing a firm diagnosis, followed by supportive therapy. Pruritic symptoms are often a challenge; Litt has summarized many alternatives to steroids[12]. Widespread acute reactions may require steroids, and some of the newer ascomycin drugs and other macrolactams may find a significant utility in the future. The controversy over steroids in various bullous eruptions continues. It has become clear that late in the evolution of a bullous eruption is not the time to begin steroids, because the process has gone beyond the point where these drugs would be effective (Figure 4). Symptomatic relief when there is widespread loss of the cutaneous envelope is mandatory; these patients often end up in a burn unit. Simple urticarial reactions and minor exanthems will respond to anti-H1 or anti-H2 and corticosteroid drugs primarily. The support of the patient and prevention of secondary infection after a widespread cutaneous drug reaction are all essential to the favorable outcome (Figure 5). In the patients with bullous eruptions, careful attention to the mucous membranes, including the conjunctiva, is essential, and these patients, as mentioned above, are candidates for the burn unit in severe cases and obviously require careful following by several specialists. Inattention to the eyes has resulted in corneal scarring and visual deterioration, so the ophthalmologist is an essential member of the consultant team.

It is essential in any given patient that the diagnosis of a specific drug allergy be pursued, so that the patient can avoid further exposure and further inconvenience or hospitalization. The dermatologist is perhaps the best equipped to carry out this monitoring.

REFERENCES

1. Bigby M, Stern RS, Arndt KA. Allergic cutaneous reactions to drugs. *Prim Care* 1989;16:713–27

2. Coi N, Fanale JF, Kronholm P. The role of medication noncompliance and adverse drug reactions in hospitalization of the elderly. *Arch Intern Med* 1990;150:841–5

3. Davies DM, ed. *Textbook of Adverse Drug Reactions*, 3rd edn. Oxford: Oxford University Press, 1985: 1–11

4. Weissman MM, Klerman GL. Sex differences and the epidemiology of depression. *Arch Gen Psychiatry* 1977;34:98–111

5. Litt JZ. *Drug Eruption Reference Manual 2000: Millennium Edition*. Casterton, UK: Parthenon Publishing, 2000

6. Millikan LE. Drug eruptions (dermatitis medicamentosa). In Moschella SL, Hurley HJ, eds. *Dermatology*. Philadelphia: WB Saunders Company, 1992:535–73

7. Breathnach SM. Drug reactions. In Champion RH, Burton JL, Ebling FJG, eds. *Textbook of Dermatology*, 6th edn. Oxford: Blackwell Scientific Publications, 1998:3349–517

8. Drake L, Dinehart SM, Farmer ER, *et al*. Guidelines of care for cutaneous adverse drug reactions. *J Am Acad Dermatol* 1996;35:458–61

9. Uno K, Yamasaku F. Application of leucocyte migration tests to detection of allergenic drugs in patients with hypersensitivity to beta-lactam antibiotics. *J Antimicrob Chemother* 1989;24:241–50

10. Shelley WB. Indirect basophil degranulation test for allergy to penicillin and other drugs. *JAMA* 1963;184:171–8

11. Sullivan JR, Shear NH. What are some of the lessons from *in vitro* studies of severe unpredictable drug reactions? *Br J Dermatol* 2000;142:203–9

12. Litt JZ. Topical treatment of itching without corticosteroids. In Bernhard JD, ed. *Itch: Mechanisms and Management in Pruritus*. New York, NY: McGraw Hill, 1994:23–5

Infections and infestations

Bacterial, rickettsial and viral diseases

23

J Carl Craft

INTRODUCTION

Epidemiological considerations of infectious diseases include sex predilection, age predilection, seasonal prevalence, incubation period, ratio of subclinical to clinical illness, distribution in the community, reservoirs and vectors. Infectious agents cannot differentiate between hosts on the basis of sex. Because of this, most infections are equally represented in both sexes. The host's exposure to the infectious agent and the host's immunoresponse can produce inequalities between sexes, but in most of these case men are the more severely affected and more frequently infected. Bacterial, rickettsial and viral infections do have manifestations or outcomes that are important to women and not of import to men. This chapter deals with the bacterial, rickettsial and viral infections involving the skin that have specific significance for women.

BACTERIAL INFECTIONS

Gram-positive cocci are the most common causes of skin infections. Skin infections caused by *Streptococcus pyogenes*[1,2] and/or *Staphylococcus aureus*[3,4] account for more than 90% of all primary pyodermas such as impetigo (Figures 1 and 2), furunculosis, erysipelas and cellulitis (Tables 1, 2 and 3). These very common infections are more often seen in men and so do not represent a specific threat to women; however, these bacteria do have a significance for women. Both *S. pyogenes* and *S. aureus* produce toxins that can cause serious cutaneous manifestations. The bacterial toxins that cause scarlet fever and toxic shock syndromes have special considerations for girls and women.

Scarlet fever

Streptococcus pyogenes, also frequently referred to as group A β-hemolytic streptococcus (GABHS), frequently produces toxins that increase the virulence of the organism[5]. These toxins result in streptococcal toxic shock syndrome and scarlet fever. After decades of decreasing virulence of streptococcal

soft-tissue infections, invasive infections with *S. pyogenes* have re-emerged[6–8]. Fatal illness with an incidence of 80% involvement of skin and soft tissues such as in necrotizing fasciitis and myositis is related to the reappearance of highly mucoid exotoxin-producing strains of GABHS[9–12]. These cases of streptococcal toxic shock syndrome do not have any particular significance for women other than that they are similar to staphylococcal toxic shock syndrome (discussed later). Scarlet fever and streptococcal pharyngitis and tonsillitis are more common in females. Three immunologically distinct erythrogenic toxins can be produced by *S. pyogenes*[13–16]. Although these toxins are frequently found in the GABHS, scarlet fever is relatively uncommon[13]. This can be explained by the need for the organism to be infected with a lysogenic bacterial phage for the toxin to be expressed[17].

Scarlet fever is a complication of streptococcal pharyngitis and is seldom seen in patients with primary pyodermas[18]. Children predominately between the ages of 2 and 10 years are affected. Bacterial pharyngitis and tonsillitis are more frequently seen in females particularly in adults. There is no proven reason for this, other than that women are the care givers in families, both as parents and as older siblings, making exposure more common. Because of this increased frequency of streptococcal pharyngitis, it is not surprising that scarlet fever is more common in women[7,8].

To develop scarlet fever, several things have to occur at the same time. First, the host must not have immunity to either the infecting strain of GABHS or the toxin. Second, the infecting strain of *S. pyogenes* must be infected with a lysogenic bacterial phage[17]. These factors can explain the low incidence of scarlet fever even during outbreaks of streptococcal pharyngitis. It is possible to have scarlet fever more than once, because there are three toxins, but this is extremely rare. During the past 50 years scarlet fever has become much less severe than it was at the beginning of the 20th century

Table 1   Gram-positive bacterial infections

Disease	Etiological agent	Eruption	Importance for women
Pyodermas			
Impetigo	*Streptococcus pyogenes* *Staphylococcus aureus*	superficial vesicular lesions, which become pustular and then crusted	no
Ecthyma	*Streptococcus pyogenes*	impetigo-like lesion, which evolves into a vesiculopustular lesion	no
Erysipelas	*Streptococcus pyogenes*	indurated erythema with red, hot, raised and well-demarcated border	no
Cellulitis	*Streptococcus pyogenes* *Staphylococcus aureus*	red, tender, swollen or indurated skin	no
Acute lymphangitis	*Streptococcus pyogenes* *Staphylococcus aureus*	ascending, tender, red streaks of the legs and arms	no
Bockhart's impetigo	*Staphylococcus aureus*	superficial follicular pustular eruption	no
Furunculosis	*Staphylococcus aureus*	perifollicular abscess or boils	no
Paronychia	*Streptococcus pyogenes* *Staphylococcus aureus*	inflammation or infection of skin folds surrounding the nails	no
Botryomycosis	*Staphylococcus aureus*	single and multiple abscesses	no
Toxic syndromes			
Scarlet fever	*Streptococcus pyogenes*	exanthem macular erythroderma with desquamation and enanthem of strawberry tongue	yes
Staphylococcal scarlet fever	*Staphylococcus aureus*	exanthem macular erythroderma with desquamation	no
Scalded skin syndrome	*Staphylococcus aureus*	diffuse macular erythroderma followed by desquamation in large, superficial wet sheets	no
Toxic shock syndrome	*Staphylococcus aureus*	diffuse macular erythroderma followed by desquamation	yes
Streptococcal toxic shock syndrome	*Streptococcus pyogenes*	diffuse macular erythroderma followed by desquamation	no

(Figure 3)[6]. More recently, severe streptococcal infections have re-emerged as a public health problem[9]. Children younger than 2 years of age do not develop scarlet fever and generally do not develop acute pharyngitis, but rather develop streptococcosis, which is not localized to the tonsil, but presents as a severe rhinorrhea.

S. *pyogenes* pharyngitis/tonsillitis has an acute onset of fever, sore throat frequently associated with nausea, vomiting, malaise, headache, chills, generalized lymphadenopathy and diffuse abdominal pain. The eruption of scarlet fever follows the pharyngitis by approximately 24–48 h. The eruption consists of both an exanthem and an enanthem. The rash begins on the head and neck, and rapidly spreads to the trunk and limbs. The lower legs are the last and least affected area of the body. The palms and soles are spared. The rash becomes generalized in 36–72 h.

The eruption of scarlet fever is composed of tiny fine papules. When stroked, they feel like sandpaper.

The cheeks of the patient are flushed with circumoral pallor. The eruption is emphasized in the axillary, antecubital, inguinal and popliteal creases, forming petechial streaks called Pastia's sign. If the rash is very intense, tiny vesicles, called miliary sudamina, appear on the trunk. The rash can vary from mild truncal erythema to the intense bright scarlet erythema of classic scarlet fever. Increased cutaneous capillary fragility and/or decreased platelets associated with the toxins can present as petechiae and purpura. Generalized lymphadenopathy is common during the height of the illness and may persist for several weeks after the rash disappears.

The enanthem of scarlet fever includes the beefy red pharynx involving the tonsils, which may have abundant pus in the tonsillar crypts. The classic white strawberry tongue with its white furred appearance is seen early in the illness. By the 4th or 5th day of illness, the tongue sloughs the white necrotic tissue and becomes bright red, producing

Table 2   Other bacterial infections

Disease	Etiological agent	Eruption	Importance for women
Gram-positive pyodermas			
Anthrax	*Bacillus anthracis*	papule progressing to vesicle to ulceration with black eschar	no
Nocardiosis	*Nocardia* species	multiple draining sinuses	no
Actinomycosis	*Actinomyces* species	abscesses with draining sinus tracts	no
Cutaneous diphtheria	*Corynebacterium diphtheriae*	pustule evolving to ulceration	no
Erysipeloid of Rosenbach	*Erysipelothrix rhusiopathiae*	purplish-red non-vesiculated inflammation with irregular raised border	no
Erythrasma	*Corynebacterium minutissimum*	brown scaling patches in the groin	
Perinatal infections			
Listeriosis	*Listeria monocytogenes*	pustules resembling miliary abscesses	yes
Mycobacterium			
Cutaneous tuberculosis	*Mycobacterium tuberculosis*	scrofuloderma, papulonecrotic tuberculia and erythema nodosum	no
Environmental mycobacterium	*Mycobacterium marinum*	swimming-pool granuloma	no
	Mycobacterium fortuitum	granulomas progressing to ulceration	
	Mycobacterium chelonae	granulomas progressing to ulceration	
	Mycobacterium ulcerans	chronic ulcerating lesions	
Leprosy	*Mycobacterium leprae*	macules, hypopigmented to hyperpigmented lesions, ulceration and scarring, lichenoid lesions, multiple papules and papulonodular lesions	no

the characteristic red strawberry or raspberry tongue. Forschheimer spots, which appear as scattered petechiae and punctate erythema on the soft palate and uvula, are seen frequently.

If scarlet fever is being considered, the diagnosis can be made by culturing *S. pyogenes* from the pharynx, tonsils, or less commonly the site of the skin infection. Rapid streptococcal tests can also be used, with results being available within minutes. If cultures are not available or if the patient has already been treated with antimicrobials, antistreptolysin O titers or the streptozyme test can be helpful. The Dick test and Schultz–Charlton test are no longer available and are not considered necessary for making the diagnosis[19].

The differential diagnosis of scarlet fever includes staphylococcal scarlet fever, toxic shock syndrome, drug reactions, early toxic epidermal necrolysis, Kawasaki disease, mononucleosis, phototoxicity reaction and sunburn.

Complications of the streptococcal infection associated with scarlet fever are tonsillar abscess, cervical adenitis, otitis media, sinusitis, osteomyelitis and rarely septicemia. Additional complications include rheumatic fever and acute glomerulonephritis, both due to an abnormal immunological response of the host to the streptococcal infection.

Treatment of the *S. pyogenes* infection can be accomplished with oral penicillin or amoxicillin therapy. Amoxicillin is generally preferred, because of higher blood levels of the antibiotic due to better gastrointestinal absorption. *S. pyogenes* remains highly susceptible to the penicillin, with no reports of resistance. In some patients penicillin may fail even though the strain is susceptible to penicillin. This may be due to β-lactamase production by the patient's normal oral flora. Alternatives to penicillin therapy include cephalosporins, which are resistant to β-lactamase activity, and macrolides such as erythromycin, clarithromycin and dirithromycin. Azithromycin, although convenient with once daily dosing for 5 days, is a poor choice, because eradication rates are less than 80% after 30 days and macrolide resistance may result. The recent trend towards short courses of therapy for streptococcal pharyngitis/tonsillitis have resulted

Table 3   Gram-negative bacterial infections

Disease	Etiological agent	Eruption	Importance for women
Pasteurella multocida infection	*Pasteurella multocida*	soft tissue swelling, pain, erythema, with serosanguinous drainage	no
Plague	*Yersinia pestis*	pustule or ulcers, developing lymphadenopathy, progressing to buboes	no
Neisseria meningitidis infection	*Neisseria meningitidis*	erythematous macules becoming papular, then vesicular to hemorrhagic	no
Haemophilus influenzae infection	*Haemophilus influenzae*	cellulitids sometimes becoming petechial	no
Salmonella infection	*Salmonella typhi* and *paratyphi*	rose spots	no
Pseudomonas infection	*Pseudomonas aeruginosa*	ecthyma gangrenosum, pyoderma, hot tub folliculitis and green nails	no
Melioidosis	*Pseudomonas psuedomallei*	nodules progressing to lymphangitis and regional lymphadenitis	no
Glanders	*Pseudomonas mallei*	nodules progressing to lymphangitis and regional lymphadenitis	no
Rat bite fever	*Streptobacillus moniliformis* *Spirillum minus*	morbilliform rash, petechial to purpuric blotchy purple macular rash	no
Bartonellosis	*Bartonella bacilliformis*	verruga peruana	no
Lyme disease	*Borrelia burgdorferi*	target lesion	no
Leptospirosis	*Leptospira* species	macules, maculopapules, urticaria and petechiae	no
Brucellosis	*Brucella* species	rare erythematous, papular, evolving vesicular	no
Tularemia	*Francisella tularensis*	ulceration and black eschar	no
Gram-negative folliculitis in acne vulgaris	many Gram-negative organisms	pustular folliculitis	

in eradication rates below 80% and a need to return to the standard 10 days of antimicrobial therapy. Supportive therapy is directed at providing adequate hydration and relief of symptoms.

Toxic shock syndrome

The first reports of toxic shock syndrome were in seven children who presented with a new syndrome of high fever, confusion, headache, conjunctival hyperemia, subcutaneous edema, scarlatiniform rash, vomiting, watery diarrhea, oliguria progressing to renal failure, hepatic abnormalities, disseminated intravascular coagulation and severe prolonged shock[20]. It was named toxic shock syndrome by James Todd and associates, who isolated *Staphylococcus aureus* related to phage group I[20,21]. In these early cases *S. aureus* was isolated from the mucosal surfaces of the patients, but no evidence of invasion was found. These strains of *S. aureus* were later found to produce an exotoxin and their effects differed

from the staphylococcal exfoliation known to produce impetigo and staphylococcal scalded skin syndrome[22].

The *S. aureus* that was isolated from patients with toxic shock syndrome was investigated for toxin production. These studies showed that at least three exotoxins were made by these isolates and that, although they were similar to streptococcal toxins, they were not the toxins associated with scarlet fever[23–26]. The first toxin to be isolated was named toxic shock syndrome toxin-1 (TSST-1) in 1984[23–26]. This exotoxin was pyrogenic and T-cell mitogenic, and increased susceptibility to endotoxin-produced shock, but was serologically distinct from scarlet fever toxins[27]. These toxins, through a novel mechanism, were found to release cytokines from immune cells and this leads to the major symptoms of toxic shock syndrome. Marrack and Kappler referred to them as superantigens[27]. The TSST-1 toxin shares three-dimensional structure similarities with

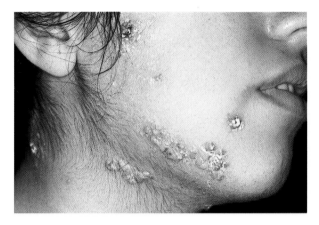

Figure 1 Impetigo developed on the chin of this girl who was also hirsute. The crusting and redness had spread from the neck to the face

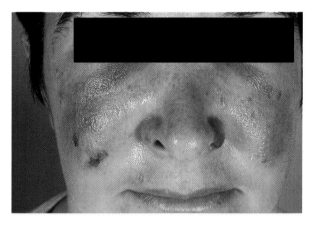

Figure 3 Erysipelas with its infiltrating redness was extremely dangerous in the preantibiotic era

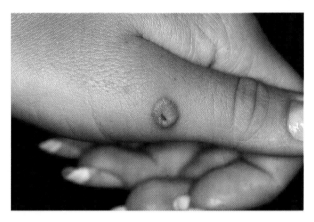

Figure 2 Bullous impetigo afflicted the hand of this woman, where the perifollicular bulla proved to be painful

staphylococcal enterotoxins and streptococcal scarlet fever toxins, all of which can cause toxic shock syndrome[27].

These reports in children were followed by an epidemic of toxic shock syndrome in young menstruating women who were using tampons[28]. The reports of the American Centers for Disease Control (CDC) from 1960 to 1982 identified 2509 cases[29]. Ninety-five per cent of these cases were in women and most of these women were young and white. Of the cases in which menstrual status was known, 89% of the women were menstruating and 99% of them were using tampons. The fatality rate was 5% for all cases, but 10% in men. Recurrences have been reported in menstrual cases varying from 25 to 64%[30]. The association with tampon use led to several investigations as to why some brands of tampon where more frequently associated with toxic shock syndrome. At first it was felt that the most absorbent brands were responsible. However, brands that were labelled 'regular' were also involved. The most likely theory to explain tampon

involvement is related to vaginal oxygen concentration. The normal vaginal environment is anaerobic[23,31]. S. aureus grows well with or without oxygen, but the toxic shock syndrome toxin (TSST) is not produced in an anaerobic condition[23,31]. In addition, the toxin is produced in neutral pH conditions, which exist during menstruation because of the buffering capacity of blood and not under the normal acid conditions of the vagina. The insertion of all tampons increases the oxygen content of the vagina, but the more absorbent tampons increase the oxygen content to a much higher degree. Another finding was that tampons composed entirely of cotton prevented the production of TSST[23]. The more widely available brands containing cotton–rayon blends are more likely to stimulate production of TSST[23]. Of these factors, the most important is the absorbency of the tampon[32]. Tampons today are labelled with their absorbency and women should be advised to use those with the lowest absorbency sufficient to control menstrual flow.

Toxic shock syndrome is an acute life-threatening multisystem disease that is best described by the CDC case definition (Table 4)[29]. Nearly all of the patients have high fevers, myalgia and a generalized scarlatiniform rash. Gastrointestinal symptoms of nausea, vomiting, diarrhea and abdominal tenderness are seen in 75–80% of cases[33–39]. The rash is a generalized scarlatiniform eruption that may resemble a sunburn. Unlike the rash of scarlet fever, it may be more prominent at the hips and thighs. Petechial and bullous changes are seen not infrequently. Mucosal involvement includes pharyngitis, and conjunctival injection (dilation of the ciliary and conjunctival vessels causing redness) is common. Strawberry tongue similar to that in

Table 4 Toxic shock syndrome: case definition

Fever (102°F; 39.9°C)

Rash (diffuse macular erythroderma)

Desquamation, 1–2 weeks after onset of illness,
   particularly of palms and soles

Hypotension (systolic blood pressure 90 mmHg for
   adults, or below the 5th centile for children under
   16 years of age, or orthostatic syncope)

Involvement of three or more of several organ systems:
   gastrointestinal (vomiting or diarrhea at onset of
      illness)
   muscular (severe myalgia or creatine phosphokinase
      level ≥ 2 times normal)
   mucous membrane (vaginal oropharyngeal
      or conjunctival hyperemia)
   renal: BUN or creatinine ≥ 2 times normal or ≥ 5
      white blood cells per high-power field in the
      absence of urinary tract infections
   hepatic: total bilirubin, SGOT or SGPT (2 times
      normal)
   hematological: platelets 100 000/mm^3 or less
   central nervous system: disorientation or alteration
      in consciousness without focal neurological signs
      (when fever and hypotension are absent)

Negative results on the following tests, if obtained:
   blood, throat, or cerebrospinal fluid cultures[*]
   serological tests for Rocky Mountain spotted fever,
      leptospirosis, or measles

BUN, blood urea nitrogen; SGOT, aspartate amino-transferase; SGPT, alanine aminotransferase. [*]Blood cultures are occasionally positive for the particular toxin-producing strains in toxic shock syndrome. Throat cultures are negative for group A β-hemolytic streptococcus but may be positive for *Staphylococcus aureus*

scarlet fever is present in over half of the patients. Vaginal hyperemia and discharge are noted in 40% of the cases in women. The skin develops a fine desquamation with prominent peeling of the hands and feet approximately 2 weeks after the initial rash. Neurological involvement is manifest by headache, confusion and depressed sensorium. Chills, rigor and arthalgia are seen early in the illness and are frequently followed by shock, oliguria, renal failure, cardiac arrhythmia and adult respiratory distress syndrome[23].

Laboratory testing is necessary to determine the extent of organ involvement. Abnormalities seen include metabolic acidosis, hypocalcemia, anemia, thrombocytopenia, leukocytosis, prolonged pro-thrombin time and partial thromboplastin time, and increased fibrin-split products. Elevated liver enzymes (aspartate aminotransferase (SGOT), ala-nine aminotransferase (SGPT) and lactate dehydro-genase (LDH)) and increased bilirubin, amylase, lipase and creatine phosphokinase (CPK) are associated with liver and muscle involvement. Increased creatinine, azotemia, proteinuria, pyuria and microhematuria are seen with kidney involve-ment. Cultures of vaginal discharge and samples from the throat and any site of obvious infection will frequently reveal *S. aureus*. Skin biopsy generally demonstrates a mild lymphohistocytic infiltrate in the mid- and upper dermis. The perivascular infil-trate is associated with edema of the papular dermis.

The differential diagnosis of toxic shock syn-drome includes Kawasaki disease, staphylococcal scarlet fever, staphylococcal scalded skin syndrome, streptococcal scarlet fever, rickettsial diseases, lep-tospirosis, Legionnaires' disease, viral exanthems and drug reactions (Figure 4). There is considerable overlap between these illnesses. In the non-menstruating female or the male, the diagnosis can be difficult.

Treatment of toxic shock syndrome is directed at eliminating the organism and providing supportive therapy, depending on the severity of the illness. The supportive therapy must return the patient to a normotensive state and correct tissue hypoxia. Antibiotic therapy for *S. aureus* should be with an agent that covers the local resistance patterns of the *S. aureus* in the community. If there is any doubt, the patient should be treated with vancomycin until the susceptibility pattern is known.

Listeriosis

Listeria monocytogenes is a small Gram-positive coc-cobacillus, an intracellular pathogen that rarely causes infections[40]. Pregnant women are particu-larly vulnerable and severe perinatal infections fre-quently result[41,42]. Listeria can also cause sporadic illness in adults and children, particularly in the immunocompromised host, such as the elderly, or patients with renal failure and other chronic ill-ness[40]. The organism is found in soil, vegetation, insects, fish, domestic and wild animals, milk and cheese[43–45]. Most infections can be traced to inges-tion of food, particularly cheese[44], except for trans-mission from mother to fetus[40,43].

Infection during pregnancy may go undetected, but most patients have a febrile flu-like syndrome. Neonatal listeriosis has two presentations: early and late disease. Early disease (granulomatosis infantisep-tica) is the result of transplacental transmission to the fetus producing chorioamnionitis and placental abscesses. Sepsis in the fetus leads to miliary granulomatous lesions. The early form has a mortality rate of 40 to 54%, mainly as stillbirths[42].

Table 5   Rickettsial infections

Disease	Etiological agent	Vector	Eruption	Importance for women
Spotted fever group				
Rocky Mountain spotted fever	*Rickettsia rickettsii*	tick	macular, maculopapular, petechial on extremities to trunk, palms and soles	no
Boutonneuse fever	*Rickettsia conorii*	tick	macular, maculopapular, petechial on trunk to extremities, face, palms, soles	no
North Asian tick typhus	*Rickettsia sibirica*	tick	eschar, maculopapular, petechial on extremities, trunk	no
Oriental spotted fever	*Rickettsia japonica*	tick	eschar, maculopapular, petechial late on extremities, trunk	no
Queensland tick fever	*Rickettsia australia*	tick	eschar, macular, papular, vesicular on trunk sometimes generalized	no
Rickettsialpox	*Rickettsia akari*	mite	eschar, macular, papular, vesicular on trunk, face, extremities	no
Typhus group				
Primary louse-borne typhus	*Rickettsia prowazekii*	louse feces	macular, maculopapular on trunk to extremities	no
Brill–Zinsser Disease (recrudescence)	*Rickettsia prowazekii*	none	macular, maculopapular on trunk to extremities	no
Murine typhus	*Rickettsia typhi*	flea	macular, maculopapular on trunk to extremities	no
Scrub typhus	*Rickettsia tsutsugamushi*	mite	eschar, macular, maculopapular on trunk to extremities	no
Q fever	*Coxiella burnetti*	none	none	no
Ehrlichiosis				
human monocytic	*Ehrlichea chaffaensis*	tick	rare rash in children	no
human granulocytic	*Ehrlichea phagocytophila*	tick	none	no
Sennetsu fever	*Ehrlichea sennetsu*		none	no
Rochalimaea-associated diseases				
Cat scratch fever	*Rochalimaea henselae*	none	lymphadenopathy, erythema nodosum	no
Trench fever	*Rochalimaea quintana*	louse	none	no

Late infection is transmitted to the infant during passage through the birth canal and presents approximately 1 week later. The meningitis or meningoencephalitis manifests as poor feeding, vomiting, diarrhea and respiratory distress syndrome.

Rare skin eruptions are seen in both early and late infections. The lesions consist of small grayish-white papules or papulopustules. The pustules resemble miliary abscesses and can also be seen on the conjunctivae and oral mucosa. Other skin lesions include petechiae, purpura, a morbilliform or roseola-like eruption and localized and generalized erythema.

Diagnosis is made by culturing skin, cerebrospinal fluid (CSF), amniotic fluid, gastric aspirate, meconium and blood. The organism can frequently be seen in Gram stains of CSF and smears of the pustules. Treatment with ampicillin and gentamycin is effective[46]. *Listeria* is resistant to all cephalosporins, and if listeriosis is considered these agents should not be used as single-agent therapy[46].

RICKETTSIAL INFECTIONS

Rickettsial diseases are caused by a variety of obligate intracellular parasites. The illness caused by *Rickettsia* can best be divided into five groups of diseases (Table 5). The spotted fever group includes the well-known disease Rocky Mountain spotted fever, but also Boutonneuse fever (Figure 5), North Asian tick typhus, oriental spotted fever, Queensland tick fever and rickettsialpox. The typhus group and the scrub typhus group are associated with wars and natural disasters, when

Table 6   Viral infections

Disease	Etiological agent	Eruption	Importance for women
Exanthems			
Enteroviruses	coxsachievirus, echovirus and enteroviruses	macular papular, vesicular, urticarial with variable distribution	no
Measles	measles virus	maculopapular maybe hemorrhagic, Koplik spots	no
Rubella	rubella virus	discrete, pink, macular papular eruption	yes
Erythema infectiosum	parvovirus B19	slapped-cheek appearance with lacy erythema of the trunk	yes
Roseola infantum	human herpesvirus-6	macular papular	no
Varicella	varicella-zoster virus	maculopapules to vesicle surrounded by a halo of erythema to scabs	no
Hemorrhagic fevers			
Dengue fever	dengue viruses	transient, macular generalized rash followed by a morbilliform, macular papular rash, can be hemorrhagic	no
Other viral hemorrhagic fever	many taxonomically different viruses	hemorrhagic lesions	no
Other integumentary viruses			
Herpes simplex viruses	HSV-1 and HSV-2	vesicles	see Chapter 26
Smallpox	smallpox virus	vesicular becoming pustular to scabs	no
Molluscum contagiosum	molluscum contagiosum virus	smooth, firm, shiny, flesh-colored to pearly white hemispheric papules with umbilicated centers	no
Papillomaviruses	human papillomaviruses	hyperkeratotic lesions	see Chapter 26

personal hygiene deteriorates, and include primary louse-borne typhus, Brill–Zinsser disease, murine typhus and scrub typhus. Ehrlichiosis and cat scratch fever have only recently been added to the infections associated with rickettsia-like organisms. They have no particular significance for women and are not discussed further.

VIRAL INFECTIONS

As already discussed under bacterial and rickettsial infections, there is no physiological reason why viruses should have a predilection for women. Viruses can have an effect on the fetus, making them of particular concern to women of childbearing potential (Table 6). The specific diagnosis of viral exanthems in pregnancy is therefore very important.

Rubella

Once a common exanthematous disease of childhood, rubella is rarely seen in the USA today because of the use of the live attenuated rubella vaccine[47,48]. Rubella (German measles, 3-day measles) produces a mild illness that would not be of importance were it not for the transmission *in utero* and the production of severe congenital infection. Rubella is a member of the Togaviridae family, genus *Rubivirus*, and only one serotype is known.

Prior to the vaccine, 60% of cases occurred in children under 10 years of age. Now the majority of cases are in adolescents and young adults. These cases are due to failure to be vaccinated. Rubella continues to be a problem in countries where vaccination is not widely available. There is no sexual predominance. The incubation period is from 12 to 23 days, with a period of communicability of 5 to 7 days before the appearance of the rash, until 3 to 5 days after its appearance. Transmission is through the respiratory route.

Rubella is a moderately contagious disease that begins insidiously and is marked by an acute exanthemous, maculopapular eruption that lasts 3 days

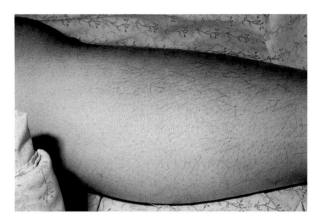

Figure 4 Toxic shock syndrome occurred in this woman who received diclofenac intramuscularly. She subsequently died. Courtesy of Arie Ingber, MD, and Leon Gilead, MD, Jerusalem, Israel

or less. Non-apparent infection may account for up to 80% of infections. A prodrome of 1–5 days before the rash consists of malaise, cough, sore throat, eye pain, headache, swollen glands, red eyes, rhinorrhea, fever, aches, chills, anorexia and nausea. There is usually tender postauricular and suboccipital lymphadenopathy.

The eruption begins on the face and progresses to the trunk and then to the extremities. It usually covers the entire body within 24 h and begins to fade on the 2nd day. The eruption may last less than 24 h or persist for 5 days or longer. The rash consists of discrete pink macules and papules, which may become confluent with a morbilliform appearance. It can be confused with scarlet fever, erythema infectiosum and roseola. Pinhead-sized rosy red macules or petechiae are seen on the soft palate and uvula (Forscheimer spots).

Arthritis and arthralgia are common complications of rubella, particularly in adult women. Joint involvement has its onset 1–6 days after the rash and most commonly affects the fingers, wrists and knees. Other rare complications include encephalitis, peripheral neuritis and thrombocytopenic purpura.

Congenital rubella syndrome was first noted in 1941 in Australia following an epidemic[49]. Fetal infection results in intrauterine growth restriction, congenital cataracts, microphthalmia, congenital heart disease, mental retardation, hearing defects, microcephaly, hypospadias and many other defects. The triad of congenital cataracts, deafness and heart diseases was considered as congenital rubella syndrome. Fortunately, today congenital rubella syndrome is seldom seen in the USA. However, as some women of reproductive age are not

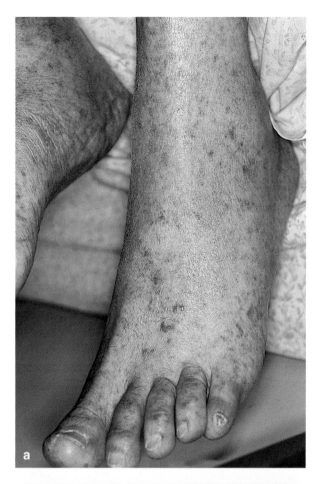

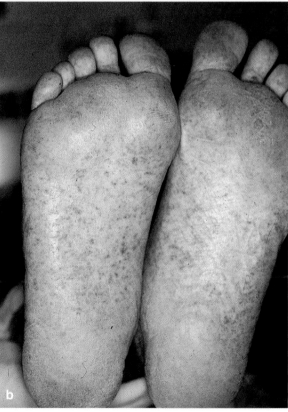

Figure 5 (a) and (b) Tick bite fever developed in this patient. *Rickettsia conorii* was identified as the pathogen

appropriately immunized, congenital rubella is still a threat[49,50].

Human parvovirus B19

Parvovirus B19 is the cause of erythema infectiosum (fifth disease), a common childhood illness. Parvoviruses are the smallest single-stranded DNA viruses infecting mammalian cells. In 1974 Cossart and co-workers found a 'serum parvovirus-like particle' while looking for hepatitis B virus[51]. This accidental discovery led to an association with hypoplastic crisis in patients with sickle cell anemia and later to the cause of erythema infectiosum. Parvovirus B19 is the only known pathogenic parvovirus in humans.

Infection with parvovirus B19 has a worldwide distribution but is more common in temperate climates particularly in the late winter and spring. Cyclic epidemics occur every 4–5 years. The virus is highly contagious, and most cases are seen in children between the ages of 4 and 11. Girls are more frequently infected than boys. Spread is primarily by the respiratory route, but spread by fomites and through the administration of infected blood can occur.

Frequently there are no clinical manifestations of infection, but in symptomatic children it is associated with fever, headache, coryza and mild gastrointestinal upset. This is followed in 2–5 days by dermatological manifestations. The typical exanthem has three stages. First, a fiery red macular erythema appears on the cheeks, giving the characteristic 'slapped-cheek' appearance on the face. Circumoral pallor may be seen in some patients. This stage is followed by discrete erythematous macules and papules on the proximal extremities spreading to the trunk. The maculopapular rash gradually evolves into the distinctive reticular lace-like erythematous eruption. The rash is difficult to recognize in black patients who may go undiagnosed.

Parvovirus B19 has a propensity for the hematopoietic system particularly the erythroid progenitor cells. White cell and platelet cell lines are less commonly affected. A mild anemia can be seen in normal patients, but this has no clinical significance. In patients with underlying chronic hemolytic processes such as sickle cell disease, thalassemia and hereditary spherocytosis, a severe anemia can result. The transient aplastic crisis seen in these patients can be fatal.

Women are more frequently infected with parvovirus B19 than men. Women are more likely to be symptomatic than children. They frequently develop a polyarthropathy affecting the hands, wrists, ankles and knees[52]. The pain, joint stiffness and swelling usually lasts 1–3 weeks[52]. In some women, these symptoms may persist for months.

Women of childbearing potential are of concern if they develop infection with parvovirus B19 during pregnancy. In up to one-third of cases, the virus is transmitted to the fetus, as detected by serology testing at birth[53,54]. Rarely, the fetus may develop a transient aplastic crisis resulting in high output failure, hydrops and fetal death[53,55–58]. Parvovirus B19 has been reported to be responsible for 10–15% of all cases of non-immune hydrops[59]. Fetal death generally occurs 4–6 weeks following maternal illness. The fetus later in pregnancy is undergoing rapid expansion of red cell volume and if there is an abrupt decrease in red cell production the fetus becomes anemic[60]. An associated viral myocarditis leads to heart failure and fetal death[61,62]. Parvovirus B19 does not appear to be teratogenic, but data are limited.

Diagnosis is generally based on the clinical presentation and characteristic rash. In the pregnant woman serological testing using an enzyme-linked immunosorbent assay for specific IgG and IgM antibodies can be used to determine infection. Culture for parvovirus B19 is not useful in the pregnant woman suspected of being infected, since the period of viremia is short.

Currently there is no treatment for parvovirus B19 infection. There are vaccines under development but none has yet proven to be effective. Because of this, women will require management decisions concerning parvovirus B19 infection. This can be divided into three presentations in a pregnant woman. The first is following exposure without evidence of infection. The second is in the pregnant woman with acute symptomatic infection with parvovirus B19. The third is when a hydropic fetus is discovered by ultrasonography. In the first two cases women should be tested for serological status. If the woman is serologically negative following an exposure, there is a less than 1% chance of fetal death. The woman with an acute infection with parvovirus B19 should be followed with serial sonograms for a period of 8–12 weeks, to detect any signs of fetal hydrops. Serology can also help to differentiate between parvovirus infection and other viral infections which may mimic erythema infectiosum. Fetal hydrops may resolve spontaneously over a 4–6-week period[63,64], but it can be treated with intrauterine blood transfusion. Even with intrauterine transfusion, 25% of fetuses died[63]. It is difficult to determine which child will benefit from transfusion.

REFERENCES

1. Peter G, Smith AL. Group A streptococcal infections of the skin and pharynx (first of two parts). *N Engl J Med* 1977;297:313–16

2. Kaplav EL. Streptococcal infections. In Katz S, Gershon AA, Hoter PJ, eds. *Krugman's Infectious Diseases of Children*, 10th edn. St Louis: Mosby, 1998:487–500

3. Sheagren JH. *Staphylococcus aureus*: the persistent pathogen. Part I. *N Engl J Med* 1984;310:1368–72

4. Sheagren JH. *Staphylococcus aureus*: the persistent pathogen. Part II. *N Engl J Med* 1984;310:1437–42

5. Wannamaker LW. Streptococcal toxins. *Rev Infect Dis* 1983;5(suppl 4):S723–32

6. Gaworzewska E, Colman G. Change in the pattern of infection caused by *Streptococcus pyogenes*. *Epidemiol Infect* 1988;100:257–69

7. Perks EM, Mayen-White RT. The incidence of scarlet fever. *J Hyg Camb* 1983;91:203–9

8. Carapetis JR, Currie BJ, Kaplan EL. Epidemiology and prevention of group A streptococcal infections: acute respiratory tract infections, skin infections, and their sequelae at the close of the twentieth century. *Clin Infect Dis* 1999;28:205–10

9. Wolf JE, Rabinowitz LG. Streptococcal toxic shock-like syndrome. *Arch Dermatol* 1995;131:73–7

10. Spencer RC. Invasive streptococci. *Eur J Clin Microbiol Infect Dis* 1995;14(suppl 1):S26–32

11. Stevens DL. Invasive group A streptococcus infections. *Clin Infect Dis* 1992;14:2–11

12. Stevens DL, Tanner MH, Winship J, *et al*. Severe group A streptococcal infections associated with a toxic shock-like syndrome and scarlet fever toxin A. *N Engl J Med* 1989;6:1–7

13. Tyler SD, Johnson WM, Huang JC, *et al*. Streptococcal erythrogenic toxin genes: detection by polymerase chain reaction and association with disease in strain isolated in Canada from 1940 to 1991. *J Clin Microbiol* 1992;30:3127–31

14. Yu CE, Ferretti JJ. Frequency of the erythrogenic toxin B and C genes (speB and speC) among clinical isolates of group A streptococci. *Infect Immun* 1991;59:211–15

15. Yu CE, Ferretti JJ. Molecular epidemiologic analysis of the type A streptococcal exotoxin (erythrogenic toxin) gene (speA) in clinical *Streptococcus pyogenes* strains. *Infect Immun* 1989;57:3715–19

16. Schlievert PM, Gray ED. Group A streptococcal pyrogenic exotoxin (scarlet fever toxin) type A and blastogen A are the same protein. *Infect Immun* 1989;57:1865–7

17. Nida SK, Ferretti JJ. Phage influence on the synthesis of extracellular toxin in group A streptococci. *Infect Immun* 1982;36:745–50

18. Shaunak S, Wendon J, Monteil M, Gordon AM. Septic scarlet fever due to *Streptococcus pyogenes* cellulitis. *Q J Med* 1988;69:921–5

19. Schlievert PM, Bettin KM, Watson DW. Reinterpretation of the Dick test: role of group A streptococcal pyrogenic exotoxin. *Infect Immun* 1979;26:467–72

20. Todd J, Fishaunt M. Toxic-shock syndrome associated with phage-group-I staphylococci. *Lancet* 1978;2:1116–18

21. Wiesenthal AM, Todd J. Toxic shock syndrome in children aged 10 years or less. *Pediatrics* 1984;74:112–17

22. Todd JK, Franc-Buff A, Lawellin DW, Vasil ML. Phenotypic distinctiveness of *Staphylococcus aureus* strains associated with toxic shock syndrome. *Infect Immun* 1984;45:339–44

23. Schlievert PM, Shands KN, Dan BB, *et al*. Identification and characterization of an exotoxin from *Staphylococcus aureus* associated with toxic-shock syndrome. *J Infect Dis* 1981;143:509–16

24. Bergdoll MS, Crass BA, Reiser RF, *et al*. A new staphylococcal enterotoxin, enterotoxin F, associated with toxic-shock syndrome *Staphylococcus aureus* isolates. *Lancet* 1981;1:1017–21

25. Schlievert PM, Bloomster DA. Production of staphylococcal pyrogenic exotoxin type C: influence of physical and chemical factors. *J Infect Dis* 1983;147:236–42

26. Kass EH, Parsonnet J. On the pathogenesis of toxic shock syndrome. *Rev Infect Dis* 1987;9(suppl 5):S482–9

27. Marrack P, Kappler J. The staphylococcus enterotoxins and their relatives. *Science* 1990;248:705–11

28. Todd JK. Toxic shock syndrome: a perspective through the looking glass. *Ann Intern Med* 1982;96:839–42

29. Reingold AL. Epidemiology of toxic-shock syndrome. United States, 1960–1984. *Morbid Mortal Weekly Rep* 1985;33:19SS

30. Fisher RF, Goodpasture HC, Pelerie JD, *et al*. Toxic shock syndrome in menstruating women. *Ann Intern Med* 1984;94:156–9

31. Todd JK, Todd BH, Franco-Buff A, *et al*. Influence of focal growth conditions on the pathogenesis of toxic shock syndrome. *J Infect Dis* 1987;155:673–81

32. Schlievert PM. Comparison of cotton and cotton/rayon tampons for effect on production of toxic shock syndrome toxin. *J Infect Dis* 1995;172:1112–14

33. Wager GP. Toxic shock syndrome: a review. *Am J Obstet Gynecol* 1983;146:93–102

34. Chesney PJ, Bergdoll MS, Davis JP, Vergeront JM. The disease spectrum, epidemiology, and etiology of toxic-shock syndrome. *Annu Rev Microbiol* 1984;38:315–38

35. Todd JK. Staphylococcus toxin syndromes. *Annu Rev Med* 1985;36:337–47

36. Broome CV. Epidemiology of toxic shock syndrome in the United States: overview. *Rev Infect Dis* 1989;11(suppl 1):S14–21

37. Reingold AL. Toxic shock syndrome: an update. *Am J Obstet Gynecol* 1991;165:1236–9

38. Steven DL. The toxic shock syndromes. *Infect Dis Clin North Am* 1996;10:727–46

39. Manders SM. Toxin-mediated streptococcal and staphylococcal disease. *J Am Acad Dermatol* 1998;39: 383–98

40. Gellin BG, Broome CV, Bibb WF, *et al.* The epidemiology of listeriosis in the United States – 1986. Listeriosis Study Group. *Am J Epidemiol* 1991;133: 392–401

41. Silver HM. Listeriosis during pregnancy. *Obstet Gynecol Surv* 1998;53:737–40

42. Lennon D, Lewis B, Mantell C, *et al.* Epidemic perinatal listeriosis. *Pediatr Infect Dis* 1984;3:30–4

43. Farber JM, Peterkin PI. Listeria monocytogenes, a food-borne pathogen. *Microbiol Rev* 1991;55: 476–511

44. Linnan MJ, Mascola L, Lou XD, *et al.* Epidemic listeriosis associated with Mexican-style cheese. *N Engl J Med* 1988;319:823–8

45. Schuchat A, Deaver KA, Wenger JD, *et al.* Role of foods in sporadic listeriosis. I. Case–control study of dietary risk factors. The Listeria Study Group. *JAMA* 1992;267:2041–5

46. Cherubin CE, Appleman MD, Heseltine PN, *et al.* Epidemiological spectrum and current treatment of listeriosis. *Rev Infect Dis* 1991;13:1108–14

47. Rosa C. Rubella and rubeola. *Semin Perinatol* 1998;22:318–22

48. Freij BJ, South MA, Sever JL. Maternal rubella and the congenital rubella syndrome. *Clin Perinatol* 1988;15:247–57

49. Menser MA, Hudson JR, Murphy AM, Upfold LJ. Epidemiology of congenital rubella and results of rubella vaccination in Australia. *Rev Infect Dis* 1985;7(suppl 1):S37–41

50. Englund J, Glezen WP, Piedra PA. Maternal immunization against viral disease. *Vaccine* 1998;16: 1456–63

51. Cossart YE, Field AM, Cant B, *et al.* Parvovirus-like particles in human sera. *Lancet* 1975;1:72–3

52. Woolf AD, Campion GV, Chishick A, *et al.* Clinical manifestations of human parvovirus B19 in adults. *Arch Intern Med* 1989;149:1153–6

53. Gratacos E, Torres P-J, Vidal J, *et al.* The incidence of human parvovirus B19 infection during pregnancy and its impact on perinatal outcome. *J Infect Dis* 1995;171:1360–3

54. Public Health Laboratory Service Working Party of Fifth Disease: prospective study of human parvovirus (B19) infection in pregnancy. *Br Med J* 1990; 300:1166–70

55. Guidozzi F, Ballot D, Ropthberg AD. Human B19 parvovirus infection in an obstetric population: a prospective study determining fetal outcome. *J Reprod Med* 1994;39:36–8

56. Kinney JS, Anderson LJ, Farrar J, *et al.* Risk of adverse outcomes of pregnancy after human parvovirus B19 infection. *J Infect Dis* 1988;157:663–7

57. Rodis JF, Quinn DL, Gary W, *et al.* Management and outcomes of pregnancies complicated by human B19 parvovirus infection: a prospective study. *Am J Obstet Gynecol* 1990;163:1168–71

58. Torok TJ, Wang Q-Y, Gary GW Jr, *et al.* Prenatal diagnosis of intrauterine infection with parvovirus B19 by the polymerase chain reaction technique. *Clin Infect Dis* 1992;14:149–55

59. Brown KE, Young NS, Lui JM. Molecular, cellular and clinical aspects of parvovirus B19 infection. *Crit Rev Oncol Hematol* 1994;16:1–31

60. Gary ES, Davidson RJC, Anand A. Human parvovirus and fetal anemia. *Lancet* 1987;1:1144

61. Naides SJ, Weiner CP. Antenatal diagnosis and palliative treatment of nonimmune hydrops fetalis secondary to fetal parvovirus B19 infection. *Prenat Diagn* 1989;9:105–14

62. Porter HJ, Quantrill AM, Fleming KA. B19 parvovirus infection of myocardial cells. *Lancet* 1988;i:535–6

63. Humphrey W, Magoon M, O'Shaughnessy R. Severe nonimmune hydrops secondary to parvovirus B19 infection: spontaneous reversal *in utero* and survival of a term infant. *Obstet Gynecol* 1991;78:900–2

64. Sheikh AU, Ernest JM, O'Shea M. Long-term outcome in fetal hydrops from parvovirus B19 infection. *Am J Obstet Gynecol* 1992;167:337–44

Superficial fungal diseases

24

Andreas D. Katsambas and Evangelia Papadavid

Fungal infections either caused by dermatophytes or yeasts are common in men and women. In addition to the geographic factors and the virulence of the infecting organism, several host factors play a significant role in the epidemiology of fungal infections including gender. Although several fungal infections are unique to women, owing to their anatomy and the presence of specific hormones, fungal infections common to both sexes may have a distinctive name and visual appearance and may even require different treatment. As an example, in HIV-immunosuppressed women, opportunistic vulvovaginal yeast infection (Figure 1) is often the first clinical expression of immunodeficiency (even before oropharyngeal involvement)[1], whereas in men the oropharynx is the most common site of mucosal candidosis. Vaginal candidosis is related to physiological aging as well as to the specific hormonal changes occurring in girls during puberty, women during pregnancy and the menopause or the cyclic variations of hormonal levels. The pathological variations in hormonal production (pathological production of steroid hormones from tumors or polycystic ovaries or by estrogen-dominant oral contraceptives) are important. *Candida* infection may also complicate mucosal tumors and pruritic and ulcerated lesions that are unique to women such as lichen sclerosus and atrophicus of the vulva. On the other hand, several factors such as moisture, warmth, friction and occlusion lead to maceration and erosion of the skin in the submammary flexures and make obese or older women more susceptible to yeast infections in this as well as other intertriginous areas. Monilial paronychia is more common in older housewives, owing to the constant immersion of their hands in water.

Terms used to describe diseases such as tinea barbae (dermatophyte infection confined to the coarse hair-bearing beard and moustache area of men) cannot be used for a female patient and therefore the term tinea faciei (Figure 2) is used instead to describe dermatophyte infection of the face in women. Additionally, men and women have traditionally had different activities. For example, because of lack of exposure of women to some

domestic animals, women had fewer anthropophilic fungal infections.

In this chapter we try to describe the more characteristic fungal infections regarding the anatomy or the hormonal changes in girls and women including mucosal, cutaneous and nail involvement, as well as the difficulties that pregnancy or breast feeding cause in terms of the treatment.

YEAST INFECTIONS

Candidosis (or candidiasis) and tinea (or pityriasis) versicolor are common yeast infections. Candidosis may affect the skin, nails, mucous membranes and gastrointestinal tract but can be systemic and affect multiple internal organs. Several of the 80 *Candida* species can be responsible for clinical disease under certain circumstances (immunosuppression, intravenous drug delivery, etc.) and most of these infections are systemic rather than localized. The species of *Candida* can be graded by descending degree of pathogenicity, as follows: *C. albicans, C. stellatoides, C. tropicalis, C. parapsilosis, C. kefyr, C. guilliermondii* and *C. krusei*. Candidosis is by far the most common fungal infection in women, and is mainly caused by the yeast *C. albicans*, but other yeasts of the genus *Candida* can occasionally be cultured (*C. tropicalis, C. glabrata, C. krusei*).

Tinea versicolor, another cutaneous yeast infection mainly caused by *Malassezia furfur* (Figure 3), does not seem to have a sex predilection and is common at an age when sebum production is high. Pregnancy is one of the predisposing factors for tinea versicolor, which also include humidity, tropical climate, immunosuppression and increased cortisone levels.

According to the anatomic location, candidal infection in girls and women can be divided as follows.

(1) Oral candidosis or thrush;

(2) Vaginal or vulvovaginal candidosis or thrush;

(3) Candidal intertrigo;

(4) Candidal nail paronychia;

(5) Candidal nail infection.

Clinical description

Oral candidosis or thrush

Candida is a regular inhabitant of the mouth, and overgrowth of *Candida* results in oral thrush or candidosis. In immunocompetent individuals free of obvious candidosis, the carrier rate for the organism is 40% with a higher prevalence in women and smokers[2]. Different types of oral candidosis are now known and several factors are implicated including the use of dentures, inadequate hygiene, diabetes mellitus and immunodeficiency. Chronic atrophic candidosis or denture stomatitis is a very common form of oral candidosis among denture wearers and more commonly affects women, with 60% older than 65 years of age[3]. The condition is characterized by chronic edema and erythema of the palatal mucosa that contacts the denture. There is pain and tenderness of the affected mucosa. In some cases, there is evidence that *Candida* plays a role in the development and maintenance of the condition[2] (Figure 4).

Vaginal or vulvovaginal candidosis

The bowel and vagina are regular hosts of *Candida*; in order for a clinical disease (candidosis) to develop, certain conditions must favor its proliferation. These include diabetes mellitus, immunosuppression, systemic therapy (antibiotics and steroids) and pregnancy, which may lower host resistance. *Candida* species are responsible for 90% of the cases (mainly *C. albicans* but also *C. glabrata*, *C. tropicalis* and *C. krusei*).

Vulvovaginitis is the most common clinical manifestation of fungal infections causing human mycoses. The condition occurs in 10% of women but during pregnancy the incidence rises to 30% of cases. This may be based on a change of the glycogen content of the vaginal mucosa, changes in the immunological status of the host, or even a local change in glycogen metabolism[4]. Pregnant patients with candidosis usually improve after delivery. In addition to the above-mentioned factors, hormonal influences may predispose to such conditions as vaginal candidosis, which usually flares immediately prior to menstruation. Recurrent vulvovaginal candidosis is due to impaired T-cell function. It may also be due to a hormonal influence in host resistance. Partial T-cell dysregulation may be exacerbated by the hormonal balance present during the follicular phase, correlating with the risk of clinical infection[5]. Vaginal symptoms include thick white vaginal discharge and soreness and burning, especially during intercourse. Vulvar signs include intense erythema and edema.

Low-grade *Candida* infection may cause only vulvar burning. Untreated infection results in a chronic vaginal discharge without symptoms.

Candidal intertigo

Candida is not a normal inhabitant of the skin and will not survive on normal dry skin. Fungal infection may develop in warm or occluded areas such as the flexures. Intertriginous areas such as the submammary folds are very frequently infected (Figure 5). Erythema surrounded by satellite pustules is the hallmark of cutaneous candidosis. Women are more predisposed to candidal intertrigo because of specific predisposing factors (e.g. obesity, heavy breasts). Chronic infection may vary from being asymptomatic to creating burning and pruritus.

Candidal nail paronychia

This is a chronic inflammatory condition resulting from invasion of the posterior and lateral nail folds by yeasts, resulting from frequent contact with moisture, recurrent trauma and destruction of the cuticle. This is common in housewives because they frequently have their hands wet, preparing food or washing up. The skin around the nail becomes erythematous and painful and the cuticle is lost. The nail may become ridged and discolored. Bacterial infections, often due to *Staphylococcus aureus* infection, may add to the pus production (Figure 6).

Candidal nail infection

Candida can also grow beneath the nail; the predisposing factor is a wet environment as found in paronychia. Other conditions of the nail plate, such as psoriasis, may be superinfected by *Candida*. A study from Italy has demonstrated that yeasts are mainly responsible for fungal nail infection of the hands and dermatophytes of the feet (59.1% of nail infections were caused by yeasts, 23.2% by dermatophytes and 17.6% by non-dermatophytic fungi). *C. albicans* was responsible for 70% of the fungal nail infections of the hand, but only 15% of those of the feet. Nail infections were more widespread in women and in both sexes over 50 years of age[6] (Figure 7).

Histopathological description

Superficial candidosis is characterized by subcorneal pustules. Organisms are not usually seen in a pustule but, by using the periodic acid–Schiff (PAS) stain, the yeast can be seen in the stratum corneum.

Essential laboratory studies

KOH examination for microscopy and culture are possible.

Oral candidosis or thrush

Diagnosis is confirmed by cytological scrapings macerated with 20% KOH and examined as a wet mount, or in smears or biopsy material stained with PAS or methenamine silver stain. A fluorescence microscopy technique using calcofluor white has also been suggested[7]. Culture technique is also available, with the potential of identifying the species and the sensitivity to antimicrobials of the particular isolate[8].

Vaginal or vulvovaginal candidosis

KOH examination of skin scrapings and wet mounts of the vaginal discharge should be taken for microscopy and a sample for culture is indicated. KOH examination will show mycelia and spores in a 'grape arbor' arrangement. *Candida* species can be identified on isolation culture media, including agar.

Candidal intertigo

KOH examination for microscopy of scrapings obtained from a satellite pustule can be performed.

Candidal nail infection and paronychia

KOH examination for microscopy of scrapings and culture are performed.

Differential diagnosis

(1) *Oral candidosis or thrush*   from leukoplakia, oral hairy leukoplakia, oral lichen planus;

(2) *Vaginal or vulvovaginal candidosis*   from bacterial, parasitic (trichomonade) and other causes of vaginitis;

(3) *Candidal intertrigo*   from erythrasma, irritant intertrigo, tinea cruris (common in men), dermatitis, seborrheic dermatitis, familial benign pemphigus, flexural Darier's disease and inverse psoriasis. The presence of the satellite pustules is characteristic of candidal infection;

(4) *Candidal nail paronychia*   from fungal nail infection (onychomycosis) and psoriasis of the nails. In these two diseases the nail plate is more prominently involved. A sample for culture has to be taken in doubt, and a nail matrix biopsy in rare cases;

(5) *Candidal nail infection*   Onychomycosis is more common in toenails than in fingernails, where *Candida* is the commonest pathogen. The nail becomes thickened, creamy white, yellow, or even black when debris enters the split nail. The material beneath the affected nail contains the fungus, which is responsible for the thickening of the nail.

Treatment

It is important in the management of candidosis to exclude the systemic causes and their role in each particular situation. It is important always to remember that systemic antifungal treatment during pregnancy has been associated with teratogenicity in animals and congenital anomalies in humans[9]. It is therefore advisable to avoid any type of oral antifungal treatment during pregnancy and breast feeding.

Oral candidosis

Topical treatment   Use topical preparations of nystatin or clotrimazole 1% or amphotericin B[2]. These topical agents are available in troches, rinses, pastilles and creams. They should be applied 2–3 times daily. If patients have dentures, these have to be brushed and washed in an antiseptic agent such as chlorhexidine.

Oral treatment   Use itraconazole 100 mg once a day (may take 3–5 weeks in chronic infection), or fluconazole 50–100 mg daily for 7–14 days.

Recurrences   These are not uncommon after discontinuation of treatment (especially when there is an underlying immunological defect) and sometimes long-term maintenance or repeated courses of these antifungals may be required.

Vaginal or vulvovaginal candidosis

In patients with confirmed cutaneous candidosis the topical application of azoles or imidazoles is usually an adequate treatment. Topical nystatin is less efficacious than a broad-spectrum antifungal[4].

In patients with both vaginal and vulvar candidosis the combined treatment of vaginal antifungal agents with topical cutaneous application is adequate.

Topical treatment   Use vaginal antifungal creams or suppositories (nystatin or azole antifungals) for

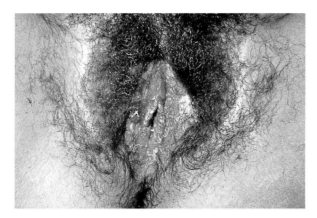

Figure 1   Vulvovaginal candidosis can be extremely discomforting as shown by the swelling and erythema in this patient

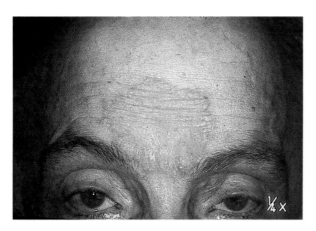

Figure 2   Topical steroids can create a much worse dermatitis – tinea incognito – as shown in this woman with tinea faciei

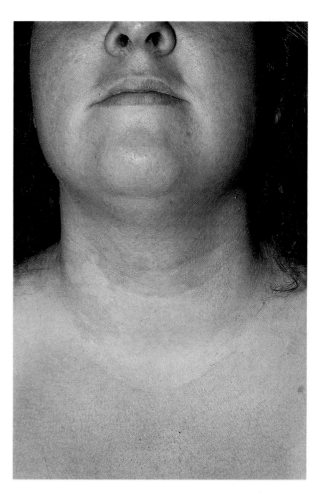

Figure 3   Tinea versicolor can be composed of both red and brown scaling

5–7 days. There is evidence to suggest that a high-dose, shorter course of therapy is as effective as the standard 7-day course[10].

Oral treatment   Use a single-day therapy with fluconazole 150 mg or a 3-day course with itraconazole 100 mg twice a day.

Treatment of partner   Oral treatment is as above.

Recurrences   (of vaginal candidosis or continuous low-grade *Candida* infection). These can be very difficult to manage. An intermittent 3-day course of oral itraconazole 100 mg twice a day followed by a single day course on the first day of menstrual cycle for 6 months or prolonged use of vaginal antifungals is recommended.

Candidal intertrigo

General measures   Avoid moisture and friction, and dry in air. It is recommended to lose weight and wear clothes that fit.

Topical treatment   Compresses of a drying agent such as potassium permaganate 1 : 40 when the skin is cracked and moist can be used. Nystatin and imidazole topical creams, and powder preparations containing nystatin are useful in moist intertriginous areas. Apply for 2–3 weeks.

Systemic treatment   If the condition is persistent (in cases of immunosuppression or in some cutaneous disorders that affect the flexures), itraconazole 100 mg twice a day for 7 days, terbinafine 250 mg daily or fluconazole 150 mg once a week for 2–4 weeks may be tried.

Candidal paronychia

General measures   Avoid damp or wet conditions. Wear gloves when washing.

Topical treatment   Use econazole or clotrimazole topical lotions (these work better than creams) once daily under the nail fold and adjacent nail until swelling subsides. Thymol 4% in chloroform or

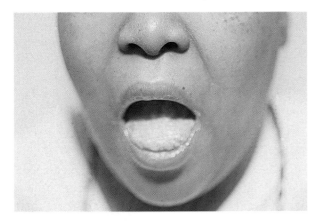

Figure 4   Thrush can occur both in immunodeficiency and with excessive use of antimicrobials, as occurred in this woman

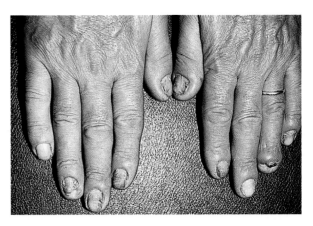

Figure 6   Once called monilial paronychia, candidal nail paronychia may be precipitated by excessive submersion in water or by over-ambitious manicuring

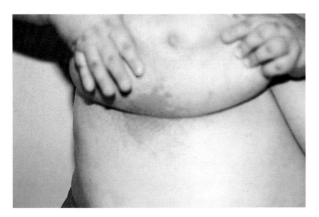

Figure 5   The submammary area is an ideal place for *Candida albicans* to proliferate, creating candidal intertrigo

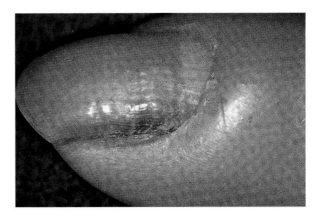

Figure 7   Candidal nail infection can result from chronic candidal infection

absolute alcohol four times a day is also helpful. This may take 3–4 months.

Oral treatment   If other organisms are implicated (staphylococci), then antimicrobials may be necessary, such as erythromycin 250 mg four times a day or flucloxacillin 250 mg four times a day for 10–14 days.

Candidal nail infection

Candida nail infection in the absence of paronychia is rare. When it occurs, topical treatment should be considered to remove the pathogen, although complete regrowth of the nail leads to elimination of the fungus.

Topical treatment   When the surface or the tip or edge of the nail only is affected, use amorfoline lacquers. Treatments take many months to have an obvious effect; toenails grow very slowly.

Oral treatment   If severe involvement of the nail plate is present, itraconazole 100 mg four times a (total 400 mg/day) for 7 days/month in a pulsed scheme is effective against *Candida albicans* and should be taken for 3 months.

DERMATOPHYTE INFECTIONS

Although *Candida* infection has a higher incidence in female patients, dermatophyte infections are present in women and girls and, according to the location, their terms vary: tinea capitis, tinea corporis, tinea unguium and manuum or tinea pedis.

Clinical description

Tinea capitis

Tinea capitis is a dermatophytosis of the scalp and is most commonly described in children. Virtually any species of *Microsporum* or *Trichophyton* may cause tinea capitis. The causative organisms are classified according to whether they can produce arthropodes outside or just under the cuticle of the hair (ectothrix) or within the hair (endothrix) and according to their host origin (anthropophilic, zoophilic, geophilic) (Table 1). Tinea capitis may resolve spontaneously but *Trichophyton* species seem to be persistent into adulthood (Figure 8).

Tinea corporis

Tinea corporis can occur in any area of the body; occupational exposure is an important risk factor. *Trichophyton rubrum* and *T. mentagrophytes* are the common pathogens but T. *rubrum* infection is more frequent. When it is due to zoophilic organisms (animal handlers), ringworm lesions are seen on exposed skin, whereas anthropophilic species cause an infection in occluded areas or in areas of trauma. Women are more susceptible to fungal infection of areas of trauma such as perifolliculitis in the legs which may be associated with leg shaving (Figure 9). Tinea cruris is mainly a male dermatophytosis.

Tinea unguium and manuum

Although the overall susceptibility to dermatophyte nail infections is higher in men than in women, the number of cases affecting toenails has increased in women[11]. Narrow shoes in women allow trauma to the toenails and the increased incidence may be explained by the differences in footwear. The most common dermatophytes are shown in Table 1. Additionally, tinea manuum may present with unilateral involvement of the palm with acute inflammation (vesicles, bullae) or in chronic cases with hyperkeratosis. It is caused by the same agents responsible for tinea pedis and tinea cruris shown in Table 1.

Tinea pedis

There are four different patterns for tinea pedis: moccasin, inflammatory, interdigitale and ulcerative. The majority of cases of tinea pedis are caused by *Trichophyton rubrum* (Table 1). *Candida albicans* may be a co-pathogen[11] (Figure 10).

Histopathological description

Hyphae are identified in the stratum corneum with the hematoxylin and eosin stain and appear basophilic. The PAS stain helps to emphasize their presence, and fungal elements appear red.

Essential laboratory studies

KOH examination for microscopy, culture and Wood's light examination are valuable for tinea capitis caused by *Microsporum* species (green fluorescence) or in the differential diagnosis from erythrasma (coral-red fluorescence).

Differential diagnosis

(1) *Tinea capitis* From other papulosquamous entities that can affect the scalp such as psoriasis, seborrheic dermatitis, pityriasis amiantacea and other conditions such as alopecia areata, trichotillomania, secondary syphilis and pseudopelade;

(2) *Tinea corporis* In particular in women, the perifolliculitis may mimic other papulosquamous entities such as psoriasis, lichen planus, nummular dermatitis, secondary syphilis, seborrheic dermatitis, pityriasis rosea, or pityriasis rubra pilaris.

(3) *Tinea unguium* From yeasts (*Candida*) and non-dermatophytic molds (*Scopulariopsis brevicaulis*,

Table 1 Common dermatophytes and skin diseases

Clinical disease	Name	Source
Tinea capitis	*Trichophyton tonsurans* (USA)	anthropophilic
	Microsporum canis (Europe)	zoophilic
	Trichophyton violaceum (Europe)	anthropophilic
Tinea corporis	*Trichophyton rubrum*	anthropophilic
	Trichophyton mentagrophytes var *interdigitale*	anthropophilic
	Trichophyton verrucosum	zoophilic
	Micropsorum canis	zoophilic
Tinea unguium–manuum	*Trichophyton rubrum*	anthropophilic
	Trichophyton mentagrophytes var *interdigitale*	anthropophilic
	Epidermophyton floccosum	anthropophilic
Tinea pedis	*Trichophyton rubrum*	anthropophilic
	Trichophyton mentagrophytes var *interdigitale*	anthropophilic
	Epidermophyton floccosum	anthropophilic

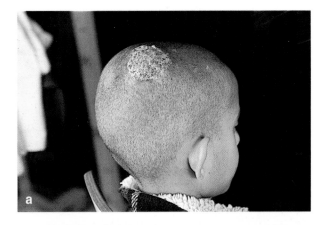

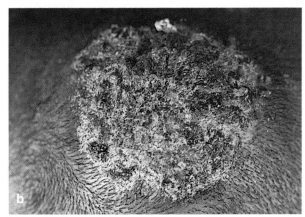

Figure 8   (a) and (b) Ringworm of the scalp, tinea capitis, can be complicated by bacterial infiltration, leading to kerion formation

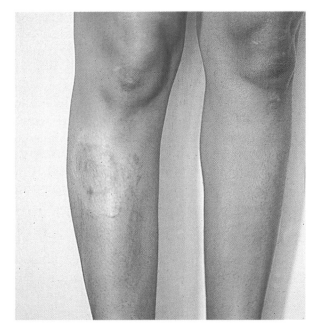

Figure 9   The redness with sharp margination of tinea corporis may be precipitated by shaving and subsequent folliculitis

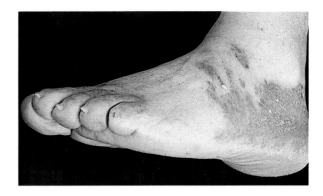

Figure 10   While athelete's foot is often thought of as involving the interdigital spaces, the redness and sharp margination of tinea pedis can be limited to the ankles

Aspergillus, Fussarium, Cephalosporium). Other diseases with nail involvement such as psoriasis, hand dermatitis, Darrier's disease, lichen planus, congenital pachyonychia and crusted scabies.

(4) *Tinea pedis*   From psoriasis, dermatitis, various keratodermas, bullous diseases, erythrasma, infections caused by *Candida albicans*, molds and bacteria.

Treatment

Any oral antifungal agent should be avoided during pregnancy and breast feeding. There are warnings by manufacturers that high doses cause toxicity and the drugs are extracted in different percentages in the breast milk. Itraconazole exhibits dose-dependent maternal toxicity and embryotoxicity[12]. Women of childbearing age should take contraceptive precautions. Griseofulvin is teratogenic in animals[13] and placental transfer has been documented. Ketoconazole is also found to cross the placenta, and terbinafine is excreted in breast milk[12].

Tinea capitis

Oral antifungals   Tinea capitis should be treated with a systemic antifungal. Griseofulvin for 40 years was the only systemic antimycotic agent curative for tinea capitis. It is still the first line for most dermatophytes but it is not effective against *Candida* infections and many infections by common dermatophytes (*Trichophyton rubrum, Trichophyton tonsurans*) do not always respond to this drug. In these cases, ketoconazole or itraconazole may be useful[14]. Frequently, the dose of griseofulvin must be doubled to see clinical improvement. It is used in children but it is teratogenic and fetotoxic in animals[13].

Because griseofulvin is the oldest established antifungal for dermatophytes, a relatively high incidence of side-effects (due to the long-time use of this drug) is recognized. Terbinafine and itraconazole are newer antimycotic agents that have been developed for systemic treatment mainly of onychomycosis and dermatomycosis. Both drugs can be used in the treatment of tinea capitis in children with success. The major disadvantage of griseofulvin over the newer antifungals is the long treatment, lasting up to 4–8 weeks or more, and the large quantity of the drug required for cure. With the recently proposed pulse schemes with terbinafine or itraconazole, no monitoring of liver enzymes and full blood count is usually necessary.

Several reports on the use of terbinafine in tinea capitis showed continuous 6-week treatment regimens to be effective in cases caused mostly by *Trichophyton* species[15]. A pulse scheme of terbinafine showed clearance in 12 out of 13 children with tinea capitis caused by *Trichophyton tonsurans* and *T. violaceum* after three pulses[16]. *Microsporum canis* shows lack of efficacy to terbinafine and prolonged courses (more than 6 weeks)[17] or more pulses may be required (Table 2).

Continuous treatment with itraconazole for 4–6 weeks is effective against *Trichopyton* species[18] and a more extended course may be necessary for *Microsporum canis* infection[19]. Pulsing is often more convenient, as well as being effective. There is also high compliance[20].

Topical treatment   This is sometimes used adjunctively with systemic treatment in some parts of the world. These include topical keratolytic agents or antifungals; the most commonly used is ketoconazole 2% shampoo.

Tinea corporis–manuum–pedis
Topical treatment   For isolated lesions topical use of imidazole or allylamine creams for a period of 3 weeks is the most effective.

Oral antifungals   These are usually necessary for treatment. For more widespread or more inflammatory lesions, oral antifungals are recommended such as itraconazole 200 mg daily for tinea corporis and 200 mg twice a day for tinea manuum and pedis for 1 week, and terbinafine 250 mg daily for 2 weeks. Griseofulvin is the oldest antifungal drug with the only disadvantage of slow cure compared to newer antifungals.

Table 2   Practical treatment regimens for common dermatophytoses

Tinea infection	Drug(s) of choice	Drug name	Dose	Treatment
Tinea capitis				
Oral treatment	griseofulvin		10–20 mg/day	4–8 weeks
	terbinafine	Lamisil®	250 mg	6 weeks
			250 mg	3 pulses*
	itraconazole	Sporanox®	100 mg	4–6 weeks
			5 mg/kg per day	3 pulses*
Topical treatment	keratolytic or antifungal shampoos			
Tinea corporis				
Topical treatment (isolated lesions)	imidazole or allylamine creams			3 weeks
Oral treatment	itraconazole	Sporanox®	200 mg	1 week
	terbinafine	Lamisil®	250 mg	2 weeks
Tinea manuum–pedis				
Oral treatment	itraconazole	Sporanox®	200 mg b.i.d	1 week
	terbinafine	Lamisil®	250 mg	2 weeks
Tinea unguium				
Oral treatment	itraconazole		200 mg b.i.d	3–4 pulses†
	terbinafine		250 mg	12 weeks
Topical treatment (limited infection)	amorolfine		once a week	6–18 months

*Each pulse lasting 1 week, with 2 weeks off between the first and second pulses, and 3 weeks off between the second and third pulses; †each pulse lasting 1 week, with 3 weeks off between pulses (see text)

Table 3 List of drugs and their generic names

Fluconazole	Diflucan
Itraconazole	Sporanox
Ketoconazole	Nizoral
Nystatin	generic
Clotrimazole	generic
Imidazole	generic
Griseofulvin	generic
Amorolfine	Loceryl
Terbinafine	Lamisil

Tinea unguium

Oral antifungals Itraconazole and terbinafine are the commonest newer antifungals used in the treatment of dermatophyte infection of the nails and can provide efficacy rates as high as with griseofulvin, with a reduced treatment duration.

Itraconazole 200 mg twice a day for 1 week is recommended in a pulse scheme (1 week on – 3 weeks off) for 3 months for fingernails and 4 months for toenails which minimizes any possible toxic side-effects. Itraconazole is also effective against *Candida* infections.

Terbinafine 250 mg daily as a continuous 6-week course is recommended for fingernails and a 12-week course for toenails. Terbinafine may not be as effective against *Candida* infections.

Topical treatment This is available in some parts of the world; it is successful on less severe fungal nail infections and should be considered in cases with limited nail involvement (up to two nails) or when systemic treatment is contraindicated. Lacquers and paints are applied directly to the infected area when the infection affects the nail surface or the edge of the nail. Apply amorolfine once a week and continue for 6 months for fingernails and 18 months for toenails.

HIV-INFECTED WOMEN AND FUNGAL INFECTIONS

Mucosal candidosis is a common complication in HIV-infected women and may develop as both oropharyngeal and vaginal candidosis. The incidence of candidosis increases with advancing immunodeficiency. It seems that candidal vaginitis is the most common initial clinical manifestation of HIV disease. This is a very distressing problem for HIV-infected women. Oropharyngeal candidosis is demonstrated by the presence of candidal pseudomycelial forms on KOH examination; isolation of *Candida* in culture is not diagnostic.

The development of oral or vaginal candidosis is dissociated, and HIV-infected women are each infected by their own unique strain of *Candida*[21]. There is a reduction in Langerhans' and plasma cells which may reflect loss of signals from CD4+ cells. This in part explains why HIV-positive women are susceptible to fungal infections even when the peripheral immune system is intact[22].

Secondary prophylactic use of fluconazole is recommended for oropharyngeal and esophageal candidosis.

In the treatment of symptomatic oropharyngeal candidosis, fluconazole is also used. The usual dosage is 50 mg once daily for 14–30 days. Sometimes, the daily dose can be increased to 100 mg. Fluconazole is more effective than ketoconazole or itraconazole in this case. The gastric pH does not affect the absorption of fluconazole[23].

CONCLUSIONS

Treatment does not vary between women and men, but pregnancy and breast feeding interfere with the use of oral antifungal drugs. Congenital anomalies have been described from the use of fluconazole during and beyond the first trimester of pregnancy. Griseofulvin is teratogenic in animals and placental transfer has been documented, as with ketoconazole. Itraconazole shows dose-dependent maternal toxicity and embryotoxicity and terbinafine is excreted in breast milk. Topical treatment should usually be the only treatment until pregnancy and breast feeding are completed.

REFERENCES

1. Imam N, Carpenter CC, Mayer KH, *et al*. Hierarchical pattern of mucosal *Candida* infections in HIV seropositive women. *Am J Med* 1990;89: 142–5
2. Gallagher GT. Disorders of mucocutaneous integument. In Fitzpatrick TB, Eisen AZ, Wolf K, *et al.*, eds. *Dermatology in General Medicine*. New York: McGraw Hill, 1993:1355–415
3. Martin AG, Kobayashi GS. Yeast infections: candidiasis and pityriasis (tinea) versicolor. In Fitzpatrick TB, Eisen AZ, Wolf K, *et al.*, eds. *Dermatology in General Medicine*. New York: McGraw Hill, 1993: 2452–66
4. Pincus S, McKay M. Disorders of the female genitalia. In Fitzpatrick TB, Eisen AZ, Wolf K, *et al.*, eds. *Dermatology in General Medicine*. New York: McGraw Hill, 1993:1463–81
5. Corrigan EM, Clancy RL, Dunkley MF, *et al*. Cellular immunity in recurrent vulvovaginal candidiasis. *Clin Exp Immunol* 1998;111:574–8

6. Mercantini R, Marsella R, Moretto D. Onychomycosis in Rome, Italy. *Mycopathologia* 1996;1136:25–32

7. Lynch DP, Gibson DK. The use of calcofluor chite in the histopathologic diagnosis of oral candidiasis. *Oral Surg* 1987;63:68–71

8. Arendorf TM, Walker DM. The prevalence and intraoral distribution of *Candida albicans* in man. *Arch Oral Biol* 1980;25:1–10

9. Pursley TJ, Blomquist IK, Abraham J, *et al.* Fluconazole-induced congential anomalies in three infants. *Clin Infect Dis* 1996;22:336–40

10. Robertson WH. A concentrated therapeutic regimen for vulvovaginal candidiasis. *JAMA* 1980;244:2549–50

11. Martin AG, Kobayashi GS. Fungal diseases with cutaneous involvement. In Fitzpatrick TB, Eisen AZ, Wolf K, *et al.*, eds. *Dermatology in General Medicine*. New York: McGraw Hill, 1993:2421–51

12. Gupta AK, Sauder DN, Shear NH. Antifungal agents: an overview. Part II. *J Am Acad Dermatol* 1994;30:911–33

13. Scott FW, LaHunta A, Schultz RD, *et al.* Teratogenesis in cats associated with griseofulvin therapy. *Teratology* 1975;11:79–86

14. Elewski BE. Superficial mycoses, dermatophytoses and selected dermatomycoses. In Elewski BE, ed. *Cutaneous Fungal Infections*. New York: Igaku-shoin, 1992:12–59

15. Jones TJ. Overview of the use of terbinafine (Lamisil) in children. *Br J Dermatol* 1995;132:683–9

16. Gupta AK, Adam P. Terbinafine pulse therapy is effective in tinea capitis. *Pediatr Dermatol* 1998;15:56–8

17. Dragos V, Lunder M. Lack of efficacy of 6-week treatment with oral terbinafine for tinea capitis due to *Microsporum canis* in children. *Pediatr Dermatol* 1997;14:46–8

18. Elewski B. Tinea capitis: itraconazole in *Trichophyton tonsurans* infection. *J Am Acad Dermatol* 1994;31:65–7

19. Greer DL. Itraconazole in the treatment of tinea capitis. *J Am Acad Dermatol* 1996;35:637–8

20. Gupta AK, Hofstader SL, Summerbell RC, *et al.* Treatment of tinea capitis with itraconazole capsule pulse therapy. *J Am Acad Dermatol* 1998;39:216–19

21. Dahl KM, Keath EJ, Fraser VJ, Powderly WG. Molecular epidemiology of mucosal candidiasis in HIV-positive women. *AIDS Res Hum Retroviruses* 1997;13:485–91

22. Olaitan A, Johnson MA, MacLean A, Poulter LW. The distribution of immunocompetent cells in the genital tract of HIV-infected women. *AIDS* 1996;10:759–64

23. Johnson RA, Dover JS. Cutaneous manifestations of human immunodeficiency virus disease. In Fitzpatrick TB, Eisen AZ, Wolf K, *et al.*, eds. *Dermatology in General Medicine*. New York: McGraw Hill, 1993:2637–85

Parasitic diseases including tropical diseases

25

Marcia Ramos-e-Silva and Nurimar Conceição Fernandes

INTRODUCTION

Cutaneous diseases are a major health problem in all underdeveloped and developing regions; it is an established fact that they receive much less attention when affecting women than men. It is also true that the effects of illnesses in general, including parasitic and tropical diseases, are different in men and women[1,2]. Parasitic diseases are most prevalent among populations with little personal hygiene who are deprived of basic sanitation (unavailability of potable water, inadequate disposal of human waste, lack of latrines) and good nutritional status. Other predisposing factors, such as a decreased level of immune protection against infectious agents, low level of education and other situations included in the overall framework of a low socio-economic level, are also features in many developing countries[3]. Characteristically, populations exposed to these factors are the ones in which women are often underprivileged[1,2].

Parasitic and tropical diseases

Parasitic diseases are widespread throughout the world and, although almost any infection-causing organism can be a parasite, only protozoa, helminthes and arthropods are considered as a cause of parasitic diseases from the clinical point of view[3]. These illnesses are also closely linked to warm and humid climates, and most of them are therefore considered tropical and subtropical diseases[4,5]. The factors that mostly influence the onset of tropical dermatoses, according to Canizares and Harman[6], are climatic, ecological, human, cultural and socio-economic. Because of these factors, such diseases are called dermatoses of the poor, of the developing and underdeveloped countries; and also dermatoses of malnutrition, illiteracy, sun radiation, humidity and insect bites.

Gender inequalities in the Third World

There has been a general lack of awareness of the effects of gender and sex on the distribution and consequences of disease. The term 'gender' encompasses the sociocultural aspects of the differences between the behavior of men and women, while the term 'sex' relates to physiological attributes, such as the influence of female hormones, menarche, pregnancy and menopause[1]. Besides the obvious sex differences, gender inequalities of health in Third World countries exist and health hazards are present at every stage of a woman's life cycle. Health issues which pose the greatest hardship to women in these countries include reproductive problems, excess female mortality in childhood, violence against girls and women, occupational and environmental hazards and cervical and breast cancer[7]. Gender, as well as sex differences, affects people's risk and response to tropical diseases, and the determinants and consequences include economic, social and personal dimensions[8].

In countries where tropical diseases are endemic – although both men and women suffer from poverty and deprivation – there is now substantial evidence that women are particularly disadvantaged owing to societal factors. Exposure to disease, intensity of infection, duration of illness, care during illness, access to and utilization of health care services, and finally the impact of illness on family life are all influenced by the significantly lower and subordinate social status of women in many countries. All these factors make them economically dependent on men, worsening their secondary role in the social group[1,9].

Feminization of poverty

The global change in the traditional social structure has led to an increase in the number of women acting as heads of households[10]. The number of aging partnerless women is increasing[11], and the treatment of dermatoses, including tropical diseases, during pregnancy is a difficult problem[2]. The rising number of women living in poverty, many of whom are mothers, poses a social and political dilemma for the 21st century[11]. Literate women are usually the first members in a household to apply their knowledge and skills to raise the levels of sanitation, nutrition and education, thus contributing to upgrading the general living standards of their homes[1]. The fact that households where women are the heads also tend to be poorer makes them more vulnerable to the effects of tropical diseases that are 'diseases of poverty'. This phenomenon has been identified as the 'feminization of poverty', a situation in which women make up the majority of the poor[12]. Tropical diseases have huge economic consequences, and although the economic effects of illness on women have not really been studied, it is a fact that when the woman in a household falls sick, there are repercussions not only for her as an individual but for the entire family group[1]. Women have mainly domestic roles in developing countries, which require them to remain indoors[13]. On the other hand and notwithstanding the fact that the home is the setting for the transmission of many vector-borne diseases[14], the voluminous clothing often worn by women in these situations protects them from insect bites[13,15]. The effects of nutritional status on tropical diseases have not been formally investigated but it has been observed that among the urban poor in India male children and adults receive the most nutritious foods[16]. It is also known that anemic adolescent girls are, for example, at greater risk of morbidity from parasitic and other infections[1]. Another very important point related to women's health is that the professionals frequently give little credibility to their experiences of symptoms, as they tend to attribute women's illnesses to psychiatric problems and treat them inappropriately. This leads to a loss of confidence in their own perceptions of illness and health[17] and explains why women prefer to consult non-professional healers, as they usually provide more easily understandable explanations[1].

There are some parasitic and tropical dermatoses that have undoubted differences in their characteristics, frequency and/or importance when affecting women as compared to men. Among them, seven diseases will be discussed in more detail, especially in their relationship to women. Leprosy shows a higher tendency to develop reactions in women although it is less frequent in them. In tuberculosis, erythema induratum tends to occur in young women; while tinea nigra and tinea capitis in adults affect women rather than men. Scabies is more often observed in young women and children, who frequently show eczematization; and schistosomiasis may lead to complications in pregnancy, among many other important features in women.

LEPROSY

Leprosy (Hansen's disease) is expected to remain a public health problem for at least the next decade.

Considerable differences exist in the registered incidence rates between the two sexes. Case detection rates are higher among men but it is assumed that risk and prevalence of infection among women is underestimated[18]. Women seem to have greater resistance to clinical leprosy and, therefore, lower incidence and less severe clinical forms, apparently associated with levels of estrogen and other female hormones; nevertheless, the effects on women are far more devastating, a phenomenon Kaur attributes to cultural reasons – what she calls women's 'greater socioeconomic vulnerability'[1,11]. Reversal reactions are more common among women, and pregnant women have a higher risk of relapse, neuritis and erythema nodosum leprosum[19]. Economic dependence on men and shame make women hide the disease, which becomes worse, while confinement to home and activities such as washing and cooking with hands that lack feeling exacerbate the disease and put women at risk[11].

Clinical description

Leprosy reactions are acute emergencies in the course of human infection by *Mycobacterium leprae*. Two types of reaction are differentiated: type 1 (reversal reaction) and type 2 (erythema nodosum leprosum) (Figures 1–4).

A patient is diagnosed as having a reversal reaction (type 1) when the following clinical signs are present: redness, swelling and sometimes tenderness of lesions; neuritis (swelling, pain, tenderness, paresthesia or nerve function impairment); edema of hands, feet or face; occasionally fever. Type 2 reaction is characterized by multiple, small, tender nodules with or without ulceration on the arms and legs; neuritis; fever, edema, iritis, or arthritis. Their etiologies are unknown and their pathogenesis poorly understood. Several studies indicate that type 1 is associated with activation of the cellular immune system but the stimulus is not known. Type 2 is generally considered to be an immune complex phenomenon[18,19].

The first appearance of leprosy, reactivation of the disease and relapse are especially likely to occur in the third trimester of pregnancy or immediately after delivery. Leprosy reactions increase during pregnancy, occurring in 32% of women with active leprosy under treatment[20]. Erythema nodosum leprosum is prevalent in the first trimester with a second peak in the third trimester to fifteen months postpartum[21-23]. During lactation erythema nodosum leprosum more commonly affects nerves and has a higher tendency to be more severe, even necrotic[23].

Histopathology

In the reversal downgrading reaction, dermal edema on skin histology is a common feature. Positive characteristics for a reversal upgrading reaction are an increased number of large Langhans giant cells, formation of discrete granulomas, fibrinoid necrosis of granulomas and reduction in the expected number of acid-fast bacilli[24].

Erythema nodosum leprosum is characterized by an influx of polymorphs, though in the late stage lymphocytes predominate. Vasculitis affecting arterioles or venules is a significant feature. The reaction is often present in the deep dermis or subcutis. In laboratory studies smears of scrapings from skin lesions, stained for acid-fast bacilli, is the standard technique used to estimate the number of *Mycobacterium leprae*. Laboratory findings may include anemia, leukocytosis, neutrophilia, elevated erythrocyte sedimentation rate and proteinuria.

Differential diagnosis

The principal criteria for the clinical diagnosis of leprosy are loss of sensation in clinically suspected skin lesions and thickening of peripheral nerves with loss of sensation in the corresponding skin area. Skin smears demonstrate acid-fast bacilli. Histopathological diagnosis is based on cellular infiltration of nerve branches and on the presence of intracellular acid-fast bacilli.

The major differential diagnosis of type 2 reaction (erythema nodosum leprosum) is erythema nodosum, which is a painful nodular syndrome which results from a hypersensitivity reaction to various possible antigenic stimuli. The painful nodules vary in number and may come together into plaques; they are red-violet in color, brilliant and located on the tibial crest, feet, knees, internal surface of the thighs, buttocks and sometimes forearms. In the regressive stage they resemble contusions and heal without scarring. These lesions never ulcerate. A septal panniculitis is the histologic feature[25].

Treatment

Pregnancy and lactation do not contraindicate standard multiple drug therapy with dapsone, rifampicin and clofazimine. These drugs should be continued without interruption during the episodes of leprosy reactions. The reversal reaction must be treated daily with 60 mg of prednisone; control of the reaction allows the dose of prednisone to be decreased and discontinued over a period of two months.

Erythema nodosum leprosum is suppressed by thalidomide, the treatment of choice, in a dosage of 100 mg three times daily. After controlling the reaction it can be tapered (100 mg weekly) to a maintenance dosage or complete withdrawal[18]. In fertile women this drug is contraindicated. Women of child-bearing age are treated with prednisone[19,24].

Conclusions

Type 1 reactions occur with significantly greater frequency in women. In pregnancy the immunological response is suppressed. Leprosy reactions are triggered by pregnancy: type 1 occurs postpartum while type 2 peaks in late pregnancy. Both types continue into lactation.

TUBERCULOSIS OF THE SKIN

Mycobacterium tuberculosis is the predominant cause of cutaneous tuberculosis (nodular vasculitis; erythema induratum) but *M. bovis*, sometimes called *M. tuberculosis* (var. *bovis*), may also infect the skin. It is classified as primary inoculation tuberculosis, reinfection tuberculosis and tuberculids. Erythema induratum is a chronic nodular eruption that usually occurs on the lower legs of young women. The disease has recently been classified as nodular vasculitis and represents a multifactorial syndrome of lobular panniculitis. The term erythema induratum should be reserved for those cases with tuberculosis etiology, while today the term nodular vasculitis is used to describe the disease in association or not with tuberculosis[26].

Clinical description

The disease manifests as recurrent crops of small, tender, erythematous, violaceous nodules that at times coalesce to form a tender plaque with or without ulceration. Most lesions affect both shins and calves and persist for several weeks; they tend to heal with scarring (Figure 5). The association with tuberculosis at an extracutaneous site (kidneys, lymph nodes, lungs and endometrium) has been described in 55.9% of patients in previous large studies[27]. More recently mycobacterial DNA has been detected on lesion biopsy specimens of erythema induratum using the polymerase chain reaction (PCR)[28].

Histopathology

Histopathology comprises lobular panniculitis with varying combinations of primary vasculitis, granulomatous inflammation, septal fibrosis and caseation necrosis. Acid-fast bacilli are rarely found in stained sections. In laboratory studies a strongly

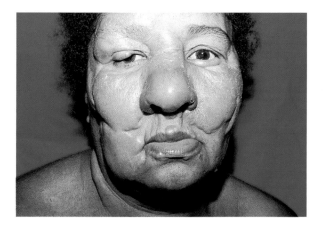

Figure 1 Reversal reaction

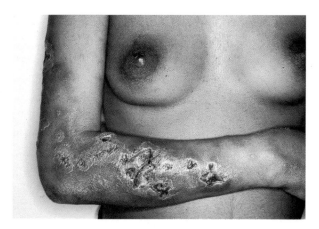

Figure 3 Erythema nodosum leprosum during lactation. Courtesy of Tania Cestari, MD, PhD, Porto Alegre, Brazil

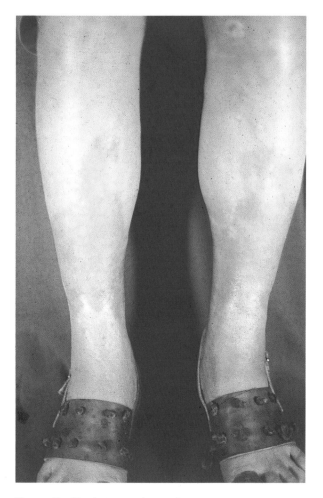

Figure 2 Erythema nodosum leprosum

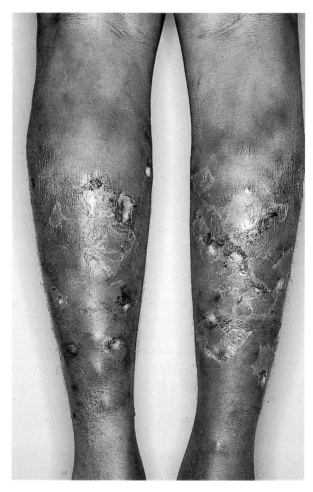

Figure 4 Erythema nodosum leprosum (patient in figure 3). Courtesy of Tania Cestari, MD, PhD, Porto Alegre, Brazil

positive tuberculin test is usually present in patients with erythema induratum.

Differential diagnosis

The following clinical features distinguish erythema induratum from erythema nodosum: a chronic recurrent course; skin lesions that involve shins and calves concentrated on the lower third of the leg; skin nodules that heal with ulcerations or depressed scars.

Treatment

The drugs currently employed in the chemotherapy of tuberculosis are rifampicin, pyrazinamide

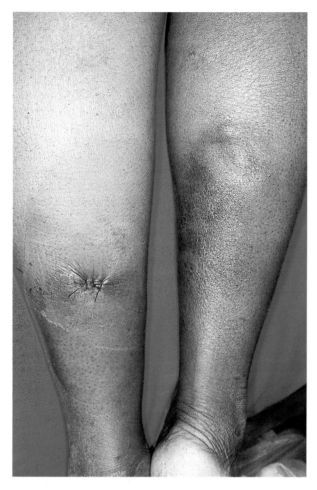

Figure 5 Erythema induratum

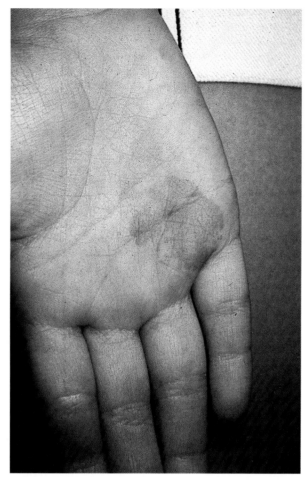

Figure 6 Tinea nigra

and isoniazid (Table 1). Response to treatment is quite variable; a good therapeutic response supports the diagnosis of tuberculosis as a cause[29]. Pregnant women with tuberculosis do not have a different course or prognosis. Rifampicin, pyrazinamide and isoniazid can be used during pregnancy with enough safety. Pyridoxine should be used (40–50 mg daily) to avoid convulsions of the newborn[29].

Conclusions

Erythema induratum is believed to represent a tuberculid. This term is applied to any group of eruption that arises in response to an internal focus of tuberculosis and is regarded as a hypersensitivity reaction to *Mycobacterium tuberculosis*. The response to treatment is quite variable, relapses are common and even periods of improvement and worsening frequently occur during the antituberculosis therapy.

The diagnosis should be made on the following presumptive criteria[29]:

(1) granuloma with caseation necrosis; or

(2) granuloma without caseation necrosis and positive tuberculin test; or

(3) established tuberculosis at another site;

(4) clinical improvement after eight weeks of exclusive antituberculosis therapy.

TINEA NIGRA

Tinea nigra – also known as keratomycosis nigricans palmaris, cladosporiosis epidermica, or microsporiasis nigra – is a superficial and benign infection of the stratum corneum caused by *Exophiala werneckii*. The fungus occurs in soil, vegetation and humus. More recently *Stenella araguata* has also been isolated as a causative agent. The infection occurs by traumatic inoculation of the agent into the skin. Women under 20 years of age are more susceptible, especially those who are hyperhydrotic[30]. It presents as brown or black nonscaly macules with a circular border on the palmar surfaces (Figure 6).

Table 1 Treatment schedule for tuberculosis

		Weight			
Phase	Drugs	< 20kg (mg/kg/day)	20–35kg (mg/day)	35–45kg (mg/day)	> 45kg (mg/day)
1 (2 months)	R	10	300	450	600
	I	10	200	300	400
	P	35	1000	1500	2000
2 (4 months)	R	10	300	450	600
	I	10	200	300	400

R, rifampicin; I, isoniazid; P, pyrazinamide

Histopathology

The stratum corneum contains dark-colored fungal elements composed of septated, branching hyphae and budding cells. Biopsy of tinea nigra is not necessary for diagnosis[31].

Laboratory study

Skin scrapings of the affected area on a slide in one or two drops of 10% potassium hydroxide solution show light brown to dark green, branched septated hyphae, 1.5–3.0 μm in diameter. Skin scales are inoculated into Sabouraud dextrose agar and kept at room temperature. In one to two weeks typical black yeast colonies are formed[30].

Differential diagnosis

The pigmented lesions simulate nevi and melanoma but these lesions uncommonly have a palmar location. Melanoma and nevi are elevated or indurated[31]. Contact dermatitis and post-inflammatory melanosis are disclosed by history and course.

Treatment

Keratolytic agents such as Whitfield's ointment, tincture of iodine, 2% salicylic acid or 3% sulfur are effective. The main topical imidazoles currently available (clotrimazole, miconazole, econazole, ketoconazole, isoconazole, tioconazole) applied twice daily for three weeks are equally effective, and safe during pregnancy[32].

Conclusion

Tinea nigra is a fungal infection that causes little discomfort to the patient. The primary clinical importance is that a correct diagnosis in the differentiation of pigmented lesions may avoid unnecessary biopsy or surgical intervention.

TINEA CAPITIS

Tinea capitis (scalp ringworm or dermatophytosis) is a dermatophyte infection of the scalp, eyebrows and eyelashes caused by species of *Microsporum* and *Trichophyton*. It is primarily a disease of children. Infection may be seen in adults, when almost invariably women rather than men are affected. All the dermatophytes usually responsible for scalp ringworm in children can also cause tinea capitis in the elderly: *M. canis*, *T. violaceum*, *T. mentagrophytes*, *T. tonsurans*. Favus is a distinctive form of scalp ringworm caused by *T. schönleinii*. The infection may also be seen in an adult woman, provoking severe scarring alopecia[33–37].

Clinical description

Tinea capitis presents with several different clinical aspects. Infected hairs often break at scalp level in anthropophilic *Trichophyton* infections (black dot). In *Trichophyton tonsurans* infection the clinical presentation is often characterized by chronic scaling and alopecia without inflammation[38]. When *T. violaceum* is isolated the following types are observed: gray patch, black dot, seborrheic, pustular inflammatory, kerion and favus[39]. When *M. canis* is isolated gray patch, seborrheic, pustular inflammatory and kerion are observed (Figure 7).

Histopathology

Hyphae are confined to the hair. In kerion celsi, a dense dermal infiltrate of lymphocytes, plasma cells, neutrophils and eosinophils is present. In folliculitis there are fungal remnants in the follicles and perifollicular inflammation[40].

Laboratory study

Broken, altered or discolored hairs should be plucked and placed in a drop of 10–20% potassium hydroxide solution, covered with a coverslip; the material on the slide may be better distributed by applying pressure to the coverslip. Clinical specimens are inoculated into Sabouraud dextrose agar and cultures are incubated for at least 15 days.

Differential diagnosis

Alopecia areata has the characteristic 'exclamation mark hairs' – hairs that are narrower at the base than the top, and that usually show a flat non-desquamative surface. Seborrheic dermatitis or psoriasis may also be confused and, in this case, it is necessary to search for lesions on the trunk or in the nails[40].

Treatment

Oral therapy is usually given for scalp disease, the usual dose of griseofulvin for an adult being between 500 and 1000 mg daily, with food. The main alternative is ketoconazole, which is more active than griseofulvin in scalp ringworm caused by *T. tonsurans*. It is given in a dose of 200 mg daily. The therapy has to be continued for 6–12 weeks until clinical and mycological cure. The other alternatives are itraconazole (100 mg daily) for six weeks and oral fluconazole (50 mg daily) for 20 days.

Pregnancy and lactation contraindicate the drugs mentioned above[41].

Conclusion

Tinea capitis is frequent in women especially during the fifth decade. Most patients reported in the literature are menopausal or postmenopausal women. Poor physiological defense in the elderly, probably due to the qualitative and quantitative differences of the sebum, could explain its higher frequency in mature women.

SCABIES

Introduction

Human scabies – also known as itch or mange – is caused by obligatory parasitic mites of the species *Sarcoptes scabiei* var. *hominis*. This agent was discovered in 1687 by Giovan Bonomo, whose findings raised great controversies and discussions at that time[42]. Its incidence throughout the world shows cyclical fluctuations that are not yet fully understood; it is often assumed that allergic sensitivity to the mite or its products plays an important role in determining the development of lesions other than burrows and in producing pruritus. *Sarcoptes scabiei* var. *hominis* is transmitted from person to person by body contact, particularly among family members and bed partners, although fomite spread can also occur since mites can survive for 2 to 3 days in bedding, clothing and house dust[43].

Clinical description

Among the skin lesions of scabies, only the burrows and vesicles are directly associated with the presence of the mite. Other lesions are the result of allergic sensitivity, scratching or secondary infection. Burrows occur most frequently on the anterior aspects of the wrists, the ulnar border of the hand and between the fingers. The points of the elbows, the anterior axillary fold, the skin around the nipples and the natal cleft are other sites often involved. In children burrows are often found on the palms; in infants under the age of two both palms and soles are often infested, presenting vesicular lesions, and eczema may be widespread and severe[44].

In adult males 85% of subjects carry mites on the hands and wrists and 63% of the vigorous feeders may be recovered from this area. The elbows, feet and ankles, and penis and scrotum each carry mites in 30–40% of subjects. Male genitalia must be examined when there is a suspicion of scabies because over 30% of infested men have penile lesions[45]. The distribution in adult women is similar but the palms are more often colonized, and the region of the nipple is often involved. Eczematous changes may follow scratching, and are particularly characteristic on the breasts of young women, with burrows near the nipple[46] (Figures 8 and 9).

The onset of pruritus is usually first noticed two weeks or longer after infestation, but earlier in subsequent infestations[44]. Type IV hypersensitivity reaction to the mites and their products begins around the first month after the infestation and results in a papular or eczematous eruption in the involved sites. At this time itching, the most obvious manifestation of scabies, is usually intensely severe and most prominent at night or after a hot bath[43,44].

In the form called crusted or Norwegian scabies a thickened horny layer hosts an enormous number of mites. The presence of huge numbers of mites is possible either because of the host's very poor hygienic conditions or by altered immune response allowing the mites to multiply. In general crusted scabies is a disease of the mentally retarded, debilitated or immunosuppressed patients[43]. Men and women are equally affected; it is rare among children and the elderly and there is no racial predilection. It is essential for clinicians to be familiar with this form of scabies because of its

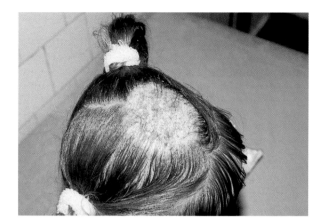

Figure 7   Kerion celsi

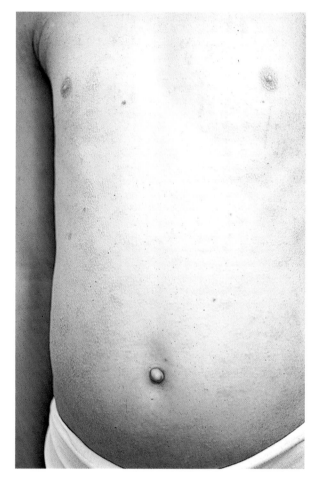

Figure 8   Scabies

highly contagious nature and unusual clinical signs, which may easily be overlooked[47,48].

Histopathology

The histological appearance of the inflammatory lesions has been regarded as non-specific, but even in the many cases which show no mites or ova in the tunnels of the horny layer that would confirm the

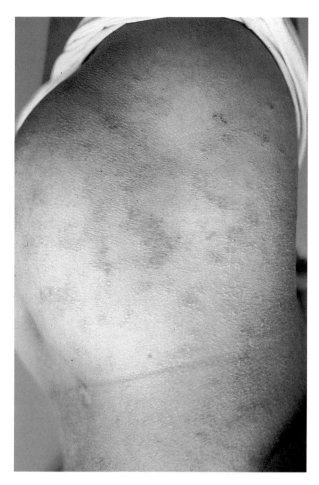

Figure 9   Scabies

diagnosis, the combination of spongiosis and vesicles in the Malpighian layer, with a dermal infiltrate, should certainly suggest scabies.

Laboratory studies

The presence of mites, eggs or fragments of eggshells under the optical microscope in material removed from burrows confirms the diagnosis. The mites are whitish and hemispherical; the male measures about 0.2×0.15 mm and the female 0.4×0.3 mm. The turtle-shaped fertilized female excavates a sloping burrow, through the stratum corneum and the granular and Malpighian layers, extending it by cytolysis by 2 mm each day, mainly during the night, and depositing two or three eggs to a total of 10–50 during her lifetime of 4–5 weeks, and then dying in the burrow[44,49]. The six-legged larvae emerge from the eggs after 3 or 4 days, wander to the skin surface and form shallow pockets in the horn of the original or a new host; they reach maturity about 14–17 days after the eggs were laid. Copulation occurs in the pocket and the female excavates her burrow, while the male soon dies[43,44].

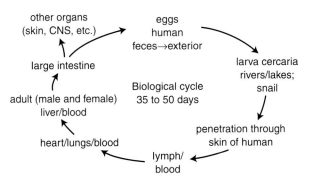

Figure 10   Life cycle of *Schistosoma mansoni*

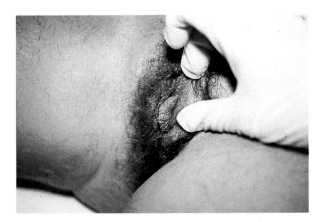

Figure 11   Schistosomiasis mansoni – left labium minora

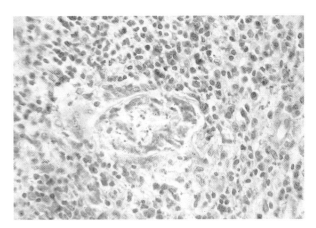

Figure 12   Histopathology of *Schistosoma mansoni* (vulval lesion in figure 11): egg of *S. mansoni* with its lateral spine (HE, 160x)

Differential diagnosis

There are various pruritic disorders that may resemble scabies, and in tropical areas it must be differentiated mainly from insect bites, pediculosis and papular urticaria.

Treatment

Several effective scabicides are available and most give very similar results: 2.5 to 10% sulfur ointment is still employed, as well as gamma benzene hexachloride (lindane), malathion, benzyl benzoate, permethin, and monosulfiram[43,44]. Oral ivermectin, an apparently safe drug, is now available and particularly useful for crusted scabies[50].

Although there are many warnings about the use of scabicides during pregnancy and breast feeding, which is understandable in view of concerns about potential toxic effects on the fetus, Burns states that there is no documented evidence that any of the available scabicides has been responsible for harmful effects in these situations. There are no data on levels of scabicides in human milk following their use on lactating women, but despite all this even nowadays many dermatologists prefer to use topical sulfur when managing scabies during both pregnancy and lactation[44].

Conclusions

This infestation shows practically no difference between its incidence in women and men, but eczematous changes following scratching are particularly characteristic on the breasts of young women. In relation to scabies in women, its treatment during pregnancy and breast feeding has been controversial up to the present.

SCHISTOSOMIASIS

Introduction

Schistosomiasis or bilharziasis is one of the most important helminthic infections because of its wide geographical distribution and extensive pathological effects[51,52]. It is a systemic disease and its causative agents are human trematodes or flukes. These trematodes affect approximately 200 million people worldwide, mainly in the tropical and subtropical latitudes, and sometimes entire communities are affected. Most infected persons experience few, if any, signs and symptoms and only a small minority develop significant disease[53].

There are three important species of the genus *Schistosoma*, known as blood flukes, that infect humans. They are: *S. haematobium*, *S. japonicum* and *S. mansoni*. *S. haematobium* is prevalent in Egypt, other parts of Africa and the Middle East, and is responsible mostly for urinary tract infections. *S. japonicum* is found in the Far East and has a predilection for the small intestine. *S. mansoni*, on the other hand, is confined to the Caribbean islands and the northeastern region of South America extending to the southeast of Brazil, and infects mostly the portal circulation and the mesenteric venules of the large intestine[52]. These three species share the same basic life cycle (Figure 10), but are unique in some aspects, such as location of adult worms, number of eggs produced, response to the ova by the host, fate of retained eggs and morphology of parasites, among other features[53].

Schistosomiasis has important implications for females. In endemic areas schistosomiasis frequently leads to complications in pregnancy including ectopic pregnancy, premature birth and abortion, as well as placental involvement causing damage to the fetus and newborn. Another consequence of schistosomiasis, particularly that caused by *S. haematobium*, is genital tract involvement, a generalized pelvic disease involving bladder, ureters, rectum and external and internal reproductive organs[54].

Different results have been found in prevalence studies of schistosomiasis. The basic requirement for infestation is contact with the contaminated waters of lakes or rivers, so regional differences depend on the habits of the local population. In most communities men show a higher prevalence rate because of their activities such as farming and fishing, but there are other regions where women have higher rates of infection owing to their washing utensils and clothes. Religious practices may also have an effect as, for example, with male Muslims, who have ablution and ritual washing several times a day[1].

Clinical description

The organs mainly affected in schistosomiasis are the urinary tract by *S. haematobium*; the small intestine by *S. japonicum*; and the large intestine and liver by *S. mansoni*[52]. Cutaneous schistosomiasis is rare and may occur in all three stages of the disease: initial penetration of the skin by the water-borne, free-living cercaria; during the immune-complex-mediated phase; or in the later stages of infection[55].

The initial cutaneous manifestation that may appear in schistosomiasis is called schistosomal dermatitis. It is characterized by pruritus, sometimes associated with a papular eruption which begins straight after contact with water and penetration of the larva (cercaria) through the skin. It usually disappears in a few hours. The immune-complex-mediated phase begins after four to eight weeks. There may be an urticarial reaction, which is particularly severe in infestation by *S. japonicum*. Sometimes there is association with malaise, fever, diarrhea, liver and spleen enlargement. Eosinophilia is a frequent feature in this phase. Late cutaneous schistosomiasis is rare and when it occurs it is usually associated with the involvement of other organs and the presence of the parasite in the stool or urine. Perigenital, paragenital or schistosomatic granuloma, especially in women, is its more common form of presentation. Ectopic cutaneous schistosomiasis may also occur[55,56].

The late manifestations are due to the deposition of adult worms and/or of eggs of *Schistosoma* in the perigenital, genital and extragenital skin of patients. The presence of eggs may also occur without any clinical manifestations, or in unrelated lesions of the skin. There can be papules, nodules, polyps, vegetations, large tumors, ulcerations, sinuses, lymphedema, elephantiasis and leukoplakia[57]. Schistosomal granuloma may be considered a potentially precancerous lesion and in one study two in twenty cases showed malignant transformation[58].

Vulval lesions are seen in greater frequency with *S. haematobium* and are an infrequent manifestation of schistosomiasis mansoni (Figure 11). The existence of venous anastomoses that communicate the mesenteric system with the pudendum plexus and the venous system of the perineum favors the production of genital lesions under normal conditions[59].

Late cutaneous schistosomiasis is diagnosed by histopathology, and its most characteristic feature is the finding of degenerated eggs inside epithelioid cell granulomas (Figure 12).

Laboratory study

Schistosomiasis is diagnosed most frequently by the presence of characteristic ova in the stool or urine, depending on the agent. The difference between the eggs of three species of *Schistosoma* is the presence and localization of a characteristic spine. *Schistosoma haematobium* shows an apical spine; *S. mansoni*, a lateral spine (Figure 12); while *S. japonicum* has no spine. The adult worm of the three human species of *Schistosoma* does not replicate within the human host. It can live as long as 33 years, although in endemic areas 2 to 5 years is normal[60].

Differential diagnosis

Cutaneous schistosomiasis, depending on its stage, may mimic an enormous number of skin diseases. From pruritus without lesion, papular and urticarial eruptions, nodules, granulomatous lesions and large tumors, skin lesions of schistosomiasis can, in general, only be diagnosed by biopsy and histopathology.

Treatment

Infections due to all three agents of schistosomiasis may be completely cured with the drug praziquantel in a single oral total dose of 40 mg/kg or divided into two of 20 mg/kg. Metrifonate in a total dose of 22.5–30 mg/kg is used for *S. haematobium*; a single dose of 7.5–10 mg/kg is given every other week three times. Oxamniquine is prescribed for *S. mansoni* in a total of 15–60 mg/kg; it may be given all at once or twice a day for two days. Good results are achieved in early infestations, however scar formation does not allow the improvement of late complications such as portal hypertension, liver fibrosis and urethral and/or ureteral stenosis[53,55,56].

Conclusion

Schistosomiasis is a tropical parasitic disease with great importance in relation to women because of its implications for pregnancy, the possible alterations of the fetus and newborn of infected mothers, and the alteration of the external and internal reproductive organs that can be caused even by the species of *Schistosoma* that affect the intestines.

CONCLUDING REMARKS

There is much evidence that skin disease occurring in women is diagnosed later than in men and there are also many skin conditions that have so far received little investigation into their pathogenesis in women[61]. Women's health as an end in itself has rarely been at the forefront of international development programs or national health planning and its attention in developing countries has been motivated largely by other concerns. Women have tended to be seen as the vehicle through which specific goals – such as family planning and child survival – could be achieved rather than as the primary beneficiaries of development programs[8].

If sustainable development is the latest challenge to the international community, then women, more than ever before, should be at the front and center of all action strategies[62]; and women's health will only be improved if the skin is included in health policy[61]. This is not a matter of social justice, nor a feminist issue; it is simple common sense[62].

REFERENCES

1. Kaur V. General considerations: tropical disease and women. *Clin Dermatol* 1997;15:171–8
2. Ryan TJ. Women in dermatology: gender and tropical diseases. *Int J Dermatol* 1995;34:226–35
3. Goldsmith R, Hegneman D. In Appleton & Lange, eds. *Tropical Medicine and Parasitology*. Prentice Hall, 1989
4. Santiso R. Effects of chronic parasitosis on women's health. *Int J Gynaecol Obstet* 1997;58:129–36
5. Chester PB, Clifton RJ, Waine EC. *Clinical Parasitology*, 9th edn. Philadelphia: Lea and Febiger, 1984
6. Canizares O, Harman R. Introduction to tropical dermatology: factors and concepts. In Canizares O, Harman RRM, eds. *Clinical Tropical Dermatology*, 2nd edn. Cambridge, MA: Blackwell Scientific Publications, 1992:1–9
7. Okojie CEE. Gender inequalities of health in the third world. *Soc Sci Med* 1994;39:1237–47
8. Vlassoff C, Bonilla E. Gender-related differences in the impact of tropical diseases on women: what do we know? *J Biosoc Sci* 1994;26:37–53
9. Rathberger E, Vlassoff C. Gender and tropical disease: a new research focus. *Soc Sci Med* 1993;37:513
10. United Nations. The World's Women 1970–1990. Trends and statistics (Social Statistics and Indicators. Series K no. 8). New York: United Nations, 1991:15–17
11. Brenner S. Introduction. *Clin Dermatol* 1997;15:1–3
12. Cook AH. International comparisons: problems and research in the industrialized world. In Koziara KS, Moskow MH, Tanner LD, eds. *Working Women: Past, Present, Future*. Washington DC: Bureau of National Affairs, 1987:342–3
13. Reuben R, Panicker KN. A study of human behaviour influencing man–mosquito contact, and of biting activity on children in a South Indian village community. *Ind J Med Res* 1979;70:723–32
14. Winch PJ, Lloyd LS, Hoemeke L, Leontsini E. Vector control at the household level: an analysis of its impact on women. *Acta Tropica* 1994;56:327–39
15. Silva KT. Malaria control through community action at grass roots: experience of the Sarvodya Malaria Control Research Project in Sri Lanka from 1980 to 1986. Geneva, WHO. *SER Project Report* no. 4, 1988:9–10
16. Khan ME, Tamang AK, Patel BC. Work pattern of women and its impact on health and nutrition – some observations form the urban poor. *J Fam Welfare* 1990;36:3–5
17. Bonilla E. La participación de la mujer en el proceso de desarrollo en Ecuador. Informe de Progreso Económico y Social del Ecuador. Washington: IDB, 1992:15–16
18. Le Grand A. Women and leprosy. A review. *Lepr Rev* 1997;68:203–11
19. Scollard DM, Smith T, Bhoopat L, *et al*. Epidemiologic characteristics of leprosy reaction. *Int J Lepr* 1994;62:559–67
20. Cestari TF. Hanseníase e gestação. In Talhari S, Neves RG, eds. Hanseníase, 3 ed. Manaus, Brazil: Grafica e Editora Tropical, 1997:83–6
21. Duncan ME. An historical and clinical review of the interaction of leprosy and pregnancy: a cycle to be broken. *Soc Sci Med* 1993;37:457–72
22. Lopes VG, Sarno EN. Hanseníase e gravidez. *Rev Assoc Med Bras* 1994;40:195–201
23. Duncan ME, Pearson JMH. The association of pregnancy and leprosy – III. Erythema nodosum leprosum in pregnancy and lactation. *Lepr Rev* 1984;55:129–42
24. Brakel WH, Khawas IB, Lucas SB. Reactions in leprosy: an epidemiological study of 386 patients in West Nepal. *Lepr Rev* 1994;65:190–203

25. Fernandes NC, Maceira J, Muniz MM. Erythema nodosum: prospective study of 32 cases. *Rev Inst Med Trop São Paulo* 1994;36:507–12

26. Wolff K, Tappeiner G. Mycobacterial diseases: tuberculosis and atypical, mycobacterial infections. In Fitzpatrick TB, Eisen A, Wolff K, Freedberg IM, Austen KF, eds. *Dermatology in General Medicine*, 3rd edn. New York: McGraw-Hill, 1987:2152–80

27. Kwang-Hyun Cho, Dong-Youn Lee, Chul-Woo Kim. Erythema induratum of Bazin. *Int J Dermatol* 1996;35:802–8

28. Schneider JW, Jordaan HF, Geiger DH, *et al.* Erythema induratum of Bazin: a clinico-pathological study of 20 cases and detection of *Mycobacterium tuberculosis* DNA in skin lesions by polymerase chain reaction. *Am J Dermatopathol* 1995;17:350–6

29. Kritski AL, Conde MB, de Souza GRM. *Tuberculose: do Ambulatório à Enfermaria*. São Paulo: Editora Atheneu, 1999:1–174

30. Mok WY. Tinea nigra. In Gatti F, De Vroey C, Persi A, eds. *Quaderni Di Cooperazione Sanitaria*. Bologna: OCSI, 1988:59–61

31. Kwon-Chung KJ, Bennett JE. *Medical Mycology*. Philadelphia: Lea & Febiger, 1992:191–7

32. Mattede MGS. Tinha negra palmar. Relato de quatro casos no Estado do Espírito Santo. *An Bras Dermatol* 1988;63:379–80

33. Severo LC, Gutierrez MJ. Tinha do couro cabeludo por *Microsporum canis* em adulto. *An Bras Dermatol* 1985;60:87–8

34. Kamalam A, Thambiah AS. Tinea capitis an endemic disease in Madras. *Mycopathologia* 1980;71:45–51

35. Aste N, Pau M, Biggio P. Tinea capitis in adults. *Mycoses* 1996;39:299–301

36. Shrum JP, Millikan LE, Batainch O. Superficial fungal infection in the tropics. *Dermatol Clin* 1994;12:687–93

37. Terragni L, Lasagni A, Oriani A. Tinea capitis in adults. *Mycoses* 1989;32:482–6

38. Ramos-e-Silva M, Trope BM, Caiuby MJ, *et al.* Tinea capitis in adult after local corticotherapy. *F Med* 1995;110:73–6

39. Venugopal PV, Venugopal TV. Tinea capitis in Saudi Arabia. *Int J Dermatol* 1993;32:39–40

40. Kwon-Chung KJ, Bennett JE. *Medical Mycology*. Philadelphia: Lea & Febiger, 1992:105–61

41. Gupta AK, Sauder DN, Shear NH. Antifungal agents: an overview. Part II. *J Am Acad Dermatol* 1994;30:911–33

42. Ramos-e-Silva M. Giovan Cosimo Bonomo (1663–1696): discoverer of the etiology of scabies. *Int J Dermatol* 1998;37:625–30

43. Plorde JJ. Scabies, chiggers, and other ectoparasites. In Wilson JD, Braunwald E, Isselbacher KJ, *et al.*, eds. *Harrison's Principles of Internal Medicine*, 12th edn. New York: McGraw-Hill, 1991:831–4

44. Burns DA. Diseases caused by arthropods and other noxious animals. In Champion RH, Burton JL, Burns DA, Breathnach SM, eds. *Rook/Wilkinson/Ebling Textbook of Dermatology*, 6th edn. Oxford: Blackwell Science, 1998:1423–81

45. Johnson CG, Mellanby K. The parasitology of human scabies. *Parasitology* 1942;34:285–90

46. Bartley WC, Mellanby K. The parasitology of human scabies (women and children). *Parasitology* 1944;35:207–8

47. Wanke NCF, Melo C, Balassiano V. Crusted scabies in a child with systemic lupus erythematosus. *Rev Soc Med Trop* 1992;25:73–5

48. Wanke NCF, Stringhini SB. Sarna crostosa: relato de quatro casos. *An bras Dermatol* 1993;68:93–4

49. Shatin H, Canizares O. Dermatoses caused by arthropods. In Canizares O, Harman RRM, eds. *Clinical Tropical Dermatology*, 2nd edn. Boston: Blackwell Scientific Publications, 1992:372–403

50. Meinking TL, Taplin D, Hermida JL, *et al.* The treatment of scabies with ivermectin. *N Engl J Med* 1995;333:26–30

51. McKee PH, Wright E, Hutt SR. Vulval schistosomiasis. *Clin Exp Dermatol* 1983;8:189–94

52. Gonzalez E. Schistosomiasis, cercarial dermatitis and marine dermatitis. *Dermatol Clin* 1989;7:291–300

53. Nash TE. Schistosomiasis. In Wilson JD, Braunwald E, Isselbacher KJ, *et al.*, eds. *Harrison's Principles of Internal Medicine*, 12th edn. New York: McGraw-Hill, 1991:813–17

54. Feldmeier H, Krantz I. A synoptic inventory of needs for research on women and tropical parasitic diseases with an application for schistosomiasis. In Wijeyaratne P, Rathgeber EM, St-Onge E, eds. *Women and Tropical Diseases*. *Manuscript Report 314e*. Ottawa: International Development Research Center, 1992:100–33

55. Bryceson ADM, Hay RJ. Parasitic worms and protozoa. In Champion RH, Burton JL, Burns DA, Breathnach SM, eds. *Rook/Wilkinson/Ebling Textbook of Dermatology*, 6th edn. Oxford: Blackwell Science, 1998:1377–422

56. Rey L. *Parasitologia*, 2 edn. Rio de Janeiro: Guanabara Koogan, 1991:351–410

57. Ramos SF. *A bilharziase cutanea*. Thesis, Lourenço Marques: [s.n.], 1971:1–248

58. El-Zawahry M. Schistosomal granuloma of the skin. *Br J Dermatol* 1965;77:344–9

59. Patrus OA. *Esquistossomose Mansoni Cutanea Ectopica*. Thesis, Belo Horizonte: Universidade Federal de Minas Gerais, 1974:1–22

60. Cook GC, Bryceson ADM. Longstanding infection with *Schistosoma mansoni*. *Lancet* 1988;i:127

61. Ryan TJ. Healthy skin for all. *Int J Dermatol* 1994;33:829–35

62. Huston P. Invisible agents for change. *World Health* 1990;April–May:29

Sexually transmitted diseases 26

Derek Freedman

The ultimate purpose of sex is the transmission of genetic information from man to woman to create a new individual and perpetuate the species. It is augmented and catalyzed by pleasure and circumscribed by social practices and mores. However, sex is also a very efficient means of transmitting infections, the consequences of which can be devastating – immune dysfunction, cancer, infertility, ectopic pregnancy, pregnancy loss, vertical transmission to the newborn and social stigmatization[1]. Women carry an unfair burden of these consequences.

This chapter is organized into two sections. The first deals with the clinical screening and examination of girls in order to diagnose, and often more importantly, to exclude a diagnosable sexually transmitted infection. Superficially, this may appear very similar to a normal gynecological examination and there is some duplication, but it is very different. The aim is to recognize the very subtle and uncertain changes wrought by infection with the background of an overwhelming appreciation that most conditions cannot be diagnosed, never mind excluded, by clinical examination alone. The patient's anxiety may be covert and she too shy to admit the possibility of infection. A certain directness is required from the physician. The second section deals with any peculiarities of presentation of sexually transmitted diseases in women and their impact upon reproduction and emotional health. Of necessity, it will be brief and only highlight these aspects which are pertinent to women; otherwise a chapter becomes a textbook.

The woman is disadvantaged in being the receptive partner with a more efficient acquisition rate for most infections. In addition, the woman has more orifices, a greater exposed surface area, both internally and externally, giving more opportunity for discontinuity to the surface epithelium. The female genitalia are not easily observed and the natural secretions and moisture tend to mask any changes arising from infections. Consequently, asymptomatic infection is the rule, rather than the exception. The first a girl may know of her infection is when her symptomatic partner informs her. This places a special responsibility on the couple to know each other's names. There is also a responsibility on an attending physician to be cognizant of this, to carry out a full examination, with a full set of screening tests to exclude infection wherever there is risk or anxiety, or when it is just good practice to screen. Sadly, this does not always occur. Wade and Buckingham found that only 15% of gynecologists and obstetricians took *Chlamydia* tests when the circumstances warranted[2]. There is hesitation and reluctance in relation to intimate examinations: too often it is more on the part of the physician than the patient. After all, it is for a professional service of the highest standard that the patient has paid the physician the compliment of attendance. The physician should repay this compliment by providing a complete and thorough professional service.

THE CLINICAL ENCOUNTER

For the woman, this is always an intrusive and invasive procedure. During the history taking it is essential to enquire about sexual relationships, both their number and nature. There is a natural inhibition to full disclosure, especially in the presence of guilt and remorse, or more particularly if the patient is made to feel disapproval from her physician. The physician must be open in nature and convey empathy to the patient.

History taking

An objective sexual history sets the scene for investigation and diagnosis, as well as realistic risk appraisal, and provides the patient with an opportunity to unburden herself. As well as the traditional presenting symptoms, medical and drug background, one needs to obtain a full, frank and explicit account of sexual encounters. It is essential to be impartial, remain unemotive and stress the complete confidentiality of the consultation to achieve this. Disclosure may initially be reluctant, so it is often necessary to stimulate the memory with direct questions on particular sexual practices, especially if they are ones that the patient feels may incur the disapproval of the physician. The tone of the consultation should be kept light, if certain encounters or practices are denied, it is often better to query 'why not', rather than passively accept a negative answer. Some demographic markers of risk of sexually transmitted diseases are shown below[3].

(1) Age 15–30 years
(2) Alcoholism
(3) Relationship disruption
(4) Drug abuse
(5) Tourism
(6) History of sexually transmitted diseases
(7) Newly living away from home
(8) History of termination of pregnancy
(9) Mobile occupation
(10) Unstable behavior and/or mental illness

If the doctor appears confident and at ease discussing sexual matters, the patient will rapidly become so and will feel able to respond.

In dermatological practice, sexually transmitted infections may form part of a hidden agenda. The patient may present with a plethora of complaints and hold the expectation that the dermatologist will uncover the latent infection as part of the normal consultation, especially as in most countries dermatologists are also trained in venereology. For this reason, it would be a wise practitioner who includes one or two questions on sexual activity, genital symptoms, contraceptive practice and recent Pap smears as part of the normal consultation. Even the simple question 'have you ever been worried about an infection' is quick and effective to yield dividends in terms of unspoken anxiety (Table 1).

The skill and confidence of doctors, the time allowed and the perception of confidentiality have been clearly demarcated in general practice as factors required for obtaining a sexual history[4]. They must equally pertain in dermatology practice.

EXAMINATION

Success in history taking leads on to the clinical examination, which can be physically as well as psychologically invasive. Empathy and tact are essential, but a fully comprehensive and professional examination is the mainstay of diagnosis. Signs may be subtle; the entire genital area should be systematically and closely inspected with reflection of all the skin folds, assessment of the perianal area, as well as passing a speculum to examine the vagina and cervix.

The patient should be examined in a warm and comfortable room, with a screen available for disrobing. In a perfect world the patient should not be left waiting on the couch, and intercoms and telephones would not ring. The examination couch

Table 1 Routine questions for screening for sexually transmitted diseases

When did you last have sex?	
Who with?	
Male/female?	Spouse/steady partner
Good friend/acquaintance	Casual/do not know?
What did you do?	
Did you enjoy it?	
Who did you have sex with before that?	
(Repeat to cover a period of 3–24 months)	
Were condoms used?	
Consistently? Throughout?	
For all forms of sexual activity	
ie: oro-genital	
Do you have any complaints?	
Soreness, discharge, lumps, dyspareunia?	
Does your partner(s) have any complaints?	
Did you see them again?	
Have you ever had an infection before?	
Have you ever been tested for infection before?	
Have you taken any medication recently?	
When was your last menstrual period?	
Have you ever had a termination of pregnancy?	

should be non-threatening with good illumination – a fiberoptic light system allows optimal illumination of the vagina and cervix. As most sexually transmitted diseases are completely asymptomatic in the woman, a full screening examination is mandatory for virtually all first consultations, and for repeat visits when further risk of exposure has taken place.

The presence of a nurse can speed the examination by assisting in specimen taking and also provide an important safeguard against any allegations of improper behavior that can so easily arise from such an intimate examination. This is not always possible in private practice, and indeed some patients seek a private consultation to ensure complete confidentiality and privacy, and may be inhibited by the presence of a nurse. In such cases it would be prudent to ensure the presence of a person who can provide chaperone protection in close proximity to the examination room, and that they have patient contact both immediately before and after the consultation, so the patient is aware of their presence.

Technically, the examination is performed most easily in a gynecological chair in the lithotomy position; however, some women feel very vulnerable and uncomfortable in this position. Examination on a couch can be equally thorough, but at the expense of stressing the physician's back!

Lymphadenopathy is sought by palpating the inguinal area. Pelvic and bladder tenderness is elicited and assessed. The pubic and adjacent areas are closely inspected for pediculosis pubis, scabies, verrucae, molluscum contagiosum, sores and blisters. The condition of the skin should be observed with particular regard for melanomas, nevae, and hair changes. In addition, those patients with a fair skin/red hair diathesis are more prone to intertrigo and expression of human papilloma virus (HPV).

The vulva and introitus are scrutinized. Obvious discharge is assessed for color, consistency and odor. The labia are systematically and thoroughly examined for any warts, ulcers, fissures, color change, thickening, scratch marks or papules. The urethral orifice is checked, as are the openings of the Bartholin's glands and Skene's glands. These glands may be palpated and any secretion collected for Gram staining and culture. The perineum and perianal area are also closely inspected.

The vagina and cervix are examined by passing a bivalve speculum. Plastic disposable ones are available which add to the patient's feeling of security. Metal reusable ones should be thoroughly cleansed and sterilized, and preferably warmed with warm water before insertion. Lubricant jelly should be avoided as it frequently contains bacteriostatic preservatives that may compromise the cultures. The speculum should be inserted obliquely to take advantage of the natural elliptical shape of the vagina. The speculum is only opened as wide as necessary to see the cervix, the patient may be warned to expect some discomfort. It is often useful, if one is using a couch instead of a chair, to ask the patient to tilt her pelvis to gain an optimal angle for insertion. A forced cough may push the cervix into view. If one fails to visualize the cervix, removal of the speculum and seeking the cervix with a finger per vaginum (PV) allows its position to be sought and sometimes mobilized to permit easier identification on reintroducing the speculum[5].

Examination and sampling proceeds systematically
The cervix

Size, shape and condition of the cervix should be noted, including the presence of tears, nodules, follicles, warts polyps or an intrauterine device (IUD). The condition of the cervical os should be closely scrutinized; presence of inflammation or mucopurulent discharge from the os, endocervicitis, is an indicator of potential infection. The position of the squamocolumnar junction and the extent of the transition zone is noted. A mucopurulent secretion from this area, an exocervicitis, is quite common and rarely indicative of infection.

Samples for Gram stain and culture of *Neisseria gonorrhoeae*

An endocervical sample is best obtained with a plastic loop, which is smeared thinly on a microscopic slide for Gram staining. If there is sufficient material, the same loop may be used to inoculate a plate of selective culture medium. A second sample should be taken if the initial one is scanty. Contamination with vaginal secretions should be avoided. If one wishes to cleanse the cervix prior to taking the sample, a cervical smear for cervical cytology should be taken first.

Cervical cytology

As well as providing opportunistic screening for cervical intraepithelial neoplasia (CIN), cervical cytology may provide additional information in relation to sexually transmitted diseases. In particular, cytological changes related to herpes simplex virus and human papilloma virus infection may be reported. The target area for cervical cytology is the squamocolumnar junction. An Aylesbury spatula is most commonly used where the squamocolumnar junction is at, or close to, the cervical os. The wider Ayre's spatula provides better coverage of a wide ectopion, but is an ineffective device for collecting endocervical cells and may give a lower yield of dyskaryosis[6]. When the squamocolumnar junction is not visible and the os is tight, a cytobrush may give optimal performance.

The end of the spatula is inserted into the os and rotated through 360° to obtain an adequate sample. This is spread onto a microscopic slide and fixed immediately with 95% alcohol. Care should be taken to mark the slide adequately for identification.

Testing for *Chlamydia trachomatis*

C. trachomatis infects the endocervical cells and is an intracellular parasite. Consequently for optimal sensitivity one must ensure adequate sampling of the endocervix. The sampling swab should be inserted and rotated in the cervical os for at least 10 seconds to ensure a good harvesting of endocervical cells. If there is a large transition zone (cervical ectopy) this should also be swabbed.

Chlamydia testing can be carried out by several techniques: culture is most specific but lacks sensitivity. Polymerase (or ligase) chain reaction (PCR/LCR) is exquisitely sensitive, but subject to contamination. Antigen detection by enzyme-linked immunosorbent assay (ELISA) is quite sensitive, but also subject to false positivity. Direct antigen detection by fluorescent antibody is very sensitive and specific, but very demanding in operator terms. Care must be taken not to use swabs that are toxic to *Chlamydia*. In particular culture systems are susceptible to inhibition by wooden swabs. For optimal results, the swab should be squeezed out in the transport medium.

More recently, urine-based PCR/LCR tests have shown sufficient sensitivity and specificity to be useful[7]. While these are valuable in population screening, their existence should not be used as an excuse to defer a full and proper pelvic examination as part of the clinical examination.

The vagina and vaginal walls

Presence of a discharge with color, consistency and odor should be noted, as well as dryness and atrophy. The vaginal walls are assessed for inflammation, ulceration and normal rugae pattern. Skin tags are noted, and specifically distinguished from warts. The application of 5% acetic acid after sample taking may assist in this.

The vaginal secretions are most effectively examined using a 10 µl plastic loop. One wishes to obtain a sample with minimal contamination from cervical secretions. If there is an obvious discharge, with pooling in the posterior fornix, that is the usual sampling area. For *Candida*, a sample of the secretion from the vaginal wall may be more sensitive. The loop is initially smeared onto a microscopic slide for Gram staining and then the remainder of the material tested for pH with narrow range pH test paper (pH 4.10–7.00). The physiological pH of the vagina is 3.5–4.5, which is maintained with candidosis, but lost with bacterial (anaerobic) vaginosis. The loop can be refreshed if necessary or mixed with a drop of normal saline to prepare a 'wet mount' covered with a cover slip. Conveniently on the same slide, a drop of 10% potassium hydroxide (KOH) is placed and mixed with a sample of vaginal secretion from the loop. This permits testing for release of the characteristic amine odor of bacterial vaginosis and also provides a further sample for screening for *Candida*. Use of the same slide is economical and saves time in labelling. The 10% KOH clears the epithelial cells and any *Candida* present stands out. Classically, a high vaginal swab is taken for culture from the posterior fornix for greater sensitivity for the identification of *Candida* and *Trichomonas*. The relevance of identification of

Candida, a vaginal commensal, by culture is questionable and a good working diagnosis of vaginitis can be made by a combination of findings on examination, amine testing, pH and initial 'wet prep' microscopy.

The speculum is gently removed, taking care that the cervix is not 'pinched' by the blades, nor pubic hair pulled[4].

Bimanual pelvic examination

This is an essential part of the examination which gives information on the size and shape of the uterus. More particularly, areas of tenderness should be sought and a specific test for 'cervical excitation' carried out by moving the cervix in all directions. If this causes pain or more discomfort than one would expect, it raises the possibility of pelvic inflammatory disease (PID). The adnexae should similarly be carefully palpated for tenderness or masses. If abnormalities in the shape or position of the uterus are suspected, or any pelvic mass noted, a pelvic ultrasound is useful for further assessment.

Urethral examination and sampling

The urethral orifice should be assessed for inflammation, and possibly 'milked' to express any secretions. Secretions are sampled with a small plastic loop (1 µl), spread onto a slide for Gram staining and inoculated on a selective culture medium for culture. The same slide as used for the cervical specimen may be used for economy, taking care to identify each specimen correctly, and if possible consistently.

Taking an additional sample from the urethra for *Chlamydia* testing enhances the sensitivity of identification of *C. trachomatis*. It may be either tested separately, or combined in the same transport medium as the cervical specimen.

Ano-rectal examination and sampling

This is particularly indicated in women who have had receptive anal intercourse, or contact with gonorrhea, or those in whom the potential for gonorrhea infection is high. Sensitivity of isolation of *N. gonorrhoeae* is increased by 3–5%.

Whilst blind sampling with a swab is adequate, use of a proctoscope allows a more thorough examination for ulcers or warts, as well as the variety of conditions that can affect the anal or perianal area, such as fissures, hemorrhoids and perianal dermatitis. A swab or loop is used for direct inoculation of a selective culture medium for *N. gonorrhoeae*. Microscopic examination of a Gram stained smear is useful to assess inflammation by detection of polymorphs. However, their significance has not been determined, even though some will treat as a 'non-specific proctitis' analogous to non-specific urethritis.

Throat swabs

These are too often omitted, but are increasingly important with the adventurous sexual practices of today. *N. gonorrhoeae* is primarily sought; transmission of gonorrhea by the oral–genital route has become increasingly important with the popularization of oral sex as a 'safe sex practice'. Safe for HIV maybe, but efficient for *N. gonorrhoeae* and herpes simplex virus. Recent political events have also brought the practice into the public domain.

Swabs are taken from the fauces and inoculated directly onto a selective culture medium[8]. Microscopy is of little use in this location, due to the large numbers of commensals of similar appearance to *N. gonorrhoeae*.

ADDITIONAL TESTING
Herpes simplex virus (HSV)

At present, most centers only test for HSV when lesions indicative of HSV are present: blisters, shallow tender ulcers or cervical lesions. The virus is shed in greatest quantity at the initial phase of the evolution of the lesions. Sensitivity can be enhanced by abrading the lesion and squeezing it to allow a serous ooze for swabbing. Marked tenderness during this procedure is characteristic of HSV infection. The swab is inoculated into viral transport medium and transported to the laboratory at 5°C.

Other tests include a direct antigen detection with a fluorescent antibody, a Tzank stain, which is of much lower sensitivity, or electron microscopy. Cytopathic changes of HSV may also be evident on cervical cytology. Increasing cognisance of atypical or non-classical HSV lesions, such as fissures or merely areas of erythema, should prompt more frequent testing for HSV.

Human papilloma virus (HPV)

Warts in most cases are clinically obvious, but increasing awareness of subclinical subtle changes caused by HPV should prompt acetowhite testing by soaking the cervix, vagina and vulva with 5% acetic acid. This coagulates protein and makes the HPV infected area appear white with a mosaic pattern under bright illumination – mosaicism. A colposcope is a useful aid to examination, providing magnification and illumination.

Syphilis

Syphilis presents with a primary chancre; traditionally every genital sore or ulcer has to have this diagnosis excluded, even though HSV is much more common in the developed world. The sore is scarified by abrading with a dry sterile gauze to induce bleeding: a clot is allowed to form before collecting serum on to a glass slide. Squeezing the base of the lesion can enhance collection of serum, as can inverting the barrel of a syringe over the lesion and inducing negative pressure by suction, which can be most efficient. Three samples are usually taken, placed on a slide and covered with a cover slip. Examination is by dark ground or phase contrast microscopy where the spirochete is seen to be mobile in all three planes. As syphilis has become increasingly rare in some areas, operator skills in dark ground microscopy have declined with a consequent reduction of sensitivity. Therefore, it is mandatory to have back up serological tests, which are repeated over a period of 3 months.

Chancroid

Chancroid is rare in the developed world, but common worldwide. Specimens for examination are obtained from ulcers or by aspirations of enlarged lymph glands (bubo). Microscopy shows the *Haemophilus ducreyi* in typical 'fish shoal' configuration. The material should also be inoculated directly on to a suitable medium and rapidly transported to the laboratory for culture. Consultation with the microbiology services is essential, as this is a most fastidious organism, which may require the preparation of special culture medium and special care. Sensitivity of culture is still only moderate at approximately 60%. In the future PCR/LCR diagnostics will greatly enhance diagnostic sensitivity and specificity.

Lympho-granuloma venereum

Pus aspirated from a bubo may be cultured for *C. trachomatis* serotypes L1–3. A specific complement fixation test usually shows positivity some 7–10 days after infection.

Granuloma inguinale

The *Calymmatobacterium granulomatis* may be identified by staining a biopsy specimen or scraping from the lesion with either Leishman or Giemsa stains.

SEROLOGICAL TESTING

All blood samples must be regarded as potentially infectious and universal precautions are essential. Care must be taken to safeguard against needlestick injuries or spillage. All syringes should be safely disposed of with a disposal bin always conveniently located. Post-exposure prophylaxis (PEP) of HIV is established and sufficient medication to promptly initiate PEP should be to hand.

Patient counseling

This is particularly centered around HIV, but the points raised are common to all sexually transmitted infections. When there was no effective therapy of HIV and where the diagnosis was associated with considerable stigma, as well as the burden of ill health, many patients questioned the usefulness of knowing their status and specifically 'did not wish to know'. The advent of effective antiretroviral therapy with three agents – Highly Active Antiretroviral Therapy (HAART) – has brought about a complete change in this philosophy. There are clear advantages to knowing one's HIV status: not only for relief of anxiety if negative, but also to allow active management and prevention of transmission if positive. By now, most people are aware of the advantages, but some, even physicians, remain trapped in the concepts of the 1980s, where HIV testing was only embarked upon with considerable pretest counseling and consideration of the answer involved.

Currently one can point out the advantages of having a HIV test, in particular in terms of reduction of anxiety with the knowledge of status, reduction of risk of transmission, not only to sex partners, but also from women to future children, and the availability of effective treatment. Negative aspects such as 'do you want to know' and the attitude of insurance companies should be mentioned. Complete confidentiality needs to be stressed and maintained. For a woman, with the potential to transmit vertically, the case for testing is overwhelming. Counseling should be directed towards those who are reluctant to be screened.

It remains essential to inform the patient what tests are taken routinely and to give them the opportunity to refuse if they so wish[9]. The 3-month 'window period' for all the serological tests should be explained with the necessity to return for followup serological screening 3 months after the risk episode(s). Serological testing is carried out for syphilis, hepatitis B and HIV.

Type-specific testing for HSV-2 has been developed and is fast becoming available. It has a particular utility for women who may wish to guard against acquisition of HSV infection in pregnancy. Where her partner has HSV-2 infection, or even a suspicion of it, they can both be tested for HSV-2 antibodies (HSV-2 ab). If she is negative and susceptible to acquisition of the infection whilst pregnant from her HSV-2 ab positive partner, then appropriate steps can be taken to reduce the potential for transmission, which can include suppressive therapy in the partner.

SEXUALLY TRANSMITTED INFECTIONS IN WOMEN

Sexually transmitted infections are conveniently divided into three generations. The first generation, the classic venereal diseases, were well described at the beginning of the 20th century, produced clinically obvious effects, and their secrets were unraveled by the scientific achievements of the 19th century, microscopy and serology. The second generation infections cause more subtle clinical effects, and require a greater understanding of the biological mechanisms of disease and the molecular methodology of the 20th century for diagnosis. The third generation infections are systemic, subtle, potentially devastating and require the most sophisticated techniques for diagnosis. They are beyond the remit of this chapter.

Special considerations

The following can only hope to note some of the more important and particular features and aspects of sexually transmitted infections in girls and women, with emphasis upon their reproductive health and emotional impact.

First generation infections

Syphilis

Syphilis has the same clinical spectrum of primary, secondary and tertiary stages in women as in men, but for the aforementioned reasons is more likely to be either asymptomatic or for its manifestations to go unnoticed. This is increasingly likely in areas of very low prevalence or when a woman attends a family or known doctor, who may be oblivious to her life style. The 'great pretender' may easily mimic acute mononucleosis and be diagnosed as the 'kissing disease'. Indeed, transmission of syphilis need not involve penetrative sex and may result from deep kissing or a bite.

Population screening gives an excellent opportunity for discovery and treatment of covert infection.

The premarital serological testing introduced in the USA following Parran's publication of *The Shadow on the Land – Syphilis*[10], as well as testing of conscripts during World War II, almost achieved elimination of the disease by the early 1950s, once penicillin was available. Today, however, marriage is seldom a prerequisite for coitus and a substantial proportion of pregnancies occur 'out of wedlock', especially in adolescence. Serological testing for syphilis is an essential part of routine antenatal care and offers the most important screening opportunity for control and discovery of covert syphilis. Routinely carried out in the first trimester of pregnancy, it should be repeated in the third trimester and at delivery in populations where infection can occur during pregnancy, i.e. intravenous drug users and prostitutes[11,12]. While today, in the developed world, the incidence of syphilis in the female population is at a record low, the epidemic seen in Russia and Eastern Europe reminds us of the perils of dismantling a good control system. A recrudescence of congenital syphilis in the USA in the 1980s reinforced the need for continuing screening and vigilance[13]. In Norway, with a maternal prevalence rate of 0.02%, the cost–benefit ratio of antenatal screening for syphilis was demonstrated to be 3.8[14]. Isolated outbreaks occur unexpectedly, as in Bristol, England[15], and demonstrate the potential for rapid spread. Isolated cases of congenital syphilis still occur, usually in the absence of antenatal testing as in late presentation of pregnancy, or unfortunately in private health care[16]. In the poorly health resourced countries, syphilis continues to cause substantial morbidity in pregnancy and in the neonate, as well as facilitating HIV transmission.

Serological testing in women   Where non-treponemal tests are relied upon for screening, caution should be exercised in case of false negative results due to prozone phenomenon[17]. False positivity is reported to occur more frequently in pregnancy[18] and there is a tendency for non-treponemal titers from previously adequately treated infection to increase non-specifically.

Treatment   It is only in pregnancy that there are any special considerations for treatment of syphilis in women. Due to the catastrophic consequences of failing to treat syphilis in pregnancy, caution, suspicion and over-treatment are recommended. Penicillin is the treatment of choice. Tetracycline is contraindicated in pregnancy. Erythromycin is the most popular alternative where there is allergy to penicillin, but has an unacceptably high failure rate which makes close follow-up of the neonate essential.

The World Health Organization additionally recommends that all infants born to mothers with a reactive serology should receive a stat dose of benzathine penicillin G (50 000 ug/kg) irrespective of whether the mother was treated in pregnancy or not[19]. This has obvious applicability to poorer countries where serological follow-up of potentially infected neonates may be unreliable, and syndromic care indicated.

Counselling and support   The diagnosis of syphilis, especially when unsuspected, causes considerable stress and angst. This is particularly magnified in pregnant women with concern for the fetus. The infection may well be a 'carry over' from a previous life style, covert from family and spouse. The potential of transmission to partner/spouse arises and must be handled with great delicacy. Tact, discretion and common sense are required, as well as the medical obligation to ensure that all those potentially at risk of infection are screened and treated. This should go hand in hand with preservation of relationships, especially in families.

Gonorrhea

The cervix, the commonest site of infection with *N. gonorrhoeae* in the woman, is concealed, and even if observed, shows either no diagnostic signs or the non-specific changes of mucopurulent cervicitis. Furthermore, there are additional sites of infection, such as the pharynx and anal canal, which are equally silent. Culture is the mainstay of diagnosis as microscopy with Gram stain is less reliable due to the great variety of commensal organisms found at these sites masking the characteristic Gram-negative intracellular diplococci of gonorrhea (Figure 1). Samples should be taken from the areas of columnar epithelium that have the potential to harbor the organism – the cervix, urethra, and also the rectal mucosa and pharynx if there is history of exposure at these sites. A high vaginal swab is insensitive for the culture of *N. gonorrhoeae*, as the organism does not grow on the vaginal epithelium. The pharyngeal swab should be taken from the tonsillar crypts for best sensitivity.

The most important complication of gonorrhea in the woman is pelvic inflammatory disease (PID). Gonococcal PID is more acute with pyrexia and pelvic symptoms, and is more likely to result in hospital admission. Bartholinitis is a common condition, that occasionally can be caused by gonorrhea.

The advent of safe sex programs for the avoidance of HIV transmission, and changes in sexual practices, has led to increased oro-genital sexual activity. Although this may be relatively safe for avoidance of HIV transmission, it remains an excellent transmission route for gonorrhea, much to the surprise of those infected. The infection is totally silent in the pharynx and a girl may be utterly dependent on contact tracing for diagnosis and treatment of her pharyngeal infection.

Chancroid

Chancroid remains a rare disease in the Western world, probably compounded by under-recognition and poor laboratory facilities. However, it remains the commonest cause of genital ulceration in several parts of the world[20]. Asymptomatic multiple ulcers at the introitus are the commonest finding, and they may merge to form serpiginous ulcers. Regional lymphadenopathy occurs, most often unilateral and painful with skin erythema. Bubo formation results when the lymph nodes develop into abscesses.

Lymphogranuloma venereum (LGV)

LGV is not widespread globally, but may cause 2–10% of genital ulcers in certain areas of India and Africa[21]. The disease is uncommon in women, who are frequently asymptomatic carriers[22]. The genital ulcer starts as a small painless papule which rapidly erodes to become a shallow ulcer, generally insignificant and unnoticed in most patients. Subsequently, in 2 to 6 weeks, acute and very painful inflammation of the lymph nodes may occur, with suppuration and even rupture. This is less commonly seen in women where the condition ends up causing chronic fibrosis and scarring of the pelvic organs, blockage of the lymphatic system with lymphedema and hypertrophic enlargement of the external genitalia (esthiomene). Pelvic scarring and adhesions increase the risk of infertility, and even if conception takes place, pelvic fibrosis may hinder delivery.

Granuloma inguinale

Caused by the bacterium *Calymmatobacterium granulomatis*, this infection is rarely seen in the Western world and is mainly found in the tropical belt that includes South America, the Caribbean, Central Africa, South East India, Northern Australia and New Guinea. The primary lesion in women is usually on the fourchette[23]. The enlarging ulcers develop friable granulation tissue with a velvety appearance. There is frequently a smooth rolled edge. The inguinal lymph glands are not usually directly involved, but become involved where

subcutaneous spread involves the area resulting in inflammation around the lymph gland, followed by ulceration and/or abscess formation.

Second generation infections

These infections give a more complex challenge; they require understanding of microbiology at the molecular level and their clinical manifestations are closely bound to the host immune reaction. Most have a silent carrier status as their commonest manifestation, require more sophisticated tests for their detection and more complex treatment for their elimination, where that is possible.

Chlamydia trachomatis and cervicitis

This is the quintessential female infection – common, silent, persistent and capable of causing long-term havoc to the reproductive system as well as infecting the neonate. *C. trachomatis* may cause a mucopurulent cervicitis in the woman, probably the commonest genital infection in women[24], especially in adolescence and early adulthood[25]. Its frequency and recurrence even among teenagers in certain areas is alarming[26].

The main site of infection, the cervix, is not readily accessible for viewing either by the woman or her sexual partner. Changes, when they occur, are quite non-specific and easily confused with the normal cyclical changes seen at the cervix and its mucous secretions. Changes of the cervical transition zone compound the issue, especially cervical ectroprion. *C. trachomatis* grows in the columnar epithelium[27], hence vaginal tissue is not a site of infection. The larger area of columnar epithelium seen in early reproductive life provides a larger target area for growth and transmission, and may provide an additional reason for the higher prevalence seen in this group, beyond excessive partner change.

Cervicitis, is the female equivalent of male urethritis. Many attempts have been made to correlate the finding of mucopurulent cervicitis (characterized by the presence of an inflamed endocervix with a yellow-green endocervical secretion), erythema, easily induced cervical bleeding, and > 30 pus cells per high field on microscopy, with the presence of a pathogen, most notably *C. trachomatis*[28], but they have not translated into clinically useful information[24]. A recent large study of more than 3000 girls found that both history and findings on examination were quite unreliable in predicting the presence of *C. trachomatis* infection[26].

That comment is focused upon *C. trachomatis* as a cause of urethritis relates to the ready availability of

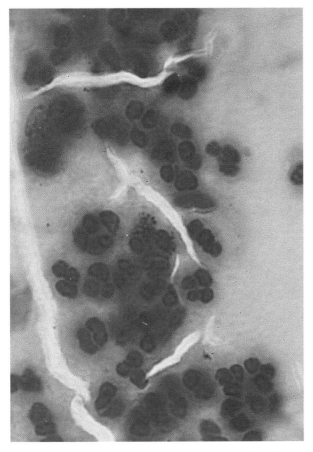

Figure 1 Cervical Gram stain showing the Gram-negative intracellular diplococci – these are visible only with close scrutiny

tests for identification of the organism and the interest that this pathogen has generated in the past two decades. Other organisms that cause urethritis in the male, such as *Mycoplasma hominis*[29], *M. genitalium*, *M. ureaplasma* and, of course, *N. gonorrhoeae*, are equally capable of producing mucopurulent cervicitis. Vaginal infections such as *Trichomonas*, candidosis and bacterial vaginosis (BV), may also produce a cervicitis, especially if long-standing[30].

Non-gonococcal urethritis in the male is treated with an appropriate antibiotic, whether a pathogen is isolated or not. This is not generally the case in women, although perhaps common sense may indicate that a syndromic approach is appropriate[31]. Schwebke *et al.*[32] noted reduced inflammation in women with *Chlamydia* and gonorrhea-negative cervicitis, who were treated with antibiotics, suggesting the involvement of other infectious agents. Increased resolution of cervicitis with a dual doxycycline and metronidazole treatment, compared with doxycycline alone, supported a role for BV-associated organisms in the causation of cervicitis.

The infections that cause cervicitis, especially *C. trachomatis*, may lead to significant complications, the most common and important being pelvic inflammatory disease and adverse pregnancy outcome[33].

Pelvic inflammatory disease

Despite the elegant recognition and description of the association of this condition with cervicitis two decades ago by Westrom and his colleagues[34,35], PID remains a diagnostic challenge due to the deep seated location of the pelvic organs and the non-specific nature of the symptoms (Table 1). It is the one area that most physicians agree on a syndromic approach[36–38] and prefer over-treatment rather than risk the consequence of infertility with a missed diagnosis. It is thought to account for over 20% of cases of infertility, and the majority of cases of avoidable infertility. That is in addition to other sequelae such as ectopic pregnancy[39], pelvic pain[40], deep dyspareunia and menstrual disorders.

Clinical presentation Textbook PID with pyrexia, bilateral abdominal pain, abnormal vaginal discharge and findings of pyosalpinx, tubo-ovarian abscess and pelvic peritonitis has become a rarity. Pyogenic bacteria, such as *N. gonorrhoeae*, as a causative organism are more likely to cause acute findings, but these agents are becoming rare today in the developed world leaving *C. trachomatis* as the major cause of PID, together with anaerobic organisms[41]. The clinical picture seen with *C. trachomatis* salpingitis is more low grade, indolent and silent and less likely to result in a hospital admission[35].

Diagnosis is classically based upon abdominal pain plus two major criteria, with increased sensitivity with presence of minor criteria (Table 2). However, it is important to note that most patients have either no symptoms or such mild symptoms that they do not present. The indication of the infection and problem only becomes apparent many years later with the resultant tubal damage[42]. This has led to more aggressive management policies with a shift to a syndromic approach[43].

Control of PID and its long-term consequences lies in control of the underlying etiological agents by primary prevention. Active screening and treatment of high-risk asymptomatic women has been shown to reduce the incidence of PID by 56% in the USA[44] and community screening programs for *C. trachomatis* have been shown to produce a reduction in the incidence of ectopic pregnancies paralleling the reduction of *C. trachomatis*[45].

Table 2   Criteria for diagnosis of pelvic inflammatory disease

Major criteria
   Lower abdominal tenderness
   Bilateral uterine and adnexal tenderness
   Cervical motion tenderness
   Signs of lower genital tract infection
Additional criteria
   Fever
   Elevated erythrocyte sedimentation rate
      or C-reactive protein
   Pus cells in high vaginal swab 'wet prep'
Syndromic criteria
   Lower abdominal tenderness
   Bilateral adnexal tenderness
   Cervical motion tenderness
   Deep dyspareunia
   Negative pregnancy test
   No competing diagnosis

Suggested areas of maximum impact to reduce this preventable cause of infertility include control and prophylaxis of PID producing sexually transmitted infections, concentration of efforts on the young (< 25 years), speedy and effective management of possible cases and treatment of couples, or more realistically all partners[46]. On an individual clinical basis, an example is the protocol developed for Accident and Emergency Department use, which ensures that questions and investigations pertinent to the diagnosis of PID are included in the standard protocol for assessment of women with abdominal pain. A dramatic improvement in clinical care can be achieved with this approach[47].

Increased public awareness of the potential of PID with non-specific symptoms, such as lower abdominal pain, and diagnoses such as 'grumbling appendix' or cystitis may lead to an increased quality of medical assessment. Cervical excitation is a difficult concept for a lay person, but deep dyspareunia is more readily understood, targets the population most at risk and is a symptom that arises close to the seat of infection.

Syndromic diagnosis may increase diagnostic sensitivity, even at the price of unnecessary antibiotic therapy[43]. The antibiotic may be used as a therapeutic trial, but the potential for other gynecological or surgical conditions remains. For a definitive diagnosis of PID, or for the differential diagnosis and treatment of the condition, the laparoscope remains the gold standard[48].

Adverse pregnancy outcome and neonatal infection

Ascending cervical infection in the intrauterine compartment in pregnancy may result in chorioamnionitis, premature rupture of membranes, amnionitis and premature delivery[48–50]. Recent attention has also focused on the role of anaerobic bacteria found in BV. Pregnant women with BV have a significantly increased incidence of intrauterine death, late miscarriage and premature birth[51–53]. Treatment of BV during pregnancy reduced the rate of premature birth by 50% in a cohort study of 1260 women[54].

Ophthalmia neonatorum is the classic neonatal infection caused by *N. gonorrhoeae* infecting the mother's cervix. A mild form, sticky eye syndrome, results from *C. trachomatis*, which incidently is also responsible for approximately 20 000 cases of neonatal pneumonia in the USA each year[55].

Human papilloma virus and warts in the woman

Vulval skin is the same as any other skin and warts grow on it; especially warts caused by HPV types 6 and 11. The vestibule and the posterior fourchette are the commonest sites affected, but warts may grow in any part of the ano-genital epithelium – the loin cloth areas. Perianal and anal canal warts may arise from indirect spread from genital lesions, especially if the woman is in the habit of wiping from front to back as advised to prevent coliform contamination and reduce the frequency of urinary tract infection. Peri-clitoral and peri-introital warts may be easily 'lost' in prominent mucosal folds: small warts covered by pubic hair are easily missed. The warts may be more clearly identified if the patient is examined in the left lateral as well as the lithotomy position. Patients may be more sensitive of the presence of warts by feel and should be invited to point out any lesions that were missed in a treatment session. Additionally asking the patient to circle the warts with a ball point pen can help ensure that a treatment session attacks all the warts present. Cervical and vaginal warts only occur in 6–10% of women with external genital warts[56,57].

Visible wart types are either exophytic acuminata types, usually found in moist areas and are papilliform or cauliflower in nature, or papular which most commonly occur in fully keratinized skin, and may have been present for longer (Figure 2).

Increased interest is being paid to subclinical infections[58,59]. Subclinical HPV associated lesions are identified by the application of 3–5% acetic acid solution to the area for 2–3 minutes followed by examination with magnification and intense light: optimally a colposcope. The aceto-white appearance derived is related to an overexpression of cytokeratin 10 in HPV infected lesions[60] as well as high protein concentration in the lesions which becomes whiter on denaturing by the acetic acid.

The diagnosis of subclinical papilloma virus infection (SPI) is based on more than acetowhitening, which can be quite non-specific. The lesions are clearly demarcated, with distinct, slightly elevated borders and have a 'thickness' with red papillary spots from hypervascularization. SPI may be associated with itching, burning and painful fissuring, and at one time was thought to be implicated in the pathogenesis of vulvodynia, but no longer[61–63].

Vestibular papillomatosis, with multiple papular or frond-like papillae on the inner surface of the labia minora is a common condition that may be confused with wart virus infection by the inexperienced (Figure 3). There are others with very pronounced hyperkeratotic vestibular filaments, who complain of itching, burning and superficial dyspareunia[64,65]. These women may have a history of previous genital warts or CIN, giving rise to a suspicion of previous HPV infection, but HPV-DNA has not been detected in excess[66–67].

Prevalence of HPV in women Carriage of HPV has been demonstrated in a considerable number of the young and sexually active. DNA hybridization techniques showed HPV sequences in 10–30% of exfoliated cervical cells more than a decade ago[68]. More sensitive DNA amplification techniques from vulval and cervical samples have shown carriage rates of up to 46% in sexually active young women[69]. Mathematical modelling of the US population estimates an overall population exposure to HPV of 75%, with 1% having visible genital warts, 5% having lesions detected by colposcopy, at least 15% showing subclinical presence of HPV as detected by HPV DNA assays, and 40–50% showing serological evidence of past human papilloma virus infection[70,71]. HPV carriage appears to be age-dependent with peak rates occurring in the sexually active aged 20–24 years, and declining thereafter[72]. More recently, studies have shown a median duration of infection of 8 months with only 9% of women remaining infected after 24 months[73]. This clearance is probably immune-mediated.

Whilst the clearance of HPV infection in the majority of cases is reassuring, and greatly lessens the psychological impact of the infection, it should not lead to complacency. Long-term persistence of HPV infection may occur in around 10% of cases; the cofactors and mediating factors are poorly understood. As it is not possible to predict who will be a long-term carrier, it is safer to counsel a patient on this possibility and the potential to transmit HPV. As this is such a common infection, this potential should not constitute a very much greater risk than one normally encounters in a new relationship, and should not cause inhibition in a sound relationship. Indeed, in the author's experience, the communication opened up by disclosure has frequently been found to enhance a relationship in the longer term.

Persistent HPV infection gives rise to a further concern – cancer. It is estimated that in excess of 500 000 new cases of cervical cancer are diagnosed per annum. These are very closely linked to the presence of high-risk types of HPV, namely HPV 16, 18, 31, 45, and HPV-associated cancer represents one of the commonest cancers affecting women[74]. The molecular mechanisms of this oncogenesis are now relatively well delineated[75] and give a fascinating insight into the complex mechanisms involved in the control of cell growth and their description in oncogenesis. Carcinoma of the cervix is a preventable cancer with screening. Up to now the screening programs have relied on relatively frequent examination of cervical cytology. Recognition of the high risk of progression with certain types of HPV[76] has led to the development of HPV type-specific detection tests in conjunction with cervical cytology. Absence of high-risk HPV has been postulated to allow a significant increase in screening intervals in a large population study with no detrimental effect[77].

Herpes simplex virus and genital herpes in women

Genital herpes is episodic; it goes through the same classical cycle of papule to blister, sore, ulcer and crusting, together with lymphadenopathy, in men and women, and recurs more frequently in genital epithelium when infection is with HSV-2 (Figure 4). Genital HSV, once thought to the provenance of HSV-2, is now increasingly due to HSV-1, especially in women, and with the popularization of oral–genital contact[78].

Classical characteristics in the woman

As the area of potential epithelium involved and supplied from an individual sensory nerve ending is larger in the woman than the man, it is no surprise that clinically the manifestations of an acute genital

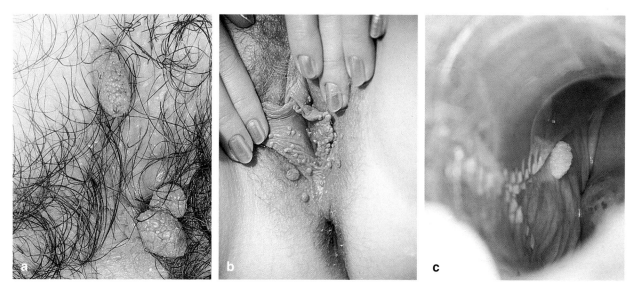

Figure 2   A medley of warts. (a) Exophytic vulval warts of recent origin; (b) hard schirrous warts of long standing; (c) vaginal wall wart

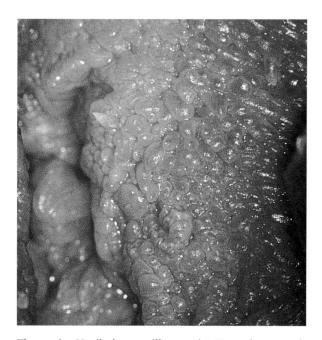

Figure 3   Vestibular papillomatosis. Note the smooth even forms of the papillae compared with warts, the absence of thickness and failure to whiten with the application of dilute acetic acid

HSV episode are more severe in the woman and may involve retention of urine due to external dysuria and feces due to tenesmus. Systemic manifestation may be present including pyrexia, headache and even meningism on occasions.

Epidemiology

The availability of type specific serology for HSV-2 has shown a 30% increase in prevalence of HSV-2 infections over the past two decades in the USA, with an excess found in women compared with men, and black populations compared with white[79]. Among teenagers, the increase has been five-fold and has doubled among those in their twenties[80]. As these data only concern HSV-2, and ignore the 20–40% of genital herpes related to HSV-1, the total burden of genital herpes is considerably understated.

These seroepidemiological studies indicate a much larger prevalence of HSV infection than was attributed to those with 'classical' episodes. Consequently, the new manta is that such clinically classical episodes are the exception rather than the rule, and that the clinical spectrum of HSV infection should be widened to include non-specific findings, such as genital skin splitting, fissures, furuncles and dysethesia, as well as pain, itch, or dermatitis. HSV may be identified by culture, antigen detection or PCR techniques[81].

Physicians as well as patients may blame non-specific causes, such as allergy, bites, physical irritation or the ubiquitous 'thrush'. The episodic nature of HSV together with a prodromal phase of dysethesia/neuritis may help clinical recognition. Lack of appreciation of the full clinical spectrum of HSV results in failure to diagnose the infection, loss of treatment opportunities and prolongs transmission potential. Consequently, any break on the skin or mucosal surface should be thoroughly evaluated for HSV.

A substantial proportion of those infected will be without any clinically recognizable manifestations and are silent carriers. They have the potential to shed the virus and be unwitting transmitters.

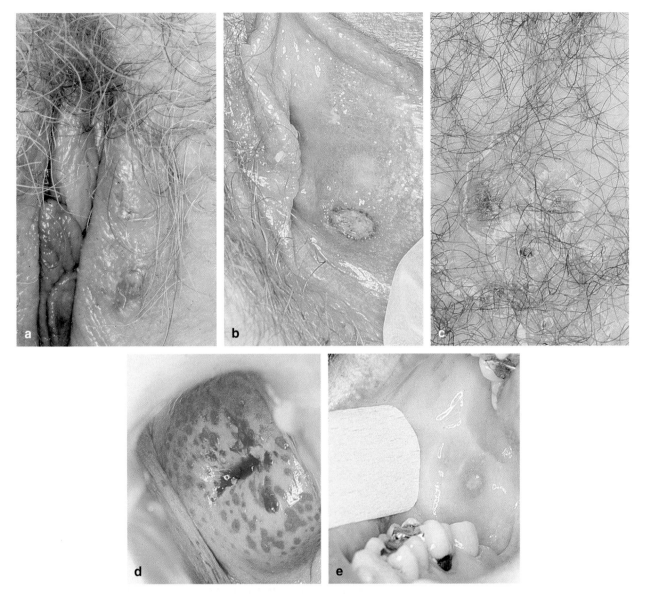

Figure 4 A crop of herpes. (a) Labial sore of herpes genitalis; (b) solitary vulval sore; (c) sore concealed in pubic hair; (d) cervical herpes; (e) oral herpes simplex virus

Viral shedding

Recent studies involving daily swabbing of the genitalia have revealed shedding of infectious virus in three-quarters of women infected with HSV-2 on 8% of the days sampled. More sensitive detection techniques showed that 95% of the women shed the virus on 28% of the days sampled[82]. This has changed the view of genital HSV infection from being an episodic latent infection to being a chronic persistent infection with classical episodes as an episodic manifestation in some cases.

Transmission of HSV

Whilst penetrative sex is frequent, transmission can occur from mere skin to skin contact. Oro-genital sex also plays a major role. On occasion, it may be acquired from auto-inoculation from a distant site. Access through fissures or micro-abrasions facilitates acquisition[83]. Transmission is more efficient from men to women, especially if the woman is seronegative for HSV-1 at exposure[84]. It is commonsense to appreciate that few people would have sexual congress in the presence of painful genital ulcers. Consequently, most transmission of HSV must take place by persons who either do not appreciate that they have the infection, or are unaware of the potential to silently shed the virus. Most subclinical shedding clusters around symptomatic episodes when present[82]; however, most people who transmit HSV are unaware of having the infection[85] and these silent carriers play a core role in spreading and perpetuating the infection. The potential widescale availability of type-specific antibody testing of HSV may help identify more of these people and induce behavior modification[86]; however, with such a widespread epidemiology, complacency could equally well be the outcome.

Genital herpes and pregnancy

Genital HSV infection in the first trimester of pregnancy is associated with spontaneous abortion, intrauterine growth restriction and prematurity. Infection near term is associated with neonatal infection. These are the most serious complications of genital HSV infection and what elevates the infection from being a trivial, if unpleasant, skin infection into an infection of consequence.

First time acquisition of genital HSV during pregnancy occurs in 2–3% of a general obstetric population surveyed in the USA[87]. Discordant couples, i.e. a HSV-2 seronegative pregnant woman who has a HSV-2 seropositive partner, result in a 13% chance of the pregnant woman acquiring HSV by onset of labor[88]. The great majority of these have no clinically recognizable symptoms or signs. Acquisition during pregnancy appears to carry a lower risk of transmission to the fetus, whereas late acquisition and incomplete seroconversion at the time of labor carries a risk as high as 40%[89].

The majority (60–75%) of HSV-2 antibody positive individuals are asymptomatic carriers in pregnancy, with reduced immune function. Symptomatic recurrences may become either apparent or more frequent. At term, 2% of HSV-2 seropositive women have a recognized symptomatic recurrence, with asymptomatic viral shedding found in 1–2% by viral culture, and in 20% using PCR[90]. For many women with a covert asymptomatic infection, as demonstrated by HSV-2 type-specific serology, their first clinical manifestation may be in pregnancy. This carries severe and traumatic psychological stress: firstly the anxiety of the infection affecting the fetus, and secondly the stress and doubt that an unexplained HSV infection can put upon a relationship. The increasing availability of HSV type-specific antibody testing will be able to answer some of the questions arising by demonstrating the prior presence of the infection.

The prevalence of neonatal HSV varies considerably from one per 2000 to one per 15 000 live births[91]. The USA appears to have a higher prevalence than Europe. It is estimated that more than 95% of the neonates acquire HSV during labor and that asymptomatic first episode infection causes 60–70% of the cases[92].

HSV type 1 transmits more often from mother to neonate than HSV-2[93], irrespective of the clinical nature of the herpes infection. Neonatal HSV-1 infection is usually limited to skin and mucous membranes, whereas HSV-2 is more frequently systemic and involves the central nervous system causing severe neurodevelopmental sequelae or death[94].

Clinical diagnosis of neonatal herpes is difficult and cases are commonly missed initially and only diagnosed when advanced and clinically evident. The mother is usually asymptomatic; the infant does not become unwell until 2–3 weeks after delivery and starts with non-specific signs. The diagnosis may only become obvious when far advanced, by which time involvement of the central nervous system is likely and sequelae inevitable.

REFERENCES

1. Cates W, Dallabella G. The staying power of sexually transmitted diseases. *Lancet* 1999;354 (Suppl):siv62
2. Wade AAH, Buckingham A. Multi-disciplinary *Chlamydia* audit project. Audit report: audit of disciplines to establish current practice in the management of *Chlamydia trachomatis* infection. Department of Genitourinary Medicine, Coventry and Warwickshire Hospital, Walsgrave Hospitals NHS Trust, Coventry, England, September 1995
3. Kinghorn, G. Screening for sexually transmitted infections. *Dermatol Clin* 1998;16:663–7
4. Robinson AJ. The clinical examination and how to obtain specimens. In Barton SE, Hay PE, eds. *Handbook of Genitourinary Medicine*. London: Arnold, 1999:5–18
5. Curtis H, Hoolaghan T, Jewitt C, eds. *Sexual Health Promotion in General Practice*. Oxford: Radcliffe Medical Press, 1995
6. Martin-Hirsch P, Lilford R, Jarvis G, *et al.* Efficacy of cervical smear collection devices: a systematic review and meta-analysis. *Lancet* 1999;354:1763–70
7. Gaydos CA, Howell MR, Pare B, *et al. Chlamydia trachomatis* in female military recruits. *N Engl J Med* 1998;339:741–4
8. Barlow D. The diagnosis of oropharyngeal gonorrhoea. *Genitourin Med* 1997;73:16–17
9. Dyer C. GP reprimanded for testing patients for HIV without consent. *Br Med J* 2000;320:135
10. Parran T. *Shadow On The Land – Syphilis*. New York: Regnal and Hitchcock, 1937
11. Van den Hoek JAR, van der Linden MMD, Coutinho RA. Increase in infectious syphilis amongst heterosexuals in Amsterdam: its relationship to prostitution and drug use. *Genitourin Med* 1990;66:31–2

12. Centers for Disease Control and Prevention. Sexually transmitted diseases treatment guidelines. *MMWR* 1998;47(RR-1):1–116

13. Centers for Disease Control and Prevention. Guidelines for the prevention and control of congenital syphilis. *MMWR* 1988;37(S1):1

14. Stray-Pederson B. Economic evaluation of maternal screening to prevent congenital syphilis. *Sex Transm Dis* 1983;10:167–72

15. Battu V, Horner P, Taylor P, *et al.* Locally acquired heterosexual outbreak of syphilis in Bristol. *Lancet* 1997;350:1100–1

16. Courtney G, Forkin C, O'Grady P, *et al.* Emergence of a cluster of new cases of syphilis: secondary to changes in donor screening in the Irish Blood Transfusion Service Board (BTSB). Oral presentation: Society for the Study of Sexually Transmissible Diseases in Ireland, April 1999

17. Berkowitz KM, Stampf K, Baxi L, *et al.* False negative screening tests for syphilis in pregnant women. *N Engl J Med* 1990;322:270–1

18. Thornton JG, Foote GA, Page CE, *et al.* False positive results of tests for syphilis and outcome of pregnancy: a retrospective case control study. *Br Med J* 1987;295:355–6

19. WHO and UNAIDS. *Management of Sexually Transmitted Diseases*. WHO/GPA/TEM/94.1 Rev 1. Geneva: WHO, 1997

20. Ndinya-Achola JO, Kihara AN, Fisher LD, *et al.* Presumptive specific clinical diagnosis of genital ulcer disease (GUD) in a primary health care setting in Nairobi. *Int J Sexual Trans Dis AIDS* 1996;7: 201–5

21. Rosen T, Dhir A. Chancroid, granuloma inguinale and lymphogranuloma venereum. In Arndt KA, LeBoit PE, Robinson JK, *et al.*, eds. *Cutaneous Medicine and Surgery. An Integrated Program in Dermatology*, vol 2. Philadelphia: WB Saunders Company, 1996:973–82

22. Engelkens HJH, Stolz E. Genital ulcer disease. *Int J Dermatol* 1993;32:169–81

23. O'Farell N. Clinico-epidemiological study of donovanosis in Durban, South Africa. *Genitourin Med* 1993;69:108–11

24. Nugent RP, Hillier SL. Mucopurulent cervicitis as a predictor of *Chlamydia* infection and adverse pregnancy outcome. *Sex Trans Dis* 1992;19:198–202

25. Aavitsland P. Survey of the treatment of *Chlamydia trachomatis* infection of the female genital tract. *Acta Obstet Gynecol Scand* 1992;71:356–60

26. Burstein GR, Gaydos CA, Diener-West M, *et al.* Incidence of *Chlamydia trachomatis* infections amongst inner city adolescent females. *JAMA* 1998;280:521–6

27. Uno M, Deguchi T, Koneda H, *et al. Mycoplasma genitalium* in the cervices of Japanese women. *Sex Transm Dis* 1997;24:284–6

28. Brunham RC, Paavonen J, Stevens CE, *et al.* Mucopurulent cervicitis: the ignored counterpart in women of urethritis in men. *N Engl J Med* 1984;311:1–7

29. Horner JP, Gilroy CB, Thomas BJ, *et al.* Association of *M. genitalium* with acute nongonococcal urethritis. *Lancet* 1993;342:582–5

30. Paavonen J. Critchlow CW, DeRoven T, *et al.* Etiology of cervical inflammation. *Am J Obstet Gynecol* 1986;154:556–64

31. Paavonen J, Miettinen A, Sterens CE, *et al. Mycoplasma hominis* in cervicitis and endometritis. *Sex Transm Dis* 1983;10:276–80

32. Schwebke JR, Schulien MB, Zajackowski M. Pilot study to evaluate the appropriate management of patients with co-existent bacterial vaginosis and cervicitis. *Infect Dis Obstet Gynecol* 1995;3:119–22

33. Rolfs RT, Galaid EI, Zaidi AA. Pelvic inflammatory disease: trends in hospitalisations and office visits 1979 through 1988. *Am J Obstet Gynecol* 1992; 166:983–90

34. Mardh P-A, Ripa KD, Svensson I, *et al. Chlamydia trachomatis* infection in patients with acute salpingitis. *N Engl J Med* 1977;296:1377–9

35. Svensson I, Westrom L, Ripa RT, *et al.* Differences in some clinical and laboratory parameters in acute salpingitis related to culture and serologic findings. *Am J Obstet Gynecol* 1980;138:1017–21

36. Larson PG, Platz-Christensen JJ, Thejls H, *et al.* Incidence of pelvic inflammatory disease after first trimester legal abortion in women with bacterial vaginosis after treatment with metronidazole: a double blind randomized study. *Am J Obstet Gynecol* 1992;166:100–3

37. Buchan H, Vessey M, Goldacre M, *et al.* Morbidity following pelvic inflammatory disease. *Br J Obstet Gynaecol* 1993;100:558–62

38. World Health Organization Task Force on the Prevention and Management of Infertility. Tubal infertility: serologic relationship to past *Chlamydia* and gonococcal infection. *Sex Transm Dis* 1995; 22:71–7

39. Weström L, Bengtsson LP, Mardh PA. Incidence, trends and risks of ectopic pregnancy in a population of women. *Br Med J* 1981;82:15–18

40. Soper DE, Brockwell NJ, Dalton HP. Observations concerning the microbial etiology of acute salpingitis. *Am J Obstet Gynecol* 1994;170:1008–17

41. Gjonnes H, Dalaker K, Anstad G, *et al.* Pelvic inflammatory disease: etiologic studies with emphasis on *Chlamydia trachomatis*. *Obstet Gynecol* 1982;59:550–5

42. Buchan H, Vessey M. Epdemiology and trends in hospital discharges for pelvic inflammatory disease in England 1975–1985. *Br J Obstet Gynaecol* 1989;396:1219–23

43. Rolfs RT, Think PID. New directions in prevention and management of pelvic inflammatory disease. *Sex Transm Dis* 1991;18:131–2

44. Scholes D, Stergachis A, Heidrich FE, *et al.* Prevention of pelvic inflammatory disease by

screening for cervical chlamydial infection. *N Engl J Med* 1996;334:1363–6

45. Egger M, Low N, Smith GD, *et al*. Screening for chlamydial infections and the risk of ectopic pregnancy in a county in Sweden: ecological analysis. *Br Med J* 1998;316:1776–80

46. Westrom L. Sexually transmitted diseases and infertility. *Sex Transm Dis* 1994;21(suppl):32–7

47. Wales NM, Barton SE, Boag FC, *et al*. An audit of the management of pelvic inflammatory disease. *Int J Sex Transm Dis AIDS* 1997;8:409–11

48. Jacobson L, Weström L. Objectivised diagnosis of acute pelvic inflammatory disease. *Am J Obstet Gynecol* 1969;105:1088–98

49. Centers for Disease Control and Prevention: 1993; Sexually transmitted diseases: treatment guidelines. *Mortal Morbid Wkly Rep* 1993;42(NoRR-14)

50. Makinen JL. Ectopic pregnancy falls in Finland. *Lancet* 1996;348:129–30

51. Hay PE, Lamont RF, Taylor-Robinson DJ, *et al*. Abnormal bacterial colonisation of the genital tract and subsequent preterm delivery and late miscarriage. *Br Med J* 1994;308:295–8

52. Kurki T, Sivonen A, Renkonen OV, *et al*. Bacterial vaginosis in early pregnancy and pregnancy outcome. *Obstet Gynecol* 1992;80:173–7

53. Hillier SL, Nugent RP, Eschenbach DA, *et al*. Association between bacterial vaginosis and preterm delivery of a low birth weight infant. *N Engl J Med* 1995;333:1772–4

54. McGregor JA, French JI, Parker R, *et al*. Prevention of premature birth by screening and treatment for common genital tract infections: results of a prospective controlled evaluation. *Am J Obstet Gynecol* 1995;173:157–67

55. Goldenberg RI, Andrews WM, Yuan AC, *et al*. Sexually transmitted diseases and adverse outcomes of pregnancy. *Clin Perinatol* 1997;24:23–41

56. Oriel JD. Natural history of genital warts. *Br J Vener Dis* 1971;47:1–13

57. Vayrynen M, Syrjanen K, Castren O. Colposcopy in women with papillomavirus lesions of the uterine cervix. *Obstet Gynecol* 1985;65:409–15

58. Jonsson M, Karlsson R, Rylander E, *et al*. The silent suffering woman: a population based study on the association between reported symptoms and past and present infections of the lower genital tract. *Genitourin Med* 1995;71:158–62

59. Bergström T, Trybala E. Antigenic differences between HSV-1 and HSV-2 glycoproteins and their importance for type-specific serology. *Intervirology* 1996;39:176–84

60. Maddox P, Szarewski A, Dyson J, *et al*. Cytokeratin expression and acetowhite change in cervical epithelium. *J Clin Pathol* 1994;47:15–17

61. Barrasso R, De Brux J, Croissant O, *et al*. High prevalence of papillomavirus-associated penile intraepithelial neoplasia in sexual partners of women with cervical intraepithelial neoplasia. *N Engl J Med* 1987;317:916–23

62. Hinchliffe SA, van Velzen D, Korporaal H, *et al*. Transience of cervical HPV infection in sexually active young women with normal cervicovaginal cytology. *Br J Cancer* 1995;72:943–5

63. Lornicz AT, Reid R, Jenson AB, *et al*. Human papillomavirus of the cervix: relative risk associations of 15 common anogenital types. *Obstet Gynecol* 1992;79:328–37

64. Bodén E, Eriksson A, Rylander E, *et al*. Clinical characteristics of papillomavirus vulvovaginitis: a new entity with oncogenic potential. *Acta Obstet Gynecol Scand* 1988;67:147–51

65. Strand A, Wilander E, Zehbe I, *et al*. Vulvar papillomatosis, aceto-white lesions and normal looking vulvar mucosa evaluated by microscopy and HPV analysis. *Gynecol Obstet Invest* 1995;40:265–70

66. Gentile G, Formelli G, Pelusi G, *et al*. Is vestibular micropapillomatosis associated with human papillomavirus infection? *Eur J Gynaecol Oncol* 1997;18:523–5

67. van Beurden M, van der Vange N, de Craen AJ, *et al*. Normal findings in vulvar examination and vulvoscopy. *Br J Obstet Gynaecol* 1997;104:320–4

68. De Villiers EM, Wagner D, Schneider A, *et al*. Human papillomavirus infections in women with and without abnormal cervical cytology. *Lancet* 1987;26:703–6

69. Bauer HM, Greer CE, Chambers JC, *et al*. Genital human papillomavirus infection in female university students as determined by a PCR-based method. *JAMA* 1991;265:472–7

70. Koutsky L. Epidemiology of genital human papillomavirus infection. *Am J Med* 1997;102(5A):3–8

71. von Krogh G. Genitoanal papillomavirus infection: diagnostic and therapeutic objectives in the light of current epidemiological observations. *Int J Sex Transm Dis AIDS* 1991;2:391–404

72. Melkert PWJ, Hopman E, van den Brule AJC, *et al*. Prevalence of HPV in cytomorphologically normal cervical smears, as determined by the polymerase chain reaction, is age dependent. *Int J Cancer* 1993;53:919–23

73. Ho GYF, Bierman R, Beardsley L, *et al*. Natural history of cervicovaginal papillomavirus infection in young women. *N Engl J Med* 1998;338:423–8

74. Guidelines for Clinical Practice and Programme Management, 2nd edn. NHS Cervical Screening Programme. Publication No. 8, December 1997

75. Saunders N, Frazer I. Simplifying the molecular mechanisms of human papillomavirus. *Dermatol Clin* 1998;16:823–7

76. Kataja V, Syrjanen S, Mantyjarvi R, *et al*. Prognostic factors in cervical human papillomavirus infections. *Sex Transm Dis* 1992;19:154–9

77. Nobbenhuis MA, Walboomers JM, Helmerhorst TJ, *et al*. Relation of human papillomavirus status to cervical lesions and consequences for cervical cancer screening: a prospective study. *Lancet* 1999;354: 20–5

78. Ross JD, Smith IW, Elton RA. The epidemiology of herpes simplex types 1 and 2 infection of the genital tract in Edinburgh 1978–1991. *Genitourin Med* 1993;69:381–3

79. Mertz G, Schmidt O, Jourden JL, *et al*. Frequency of acquisition of first-episode genital infection with herpes simplex virus from symptomatic and asymptomatic source contacts. *Sex Transm Dis* 1985;12: 33–9

80. Fleming DT, McQuillan GM, Johnson RE, *et al*. Herpes simplex virus type 2 in the United States, 1976–1994. *N Engl J Med* 1997;337:1105–11

81. Koutsky LA, Stevens CE, Holmes KK, *et al*. Underdiagnosis of genital herpes by current clinical and viral isolation procedures. *N Engl J Med* 1992;326:1533–9

82. Wald A, Corry L, Cone R, *et al*. Frequent genital herpes simplex virus 2 shedding in immunocompetent women: effect of acyclovir treatment. *J Clin Invest* 1997;99:1092–7

83. McCormack S. The diagnosis and management of genital ulceration. In SE Barton, PE Hay, eds. *Handbook of Genitourinary Medicine*. London: Arnold, 1999:97–122

84. Mertz GJ, Benedetti J, Ashley R, *et al*. Risk factors for the sexual transmission of genital herpes. *Ann Intern Med* 1992;116:197–202

85. Mertz G, Schmidt O, Jourden J, *et al*. Frequency of acquisition of first-episode genital infection with herpes simplex virus from symptomatic and asymptomatic source contacts. *Sex Transm Dis* 1985; 12:33–9

86. Slomka M, Ashley R, Cowan F, *et al*. Monoclonal antibody blocking tests for the detection of HSV-1 and HSV-2 specific humoral responses: comparison with Western blot assay. *J Virol Methods* 1995; 55:27–35

87. Brown Z, Selke S, Zeh J, *et al*. The acquisition of herpes simplex virus during pregnancy. *N Engl J Med* 1997;337:509–15

88. Brown ZA, Annholm A, Ashley R, *et al*. HSV serology discordancy among sexual partners and rates of seroconversion during pregnancy. In *Program and Abstracts of the Infectious Disease Society for Obstetrics and Gynecology*. Stowe, VT, August 1993

89. Brown ZA. Genital herpes complicating pregnancy. *Dermatol Clin* 1998;16:805–10

90. Cone RW, Hobson AC, Brown ZA, *et al*. Frequent detection of genital herpes simplex virus DNA by polymerase chain reaction amongst pregnant women. *JAMA* 1994;272:792–6

91. Hensleigh P, Andrews W, Brown Z, *et al*. Genital herpes during pregnancy: inability to distinguish primary and recurrent infections clinically. *Obstet Gynecol* 1997;89:891–5

92. Brown ZA, Benedetti J, Ashley R, *et al*. Neonatal herpes simplex virus infection in relation to asymptomatic maternal infection at the time of labor. *N Engl J Med* 1991;324:1247–52

93. Brown Z, Hume RF, Selke S, *et al*. Subclinical shedding of herpes simplex virus at the time of labor. Presented at the annual meeting of the Society of Perinatal Obstetricians. Miami Beach, FL, February 1998

94. Whitley R, Arvin A, Prober C, *et al*. Predictors of morbidity and mortality in neonates with herpes simplex virus infections. *N Engl J Med* 1991;324: 450–4

AIDS
27

John D. Stratigos, Andreas D. Katsambas and Alexander C. Katoulis

INTRODUCTION

Acquired immunodeficiency syndrome (AIDS) was first recognized as a new, distinct entity in 1981. With the outburst of a global pandemic a few years later, human immunodeficiency virus (HIV)/AIDS became one of the ten leading causes of death worldwide, tending to be included among the top five[1]. However, in the USA, after the introduction of combined antiretroviral therapy in 1996, AIDS dropped into the second place of causes of death for people aged 25–44 years for the first time since 1992[2].

HIV infection in women is exceedingly important: first, because of the rapidly increasing incidence of HIV infection in women who acquire the virus through heterosexual contact; and second, because of the devastating impact of vertical transmission from the HIV-infected mother to the newborn during pregnancy, labor, or breast feeding.

In general, the natural history, clinical course, treatment and prognosis are similar in HIV-infected men and women. On the other hand, there are some differences by gender, which are discussed below.

EPIDEMIOLOGY

Worldwide, the risk of HIV infection for women is increasing dramatically. By the end of 1997, of the 30.6 million cumulative HIV/AIDS cases, 12.2 million were women and 1.1 million were children under 15 years of age[2]. Women now comprise approximately 40% of all HIV-infected adults, with the vast majority of them living in developing countries[3,4]. Southeast Asia is experiencing the steepest increase in HIV/AIDS incidence, remaining second only to sub-Saharan Africa[5].

In the USA, women represent the fastest growing group of adults with AIDS. The percentage of HIV-infected women has risen from nearly 0% in 1981 to almost 20% in 1997[6,7]. Currently, almost half of all new HIV infections are being reported in women[4]. Minorities bear a disproportionate burden of HIV infection: approximately 50% of HIV-seropositive women are African-Americans and 20% are Hispanics[8].

In Africa, where the epidemic has matured, women tend to become infected at higher rates and at younger ages in comparison with men[4]. In the developed countries, the average age at which HIV infection occurs seems to be declining. In the USA, the majority of newly infected persons are aged 20 to 29 years, whilst one-quarter of all new infections occur in persons less than 21 years of age[9]. In a comparison between men ($n = 3799$) and women ($n = 768$) enrolled in a multicenter study from 1990 to 1993, women were younger (women usually have relationships with older men), more likely to have used injectable drugs and more likely to be of color[10]. Rates of HIV infection are highest for women in urban areas; nevertheless, the epidemic is spreading to suburban and rural areas[11].

Worldwide, since the beginning of the epidemic, 3.9 million women have died of AIDS, 800 000 in 1997 alone[2]. The overall HIV seroprevalence in the USA is estimated to be 1.1–1.4 per 1000 women of reproductive age[12]. AIDS is the third leading cause of death for women aged 18–44 years in the USA and, since 1990, the leading cause of death for black women of this age group[13].

TRANSMISSION

On a global basis, unprotected sexual intercourse is the major route of transmission of HIV in adolescent and adult women[4]. In the developed world, heterosexual transmission is increasing at the fastest rate[8,14,15]. In the USA, since 1993, heterosexual contact has become the leading mode of transmission, accounting for more than one-third of cases in women[8,14–16]. Data suggest that HIV is transmitted more easily from men to women than from women to men[4,8,16]. Studies of discordant couples have demonstrated that male to female transmission (estimated rate 20–30%) is 2–4 times more efficient than the opposite[17,18]. This may be attributed, in part, to the large area of exposed mucosa in the vagina and to the higher concentration of HIV in semen compared to that in vaginal secretions[3]. HIV is isolated from vaginal secretions throughout the menstrual cycle; therefore, it can be transmitted independently of menstrual bleeding[19].

Factors associated with increased risk of heterosexual transmission include[20]: unprotected sexual intercourse, particularly anal intercourse; a history of sexually transmitted diseases (STDs), especially those associated with genital ulcers[21,22] (however, it is unclear whether STDs are markers for high-risk behavior or co-factors for transmission); illegal drug use; and symptomatic or advanced HIV disease of the partner (CD4 count < 400 cells/mm^3, detectable serum p24 antigen).

The role of hormonal contraception in HIV transmission is uncertain. Theoretically, hormonal contraceptives may increase the risk by increasing cervical ectopy, modifying menstrual patterns, inducing changes in cervical mucus or by local effects of progesterone on the vaginal epithelium[23]. Most human studies on the subject are inconclusive; it is therefore important to promote the use of condoms for both contraceptive and preventive purposes[4].

Illicit intravenous drug use still accounts for the majority of cumulative cases among women, because it was the leading mode of transmission in the USA and Europe prior to 1993[16]. Factors that may be important for transmission include the sharing of contaminated needles and high-risk sexual behaviors with infected drug-using partners due to disinhibition. Exchange of sex for money or drugs by women who use crack cocaine has been shown to account for a significant part of the high seroprevalence reported in urban areas[24].

Of the HIV-seropositive women, 3–5% are infected secondary to transfusion of contaminated blood products[8,14]. Fortunately, this percentage is declining steadily.

NATURAL HISTORY

The causative agent of HIV/AIDS is the human immunodeficiency virus, type 1 or 2, of the retrovirus group.

The CD4 antigen is an important component of the viral receptor, which is required for cell entry, rendering cells susceptible to infection by HIV. HIV infects cells that display the CD4 molecule, namely helper/inducer (CD4 +) T lymphocytes, monocytes, macrophages and some B lymphocytes[7,25]. Depletion or impaired function of CD4 lymphocytes, which play a pivotal role in the immune response, is the primary immune abnormality in HIV disease, resulting in progressive immunodeficiency. After the initial infection, continuous high-level viral replication causes dissemination throughout the body, including lymphoid tissues, the central nervous system (CNS) and the genital tract. A hundred million to ten billion new HIV virions are produced each day[26]. In addition, mutations in the viral DNA select viral phenotypes resistant to drug therapy.

The immune system mounts a CD8 T lymphocyte- and a B cell-produced antibody response to reduce the HIV levels. Both cytolytic and non-cytolytic suppression are employed to kill HIV-infected cells. The clinical course is determined by the interaction of persistent HIV multiplication/cell infection and the host's immune response. Ultimately, the virus overcomes the immune system, leading to progressive collapse and the host's death[27].

The natural history of HIV infection evolves in three clinical stages:

(1) *Acute infection*   After 3–30 days from exposure, 70% of infected persons experience flu-like symptoms or a mononucleosis-like syndrome (fever, malaise, myalgia, pharyngitis, lymphadenopathy, measles-like rash) and, occasionally, aseptic meningitis. Symptoms may last for 1–4 weeks.

(2) *Asymptomatic period*   This is characterized by active viral replication within lymph nodes and progressive depletion of CD4 T lymphocytes. One-third of HIV-infected patients may have persistent generalized lymphadenopathy. This stage may last for 3–10 years.

(3) *Symptomatic disease*   Intermittent or persistent non-specific constitutional symptoms develop, including fever, night sweats, diarrhea and weight loss. Minor opportunistic infections and skin or mucosal manifestations may also ensue (oral candidosis, oral hairy leukoplakia, herpes zoster, recurrent HSV infection, seborrheic dermatitis (Figure 1), folliculitis, tinea infections). This group of signs and symptoms is referred to as symptomatic non-AIDS or AIDS-related complex.

AIDS is defined by the presence of one or more indicator diseases (Table 1) in the absence of another cause of immunodeficiency[25], or with laboratory evidence of HIV infection. In 1993, the Centers for Disease Control (CDC) extended the definition of AIDS to include all patients who were severely immunosuppressed (CD4 cell count < 200/mm^3). The CD4 cell level of individual patients can help to predict which malignancies and opportunistic infections will develop.

PROGRESSION AND SURVIVAL

Based on several large cohort studies of adults in the USA and Europe, the average interval from the onset of infection to clinical AIDS was estimated to be approximately 10 years[28,29]. However, 10–15% of patients exhibiting an even slower rate of progression with no clinical signs after 10–15 years[30]. In a smaller subset the disease progressed quickly to AIDS and death in less than 5 years. After AIDS diagnosis, the current median survival for women receiving antiretroviral therapy has been reported to be 22–28 months (range 1–5 years)[31]. In Africa, the time to AIDS diagnosis is much shorter (5 years or less). Tuberculosis causes significant morbidity and mortality in these settings.

Disease progression in both men and women has been associated with older age, symptomatic disease, lower CD4 counts at entry or rapid decline in CD4 counts[32]. In recent years, survival after AIDS diagnosis has improved, particularly for those receiving antiretroviral therapy[4,28]. Additional predictors of poor survival after AIDS diagnosis are: HIV dementia, disseminated tuberculosis, hemoglobin levels of < 8 g/dl, albumin levels of < 3 g/dl and evidence of *Mycobacterium avium* complex (MAC).

Whether gender influences the progression and survival of HIV disease is still a matter of debate. It seems plausible that HIV may behave differently in men and women. In the general population, CD4 lymphocyte counts are slightly higher in females than in their male counterparts. CD4 lymphocyte counts decline with age in both sexes[33] and women are younger than men at the time of AIDS diagnosis. Estrogens influence immune functions[33]. Furthermore, women may show increased susceptibility to certain micro-organisms.

Early reports suggested a less favorable prognosis for HIV-infected women in comparison with men[4,10,34]. Women were diagnosed at a later stage, they had increased risk of dying from pneumonia and their overall survival was lower[35]; however, it was thought that this may reflect decreased access to care among HIV-infected women, due to their lower socioeconomic status, rather than reflecting a true biological difference[14]. In addition, more recent evidence, especially from Europe, supports the speculation that progression and survival in HIV-infected men and women are not significantly different after control for socioeconomic factors, CD4 counts at diagnosis and the use of antiretroviral or other therapy[4,14,35,36]. Several ongoing studies may elucidate this controversial issue.

Most HIV-infected women are poor and of color. Socioeconomic factors influence the access to and quality of health care, as well as the survival rates. Debate exists about whether possible survival differences are due to biological factors related to race or whether race serves as a marker of lower socioeconomic status[7]. The results of recent studies lead to the conclusions that race and ethnicity are not

Table 1 Diseases diagnostic of AIDS if laboratory evidence of HIV exists

Pneumocystis carinii pneumonia
Cerebral toxoplasmosis
Herpex simplex virus infection – mucocutaneous ulceration lasting more than 1 month, or pulmonary, or esophageal infection
Cytomegalovirus retinitis
Cytomegalovirus disease – not in the liver, spleen or lymph nodes
Candidosis – pulmonary, esophageal
Coccidioidomycosis – disseminated
Cryptococcosis – pulmonary
Cryptosporidiosis – with diarrhea persisting more than 1 month
Histoplasmosis – disseminated
Isosporiasis – with diarrhea persisting more than 1 month
Mycobacterial tuberculosis – extrapulmonary, pulmonary
Disseminated mycobacteriosis – *Mycobacterium avium*
Recurrent pneumonia within a 12-month period
Recurrent/multiple bacterial infections – child aged under 13 years
Lymphoid interstitial pneumonia – child aged under 13 years
Kaposi's sarcoma
Non-Hodgkin's lymphoma – Burkitt's or immunoblastic
Primary cerebral lymphoma
Invasive cervical carcinoma
HIV encephalopathy
Progressive multifocal leukoencephalopathy

predictive of disease progression and that differences are most likely to be due to a delay of diagnosis and entry to treatment as a result of less access to care[32,34,37].

CLINICAL MANIFESTATIONS

Although clinical features and course of the HIV disease are similar for both men and women, there are some gender differences, especially regarding the prevalence of certain AIDS-related conditions[3,4,7]. HIV-infected women appear to have increased rates of esophageal candidosis, bacterial pneumonia and herpes simplex virus (HSV) ulcerations. Diseases of the female genital tract, including recurrent vaginitis and cervical intraepithelial neoplasia, are more frequent in HIV-infected women compared with those not infected and of similar socioeconomic background. In contrast, Kaposi's sarcoma is rare among HIV-infected women, with rates similar to those of HIV-infected heterosexual men. In addition, HIV-seropositive women face non-HIV-related clinical problems, such as chemical dependency and its sequelae and mental health problems. Referrals to specialists and programs that address the gender-specific issues of these problems are most likely to be successful.

Opportunistic infections

Women with HIV disease are at equal risk with their male counterparts of acquiring most opportunistic infections, including *Pneumocystis carinii* pneumonia (PCP), tuberculosis, toxoplasmosis, cytomegalovirus (CMV) infections and cryptococcal meningitis[38,39]. The CD4 count is the most important predictor of this risk; however, gender differences have been reported for esophageal candidosis and HSV infections (see below).

PCP is one of the most common opportunistic infections in HIV-infected men and women[40]. According to some authors, it is the most common AIDS-defining diagnosis in women. Data from the Centers for Disease Control and Prevention (1981–91) indicated that esophageal candidosis was the leading initial opportunistic infection in women, followed by PCP[41].

Candidosis

Mucosal candidosis occurs in over 90% of HIV-infected individuals, thus being one of the most common manifestations of HIV disease. The pattern of *Candida* infections in HIV-seropositive women is linked to the stage of infection[42]. Vaginal candidosis occurs with CD4 counts above 500/mm^3. Oropharyngeal candidosis is observed when CD4 counts are less than 500 cells/mm^3, while esophageal candidosis occurs when CD4 counts are less than 100 cells/mm^3.

Vulvovaginal candidosis is often the earliest presenting symptom of HIV infection[42]. The prevalence of recurrent vaginal candidosis has been reported to be 24–50% among HIV-infected women in various studies, but it is not clear whether this is higher than in the general population[43]. HIV infection should always be considered in the differential diagnosis of recurrent vulvovaginal candidosis. *Candida albicans* accounts for 85–90% of the cases. Non-albicans vaginal candidosis represents 10–15% of the cases, being much more frequent in HIV-infected than in non-infected women[44]. The clinical picture is independent of the HIV status and includes vulvar pruritus and burning, erythema and increased white, non-frothy vaginal discharge with a pH generally less than 4.5. Vaginal candidosis in HIV patients is

difficult to eradicate[42,43]. Standard therapy with topical imidazoles or nystatin is often ineffective[38]. Longer courses or oral therapy with ketoconazole, itraconazole, or fluconazole may be required[42]. Recurrences are common. In patients with severe or recurrent vaginitis, suppressive therapy with fluconazole (100–200 mg daily, orally) or ketoconazole may be of benefit.

Oropharyngeal candidosis has been associated with progressive immunosuppression. Four clinical patterns have been described: pseudomembranous (thrush), erythematous (atrophic), hyperplastic and angular cheilitis.

Several studies have demonstrated esophageal candidosis as the most frequent AIDS-defining illness among HIV-infected women[3,31,38]. Clinically, candida esophagitis is manifested by retrosternal burning and odynophagia. KOH preparation and culture are key in confirming the diagnosis, especially in order to isolate non-albicans species. For treatment, oral antifungals (fluconazole or itraconazole) are necessary. Long-term prophylactic therapy with fluconazole has been widely used, but is has been associated with the development of resistant *Candida* species[3].

Herpes simplex virus infections

HSV infections are common in HIV disease, usually resulting from reactivation of latent infection. With the impairment of the immune system, these infections become chronic, progressive and recalcitrant to treatment[14,38]. Painful erosions or giant ulcers may appear on the genital or the orofacial regions (Figure 2). An HSV ulcer persisting for longer than 1 month is an AIDS-defining condition.

Recurrent herpes labialis infection is extremely common. Oropharyngeal HSV occurs with increased frequency in HIV disease and may progress to involve the esophagus or the lower respiratory tract[45]. Herpes genitalis is exceedingly common in HIV-infected women, increasing the risk for sexual transmission of HIV[14]. Herpetic whitlow may exhibit atypical presentation with chronic ulcers and multiple finger involvement, resulting in digital necrosis.

Antivirals, such as acyclovir or famciclovir, are usually effective, but higher than standard doses, longer courses or intravenous administration may be needed. Valacyclovir should be used with caution, owing to the reported adverse effects (hemolytic–uremic syndrome, thrombotic thrombocytopenic purpura (Figure 3)) in patients with severe immunosuppression[14]. Suppressive therapy with acyclovir

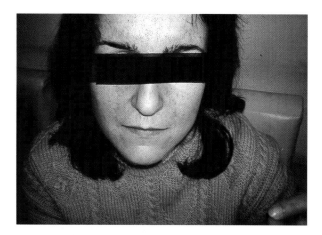

Figure 1 Seborrheic dermatitis

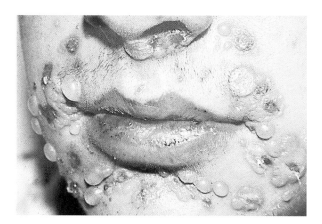

Figure 2 Herpes simplex virus infection

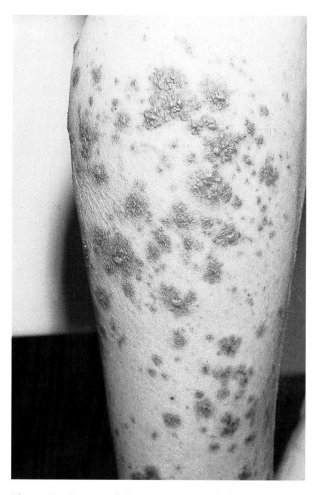

Figure 3 Purpura following antiretroviral treatment

(400 mg twice a day) may select resistant strains that nevertheless respond to foscarnet[3,38].

Human papilloma virus infections

Human papilloma virus (HPV) infections occur at high rates in HIV patients. The clinical spectrum includes common warts, condylomata acuminata, bowenoid papulosis, epidermodysplasia verruciformis and cervical intraepithelial neoplasia (CIN).

Genital warts and CIN are more prevalent in HIV-infected women compared to uninfected women, and tend to be more persistent and severe[40,46]. Almost half of the HIV-infected women have CIN[47]. Persistent HPV infection by oncogenic strains, especially 16 or 18, has been associated with increased risk for CIN. Local immune impairment, as evidenced by a decrease in endometrial CD4 cells (independent of blood CD4 counts) and Langerhans cells in HIV-positive women, may also play a part[48]. The prevalence, severity and rate of progression of CIN are directly related to the immunodeficiency state[49]. A synergistic effect of HPV and HIV, in the setting of immunodeficiency, has been suggested, inducing cervical dysplasia or neoplasia development. Some authors claim that cytological screening alone may be inadequate, because CIN is often missed, and they recommend colposcopy as a routine diagnostic procedure for HIV-seropositive women[50]. Papanicolaou (Pap) smears should be performed on a 6–12-month basis in HIV-infected women. Treatment of CIN with cervical conization or cryotherapy has been associated with high level of recurrence[14].

Invasive cervical cancer has been added to the list of AIDS-defining conditions. Despite the evidence of increased risk for CIN in HIV/AIDS, the decline in the incidence rates of invasive cervical cancer after the dramatic increase of HIV/AIDS among women argues for a pathogenetic link between HIV and invasive cervical cancer[51].

Neoplasms

Of HIV-infected individuals, 40% have cancer as a source of morbidity or mortality[52]. For certain conditions, HIV-infected men and women appear to be at different risks. Malignancies and precancerous

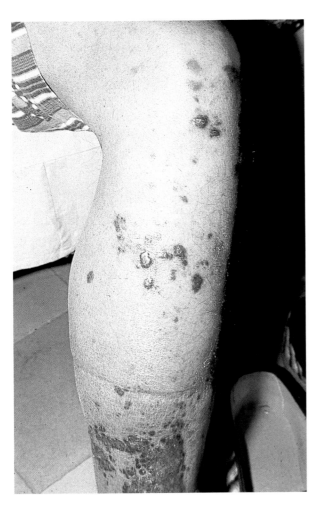

Figure 4   Kaposi's sarcoma

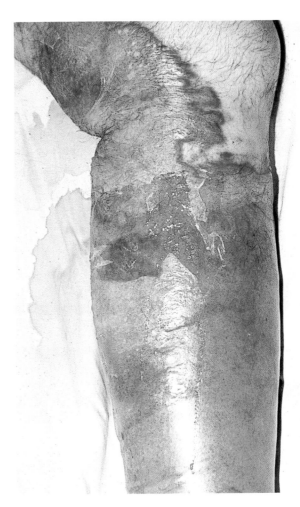

Figure 5   Erysipelas

conditions in HIV-infected women result from infection with oncogenic γ-herpes viruses (EBV, HHV-8) or HPV.

Kaposi's sarcoma (KS) is a multifocal angiomatous tumor (Figure 4). It is an AIDS-defining condition and by far the most common malignancy associated with HIV disease[53]. KS may occur at any stage of HIV/AIDS, but more often with CD4 counts less than 500 cells/mm[3 54]. Population data from the USA show an increased incidence of KS in women, consistent with the introduction of HIV into the population during the past decade. By 1988, the incidence rate was 1.8 cases per 100 000 per year for black women and 0.8 cases per 100 000 per year for white women in New York City[51]. KS is much less common in HIV-infected females (< 1%) compared with their male counterparts[7]. It is noteworthy that most women with AIDS-associated KS have acquired HIV through sexual contact with a bisexual male[55]. European data show that women, intravenous drug users and heterosexual males have an equal proportion KS as their initial AIDS-defining illness[4].

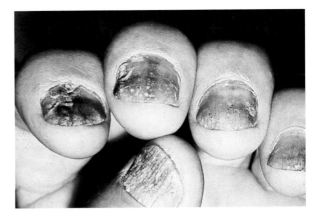

Figure 6   Brownish discoloration of nails as a side-effect of zidovudine treatment

Epidemiological evidence supports the theory that KS may be due to an unknown, probably sexually transmitted, infectious agent[56]. Recently, DNA sequences of a new herpes virus (HHV-8) have been detected in all clinical forms of KS[57,58]. However, its causal role is still a matter of controversy. It is of interest that low serum estrogen levels have been observed in female patients with KS, suggesting that female sex hormones may act prophylactically in KS development[14,56].

KS causes disturbing symptoms, such as pain and dysphagia, and produces significant cosmetic disfigurement. Visceral and lymph node involvement is not uncommon, but KS-associated mortality is only 10–20%. Some studies suggest that KS in women is associated with a more aggressive course and more profound immunodeficiency[59].

Wasting syndrome

According to some studies, the wasting syndrome occurs more frequently in women[60]. No difference by gender was noted after controlling for socioeconomic status.

Oral hairy leukoplakia

This is an oral manifestation of EBV infection that occurs almost exclusively in HIV disease and often predicts the rapid onset of AIDS[61]. The prevalence of oral hairy leukoplakia is reported to be higher in heterosexually infected women than in those infected by intravenous drug use[62]. Topical podophyllin or tretinoin 0.05% solution are effective, as is oral acyclovir, but recurrences are the rule[3].

Non-opportunistic infections and other conditions

A higher rate of bacterial pneumonia, especially with encapsulated organisms, has been observed in women who are injecting drug users compared with homosexual men[63]. Other bacterial infections, such as erysipelas (Figure 5) may also ensue.

Thrombocytopenia and skin diseases are reported to be less common, while urinary tract infections are more common in HIV-infected women than in their male counterparts[14,35].

Gynecological manifestations

These are more frequent and more severe in HIV-infected women[14]. Abnormal uterine bleeding is common, as it is in the general female population. Among HIV-infected persons, the most frequent causes include infection with *Chlamydia trachomatis*, *Neisseria gonorrhoeae*, cytomegalovirus or HSV; bleeding disorders; hormonal imbalance; fibroids; and cervical or endometrial cancer[40].

Menstrual abnormalities, which are common among HIV-infected women, are of great importance, because they make it difficult to predict ovulation and to prevent conception, as well as to protect the sexual partner from exposure to blood[64]. In one study, amenorrhea was found more often in seropositive than in seronegative women[14]. Secondary amenorrhea may be related to significant weight loss, which may suppress the surge of luteinizing hormone and the menstrual cycle.

Pelvic inflammatory disease (PID) is more frequent and pursues a more severe clinical course in HIV-infected women[65]. Organisms cultured do not differ for HIV-seronegative females. There are high rates of syphilis, gonorrhea and trichomoniasis in HIV-patients. Laboratory screening for sexually transmitted diseases is highly advisable[40]. Prolonged fever and tubo-ovarian abscess is not uncommon, often requiring surgical treatment[66]. Alarming signs include pelvic pain (with or without fever), abnormal cervical discharge, cervical motion tenderness and adnexal tenderness. It is noteworthy that leukocytosis may be absent in HIV patients with PID[66]. Treatment with intravenous antibiotics and hospitalization are often necessary[40].

Syphilis

Syphilis is not uncommon in HIV patients and it is associated with increased risk for HIV transmission[21]. The course is often more aggressive, requiring increased therapy to achieve eradication.

Psychologic issues

HIV-infected women face serious socioeconomic problems even prior to their infection. Their emotional distress originates not only from their own disability and fear of death, but also from those of their partners. They are often unable to provide appropriate protection and care for their children[38,67].

Major psychiatric disease is rare at the time of seroconversion. Psychiatric diagnoses become more common on follow-up. Depression, sexual dysfunction and alcohol or drug abuse are not unusual[68].

Pregnancy

Concerns have been raised as to whether pregnancy could accelerate the progression of HIV disease. Previous studies have reported a decline in CD4 counts in HIV-infected pregnant women, at a rate (2% per month) higher than that in HIV-positive men (0.5–1.0% per month), as well as an increase in CD8 cells that did not recover postpartum[69,70]. Elevated levels of progesterone during pregnancy may be implicated. An increased risk of opportunistic infections, AIDS-related symptoms and bacterial pneumonia has been reported for HIV-positive pregnant women compared with matched HIV-negative controls[71]. A recent prospective study of 145 women in the UK concluded that pregnancy had no adverse effect on the immunological markers of HIV disease[72]. Overall, the weight of evidence suggests that, although pregnancy is generally associated with immunosuppression, it does not lead to faster progression of HIV/AIDS[3,73].

Rates of vertical transmission vary considerably between studies, with the most accepted estimate at 25–30%[3,74]. Increased immunosuppression (as indicated by decreased CD4 counts and increased CD8 counts), increased plasma viremia (marked by increased p24 antigens) and symptomatic disease have been linked with elevated risk of transmission[74,75]. Zidovudine therapy has been shown to decrease vertical HIV transmission (8.3% for the zidovudine arm vs. 25.5% for the placebo arm)[76]. In France and in the USA, where zidovudine therapy for the pregnant woman and the newborn is widely utilized, less than 5% of babies born to HIV-positive women in 1997 were infected[77]. Consequently, it is crucial to perform HIV testing on all pregnant women in order to initiate zidovudine therapy in those infected with HIV[40].

HIV transmission may occur at delivery, so the route of delivery is important[78]. Cesarean delivery has been associated with a lower frequency of vertical transmission, particularly in premature infants, premature membrane rupture or mother's CD4 count less than 200 cells/mm^3 [74]. Other studies have shown no difference between Cesarean section and vaginal delivery[78,79]. Transmission via breast feeding has been documented; therefore, breast feeding should be avoided[80].

Data on the effect of HIV disease on the outcome of pregnancy are limited. In an American cohort, no significant impact was noted[81]. In contrast, studies from Africa have shown an increased risk of low birth weight, stillbirth and prematurity in infants born to HIV-positive mothers[82]. Contrasting results may reflect differences in confounding factors in the study populations. There is some evidence of decreased fertility and high rate of spontaneous first-trimester abortions in HIV-infected women[83].

For zidovudine antiretroviral therapy of the pregnant and the newborn, see Treatment. Possible adverse effects of zidovudine on the fetus remain unknown. Concurrently with zidovudine treatment, pregnant women with CD4 counts less than 200 cells/mm^3 should receive PCP prophylaxis with trimethoprim–sulfamethoxazole. Alternatively, dapsone and aerosolized pentamidine can be used.

LABORATORY STUDIES

Sophisticated serological techniques have been developed in order to establish or, quantitatively, to assess HIV infection. Antibody tests are utilized to screen and confirm HIV seropositivity. Viral measurement assays are employed to diagnose acute infection, to follow the course of the disease and to evaluate the response to therapy. Finally, immunological markers are the cornerstone for HIV patients' staging, prognosis and management.

Owing to the potentially significant medical, social and psychological consequences, an HIV screening test requires informed consent. Both pre- and post-test counseling are necessary[84]. Pretest counseling aims to assess an individual's risk for acquiring HIV, to educate on HIV infection prevention and to provide information about the test. The objectives of post-test counseling include the interpretation of the results, emotional support, referrals and guidance for appropriate follow-up (in case of seropositivity) or discussion on how to minimize the risk for infection.

HIV testing is recommended in the following situations[84,85]:

(1) After individual voluntary request, even in the apparent absence of risk factors;

(2) In high-risk populations, i.e. anyone engaged, since 1975, in high-risk activities, namely, use of injected drugs, sharing of needles or having sexual intercourse with injecting drug user, male homosexual activity, exchange of sex for money or drugs, blood product transfusion or organ transplantation between 1975 and 1985;

(3) History of symptoms and signs suggestive of HIV disease (unexplained weight loss, generalized lymphadenopathy or oral candidosis, atypical pneumonia not responding to standard therapy, etc.);

(4) Conditions strongly associated with HIV such as tuberculosis, HBV or HCV infection or STDs acquired after 1975.

Regarding screening in women, the CDC recommendations suggest HIV testing for women with one or more of the following risk factors (apart from those mentioned above): history of prostitution, sexual partners who are HIV-infected or at high risk of HIV infection and being from areas with a high rate of HIV infection among women[14]. Most authorities strongly encourage voluntary testing of pregnant women. Arguments in favor include allowing women to make informed reproductive decisions after assessing the risk of vertical transmission, preventing transmission by breast feeding, earlier diagnosis of infected women and administration of zidovudine to the pregnant mother and the newborn[12,14,86].

The detection of antibodies that react against HIV represents the most common method for diagnosing HIV infection. Measurements in serum are more sensitive than in saliva or urine. After infection with HIV, 50% of patients will develop antibody by 3 months and more than 95% by 6 months[87]. Enzyme immunoassays (EIA) detect antibodies to HIV viral proteins in a quantitative manner, with a specificity and sensitivity greater than 99%. However, the positive predictive value ranges from 20 to > 95%, being lower in populations with low HIV prevalence. To ensure that the antibody reaction is specific for HIV, a confirmatory assay, more often Western blot or immunofluorescence assay (IFA) is mandatory. Western blot, the most widely used technique, detects serum antibodies directed against specific HIV-1 proteins of various molecular weights. The CDC has defined as a positive test the presence of two or three of the following antibody bands: p24, gp41 and gp120/160[88].

During the 'window period', which may last for weeks or months after the infection, anti-HIV antibody may not be detected. To document the diagnosis, tests that detect viral antigen (p24 antigen), nucleic acid (by the polymerase chain reaction (PCR)) or isolation of the virus in culture can be employed. PCR is preferred for diagnosis of acute HIV infection. HIV p24 antigen, an HIV core protein, can be found in plasma or in serum, using an enzyme-linked immunosorbent assay (ELISA) technique, in all stages of HIV infection, but it is more often detected in those with advanced HIV disease or those undergoing acute seroconversion[89]. HIV may be cultured either from peripheral blood monocytes or from plasma. The likelihood of positive HIV culture increases with advancing HIV disease.

Methods to detect and, most importantly, to quantitate HIV infection include[90]:

(1) Reverse transcriptase PCR, an extremely sensitive method that detects HIV proviral DNA in cells or HIV viral DNA in plasma. It assists diagnosis of HIV infection in the newborn and in the newly infected prior to seroconversion.

(2) Branched chain DNA amplification, a technique that quantifies HIV RNA. It has been shown that HIV RNA levels have a predictive value. Higher levels of HIV RNA have been correlated with a more rapid decline in CD4 cell counts, more rapid progression to AIDS and decreased

survival[91]. Successful treatment produces a significant decrease in HIV RNA levels[92].

(3) Nucleic acid sequence-based amplification (NASBA). Quantitative measurements of HIV RNA are recommended in the following circumstances: prior to initiating antiretroviral therapy (two measurements within 2 weeks), 4 weeks after starting a new antiretroviral regimen (therapy should decrease HIV RNA measurement at least three-fold), and every 3–4 months during antiretroviral therapy (return of HIV RNA to within 0.5 log of pretreatment values suggests failure)[93].

CD4 cells are the major cell type infected by HIV. They are measured in three ways: absolute CD4 cell count, CD4 percentage of total lymphocytes and the CD4/CD8 ratio[90]. The absolute CD4 cell count and its rate of decline have prognostic value[94,95]. Most therapeutic recommendations and treatment evaluations are based on CD4 counts. Routine periodic monitoring is recommended every 6 months for patients with CD4 counts of > 500 cells/mm^3 or every 3 months when CD4 counts are < 500 cells/mm^3. Shortening of intervals is necessary in patients with an unpredictable rate of decline. Combining viral load information with CD4 measurements may give a clearer picture of the clinical outcome of HIV infection for the individual patient[7,95,96].

β_2-Microglobulin is the light chain protein of the class I major histocompatibility complex (MHC), which is present on all nucleated cell membranes. Lymphocyte activation or destruction results in elevated serum levels. Increased β_2-microglobulin indicates increased probability of progression to AIDS, new complications, or death[90]. Neopterin is an intermediate product of GTP metabolism that is released in the serum by stimulated macrophages and monocytes. Neopterin levels increase with advancing disease[97]. In conjunction with CD4 counts, neopterin provides a slightly better correlation with disease stage. Neither of the aforementioned tests are specific for HIV infection.

In all HIV patients a detailed history should be obtained and a complete physical examination should be performed. Laboratory investigation (apart from HIV serology and CD4 counts) includes complete blood count, erythrocyte sedimentation rate, serum chemistries and liver function tests, toxoplasma IgG, hepatitis antigen and antibody, PPD skin testing, syphilis serology and chest radiograph.

HIV-infected women should have a Pap smear every 6–12 months. When CD4 count falls below

200 cells/mm³ or if atypia or CIN is reported on the Pap smear, colposcopy is indicated. Sexually active HIV-infected women should undergo a complete STD work-up every 6–12 months, which includes pelvic examination, cervical Gram stain, cervical culture for gonorrhea and chlamydia, vaginal wet mount and serum VDRL[40].

TREATMENT

The therapeutics of HIV infection is a rapidly evolving field. Current therapeutic modalities can significantly alter or halt the progression of HIV infection, but do not offer definitive cure[98,99]. Intensive research provides new agents and new interventions that will probably further improve the prognosis for HIV patients in the near future.

Treatment of HIV infection can be divided into etiological and symptomatic therapy. Antiretroviral (etiological) therapy is the backbone of the HIV patient's management. At the time of writing, three major classes of antiretroviral drugs are licensed[100]: Nucleoside analog or non-nucleoside analog reverse transcriptase inhibitors (reverse transcriptase is the virally encoded enzyme that converts single-stranded HIV RNA into double-stranded DNA) and protease inhibitors. HIV protease cleaves viral polyprotein precursors into individual functional proteins. Protease inhibition results in the formation of less infectious HIV particles. Antiretroviral agents can be used as monotherapy, combination therapy or alternating therapy[100,101]. Approved antiretroviral agents are listed in Table 2.

Although there are no rigid guidelines, initiation of antiretroviral therapy is recommended for the following categories of HIV-positive patients[102,103]:

(1) Those with acute (primary) HIV infection or recent (less than 6 months ago) seroconversion, regardless of CD4 counts or HIV RNA measurements;

(2) Symptomatic patients with AIDS-related complex or AIDS, regardless of CD4 counts or HIV RNA measurements;

(3) Asymptomatic patients with CD4 counts less than 500 cells/mm³ (two measurements during a 2-week period) or HIV RNA with more than 10 000 copies/ml of plasma (measured by branched-chain DNA amplification) or more than 20 000 copies/ml (measured by reverse transcriptase-PCR) in two measurements within 2 weeks. For patients with CD4 counts of 350–500 cells/mm³ and HIV RNA measurements lower than the above levels, initiation of aniretroviral therapy is still a matter of debate. On the other hand, some experts recommend immediate initiation of treatment of all asymptomatic seropositve individuals even with CD4 counts greater than 500 cells/mm³. However, this is not generally accepted;

(4) HIV-positive pregnant women and infants born to HIV-infected mothers, to prevent vertical or perinatal transmission;

(5) Individuals exposed to HIV, e.g. injured by contaminated needles, as post-exposure prophylaxis. Prophylaxis for other forms of exposure has also been considered.

Initial antiretroviral therapy

Studies and clinical trials show significant improvement of prognosis for HIV patients receiving early combination antiretroviral therapy[98,99,104]. In contrast, there are insufficient data to support the use of monotherapy or alternating therapy. A combination of three agents, preferably two nucleoside reverse transcriptase inhibitors (NRTIs) and one protease inhibitor is strongly recommended[105,106]. Suggested NRTI pairs include: zidovudine plus didanosine, stavudine plus didanosine, zidovudine plus zalcitabine, zidovudine plus lamivudine and stavudine plus lamivudine. In addition, a protease inhibitor, such as indinavir, neflinavir, saquinavir or ritonavir, can be used. Alternatively, two NRTIs, as described above, plus one non-nucleoside reverse transcriptase inhibitor (NNRTI), such as nevirapine or delavirdine, may be given to the patient.

Table 2 Antiretroviral agents

Nucleoside analogs	Non-nucleoside analogs	Protease inhibitors	Nucleotide analog
zidovudine/AZT	nevirapine	ritonavir	adefovir
zalcitabine/DDC	delavirdine	indinavir	
didanosine/DDI	efavirenz	nelfinavir	
stavudine/d4T		saquinavir	
lamivudine/3TC		amprenavir	
abacavir			

Treatment failure

Treatment failure is regarded as failure to sustain HIV RNA by at least 1 log after 4 weeks of therapy; or to reduce it to undetectable levels (< 50 copies/ml) after 6 months of therapy; or a marked decline of CD4 cell counts (more than 50%); or CD4 counts under 100 cells/mm³; or the occurrence of a new or recurrent opportunistic illness[107,108]. Under these circumstances, the antiretroviral regimen should be changed. Change of regime is also indicated in case of adverse effects (Figure 6) or serious problems with adherence to the regime. Ideally, all agents already given should be replaced or at least two new agents should be administered. Whenever viral resistance data are available, these may be of help in decision making, especially after the failure of the second or the third regime[109].

Prevention of vertical transmission

Antiretroviral therapy with zidovudine has been shown to reduce HIV transmission significantly during pregnancy or delivery[76,110]. Because the safety of antiretrovirals has not yet been documented, it is wise to postpone the initiation of therapy or temporarily to interrupt antiretroviral therapy until the end of the 14th week of pregnancy. If there is no other indication for starting antiretroviral therapy, monotherapy with zidovudine is the treatment of choice[40] (300 mg twice a day or 200 mg three times a day or 100 mg five times a day, orally, throughout pregnancy). If the patient is already receiving antiretroviral therapy, or combination therapy is indicated, the regimen should also include zidovudine. During labor, zidovudine should be administered intravenously (loading infusion of 2 mg/kg for 1 h, followed by continuous infusion of 1 mg/kg per hour until delivery)[40]. Zidovudine should also be given to the newborn at 2 mg/kg, orally, every 6 h for the first 6 weeks of life, beginning 8–12 h after birth[111]. If resistance to zidovudine is present, stavudine may be used.

Post-exposure prophylaxis

Following accidental exposure to HIV, the exposed skin or mucous membrane should be thoroughly washed. Blood specimens from both the source person and the exposed person should be obtained to determine the HIV status. The risk depends on the contaminated material, the nature of the injury, the integrity of the exposed area and the HIV status of the source person. Prophylaxis should be started immediately, preferably within 1–2 h from exposure. A combination of zidovudine, lamivudine and indinavir or neflinavir should be administered over a period of 4 weeks[112].

PREVENTION

'To prevent is better than to treat', as taught by Hippocrates 2500 years ago, is even more valid regarding HIV infection. The medical, psychological, social, ethical and financial cost for every HIV patient is so high that, as has been rightly said, every infection that is prevented represents an enormous public health victory[7].

Unfortunately, despite tireless research efforts, an effective vaccine is not currently available. Emphasis should therefore be placed on the education of the population regarding the modes of transmission, factors that increase the risk of the transmission and methods of effective prevention. As far as women are concerned, preventive strategies should be targeted to the whole female population, particularly to sexually active women and those at high-risk, i.e. commercial sex workers, injecting drug users or partners of injecting drug users, and those engaged in unprotected high-risk sexual behaviors[14,38]. Messages may carry more weight if they come from members of the same high-risk group[113].

Programs to reduce sexual transmission should aim, first, to educate women who may be at risk and, second, to enhance safer sex practices. Latex condoms represent an effective mechanical barrier to HIV, and their use should be encouraged[8,114,115]. The female condom may be an alternative that allows women to have control over safe sex practices[116]. It is of interest that, among African-American or Hispanic women in the USA, negative attitudes toward condoms or association with prostitution and 'loose' sexual behaviors are the main arguments for not using condoms[117]. To reduce transmission via injected drug use, referrals to chemical dependency treatment programs and access to needle exchange programs may be of help. Drug users who enter methadone treatment are significantly less likely to become HIV infected[118]. Screening of pregnant women for HIV, zidovudine therapy during pregnancy and recommendations to avoid breast feeding can dramatically reduce the risk of mother-to-child transmission.

CONCLUSION

Strategies for effective primary prevention of HIV must be a top public health priority.

REFERENCES

1. UNAIDS. *WHO Report on the Global HIV/AIDS Epidemic*. Geneva: WHO, 1997

2. Stratigos JD, Tzala E. Global epidemiology of HIV infection and AIDS. *Clin Dermatol* 2000; in press

3. Wright SW, Johnson RA. Human immunodeficiency virus in women. Mucocutaneous manifestations. *Clin Dermatol* 1997;5:93–111

4. Fowler MG, Melnick SL, Mathieson BJ. Women and HIV. Epidemiology and global overview. *Obstet Gynecol Clin North Am* 1997;24:705–29

5. The Global Aids Policy Coalition. *Status and Trends of HIV/AIDS Pandemic as of January 1996*. Cambridge: Harvard School of Public Health, 1997

6. Centers for Disease Control and Prevention. *HIV/AIDS Surveillance Report 7 (no. 2)*. Atlanta: Centers for Disease Control and Prevention, 1995

7. Cohen M. Natural history of HIV infection in women. *Obstet Gynecol Clin North Am* 1997;24:743–58

8. Novello AC. The HIV/AIDS epidemic: a current picture. *J Acquir Immune Defic Syndr* 1993;6:645–54

9. Rosenberg PS, Biggar R, Goedert JJ. Declining age at HIV infection in the United States. *N Engl J Med* 1994;330:789–90

10. Melnick SL, Sherer R, Louis TA, *et al.* Survival and disease progression according to gender of patients with HIV infection. *JAMA* 1994;272:1915–21

11. Wasser SC, Gwinn M, Fleming P. Urban–nonurban distribution of HIV infection in childbearing women in the United States. *J Acquir Immune Defic Syndr* 1993;6:1035–42

12. Gwinn M, Pappaioannou M, George JR, *et al.* Prevalence of HIV infection in childbearing women in the United States. Surveillance using newborn blood samples. *JAMA* 1991;265:1704–8

13. Selik RM, Chu SY, Buehler JW. HIV infection as leading cause of death among young adults in US cities and states. *JAMA* 1993;269:2991–4

14. Coodley GO, Coodley MK, Thompson AF. Clinical aspects of HIV infection in women. *J Gen Intern Med* 1995;10:99–110

15. Steel E, Haverkos HW. Increasing incidence of reported cases of AIDS. *N Engl J Med* 1991;325:65–6

16. Centers for Disease Control and Prevention. Update: AIDS among women – United States, 1994. *Morbid Mortal Weekly Rep* 1994;44:81

17. Vincenzi I, European Study Group on Heterosexual Transmission of HIV. A longitudinal study of human immunodefiency virus transmission by heterosexual partners. *N Engl J Med* 1995;331:341–6

18. European Study Group on Heterosexual Transmission of HIV. Comparison of female to male and male to female transmission in 563 stable couples. *Br Med J* 1992;304:807–13

19. Vogt MW, Witt DJ, Craven DE, *et al.* Isolation patterns of the HIV virus from cervical secretions during the menstrual cycle of women at risk for the acquired immunodeficiency syndrome. *Ann Intern Med* 1987;106:380–2

20. European Study Group. Risk factors for male to female transmission of HIV. *Br Med J* 1989;82:411–15

21. Stamm WE, Handsfield HH, Rompalo AM, *et al.* The association between genital ulcer disease and acquision of HIV infection in homosexual men. *JAMA* 1988;260:1429–33

22. Laga M, Manoka AT, Kivuvru M, *et al.* Non-ulcerative sexually transmitted diseases as risk factors for HIV-transmission in women. Results from a cohort study. *AIDS* 1993;7:95–102

23. Daly CC, Helling-Giese GE, Mati JK, *et al.* Contraceptive methods and the transmission of HIV. Implications for family planning. *Genitourin Med* 1994;70:110–17

24. Edlin BR, Irwin KL, Faruque S. Intersecting epidemics – crack cocaine use and HIV infection among inner-city young adults. *N Engl J Med* 1994;331:1422–7

25. Weller I, Williams I. AIDS. In Adler WM, ed. *ABC of Sexually Transmitted Diseases*, 3rd edn. London: BMJ Publishing Group, 1995:32–9

26. Wei X, Ghosh SK, Taylor ME. Viral dynamics in human immunodeficiency virus type I infection. *Nature (London)* 1995;373:117–22

27. Sheffield JVL, Root RK. Natural history. In Spach DH, Hooton TM, eds. *The HIV Manual. A Guide to Diagnosis and Treatment*. New York: Oxford University Press, 1996:34–41

28. Moore RD, Hidalgo J, Sugland BW, *et al.* Zidovudine and the natural history of the acquired immunodeficiency syndrome. *N Engl J Med* 1991;324:1412–16

29. Rutherford GW, Lifson AR, Hessol NA. Course of HIV-1 infection in a cohort of homosexual and bisexual men: an 11-year follow-up study. *Br Med J* 1990;301:1183–8

30. Buchbinder SP, Katz BZ, Hessol NA, *et al.* Long-term HIV-1 infection without immunologic progression. *AIDS* 1994;8:1123–8

31. Sha BE, Benson CA, Pottage JC, *et al.* HIV infection in women. An observational study of clinical characteristics, disease progression and survival for a cohort of women in Chicago. *J Acquir Immune Defic Syndr* 1995;8:486–95

32. Clark PA, Plakley SA, Rice J, *et al.* Predictors of HIV disease progression in women. *J Acquir Immune Defic Syndr* 1995;9:43–7

33. Schuurs AHWM, Verheul HAM. Effects of gender and sex steroids on the immune response. *J Steroid Biochem* 1990;35:157–72

34. Lepri AC, Pezzotti P, Dorucci M, *et al.* HIV disease progression in 854 women and men infected through injecting drug use and heterosexual sex

and followed for up to nine years from serono-version. *Br Med J* 1994;309:1537–42

35. Brettle RP, Leen CLS. The natural history of HIV and AIDS in women. *AIDS* 1991;5:1283–92

36. Chang HH, Morse DL, Noonan C. Survival and mortality patterns of an acquired immunodeficiency syndrome (AIDS) cohort in New York State. *Am J Epidemiol* 1993;138:341–9

37. Chaisson RE, Keruly JC, Moore RD. Race, sex, drug use and progression of human immunodeficiency virus disease. *N Engl J Med* 1995;333:751–6

38. Carpenter CCJ, Meyer KH, Stein MD, *et al.* Human immunodeficiency virus infection in North American women: experience with 200 cases and a review of the literature. *Medicine* 1991;70:307–25

39. Smith E, Orholm M. Trends and patterns of opportunistic disease in Danish AIDS patients 1980–1990. *Scand J Infect Dis* 1990;22:665–72

40. Celum CZ, Watts DH. HIV and women. In Spach DH, Hooton TM, eds. *The HIV Manual. A Guide to Diagnosis and Treatment*. New York: Oxford University Press, 1996:120–7

41. Fleming PL, Ciesielski CA, Byers RH, *et al.* Gender differences in reported AIDS – indicative diagnoses. *J Infect Dis* 1993;168:61–7

42. Imam N, Carpenter CCJ, Mayer KH, *et al.* Hierarchial pattern of mucosal candida infections in HIV-seropositive women. *Am J Med* 1990;89:142–6

43. Rhoads JL, Wright DC, Redfield RR, Burke DS. Chronic vaginal candidiasis in women with human immunodeficiency virus infection. *JAMA* 1987;257:3105–7

44. Spinillo A, Michelone G, Cavanna C. Clinical and microbiological characteristics of symptomatic vulvovaginal candidiasis in HIV seropositive women. *Genitourin Med* 1994;70:268–72

45. Sacks SL, Wanklin RJ, Reece DE, *et al.* Progressive esophagitis from an acyclovir-resistant herpes simplex. Clinical roles for DNA polymerase mutants and viral heterogeneity? *Ann Intern Med* 1989;111:893–9

46. Byrne MA, Taylor-Robinson D, Munday PE, Harris JRW. The common occurrence of human papillomavirus infection and intraepithelial neoplasia in women infected by HIV. *AIDS* 1989;3:379–82

47. Feingold AR, Vermund SH, Burk RD, *et al.* Cervical cytologic abnormalities and papillomavirus in women infected with human immunodeficiency virus. *J Acquir Immune Defic Syndr* 1990;3:896–903

48. Spinillo A, Tenti P, Zappatore R, *et al.* Langerhans' cell counts and cervical intraepithelial neoplasia in women with human immunodeficiency virus infection. *Gynecol Oncol* 1993;48:210–13

49. Schafer A, Friedmann W, Mielke M, *et al.* The increased frequency of cervical dysplasia/neoplasia in women infected with the human immunodeficiency virus is related to the degree of immunosuppression. *Am J Obstet Gynecol* 1991;164:593–9

50. Spurrett B, Jones DS, Stewart G. Cervical dysplasia and HIV infection. *Lancet* 1988;1:237–8

51. Rabkin CS, Biggar BJ, Baptiste MS, *et al.* Cancer incidence trends in women at high risk of human immunodeficiency virus (HIV) infection. *Int J Cancer* 1993;55:208–12

52. Levine AM. AIDS-related malignancies. The emerging epidemic. *J Natl Cancer Inst* 1993;85:1382–97

53. Stavrianeas NG, Polydorou D, Paparizos V, *et al.* Systemic treatment for AIDS-associated Kaposi's sarcoma. The experience of Athens University Hospital for Skin and Venereal Diseases. *Skin Cancer* 1996;11:95–101

54. Tappero JW, Conant MA, Wolfe SF, *et al.* Kaposi's sarcoma: epidemiology, pathogenesis, histology, clinical presentation, staging criteria and therapy. *J Am Acad Dermatol* 1993;28:371–95

55. Serraino D, Franceschi S, Dal Maso L, *et al.* HIV transmission and Kaposi's sarcoma among European women. *AIDS* 1995;9:791–4

56. Stratigos JD, Potouridou I, Katoulis AC, *et al.* Classic Kaposi's sarcoma in Greece. A clinico-epidemiological profile. *Int J Dermatol* 1997;36:735–40

57. Chang Y, Cesarman E, Pess MS, *et al.* Identification of herpes virus-like DNA sequences in AIDS-associated Kaposi's sarcoma. *Science* 1994;266:1865–9

58. Moore PS, Chang Y. Detection of herpesvirus-like DNA sequences in Kaposi's sarcoma in patients with and without HIV infection. *N Engl J Med* 1995;332:1181–5

59. Lassoued K, Chauvel J, Fegneux S, *et al.* AIDS-associated Kaposi's sarcoma in female patients. *AIDS* 1991;5:877–80

60. Nahlen BL, Chu SY, Nwanyanwu O, *et al.* HIV wasting syndrome in the United States. *AIDS* 1993;7:183–8

61. Resnick L, Herbst JS, Raab-Traub N. Oral hairy leucoplakia. *J Am Acad Dermatol* 1990;22:1278–82

62. Shiboski CH, Hilton JF, Greenspan D, *et al.* HIV related oral manifestations in two cohorts of women in San Francisco. *J AIDS* 1994;7:964–71

63. Witt DJ, Craven DE, McCabe WR. Bacterial infections in adult patients with the acquired immunodeficiency syndrome (AIDS) and AIDS-related complex. *Am J Med* 1987;82:900–6

64. Shah PN, Smith JR, Iatrakis GM, *et al.* Kitchen vs HIV infection and menstrual abnormalities. *Genitourin Med* 1992;68:425–6

65. Safrin S, Dattel BJ, Hauer L, Sweet PZ. Seroprevalence and epidemiologic correlates of human immunodeficiency virus infection in women with acute pelvic inflammatory disease. *Obstet Gynecol* 1990;75:666–70

66. Hoegsberg B, Abulafia O, Sedlis A, *et al.* Sexually transmitted diseases and human immunodeficiency virus infection among women with pelvic inflammatory disease. *Am J Obstet Gynecol* 1990;163:1135–9

67. Pizzi M. Women, HIV infection and AIDS: tapestries of life, death and empowerment. *Am J Occup Ther* 1992;46:1021–7

68. Brown GR, Rundell JR. A prospective study of psychiatric aspects of early HIV disease in women. *Gen Hosp Psychiatry* 1993;15:139–47

69. Biggar RJ, Pahwa S, Minkoff H, *et al.* Immunosuppression in pregnant women infected with human immunodeficiency virus. *Am J Obstet Gynecol* 1989;161:1239–44

70. Kell PD, Johnston FD (reply). Survival time after AIDS in pregnancy (letter). *Br J Obstet Gynaecol* 1993;100:397–8

71. Minkoff HL, Willoughby A, Mendez H, *et al.* Serious infections during pregnancy among women with advanced immunodeficiency virus infection. *Am J Obstet Gynecol* 1990;162:30–4

72. Brettle PP, Raab GM, Ross A, *et al.* HIV infection in women: immunologic markers and the influence of pregnancy. *AIDS* 1995;9:1177–84

73. Deschamps M, Pape JW, Devarieux J, *et al.* A prospective study of HIV-seropositive asymptomatic women of childbearing age in a developing country. *J Acquir Immune Defic Syndr* 1993;6:446–51

74. Newell ML, Dunn D, Peckham CS, *et al.* Risk factors for mother-to-child transmission of HIV-1. *Lancet* 1992;339:1007–12

75. St Louis ME, Kamenga M, Brown C, *et al.* Risk for perinatal HIV-1 transmission according to maternal immunologic, virologic and placental factors. *JAMA* 1993;269:2853–9

76. Connor EM, Sperling RS, Gelber R, *et al.* Reduction of maternal–infant transmission of human immunodeficiency virus type 1 with zidovudine treatment. *N Engl J Med* 1994;331:1173–80

77. Bulterys M, Lepage P. Mother-to-child transmission of HIV. *Curr Opin Pediatr* 1998;10:143–50

78. Goedert JJ, Duliege A, Amos CL, *et al.* High risk of HIV-1 infection for first-born twins. *Lancet* 1991;338:1471–5

79. Connor E, Bardeguez A, Apuzzio J. The intrapartum management of the HIV-infected mother and her infant. *Clin Perinatol* 1989;16:899–908

80. Minkoff HL. Care of pregnant women infected with human immunodeficiency virus. *JAMA* 1987;258:2714–17

81. Minkoff HL, Henderson C, Mendez H, *et al.* Pregnancy outcomes among mothers infected with human immunodeficiency virus and uninfected control subjects. *Am J Obstet Gynecol* 1990;163:1598–604

82. Ryder RW, Nsa W, Hassig SE, *et al.* Perinatal transmission of the human immunodeficiency virus type 1 to infants of seropositive women in Zaire. *N Engl J Med* 1989;320:1637–41

83. Langston C, Lewis DE, Hammill HA, *et al.* Excess intrauterine fetal demise associated with maternal human immunodeficiency virus infection. *J Infect Dis* 1995;172:1451–60

84. Goldbaum GM, Chafee F. Counseling, testing and risk reduction. In Spach DH, Hooton TM, eds. *The HIV Manual. A Guide to Diagnosis and Treatment.* New York: Oxford University Press, 1996:20–7

85. Centers for Disease Control and Prevention. *HIV Counseling, Testing and Referral Standards and Guidelines.* Atlanta, GA: US Department of Health and Human Services, 1994

86. Goldberg DJ, Johnstone FD. Universal named testing of pregnant women for HIV. *Br Med J* 1993;306:1144–5

87. Gaines H, Sydow MV, Sonnerborg A, *et al.* Antibody response in primary human immunodeficiency virus infection. *Lancet* 1987;1:1249–53

88. Celum CL, Coombs RW. Laboratory diagnosis of HIV. In Spach DH, Hooton TM, eds. *The HIV Manual. A Guide to Diagnosis and Treatment.* New York: Oxford University Press, 1996:28–33

89. MacDonell KB, Chmiel JS, Poggensee L, Phair JP. Predicting progression to AIDS: combined usefulness of CD4 lymphocyte counts and p24 antigenemia. *Am J Med* 1990;89:706–12

90. Cavert W, Coombs RW. Laboratory markers of HIV infection. In Spatch DH, Hooton TM. *The HIV Manual. A Guide to Diagnosis and Treatment.* New York: Oxford University Press, 1996:53–9

91. Mellors JW, Kingsley LA, Rinaldo CR, *et al.* Quantitation of HIV-1 RNA plasma predicts outcome after seroconversion. *Ann Intern Med* 1995;122:573–9

92. Coombs RW. HIV-1 burden as a marker of disease progression and clinical response to therapy in AIDS. *Clin Lab Med* 1994;14:301–11

93. Saag MS, Holodniy M, Kuritzkes RD, *et al.* HIV viral load markers in practice. *Nature Med* 1996; 2:625–7

94. Stein DS, Korvick JA, Vermund SH. CD4 + lymphocyte cell enumeration for prediction of clinical course of human immunodeficiency virus disease: a review. *J Infect Dis* 1992;165:352–63

95. O'Brien WA, Hartigan M, Martin D, *et al.* Changes in plasma HIV-1 RNA and CD4 + lymphocyte-counts and the risk of progression to AIDS. *N Engl J Med* 1996;332:209–16

96. Cao Y, Qin I, Zhang L, *et al.* Virologic and immunologic characterization of long-term survivors of human immunodeficiency virus type 1 infection. *N Engl J Med* 1995;332:201–8

97. Reddy MM, Grieco MH. Neopterin and alpha and beta interleukin-1 levels in sera of patients with human immunodeficiency virus infection. *J Clin Microbiol* 1989,27:1919–23

98. Hogg RS, Heath KV, Yip B, *et al.* Improved survival among HIV-infected individuals following initiation of antiretroviral therapy. *JAMA* 1998;279:450–4

99. Palella JF Jr, Delaney KM, Moorman AC, *et al.* Declining morbidity and mortality among patients

with advanced human immunodeficiency virus infection. HIV Outpatient Study Investigators. *N Engl J Med* 1998;338:853–60

100. Chaudry MN, Shepp DH. Antiretroviral agents. Current usage. *Dermatol Clin* 1997;15:319–29

101. Carpenter CC, Fischl MA, Hammer SM, *et al.* Antiretroviral therapy for HIV infection in 1996. Recommendations of an international panel. International AIDS Society – USA. *JAMA* 1996; 276:146–54

102. Guidelines for the use of antiretroviral agents in HIV-infected adults and adolescents. Department of Health and Human Services and Henry J. Kaiser Family Foundation. *Morbid Mortal Weekly Rep* 1998;47:43–82

103. Antiretroviral therapy for HIV infection in 1998. Updated Recommendations of the International AIDS-SOCIETY–USA Panel. *JAMA* 1998;280: 78–86

104. Brettle RP, Wilson A, Povey S, *et al.* Combination therapy for HIV: the effect on inpatient activity, morbidity, and mortality of a cohort of patients. *Int J Sex Transm Dis AIDS* 1998;9:80–7

105. Schmit JC, Weber B. Recent advances in antiretroviral therapy and HIV infection monitoring. *Intervirology* 1997;40:304–21

106. Moyle GJ, Gazzard BG, Cooper DA, Gatell J. Antiretroviral therapy for HIV infection. A knowledge-based approach to drug selection and use. *Drugs* 1998;55:383–404

107. Fatkenheuer G, Theisen A, Rockstroh J, *et al.* Virological treatment failure of protease inhibitor therapy in an unselected cohort of HIV-infected patients. *AIDS* 1997;11:113–16

108. d'Arminio Monforte A, Testa L, Adorni F, *et al.* Clinical outcome and predictive factors of failure of highly active antiretroviral therapy in antiretroviral-experienced patients in advanced stages of HIV-1 infection. *AIDS* 1998;13:1631–7

109. Hirsch MS, Conway B, d'Aquila RT, *et al.* Antiretroviral drug resistance testing in adults with HIV infection. Implications for clinical management. *JAMA* 1998;279:1984–91

110. Conner EM, Sperling RS, Gelber R, *et al.* Reduction of maternal–infant transmission of human immunodeficiency virus type 1 with zidovudine treatment. *N Engl J Med* 1994;331:1173–80

111. Taylor GP, Lyall H, Mercey D, *et al.* British HIV Association guidelines for prescribing antiretroviral therapy in pregnancy, 1998. In Gazzard B, ed. *Chelsea and Westminster Hospital AIDS Care HandBook.* London: Mediscript Ltd Medical Publishers, 1999

112. Pinkerton SD, Holtgrave DR, Bloom FR. Cost-effectiveness of post-exposure prophylaxis following sexual exposure to HIV. *AIDS* 1998;12: 1067–78

113. Mondanaro J. Strategies for AIDS prevention: motivating health behavior in drug dependent women. *J Psychoactive Drugs* 1987;19:143–9

114. Feldblum PJ, Fortney JA. Condoms, spermicides and the transmission of human immunodeficiency virus: a review of the literature. *Am J Public Health* 1988;78:52–4

115. Plummer FA, Simonsen JN, Cameron DW, *et al.* Cofactors in male–female sexual transmission of human immunodeficiency virus type 1. *J Infect Dis* 1991;163:233–9

116. Gollub EL, Stein ZA. The new female condom – item 1 on a women's AIDS prevention agenda. *Am J Public Health* 1993;83:498–500

117. Hinkle YA, Johnson EH, Gilbert D, *et al.* African-American women who always use condoms: attitudes, knowledge about AIDS and sexual behavior. *J Am Med Wom Assoc* 1992;47:230–7

118. Metzger DS, Woody GE, McLellan AJ, *et al.* Human immunodeficiency virus seroconversion among intravenous drug users in- and out-of-treatment: an 18 month prospective follow-up. *J Acquir Immune Defic Syndr* 1993;6:1049–56

Topographic dermatology

Diseases of the breast

28

Diane Roseeuw and Jean-Pierre Hachem

Women's breasts are the site of many physiological and morphological changes during life and can therefore be the nidus of many pathological manifestations. Although most women seek the advice of a gynecologist concerning abnormal findings on the breast, the dermatologist should be aware of breast diseases that may involve or manifest symptoms on the skin and the nipple–areolar region. The skin of the breast may show retraction, redness or edema (Table 1).

Retraction may indicate the presence not only of a carcinoma but also of benign lesions such as mammary duct ectasia, fat necrosis, or Mondor's disease. If cutaneous erythema is present, the possibility of acute or chronic inflammation, or even inflammatory carcinoma, should be considered. Skin edema may be due to infection or possibly carcinoma. The dermatologist may also observe changes of the nipple–areolar complex (Table 2), which enables a distinction to be made between physiological and pathological conditions. Nipple inversion, retraction, flattening, broadening and deviation may indicate the involvement of breast cancer. Alternatively, these manifestations may be acquired without any associated pathologies. The skin of the nipples and areolas can be thickened, red or eroded, indicating disorders such as Paget's disease, contact dermatitis, erosive adenomatosis of the nipple, or cracked nipples of the lactating mother.

With a view to imparting a detailed understanding of the various physiological and pathological conditions of the female breast, a short description of the developmental course of the breast follows.

The human breast begins to develop in the 6th week of fetal life with the formation of a symmetrical ectodermal thickening called the 'milk line', joining the axilla to the inguinal region. Further mammary gland development may occur along this milk line, with the number and location of these glands being specific for the species (Figure 1). In human beings, one pair of breasts start to form in the fourth intercostal space with the disappearance of the major part of the milk line during the 3rd month. The mammary gland is formed in the 8th month of development[1]. At birth, the human breast is undeveloped.

The areola forms a slightly pigmented thickening of skin with few rudimentary glands around a slightly elevated nipple. No demonstrable differences can be observed between boys and girls. Later on, sweat glands and specialized sebaceous glands develop. During pregnancy, these sebaceous glands produce oily secretions that protect the skin of the areola and nipple during lactation. No hair grows on the areolar surface, but hair may be present on the surrounding skin.

INFANCY

Most breast diseases that dermatologists encounter in neonates are malformations and abscesses.

Amastia

Amastia, or absence of the breast and the nipple, is a very rare condition. Small rudimentary breasts are not as rare. Usually there is associated underdevelopment or absence of the shoulder girdle structures, the chest or the arm. This condition has been reported in the AREDYLD syndrome, which consists of ectodermal dysplasia, lipoatrophy and diabetes mellitus[2], as well as in Poland's disease, which is characterized by the absence of the pectoralis major and minor and a homolateral brachysyndactyly[3]. Cosmetic surgery is required in adulthood, with a complete evaluation of the disorder.

Neonatal mammary hyperplasia

Neonatal mammary hyperplasia is a physiological condition occurring in 70% of newborns[4]. It is characterized by the sudden onset of unilateral or bilateral mammary development and in 50% of cases is accompanied by colostrum secretion ('witch's milk'). Physiological hyperplasia occurs by the 4th day of birth and regresses spontaneously after 3 weeks. This phenomenon is considered to be a response to elevated levels of maternal hormones in the infant's blood. Its involution is more complete in boys than in girls. The absence of a palpable gland is considered to be a criterion of prematurity.

Table 1   Skin symptoms associated with breast diseases

Retraction
Duct ectasia
Fat necrosis
Mondor's disease
Carcinoma

Redness
Acute inflammation
Chronic infection
Carcinoma
Paget's disease

Edema or thickening
Infection
Carcinoma
Paget's disease

Table 2   Nipple–areolar diseases

Physiological
Supernumerary nipples
Inverted nipples
Jogger's irritation
Cracked nipple of lactating women

Pathological
Contact dermatitis
Paget's disease
Hyperkeratosis
Erosive adenomatosis

Supernumerary nipples (polythelia) or breasts (polymastia)

In 90% of cases, the 'milk line' is the preferred site of supernumerary nipples and, less frequently, of supernumerary breasts[5]. The supernumerary nipple is considered to be a minor condition, and affects more women (2–4%) than men. Both hereditary cases and correlation with familial alcoholism have been reported[6]. Cases of supernumerary nipples have been discussed in association with Becker's nevus[7], aplasia cutis congenita, Hay–Wells syndrome, neurofibromatosis type 1, Bannayan–Riley–Ruvacalba syndrome, Simpson–Golabi–Behmel syndrome, Birt–Hogg–Dubé syndrome, incontinentia pigmenti[8], skeletal anomalies[9] and renal anomalies[10]. The last-named is characterized by a higher prevalence of urological malformations such as obstructive uropathy[11] and malignancies[12], as seen in Caucasian children. There is no evidence of a significant correlation between supernumerary nipples and renal abnormalities, which makes the routine urinary tract examination of newborns with a supernumerary nipple controversial[13,14]. The examination of newborns with supernumerary nipples should be done carefully, however, in order to exclude any other malformation.

Clinically, the supernumerary nipple with or without the areola or breast glands usually appears on the chest wall, although other locations are possible. In most cases, the supernumerary nipple manifests itself as a brownish papule and can easily be confused with a pigmented nevus (Figure 2).

The diagnosis of supernumerary breasts can be difficult, because the condition can be confounded with tumors, especially if it develops during puberty or pregnancy. For example, the axillary tail of Spence is characterized by breast tissue expansion to the axillary region and sometimes manifests itself through pain and swelling during puberty or pregnancy. If the clinical diagnosis is difficult to establish, fine needle aspiration may help to identify breast tissues.

As these structures have pathological degeneration potential, long-term follow-up is indicated. Simple excision of the supernumerary mammary tissue can be performed as a symptomatic, cosmetic, or preventive measure.

Neonatal breast abscess

Breast abscesses occur mainly in the 3rd or 4th week of life and seem to affect more girls than boys[15]. Neonatal mammary hyperplasia constitutes a possible risk factor. It does not concern the premature newborn, owing to the lack of mammary tissue development. Sometimes, staphylococcal epidemics in newborn nurseries are observed with the onset of breast abscesses[16].

The most frequent presentation is a unilateral swelling with warmth, erythema and pain. In some cases, only swelling might be present. Fever is observed in only 25% of cases[15]. Complications are rare, but the literature reports necrotizing fasciitis following a breast abscess[17]. A few girls maintain abnormal tissue development of the affected area into adulthood. The diagnosis is mainly clinical, but in some cases a needle aspiration can help to differentiate this entity from neonatal mammary hyperplasia.

For some authors, incision and drainage followed by antibiotics[18] (methicillin, amoxycillin–clavulinic acid) is needed. For others, the surgical incision can be avoided through early antimicrobial therapy[16].

ADOLESCENCE

Between the ages of 8 and 14, the development of the breast constitutes the first sign of female puberty (thelarche). In general, it is believed that estrogen influences the development of the nipple, the adipose tissue and the duct system[19]. Progesterone is required for alveolus maturation. Insulin, adrenal glucocorticoids, growth hormones and prolactin play a role in protein metabolism[20,21]. The breast continues its maturation until the age of 16 to 18, showing various morphological aspects[22]. Premature thelarche consists of the development of the breast before the age of 8 years without the concomitant evolution of the other secondary sexual characteristics. In these children, a maturational defect of the hypothalamic–pituitary–gonadal axis, with elevated levels of serum follicle stimulating hormone (FSH), seems to be the cause. Therefore, any girl with premature breast development must undergo a complete endocrinological evaluation to rule out an active tumor, the ingestion of estrogenic substances, or true isosexual precocious puberty[1].

In this section we discuss mainly the anomalies of breast aspects that can affect adolescent women.

Hypoplasia

Varying degrees of hypoplasia can affect young women. The size of the breasts depends not only on the gland components but also on the development of adipose tissue (Figure 3). Racial differences also play a role and are common. In the majority of cases, underdevelopment is observed with thin women. Fifty per cent of women with hypomastia presented mitral valve prolapsus as compared with an incidence of 6% in a normal control group[23,24].

Cardiac examination is recommended in these women to exclude bacterial endocarditis and arrhythmias. Estrogen treatment can be useful in Turner's syndrome, but has no effect in the treatment of idiopathic hypoplasia. In such circumstances, plastic surgical reconstruction (prostheses, fat grafts) is indicated.

The craniofrontonasal syndrome is an X-linked disease affecting mainly women. In 11% of cases it includes hair anomalies, anterior cranium bifidum, axillary pterygia, asymmetric lower limb shortness and postpubertal unilateral breast hypoplasia[25]. Hypomastia can be acquired as a consequence of other diseases, such as anorexia nervosa, tuberculosis and morphea[26].

Breast asymmetry

Just like other organs, the two breasts can never be identical. The degree of asymmetry can be evaluated only after complete development (Figure 4). When an important asymmetry is present, patients may complain of pain in the breast, shoulders, back or neck. They may be emotionally distressed. The cause may be due to a varying sensitivity of the target cells to hormones. Plastic surgery is often indicated, and hormonal treatment should be avoided.

Hypertrophy of the breast

Breast hypertrophy generally occurs during puberty; sometimes the breasts grow very rapidly in the space of a year, reaching a weight of up to 6–13 kg. The overlying skin may show inflammatory and edematous reactions. The skin is tender, and has striae and ulcerations. Associated symptoms are lumbar lordosis with frequent psychological implications. No 'target estrogen organ' activity has been correlated with hypertrophy. In fact, the estrogen receptors remained undetectable in 25 patients with breast hypertrophy[27]. A familial pattern is rarely reported, but in most cases the condition occurs as virginal bilateral breast hypertrophy (rarely unilateral). Reduction mammoplasty has proven efficacious in relieving rheumatological pain and may be helpful when it comes to psychological problems[28].

ADULT WOMEN

In this section we describe the various problems that may affect women during adulthood. Benign dermatoses, malignant diseases and iatrogenic disorders are discussed.

Jogger's nipple

Jogger's nipple dermatosis may be a difficult diagnosis to make, but it should be kept in mind with reference to long-distance joggers who do not wear a bra. It appears as a painful erosion that sometimes bleeds, but diminishes during sedentary periods. Jogger's nipples can be prevented by the application of tape to the nipples and areolas during jogging. It can also be avoided by the wearing of a bra and a silk or semi-synthetic T-shirt[29,30].

Inverted nipple

The inverted nipple is a common finding in adult women (Figure 5). This benign condition is caused by the lack of development of the fibrous bands

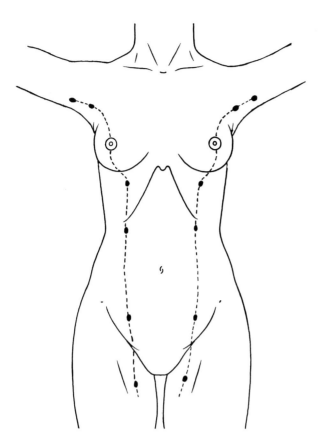

Figure 1   The milk line or the distribution of the supernumerary nipples and breasts

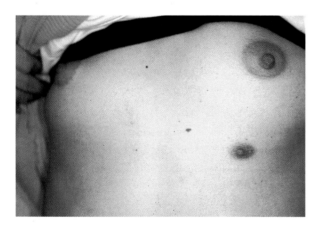

Figure 2   Supernumerary nipple on the chest wall of a young woman. Courtesy of P. Wylock, MD, Brussels, Belgium

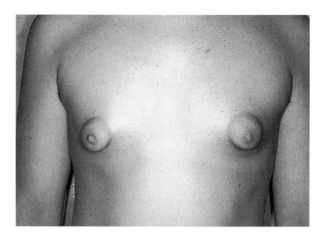

Figure 3   Breast hypoplasia. Only rudimentary mammary tissue is present. Courtesy of P. Wylock, MD, Brussels, Belgium

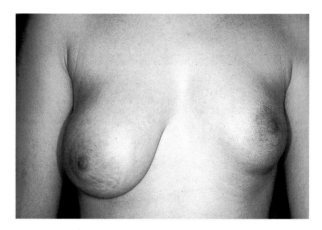

Figure 4   Breast asymmetry in a young woman. Courtesy of P. Wylock, MD, Brussels, Belgium

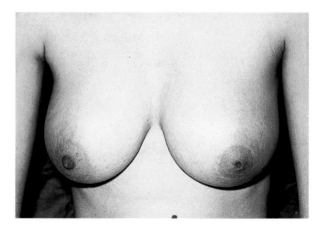

Figure 5   Nipple inversion of the left breast. The normal anatomy of the nipple can be observed on the right breast of the patient. Courtesy of P. Wylock, MD, Brussels, Belgium

that fix the nipple to the underlying fascia. Sometimes, spontaneous improvements are noted during pregnancy. On the other hand, if the condition does not improve, breast feeding may be seriously compromised.

Acquired inversion of the nipple should be investigated for the possibility of underlying cancer (namely, breast cancer).

While plastic surgery corrects the esthetic aspect of the nipple, it causes the destruction of the breast function and is therefore not advised in young women[31]. New non-aggressive methods, such as use of suction devices, have given good results when carried out as a daily exercise. These devices apply a negative pressure to the nipple in order to draw it out[32].

Nipple discharge and galactorrhea

Galactorrhea is a spontaneous nipple secretory discharge having a milky aspect and occurring in non-pregnant or non-lactating women.

Normal nipple discharge is physiologically acceptable in the following situations: in patients taking oral contraceptives, during the second and third trimesters of pregnancy, in those with breast engorgement during menstruation and in women nearing the menopause[33].

Abnormal nipple discharge as galactorrhea in non-pregnant, non-lactating women can be provoked by multiple causes (Table 3).

In the idiopathic form, circulating prolactin levels are normal, but regular control of the prolactin level is important. If concomitant hyperprolactinemia is found, a complete evaluation by an endocrinologist should be carried out to exclude central nervous system lesions or other endocrine disturbances. Drugs and trauma are also known to be a possible cause of galactorrhea[1].

Discharge may be bloody or serous. For the majority (75%) of patients, serous or bloody nipple discharge is due to mammary duct ectasia (see below) or intraductal papilloma. A biopsy may be necessary to exclude a carcinoma if a palpable mass is detected. Black galactorrhea is of special interest in a dermatology practice and is discussed in connection with iatrogenic disorders of the breast.

Erosive adenomatosis of the nipple

Erosive adenomatosis of the nipple is also known as papillary adenoma of the nipple, florid papillomatosis of the nipple ducts, subareolar duct papillomatosis and benign papillomatosis of the nipple. This pathology consists of a complex benign proliferation of the epithelium of the lactiferous ducts and the milk sinuses. It affects mainly adult women.

The onset of the clinical course may be insidious and usually starts on one side with a serous or bloody discharge, associated with a crusted eroded or eczematous nipple. Premenstrual worsening is observed[34]. Occasionally, a nodule that adheres to the skin but that migrates across the mammary gland is palpable (Figure 6). The cutaneous lesion may be accompanied by itching, irritation, or pain. Differential diagnoses include atopic dermatitis, Paget's disease, or a sweat gland tumor.

Table 3 Causes of galactorrhea

Idiopathic
Induced
Drugs
oral contraceptives
neuroleptica
imipramine
reserpine
methyldopa
amphetamine
Infections
herpes zoster
Trauma
head
thoracotomy
Central nervous system lesions
Hypothalamic–pituitary tumors
Empty sella
Endocrinological diseases
Cushing's disease
Hepatic cirrhoses
Hypothyroidism
Chronic diseases
Chronic renal failure
Schuller–Christian disease
Sarcoidosis

A diagnosis of erosive adenomatosis of the nipple can be established only by histological examination. The histopathology is characterized by tubes and papillae lined by a double layer of epithelial and myoepithelial cells: the adluminal layer consists of cylindrical cells showing an apocrine differentiation; the myoepithelial cells are cuboidal and separate the epithelium from the connective tissues. Papillomatosis and adenomatosis are observed separately and may coexist. Infiltrate contains eosinophils and in some cases giant cells. The overlying epidermis may show acanthosis and hyperkeratosis as well as ulcerations[34,35].

The differential diagnosis with Paget's disease should be ruled out by skin biopsy[36] or fine needle aspiration cytology[37] in order to avoid unnecessary radical surgery. In fact, non-mutilating limited excision can be performed. The treatment of choice is a limited local excision. The excision, however, has to be complete; otherwise there can be a recurrence.

As the nipple and areola are an important cosmetic anatomic area, complete but minimal excision of the lesion is important and micrographic surgery is recommended in these cases[38]. Later, if necessary, reconstructive surgery would be easier to perform.

Hyperkeratosis of the nipple and areola

Hyperkeratosis of the nipple is a rare dermatosis[39], usually affecting women between the second and the third decades of life. Clinically, it appears as a dark brownish verrucous thickening of the nipple and areola and is usually bilateral. Sometimes only the nipple or only the areola is affected. Accentuation is possible during pregnancy, making lactation impossible. Microscopic examination of the skin shows hyperkeratosis, acanthosis and papillomatosis[40].

This condition has been associated with various diseases[41,42], such as Darier's disease, acanthosis nigricans, ichthyosiform erythroderma and ichthyosis. The most frequently reported combination is with T-cell lymphoma and mycosis fungoides[41]. Clinical examinations for the purpose of searching for a possible underlying disease should be undertaken.

If the hyperkeratosis is unilateral, it may be part of an epidermal nevus[42]. Because hyperkeratosis of the nipple and areola, as mentioned in the literature, is mostly associated with other diseases, diagnosis and treatment of the underlying condition are imperative if the hyperkeratosis is to be relieved. Additional treatment with keratolytic agents or cryotherapy may help. The topical use of 12% lactic acid lotion has been reported to resolve the situation within 6 months[41]. Retinoid therapy seems to be ineffective[43].

Dermatitis

In dermatological practice, eczema of the breasts and nipples is mainly observed during lactation and in atopic patients. In reality, it is the treatment of infected lactating nipples that regularly induces contact dermatitis. In atopic adult patients, eczema of the nipples is due to mechanical irritation. The position of the breast is believed to play a role in the onset of eczema[44–46]. Mild cortisone cream can resolve the situation in both conditions, but long-term skin hydration should be initiated to prevent relapse. The use of cotton bras is recommended for atopic patients.

Infectious diseases of the skin must sometimes be excluded. This could be the case with scabies, which may infest the mammary area and the nipples. A history of night itching spreading to the rest of the family is typical of scabies. Physical examination also discloses other nidi of the parasite.

Candida is often implicated in breast intertrigo and may clinically mimic eczema. Occasionally

Paget's disease can be misdiagnosed as eczema, especially if it presents as a round, unilateral erythematous lesion of the nipple in older women. In this case, a biopsy is advisable in order to exclude a malignancy (i.e. Paget's disease).

Hair sinus of the breasts

Hair sinus is mainly observed as an occupational dermatitis affecting the interdigital spaces and nail edges of barbers, but it can also be observed on the breasts of women shepherds (sheep shearing)[47], in dog groomers and in hairdressers[48]. It may cause mastalgia and recurrent infections and abcesses. As a preventive measure, a protective bra can be worn. Treatment consists of total excision of the sinus.

Mastitis

Mastitis presents as an erythematous inflammatory infiltration of the skin and manifests general symptoms, depending on the cause. Mastitis may, in fact, be due to either infectious agents (puerperal mastitis, extrapuerperal mastitis) or non-infectious pathogens (carcinomatous mastitis, granulomatous mastitis, B-lymphocytic mastitis). Mastitis is rare and often occurs subsequent to carcinomatous invasion of an underlying breast cancer[49]. If mastitis symptoms are observed in non-pregnant women, the investigation should be oriented towards excluding the possibility of breast cancer through a skin biopsy and mammography[50].

Puerperal mastitis and carcinomatous mastitis are discussed further on in this chapter; in this section we describe extra- or non-puerperal mastitis, tuberculosis and syphilitic mastitis, granulomatous mastitis and B-lymphocytic mastitis (Table 4).

Infectious mastitis

Extrapuerperal mastitis   This is relatively rare; the infection of the breast is accompanied by general symptoms such as fever with chills, fatigue, tachycardia, headache, malaise and anorexia. The involvement is usually unilateral. Cutaneous findings consist of erythema, tenderness and induration of the skin and breast. By far the most common organism associated with breast infections is *Staphylococcus aureus*.

Extrapuerperal mastitis can easily be misdiagnosed as inflammatory carcinoma, erysipelas of the breast region, or carcinoma erysipelatoides. Leukocytosis is an indication of an acute inflammatory reaction. Non-puerperal mastitis is often due to rare or obscure organisms. If not treated in time

Table 4 Different types of mastitis, etiologies and a few typical characteristics

Mastitis	Etiology	Characteristics
Puerperal mastitis	infections	lactating women
Extrapuerperal mastitis	infections	no underlying breast cancer
Tuberculosis	infections	young pregnant women with history of tuberculosis
Syphilis	infections	serology reactive
Granulomatous mastitis	idiopathic, rarely infectious	young women
Erysipeloides carcinoma	breast cancer, idiopathic	underlying breast cancer
B-lymphocytic mastitis	systemic involvement	insulin-dependent
Systemic disease-associated mastitis		sarcoidosis, Rosai–Dorfman disease

and with appropriate antimicrobials, the infection may become chronic.

Abscess Infectious mastitis can progress to abscess formation. It presents as a discharging abscess. Attention should be focused on the recurring prior subareolar abscess, which produces repeated episodes of inflammation and abscesses[51]. Fistula formation from the areola or periareolar skin into a lactiferous duct is possible. It usually develops in young women but is unrelated to lactation. Cutaneous redness, pain and warmth are seen in the beginning of the disease, with evolution to the formation of a small abscess. The pathology is an infection in the terminal portion of the main collecting ducts. It has been shown that cigarette smoking may be a predisposing factor in the development of mammillary fistulas and breast abscesses with anaerobic infections in the non-lactating woman[52].

Through appropriate treatment with antibiotics, an unnecessary mastectomy may be avoided in patients with frequent recurrences. If there is currently an abscess formation, antibiotics and incision may resolve the acute situation, but in some chronic cases of mastitis, excision of the affected ducts is necessary in a second phase in order to prevent relapse (Figure 7). Aspiration under the control of ultrasonographic imaging is an effective alternative to incision in abscess-forming mastitis[53].

Tuberculosis Breast tuberculosis is a rare entity throughout the world, and young pregnant women seem to be more predisposed. It may appear in a diffuse or nodular pattern. Differential diagnosis is sometimes difficult, mainly because of the mammary edema due to lymph node compression of the axillary veins. It is accompanied by neither pain nor tenderness and is usually secondary to extensive involvement of the mediastinal, cervical, or supraclavicular nodes[54]. Incision of the focus of infection

with initiation of antituberculosis therapy may resolve the problem.

Syphilis The skin of the breast and the nipple can be involved by a chancre or a gumma. The symptoms are classic, such as a painless ulcer with rolled edges and an indurated base in the case of primary syphilis. Ulceration with serous discharge that may extend or heal with an atrophic scar indicates a gumma of tertiary syphilis. Although these conditions are rare, differential diagnoses must be made when the physician initially considers Paget's disease of the nipple or a pyoderma gangrenosum of the breast[55].

Non-infectious mastitis

Non-infectious mastitis constitutes a group of breast inflammatory disorders that seem to be more frequent than classical puerperal mastitis[56]. It includes granulomatous mastitis, B-lymphocytic mastitis and systemic diseases with inflammatory breast involvement.

Granulomatous diseases These can cause inflammatory breast lesions but they do so infrequently. These lesions can be due to infectious disease[57] such as tuberculosis, syphilis and deep fungal infections[58], or to non-infectious conditions, such as granulomatous mastitis, sarcoidosis, perforating granuloma annulare, necrobiosis lipoidica, idiopathic lobular panniculitis and factitial panniculitis.

The etiology of non-infectious granulomatous mastitis remains unclear and controversial, but it is likely to be idiopathic[59]. Clinically resembling the other mastitis described above, granulomatous mastitis occurs mainly in young women with a history of childbirth and oral contraceptives.

Wegener granulomatous disease of the breast is rare. Except for one case, however, all cases reported to date have involved the breast of women.

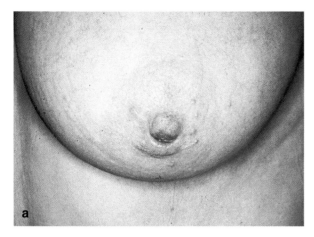

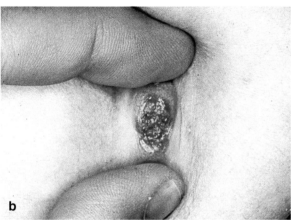

Figure 6 Patient with erosive adenomatosis of the nipple. (a) The nipple–areola complex appears almost normal, (b) but careful clinical examination shows erosion under the nipple. Courtesy of J. Delescluse, MD, Brussels, Belgium

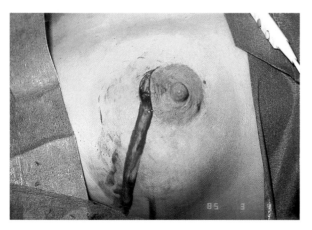

Figure 7 Abscess excision and drainage of the infected breast. Courtesy of P. Wylock, MD, Brussels, Belgium

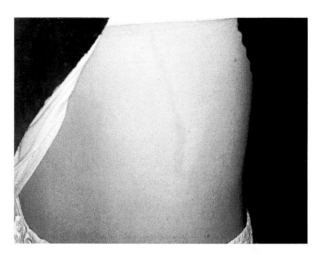

Figure 8 Retraction of the skin showing a puckered groove on the chest wall of a patient following Mondor's disease. Courtesy of J. Delescluse, MD, Brussels, Belgium

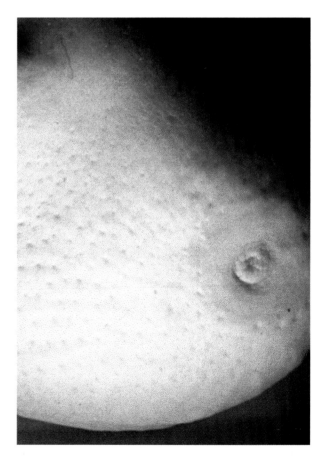

Figure 9 Typical skin signs in a patient with breast cancer. The *peau d'orange* sign and nipple retraction are observed. Courtesy of R. Sacré, MD, Brussels, Belgium

Predominantly, they present a unilateral breast involvement consisting of nodular lesions, thickening, erythema and ulcerations of the skin, nipple retraction and discharge[60].

After carcinomatous mastitis has been ruled out, other types of mastitis constitute a possible differential diagnosis (Table 4). Biopsy specimens or otherwise fine needle aspirates have been helpful

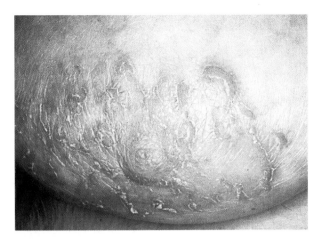

Figure 10 Paget's disease of the breast with scaling and erythema. Courtesy of J. Delescluse, MD, Brussels, Belgium

in establishing the correct diagnosis of carcinoma but not always of granulomatous mastitis[61].

Granulomatous mastitis responds to systemic corticoids, but long-term follow-up should be considered because of the high incidence of relapse[59].

B-Lymphocytic autoimmune mastitis This is also called diabetic mastopathy. It is observed in 13% of insulin-dependent diabetics[62] and affects both men and women. Histological examination of lymphocytic mastitis reveals periductal and perivascular infiltration of B lymphocytes and focal homogeneous fibrosis[63].

Systemic diseases associated with mastitis Various diseases may show breast involvement, such as sarcoidosis, perforating granuloma annulare, necrobiosis lipoidica, idiopathic lobular panniculitis and factitial panniculitis. It should be noted that in sarcoidosis the mastitis is of the granulomatous type. In other words, the presence of systemic involvement with a granulomatous mastitis sarcoidosis should be suspected[64]. Rosai–Dorfman disease has also been reported to present breast involvement[65].

Distinctions between these diseases can be made on the basis of history, clinical examination, histopathology with special staining procedures for the detection of micro-organisms, polarization microscopy and tissue cultures.

The presence of a disseminated disease and of other organ involvement facilitates the diagnosis.

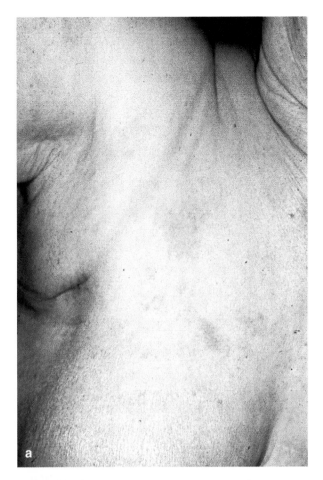

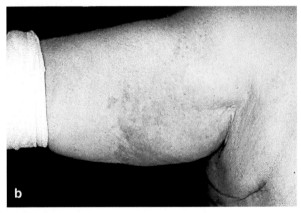

Figure 11 (a) Carcinoma erysipeloides of the breast and the chest wall. (b) The lymphatic involvement has spread to the arm of the patient

Fat necrosis

Fat necrosis is a benign condition occurring mainly in women because of the unprotected position and protrusion of the breast. A history of trauma is reported in 52% of cases[66]. This disorder has also been observed after cyst aspiration, biopsy, lumpectomy, radiation therapy, reduction mammoplasty, breast reconstruction with a transverse rectus abdominis myocutaneous flap, implant removal and anticoagulant therapy[67]. It presents as an enlarging hard mass with irregular borders. Sometimes skin retraction and a mild cutaneous inflammatory reaction are observed. Mammography is indicated and it may show lipid cysts, microcalcifications, spiculated high-density areas and focal masses[68].

Owing to the worrisome clinical and mammographic features, which can be confused with breast cancer, a biopsy of the tumor is highly recommended if no history of trauma is reported[69]. Histological features consist of fat saponification and adipocyte degeneration, giant cells and lymphocytes in the central part[66], while foamy macrophages and fibrosis are observed in the outer part of the lesion. If the diagnosis is obvious, a 2-week follow-up is recommended.

Mondor's disease

Mondor's disease, or sclerosing periphlebitis of the chest wall, affects more women (63%) than men and is due to the obstruction of thoracic veins[70]. Pain (51%) and tension sensation (28.9%) are possible complaints, but often no symptoms are reported by the patient[71]. On physical examination, a linear reddish cord spreading from the abdomen to the lateral thorax is detected.

This cord, which ranges from a few centimeters to 40 cm in length, may persist for periods ranging from several weeks to 7 months and then retract, leaving a puckered groove along the breast (Figure 8). Usually no cause is found; however, a history of infectious diseases, carcinoma, surgical trauma or muscular stress has been reported. Consequently, a mammography is recommended to exclude an underlying carcinoma[72]. The situation resolves without complications within 2–8 weeks of onset. Non-steroidal anti-inflammatory drugs may be helpful in coping with pain[73].

Breast cancers

Skin manifestations of breast cancers

Strictly speaking, breast cancer is not a dermatological topic, but some visible skin signs may be predictive of underlying breast carcinoma. The signs include *peau d'orange* and inverted nipples[74], which are caused by skin retraction (Figure 9). Although these signs are clinically discreet, they frequently indicate well-developed tumors.

Other possible signs are: dilated subcutaneous veins, red skin, edematous skin, erosions and ulcerations. Nodules on the skin may be observed by stoma infiltration of underlying breast cancer.

In any case, whether the skin manifestation is obvious or not, careful breast and axillary palpation is necessary, as is mammography. A skin biopsy can establish the diagnosis if carcinomatous mastitis is suspected. Lymphatic invasion of the breast presents as an infiltrating erythema mimicking erysipelas and is discussed under Carcinoma erysipeloides, below.

Paget's disease

Usually Paget's disease of the breast affects middle-aged women and presents clinically as a scaling red lesion that imitates nipple dermatitis[75] (Figure 10). Both its course and its unilateral onset (although bilateral forms are reported[76]) may distinguish it from contact dermatitis. Consequently, a skin biopsy should be performed so that any unilateral dermatitis of the nipple can be found.

Histological examination shows large cells, with abundant and pale-staining cytoplasm infiltrating the nipple epithelium. The nuclei of Paget cells show a vesicular chromatin design and identifiable nucleoli.

A non-invasive screening method for eczematous lesions of the nipple based on scrape–smear cytology has been described and is believed to be reliable[77-79]. Specific staining methods have been described for making a differential diagnosis between erosive adenomatosis[80], Bowen's disease of the nipple, skin carcinoma and pseudoxanthoma elasticum (Table 5)[81].

The pathogenesis of Paget's disease is controversial, but PAS-positive staining and its diastase-resistant nature support the hypothesis of a glandular origin[82]. In other words, Paget's disease

Table 5 Immunohistochemical staining techniques that can help to establish a diagnosis between Paget's disease, erosive adenomatosis of the nipple, dermatitis and Bowen's disease

	Paget's disease	Erosive adenomatosis	Dermatitis	Bowen's disease
EMA	positive	positive	negative	negative
C-erbB2	positive	negative	negative	negative

EMA, epithelial membrane antigen; C-erbB2, immunoperoxidase staining for C-erbB2 oncoprotein

is nearly always associated with breast cancer, although the latter is undetectable in 40% of cases[83]. Because of this association, total mastectomy is the treatment of choice[84].

Carcinoma erysipeloides

Carcinoma erysipeloides, also called inflammatory carcinoma, is a form of skin metastasis, complicating 1–2% of malignant breast cancers[85].

Carcinoma erysipeloides presents as an inflammatory, rapidly growing unilateral erythema of the chest wall, characterized by an erysipela-like border. Upon palpation the skin is warm and tenderness is elicited (Figure 11). The patient exhibits no abnormal temperature or other signs of infectious disease. The term 'carcinoma telangiectatica' is a clinical term to describe the presence of purpuric plaques within the carcinoma erysipeloides. Carcinoma *en cuirasse* refers to the *peau d'orange* changes due to the progression into marked thickening and fibrosis. Carcinoma erysipeloides complicates homolateral and heterolateral breast cancers, but has also been described with melanoma and lung, ovary, colon and pancreatic tumors. In fact, the clinical features are secondary to the lymphatic obstruction by the metastatic cells of the primary tumor. Therefore, the histological characteristics of carcinoma erysipeloides are the invasion of the dermal lymphatics by tumor cells[86] accompanied by edema and perivascular infiltrate. The nature of the tumor cells may be indicative of its origin since associations with occult cancers are possible[87]. Mammography is indicated and may give evidence of an underlying breast cancer.

The average life expectancy is 2 years from the time of diagnosis. Surgery is useless, because of the immediate skin recurrences due to the diffuse lymphatic invasion. Chemotherapy is very often given, however, without influence on life prognosis.

Iatrogenic disorders of the breasts

Complications of plastic surgery

The complications of plastic surgery of the nipple are more frequently observed because of the proliferation of breast reconstruction techniques worldwide (Figure 12). In addition, fat necrosis (see above), keloids, or hypotrophic scars are usually observed.

Silicone implants

The complications of breast silicone implants are currently a highly controversial subject[88]. Generally, two direct complications are reported: capsular contracture and induction of systemic diseases.

According to the latest studies, it seems that the capsular contracture side-effect depends on the texture of the implant[89,90]: smooth-textured implants are much more frequently associated with contraction (59%) than textured implants (11%). Others have reported that silicone diffusion around the implant does not induce the contraction[91]. Existing risk factors, such as previous radiotherapy on the implanted breast and racial differences, seem to play a role.

The controversy concerns systemic disease implications[92]. Silicone diffuses to the body tissue through envelope rupture, gel bleed, elastomer fragmentation or simple diffusion. Consequently, the search for autoantibodies in the sera of women with breast implants has disclosed different types of anticollagen antibodies in healthy patients and antinuclear antibodies in patients with silicone-associated rheumatic diseases[93,94]. On the other hand, other studies have demonstrated no evidence of a relationship between silicone implants and systemic diseases[93–95]. One point on which all scientists agree is the need for further epidemiological studies[96].

Black galactorrhea

Minocycline, which is widely prescribed by dermatologists for acne vulgaris, is known to produce skin pigmentation and phototoxic reactions. It has also been reported to be responsible for black galactorrhea, which is probably due to the iron chelate of minocycline[97]. Phenothiazine has also been related to this side-effect[98].

Other breast involvements

Other conditions can involve the skin of the breast, but are not specific to the location of the female breast. Local morphea[99], neurofibromas and vitiligo are sometimes observed in daily dermatology practice.

PREGNANCY, LACTATION AND SUBSEQUENT COMPLICATIONS

During pregnancy, breasts enlarge under the stimulation of estrogen and progesterone. These hormones stimulate the ducts and the acini, respectively. On the other hand, milk is secreted only after the placenta is delivered, which stops estrogen inhibition

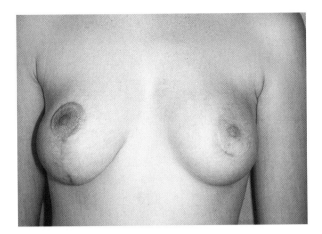

Figure 12 Hypertrophic scar after surgical reconstruction of the breast. Courtesy of P. Wylock, MD, Brussels, Belgium

of the pituitary glands. Afterwards, prolactin initiates milk secretion and is maintained by nipple-suckling stimulation.

Cracked nipple

Cracked nipples are a possible complication after delivery and may lead the mother to discontinue lactation. The nipple becomes very painful, showing deep fissures and superficial ulcers. Lack of milk in the breast may cause the baby to suck energetically, thereby bringing about nipple erosions. If the mother does not depress the breast while lactating, the baby has to drop the breast repeatedly, which causes nipple soreness. Infections may also cause painful cracked nipples.

Candida is frequently implicated in the infection of cracked, painful nipples in lactating women. The breast and nipple are painful during and after breast feeding. They may sting and burn throughout and after feeding. The nipples and areolas may appear inflamed, bright pink or shiny, or they may flake or peel. Sometimes there is an itching sensation on the nipple or inside the breast. Fissures of the nipples may be colonized by *Staphylococcus aureus*[100].

In an attempt at healing, the cracked nipple should be given a rest and treated with a topical antiseptic or nystatin cream that does not remove the newly formed epithelium. Topical greasy creams should be prescribed. In order to prevent relapses it is also recommended to empty the breast of milk while the crack is healing, and afterwards, in the beginning, to let the baby suck on the nipple for only a few minutes[101]. Oral antifungals can be given if lactation is discontinued.

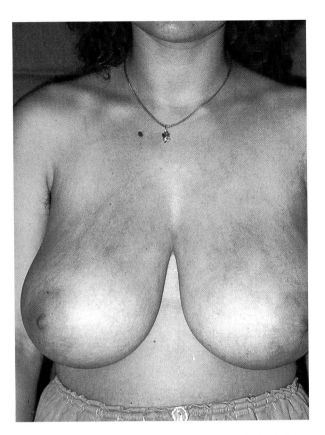

Figure 13 Pendulous breast. Courtesy of P. Wylock, MD, Brussels, Belgium

Puerperal mastitis

Acute puerperal mastitis is an infectious breast disease occurring 2–3 weeks after delivery, and is caused mainly by *Staphylococcus aureus*. The reported incidence varies between 2.9% and 24%[102,103]. Breast irritation during lactation and concomitant skin infection of the baby are thought to be the causal events. Tenderness is the initial symptom, usually accompanied by erythema adjacent to the areolar margin. Induration and edema of the breast follow.

The clinical signs may vary from cellulitis to erysipelas, accompanied by fever and an infectious syndrome as the infection continues. Breast feeding should be interrupted and an antibiotic therapy with dicloxacillin 500 mg four times a day[104] or clarithromycin 500 mg twice a day[105] given until bacterial sensitivity reports are available. Targeted therapy is then initiated if the pathogenic agent resists the antimicrobial. If the mastitis is not treated in time, a breast abscess may develop. The erythema becomes marked, the tenderness and induration increase, and the breast becomes enlarged and edematous. A mass that is painful to the touch and flucturant may be palpable in the breast. In this situation, besides interruption of breast feeding, the patient is given 2.5 mg of bromocriptine twice daily in order to suppress lactation[101]. Abscess incision and drainage are performed and this is followed by antimicrobial therapy[106].

Pendulous breasts

Although age and obesity may play a role, pendulous breasts usually develop after pregnancy and lactation (Figure 13). It is thus advisable to support the breast and encourage pectoral exercises immediately after lactation[22]. In well-defined conditions, plastic surgery is recommended. Pendulous breasts have also been described as a predisposing factor for Mondor's disease[107].

POSTMENOPAUSAL BREAST DERMATITIS

Skin aging is a normal process that occurs in elderly skin and naturally affects the breasts. Normal aging of the skin may be accompanied by photo-damage, characterized by elastotic degeneration and the wrinkling typical of it. Also, glandular tissue of the breast becomes atrophic and thin.

Mammary duct ectasia

Mammary duct ectasia is considered to be a pathology affecting postmenopausal women, aged between 50 and 60 years of age. It is a benign condition characterized by inflammatory reactions in the collecting ducts. Pathogenically, it starts as dilatation of the terminal tubules, which are filled with lipid-containing material. At this stage, no signs are generally observed except for a spontaneous intermittent nipple discharge that is bloody or serous. Because glandular atrophy takes place after the menopause, disruption of the epithelium due to collection of lipid-like material in the stroma is possible. In this phase, the breast shows inflammation with nipple discharge and retraction in addition to pain, erythema and edema; fistula formation and subareolar tumor, and abscess formation together with general symptoms and axillary lymph nodes may be present[108,109]. Surgical excision of the entire focus and corresponding duct seems to be the best curative treatment[109,110]. Surgical excision of the ducts is necessary for the treatment.

REFERENCES

1. Shirley RL. The endocrinology of the mammary gland. In Hindle WH, ed. *Breast Diseases for Gynecologists*. Norwalk, CT: Appelton & Lange, 1989;3:21–9

2. Breslau-Siderius EJ, Toonstra J, Baart JA, *et al.* Ectodermal dysplasia, lipoatrophy, diabetes mellitus and amastia – a second case of the AREDYLD syndrome. *Am J Med Genet* 1992;44:374–7
3. David TJ. Nature and etiology of the Poland anomaly. *N Engl J Med* 1972;287:487–9
4. Kissane JN, Smith MG. *Breast Pathology of Infancy and Childhood*. St Louis: Mosby Company, 1976:1038
5. Shewmake SW, Izuno GT. Supernumerary areola. *Arch Dermatol* 1997;113:823–5
6. Cellini A, Offidani A. Familial supernumerary nipples and breast. *Dermatology* 1992;185:56–8
7. Urbani CE, Betti R. Supernumerary nipples occurring together with Becker's naevus: an association involving one common paradominant trait. *Hum Genet* 1997;100:388–90
8. Cohen PR, Kurzrock R. Miscellaneous genodermatosis: Beckwith–Wiedemann syndrome, Birt–Hogg–Dube syndrome, familial atypical multiple mole melanoma syndrome, hereditary tylosis, incontinentia pigmenti, and supernumerary nipples. *Dermatol Clin* 1995;13:211–29
9. Zohar Y, Laurian N. Bifid condyl of the mandible with associated polythelia and manual anomalies. *J Laryngol Otol* 1987;101:1315–19
10. Meggyessy V, Mehes K. Association of supernumerary nipples with renal anomalies. *J Pediatr* 1987;111:412–13
11. Kenney RD, Flippo JL, Black EB. Supernumerary nipples and renal anomalies in neonates. *Am J Dis Child* 1987;141:987–8
12. Mehes K, Szule E, Torzsok F, Meggyessy V. Supernumerary nipples and urologic malignancies. *Cancer Genet Cytogenet* 1987;24:185–8
13. Jojart G, Seres E. Supernumerary nipples and renal anomalies. *Int Urol Nephrol* 1994;26:141–4
14. Armori M, Filk D, Schlesinger M. Accessory nipples, any relationship to urinary tract malformation? *Pediatr Dermatol* 1992;9:239–40
15. Scaffer AJ, Avery ME. *Diseases of the Newborn*, 4th edn. Philadelphia: WB Saunders Company, 1977;85:773–7
16. Efrat M, Mogilner JG, Iujtman M, *et al.* Neonatal mastitis – diagnosis and treatment. *Isr J Med Sci* 1995;31:558–60
17. Moss RL, Musemeche CA, Kosloske AM. Necrotizing fasciitis in children: prompt recognition and aggressive therapy improve survival. *J Pediatr Surg* 1996;31:1142–6
18. Rudoy RC, Nelson JD. Breast abscess during the neonatal period: a review. *Am J Dis Child* 1975;129:1031–4
19. Styne DM, Kaplan SL. Normal and the abnormal puberty in the female. *Pediatr Clin North Am* 1979;26:123
20. Guyton AC, Hall JE. *Textbook of Medical Physiology*. Philadelphia: WB Saunders Company, 1996:1044

21. Lyons WR, Lee LH, Johnson RE. The hormonal control of mammary growth and lactation. *Recent Prog Horm Res* 1958;14:219

22. Tindall UR. Breast function and disorders. *Jeffcoate's Principles of Gynaecology,* 5th edn. London: Butterworths, 1987;8:122–30

23. Barnett HJM, Derek R, Boughner DR. Further evidence relating mitral-valve prolapse to cerebral events. *N Engl J Med* 1980;302:139–44

24. Deveraux RB. Mitral valve prolapse. *Circulation* 1976;54:3–14

25. Saavedra D, Richieri Costa A, Guion-Almeida ML, *et al.* Craniofrontonasal syndrome: study of 41 patients. *Am J Med Genet* 1996;61:147–51

26. Kupfer D, Dingman D, Broadbest R. Juvenile breast hypotrophy: report of a familial pattern and review of the literature. *Plast Reconstr Surg* 1992;90:303–9

27. Jabs AD, Frantz AG, Smith Vaniz A, *et al.* Mammary hypertrophy is not associated with increased oestrogen receptors. *Plast Reconstr Surg* 1990;86:64–6

28. Fouquet B, Goupilli P, Rouif M, *et al.* Breast hypertrophy and dorso lumbar spine prognostic influences on lumbar cordons: preliminary results. *Rhum Mal Osteostic* 1991;58:453–7

29. Levit F. Jogger's nipples. *N Engl J Med* 1977;297:1127

30. Conklin RJ. Common cutaneous disorders in athletes. *Sports Med* 1990;9:100–9

31. Aiache A. Surgical repair of the inverted nipple. *Ann Plast Surg* 1990;25:457–60

32. McGeorge DD. The 'Niplette': an instrument for non-surgical correction of inverted nipples. *Br J Plast Surg* 1994;47:46–9

33. Hindle WH. *Diagnosis and Treatment of Benign Lesions of the Breast.* Norwalk, CT: Appleton & Lange, 1989;16:193–201

34. Erosive adenomatosis of the nipple: histology, immunhistology and differential diagnosis. *Mod Pathol* 1992;5:179–84

35. Bourlond J, Bourlond-Reinert L. Erosive adenomatosis of the nipple. *Dermatology* 1992;185:319–24

36. Pierard G. Paget's disease or erosive adenomatosis of the nipple? *Dermatologica* 1990;180:55

37. Pinto RG, Mandreker S. Fine needle aspiration cytology of adenoma of the nipple. A case report. *Acta Cytol* 1996;40:789–91

38. Van Mierlo PL, Geelen GM, Neumann HAM. Mohs micrographic surgery for an erosive adenomatosis of the nipple. *Dermatol Surg* 1998;24:681–3

39. Alpsoy E, Yilmaz E, Aykol A. Hyperkeratosis of the nipple: report of two cases. *J Dermatol* 1997;24:43–5

40. Schwartz RA. Hyperkeratosis of the nipple and areola. *Arch Dermatol* 1978;114:1844–5

41. Ahn SK, Chung J, Soo Lee W, *et al.* Hyperkeratosis of the nipple and areola simultaneously developing with cutaneous T cell lymphoma. *J Am Acad Dermatol* 1995;32:124–5

42. English JC III, Coots NV. A man with nevoid hyperkeratosis of the areola. *Cutis* 1996;57:354–6

43. Ortonne JP, El Baze P, Juhlin L. Nevoid hyperkeratosis of the nipple and areola mammae: ineffectiveness of etretinate therapy. *Acta Derm Venereol (Stockhol)* 1986;66:175–7

44. Nagaraja, Kanwar AJ, Dhar S, Singh S. Frequency and significance of minor clinical features in various age-related subgroups of atopic dermatitis in children. *Pediatr Dermatol* 1996;13:10–13

45. Kanwar AJ, Dhar S, Kaur S. Evaluation of minor clinical features of atopic dermatitis. *Pediatr Dermatol* 1991;8:114–16

46. Rudzki E, Samochocki Z, Litewska D, *et al.* Clinical features of atopic dermatitis and a family history of atopy. *Allergy* 1991;46:125–8

47. Bowers PW. Roustabouts' and barbers' breasts. *Clin Exp Dermatol* 1982;7:445–7

48. Baneerjee A. Pilonidal sinus of the nipple in canine beauticians. *Br Med J* 1985;291:1787

49. Parades-Lopez A, Moreno G. Non puerperal mastitis: a study of 30 patients. *Gynecol Obstet Mex* 1995;63:226–30

50. Lequin MH, van Spengler J, Van Pel R, *et al.* Mammographic and sonographic spectrum of non puerperal mastitis. *Eur J Radiol* 1995;21:138–42

51. Schwartz GF. Benign neoplasms and inflammations of the breast. *Clin Obstet Gynecol* 1982;25:373–85

52. Bundred NJ, Dover MS, Coley S, Morrison JM. Breast abscesses and cigarette smoking. *Br J Surg* 1992;79:58–9

53. Berna JD, Garcia-Medina V, Madrigal M, *et al.* Percutaneous catheter drainage of breast abscesses. *Eur J Radiol* 1996;21:217–19

54. Goksoy E, Duren M, Durgun V, Uygun N. Tuberculosis of the breast. *Eur J Surg* 1995;161:471–3

55. Stehman FB. Infection and inflammations of the breast. In Hindle WH, ed. *Breast Diseases for Gynecologists.* Norwalk, CT: Appelton & Lange, 1989;11:151–4

56. Bassler R. Mastitis. Classification, histopathology and clinical aspects. *Pathologe* 1997;18:27–36

57. Binelli C, Lorimier G, Bertrand G, *et al.* Granulomatous mastitis and corynebacteria infection. Two case reports. *J Gynecol Obstet Biol Reprod Paris* 1996;25:27–32

58. Moreira MA, de-Freitas-Junior R, Gerais BB. Granulomatous mastitis caused by sparganum. A case report. *Acta Cytol* 1997;41:859–62

59. Imoto S, Kitaya T, Kodama T, *et al.* Idiopathic granulomatous mastitis. Case report and review of the literature. *Jpn J Clin Oncol* 1997;27:274–7

60. Trüeb RM, Pericin M, Kohler E, *et al.* Necrotizing granulomatosis of the breast. *Br J Dermatol* 1997;137:799–803

61. Martinez-Parra D, Nevado Santos M, Melendez Guerrero B, *et al.* Utility of the fine needle aspiration

in the diagnosis of granulomatous lesions of the breast. *Diagn Cytopathol* 1997;17:108–14

62. Hunfeld KP, Bassler R. Lymphocytic mastitis and fibrosis of the breast in long standing insulin-dependent diabetes. A histopathologic study on diabetic mastopathy and report of ten cases. *Gen Diagn Pathol* 1997;143:49–58

63. Hunfeld KP, Bassler R, Kronsbein H. 'Diabetic mastopathy' in male breast – a special type of gynecomastia. A comparative study of lumphocytic mastitis and gynecomastia. *Pathol Res Pract* 1997;193:197–205

64. Petit M, Wasserman K, Vierbuchen M, *et al.* Non puerperal granulomatous mastitis: sarcoidosis or non-specific inflammatory reaction? *Med Klin* 1992;15:663–6

65. Green I, Dorfman RF, Rosai J. Breast involvement by extranodal Rosai–Dorfman disease: report of seven cases. *Am J Surg Pathol* 1997;21:664–8

66. Harrisson RL, Britton P, Warren R, *et al.* Can we be sure about a radiological diagnosis of fat necrosis of the breast? *Clin Radiol* 2000;55:119–23

67. Hogge JP, Robinson RE, Magnant CM, Zuurbier RA. The mammographic spectrum of fat necrosis of the breast. *Radiographic* 1995;15:1347–56

68. Pignatelli V, Basolo F, Bagnolesi A, *et al.* Hematoma and fat necrosis of the breast: mammographic and echographic features. *Radiol Med Torino* 1995;89:36–41

69. Rasa G, Veroux P, Tumminelli MG, *et al.* Contribution to the knowledge of the pseudoneoplastic pathology of the breast. Cytosteatonecrosis. *Ann Ital Chir* 1996;67:637–45

70. Farinella M. Mondor's disease. Thrombophlebitis of the lateral thoracic and thoraco-epigastric vein. *Minerva Cardioangiol* 1986;34:333–6

71. Bartolo M, Spigone C, Antignani P. Contribution to the recognition of Mondor's phlebitis. *J Mal Vasc* 1983;8:253–6

72. Verburg GP, Perre CI, Perenboom RM. Mondor's disease. *Ned Tijdschr Geneeskd* 1989;133:2035–7

73. Nasr FW, Mufarrij AA, El-Ashkar K. Mondor's disease. A forgotten case of chest pain. *J Med Liban* 1996;44:41–3

74. Neville EM, Freeman AH, Adiseshiah M. Clinical significance of recent inversion of the nipple: a reappraisal. *J R Soc Med* 1982;75:111–13

75. Von Dach B, Neuweiller J, Haller U. Differential diagnosis of breast tumors with eczematous breast changes: two rare cases. *Helv Chir Acta* 1992;59:217–20

76. Markopoulos C, Gogas H, Sampalis F, Kyriakou B. Bilateral Paget's disease of the breast. *Eur J Gynaecol Oncol* 1997;18:495–6

77. Gupta RK, Simpson J, Dowle C. The role of cytology in the diagnosis of Paget's disease of the nipple. *Pathology* 1996;28:248–50

78. Pinto RG, Mandreker S. Fine needle aspiration cytology of adenoma of the nipple. A case report. *Acta Cytol* 1996;40:789–91

79. Samarasinghe D, Frost F, Sterrett G, *et al.* Cytological diagnosis of Paget's disease of the nipple by scrape smears: a report of five cases. *Diagn Cytopathol* 1993;9:291–5

80. Miller L, Tyler W, Maroon M, Miller OF III. Erosive adenomatosis of the nipple: a benign imitator of malignant breast disease. *Cutis* 1997;59:91–2

81. Viehl P, Validire P, Kheirallah S, *et al.* Paget's disease of the nipple without clinically and radiologically detectable breast tumors. Histochemical and immunohistochemical study of 44 cases. *Pathol Res Pract* 1993;189:150–5

82. Jamali FR, Ricci A Jr, Deckers PJ. Paget's disease of the nipple areola complex. *Surg Clin North Am* 1996;76:365–81

83. Bhave S, Saxena R, Jambhekar N. Paget's disease of the breast: a study of 43 cases. *Indian J Cancer* 1992;29:90–5

84. Napoli L, Pagono A, Comparetto S, *et al.* Paget's disease of the breast. *Minerva Chir* 1997;52:927–31

85. Zala I, Jenni C. Das carcinoma erysipelatoides. *Dermatologica* 1980;160:80–9

86. Lever LR, Holt PJ. Carcinoma erysipeloides. *Br J Dermatol* 1991;124:279–82

87. Lucas FV, Perez-Meza C. Inflammatory carcinoma of the breast. *Cancer* 1978;41:1595–605

88. Jenkins ME, Friedman HI, von Recum AF. Breast implants: facts, controversy and speculation for future research. *J Invest Surg* 1996;9:1–12

89. Coleman DJ, Foo IT, Sharpe DT. Textured or smooth implants for breast augmentation? A prospective controlled trial. *Br J Plast Surg* 1991;44:444–8

90. Malata CM, Feldberg C, Coleman DJ, *et al.* Textured or smooth implants for breast augmentation? Three year follow up of a prospective randomised controlled trial. *Br J Plast Surg* 1997;50:99–105

91. Jennings DA, Morykwas MJ, De Franzo AJ, Argenta LC. Analysis of silicon in human breast and capsular tissue surrounding prostheses and expanders. *Ann Plast Surg* 1991;27:553–8

92. Aljatas-Reig J, Garcia-Domingo MI. Silicone and autoimmune diseases. *Ann Med Interna* 1998;15:276–83

93. Sever CE, Leith CP, Appenzeller J, Foucar K. Kiluchi's histiocytic necrotizing lymphadenitis associated with ruptured silicone breast implants. *Arch Pathol Lab Med* 1996;120:380–5

94. Rowley MJ, Cook AD, Mackay IR, *et al.* Comparative epitope mapping of anti-bodies to collagen in women with silicone breast implants, systemic lupus erythematosus, and rheumatoid arthritis. *Curr Top Microbiol Immunol* 1996;210:307–16

95. Weinzweig J, Schnur PL, Mcconnell JP, *et al.* Silicon analysis of breast and capsular tissue from patients

with saline and silicone gel breast implants. Correlation with connective tissue disease. *Plast Reconstr Surg* 1998;101:1836–41

96. Liang MH. Silicone breast implants and systemic rheumatic diseases. Some smoke but little fire to date (editorial). *Scand J Rheumatol* 1997;26: 409–11

97. Hunt MJ, Salisbury EL, Grace J, Armati R. Black breast milk due to minocycline therapy. *Br J Dermatol* 1996;134:943–4

98. Booler RSW, Lynch PY. Black galactorrhea as a consequence of minocycline and phenothiazine therapy. *Arch Dermatol* 1985;121:417–18

99. Treiber ES, Goldberg NS. Breast deformity produced by morphea in a young girl. *Cutis* 1994;54:267–8

100. Amir LH, Garland SM, Dennerstein L, Farish S. *Candida albicans*: is it associated with nipple pain in lactating women? *Gynecol Obstet Invest* 1996;41:30–4

101. Lewis TLT, Chamblerain GPV. Abnormal puerperum. *Obstetrics by 10 teachers*, 15th edn. London: Edward Arnold, 1990;7:260–2

102. Peters F, Flick-Fillies D, Ebel S. Hand disinfection as the central factor in the prevention of puerperal mastitis. Clinical study the results of a survey. *Geburtshilfe Frauenheilk* 1992;52:117–20

103. Jonsson S, Pulkkinen MO. Mastitis today: incidence prevention and treatment. *Ann Chir Gynaecol Suppl* 1994;208:84–7

104. Johnson PE, Hanson KD. Acute puerperal mastitis in the augmented breast. *Plast Reconstr Surg* 1996;98:723–5

105. Sedlmayr T, Peters F, Raash W, Kees F. Clarithromycine a new macrolide antibiotic. Effectiveness in puerperal infections and pharmacokinetics in breast milk. *Geburtshilfe Frauenheilk* 1993;53: 448–91

106. Krause A, Gerber B, Rhode E. Puerperal and non puerperal mastitis. *Zentralbl Gynacol* 1994;116: 488–91

107. Hacher SM. Axillary string phlebitis in pregnancy: a variant of Mondor's disease. *J Am Acad Dermatol* 1994;31:636–8

108. Petersen L, Graversen HP, Andersen JA, *et al.* The duct ectasia syndrome: an overlooked disease entity. *Ugeskr Laeger* 1993;155:1540–5

109. Petersen L, Graversen HP, Andersen JA, *et al.* The duct ectasia syndrome. A prospective clinical study of patients with breast diseases. *Ugeskr Laeger* 1993;155:1545–9

110. Hartley MN, Stewart J, Benson EA. Subareolar dissection for duct ectasia and periareolar sepsis. *Br J Surg* 1991;78:1187–9

Oral lesions

29

Marilyn G. Liang, Stella D. Calobrisi and Roy S. Rogers III

Some oral lesions occur in girls and women at a prevalence greater than in boys and men. The increased prevalence may represent a genetic predisposition, the effect of female sex hormones, other factors, or a combination of one or more factors. The clinician should be aware of these oral lesions as they care for female patients.

TUMORS
Congenital epulis

A congenital epulis or gingival granular cell tumor of the newborn is a rare solid tumor that occurs predominantly in female neonates[1,2]. These pedunculated or sessile growths are usually located on the anterior or lateral alveolar ridges along the maxillary more than the mandibular arch, and are composed of neuroectodermal granular cells probably of Schwann cell origin. These benign, single or multiple tumors commonly regress, even following incomplete excision, suggesting a reactive pathogenesis.

Granular cell tumors

Granular cell tumors arise in adults 30–60 years of age with a 2 : 1 predilection for women[3]. Granular cell tumors are commonly found on the tongue, which is the site of one in three lesions[4], but they may be found at any site. Multiple tumors are extremely rare. Lesions present as solitary, firm, flat nodules, which may be painful. Local recurrence is uncommon unless the tumor is infiltrative. Granular cell tumors arise from Schwann cells of the nerve sheath. Histologically, the overlying epithelium has been found to exhibit pseudoepitheliomatous hyperplasia in 50% of patients. This may cause confusion with squamous cell carcinoma. Malignant granular cell tumors are rare. Features suggestive of malignancy include large nodules > 5 cm in size, rapid growth, vascular invasion, necrosis and pleomorphism[5].

Nasolabial cysts

Nasolabial cysts are uncommon asymptomatic tumors of the lateral aspect of the upper lip which may be associated with distortion of the lip–ala interface[6]. They are thought to arise from aberrant nasal lacrimal duct epithelium. Nasolabial cysts occur in adults with a 3 : 1 female prevalence. They are treated by surgical excision. Recurrences are uncommon.

Hemangiomas

Hemangiomas are the most common neoplasms of the oral cavity[7]. Hemangiomas are benign vascular tumors that typically present at birth or develop within the first month of life. Women are more commonly affected, at a 3 : 1 ratio. The tumors proliferate rapidly during the first several months of life, then involute over years; this distinguishes them from vascular malformations, which remain static over time. Hemangiomas may be superficial, deep, or mixed within the lips, tongue, buccal mucosa and bone. Ulceration, infection and hemorrhage may occur and may cause interference with speech and sucking. Treatment is predicated on the size and location of the lesion, complications and the cosmetic concerns of the patient and family. Laser ablation with the pulsed dye laser is effective treatment for ulcerated hemangiomas or early thin superficial hemangiomas. If the hemangioma is interfering with vital functions such as feeding or breathing, more aggressive therapy with intralesional or systemic corticosteroids or interferon may be indicated.

Pyogenic granulomas

Pyogenic granulomas often follow minor trauma or infection. Some patients develop lesions at the end of the first trimester of pregnancy which persist or expand in the ensuing months. When present on the gingiva, these lesions are called epulis of pregnancy[8]. Pyogenic granulomas present as bleeding, fragile, sessile or pedunculated papules, which may grow rapidly. The most common location is the maxillary anterior attached gingivae. They may be surgically excised or destroyed by cryosurgery or electrodesiccation with or without curettage. Recurrence after surgery is not uncommon.

GEOGRAPHIC TONGUE

Benign migratory glossitis or geographic tongue is a common condition affecting 2% of the general population[9]. It affects all age groups but is more prevalent in children and women. Clinical manifestations include one or many annular patches with a white, raised, hyperplastic border surrounding a red, depressed, atrophic center in which the filiform papillae are absent and the larger fungiform papillae stand out in bas relief (Figure 1). These patches characteristically involve the lateral and dorsal tongue surfaces and may occasionally involve other oral mucosae such as the ventral surface of the tongue and labial and buccal mucosal surfaces. Geographic tongue changes usually appear suddenly and may be short-lived for a few weeks or months. Some patients' disease can persist for several years.

Geographic tongue is a disturbance of the physiology of filiform papillae with desquamation in the atrophic center and hyperplasia of the stratum corneum at the borders. Most patients are asymptomatic and accept reassurance that the condition is benign and does not imply a systemic disease. Symptomatic therapy with frequent application of fluorinated corticosteroids to the patches can be helpful. The geographic tongue condition may persist for months or years before undergoing a remission.

CONNECTIVE TISSUE DISEASES

Lupus erythematosus

Patients with cutaneous and/or systemic lupus erythematosus may present with lesions affecting the oral mucosa but without skin lesions[10,11]. Clinical features include erythematous plaques with irregular borders and hypopigmented, radiating striae (Figure 2). These plaques may ulcerate. Lupus erythematosus is more prevalent in women, and adults are more commonly affected than children. The oral lesions of lupus erythematosus may be symptomatic when active or ulcerated. Topical or intralesional corticosteroid therapy is indicated. The lesions may improve with systemic therapy, but usually require local treatment for clearing.

Sjögren's syndrome

Sjögren's syndrome is an autoimmune disease characterized by dryness of the mucous membranes of the eyes, mouth, skin, vagina and other mucosal surfaces. This occurs most commonly in women (9 : 1 female/male ratio)[12]. The condition may affect 3% of women under 55 years of age. Oral findings include burning tongue, altered taste, xerostomia (Figure 3), swollen salivary glands, angular cheilitis (Figure 4) and dental caries on root surfaces

adjacent to the gingival margins. Some patients have xerostomia and xerophthalmia with associated medical conditions. This is often described as the 'sicca complex'. Sjögren's syndrome is often associated with connective tissue diseases. Systemic involvement reflects the associated rheumatological diseases such as rheumatoid arthritis, systemic lupus erythematosus, systemic scleroderma and dermatomyositis. Sjögren's syndrome may also occur secondary to chronic active hepatitis, graft-versus-host disease or other autoimmune diseases. Anti-Ro (SS-A) antibodies are positive in 40–45% of patients and anti-La (SS-B) antibodies are positive in 20% of patients with sicca complex[13,14]. Therapy is directed towards the autoimmune disease if present. Oral candidosis is common in patients with xerostomia. Xerostomia is treated palliatively with increased intake of fluid, oral rinses or saliva substitutes, with careful oral hygiene and dental care including fluoride treatments to prevent dental caries. These patients should see their dentist every 3 months. Some patients may require systemic pilocarpine therapy to ameliorate their symptoms.

Juvenile dermatomyositis

Juvenile dermatomyositis is an angiopathy of the microvasculature. In children younger than 10 years of age, there is an equal race and gender distribution. In early teenage years, young women predominate, at a ratio of 10 : 1[15]. In dermatomyositis, black women are most commonly affected at the ages of 20–44 years, and among patients age 60 and over white women predominate. The clinical presentation includes symmetric proximal limb weakness due to non-suppurative myositis and characteristic violaceous erythema over the eyelids and extensor surfaces. With severe disease, erythroderma or ulcerations involving the large areas of cutaneous surface may be encountered. In children, mucosal ulcerations can occur in any part of the gastrointestinal tract with hemorrhage. Other oral lesions include soft tissue calcification, tooth root formation anomalies and arrested tooth root resorption[16].

LICHEN PLANUS

Lichen planus (LP) is an inflammatory disorder affecting the skin and mucosal surfaces. Approximately one-third of patients with oral LP have skin lesions. Approximately one-half of patients with cutaneous LP have oral lesions. Women are more commonly symptomatic than men, and patients usually present in the sixth decade of life[17]. A lichenoid tissue reaction or LP-like eruption can be

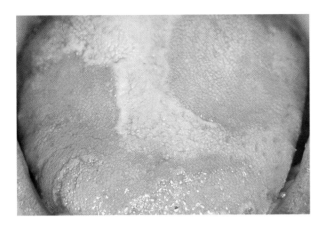

Figure 1 Geographic tongue. Red atrophic or 'bald' patches adjacent to the white hypertrophic patches on the dorsum of the tongue

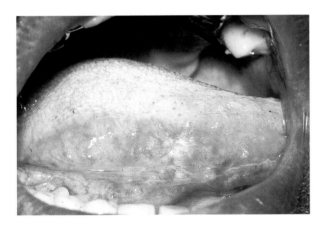

Figure 2 Oral lupus erythematosus. White hyperkeratotic plaque with radiating white striae on the lateral surface of the tongue

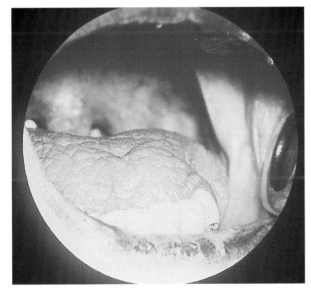

Figure 3 Sjögren's syndrome. Dry oral mucosa with the thickened and fissured tongue. These patients have difficulty masticating and swallowing a cracker without supplemental fluid

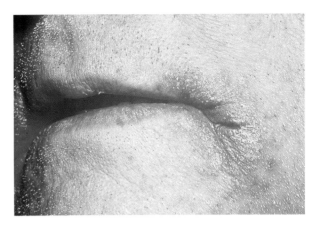

Figure 4 Angular cheilitis. Dry skin and fissuring at the labial commissure. Secondary colonization with bacteria and/or yeast can exacerbate this condition

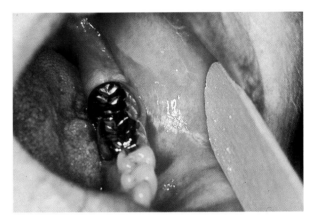

Figure 5 Oral lichen planus. Linear white plaque with reticulated, radiating white striae (Wickham's striae) of the buccal mucosa

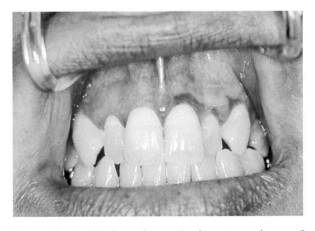

Figure 6 Oral lichen planus. Erythematous plaque of the marginal attached gingivae in this patient with oral lichen planus

seen in association with certain drugs, dental materials and hepatitis. Oral findings include typical reticular, white striae (Wickham's striae) and non-erosive (linear, papular, plaques) (Figure 5) or erosive (atrophic, erosive, bullous, ulcers) lesions. Characteristically, oral LP is seen on the buccal

Table 1 Drugs implicated in oral lichen planus

Antirheumatic drugs
d-Penicillamine
Gold
Antihypertensive drugs
Thiazide diuretics
α-Methyldopa
Antimalarial drugs
Quinine
Quinidine
Chloroquine
Antibiotics
Tetracycline
Para-amino salicylic acid

mucosa in almost all patients. The tongue is the next most common site. LP, when involving the gingivae, presents as erythematous plaques of the marginal gingivae (Figure 6). Although this is somewhat controversial, most authors believe that oral LP is a premalignant lesion with a 1% incidence of malignant transformation. Management includes symptomatic treatment with topical fluorinated corticosteroids. Avoiding drugs that are a possible cause is a reasonable approach (Table 1). Replacement of dental restorations in direct apposition to symptomatic lesions is indicated when contact hypersensitivity is confirmed by patch testing.

A special variant of erosive LP is the vulvovaginal gingival form (Figures 6 and 7) described initially by Pelisse and colleagues[18] and expanded by Pelisse[19] and Eisen[20]. Eisen recommends that all patients with oral LP have a careful history taken and examination for involvement of other mucosal surfaces. We have presented 25 Mayo Clinic patients with erosive orogenital LP[21]. The mean age at onset was 52 with a range of 18–78 years. Oral lesions began first in 13, oral and genital simultaneously in 11, and genital lesions first in one. Most (19) were menopausal or postmenopausal. Skin lesions were present in nine, scalp lesions in four and nail involvement in four. Several patients had desquamative vaginitis with adhesions; three underwent surgical procedures. Both light and immunofluorescence microscopy revealed LP or lichenoid tissue reactions. Light microscopic studies of oral mucosal biopsy specimens revealed LP in 13 out of 22, a lichenoid tissue reaction in five out of 22 and non-specific findings in four out of 22 patients. Cutaneous biopsy specimens were positive for LP in four out of four patients. Genital biopsy specimens revealed LP in seven out of 13, a lichenoid tissue reaction in five out of 13, and non-specific findings in one out of 13. Immunofluorescence studies revealed a pattern typical of LP or a lichenoid tissue reaction in 14 out of 15 oral, two out of two cutaneous and five out of five genital biopsy specimens. Therapy with systemic and topical corticosteroids was palliative. Hydroxychloroquine was beneficial in some patients. Effective therapy with other anti-inflammatory drugs was limited: griseofulvin (none out of six), dapsone (one out of one), systemic retinoids (one out of three) and tetracycline (none out of two). The erosive orogenital variant of LP in women is a chronic disease for which control remains the chief therapeutic goal.

BLISTERING DISEASES
Mucous membrane pemphigoid

Mucous membrane (cicatricial) pemphigoid is a chronic autoimmune subepithelial blistering disease characterized by bullae and erosions of the mucous membranes and skin, resulting in scarring. Women are affected twice as often as men[22,23]. Mucous membrane pemphigoid is predominantly a disease of the elderly. Lesions commonly involve the oral mucosa (Figure 8) and conjunctiva (Figure 9). Blisters occur within the lamina lucida of the basement membrane zone. Direct immunofluorescence testing shows continuous linear deposition of immunoreactants, particularly IgG (IgG$_4$) and C3, along the basement membrane zone of mucosal specimens. Indirect immunofluorescence testing is positive for IgG anti-basement membrane autoantibodies in < 5% of patients. Indirect immunofluorescence on salt split skin reveals epidermal and/or dermal binding, suggesting that mucous membrane pemphigoid is a phenotype associated with several different autoantibodies. The best characterized autoantigens are bullous pemphigoid antigen 2 and laminin 5[24].

Some patients with mucous membrane pemphigoid present with oral or gingival (Figure 10) lesions only. Others present with ocular lesions only. The rest may have multiple mucosal or cutaneous sites involved[22,23]. Those patients with a single site such as oral or ocular involvement tend to have a less aggressive form of mucous membrane pemphigoid and appear to be more responsive to treatment[24].

Treatment of mucous membrane pemphigoid is challenging. For extensive or rapidly progressive disease, prednisone and a corticosteroid-sparing, immunosuppressive agent such as azathioprine or cyclophosphamide is often indicated[23,25]. For less extensive and milder disease, dapsone and sulfapyridine are good treatment options[25–27]. Some authors recommend tetracycline and niacinamide as an effective combination therapy.

Erythema multiforme

Oral erythema multiforme is most common in young adults. Women are slightly more often affected than men[28]. The disease may be recurrent or persistent with an average duration of 4–7 years. Skin or genital involvement occurs in 25% of patients (Figure 11). Etiologies include herpes simplex virus (HSV) infections, other infections, drugs, contact hypersensitivity and chronic or recurrent candidosis. Treatment is directed at the presumed cause such as antiviral therapy for recurrent HSV infections. Palliative therapy with systemic corticosteroids and corticosteroid-sparing agents such as dapsone are often necessary to control signs and symptoms of recurrent oral erythema multiforme.

GLOSSODYNIA

Glossodynia or burning mouth syndrome frequently occurs in postmenopausal women and is characterized by mouth pain with normal findings on oral examination[29–31].

Glossodynia is one of the most vexing complaints in medicine, both to the patient and to the clinician. Many patients seek help because of the distracting symptoms of the condition. Some patients will consult ten or more clinicians including primary care clinicians and dentists, dental specialists, allergists, ear, nose and throat physicians, neurologists and dermatologists. The clinician should take a careful history and perform a thorough examination, seeking an organic cause or causes for the burning mouth syndrome.

We have emphasized the identification of correctable causes[29]. (Table 2). The most frequent association in the Mayo series was psychiatric disease (one out of three), most commonly depression. Nutritional deficiencies were present in approximately 20% of patients, and positive patch tests for potentially relevant allergens were noted in 13% of patients. Some patients have a tongue-thrusting habit (Figure 12). The diagnosis and treatment are best accomplished by a multidisciplinary approach. The clinician should identify one or more causes and treat each simultaneously in order to enhance the likelihood of a positive outcome. Most patients (72%) will improve with individualized treatment on the basis of the proposed cause or causes (Table 3).

ALLERGIC REACTIONS

Angioedema and urticaria are common, with the highest incidence in young adults. Recurrent episodes lasting more than 12 weeks are more

Table 2   Recommended work-up of the burning or sore mouth (from reference 29)

Thorough history
Oral examination
General medical examination
Laboratory tests
    complete blood cell count
    iron, total iron-binding capacity, iron saturation,
        ferritin
    vitamin B_{12} and folate
    zinc
    glucose and glycosylated hemoglobin
Biopsy (if indicated on the basis of oral examination)
Culture for *Candida*
Patch testing (as indicated by patient history)
Further consultation if indicated
    dentistry
    psychiatry
    neurology
    otorhinolaryngology

Table 3   Management strategies for the burning or sore mouth. Treatment is tailored to the suspected causal factor or factors. From reference 29

Denture adaptation
Control of oral habits
Vitamin and mineral replacement
Avoidance of allergens
Avoidance of irritants
Antifungal agents
Sialagogs
Appropriate psychiatric medications or therapy
    (or both)
Discontinuation of medications leading to xerostomia
Low doses of tricyclic antidepressants (chronic pain
    protocol)
Reassurance that cancer is not present

prevalent in women[32]. Lesions of the lips and perioral tissues may be chronic or recurrent. Urticaria and angioedema may be idiopathic or due to various immunological and inflammatory mechanisms (Table 4).

Allergic contact cheilitis results in erythema, dryness, scaling and vesiculation often extending onto adjacent skin (Figure 13). Contact cheilitis affects women more often than men, because lipsticks and lip salves are among the common culprits[33]. Sensitivities may also be noted to lanolin and photoprotectants such as oxybenzone. Identification of the sensitizing agent through patch testing is helpful in eliminating recurrences.

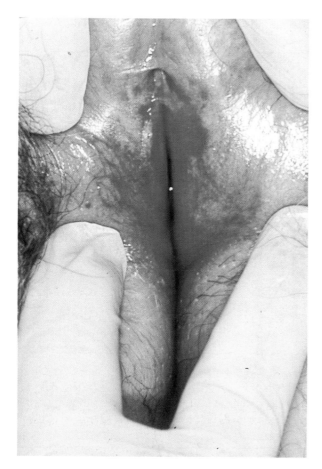

Figure 7 Vulvovaginal lichen planus. Erosive erythematous plaques involving the introitus

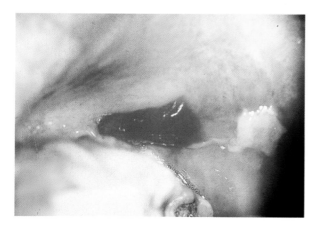

Figure 8 Mucous membrane pemphigoid. Involvement of the buccal mucosa with a hemorrhagic subepithelial blister posteriorly and an erosive lesion covered by a yellowish fibromembranous slough anteriorly

APHTHOUS STOMATITIS

Recurrent aphthous stomatitis (RAS) is also known as canker sores. Many patients confuse RAS with recurrent herpes simplex virus infections and believe that RAS is a 'herpes infection'. They are two distinct and separate conditions, both of which

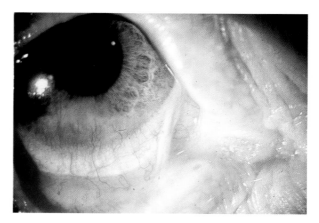

Figure 9 Mucous membrane pemphigoid. Involvement of both the palpebral and bulbar conjunctiva with the development of a scar band (symblepharon). Note the absence of eyelashes from previous epilating surgical procedures to treat trichiasis

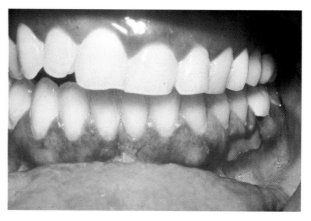

Figure 10 Mucous membrane pemphigoid. Erythema and edema of attached gingivae with desquamation of the lower attached gingivae. This form of desquamative gingivitis, a reaction pattern, is gingival pemphigoid

commonly affect young patients. RAS is the most common inflammatory ulcerative condition of the oral mucosa in North American patients[34].

The lesions of RAS are localized, painful, shallow, round to oval ulcers often covered by a gray to tan fibromembranous slough and surrounded by an erythematous halo. Lesions of RAS typically afflict the non-masticatory, soft mucosa of the oral cavity, largely sparing the masticatory mucosa of the hard palate and maxillary and mandibular alveolar ridges (Figure 14). Sites of predilection include the undersurface of the tongue and the floor of the mouth as well as the buccal, lingual (Figure 15), labial, sulcular, soft palatal and oropharyngeal mucosal surfaces. The ulcers of RAS are self-limited, persisting for 1–2 weeks, resolving with or without scarring and recurring after periods of remission.

The lesions of RAS are usually noted in childhood or adolescence and recur with decreasing

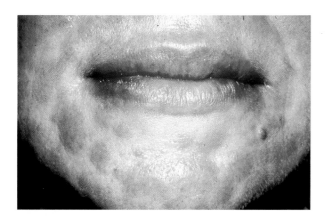

Figure 11 Erythema multiforme. Note the bright red edematous plaques of the face and the swollen lips. Note also the crusted erosion of the right lower lip representing a resolving herpes labialis infection. The recurrent herpes simplex virus infection was the trigger for erythema multiforme

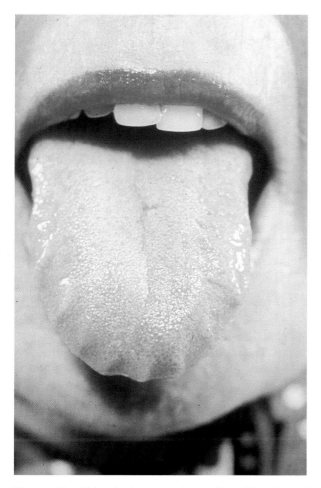

Figure 12 Glossodynia. Note the scalloped borders of the enlarged tongue. The persistent paresthesias of the tongue have caused a tongue-thrusting habit to alleviate the sensation

frequency and severity with age. The prevalence of RAS varies with the population studies, ranging from 5 to 50%. It is estimated that 20% of the

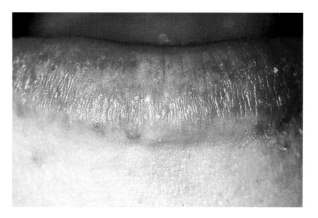

Figure 13 Allergic contact cheilitis. Erythema and papulovesicles of the lower lip vermilion of this patient with allergic contact cheilitis

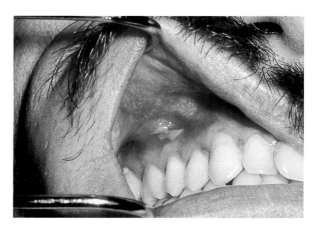

Figure 14 Recurrent aphthous stomatitis. Small oral erosions covered by a tan fibromembranous slough in the right maxillary sulcus. These minor aphthous ulcers are the type seen in patients with simple aphthosis

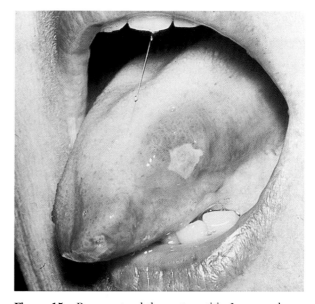

Figure 15 Recurrent aphthous stomatitis. Large oral erosion surrounded by an erythematous halo on the lateral border of the tongue. These larger, painful, slow-healing ulcers are the type seen in patients with complex aphthosis

Table 4 Classification of urticaria and angioedema. From reference 32

Immunological IgE- and IgE receptor-dependent
urticaria/angioedema
Atopic diathesis
Specific antigen sensitivity (foods, drugs, therapeutic
    agents, aeroallergens, *Hymenoptera* venom, helminths)
Physical urticaria/angioedema
Contact urticaria
Autoimmune urticaria
Urticaria/angioedema mediated by
complement system and other plasma effector systems
Hereditary angioedema with C1 esterase inhibitor
    deficiency and malignant disorders or autoantibody
Necrotizing venulitis
Serum sickness
Reactions to blood products
Infections
Angiotensin-converting enzyme inhibitors
Urticaria/angioedema after direct mast cell degranulation
Opiates
Analgesics
Polymyxin B
Curare
D-tubocurarine
Radiocontrast media
Urticaria/angioedema relating to abnormalities of arachidonic
acid metabolism
Aspirin and non-steroidal anti-inflammatory agents
Azo dyes and benzoates
Idiopathic urticaria/angioedema
Idiopathic
Cyclical episodic angioedema

Table 5 Classification of recurrent aphthous stomatitis

Simple aphthosis	Complex aphthosis
Episodic	episodic or continuous
Short-lived	persistent
Few ulcers	few to many ulcers
3–6 episodes/year	continuous ulcers
Heals quickly	slow healing
Minimal pain	marked pain
Little disability	disabling
Limited to oral cavity	may have genital lesions

Successful management of patients with lesions of RAS is dependent on an accurate diagnosis, classification of the disease, recognition of possible causative factors and the identification of associated systemic disorders that contribute to the disability, treatment and prognosis of RAS[34].

general population will have RAS during their childhood or early adult life. Women are afflicted more commonly than men.

Although some patients have infrequent recurrences, two to four times each year (simple aphthosis), other patients may have almost continuous disease activity with new lesions developing as older lesions heal (complex aphthosis) (Table 5). Simple aphthosis represents the common presentation of a few lesions that heal in 1–2 weeks and recur infrequently. Complex aphthosis, on the other hand, represents a complicated clinical picture of severe disease, numerous large or deep ulcers, new ulcers developing as older ones heal (continuous ulcerations), marked pain or disability and, occasionally, associated genital or perianal lesions[35,36]. The presence of anogenital aphthae does not confirm the diagnosis of Behçet's disease, as some patients with complex aphthosis will have occasional genital aphthae but never develop Behçet's disease[34].

REFERENCES

1. Dela Monte SM, Radowsky M, Hood AF. Congenital granular cell neoplasms: an unusual case report with ultrastructural findings and a review of the literature. *Am J Dermatopathol* 1986;8:57–63
2. Tucker MC, Rusnock EJ, Azumi N, *et al.* Gingival granular cell tumors of the newborn. An ultrastructural and immunohistochemical study. *Arch Pathol Lab Med* 1990;114:895–8
3. Khansur R, Balducci L, Tavassoli M. Granular cell tumor. Clinical spectrum of the benign and malignant entity. *Cancer* 1987;60:220–2
4. Papageorgiou S, Litt JZ, Pomeranz JR. Multiple granular cell myoblastomas in children. *Arch Dermatol* 1967;96:168–71
5. Gokaslan ST, Rerzakis JA, Santagada EA. Malignant granular cell tumor. *J Cutan Pathol* 1994;21:263–70
6. Kuriloff DB. The nasolabial cyst – nasal hamartoma. *Otolaryngol Head Neck Surg* 1987;96:268–72
7. Silverman RA. Hemangiomas and vascular malformations. *Pediatr Clin North Am* 1991;38:811–34
8. Butler EJ, Macintyre DR. Oral pyogenic granulomas. *Dent Update* 1991;18:194–6
9. Halperin V, Kolas S, Jefferis KR, *et al.* The occurrence of Fordyce spots, benign migratory glossitis, median rhomboid glossitis and fissured tongue in 2478 dental patients. *Oral Surg* 1953;6:1072–7
10. Schiodt M. Oral manifestations of lupus erythematosus. *Int J Oral Surg* 1984;13:101–47
11. Jorizzo JL, Salisbury PL, Rogers RS III, *et al.* Oral lesions in systemic lupus erythematosus: do ulcerative lesions represent a necrotizing vasculitis? *J Am Acad Dermatol* 1992;27:389–94
12. Pavlidis NA, Karsh J, Moutsopoulos HM. The clinical picture of primary Sjogren's syndrome: a retrospective study. *J Rheumatol* 1982;9:685–90

13. Alexander EL, Hirsch TJ, Arnett FC, *et al*. Ro(SSA) and la(SSB) antibodies in the clinical spectrum of Sjogren's syndrome. *J Rheumatol* 1982;9:239–46

14. Harley JB, Alexander EL, Bias WB, *et al*. Anti-Ro (SSA) and anti-La (SSB) in patients with Sjogren's syndrome. *Arthritis Rheum* 1986;29:196–206

15. Oddis CV, Conte CG, Steen VD, Medsger TA. Incidence of polymyositis–dermatomyositis: a 20-year study of hospital diagnosed cases in Allegheny County, PA 1963–1982. *J Rheumatol* 1990;17:1329–34

16. Hamlin C, Shelton JE. Management of oral findings in a child with an advanced case of dermatomyositis: clinical report. *Pediatr Dent* 1984;6:46–9

17. Silverman S, Borsky M, Lozada-Nur F, *et al*. A prospective study of findings and management in 214 patients with oral lichen planus. *Oral Surg* 1991;72:665–70

18. Pelisse M, Leibowitch M, Sedel D, Hewitt J. Un noveau syndrome vulvo-vagino-gingival. Lichen plan erosif plurimuqueux. *Ann Dermatol Venereol* 1982;109:797–8

19. Pelisse M. The vulvo-vaginal-gingival syndrome. A new form of erosive lichen planus. *Int J Dermatol* 1989;28:381–4

20. Eisen D. The vulvovaginal–gingival syndrome of lichen planus. *Arch Dermatol* 1994;130:1379–82

21. Rogers RS III. Erosive orogenital lichen planus in women (vulvo-vaginal syndrome). Presented at the *19th World Congress of Dermatology*, (abstr). *Aust J Dermatol* 1997;38(suppl):104

22. Hanson RD, Olsen KD, Rogers RS III. Upper aerodigestive tract manifestations of cicatricial pemphigoid. *Ann Otol Rhinol Laryngol* 1988;97:493–9

23. Ahmed AR, Kurgis FS, Rogers RS III. Cicatricial pemphigoid. *J Am Acad Dermatol* 1991;24:987–1001

24. Mobini N, Nagarwalla N, Ahmed AR. Oral pemphigoid: subset of cicatricial pemphigoid? *Oral Surg Oral Med Oral Pathol Oral Radiol Endod* 1998;85:37–43

25. Rogers RS III, Mehregan DA. Dapsone therapy of cicatricial pemphigoid. *Semin Dermatol* 1988;7:201–5

26. Rogers RS III. Dapsone and sulfapyridine therapy in pemphigoid diseases. *Aust J Dermatol* 1982;21:51–7

27. Rogers RS III, Seehafer JR, Perry HO. Treatment of cicatricial (benign mucous membrane pemphigoid) with dapsone. *J Acad Dermatol* 1982;6:215–23

28. Lozada-Nur F, Gorsky M, Silverman S. Oral erythema multiforme: clinical observations and treatment of 95 patients. *Oral Surg Oral Med Oral Pathol* 1989;67:36–40

29. Drage LA, Rogers RS. Clinical assessment and outcome in 70 patients with complaints of burning or sore mouth symptoms. *Mayo Clin Proc* 1999;74:223–8

30. Basker RM, Strudee DW, Davenport JC. Patients with burning mouths. *Br Dent J* 1978;145:9–16

31. Lamey PJ. Burning mouth syndrome. In Miles DA, Rogers RS III, eds. *Disorders Affecting the Oral Cavity*. Philadelphia: WB Saunders, 1996:339–54

32. Soter NA. Urticaria and angioedema. In Freedberg IM, Eisen AZ, Wolff K, *et al.*, eds. *Dermatology in General Medicine*. New York: McGraw-Hill, 1999:1409–19

33. Rogers RS III, Bekic M. Diseases of the lips. *Semin Cutan Med Surg* 1997;16:328–36

34. Rogers RS III. Recurrent aphthous stomatitis: clinical characteristics and associated systemic disorders. *Semin Cutan Med Surg* 1998;16:278–83

35. Jorizzo JL, Taylor RS, Schmalsteig FC, *et al*. Complex aphthosis: a forme fruste of Behçet's syndrome? *J Am Acad Dermatol* 1985;13:80–4

36. Ghate JV, Jorizzo JL. Behçet's disease and complex aphthosis. *J Am Acad Dermatol* 1999;40:1–18

Disorders of the perineum and perianal region

30

Michael Camilleri and Joseph L. Pace

There is a wide variety of disorders (Table 1) that affect perineal and perianal regions in girls and women. Many are dermatoses that also involve the external genitalia and at times the mucocutaneous surfaces. These disorders encompass a wide variety of conditions ranging from the mundane (seborrheic dermatitis) to the unusual (Behçet's disease), from the exclusively cutaneous (contact dermatitis) to serious systemic disorders (Crohn's disease and ulcerative colitis), from the benign (lichen simplex) to the malignant neoplasm.

These disorders usually but not invariably present with one or more related symptoms and signs (Tables 2 and 3): in particular, pruritus ani, perianal pain, rectal bleeding, or changes in bowel habit or complaints of papules/nodules, sore cracked skin and perhaps perianal 'tightness'.

It is clear that, in management, consideration will be given to:

(1) Age, for example, in diaper dermatitis, zinc deficiency and Kawasaki's disease, the condition will occur in a very young age group;

(2) Other signs of cutaneous disease, e.g. psoriasis, lichen sclerosis et atrophicus, blistering in the mouth or on the skin (pemphigus, cicatricial pemphigoid, Behçet's disease);

(3) The presence of known systemic disease such as uncontrolled diabetes, of the patient being pregnant or on oral contraceptives. These may all suggest the likelihood of candidosis;

(4) Systemic disorders such as Crohn's disease or ulcerative colitis or immunosuppressive medication the patient may be taking for these or other conditions;

(5) Tuberculosis in immunosuppressed persons or those suffering from poor nutrition (immigrants). This is making strong inroads and would need consideration;

(6) Sexual preferences and practices when sexually transmitted diseases are a strong possibility.

The diagnosis and treatment may often be straightforward, but on other occasions the clinician may need to be aware of systemic diseases and utilize sophisticated investigations. Such diseases are likely to increase, as more patients will lead longer lives sustained for one reason or another by powerful immunosuppressive therapy, which may modify quite significantly both the appearance and the natural progression of infectious and neoplastic processes. Consultation with colleagues specializing in gynecology, gastroenterology, infectious diseases, oncology and immunology will provide a wider clinical and diagnostic base than has hitherto seemed necessary.

INFLAMMATORY DISEASES
Contact dermatitis
Contact irritant dermatitis

Contact irritant dermatitis of the perineum and perianal area is seen in various clinical settings. It is commonly seen in infants or any other individual who wears diapers, where the resulting increased dampness, exacerbated by the retention of urine and feces, results in maceration and irritation of the covered skin[1]. Chronic contact irritant dermatitis may rarely result in either of two perianal complications: granuloma gluteale infantum; and perianal pseudoverrucous papules and nodules. The former is characterized by violaceous nodules on the convexities of the diaper area that especially occur with the use of potent fluorinated topical steroids[2]. The latter is characterized by multiple shiny red papules in the perianal and perineal regions[3].

Contact irritant dermatitis can also result from rectal discharge or fecal soiling in association with chronic constipation or chronic diarrhea or anorectal disease, such as proctitis, perianal fissures and fistulae, anorectal tumors and hemorrhoids[4].

Contact allergic dermatitis

This is commonly seen as a result of allergies to topical medications applied to the perianal area for various reasons. One study showed neomycin, caine mix, quinolines, lanolin and ethylenediamine to be the commonest sensitizers in the perianal area. The risk of contact allergic dermatitis in

362

Table 1 Disorders of the perineal and perianal regions

Inflammatory conditions
Contact dermatitis
Seborrheic dermatitis
Neurodermatitis
Psoriasis
Lichen sclerosis et atrophicus
Lichen planus
Cicatricial pemphigoid
Hidradenitis suppurativa
Kawasaki's disease
Recurrent toxin-mediated perineal erythema
Behçet's disease
Inflammatory bowel disease
Necrolytic migratory erythema
Zinc deficiency
Langerhans cell histiocytosis
Drug reactions
Infections
Bacterial infections
Mycotic infections
Viral infections
Parasitic infections
Neoplastic conditions
Premalignant neoplasms
Malignant neoplasms

Table 2 Symptoms by which perineal and perianal disease present

Pruritus ani
Perianal or perineal pain
Rectal bleeding
Changes in bowel habit

the perineal area is increased with fissuring and excoriations. Associated hand dermatitis may also be seen, secondary to contact of the hands with the allergens[4].

Treatment of contact dermatitis in general includes avoidance of known sensitizers, adequate moisturizing of the area and use of low-potency topical steroids and antimicrobials. Care should be taken to use topical preparations with the least amount of irritants and potential sensitizers[4].

Seborrheic dermatitis

Seborrheic dermatitis may also affect the perineal and perianal area. It is characterized by the typical brownish red, greasy scales that also affect other areas of the body including the scalp, other flexural areas and central portions of the trunk. This is treated with a low-potency topical steroid and an anti-yeast preparation[5].

Table 3 Physical signs by which perianal and perineal disease present

Perianal/perineal erythema
Perianal/perineal fissuring or ulcerations
Perianal papules or nodules
Perianal stenosis

Neurodermatitis

The perianal and the perineal regions are some of the commonest sites of neurodermatitis or lichen simplex chronicus. This is characterized by a discrete area of lichenification, typically unilateral and resulting from chronic pruritus and scratching of this area. It may be difficult to distinguish clinically from psoriasis, but the latter tends to be bilateral and there are usually other signs of psoriasis elsewhere. Treatment involves adequate moisturization, low- to mid-potency topical steroids and, sometimes, the tricyclic antidepressant doxepin, which also has strong anti-histaminic properties[4].

Psoriasis

Perianal and perineal psoriasis is a common manifestation of inverse psoriasis, especially in young infants[6]. It is characterized by perianal, erythematous plaques with distinct borders and fissures and lacks scale. Other signs of psoriasis, including extensor plaques and nail changes will assist in confirming the diagnosis. A KOH preparation will help to differentiate this from mycotic infections.

Treatment involves low-potency topical steroids, such as hydrocortisone or desonide. A short initial 2–3-week course of a topical anti-yeast preparation, such as miconazole or ketoconazole cream, will be helpful to clear any secondary yeast infection. Unfortunately, non-steroid preparations such as calcipotriene or tazoratene are too irritating to apply on the perianal region. Recently, some workers have achieved good results even in 'delicate' areas by applying a low-potency steroid and calcipotriene cream either in succession or in combination. Indeed, such a combined preparation is scheduled for early release. Tar preparations and low-strength anthralin, although also irritating, are more tolerated[7].

Lichen sclerosis et atrophicus

Lichen sclerosis et atrophicus (LSA) is a fairly common inflammatory dermatosis that more often affects girls and women, especially in the prepubertal, perimenopausal and postmenopausal periods. The exact cause of this condition is unknown.

It mainly affects the genital area, but there is also extragenital involvement (Figure 1). The perineal and perianal regions of the skin can also be affected, although rarely on their own. This is usually seen in two-thirds of cases of vulvar LSA. The early lesions are characterized by white polygonal papules that coalesce into plaques, which may fissure in the perineum midline. Occasionally, hemorrhagic bullae may also form. In later lesions there is a fibrotic plaque that forms a figure-of-eight pattern (also known as the keyhole, hourglass, butterfly or lotus flower pattern). LSA exhibits the Koebner phenomenon, where warmth and moisture, low-grade infection or tight nylon underwear may all contribute to the development of the lesions.

Multiple reports of squamous cell carcinoma (SCC) developing in areas of LSA at genital sites have been noted, but there has been only one report of the development of perianal SCC in perianal LSA[8].

Diagnosis is confirmed by biopsy for histopathological evaluation, which shows the characteristic papillary dermal edema and homogenization with associated epidermal changes (atrophy, hyperkeratosis and basal cell vacuolization) and a lymphocytic infiltrate just beneath the altered papillary dermis.

Treatment of LSA is with a short burst of high-potency topical steroids (clobetasol propionate) for 1–2 weeks followed by lower-potency steroids[9].

Lichen planus

Lichen planus (LP) is an idiopathic, usually self-limiting inflammatory dermatosis that affects women preferentially, usually in their 5th to 6th decade of life (Figure 2). LP can affect the mucosal anal surface, usually manifesting as confluent, violaceous and leukohyperkeratotic papules with fissures and erosions. These lesions are very itchy. Mucosal anal LP can occur alone or with other mucocutaneous involvement.

When it is solitary, the diagnosis is made by histopathological examination and direct immunofluorescence of a biopsy specimen. Treatment includes low- to mid-potency topical steroids. In recalcitrant cases or in more generalized cases, systemic medications can be used, including corticosteroids, dapsone, griseofulvin and retinoids[10].

Cicatricial pemphigoid

Also known as benign mucosal pemphigoid or ocular pemphigus or scarring pemphigoid, this is a rare chronic immunobullous disorder of the mucosa and skin, more commonly affecting women in late middle to old age (Figure 3). It is characterized by permanent scarring following blistering of the affected areas. The target antigens are the same as the bullous pemphigoid antigens, BP 180 and BP 230, as well as other antigens including the α-subunit of laminin 5 (epiligrin) and other less well characterized antigens of 120, 160 and 45 kDa.

The characteristic clinical manifestations of cicatricial pemphigoid are blisters that commonly affect the mucosal surfaces and the periorificial skin, which characteristically heal with scarring. It may affect any mucosal surface and periorificial site, including the anal mucosa and perianal skin. The anal involvement results in anal fissures with painful defecation and rectal bleeding. Eventually the fissures heal by scarring, resulting in anal stenosis and constipation.

The diagnosis is made by biopsy, where hematoxylin and eosin preparations show a subepidermal separation with a lymphohistiocytic and eosinophilic inflammatory infiltrate, and later healing by fibrosis. Direct immunofluorescence shows a linear basement membrane zone deposition of IgG and C3.

Treatment of cicatricial pemphigoid includes topical potent steroids and a number of systemic treatments alone or in combination. Systemic agents found to be effective in cicatricial pemphigoid include systemic steroids, dapsone, sulfapyridine, tetracycline combined with nicotinamide, azathioprine, cyclophosphamide and cyclosporine A[11,12].

Hidradenitis suppurativa

Hidradenitis suppurativa is a chronic, inflammatory follicular scarring disorder of the apocrine gland-bearing skin, which is associated with two other follicular occlusion disorders – acne conglobata and dissecting cellulitis of the scalp. All three conditions are collectively known as the follicular triad. It is more common in women in their 2nd and 3rd decades (Figure 4). The cause of hidradenitis suppurativa is unknown, although a hyperandrogenic state and obesity seem to play a role. It affects mainly the intertriginous areas, including the perianal and the buttock area. The clinical manifestations are the same in all sites and go through three clinical stages:

(1) Stage I. Abscesses;
(2) Stage II. Abscesses with sinus tract formation and scarring;
(3) Stage III. Broad area of abscesses with multiple interconnected sinus tracts and scarring.

Complications of perianal hidradenitis suppurativa include secondary infection, anal fistulae, anal strictures and SCC. SCC arising from hidradenitis suppurativa is most common in the perianal area and tends to behave aggressively with local invasion and metastasis. Treatment includes intralesional steroids, incision and drainage of abscesses, systemic antibiotics, systemic steroids (in severe inflammation), isotretinoin, ethinylestradiol with cyproterone acetate, cyclosporine, local excision and CO_2 ablation. Care must be taken with surgery in the perianal area, owing to the risk of traumatization of the anal sphincter[13].

Kawasaki's disease

Kawasaki's disease is a multisystem disorder, mainly affecting children under 5 years of age and commonly seen in winter and early spring. Although the exact cause is uncertain it is thought to be related to an infectious agent, possibly a manifestation of a toxin-mediated, superantigen-driven process derived from toxin-producing bacteria such as *Staphylococcus aureus* or *Streptococcus pyogenes*.

Among its various mucocutaneous manifestations, a prominent feature is an erythematous, desquamating perineal erythema that usually appears within 6 days of the first symptom. The other features of Kawasaki's disease include bilateral conjuctival injection, erythematous or fissured lips, strawberry tongue, pharyngeal erythema, edema and erythema of the hands and feet, a morbilliform eruption, cervical adenopathy and coronary artery aneurysms.

Treatment of Kawasaki's disease includes aspirin or dipyramidole with intravenous immunoglobulin[14,15].

Recurrent toxin-mediated perineal erythema

Recurrent toxin-mediated perineal erythema is a recently described toxin-mediated illness characterized by a diffuse, macular perineal erythema, occurring within 24–48 h after a bacterial pharyngitis with either *Streptococcus pyogenes* or *Staphylococcus aureus*. There may be associated erythema, edema and desquamation of the hands and feet, strawberry tongue and diarrhea. This condition may be recurrent[15].

Inflammatory bowel disease

Inflammatory bowel disease consists of two main conditions: Crohn's disease and ulcerative colitis. A common manifestation, especially in Crohn's disease, is perianal disease. The manifestations of perianal inflammatory bowel disease include perianal and ischiorectal abscesses, perianal fistulae, anal ulcers and strictures and florid, multiple inflammatory perianal skin tags. Perineal granulomas may occasionally be found as well. Biopsy of these inflamed areas will usually show non-caseating granulomas. The importance of perianal disease in inflammatory bowel disease, particularly in Crohn's disease, is that often Crohn's disease may present with severe perianal disease months to years before its other symptoms appear. Chronic perianal disease due to inflammatory bowel disease predisposes to anal SCC. Treatment of perianal Crohn's disease includes metronidazole and surgical treatment in more severe cases[16].

Behçet's disease

Behçet's disease is a multisystem inflammatory disorder of unknown etiology, mainly seen in the 2nd to 4th decades with a slight male preponderance. It is characterized by orogenital aphthosis in association with anterior and posterior uveitis, erythema nodosum, central nervous system involvement, arteriovenous thrombosis and ulcerations of the entire gastrointestinal tract. It can occasionally present with multiple shallow ulcerations and fissures of the anal margin. Treatment may include topical steroids and systemic treatments that include dapsone, colchicine, thalidomide, systemic steroids, low-dose methotrexate and interferon-α[17].

Necrolytic migratory erythema

Necrolytic migratory erythema is a cutaneous manifestation of the glucagonoma syndrome, thought to result from nutritional deficiencies (zinc, amino acids or essential fatty acids) (Figure 5). It is manifested by a migratory, figurate erythema, followed by erosions, crusting and eventual superficial cutaneous necrosis that tends to affect the periorificial regions, including the perineal areas. There may be associated stomatitis, angular cheilitis, glossitis, alopecia, brittle nails, diarrhea, weight loss and diabetes mellitus.

The diagnosis is made by the detection of high serum glucagon levels and the detection of a pancreatic mass, which on biopsy proves to be a glucagonoma.

The treatment of necrolytic migratory erythema includes surgical excision of the tumor, but if for some reason surgery is contraindicated, intravenous amino acid or essential fatty acid infusions, zinc supplementation, or octreotide (a somatostatin analog) may clear the eruption.

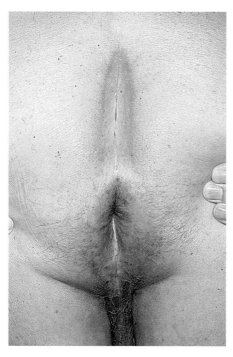

Figure 1 Lichen sclerosis et atrophicus. Courtesy Department of Dermatology, Mayo Clinic, Rochester, MN

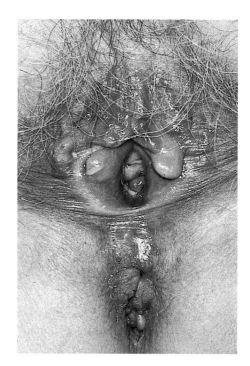

Figure 3 Cicatricial pemphigoid. Courtesy Department of Dermatology, Mayo Clinic, Rochester, MN

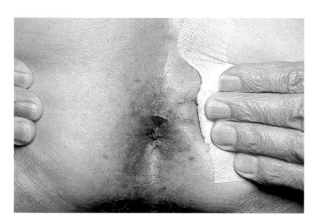

Figure 2 Lichen planus. Courtesy Department of Dermatology, Mayo Clinic, Rochester, MN

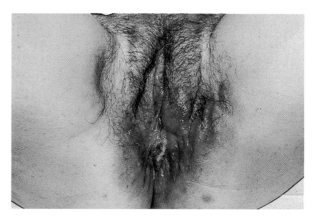

Figure 4 Hidradenitis suppurativa. Courtesy Department of Dermatology, Mayo Clinic, Rochester, MN

Cases of necrolytic migratory erythema without glucagonoma, but associated with other gastrointestinal disease, have been observed. Other associations include liver cirrhosis, Crohn's disease, chronic pancreatitis and celiac disease[18].

Zinc deficiency

Zinc deficiency due to a variety of causes may result in a periorificial and acral eruption similar to necrolytic migratory erythema. Zinc deficiency is commonly caused by an autosomal recessive genetic defect of zinc absorption – acrodermatitis enteropathica (Figure 6), a diet exclusively of breast milk, prematurity, hyperalimentation without zinc supplementation and malabsorption syndromes,

especially celiac disease, or cystic fibrosis and Crohn's disease.

Treatment includes zinc supplementation, local skin care with moisturizers and topical steroids and treatment if possible of any underlying cause[1].

Langerhans cell histiocytosis

Langerhans cell histiocytosis is a reactive hyperplasia of Langerhans cells commonly presenting with perianal disease with nodules and ulcerations (Figure 7). The diagnosis is confirmed by histopathological examination of a skin biopsy. Treatment includes topical nitrogen mustard, CO_2 laser and thalidomide[19].

Drug reactions

Drug reactions may affect the perineum and perianal skin. These include:

(1) Fixed drug eruption, commonly seen with phenolphthalein, oral contraceptives, sulfonamides, tetracycline and non-steroidal anti-inflammatory drugs.

(2) Stevens–Johnson syndrome with associated erythema multiforme and orogenital ulcerations, and commonly seen with sulfonamides, phenytoin, allopurinol and carbamazepine.

(3) Part of an exfoliative dermatitis or exanthem.

INFECTIONS

Bacterial infections

Perianal streptococcal dermatitis/cellulitis

This is a fairly common perianal infection, mainly affecting males of 3–4 years of age, but it may affect females and any age group. This infection is caused by the group A β-hemolytic streptococcus (GABHS), which is thought to be transmitted by a contaminated digit from another infected area, such as the oropharynx. The oropharynx harbors GABHS in most cases of perianal streptococcal cellulitis.

The condition can present in three main ways: bright pink erythema; beefy red erythema with superficial peripheral crusts; and minimal erythema but with fissuring and dried mucous secretions. The condition presents with pruritus ani, rectal bleeding and pain on defecation with fecal retention. It is commonly associated with acute flares of guttate psoriasis.

Diagnosis is confirmed by culture of GABHS from a swab of the affected area. Treatment is with a combination of oral penicillin V or erythromycin (in penicillin-sensitive individuals) with topical mupirocin, twice a day, for a total of around 15 days each[20].

Sexually transmitted bacterial infections

Most bacterial sexually transmitted disease can affect the perianal area as a result of anal intercourse.

Syphilis This is caused by the spirochete *Treponema pallidum*. Primary syphilis is characterized by the anal chancre with anal fissures especially occurring in the posterior midline, and usually associated with bilateral inguinal adenopathy. Secondary syphilis is manifested by condyloma lata, characterized by exuberant perianal nodules, and is associated with a more systemic disease with a generalized eruption, systemic upset, hepatosplenomegaly and meningitis. The diagnosis is made with dark field microscopy of the surface exudate in primary syphilis and serological testing in secondary syphilis. Treatment is with penicillin or erythromycin in penicillin-sensitive individuals[4,21].

Lymphogranuloma venereum (LGV) This is caused by the chlamydial organism *Chlamydia trachomatis*, of which there are three subtypes – LGV 1–3. Perianal LGV seems to be more common in women, where it is thought to reach the perianal and perirectal area via the internal lymphatic drainage of the proximal two-thirds of the vagina. Acute perianal LGV is characterized by an acute proctitis with pain and a serosanguinous anal discharge, with late complications including scarring, fistulae, ulceration and elephantiasis of the perineum, called esthiomene. The diagnosis is made with a complement fixation test. Treatment is with tetracycline or sulfisoxazole, with consideration of surgical treatment in late cases[4,22].

Gonorrhea This is caused by the Gram-positive diplococcus *Neisseria gonorrhoeae*, and may also affect the perianal region by anal discharge secondary to gonococcal proctitis, or by anal inflammation, manifest as perianal erythema with fissures and erosions. The diagnosis is made with Gram stain and culture of the anal discharge. Treatment is with intramuscular ceftriaxone[4,23].

Chancroid This is caused by the Gram-negative bacillus *Haemophilus ducreyi*, and may also affect the perianal region, resulting in extremely painful anal ulcers. The diagnosis is made with Gram stain and culture of a swab of these ulcerations. Treatment is with intramuscular ceftriaxone or oral erythromycin[4,24].

Granuloma inguinale This is caused by the Gram-negative bacillus *Calymmatobacterium granulomatis*, and in the perianal region causes an ulcerated papule that may result in an anal stricture. Diagnosis is by identification of Donovan bodies (organisms in vacuoles within macrophages) on biopsy or a crush specimen. Treatment is with tetracycline or sulfamethoxazole/trimethoprim[4,25].

Other bacterial infections

Other perianal and perineal bacterial infections include the following.

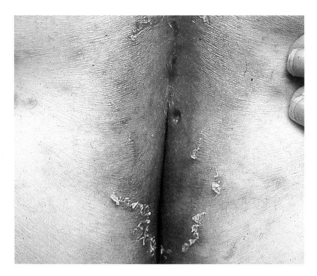

Figure 5 Necrolytic migratory erythema. Courtesy Department of Dermatology, Mayo Clinic, Rochester, MN

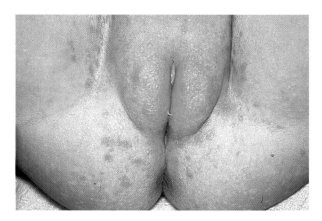

Figure 7 Langerhans cell histiocytosis. Courtesy Department of Dermatology, Mayo Clinic, Rochester, MN

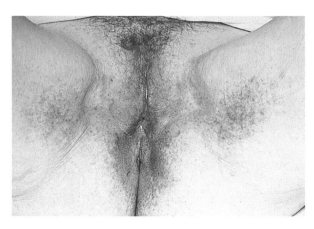

Figure 8 Perianal candidosis. Courtesy Department of Dermatology, Mayo Clinic, Rochester, MN

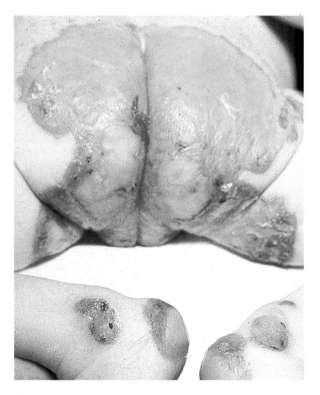

Figure 6 Acrodermatitis enteropathica. Courtesy Department of Dermatology, Mayo Clinic, Rochester, MN

Gangrenous, necrotizing bacterial infections Secondary to both aerobic and anaerobic organisms, these are commonly seen in the anorectal and perineal areas. These commonly follow surgery (gynecological in women) or trauma in the area, as well as resulting from immunosuppression, especially in diabetics and leukemia patients, or malignancy of the perineal area. These infections mainly involve the subcutaneous tissue or fascia. They can be of various types including gas gangrene (usually clostridial infections), ecthyma gangrenosum (usually *Pseudomonas aeruginosa* and other Gram-negative organisms, cellulitis and myositis (streptococci and staphylococci), necrotizing fasciitis (polymicrobial), Fournier's gangrene (polymicrobial) and synergistic gangrene (polymicrobial).

The clinical manifestations of perianal/perineal necrotizing infections include severe pain with dusky red erythema that spreads rapidly and may be accompanied by crepitus, gangrenous ulceration and discharging pus. Diagnosis is made with Gram stain and culture of any discharging fluid and the blood. Treatment includes antimicrobials (penicillin G and an aminoglycoside or a cephalosporin with anaerobic coverage – clindamycin or metronidazole) and more importantly early, rapid and extensive debridement, with a colostomy sometimes being necessary[4,26].

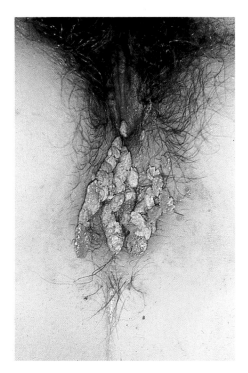

Figure 9 Condyloma acuminata. Courtesy Department of Dermatology, Mayo Clinic, Rochester, MN

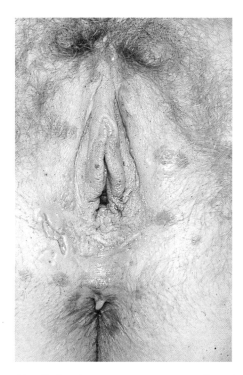

Figure 10 Perianal verrucous squamous cell carcinoma. Courtesy Department of Dermatology, Mayo Clinic, Rochester, MN

Tuberculosis   This must be included in the differential diagnosis of chronic perianal disease with painful fissures, fistulae and abscesses (orificial tuberculosis); of verrucous lesions (tuberculosis verrucosa cutis); and of granulomatous plaques (lupus vulgaris). The diagnosis is made with histopathological examination and culture of a biopsy specimen. Treatment is the same as with all other forms of tuberculosis with quadruple therapy (rifampicin, isoniazid, ethambutol and pyrazinamide)[27].

Fungal infections

Candidosis

Candidosis is a common mycotic infection that affects girls and women, primarily in the vulvovaginal area, but with spreading to the perineum and the perianal region (Figure 8). The main predisposing factors include extremes of age, pregnancy, menses, use of oral contraceptives, use of broad-spectrum antibiotics, diabetes and immunosuppression. It may also be sexually transmitted. In infants the source of the yeast is the gastrointestinal tract, with the eruption starting perianally and spreading to the perineum and genitocrural folds, resulting in a diaper eruption.

It is mainly characterized by pruritic, macerated, erythematous plaques with satellite vesicopustules. The diagnosis is confirmed by a KOH preparation

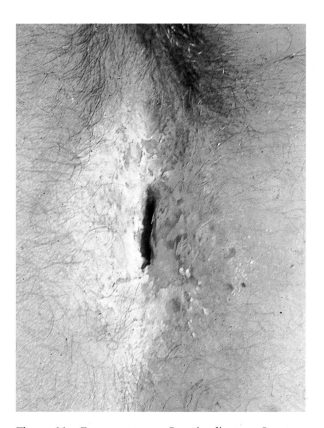

Figure 11 Extramammary Paget's disease. Courtesy Department of Dermatology, Mayo Clinic, Rochester, MN

that will show pseudohyphae and spores. Treatment is usually achieved with topical antifungal agents (miconazole or ketoconazole), and oral nystatin to clear the gastrointestinal colonization, when this is the suspected source[4].

Dermatophytosis

Tinea cruris may affect the perianal area, especially with *Trichophyton rubrum* infection, but to a lesser extent with *Epidermophyton floccosum*. It is characterized by an advancing, erythematous papulovesicular border with central clearing. The diagnosis is confirmed with a KOH preparation of skin scrapings. Treatment is usually with topical antifungals (miconazole or ketoconazole), but if it is severe and/or widespread a systemic antifungal may also be used (griseofulvin, terbinafine or itraconazole)[4,28].

Viral infections

Condyloma acuminatum

Perianal condyloma acuminatum can be transmitted sexually via anal intercourse, but it can also be non-venereal (Figure 9). It is usually caused by the human papilloma virus (HPV) types 6 and 11. Types 16, 18, 31 and 33–35 also cause condyloma acuminatum and are associated with dysplasia and carcinoma. The condition is characterized by multiple, variably sized, skin-colored, filiform papules that may enlarge into exophytic masses, especially in the immunosuppressed. The warts may extend internally into the rectal epithelium. Treatment of perianal condyloma acuminatum may include topical imiquimod or podophyllotoxin, intralesional interferon-α, or destructive therapies (cryotherapy, electrodesiccation, surgical excision, or CO_2 laser). Management should include proctoscopy and colposcopy to detect rectal and cervical involvement[29].

Herpes simplex

Perianal herpes simplex infection is usually caused by herpes simplex virus type 2, which is usually transmitted sexually by anal intercourse. It is characterized by painful, itchy vesicles on an erythematous base which usually erode. In immunosuppressed individuals the erosions become deep ulcers and tend to be more extensive and chronic. The diagnosis is confirmed with a Tzanck smear and culture of vesicle fluid. Treatment is with systemic antivirals such as acyclovir, valaciclovir, or famciclovir, with use of foscarnet in resistant cases, usually seen in immunocompromised individuals[30].

Herpes zoster

Herpes zoster of the S2-S4 dermatomes results in anogenital zoster, which is characterized by unilateral involvement and severe pain, and can be associated with bladder and anal dysfunction. Treatment is with antiviral agents as for perianal herpes simplex, but at higher doses[4].

Cytomegalovirus

Cytomegalovirus infection may be a cause of perianal vesicles, ulcers and inflammation in the immunocompromised, particularly in infants with HIV infection. Diagnosis is made by culture from the vesicle fluid. Treatment is with various systemic antiviral agents, including ganciclovir, foscarnet or cidifovir[31].

Parasitic infections

Amebiasis

This is an infection caused by the protozoan *Entamoeba histolytica*, and normally causes colitis, but there may be perianal cutaneous involvement secondary to direct extension of rectal involvement. The lesion is usually a pustule that quickly breaks down into a painful ulcer with an erythematous halo. The diagnosis is made by finding trophozoites on skin scrapings or skin biopsy. Treatment is with metronidazole or tinidazole[4].

Schistosomiasis

This is caused by the trematode of *Schistosoma* species. The perianal manifestations of schistosomiasis are painless, skin-colored, erosive papules, which may be verrucous. The diagnosis is made by detecting ova on biopsy of the lesions. Praziquantel is the treatment of choice for schistosomiasis[4].

Enterobiasis

This is an intestinal infestation caused by the nematode *Enterobius vermicularis*, and is transmitted by the feco-oral route. It results in nocturnal perianal pruritus that can result in secondary infection. The diagnosis is made by identification of the eggs in the perianal area. Treatment is with various antihelminthics, including mebendazole or albendazole[32].

NEOPLASTIC DISEASES
Premalignant neoplasms

Bowen's disease

Bowen's disease is a SCC *in situ*, and can affect the perianal region, where it manifests as a verrucous or erythroplakic patch. In 38% of women with anogenital Bowen's disease, it is associated with cancer of the genitourinary tract, thus necessitating a gynecological examination. Treatment is usually with surgical excision[33].

Bowenoid papulosis

Bowenoid papulosis is a low-grade SCC *in situ* that is caused by the human papilloma virus, usually types 16 (particularly in women), 18, 31, 32 and 34. It is slightly more common in women. It is characterized by reddish-brown to violaceous papules. Diagnosis is made with histopathological examination of a biopsy specimen. Treatment is by destructive methods such as cryotherapy or electrodesiccation[33].

Malignant neoplasms

Anal squamous cell carcinoma

Anal SCC is the commonest malignant neoplasm of the anal region, accounting for about 55% of anal carcinomas (Figure 10), the rest being basal cell carcinoma, adenocarcinoma or melanoma. It seems that there has been an increase in the incidence of anal SCC. It is slightly more common, but less aggressive, in women. A number of predisposing factors are implicated in the causation of SCC, these including previous human papilloma virus infection, a previous history of cervical intraepithelial neoplasia (Buschke–Lowenstein tumor), chronic inflammatory conditions (lichen sclerosis et atrophicus, Crohn's disease, lymphogranuloma venereum), smoking and radiotherapy for gynecological malignancy.

Anal SCC presents with rectal bleeding or pain, constipation, an indurated and ulcerated perianal nodule, and inguinal adenopathy. The diagnosis is confirmed by histopathological examination of a biopsy specimen.

Treatment involves surgical excision and inguinal lymphadenectomy. Radiotherapy is also used as adjuvant therapy or when surgery is contraindicated[4].

Extramammary Paget's disease

Extramammary Paget's disease is an intraepithelial adenocarcinoma that may affect the perianal regions, amongst other regions (Figure 11). It is characterized clinically by a pruritic, bleeding, scaly, erythematous plaque, which may ulcerate. The diagnosis is confirmed by histopathological examination of a biopsy specimen. It may or may not be associated with an adnexal carcinoma or a visceral carcinoma (usually genitourinary or gastrointestinal). It seems that the perianal condition is more likely to be associated with an underlying adnexal or visceral carcinoma, thus warranting a search for an underlying visceral cancer. Treatment is usually with surgical excision (including Mohs micrographic surgery) preceded by topical 5-fluorouracil. The prognosis is worse with underlying adnexal or visceral cancer[34].

REFERENCES

1. Sires UI, Mallory SB. Diaper dermatitis. *Postgrad Med* 1995;98:79–86
2. Konya J, Gow E. Granuloma gluteale infantum. *Australas J Dermatol* 1996;37:57–8
3. Goldberg NS, Esterly NB, Rothman KF, *et al.* Perianal pseudoverrucous papules and nodules in children. *Arch Dermatol* 1992;128:240–2
4. Ive FA. The umbilical, perianal and genital regions. In Champion RH, Burton JL, Burns DA, Breathnach SM, eds. *Textbook of Dermatology*, 6th edn. Oxford: Blackwell Science, 1998:3169–81
5. Schopf R. Seborrheic eczema. In Marks R, ed. *Eczema*, 1st edn. London: Martin Dunitz, 1992: 129–48
6. Farber EM, Mullen RH, Jacobs AH, *et al.* Infantile psoriasis: a follow-up study. *Pediatr Dermatol* 1986;3:237–43
7. Christophers E, Mrowietz U. Psoriasis. In Freedberg I, Eisen AZ, Wolff K, Austen KF, eds. *Dermatology in General Medicine*, 5th edn. New York: McGraw-Hill, 1999:495–521
8. Sloan PJM, Goepel J. Lichen sclerosis et atrophicus and perianal carcinoma. *Clin Exp Dermatol* 1981;6: 399–402
9. Meffert JL, Davis BM, Grimwood RE. Lichen sclerosis. *J Am Acad Dermatol* 1995;32:393–416
10. Boyd AS, Neldner KH. Lichen planus. *J Am Acad Dermatol* 1991;25:593–619
11. Mutasim DF, Pelc NJ, Anhalt GJ. Cicatricial pemphigoid. *Dermatol Clin* 1993;11:499–510
12. Wojnarowska F, Eady RAJ, Burge M. Bullous eruptions. In Champion RH, Burton JL, Burns DA, Breathnach SM, eds. *Textbook of Dermatology*, 6th edn. Oxford: Blackwell Science, 1998:1817–97
13. Daoud MS, Dicken CH. Apocrine glands. In Freedberg IM, Eisen AZ, Wolff K, Austen KF, eds. *Dermatology in General Medicine*, 5th edn. New York: McGraw-Hill, 1999:810–17
14. Friter BS, Lucky AW. The perineal eruption of Kawasaki syndrome. *Arch Dermatol* 1988;124: 1805–10
15. Manders SM. Toxin-mediated streptococcal and staphylococcal disease. *J Am Acad Dermatol* 1998; 39:383–98
16. Weismann K, Graham RM. Systemic disease and the skin. In Champion RH, Burton JL, Burns DA,

Breathnach SM, eds. *Textbook of Dermatology*, 6th edn. Oxford: Blackwell Science, 1998:2703–57

17. Ghate JV, Jorizzo JL. Behçet's disease and complex aphthosis. *J Am Acad Dermatol* 1999;40:1–18

18. Thorisdottir K, Camisa C, Tomecki KJ, *et al.* Necrolytic migratory erythema. *J Am Acad Dermatol* 1994;30:324–9

19. Chu AC. Histiocytoses. In Champion RH, Burton JL, Burns DA, Breathnach SM, eds. *Textbook of Dermatology*, 6th edn. Oxford: Blackwell Science, 1998: 2311–36

20. Kokx NP, Comstock J, Facklam RR. Streptococcal perianal disease in children. *Pediatrics* 1987;80: 659–63

21. Sanchez MR. Syphilis. In Freedberg IM, Eisen AZ, Wolff K, Austen KF, eds. *Dermatology in General Medicine*, 5th edn. New York: McGraw-Hill, 1999: 2551–81

22. Rothenberg RB. Lymphogranuloma venereum. In Freedberg IM, Eisen AZ, Wolff K, Austen KF, eds. *Dermatology in General Medicine*, 5th edn. New York: McGraw-Hill, 1999:2591–4

23. Feingold DS, Peacocke M. Gonorrhea. In Freedberg IM, Eisen AZ, Wolff K, Austen KF, eds. *Dermatology in General Medicine*, 5th edn. New York: McGraw-Hill, 1999:2598–603

24. Eichmann AR. Chancroid. In Freedberg IM, Eisen AZ, Wolff K, Austen KF, eds. *Dermatology in General Medicine*, 5th edn. New York: McGraw-Hill, 1999:2587–91

25. Rothenberg RB. Granuloma inguinale. In Freedberg IM, Eisen AZ, Wolff K, Austen KF, eds. *Dermatology in General Medicine*, 5th edn. New York: McGraw-Hill, 1999:2595–8

26. Green RJ, Dafoe DC, Raffin TA. Necrotizing fasciitis. *Chest* 1996;110:219–28

27. Gawkrodger DJ. Mycobacterial infections. In Champion RH, Burton JL, Burns DA, Breathnach SM, eds. *Textbook of Dermatology*, 6th edn. Oxford: Blackwell Science, 1998:1181–214

28. Martin AG, Kobayashi GS. Superficial fungal infections: dermatophytosis, tinea nigra, piedra. In Freedberg IM, Eisen AZ, Wolff K, Austen KF, eds. *Dermatology in General Medicine*, 5th edn. New York: McGraw-Hill, 1999:2337–57

29. Lowy DR, Androphy EJ. Warts. In Freedberg IM, Eisen AZ, Wolff K, Austen KF, eds. *Dermatology in General Medicine*, 5th edn. New York: McGraw-Hill, 1999:2484–97

30. Crumpacker CS. Herpes simplex. In Freedberg IM, Eisen AZ, Wolff K, Austen KF, eds. *Dermatology in General Medicine*, 5th edn. New York: McGraw-Hill, 1999:2414–26

31. Thiboutot DM, Beckford A, Mart CR, *et al.* Cytomegalovirus diaper dermatitis. *Arch Dermatol* 1991;127:396–8

32. Lucchina LC, Wilson ME. Cysticercosis and other helminthic infections. In Freedberg IM, Eisen AZ, Wolff K, Austen KF, eds. *Dermatology in General Medicine*, 5th edn. New York: McGraw-Hill, 1999:2619–54

33. Schwartz RA, Stoll HL. Epithelial precancerous lesions. In Freedberg IM, Eisen AZ, Wolff K, Austen KF, eds. *Dermatology in General Medicine*, 5th edn. New York: McGraw-Hill, 1999:2595–8

34. Connolly MS. Mammary and extramammary Paget's disease. In Freedberg IM, Eisen AZ, Wolff K, *et al.*, eds. *Dermatology in General Medicine*, 5th edn. New York: McGraw-Hill, 1999:919–24

Dermatological diseases of the vulva

31

Jivko A. Kamarashev and Snejina G. Vassileva

INTRODUCTION

Vulvar pathology represents a complex matter due to the organ's morphology and variety of functions throughout the life cycle of a woman. This raises diffculties for outlining and classifying the spectrum of dermatological diseases of the vulva often faced by different medical specialties. The vulva can be affected in the course of many systemic dermatitides such as psoriasis, lichen planus, vitiligo, benign familial pemphigus, acquired autoimmune bullous disorders, seborrheic dermatitis, atopic dermatitis and even adverse cutaneous drug reactions. Other diseases including vulvodynia, cyclic vulvitis, vulvar vestibulitis and vestibular papillomatosis are essentially confined to the vulva. The vulvar region may be also involved by disorders of the internal organs, as in the case of the inflammatory bowel syndrome. Regardless of their origin, dermatological diseases of the vulva merit careful attention and clinical competence to counteract the patient's timidity and psychological distress and to prevent possible sexual dysfunction.

In very young girls, malformations, nevi and vascular tumors are rare but may cause morbidity and sequelae, while intercurrent conditions such as napkin dermatitis, intertrigo and non-venereal vulvovaginitis, although common, are easily managed. Certain dermatoses such as vulvar lichen sclerosus and localized vulvar cicatricial pemphigoid relatively often affect prepubertal girls and can become a subject of great parental concern. Sexually transmitted diseases and traumatic lesions in this age group are suggestive of child sexual abuse, but extreme caution is required in the differential diagnosis of such cases, because of the grave social consequences.

In the sexually active period, the female genitalia are subjected to significant hormonal influences and fulfil important functions. A major proportion of vulvar pathology during that period is contributed by sexually transmitted diseases, which are developed in a separate chapter of this book. A number of premalignant and malignant diseases may affect the vulva including genital Bowen's disease, Paget's disease, squamous cell carcinoma, basal cell carcinoma and malignant melanoma, raising the issue of finding the optimal balance between radicality of therapy and preservation of functions, which is important for minimally affecting the quality of life. Although most such lesions are observed after the menopause, some of them can also be encountered in younger women.

In this brief overview several items are evoked only to illustrate the diversity and complexity of the matter. Selected issues are addressed, which we feel are of particular importance to the clinical dermatologist, and the understanding of which has undergone significant development in recent years.

VULVOVAGINAL CANDIDOSIS

Vulvovaginal candidosis (VVC) is a common problem in dermatological and gynecological practice of panglobal distribution. Epidemiological data suggest that its incidence is on the rise. Seventy-five per cent of women are thought to experience at least one episode of VVC in their childbearing period[1]. Forty to fifty per cent of these suffer a second attack. A small proportion of patients are prone to many recurrences for years on end. Recurrent VVC has proved to be stubbornly refractory to the wide spectrum of modern antifungals. On the other hand *Candida albicans* has been isolated from 15–20% of asymptomatic women and for pregnant women this figure rises to 30–45%[2].

The vulva and vagina can each be separately affected by candidosis but concurrent involvement is far more common. The most often encountered symptom is vulvar pruritus, followed by vaginal discharge, vulvodynia, vaginal soreness and dyspareunia. On physical examination there are mucosal erythema and edema, with numerous fragile pustules and satellite lesions. Small erosions and fissures in the natural folds may additionally be detected. In non-treated cases the infection may spread to the genitocrural folds and the perianal region (Figure 1), to the urethra and even the urinary bladder.

The pathogenesis of VVC and particularly the pathogenicity determinants, predisposing factors and host–microorganism interactions have been intensively studied in the past decade. Today it is generally accepted that *Candida* species different from *Candida albicans* are capable of causing disease. These include *C. glabrata, c. tropicalis, C. kefyr, C. parapsilosis* and *C. kruzei*, some of which have been shown to be significantly more resistant to therapy[3,4]. The extensive use of antifungal agents may account for the well-documented rise in prevalence of non-*albicans* species, which was 9.9% in the 1970s and climbed to 21.3% in the 1980s[5]. A major problem that still remains to a significant extent unsolved is recurrent VVC – a source of anxiety and frustration for both patients and physicians. In patients with current candidosis a provoking factor is usually detectable, which is not the case in patients with recurrent VVC. The intestinal reservoir[6], contaminated underwear[7] and sexual transmission[8] have all been proposed as sources of reinfection, but the importance of their role has been seriously challenged. Views have significantly shifted in the past few years in the direction of the vaginal relapse theory. It is suspected that, regardless of therapy, low numbers of yeasts may persist in the vagina and eventually cause recurrences[5].

Host defense mechanisms are most probably inadequate in patients with recurrent VVC, although the nature of their impairment remains debatable. Humoral immunity mechanisms do not seem to be responsible, because both serum and secretory anti-*Candida* antibodies can be detected in most if not all patients, provided a sensitive serological method is applied[9].

Suppression of cell-mediated immunity, on the other hand, correlates very well with systemic candidosis and has been suspected to be involved in recurrent VVC. Reduced T-cell proliferative responses to *C. albicans* have been demonstrated *in vitro*; these have been attributed to the production of *Candida*-specific suppressor T lymphocytes and a soluble inhibiting factor[10]. It has been suggested that immunosuppression can be caused by a toxin/gliotoxin produced by *C. albicans*. Significant levels of gliotoxin have been detected in vaginal samples of patients with vaginal candidosis but not in control samples of healthy women[11].

A hypersensitivity mechanism has also been proposed as a plausible explanation for at least some cases of recurrent VVC. It has been noted that the number of yeasts in recurrent infection may be much smaller than is necessary to induce an initial attack. *C. albicans*-specific antibodies of the IgE class have been detected in the vaginal secretions of one-third of patients with recurrent VVC by means of a radioallergosorbent test (RAST) or enzyme-linked immunosorbent assay (ELISA)[12]. Conversely, IgE antibodies were not detected in any of the healthy controls. Almost half of the patients with IgE antibodies to *C. albicans* also had eosinophils in their vaginal smears.

The complexity and divergence of pathogenesis has motivated Monif[13] to propose a classification of VVC (Table 1).

Diagnosis of VVC is based on clinical findings, microscopic examination (wet mount, 10% KOH preparation, methylene blue or Gram stain) and cultural methods. An advance in the diagnosis of VVC has been the introduction of a latex agglutination test based on the detection of a yeast antigen (mannan) in vaginal swabs. The test's sensitivity has been reported to be 71.8%, compared to 38.5% sensitivity of microscopic examination, while specificity is similar for both methods[14]. Strain determination techniques should be reserved for the proper diagnosis and management of recurrent VVC.

In most cases, therapy of VVC is not problematic. In the past two decades, polyenes have largely been replaced by azole derivatives, because of greater efficacy. A tendency has developed for the local application of larger doses for shorter periods of time. Ever since ketoconazole was introduced in the beginning of the 1980s, the question has arisen whether VVC should be treated locally or orally. This dilemma has become even more debatable since the triazoles fluconazole and itraconazole became available, providing the opportunity for single-day treatment. There is little doubt that patient preference lies with oral therapy. On the

Table 1 Monif's classification of vulvovaginal candidosis. From reference 13

Genesis I. Primary candidal vulvovaginal candidosis
A. Vulvitis
B. Vulvovaginitis with predominantly
  vulvar involvement
C. Vaginitis with relatively minimal involvement
Genesis II. Antibiotic
A. Resulting from systemic therapy for
  non-vulvovaginal infection
B. Resulting from local or systemic therapy for
  vaginal infection
Genesis III. Systemically influenced vulvovaginal candidosis
A. Pregnancy, high-dose estrogen and contraceptives
B. Steroids
C. Diabetes mellitus
D. T-cell dysfunction
  congenital
  acquired

other hand, topical formulations are the only alternative during pregnancy, and should be preferred in cases of extensive vulvar involvement.

Recurrent VVC is still a major therapeutic problem, for which oral treatment and long-term prophylactics seem a more logical approach, because this provides the additional opportunity for elimination of extravaginal *Candida* species. Although no ultimate treatment of chronic VVC is available at this point, low-dose monthly prophylaxis with itraconazole for 6 months has been shown to reduce symptomatic episodes effectively and safely[15].

VULVODYNIA

Vulvodynia or vulvar 'burning' syndrome is a descriptive term reserved for cases of refractory vulvar pain in the absence of defined dermatological disease or obvious physical abnormalities. The first description of vulvar pain syndrome dates back to the end of the 19th century, but a greater body of understanding, diagnostic procedures and treatment modalities has been accumulated only after 1983, when the International Society for Study of Vulvar Diseases was established, and a new nomenclature and classification were introduced[16].

Vulvodynia is currently regarded as a group of diseases characterized by the patient's complaint of vulvar burning, stinging, irritation, or rawness in the absence of pruritus. In the majority of cases, vulvodynia has an acute onset but later takes a chronic course lasting months to years. Physical discomfort, dyspareunia, sexual disability and psychological disturbances are common resulting features. Some patients may be embarrassed to report their vulvar symptoms and sexual dysfunctions, while others continuously see multiple practitioners. They try all kinds of remedies in the hope of finding a diagnosis and relief from pain. They often fear cancer or communicable disease. Until recently, vulvodynia was thought to be solely a psychosomatic syndrome. Within the past decade, however, the initial insistence on a major role for psychological factors has gradually given way to sophisticated searches for other factors in the etiology and pathogenesis of the 'burning' vulva syndrome.

According to current concepts vulvodynia is a multifactorial disease spectrum[16], comprising several clinical conditions:

(1) Morphologically defined and recognizable vulvar dermatoses, such as vulvovaginal candidosis, papilloma virus infection, lichen sclerosus, erosive lichen planus, contact dermatitis and bullous dermatoses;

(2) Cyclic vulvitis;

(3) Vulvar vestibulitis;

(4) Vestibular papillomatosis;

(5) Essential (dysesthetic) vulvodynia.

Each of these subtypes of vulvodynia has specific etiological and diagnostic considerations and their recognition is mandatory for the treatment of patients' complaints. On the other hand, vulvodynia may be primarily associated with only one factor, but simultaneously or consequently several factors may coexist and overlap. It is therefore mandatory to investigate all potential factors in every patient with vulvodynia. Patient evaluation should comprise several steps. A thorough history should be taken, especially with regard to underlying dermatoses, candidosis, condylomata, cleansing methods and the use of topical and systemic medications. Diagnostic tests should be directed towards ruling out infection and should include a vaginal smear, culture for *Candida*, whitening with acetic acid and patch-testing in suspected contact dermatitis. Biopsies should be performed in any questionable areas. Evaluation of patients' psychological profile through appropriate psychometric instruments would reveal several disturbances, such as anxiety, depression, hypochondriasis, obsessive–compulsive behaviors, etc., which also have to be treated.

Cyclic vulvitis

This denomination refers to cases of variable vulvodynia, characterized by periodic exacerbations or alternatively by symptom-free intervals with a patient-specific pattern regarding the menstrual cycle. In some women it may be associated with episodic vulvar erythema, pruritus, discharge and a sensation of tumification of the vulva. An association between *Candida* infection and cyclic vulvitis has been hypothesized but remains unproved, because of inconsistent microscopic and culture yields. Long-term topical or systemic antifungal therapy has been reported to result in significant symptom alleviation in a group of patients with cyclic vulvitis, regardless of preliminary culture results. On the basis of these data it has been suggested that, in everyday practice, a history of a variable vulvodynia pattern may be sufficient reason to initiate long-term anticandidal therapy.

Vulvar vestibulitis

As a separate entity, vulvar vestibulitis has attracted considerable attention. The same condition has also been referred to in the literature as 'minor

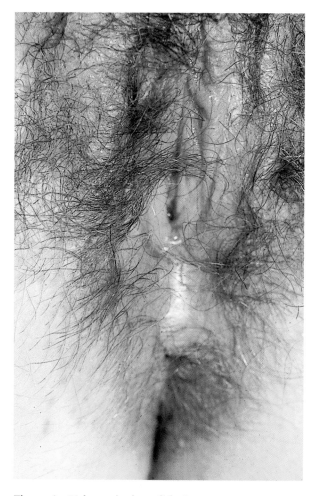

Figure 1 Vulvovaginal candidosis

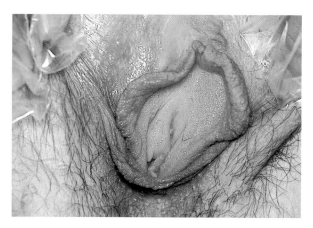

Figure 2 Vestibular papillomatosis

vestibular gland syndrome', 'focal vulvitis', 'vulvar vestibulitis' syndrome and 'periglandular vestibulitis'. It involves[17]:

(1) Severe pain on vestibular touch or attempted vaginal entry;

(2) Tenderness to pressure localized within the vulvar vestibule;

(3) Physical findings consisting of vulvar erythema of various degrees.

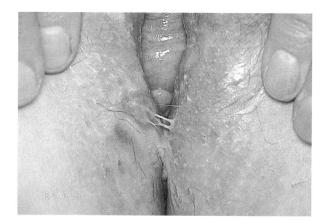

Figure 3 Cicatricial pemphigoid – vulvar involvement

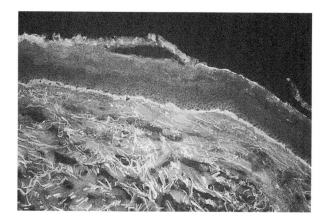

Figure 4 Cicatricial pemphigoid (same patient as in Figure 3). Direct immunofluorescence revealing linear IgG at the dermal–epidermal junction

Most patients are sexually active women in their twenties or thirties. A marked predominance of Caucasians has been noted[18]. Every third patient in one series had at least one relative with dyspareunia or tampon intolerance, suggesting a genetic predisposition[19]. The etiology is unclear. Subclinical human papilloma virus (HPV) infection has been suspected as a causal factor by some[20], but others have failed to demonstrate an increased frequency of HPV in patients with vulvar vestibulitis when compared to control groups[21–23]. Some have attributed the syndrome to an autoimmune cross-reactivity response elicited by *C. albicans*[24]. Other infections have also been incriminated, but to date there is no proof that any of these are related to vulvar vestibulitis, and serious doubts exist that pathogenic micro-organisms are relevant to this syndrome[25]. Chemical and destructive therapeutic agents (cryosurgery, podophyllin, laser treatment) have also been suggested as causative factors. Severe cases have been reported after use of fluorouracil cream[19]. Metabolic factors, such as periodic hyperoxaluria and persistent pH alterations, have been shown to be of importance in some cases[26,27].

Cases in which vulvar vestibulitis was associated with interstitial cystitis have suggested that the two conditions may be manifestations of a generalized disorder of urogenital sinus-derived epithelium[28]. Ulcerations[29] and acute vasculitis[18] may sometimes be detected and raise the possibility of a connection to Behçet's disease.

The relative risk for the development of vulvar vestibulitis in women who had started using oral contraceptives before the age of 17 has been reported to be 11 times greater than that for women who had never been on the pill. This indicates a possible contribution of hormonal factors to the etiology of the disorder.

Increased urethral pressure variability, probably attributed to variation in muscular tone of the urethra, has been detected in patients with vulvar vestibulitis[30], although its importance in the pathogenesis is uncertain. Deviations in pelvic floor muscle parameters have been recorded by computerized electromyographic evaluation; recently, electromyographic biofeedback has shown promising therapeutic results[31]. Cases with vulvodynia in association with delayed pressure urticaria and dermographism have been described, and an immunological basis mediated by IgE antibodies has been suggested[32]. Treatment with H1 antagonists has proven to be effective. Finally, psychosexual and relational aspects have been considered[33,34].

The main presenting complaint is superficial dyspareunia. The onset is usually sudden, rarely gradual. As a rule the pain is well localized to one or several spots on the vestibule and is severe enough to force the majority of patients to relinquish sexual activity. Tampon installation or even the wearing of tight underwear have been reported as additional pain-provoking factors.

Physical examination reveals minute spots of erythema around the small vestibular glands, ranging in size from 2 to 7 mm. The number of such lesions ranges from one to 11 (median 3)[30]. Small ulcerations may rarely be noted. Lesions are predominantly situated in the lower half of the vestibule, which may in some instances be diffusely reddened. Palpation with a cotton swab around the base of the hymeneal ring and the posterior fourchette reveals exquisite point tenderness of the lesions.

Histologically a chronic inflammatory infiltrate is found consisting predominantly of T lymphocytes and a smaller number of B lymphocytes and an admixture of plasma cells, mast cells and occasional monocytes[23,35]. Immunohistochemically the predominance of IgG-positive plasma cells was identified, suggesting a chronic irritation, but an autoimmune mechanism cannot be excluded. The infiltrate is situated in the mucosal lamina propria and in the periglandular periductal connective tissue. Foci of squamous metaplasia of the minor vestibular glands are a regular finding. In some cases nodular hyperplasia ('adenoma') of vestibular glands is observed[23,36].

Numerous therapeutic approaches have been tried, with variable success. In all cases with an identifiable causal factor, etiological treatment has to be attempted. Spontaneous resolution has been reported in up to 50% of cases[30], underlining the importance of conservative treatment aimed at symptom alleviation. Topical application of lidocaine in the form of a solution or gel has been recommended. Topical and intralesional corticosteroids can be tried. In cases persisting for more than 6 months, interferon treatment has been recently recommended as a first-line approach. Good results in HPV infection associated with vulvar vestibulitis have been reported with intramuscular injections of interferon-β[37,38]. Intralesional recombinant interferon-α has been shown to be cost effective in the management of vulvar vestibulitis persisting for at least 6 months, and has been advocated as a first-choice treatment[39]. Surgical excision without or with vaginal advancement should be reserved as a least resort in recalcitrant vulvar vestibulitis. The role of psychological support, counseling and patient education should not be underestimated.

Vestibular papillomatosis

Vestibular papillomatosis (synonyms pseudocondylomata, pruritic vulvar squamous papillomatosis, benign squamous papillomatosis, hirsutoid papillomas of vulvae, vestibular micropapilloma) was first described in the early 1980s[40]. Vestibular papillomatosis is by no means rare, and a recent study[41] has shown a prevalence of 1% among unselected outpatients attending a genitourinary medicine clinic.

Vestibular papillae appear as numerous, smooth, pearly white, soft excrescences, providing a grainy appearance of the affected sites, although they may sometimes be digitiform or even filiform, reaching a length of 6–8 mm. The inner aspects of the labia minora, the vulvar vestibule and the fourchette are the typical localizations (Figure 2). The pattern of distribution is predominantly bilateral, often symmetrical, and sometimes linear. In the majority of cases vestibular papillae are an incidental asymptomatic finding. In some patients, however, they may be associated with pruritus, vulvodynia, superficial dyspareunia and postcoital irritation of variable intensity.

There is no universal agreement as to their etiology. They have been regarded as a normal anatomical variant and later as a 'subclinical' manifestation of an HPV infection[42,43]. In one series of 20 patients[44], all had histopathological changes suggestive of HPV infection and 16 (80%) of specimens contained DNA sequences homologous to HPV probes. On the other hand, follow-up for more than 18 months showed that vestibular papillae remained unchanged in appearance and distribution and no HPV-associated lesions were detected in any male partner. On the basis of these observations the authors concluded that 'HPV16 is frequently associated with vestibular papillae but does not support a productive infection'. In another study[41], 17 of 18 cases (94%) had histological features consistent with HPV infection and HPV16 was found by DNA hybridization studies or polymerase chain reaction in seven cases (39%). This association, however, is far from universally accepted. Vestibular papillae are in most cases easily distinguished from condylomata acuminata on the basis of their regular distribution pattern, uniform color, soft consistency and lack of a tendency to coalesce. Numerous studies have failed to establish a cause–effect relationship between vestibular papillomatosis and HPV infection, from histological and virological data[45–49]. Despite the controversy, at this point most authors agree that patients with symmetrically distributed vulvar papillae of long duration need not be treated but should be followed up.

Essential vulvodynia

The exclusion of the above subsets of vulvodynia in some patients makes plausible the diagnostic denomination 'essential' or 'dysesthetic' vulvodynia. The patients, often postmenopausal women, complain of constant unremitting burning localized to the vulva, but do not show any significant changes on physical examination. Other symptoms such as dysesthesia, hyperesthesia, hyperalgesia and allodynia are frequently reported. This syndrome could therefore be compared to other idiopathic pain syndromes, including post-zoster neuralgia, glossodynia (burning tongue) and sympathetic reflex dystrophy. An involvement of the primary afferent fibers (PAFs) has been postulated as playing a role in the pathogenesis and maintenance of essential vulvodynia. The results of a recent study have shown that the pain threshold to acid solutions is decreased in essential vulvodynia cases, probably in relation to increased sensitivity of PAFs and release of substance P[50].

Psychological evaluation, comparing patients with essential vulvodynia and vulvodynia of other subtypes, has retrieved several common personality traits in the first studied group. Patients with essential vulvodynia were more anxious, more suggestible and more distressed than patients with vulvodynia with other physical causes[51]. Treatment with low-dose amitriptyline (40–60 mg daily) has proven to be effective in many cases[52]. Further psychological support is required in the management of this chronic debilitating disorder.

VULVITIS CIRCUMSCRIPTA PLASMACELLULARIS (ZOON'S VULVITITS)

The initial report of this entity belongs to Garnier and dates back to 1954[53]. It is much rarer than its male counterpart – balanitis circumscripta plasmacellularis – and until the mid-1980s only ten cases had been reported[54]. At least 17 additional case reports have been published in the past 10 years[55–62]. This is most probably due to a better awareness of the problem rather than to an actual rise in prevalence.

The reported age of patients varies between 28 and 89 years. Any part of the vulva may be affected. Lesions are less striking than in Zoon's balanitis and in typical cases present as shiny, glazed erythematous patches with an orange hue. Often, multiple pinpoint purpuric 'cayenne pepper spots' are conspicuous. Painful shallow erosions can be present. Symptoms vary from patient to patient from non-existent to pronounced, pruritus, burning, soreness and dyspareunia. Clinical diagnosis, however, is unreliable, and differentiation from lichen planus, genital Bowen's disease, extramammary Paget's disease, syphilis, fixed drug eruption or candida vulvitis may be difficult.

Histological findings are quite characteristic[63]. Typical epidermal changes are atrophy with loss of rete ridges, spongiosis and elongated 'lozenge' keratinocytes. Scattered dyskeratotic cells may be observed, but atypia and mitoses are lacking. A dense lichenoid infiltrate is present in the upper and mid-dermis, consisting largely of plasma cells, intermingled with lymphocytes, mast cells, scarce neutrophils and eosinophils. Vascular proliferation, erythrocyte extravasation and hemosiderin deposition are other helpful clues for establishing the histological disgnosis of Zoon's vulvitis. Direct immunofluorescence (DIF) may be negative[55], or might reveal staining of plasma cells with anti-IgA[61] or with anti-IgE[64] hyperimmune sera.

The etiology is unknown. Chronic irritation due to warmth, friction, poor personal hygiene or persistent infection has been suggested as a possible provoking factor. This might be a pattern of inflammation characteristic of all periorificial sites, since cases of oral mucosa and conjunctiva involvement have been reported and the term 'circumorificial plasmacytosis' has been proposed[65]. The importance of the vascular changes has been stressed. Therapy is difficult. The effect of topical corticoids is inconsistent. Interferon-α proved successful in one case[56]. Excellent results were reported after 3 months of topical cyclosporin application in another[61].

BULLOUS DISEASES

Many bullous dermatoses may affect the female genitalia. Pemphigus vulgaris may involve not only the vulva, but also the vagina and even the cervix[66]. Dermatitis herpetiformis and epidermolysis bullosa acquisita may also spread to this area and cicatricial pemphigoid has been reported to affect the genitalia in 19% of cases[67]. Pemphigoid gestationis has a certain predilection for the vulva.

Localized bullous pemphigoid may be confined to the female genitalia[68,69]. Most commonly this is the case of mucous membrane or cicatricial pemphigoid, primarily observed in elderly women. The chronic progressive course of the disease with recurrent bullae, which heal with scars and synechiae, frequently results in introital and vaginal atresia (Figure 3)[70]. In 1985 De Castro and colleagues[71] first described a childhood variant of localized vulvar pemphigoid. Several additional cases have been reported[72–74], confirming the affiliation of this condition to the bullous pemphigoid spectrum. Despite its rarity, it deserves a high level of awareness, since it is part of the most unfortunate group of dermatological diseases (including mongolian spots, phytophotodermatitis, chronic bullous dermatosis, allergic contact dermatitis and lichen sclerosus)[75,76], which may be and have been misdiagnosed as child sexual abuse. Of the reported cases to date the youngest was in a 3-year-old girl[73]. Lesions typically consist of tense clear or hemorrhagic bullae overlying normal or erythematous skin. Upon rupture, painful erosions are formed which heal without scarring or milia formation. The correct diagnosis is established by histological, immunofluorescent (Figure 4), ultrastructural and immunoblotting methods. Topical corticosteroids are mostly effective, but recurrences may be expected after cessation of therapy[74].

LICHEN PLANUS

Lichen planus (LP) is well known for afflicting the oral mucosa. Genital lesions occur in up to 25% of men with LP[77], while the general conviction that vulvovaginal involvement is rare has led to underestimation of the problem and undue delay in diagnosis and treatment of such patients.

Vulvar lesions present as whitish, slightly elevated, reticulated papules and plaques, which are a source of pruritus of variable intensity. Pronounced erythema and erosions are sometimes observed, associated with burning, pain, dyspareunia and postcoital bleeding[78,79]. The erosions, which may be extensive and may dominate the clinical picture, are in most cases rimmed by white lacy epithelial lesions, providing a valuable diagnostic clue. In severe cases scarring and mutilation of the vulva may result. Patients with erosive lichen planus of the vulva often have concurrent desquamative or frankly erosive vaginitis, and in some cases even the cervix may be affected. Vaginal involvement may result in adhesions and stenosis, rendering intercourse impossible[80].

The association of erosive lichen planus of the vulva and vagina with desquamative gingivitis was first recognized in the early 1980s[81]. The new vulvovaginal–gingival syndrome is considered to be a variant of mucosal lichen planus comprising erosions and desquamation of the vulva, vagina and gingiva. Associated skin lesions are a rare finding in this plurimucosal variant of the disease. Several series of patients with the syndrome have been published to date[78,81,82].

Vulvar lesions of lichen planus have to be differentiated from those of pemphigus vulgaris, bullous and cicatricial pemphigoid, epidermolysis bullosa acquisita, bullous lichen sclerosus and vulvitis circumscripta plasmacellularis.

Typical histology and the demonstration of colloid bodies by direct immunofluorescence are of major value for the diagnosis of vulvar LP. A biopsy specimen should be obtained from the whitish reticulated periphery, since findings in material from eroded sites are often non-specific.

A recent report of two cases of squamous cell carcinoma arising in vulvar LP[83] has raised the issue that the condition should be regarded as a precancerosis. It has been suggested that such patients should be subjected to regular follow-up,

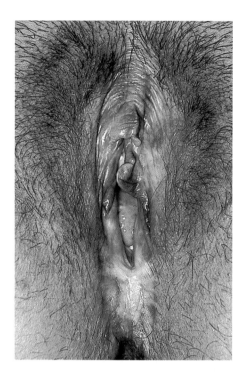

Figure 5   Lichen sclerosus

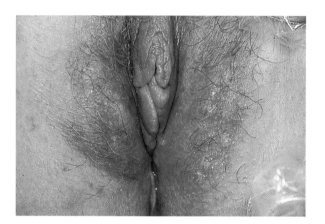

Figure 6   Papuloerosive diaper dermatitis in a 73-year-old woman with urinary incontinence

and serial biopsies of any atypical lesions should be performed to exclude the development of malignancy.

Mucosal LP represents a major therapeutic problem, and genital lesions are even more refractory than oral ones. Topical and systemic corticosteroids, systemic retinoids, griseofulvin, dapsone and cyclosporin-A have all been used with variable benefit in this chronic, debilitating condition, which is unlikely to undergo spontaneous remission. Recently, encouraging results have been reported in some cases of vulvar LP with topical cyclosporin[84,85].

LICHEN SCLEROSUS

Lichen sclerosus (LS) is an inflammatory dermatosis of unknown etiology and incompletely

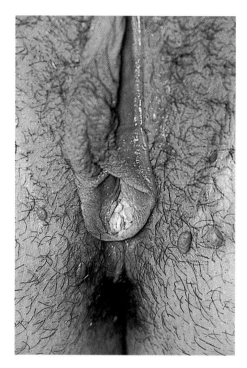

Figure 7   Nevi, Bowenoid papulosis, and condylomata acuminata (note acetowhitening in the posterior commissure)

understood complex pathogenesis with characteristic clinical and consistent histopathological findings. In the dermatological, gynecological, urological and pediatric literature this condition has been reported under various names, and the different specialities have focused on different aspects, rendering the available epidemiological data not very reliable. Women are affected more often than men, but the exact prevalence is unknown and probably higher than suspected in both sexes. A review of 5207 cases revealed a female/male ratio of 6.2 : 1[86]. Caucasians are most susceptible to LS, but it has been reported in all races. All age groups can be affected, but most cases are observed in peri- and postmenopausal women. It is hard to determine the ratio of genital versus extragenital LS and LS with both localizations, since gynecologists seldom look for the extragenital manifestations, which could be very helpful to establish what is not always an easy diagnosis; dermatologists often refrain from performing a thorough examination of the genitalia. Nevertheless, it is recognized that the vulva is far more often affected than not, and in many cases genital lesions are the sole manifestation of the disease. It is not accidental that the first description of what is now recognized as LS, made by Breisky[87], appeared in the gynecological literature and preceded Hallopeau's report[88].

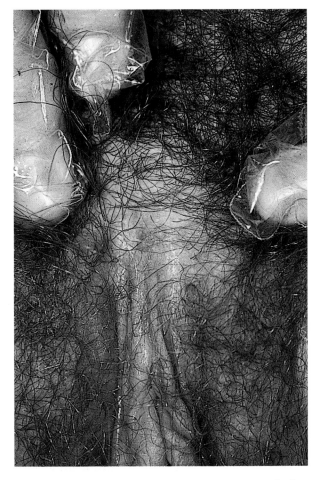

Figure 8 Vulvar syringomas appearing during pregnancy

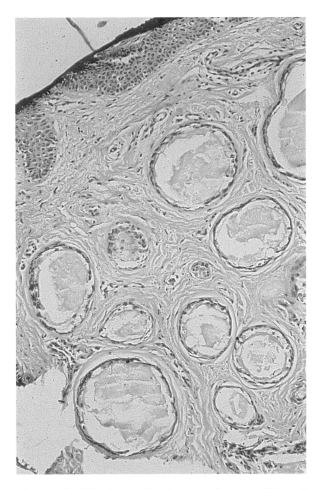

Figure 10 Histology of syringoma (hematoxylin and eosin)

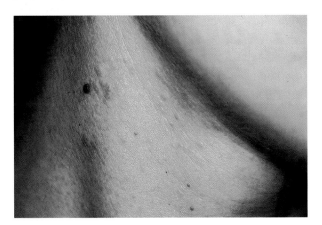

Figure 9 Eruptive syringoma on the neck (same patient as Figure 8), preceding the vulvar involvement

The labia majora, labia minora, clitoris, perineum and perianal skin may all be affected, usually symmetrically, resulting in what is usually described as a 'key hole', 'hourglass' or 'figure 8' configuration of the lesions. The initial small, flat, angular papules, off-white or ivory in color, with a shiny, translucent appearance, coalesce to form plaques (Figure 5). Dark follicular comedo-like horny plugs

often provide a helpful clue to the diagnosis. Edema of the clitoral foreskin with subsequent phimosis may be an early sign. Telangiectases, hemorrhagic lesions and bullae can also occur[89]. The epidermal atrophy gives the fully developed lesions a parchment-like, wrinkled appearance. Lichenification may result from scratching. The development of sclerosis and the ensuing loss of elasticity provide for the occurrence of fissures. In extreme cases the labia minora may disappear and the introitus may become so narrow as to make sexual intercourse impossible. LS may affect not only the skin, but also the mucosa, which then becomes whitish often with hemorrhages, telangiectases or bullae.

The most common subjective symptom is pruritus, which can be frustrating and differentiates LS of the vulva from extragenital LS. Patients with LS may experience vulvodynia, dysuria, dyspareunia, painful defecation and anogenital bleeding.

The Koebner phenomenon has been reported in LS. Wearing of tight underwear, friction, trauma and pinworm infection have all been suggested as predisposing factors for the development of vulvar LS. The isomorphic phenomenon is also suspected to contribute to the often observed recurrences after surgical treatment of LS[90].

Up to 15% of patients with LS are children[86], with a definite prevalence of girls, with genital localization of the disease[91,92]. The clinical presentation and histological findings are analogous to those in older women, but the course and prognosis are rather more favorable. Spontaneous resolution with few residual changes can be expected by the onset of puberty in up to two-thirds of those patients. This is most probably due to the significant hormonal alterations in adolescence.

The bruised appearance of anogenital LS lesions in children with a variable amount of hemorrhagic blistering, fissuration, anal and vulval bleeding, together with the often encountered dysuria and painful defecation may be mistaken for trauma inflicted through sexual abuse[93,94]. This is associated with a high level of anxiety on the part of the parents and their unwillingness to seek medical help. It also necessitates awareness of the clinical features of LS by people in the medical profession, which could prevent unnecessary intervention by police and social workers and spare the family of the child undeserved tribulation.

Histological features include hyperkeratosis with follicular plugging, atrophy of the stratum malpighii and hydropic degeneration of the basal layer, which when extreme may lead to bulla formation. Most specific are the alterations observed in the upper dermis, which becomes edematous, homogenized and subsequently sclerotic. Histochemical and ultrastructural studies have demonstrated degeneration to complete absence of elastic fibers, substantial changes in collagen metabolism and increased ground substance[95,96]. This zone is demarcated from beneath by an inflammatory infiltrate, consisting mainly of lymphoid cells with some histiocytes. The infiltrate is often band-like and is usually found in the mid-dermis. In very early lesions and at the periphery of older ones it may be more superficial.

The relation of LS to vulvar malignancy has been a source of debate over many decades. It seems now justified to state that LS is not a premalignant condition *per se*. Nevertheless, it may be complicated by other dystrophic disorders with malignant potential, in which case squamous cell carcinoma may subsequently develop. In the often-cited report of Wallace[97] this was documented in 4% of cases and it has been suggested that the rate may be higher[98]. Many approaches have been tried over the years for the management of vulvar LS. In the past, most patients were subjected to vulvectomy or radiotherapy, but these aggressive modalities have been relinquished in favor of conservative therapy. Topical corticosteroids are widely used currently for the treatment of vulvar LS. However, preparations with mild or moderate potency often fail to control disease effectively. A 3-month course of clobetasol propionate 0.05% cream twice daily has been shown substantially to improve the clinical manifestations, histopathological features and immunochemical parameters[99,100], and is not associated with a higher risk of vulvar infection or skin atrophy. After completion of the 3-month course, maintenance therapy is much easier with a moderately potent topical steroid[101]. Topical testosterone provides a therapeutic alternative, but recently its superiority over emollients has been challenged[102]. Virilization is a serious and not uncommon side-effect[103], because of which it cannot be applied in children and young women. No significant effect has been achieved with topical cyclosporin, although some response of the immunohistological profile has been noted[104]. Both etretinate and acitretin have been shown to be beneficial in vulvar LS, leading to regression of the clinical manifestations and some histological abnormalities[105,106].

CONTACT DERMATITIS

Certain physiological particularities of vulvar skin as well as the course of dermatoses affecting it, which is often protracted and necessitates prolonged medication, are factors contributing to the occurrence of intolerance reactions, precipitated through irritant and allergic mechanisms. The clinical manifestations of such intolerance become superimposed on those of the underlying disease, thus blurring the picture and creating serious diagnostic and management problems. Barrier function of vulvar skin is substantially weaker than at other anatomical sites. Comparative studies have demonstrated that transepidermal water loss of labia majora skin is significantly higher than in forearm skin[107,108]. The same applies for hydrocortisone percutaneous penetration[109]. These findings suggest that the vulvar skin may be more susceptible to irritant offense. Vulvar skin was shown to be more reactive to benzalkonium chloride and maleic acid than forearm skin, judged by the intensity of erythema and subjective perceptions[110], although, when tested with sodium lauryl sulfate, vulvar skin was not more susceptible to irritation than forearm skin[111,112]. Increased vulvar reactivity does not extend to all irritants. Moisture, friction, urine and vaginal discharge all contribute to vulvar irritation. Potential external irritants include cosmetics, cleansing products, topical medications, spermicidal preparations, underwear and vulvar pads. Three main clinical types of response to irritants are recognized: acute irritant dermatitis, chronic (cumulative) irritant dermatitis and sensory irritation[113]. The acute type develops as a result of exposure to a potent irritant and is equivalent to a chemical burn. The cumulative type is elicited by repeated exposure to weak irritants when the intervals between offenses are insufficient for restoration ad integrum. Sensory irritation is characterized by subjective sensations of stinging and burning provoked by chemical exposition, and lack of detectable objective skin changes. Chronic irritant dermatitis is often encountered in overscrupulous women with exaggerated hygienic needs and fears of infection. It may also arise as a complication of prolonged topical application of medications containing alcohol, propylene glycol, sodium lauryl sulfate or other potential irritants. A particular form of irritant diaper dermatitis, called 'nappy rash of neglect', presents with well-demarcated papular, centrally eroded lesions confined to the convexed parts of vulvar labia majora and the perineal regions. This condition, known as Sevestre and Jacquet syphiloid erythema (erythème papulo-erosif de Sevestre et Jacquet) is typically encountered in neglected children, but it may also be diagnosed in elderly women with urinary incontinence (Figure 6)[114]. Friction, maceration, occlusion from disposable napkins, increased skin humidity, alteration in cutaneous pH in the presence of urine and fecal matter, and superimposed microorganisms are the main responsible factors.

Allergic contact dermatitis is a manifestation of a cell-mediated immunological reaction in sensitized individuals. Antigen-presenting Langerhans' cells, T lymphocytes and numerous cytokines all participate in the pathogenesis of allergic contact dermatitis. The occurrence of sensitization is determined by the complex interaction of factors concerning the chemical structure of the allergen (potent and weak allergens), the individual (genetic predisposition, age) and the conditions under which the contact takes place (duration of contact, pre-existing epidermal injury, etc.). Since the elicitation phase of the allergic reaction requires one to several days, the cause–effect relationship between the allergen exposure and the development of dermatitis may not be easily recognized. This is especially relevant to a subset of patients, who apply different, often numerous topical preparations for the treatment of a pre-existing dermatological disease of the vulva, over long periods of time. Curiously, this problem has been largely ignored

and the first large-scale study was published only within recent years. Patch-test results were reviewed[115] in 135 patients with persistent vulval symptoms in whom therapy for a specific vulvar dermatosis had not met expectations or in whom no particular diagnosis could be established. Sixty-three patients (47%) had at least one positive reaction. In 39 patients (29%) positive results were assessed to be relevant to their clinical condition. Relevant medicament hypersensitivity was detected in 37 patients. The most frequent offenders were ethylenediamine, neomycin, framycetin and clobetasol propionate. This exemplary study has demonstrated that patients with chronic dermatological diseases of the vulva comprise a high-risk group for the development of contact hypersensitivity, especially to topically applied medicaments[115].

While irritant or allergic contact dermatitis are complications of topical therapy, systemic drug intake may result in the development of erythema fixum, Stevens–Johnson syndrome or toxic epidermal necrolysis – conditions which often affect the vulva and require adequate care to avoid adhesion formation and other sequelae which may lead to serious functional impairment.

TUMORS OF THE VULVA

Multiple benign and malignant tumors of varying tissue origins can arise in the vulva. The proper evaluation of these lesions requires a background in general dermatology and an understanding of the special nature of many vulvar conditions. The variability in clinical appearance of vulvar tumors and the overlap between the clinical features of benign conditions and malignant neoplasms suggests that biopsy confirmation should be obtained on all lesions for which there is the least doubt regarding the diagnosis.

Benign tumors and 'dark lesions' accounted for 22% of vulvar diseases diagnosed in one vulvar clinic over an 8-year period[116]. The reported order of frequency of the lesions is: epidermal inclusion cysts, lentigo, Bartholin's duct obstruction, carcinoma in situ, melanocytic nevi, acrochordon, mucous cyst, hemangiomas, postinflammatory hyperpigmentation, seborrheic keratoses, varicosities, hidradenomas, verruca, basal cell carcinoma, unusual tumors such as neurofibromas, ectopic tissue, syringomas and abscesses.

Bowenoid papulosis

Bowenoid papulosis is a common problem in young adult women. It appears as asymptomatic or occasionally pruritic, papular, pigmented or skin-colored lesions or flat verruciform papules, located in the groin and on the genitalia[117]. Lesions may frequently be precipitated by pregnancy. More exophytic forms can be confused with fibromata or condylomata accuminata, but coexistence of those conditions may also be observed (Figure 7).

Successful treatment is performed by electrodesiccation or cryotherapy.

Vulvar syringoma

In contrast to syringomas of the eyelids and cheeks, which are well known and defined, vulvar syringomas are only occasionally observed and can therefore be easily misdiagnosed. Vulvar localization is seldom unique, but there are several cases of localized vulvar syringomas reported in the literature[118–120]. The tumors appear as dermal skin-colored round papules measuring up to 5 mm in diameter. They may be localized around the clitoris, the labia majora and the perigenital areas and are usually asymptomatic or mildly pruritic. There are isolated reports of vulvar syringoma appearing during pregnancy[121], as was the case of a 27-year-old patient observed by us (Figures 8 and 9). The differential diagnosis in cases limited to the vulva includes Fox–Fordyce disease, small epidermal cysts, steatocystoma multiplex and adenocarcinoma. When distant cutaneous lesions are present, they are suggestive for the clinical diagnosis, but microscopic examination would reveal the characteristic structure of the tumor (Figure 10). The treatment consists of tumor excision or laser destruction.

Squamous cell carcinoma

Squamous cell carcinoma (SCC) of the vulva is a rare disease, mainly seen in elderly women. Lately, younger age groups are increasingly affected. The overall incidence has been reported to be 1–2 per 100 000 women per year. Among women more than 75 years of age, the incidence is at least ten times higher. The cause of vulvar carcinoma is not known. Risk factors include advanced age, an immunocompromised status, smoking, long-standing vulvar dystrophy, vulvar intraepithelial neoplasm (VIN), a history of vulvar HPV infection and a history of cervical cancer[122].

Epidemiological and virological evidence suggests that invasive SCC of the vulva is etiologically heterogeneous. Two subtypes have been recognized, distinguished by their association with HPV infection and patient demographics. Basaloid or warty SCC and VIN are linked to HPV infections in younger women, while keratinizing SCC is a non-HPV-associated malignancy in older patients, often preceded by vulvar dystrophy.

Vulvar cancer can be regarded as a skin tumor and detection is possible at an early stage, which is essential for the outcome. Unfortunately, due to delay on the patient's or the physician's side in 30% of the cases, the diagnosis is first made at a late stage (stage III or IV)[123]. Introducing symptoms include pruritus, vulvar mass, local discomfort, discharge, bleeding and groin mass[124].

At physical examination, SCC presents most often as an ulcerating lesion with an indurated edge. It may also appear as an exophytously growing verrucous tumor. In a proportion of the younger patients the lesions are multifocal. The tumor produces mainly lymphatogenic metastases to the inguinal lymph nodes.

Tumor localization, tumor size, lymph node status and especially the depth of invasion are the important prognostic factors in vulvar cancer. A relative decrease in survival in smokers has been reported, despite younger age and fewer positive nodes at diagnosis compared to non-smokers. The most accurate prognostic information is presented by the staging systems (Table 2). Numerous comparative retrospective studies have shown that the procedure widely practiced in the past – radical vulvectomy – 'en bloc' has no advantage over radical local excision as far as survival rates are concerned[125–127]. The better current understanding of the prognostic factors of every tumor correlated with the patient's age allows the performance of individualized, adequate radical surgery without the large mutilations of the past, thus providing for a rapid recovery, fewer complications and an improved quality of life for the patients.

Basal cell carcinoma

Basal cell carcinoma (BCC), although a rare neoplasm, deserves special attention because it often demonstrates aggressive biological behavior and may metastasize[128]. BCC accounts for 2–3% of all vulvar malignancies[129–131]. Patients are as a rule in the eighth or ninth decade of life. Patients typically present with an irritation or soreness, with symptom duration ranging from a few months to several years[132]. This tumor can present as a unifocal or multifocal lesion[133]. Most lesions are confined to the anterior half of the vulva. The clinical appearance can be deceptively innocent. The timely accurate diagnosis relies upon a high index of suspicion and

Table 2 Vulvar squamous cell carcinoma staging system according to the International Federation of Gynecology and Obstetrics (FIGO) (modified)

	Description	Size	Lymph node involvement
Stage IA	tumor confined to vulva/perineum	maximum diameter 2 cm, depth of invasion < 1 mm	groin lymph nodes not palpable
Stage I	tumor confined to vulva/perineum	maximum diameter 2 cm	groin lymph nodes negative
Stage II	tumor confined to vulva/perineum	diameter > 2 cm	groin lymph nodes negative
Stage III	tumor of any size with adjacent spread to the lower urethra and/or vagina, or the anus		unilateral regional lymph node metastasis
Stage IVA	tumor of any size with spreads to upper urethra, bladder mucosa, rectal mucosa, pelvic bone		bilateral regional lymph node metastasis
Stage IVB	tumor of any size and any lymph node spread with any distant metastasis, including pelvic lymph node metastasis		

histological evaluation. The therapy of choice is wide local excision and continued follow-up.

Extramammary Paget's disease of the vulva

In 1874 Sir James Paget[134] described a cutaneous disease of the mammary area, associated with a cancer of the mammary gland, which became known as Paget's disease of the breast. Paget's disease occurs less frequently in extramammary sites, typically involving the anogenital region. Extramammary Paget's disease (EMPD) of the vulva affects predominantly elderly women in the seventh decade and represents 1–2% of all vulvar malignancies. The introducing symptom is usually pruritus, which precedes diagnosis by months to years. Clinically, EMPD of the vulva appears as an erythematous exudative dermatitis, usually with a well-defined margin. Histology shows large, pale cells within the epidermis; in these cells the cytoplasm is abundant and vacuolated, the nucleus is large and the nucleolus is frequently prominent. Apart from the suprabasal epidermis, such cells may also be detected in the cutaneous appendages. The periodic acid–Schiff test is positive and diastase-resistant cytoplasmatic granules are a persistent finding helping to differentiate these cells from those of Bowen's disease or melanoma.

The histogenesis of EMPD of the vulva is uncertain. There is a long history of controversies about its derivation, with eccrine, apocrine and supernumerary mammary glands or related pluripotent germinative cells suggested as possible sources. Recently a special type of anogenital sweat gland has been identified, which is histologically different from eccrine, apocrine and mammary glands and shares features of them all[135]. Initially named 'anogenital sweat gland', this gland has a striking microscopic resemblance to mammary glands, for which reason the term 'mammary-like glands' (MLG) is now preferred. A concept has been put forward, according to which EMPD of the vulva arises in these glands[136].

EMPD of the vulva may occur alone or in association with other malignancies. The malignancies reported to occur with it include: carcinoma of Bartholin's gland; carcinoma of the ureter, bladder and urethra; carcinoma of the cervix; and adenocarcinoma of the ovary[137]. It is considered as an intraepithelial carcinoma with an invasive potential that should not be underestimated. Surgical excision is the treatment of choice. A major goal of conservative surgery is to preserve sexual function, normal anatomy and body image. This, however, is not always easy. The lesions are often multifocal and Paget's cells may be present far from the clinical border of the lesion[138]. This accounts for the quite high rate of recurrence. Some one-third of the patients with EMPD of the vulva are reported to experience local recurrence[139]. This necessitates a close follow-up for a longer period of time, to exclude recurrence.

Vulvar malignant melanoma

Vulvar malignant melanoma (VMM) is a rare but aggressive tumor. Malignant melanoma of the vulva and vagina is 100-fold less common than malignant melanoma of non-genital skin[140]. The mean age for developing VMM is reported to be 66 years[140]. VMM, though in general rare, is actually the second most common neoplasm of the vulva after squamous cell carcinoma. Overall melanomas of the vulva account for 2–10% of all malignancies of the female external genitalia[141]. VMM appears to behave similarly to truncal melanoma, but its later diagnosis, owing to its less accessible and less visible site, gives the false impression of more aggressive behavior. In spite of that, the survival, stage by stage, is not markedly different from that of truncal melanoma[142]. Clinical symptoms appear late and consist of bleeding, pruritus or a tumor mass, or change in a pre-existing mole[143]. There is a preference for the labia minora. The majority of the lesions show a histology characteristic of the mucosal-lentiginous type of malignant melanoma, but nodular melanomas, as well as desmoplastic melanomas, with or without neurotropismus, have been reported[144]. The differential diagnosis of pigmented lesions is quite broad. Pigmented vulvar lesions, including diffuse hyperpigmentation, are observed in 10 to 12% of Caucasian women. About 2% of these lesions are nevocellular nevi[145]. In general, nevi on the vulva share the morphological and histopathological criteria of truncal nevi, with the exception of a small subset of nevi in younger women. Nevi in this subset have the striking features of enlarged junctional nests that are variable in size, shape and position. It is exactly this subset of nevi that creates most problems in the differential diagnosis of malignant melanoma. Other benign pigmented lesions include melanosis, lentigines, post-inflammatory hyperpigmentation, seborrheic keratoses and warts.

The 5-year survival has been reported to be between 30 and 50%[140,141,146,147]. Parameters such as age, Breslow's thickness, Clark's level of invasion, lymph node involvement, anatomic site and post-operative stage are prognostic factors for survival.

As with SCC, recent years have brought about a critical re-evaluation of surgical treatment and it has been shown that less radical procedures offer equal results with decreased morbidity.

CONCLUSIONS

The past decade has witnessed significant advances in the study of vulvar pathology. Efforts have been made to unify the nomenclature in order to overcome the confusion of terms used in the dermatological and gynecological literature. Important insights have been made in the etiology and pathogenesis of many vulvar dermatoses. New approaches have been introduced, and a general tendency has evolved for the substitution of aggressive surgical methods by conservative treatment modalities.

Many problems, however, still remain unresolved, and further efforts are needed for the better understanding and more effective management of these disorders, which often result in low self-esteem and poor quality of life on the part of the affected patients.

REFERENCES

1. Berg AO, Heidrich FE, Fihn SD, *et al*. Establishing the course of genitourinary symptoms in women in a family practice. Comparison of clinical examination and comprehensive microbiology. *JAMA* 1984;251:620–5
2. Evans EGV. Diagnostic laboratory techniques in vaginal candidosis. *Br J Clin Pract* 1990;44 (suppl 71):70–2
3. Kerridge D, Nicholas RO. Drug resistance in the opportunistic pathogens. *Candida albicans* and *Candida glabrata*. *J Antimicrob Chemother* 1986;18 (suppl B):39–40
4. Horowitz BJ, Edelstein SW, Lippman L. *Candida tropicalis* vulvovaginitis. *Obstet Gynecol* 1985;66:229–32
5. Odds FC. *Candida and Candidosis*, 2nd edn. London: Ballière Tindall, 1988
6. Miles MR, Olsen L, Rogers A. Recurrent vaginal candidiasis. Importance of an intestinal reservoir. *JAMA* 1977;238:1836–7
7. Rashid S, Collins M, Kennedy RJ. A study of candidosis: the role of fomites. *Genitourin Med* 1991;67: 137–142
8. Horowitz BJ, Edelstein SW, Lippman L. Sexual transmission of *Candida*. *Obstet Gynecol* 1987;69:883–6
9. Gough PM, Warnock DW, Richardson MD, *et al*. IgA and IgG antibodies to *Candida albicans* in the genital tract secretions of women with or without vaginal candidosis. *Sabouraudia: J Med Vt Mycol* 1984;22:265–71
10. Witkin SS, Yu IR, Ledger WJ. Inhibition of *Candida albicans*-induced lymphocyte proliferation by lymphocytes and sera from women with recurrent vaginitis. *Am J Obstet Gynecol* 1983;147:809–11
11. Shah DT, Glover DD, Larsen B. *In situ* mycotoxin production by *Candida albicans* in women with vaginitis. *Gynecol Obstet Invest* 1995;39:67–9
12. Witkin SS, Jeremias J, Ledger WJ. Vaginal eosinophils and IgE antibodies to *Candida albicans* in women with recurrent vaginitis. *J Med Vet Mycol* 1989;27:57–8

13. Monif GRG. Classification and pathogenesis of vulvovaginal candidiasis. *Am J Obstet Gynecol* 1985;152:935–9

14. Rajakumar R, Lacey CJN, Evans EGV, Carney JA. Use of slide latex agglutination test for rapid diagnosis of vaginal candidosis. *Genitourin Med* 1987;63: 192–5

15. Merkus JMWM, van Heusden AM. Chronic vulvovaginal candidosis: the role of oral therapy. *Br J Clin Pract* 1989;44(suppl 71):81–4

16. McKey M. Vulvodynia: a multifactorial clinical problem. *Arch Dermatol* 1989;125:256–62

17. Friedrich EG Jr. Vulvar vestibulitis syndrome. *J Reprod Med* 1987;32:110–14

18. Furlonge CB, Thin RN, Evans BE, McKee PH. Vulvar vestibulitis syndrome: a clinicopathological study. *Br J Obstet Gynaecol* 1991;98:703–6

19. Goetsch MF. Vulvar vestibulitis: prevalence and historic features in a general gynecologic practice population. *Am J Obstet Gynecol* 1991;164:1609–14

20. Turner ML, Marinoff SC. Association of human papillomavirus with vulvodynia and the vulvar vestibulitis syndrome. *J Reprod Med* 1988;33:533–7

21. Wilkinson EJ, Guerrero E, Daniel R, *et al.* Vulvar vestibulitis is rarely associated with human papillomavirus infection types 6, 11, 16, or 18. *Int J Gynecol Pathol* 1993;12:344–9

22. Bergeron C, Moyal Barracco M, Pelisse M, Lewin P. Vulvar vestibulitis. Lack of evidence for a human papillomavirus etiology. *J Reprod Med* 1994;39: 936–8

23. Prayson RA, Stoler MH, Hart WR. Vulvar vestibulitis. A histopathologic study of 36 cases including human papillomavirus *in situ* hybridization analysis. *Am J Surg Pathol* 1995;19:154–60

24. Ashman RB, Ott AK. Autoimmunity as a factor in recurrent vaginal candidosis and the minor vestibular gland syndrome. *J Reprod Med* 1989;34:264–6

25. Bazin S, Bouchard C, Brisson J, *et al.* Vulvar vestibulitis syndrome: an exploratory case–control study. *Obstet Gynecol* 1994;83:47–50

26. Solomons CC. Calcium citrate for vulvar vestibulitis. A case report. *J Reprod Med* 1991;36:879–82

27. Baggish MS, Sze EH, Johnson R. Urinary oxalate excretion and its role in vulvar pain syndrome. *Am J Obstet Gynecol* 1997;177:507–11

28. Fitzpatrick CC, DeLancey JO, Elkins TE, McGuire EJ. Vulvar vestibulitis and interstitial cystitis: a disorder of urogenital sinus-derived epithelium? *Obstet Gynecol* 1993;81:860–2

29. Peckham BM, Maki DG, Patterson JJ, Hafez GR. Focal vulvitis: a characteristic syndrome and cause of dyspareunia. Features, natural history, and management. *Am J Obstet Gynecol* 1986;154: 855–64

30. Foster DC, Robinson JC, Davis KM. Urethral pressure variation in women with vulvar vestibulitis syndrome. *Am J Obstet Gynecol* 1993;169:107–12

31. Glazer HI, Rodke G, Swencionis C, *et al.* Treatment of vulvar vestibulitis syndrome with electromyographic biofeedback of pelvic floor musculature. *J Reprod Med* 1995;40:283–90

32. Lambiris A, Greaves MW. Dyspareunia and vulvodynia are probably common manifestations of factitious urticaria. *Br J Dermatol* 1997;136:140–1

33. Schover LR, Youngs DD, Cannata R. Psychosexual aspects of the evaluation and management of vulvar vestibulitis. *Am J Obstet Gynecol* 1992;167:630–6

34. de Jong JM, van Lunsen RH, Robertson EA, Stam LN, Lammes FB. Focal vulvitis: a psychosexual problem for which surgery is not the answer. *J Psychosom Obstet Gynecol* 1995;16:85–91

35. Chadha S, Gianotten WL, Drogendijk AC, *et al.* Histopathologic features of vulvar vestibulitis. *Int J Gynecol Pathol* 1998;17:7–11

36. Axe S, Parmley T, Woodruff JD, Hlopak B. Adenomas in minor vestibural glands. *Obstet Gynecol* 1986;68:16–18

37. Bornstein J, Pascal B, Abramovici H. Treatment of a patient with vulvar vestibulitis by intramuscular interferon beta; a case report. *Eur J Obstet Gynecol Reprod Biol* 1991;42:237–9

38. Bornstein J, Pascal B, Abramovici H. Intramuscular beta-interferon treatment for severe vulvar vestibulitis. *J Reprod Med* 1993;38:117–20

39. Marinoff SC, Turner ML, Hirsch RP, Richard G. Intralesional alpha interferon. Cost-effective therapy for vulvar vestibulitis syndrome. *J Reprod Med* 1993;38:19–24

40. Altmeyer P, Chilf GN, Holzman H. Pseudokondylome der vulva. *Geburtshilfe Frauensheilkd* 1981; 41:783–6

41. Welch JM, Nayagam M, Parry G, *et al.* What is vestibular papillomatosis? A study of its prevalence, etiology and natural history. *Br J Obstet Gynaecol* 1993;100:932–42

42. Growdon WA, Fu YS, Lebherz TB, *et al.* Pruritic vulvar squamous papillomatosis: evidence for human papillomavirus infection. *Obstet Gynecol* 1985;66:564–8

43. Manoharan V, Sommerville JM. Benign squamous papillomatosis: case report. *Genitourin Med* 1987; 63:393–5

44. Costa S, Rotola A, Terzano P, *et al.* Is vestibular papillomatosis associated with human papillomavirus? *J Med Virol* 1991;35:7–13

45. Moyal-Barraco M, Leibowitch M, Orth G. Vestibular papillae of the vulva. Lack of evidence for human papillomavirus etiology. *Arch Dermatol* 1990;126: 1594–8

46. Ferenczy A, Mitao M, Nagai N, *et al.* Latent papillomavirus and recurrent genital warts. *N Engl J Med* 1985;313:784–8

47. Potkul RK, Lancaster WD, Kurman RJ, *et al.* Vulvar condylomas and squamous vestibular micropapilloma. Differences in appearance and response to treatment. *J Reprod Med* 1990;35:1019–22

48. Xia MY, Zhu WY, Li HX, *et al.* Hirsutoid papilloma of vulvae: absences of human papilloma virus DNA by the polymerase chain reaction. *J Dermatol Sci* 1994;7:84–8

49. Fimiani M, Mazzatenta C, Biagioli M, Andreassi L. Vulvar squamous papillomatosis and human papillomavirus infection. A polymerase chain reaction study. *Arch Dermatol Res* 1993;285:250–4

50. Sonni L, Cattaneo A, De Marco A, *et al.* Idiopathic vulvodynia. Clinical evaluation of the pain threshold with acetic acid solutions. *J Reprod Med* 1995;40:337–41

51. Stewart DE, Reicher AE, Gerulath AH, Boydell KM. Vulvodynia and psychological distress. *Obstet Gynecol* 1994;84:587–90

52. McKay M. Dysesthetic ('essential') vulvodynia. Treatment with amitriptyline. *J Reprod Med* 1993; 38:9–13

53. Garnier G. Vulvite érythémateuse circonscrite bénigne à type érythroplasique. *Bull Soc Fr Dermatol Syphilol* 1954;61:102–4

54. Davis J, Shapiro L, Baral J. Vulvitis circumscripta plasmacellularis. *J Am Acad Dermatol* 1983;8:413–16

55. Nedwich JA, Chong KC. Zoon's vulvitis. *Aust J Dermatol* 1987;28:11–13

56. Morioka S, Nakajima S, Yaguchi H, *et al.* Vulvitis circumscripta plasmacellularis treated succesfully with interferon alpha. *J Am Acad Dermatol* 1988;19: 947–50

57. Woodruff JD, Sussman J, Shakfeh S. Vulvitis circumscripta plasmocellularis. A report of four cases. *J Reprod Med* 1989;34:369–72

58. McCreedy CA, Melski JW. Vulvar erythema. Vulvitis chronica plasmacellularis (Zoon's vulvititis). *Arch Dermatol* 1990;126:1352–6

59. Kavanagh GM, Burton PA, Kennedy CT. Vulvitis chronica plasmacellularis (Zoon's vulvitis). *Br J Dermatol* 1993;129:92–3

60. Scurry J, Dennerstein G, Brenan J, *et al.* Vulvitis circumscripta plasmacellularis. A clinicopathologic entity? *J Reprod Med* 1993;38:14–18

61. Hautmann G, Geti V, Difonzo EM. Vulvitis circumscripta plasmacellularis. *Int J Dermatol* 1994;33: 496–7

62. Yoganathan S, Bohl TG, Mason G. Plasma cell balanitis and vulvitis (of Zoon). A study of 10 cases. *J Reprod Med* 1994;39:939–44

63. Souteyrand P, Wong E, McDonald DM. Zoon's balanitis (balanitis circumscripta plasmacellularis). *Br J Dermatol* 1981;105:195–9

64. Nishimura M, Matsuda T, Muto M, Hori Y. Balanitis of Zoon. *Int J Dermatol* 1990;29:421–3

65. Scuermann H. Plasmocytosis circumorificialis. *Deut Zahnärztl Z* 1960;15:601–10

66. Bourgeois Droin C, Granier F, Pedreiro J, *et al.* Localisations vulvovaginales et du col utérin révélatrices d'un pemphigus vulgaire. Efficacité des sels d'or. *Ann Dermatol Venereol* 1990;117:894–5

67. Lever WF. Pemphigus and pemphigoid – a review of the advances made since 1964. *J Am Acad Dermatol* 1979;1:2–31

68. Haustein UF. Localized nonscarring bullous pemphigoid of the vagina. *Dermatologica* 1988;176: 200–1

69. Rupprecht M, Stäbler A, Hornstein OP. Genitale Schleimhautmanifestation eines lokalisierten bullösen Pemphigoids. *Hautarzt* 1991;42:183–5

70. Marren P, Walkden V, Mallon E, Wojnarowska F. Vulval cicatricial pemphigoid may mimic lichen sclerosus. *Br J Dermatol* 1996;134:522–4

71. De Castro P, Jorizzo JL, Rajaraman S, *et al.* Localized vulvar pemphigoid in a child. *Pediatr Dermatol* 1985;2:302–7

72. Oranje AP, Vuzevski VD, Van Joast T, *et al.* Bullous pemphigoid in children. *Int J Dermatol* 1991;30: 339–42

73. Levine V, Sanchez M, Nestor M. Localized vulvar pemphigoid in a child misdiagnosed as sexual abuse. *Arch Dermatol* 1992;128:804–6

74. Saad RW, Domloge-Hultsch N, Yancey KB, *et al.* Childhood localized vulvar pemphigoid is a true variant of bullous pemphigoid. *Arch Dermatol* 1992;128:807–10

75. Saulsbury FT, Hayden GF. Skin conditions simulating child abuse. *Pediatr Emerg Care* 1985;1:147–50

76. Herman-Giddens ME, Berson NL. Dermatologic conditions misdiagnosed as evidence of child abuse. *JAMA* 1989;261:3546–7

77. Arndt KA. Lichen planus. In Fitzpatrick TB, Eisen AZ, Wolff K, *et al.*, eds. *Dermatology in General Medicine*, 3rd edn. New York: McGraw-Hill International Book Co; 1987:967–73

78. Edwards L. Vulvar lichen planus. *Arch Dermatol* 1989;125:1677–80

79. Soper DE, Patterson JW, Hurt WG, *et al.* Lichen planus of the vulva. Obstet Gynecol 1988;72:74–6

80. Pelisse M, Leibowitch M, Sedel D, Hewitt J. Un nouveau syndrome vulvo-vagino-gingival: lichen plan érosif plurimuqueux. Ann Dermatol Venereol 1982;109:797–8

81. Pelisse M. The vulvo-vaginal-gingival syndrome: a new form of erosive lichen planus. *Int J Dermatol* 1989;28:381–4

82. Eisen D. The vulvovaginal–gingival syndrome of lichen planus: the clinical characteristics of 22 patients. *Arch Dermatol* 1994;130:1379–82

83. Lewis FM, Harrington CI. Squamous cell carcinoma arising in vulval lichen planus. *Br J Dermatol* 1994;131:703–5

84. Bécherel PA, Chosidow O, Boisnic S, Reigneau O. Topical cyclosporine in the treatment of oral and vulvar erosive lichen planus: a blood level monitoring study. *Arch Dermatol* 1995;131:495–6

85. Borrego L, Ruiz-Rodriguez R, Ortiz de Frutos J, *et al.* Vulvar lichen planus treated with topical cyclosporine. *Arch Dermatol* 1993;129:794

86. Meffert JJ, Davis BM, Grimwood RE. Lichen sclerosus. *J Am Acad Dermatol* 1995;32:393–416

87. Breisky A. Über Kraurosis vulvae. *Z Heilkr* 1885; 6:69

88. Hallopeau H. Lichen plan atrophique. *Ann Dermatol Syphilol* (*Paris*) 1887;8:790

89. Di Silverio A, Serri F. Generalized bullous and haemorrhagic lichen sclerosus et atrophicus. *Br J Dermatol* 1975;93:215–17

90. Barker LP, Gross P. Lichen sclerosus et atrophicus of the female genitalia. *Arch Dermatol* 1962;85:362–71

91. Berth Jones J, Graham Brown RA, Burns DA. Lichen sclerosus et atrophicus: a review of 15 cases in young girls. *Clin Exp Dermatol* 1991;16:14–17

92. Loening Baucke V. Lichen sclerosus et atrophicus in children. *Am J Dis Child* 1991;145:1058–61

93. Jenny C, Kirby P, Fuquay D. Genital lichen sclerosus et atrophicus mistaken for child sexual abuse. *Pediatrics* 1989;83:597–9

94. Young SJ, Wells DL, Ogden EJ. Lichen sclerosus, genital trauma, and child sexual abuse. *Aust Fam Physician* 1993;22:729–33

95. Frances C, Wechsler J, Meimon G, *et al.* Investigation of intercellular matrix macromolecules involved in lichen sclerosus. *Acta Derm Venereol* (*Stochk*) 1983;63:483–90

96. Panizzon R, Vuorio T, Bruckner-Tuderman L. Collagen biosynthesis and type I and type II procollagen mRNA in lichen sclerosus et atrophicus. *Arch Dermatol Res* 1990;282:480–3

97. Wallace HJ. Lichen sclerosus et atrophicus. *Trans St Johns Hosp Soc* 1971;57:9–30

98. Rodke G, Friedrich EG, Wilkinson EJ. Malignant potential of mixed vulvar dystrophy (lichen sclerosus associated with squamous cell hyperplasia). *J Reprod Med* 1988;33:545–50

99. Dalziel KL, Millard PR, Wojnarowska F. The treatment of vulval lichen sclerosus with a very potent topical steroid (clobetasol propionate 0.05%) cream. *Br J Dermatol* 1991;124:461–4

100. Carli P, Cattaneo A, Giannotti B. Clobetasol propionate 0.05% cream in the treatment of vulvar lichen sclerosus: effect on the immunohistological profile. *Br J Dermatol* 1992;127:542–3

101. Dalziel KL, Wojnarowska F. Long-term control of vulval lichen sclerosus after treatment with a potent steroid cream. *J Reprod Med* 1993;38:25–7

102. Sideri M, Origoni M, Spinaci L, Ferrari A. Topical testosterone in the treatment of vulvar lichen sclerosus. *Int J Gynaecol Obstet* 1994;46:53–6

103. Ayhan A, Urman B, Yuce K, *et al.* Topical testosterone for lichen sclerosus. *Int J Gynaecol Obstet* 1989;30:253–5

104. Carli P, Cattaneo A, Taddei G, Giannotti B. Topical cyclosporine in the treatment of vulvar lichen sclerosus: clinical, histologic, and immunohistochemical findings. *Arch Dermatol* 1992;128: 1279–80

105. Mork NJ, Jensen P, Hoel PS. Vulval lichen sclerosus et atrophicus treated with etretinate (Tigason®). *Acta Derm Venereol* (*Stockh*) 1986;66:363–5

106. Buosema MT, Romppanen U, Geiger JM, *et al.* Acitretin in the treatment of severe lichen sclerosus et atrophicus of the vulva: a double-blind, placebo-controlled study. *J Am Acad Dermatol* 1994;30: 225–31

107. Elsner P, Wilhelm D, Maibach HI. Physiological skin surface water loss dynamics of human vulvar and forearm skin. *Acta Derm Venereol* (*Stockh*) 1990; 70:141–4

108. Elsner P, Maibach HI. The effect of prolonged drying on transepidermal water loss, capacitance and pH of human vulvar and forearm skin. *Acta Derm Venereol* (*Stockh*) 1990;70:105–9

109. Britz MB, Maibach HI. Human percutaneous penetration of hydrocortisone: the vulva. *Arch Dermatol Res* 1980;267:313–16

110. Britz MB, Maibach HI. Human cutaneous vulvar reactivity to irritants. *Contact Dermatitis* 1979;5:375–7

111. Elsner P, Wilhelm D, Maibach HI. The effect of low-concentration sodium lauryl sulfate on human vulvar and forearm skin: age-related differences. *J Reprod Med* 1990;36:77–81

112. Elsner P, Wilhelm D, Maibach HI. Study on sodium lauryl sulfate-induced irritant contact dermatitis in vulvar and forearm skin of pre- and postmenopausal women. *J Am Acad Dermatol* 1990;23: 648–52

113. Elsner P, Maibach HI. Irritant and allergic contact dermatitis. In Elsner P, Martius J, eds. *Vulvovaginitis*. New York: Marcel Decker, 1993:61–82

114. Virgil A, Corazza M. Erytheme syphiloide de Sevestre et Jacquet. *Ann Dermatol Venereol* 1992; 119:744–5

115. Marren P, Wojnarowska F, Powell S. Allergic contact dermatitis and vulvar dermatoses. *Br J Dermatol* 1992;126:52–6

116. Hood AF, Lumadue J. Benign vulvar tumors. *Dermatol Clin* 1992;10:371–85

117. Wade TR, Kopt AW, Ackerman AB. Bowenoid papulosis of genitalia. *Arch Dermatol* 1979;115:306–8

118. Thomas J, Majmudar B. Syringoma localized to the vulva. *Arch Dermatol* 1979;115:95–6

119. Tay YK, Tham SN, Teo R. Localized vulvar syringomas – an unusual cause of pruritus vulvae. *Dermatology* 1996;192:62–3

120. Belardi MG, Maglione MA, Vighi S, di Paola GR. Syringoma of the vulva. A case report. *J Reprod Med* 1994;39:957–9

121. Turan C, Ugur M, Kutluay L, *et al.* Vulvar syringoma exacerbated during pregnancy. *Eur J Obstet Gynecol Reprod Biol* 1996;64:141–2

122. Ansink A. Vulvar squamous cell carcinoma. *Semin Dermatol* 1996;15:51–9

123. Cavanagh D, Fiorica JV, Hoffman MS, *et al.* Invasive carcinoma of the vulva. Changing trends

in surgical management. *Am J Obstet Gynecol* 1990;163:1007–15

124. Ansink AC, van Tinteren H, Aartsen EJ, Heintz AP. Outcome, complications and follow-up in surgically treated squamous cell carcinoma of the vulva 1956–1982. *Eur J Obstet Gynecol Reprod Biol* 1991; 42:137–43

125. Berman ML, Soper JT, Creasman WT, Olt GT, DiSaia PJ. Conservative surgical management of superficially invasive stage I vulvar carcinoma. *Gynecol Oncol* 1989;35:352–7

126. Burke TW, Stringer CA, Gershenson DM, *et al.* Radical wide excision and selective inguinal node dissection for squamous cell carcinoma of the vulva. *Gynecol Oncol* 1990;38:328–32

127. Hacker NF, Berek JS, Legasse LD, *et al.* Individualization of treatment for stage I squamous cell vulvar carcinoma. *Obstet Gynecol* 1984; 63:155–62

128. Gleeson NC, Ruffolo EH, Hoffman MS, Cavanagh D. Basal cell carcinoma of the vulva with groin node metastasis. *Gynecol Oncol* 1994;53:366–8

129. Hoffman MS, Roberts WS, Ruffolo EH. Basal cell carcinoma of the vulva with inguinal lymph node metastases. *Gynecol Oncol* 1988;29:113–19

130. Mizushima J, Ohara K. Basal cell carcinoma of the vulva with lymph node and skin metastasis – report of a case and review of 20 Japanese cases. *J Dermatol* 1995;22:36–42

131. Perrone T, Twiggs LB, Adcock LL, Dehner LP. Vulvar basal cell carcinoma: an infrequently metastasizing neoplasm. *Int J Gynecol Pathol* 1987;6:152–65

132. Benedet JL, Miller DM, Ehlen TG, Bertrand MA. Basal cell carcinoma of the vulva: clinical features and treatment results in 28 patients. *Obstet Gynecol* 1997;90:765–8

133. Goldberg DJ. Multiple basal-cell carcinoma of the vulva. *J Dermatol Surg Oncol* 1984;10:615–17

134. Paget J. Disease of the mammary areola preceding cancer of the mammary gland. *St Bartholomew's Hosp Rep* 1874;10:87–9

135. van der Putte SC. Anogenital 'sweat' glands. Histology and pathology of a gland that may mimic mammary glands. *Am J Dermatopathol* 1991; 13:557–67

136. van der Putte SC, van Gorp LH. Adenocarcinoma of the mammary-like glands of the vulva: a concept unifying sweat gland carcinoma of the vulva, carcinoma of supernumerary mammary glands and extramammary Paget's disease. *J Cutan Pathol* 1994;21:157–63

137. Powell FC, Bjornsson J, Doyle JA, Cooper AJ. Genital Paget's disease and urinary tract malignancy. *J Am Acad Dermatol* 1985;13:84–90

138. Curtin JP, Rubin SC, Jones WB, *et al.* Paget's disease of the vulva. *Gynecol Oncol* 1990;39:374–7

139. Kodama S, Kaneko T, Saito M, *et al.* A clinicopathologic study of 30 patients with Paget's disease of the vulva. *Gynecol Oncol* 1995;56:63–70

140. Weinstock MA. Malignant melanoma of the vulva and vagina in the United States: patterns of incidence and population-based estimates of survival. *Am J Obstet Gynecol* 1994;171:1225–30

141. Raber G, Mempel V, Jackisch C, *et al.* Malignant melanoma of the vulva. Report of 89 patients. *Cancer* 1996;78:2353–8

142. Woolcott RJ, Henry RJ, Houghton CR. Malignant melanoma of the vulva. Australian experience. *J Reprod Med* 1988;33:699–702

143. Ariel IM. Malignant melanoma of the female genital system. In Ariel IM, ed. *Malignant Melanoma.* New York: Appleton & Rycrofts, 1981: 489–97

144. Mulvany NJ, Sykes P. Desmoplastic melanoma of the vulva. *Pathology* 1997;29:241–5

145. Rock B. Pigmented lesions of the vulva. *Dermatol Clin* 1992;10:361–70

146. Bradgate MG, Rollason TP, McConkey CC, Powell J. Malignant melanoma of the vulva: a clinicopathological study of 50 women. *Br J Obstet Gynaecol* 1990;97:124–33

147. Ragnarsson Olding B, Johansson H, Rutqvist LE, Ringborg U. Malignant melanoma of the vulva and vagina. Trends in incidence, age distribution, and long-term survival among 245 consecutive cases in Sweden 1960–1984. *Cancer* 1993;71:1893–7

Diseases and conditions limited to girls and women

Menstrually-related conditions **32**

Susan Swiggum and John Adam

THE MENSTRUAL CYCLE

The menstrual cycle[1] (Figure 1) can be divided into:

(1) A follicular phase or preovulatory phase;

(2) An ovulatory phase;

(3) A luteal phase or postovulatory phase.

Follicular phase

During the course of a normal ovulatory cycle, follicle stimulating hormone (FSH) stimulates the maturation of an ovarian follicle. The responding ovarian follicle secretes increasing quantities of 17β-estradiol. Luteinizing hormone (LH) completes the maturation of the follicle.

Ovulatory phase

When the plasma concentration of 17β-estradiol reaches the threshold level necessary to induce an LH surge, ovulation follows and the follicle is transformed into a corpus luteum.

Luteal phase

During a normal ovulatory cycle, the corpus luteum that forms at the site of the ovarian follicle begins secreting progesterone. Progesterone acts on the endometrium to suppress the mitogenic action of 17β-estradiol and converts the proliferative endometrium into secretory endometrium. The endometrial glands and stroma then deteriorate.

If fertilization and implantation of the ovum do not occur, the corpus luteum fails approximately 12 days after it is formed. With corpus luteum regression, estradiol and progesterone production decline, hormonal stimulation of the endometrium is withdrawn and menstruation begins.

After hormonal withdrawal from the endometrium at the end of corpus luteum function, the concentration of prostaglandins (PGE_2 and PGF_2) increases. The prostaglandins induce epithelial ischemia, with subsequent necrosis and shedding[2].

Androgen synthesis by the normal ovary is cyclic. Androstenedione and 17α-hydroxyprogesterone production reach a peak at the preovulatory phase, while peak production of dehydroisandrosterone and 17α-hydroxypregnenolone occurs at the midluteal phase.

SKIN CHANGES DURING THE MENSTRUAL CYCLE

The rise in estrogen levels during the preovulatory phase of the menstrual cycle, followed by a rise in progesterone levels during the postovulatory phase of the menstrual cycle, may result in a variety of physiological effects. These may be estrogen dependent, progesterone dependent, or androgen depedent.

Epidermis

Estrogen may have a tendency to halt epidermal atrophy in oophorectomized women[3], and it may stimulate the reticuloendothelial system[4].

Dermis

Estrogen increases dermal hyaluronic acid levels, resulting in an increase in dermal water content[5]. Hyaluronic acid can hold up to a thousand times its weight in water[6]. The rate of diffusion of substances injected intradermally, such as tuberculin and other intradermal tests, may be attenuated during the premenstrual phase and on the first day of menstruation, owing to the estrogen-induced increase in the hyaluronic acid content of the dermis[7]. Estrogen may also decrease the breakdown of collagen[8].

Appendages

Sebaceous gland activity is suppressed during the estrogen preovulatory phase, but is increased

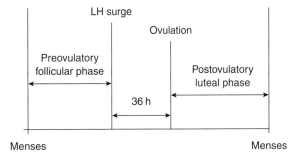

Figure 1 The menstrual cycle

during the postovulatory or progesterone phase[9]. There appears to be no effect on apocrine glands.

Blood vessels

The vascularity of the skin is increased by estrogens, reaching its peak premenstrually[10].

Mucosa

The mucous membranes of the vagina thicken during the follicular–preovulatory phase and then regress and desquamate throughout the luteal–postovulatory phase. Vaginal smears can be interpreted for clinical diagnosis, as they will reflect the patient's endocrine status[11]. Although oral mucosal lesions are seldom recognized during the cycle, intermenstrual gingivitis coinciding with ovulation can occur[11].

Pigmentation

Cyclical variation can occur in up to 50% of women[12]. Estrogen can enhance pigmentation premenstrually[13,14], especially around the eyes and on the nipples.

Fluid retention

Retention of salt and water occurs during the premenstrual phase and may result in an increase of several pounds in weight[11]. The degree of water retention is extremely variable.

Temperature

There is frequently a rise in temperature during the preovulatory follicular phase, with an abrupt drop just before ovulation, and a rise again until 1 or 2 days before the start of menstruation[11].

Immunological

Estrogens may decrease the cutaneous response in delayed hypersensitivity reactions and may have direct anti-inflammatory effects[11,15,16]. On the other hand, elevated levels of progesterone in the premenstrual phase of the cycle could exacerbate hypersensitivity reactions of types I and IV[17]. Progesterone may impair cell-mediated immunity through increased suppressor T-cell activity when T cells are stimulated by concanavalin A[18]. Progesterone may also have a stimulatory effect on immune function by increased T-cell rosetting, monocyte phagocytosis[19] and monocyte interleukin-1 production[20] at some concentrations (10^{-9} mol/1), but with inhibition at other concentrations (above 10^{-7} mol/1). Progesterone may also increase leukocyte binding to endothelial cells[21], which may help explain the increase in cutaneous delayed-type hypersensitivity[8].

CLINICAL CHANGES

Many otherwise healthy women experience clinical and psychological changes during the premenstrual and menstrual phase of their cycle[22]. This so-called premenstrual syndrome (PMS) has generally been attributed to increasing levels of progesterone.

The physical symptoms of abdominal bloating, breast tenderness and food craving, and the mood symptoms of anger, depression and irritability, have been used by Kemmett and Tidman to define PMS[23]. Edema of the hands, feet and occasionally the face can also occur. In other women emotional tension headaches and a variety of abdominal and urinary symptoms may occur[11]. Mood changes of PMS have been postulated to be due to an abnormality of neurotransmitters such as endorphins[24].

PMS can be improved with short courses (6 months) of contraceptives. This often regulates the cycle, and when the patient is no longer receiving oral contraceptives the PMS is less severe. The cramping and pain of PMS are helped by non-steroidal anti-inflammatory drugs. The bloating and edema can be decreased with a short course of hydrochlorothiazide during the premenstrual period.

If we accept the general concept that androgens stimulate and estrogens depress sebaceous glands, then we can appreciate that up to 70% of women get an acne flare and 35% complain of greasy hair premenstrually. Others have suggested that the flare of acne 2–7 days premenstrually is secondary to changes in the hydration of the pilosebaceous epithelium[11]. In spite of this generalization, about 18% of women complain that their hair becomes drier than normal.

Treatment for acne is usually helpful with the normal acne regimens that are currently available. In some women, antibiotic doses need to be increased premenstrually to control flare-ups, and reduced during the rest of the monthly cycle. The premenstrual flare of acne is often helped by certain contraceptives. Antiandrogens are also used to treat acne.

Severe dysmenorrhea with premenstrual depression and acne with hirsutism may also be due to increased testosterone, as might be seen with polycystic ovaries[11].

Many pre-existing dermatoses may become more active during the premenstrual period. Rosacea, acne, lupus erythematosus, psoriasis, lichen planus, anogenital pruritus, hidradenitis suppurativa and many forms of eczema may show some degree of exacerbation.

A survey was carried out of 150 women with atopic dermatitis: 33% noticed a premenstrual deterioration in their symptoms and improvement in the week after menstruation[23]. The premenstrual deterioration correlated significantly with the somatic and psychological symptoms of PMS. A menstrual variation in the itch/pain threshold has been shown to occur, being lower in the postovulatory phase[25]. Similarly, the cutaneous erythema response to histamine varies with menstruation, being highest on the first day of menstrual flow[26]. These may be contributing factors in the premenstrual flaring of atopic dermatitis[23] as well as other itching dermatoses. In these patients more potent topical steroids or increased frequency of application of their normal topical steroid may need to be carried out during this phase of the cycle.

Some women develop a premenstrual urticarial and/or erythema multiforme type of eruption with bullae. Hart[27] described this condition, calling it autoimmune progesterone dermatitis. It was implied that exposure to an oral progesterone sensitized the patients to progesterone-secreting cells in their own corpus luteum. The rash completely resolved with estrogen therapy.

The etiological role of progesterone in premenstrual urticaria was confirmed[28]. In another patient reported by Mayou and colleagues[29], it was postulated that the patient's recurring premenstrual urticaria was estrogen- rather than progesterone-dependent. Her symptoms were controlled by suppression of ovulation, and finally by bilateral oophorectomy and hysterectomy. Challenge with conjugated estrogens 2 months postoperatively induced an exacerbation of the rash after 2 days.

The concept of an autoimmune basis for progesterone-induced urticaria was challenged by Wilkinson and co-workers[17]. They agreed that systemic administration of progesterone in their patients caused a flare, but they were not able to confirm that there was an immunological reaction to endogenous progesterone or estrogen. They concluded that in some patients there may be an immunological reaction to the hormone; in others, non-immunological mechanisms may play a role.

Schofield and associates[30], in a paper on recurring erythema multiforme, had one patient with no predisposing precipitating factors other than her menstrual period.

The relationship of autoimmune diseases and the menstrual cycle has not as yet been clearly elucidated. Lupus erythematosus[31] and psoriasis can flare premenstrually. In patients with severe lupus erythematosus, cessation of menses for 3–6 months is not uncommon, but they usually return to normal as the disease goes into remission[32].

It is important for clinicians to recognize the cyclical variations in female dermatological problems related to the menstrual cycle.

REFERENCES

1. Yen SSC, Jaffe RB. *Reproductive Endocrinology*, 2nd edn. Philadelphia: WB Saunders, 1986:200–36
2. Rivlin ME, Martin RW. *Manual of Clinical Problems in Obstetrics and Gynecology*, 4th edn. Toronto: Little, Brown, 1994:398–9
3. Punnonen R. Effect of castration and peroral estrogen therapy on the skin. *Acta Obstet Gynecol* 1972;21 (suppl):3–4
4. Nicol T, Bilbey DL, Charles LM, *et al*. Oestrogen: the natural stimulant of body defense. *J Endocrinol* 1964;30:277–91
5. Green R, Dalton K. Premenstrual syndrome. *Br Med J* 1953;1:1007–14
6. Maddin S. *Skin Therapy Letter*, 1998;3:5
7. Seeberg G. Cutaneous absorption during menstrual cycle and its influence on intradermal reactions of delayed type. *Acta Derm Venereol (Stockh)* 1950;30: 231–48
8. Katz FU, Kappas A. Influence of estradiol and estriol on urinary excretion of hydroxyproline in man. *J Lab Clin Med* 1968;71:65
9. Burton JL, Cartlidge M, Suster S. Variations in sebum excretion during the menstrual cycle. *Acta Derm Venereol (Stockh)* 1973;53:81–4
10. Edwards EA, Dontley SQ. Cutaneous vascular changes in women in reference to menstrual cycle and ovariectomy. *Am J Obstet Gynecol* 1949;57: 501–9
11. Graham-Brown RAC, Ebling FJG. The ages of man and their dermatoses. In Rook A, Wilkinson DS, Ebling FJG, *et al*., eds. *Textbook of Dermatology*, 5th edn. Oxford: Blackwell Scientific, 1984:2885–6
12. McGuines BW. Skin pigmentation and the menstrual cycle. *Br Med J* 1961;5251:563–5
13. Resnick S. Melasma induced by oral contraceptive drugs. *JAMA* 1967;199:601
14. Snell RS, Bischitz PG. The melanocyte and melanin in human abdominal wall skin. *J Anat* 1963; 97:361
15. Bodel P. Anti inflammatory effects of estradiol on human blood leukocytes. *J Lab Clin Med* 1972; 80:737

16. Marks R, Shahrad P. Skin changes at the time of the climacteric. *Clin Obstet Gynecol* 1977;4:207–26

17. Wilkinson SM, Beck MM, Kingston TP. Progesterone induced urticaria – need it be autoimmune? *Br J Dermatol* 1995;133:792–4

18. Holdstuck G, Chastenay BF, Kranitt EL. Effects of testosterone, estradiol and progesterone on immune regulation. *Clin Exp Immunol* 1982;47:449–56

19. Wybran J, Goraerts A, Van Dam D, Appleboem T. Stimulating properties of lynestral on normal human blood, T lymphocytes and other leukocytes. *Int J Immunopharmacol* 1979;1:151–5

20. Polan ML, Daniele A, Kuo A. Gonadal steroids modulate human monocyte interleukin activity. *Fertil Steril* 1998;49:964–8

21. Cid MC, Kleinman HK, Grant DS, et al. Estradiol enhances leukocyte binding. *J Clin Invest* 1994;93:17–25

22. Coppen A, Kessel N. Menstruation and personality. *Br J Psychiatry* 1963;109:711–21

23. Kemmett D, Tidman MJ. The influence of the menstrual cycle and pregnancy on atopic dermatitis. *Br J Dermatol* 1991;125:59–61

24. Reid RL, Yen SSC. Premenstrual syndrome. *Am J Obstet Gynecol* 1981;139:85–104

25. Procacci P, Buzzelli G, Passeri I, et al. Studies on the cutaneous pricking pain threshold in man, cercadian and circatrigintan changes. *Res Clin Stud Headache* 1972;3:260

26. McGovern JP, Smolensky MH, Reinberg A. Circadian and circamenstrual rhythmicity in cutaneous reactivity to histamine and allergenic extracts. In McGovern JP, Smolensky MH, Reinberg I, eds. *Chronobiology in Allergy and Immunology.* Springfield, IL: Charles C Thomas, 1997:79–116

27. Hart R. Autoimmune progesterone dermatitis. *Arch Dermatol* 1997;113:426–30

28. Farah FS, Shbakluz Z. Autoimmune progesterone urticaria. *J Allergy Clin Immunol* 1971;48:257–61

29. Mayou SC, Charles-Holmes R, Kenney A, Black MM. A premenstrual urticarial eruption treated with bilateral oophorectomy and hysterectomy. *Clin Exp Dermatol* 1988;13:114–16

30. Schofield JK, Tatnall FM, Leigh IM. Recurrent erythema multiforme: clinical features and treatment in a large series of patients. *Br J Dermatol* 1993;128:542–5

31. Pardo JA, Gourley MF, Wilder RL, et al. Hormonal supplementation as treatment of cyclic rashes in patients with systemic lupus erythematosus. *J Rheumatol* 1995;22:2159–62

32. Fitzpatrick JB, Eisen AZ, Wolff K, et al. *Dermatology in General Medicine,* 3rd edn. New York: McGraw-Hill, 1987:1831

Pregnancy-related conditions

33

Samantha A. Vaughan Jones and Martin M. Black

During pregnancy, immunological, endocrine, metabolic and vascular changes occur which make the pregnant woman particularly susceptible to skin changes, both physiological and pathological. These changes result in a group of disorders now referred to as the pregnancy dermatoses. Pre-existing skin disease can be either improved or exacerbated as a result of pregnancy. In addition, there are five conditions with characteristic features that have been well described that are seen almost exclusively during pregnancy or in the immediate postpartum period (the specific dermatoses of pregnancy).

This chapter describes the following points:

(1) Physiological skin changes in pregnancy;
(2) Dermatoses exacerbated by pregnancy;
(3) Dermatoses occurring only in pregnancy;
(4) Specific dermatoses of pregnancy.

PHYSIOLOGICAL SKIN CHANGES IN PREGNANCY

During pregnancy, a number of physiological skin changes can occur (Table 1). One of the commonest of these changes and perhaps the most distressing is pruritus gravidarum, the etiology of which is probably multifactorial. It is thought that estrogen impairs the transport of bile to the bile canaliculi, leading to an increase in circulating bile salts, while prostaglandins reduce the threshold for pruritus[1]. However, in severe cases of pruritus gravidarum, obstetric cholestasis should be excluded by analysis of serum liver function tests and bile acids, as this is the most important differential diagnosis. The treatment of pruritus gravidarum is antihistamine therapy (e.g. chlorpheniramine), while soothing emollients such as aqueous cream can also be helpful.

Hyperpigmentation occurs in up to 90% of pregnant women and is thought to be due to elevated levels of melanocyte stimulating hormone (MSH), estrogen and possibly progesterone[2]. This is usually mild and generalized but is accentuated on the areolae, in the linea nigra (Figure 1) and on the genital skin. Pre-existing freckles and moles may also darken, although these pigmentary changes tend to regress postpartum.

A related phenomenon is melasma, which is seen both in pregnancy and with oral contraceptive therapy. This commonly involves the cheeks, forehead, nose and chin, and often follows a malar distribution. Histologically, excessive melanin deposition is seen either in the epidermis or in dermal macrophages[3]. This condition is exacerbated by excessive sun exposure; treatment should therefore include potent sunscreens.

Hirsutism is seen in pregnancy to a varying degree, most commonly involving the face, arms, legs and back. On the scalp the conversion from anagen to telogen hairs is slowed during pregnancy, creating thicker hair growth. This process is altered postpartum with a greater number of hairs entering the telogen phase and consequent shedding[2]. Nail changes during pregnancy include grooving, brittleness and distal onycholysis. Vascular proliferation can result in the development of spider nevi, particularly on the face and upper chest (Figure 2).

Striae distensae develop in both puberty and pregnancy and are often preceded by stretching of the skin or rapid weight gain (Figure 3). They are seen in up to 90% of pregnant women[2]. These pink atrophic bands of tissue develop on the abdomen and less commonly on the thighs, breasts and inguinal areas later in pregnancy. Stress-induced rupture of the connective tissue was proposed as a possible explanation[4], although other studies have shown dense elastic tissue deposition compatible with scar formation[5]. Another suggestion was that they result from increased adrenocortical activity rather than increased abdominal size. Postpartum, they fade to persistent pale atrophic lines. Other vascular changes during pregnancy include proliferation of vessels (such as spider nevi), palmar erythema, flushing due to vasomotor instability and an increase in venous varicosities resulting from increased venous pressure in femoral and pelvic vessels.

Eccrine gland activity is increased in pregnancy, leading to an increase in hyperhidrosis and dyshidrotic eczema, while apocrine gland activity is reduced, so that hidradenitis suppurativa tends to improve.

Table 1   Physiological changes in skin, nails and hair

Striae
Vascular changes
Decreased apocrine gland activity
Increased sebaceous gland activity
Increased eccrine gland activity
Pruritus gravidarum
Hyperpigmentation
Melasma
Hirsutism
Nail changes

Table 2   Dermatoses exacerbated by pregnancy. From reference 6

Inflammatory
Psoriasis
Atopic dermatitis
Acne vulgaris
Urticaria
Lichen planus
Erythema nodosum
Infective
Viral (herpes simplex, zoster)
Bacterial (impetigo, tuberculosis, leprosy)
Fungal (*Candida, Pityrosporum* spp.)
Autoimmune
Lupus erythematosus
Systemic sclerosis
Polymyositis/dermatomyositis
Pemphigus vulgaris/foliaceus
Metabolic
Porphyria cutanea tarda
Acrodermatitis enteropathica
Connective tissue
Ehlers–Danlos syndrome
Pseudoxanthoma elasticum
Miscellaneous
Erythrokeratoderma variabilis
Mycosis fungoides
Neurofibromatosis
Acquired immune deficiency syndrome
Skin tumors
Nevi
   melanoma
Vascular
   pyogenic granuloma
   hemangioma
Others
   dermatofibroma
   keloid
   leiomyoma

Sebaceous gland activity tends to increase, particularly in the third trimester, so that acne vulgaris may either be exacerbated or develop for the first time.

DERMATOSES EXACERBATED BY PREGNANCY

These can largely be subdivided into inflamatory, infective, autoimmune, metabolic, miscellaneous skin disorders and skin tumors[6] (Table 2). The inflammatory disorders such as eczema, psoriasis and acne vulgaris appear to behave unpredictably in pregnancy. In those cases with pre-existing skin disease there may be relative remission during pregnancy, but in the majority of cases there is exacerbation of disease or, indeed, these disorders may appear for the first time during pregnancy in individuals not previously affected.

Psoriasis

Psoriasis affects 1.5–2% of the normal population and is characterized by inflammatory scaly plaques on the skin surface, accompanied by a seronegative arthropathy in up to 7% of cases. Trauma or injury to the skin often results in localized psoriasis at the injury site (Koebner phenomenon). Psoriasis has several distinct clinical types. The commonest of these is the plaque type, with characteristic silvery scaly plaques on the extensor aspects of the limbs, sacrum and scalp. The guttate form consists of small scattered pink papules occurring in crops mainly on the trunk. It often follows an upper respiratory tract infection, particularly with streptococci. In erythrodermic psoriasis there is widespread erythema and a fine scale present, often over the entire skin surface. Finally, in pustular psoriasis there are small sterile pustules occurring either in pre-existing plaques or *de novo* on the skin surface. The effect of pregnancy on psoriasis is unpredictable, and in up to 15% of patients the condition may deteriorate[7]. Management is

particularly difficult, as systemic agents such as methotrexate, etretinate and PUVA are all specifically contraindicated. The use of ultraviolet B therapy, topical corticosteroids and dithranol, however, appears to be safe. Impetigo herpetiformis is a very rare acute pustular form of psoriasis precipitated by pregnancy, often with no prior history of psoriasis, and should be included in the differential diagnosis of pustular psoriasis (see later).

Atopic dermatitis

Atopic dermatitis is a chronic relapsing pruritic dermatosis affecting 1–5% of the general population, and in many cases accompanied by other atopic features (asthma or hay fever). It often improves during pregnancy, but can deteriorate owing to excessive excoriation from pruritus gravidarum[8] (Figure 4). It may present for the first time during pregnancy (Figure 5). Management should include liberal emollients and mild to moderately potent topical corticosteroids (clobetasone butyrate 0.05% or betamethasone valerate 0.1%). Topical corticosteroid ointments should be applied to all affected areas twice daily, preferably with emollients used beforehand. Soap and detergents should be avoided and a soap substitute such as aqueous cream or emulsifying ointment used instead. Antihistamines such as chlorpheniramine, which are safe in pregnancy, can be effective in reducing pruritus and assisting sleep, but the newer non-sedating antihistamines are contraindicated in pregnancy[9]. Occasionally systemic corticosteroids such as prednisolone are required for a short time. Although fetal cleft palate has been reported in pregnancy when prednisolone is used in the first trimester, prednisolone can be used when indicated in the later stages of pregnancy and during breast feeding. Prednisolone is the steroid of choice because it has been well described during pregnancy. Particular attention should be placed on screening for pregnancy-induced glucose intolerance, hypertension and delayed fetal growth[10]. Breast feeding has been found to be safe, with clinically insignificant amounts of the drug being concentrated in breast milk.

Nipple dermatitis can be provoked by breast feeding, with dry cracked skin and fissures that become secondarily infected with *Staphylococcus aureus*. This can be treated with frequent moisturizers and a mild topical corticosteroid such as hydrocortisone, combined with a topical antibiotic such as fucidin if infected.

Hand dermatitis is often exacerbated in the puerperium because of the constant exposure to irritants used in the care of the young infant. Prophylactic measures such as the protection of hands using gloves and liberal emollients can be effective. As there is a higher incidence of contact dermatitis during pregnancy, rubber gloves should be avoided and should be replaced with vinyl gloves. Moderately potent or potent topical corticosteroids (betamethasone valerate 0.1%) can also be used and, again, these should be used in conjunction with liberal emollients and soap substitutes such as aqueous cream or emulsifying ointment.

Acne vulgaris

Acne vulgaris can improve during pregnancy but is occasionally exacerbated. As most of the systemic antiacne drugs are teratogenic, treatment should be with topical therapy such as benzoyl peroxide (2.5–10% cream, lotion or gel) or topical antibiotics such as clindamycin or erythromycin. Oral tetracyclines should be avoided in treatment, as they may lead to yellow discoloration of developing teeth. Oral erythromycin is safe during pregnancy and can be used systemically as a treatment for acne. Treatments for severe acne (isotretinoin and cyproterone acetate) are specifically contraindicated in pregnancy at any stage. Isotretinoin is teratogenic, and the antiandrogen cyproterone acetate can produce feminization of a male fetus.

Erythema nodosum

This is an inflammatory process involving the subcutaneous fat; it can be precipitated by a number of systemic conditions (streptococcal infection, tuberculosis, leprosy, sarcoidosis, inflammatory bowel disease) or drugs (sulfonamides and oral contraceptives). However, it can also present in pregnancy for the first time, with tender symmetrical erythematous nodules or plaques, classically on the anterior shins[11]. It can be associated with fever and arthralgia and usually resolves over a period of 6–8 weeks. Treatment in pregnancy should consist of bed rest and mild analgesics such as paracetamol. Non-steroidal inflammatory agents must be avoided in pregnancy, as they may cause premature closure of the ductus arteriosus *in utero*.

Systemic lupus erythematosus

With the advent of more conservative treatments for systemic lupus erythematosus (SLE), pregnancy is now commoner among SLE patients. It is thought that disease flares occur no more commonly than in the non-pregnant state, although several reports have shown conflicting data. One recent retrospective study compared the frequency of flare in pregnant and non-pregnant controls using logistic regression analyses to assess the role of prepregnancy disease activity as a prognostic factor for flare during pregnancy or the postpartum period[12]. The authors found no significant difference between pregnant patients and controls, but showed that inactive disease at the onset of pregnancy in SLE provided optimun protection against the incidence of flare during pregnancy. However, a recent case–control study compared 68 pregnant SLE patients with 50 consecutive age-matched non-pregnant SLE patients and found a significant difference in the incidence of disease flares between the two groups: 65% of the patients flared during pregnancy and

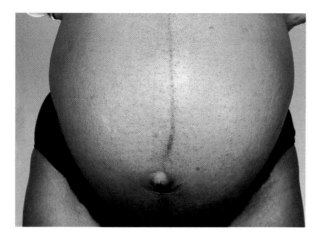

Figure 1   Linea nigra on the abdomen caused by hyper-pigmentation of the linea alba during pregnancy

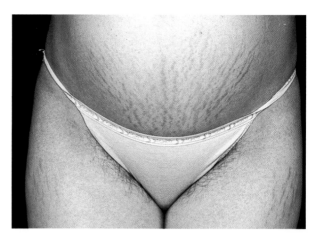

Figure 3   Striae distensae gravidarum on the lower abdomen and upper thighs

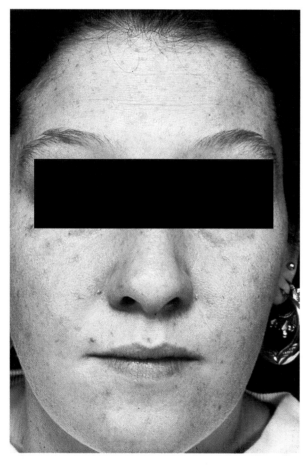

Figure 2   Multiple spider nevi on the face in early pregnancy due to vascular proliferation

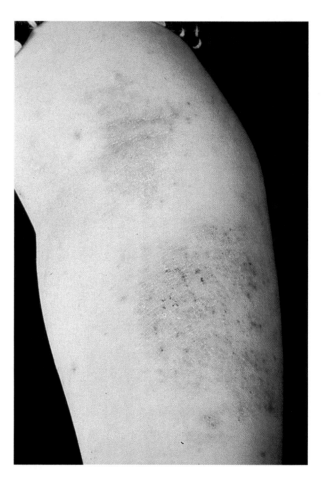

Figure 4   Excoriated patch of dermatitis on the elbow flexure in a pregnant women with a history of atopy in childhood

42% flared in the control group[13]. They concluded that SLE tends to flare during pregnancy, and found that flares were maximal in the second and third trimesters and the puerperium, but were not prevented by the administration of systemic prednisolone. Similar results were found in a comparison of the flare rate during and after pregnancy in

36 SLE patients[14]. Approximately 25% of liveborn infants whose mothers have SLE will be small for gestational age, presumably because of placental dysfunction as a result of immunoglobulin and complement deposition[15]. Neonatal lupus erythematosus is seen in babies of mothers with circulating anti-Ro antibodies and can lead to congenital heart block.

Cutaneous flares of lupus erythematosus appear to be the most common, followed by arthritic flares, often presenting with morning stiffness. A common cutaneous presentation is that of lupus vasculitis seen classically on the palms and soles. Treatment should be tailored to the disease severity, although systemic prednisolone is probably the safest.

Pemphigus vulgaris

Pemphigus vulgaris reported during pregnancy is extremely rare and usually requires treatment with systemic corticosteroids or other immunosuppressive agents. It is caused by an autoantibody directed against desmosomal antigens (130-kDa desmoglein 3 in the case of pemphigus vulgaris and 160-kDa desmoglein 1 in pemphigus foliaceus). Exacerbation of pre-existing disease can also occur during pregnancy, generally in the first or second trimester. As in the non-pregnant individual, it presents with non-healing erosions on the trunk and limbs and associated mucosal lesions. Differential diagnosis from pemphigoid gestationis is important; direct and indirect immunofluorescence (IMF) confirm the diagnosis, with an intercellular pattern of IgG deposition between the keratinocytes of the epidermis. There is a reported increase in fetal morbidity and mortality, although some authors have reported cases with normal prognosis[16–18]. During pregnancy, immunosuppressants (cyclophosphamide, azathioprine, methotrexate and gold) should all be avoided, to minimize possible teratogenicity. Antibody titers (indirect IMF) may be helpful as a guide to disease activity and response to treatment. Control of disease with corticosteroids only is preferable, and this can be continued while breast feeding.

The trauma of vaginal delivery can result in worsening of erosions, and cesarean section delivery provides an alternative if there is already severe vulval involvement. Neonatal pemphigus can occur, owing to transplacental transfer of IgG autoantibodies. Most neonates who have symptoms do not require therapy, and blisters generally resolve within 2–3 weeks. Breast feeding is not contraindicated, although local blister formation may occur and passive transfer of antibodies to the infant via breast milk is a potential risk[18].

Malignant melanoma

The influence of pregnancy on the prognosis in malignant melanoma is extremely controversial. As in non-pregnant individuals, it appears that the prognosis should be based on tumor thickness. In 1991, Mackie and colleagues[19] reported the results of an epidemiological study of 388 women treated for stage I primary cutaneous disease during their childbearing years. They showed that melanomas that are diagnosed during pregnancy tend to be thicker than those in women of a similar age who develop melanoma not associated with pregnancy ($p = 0.002$). When controlled for tumor thickness, however, pregnancy did not alter the prognosis of melanoma, as might be expected. The authors concluded that women with melanoma should be advised about pregnancy on the basis of thickness and site of the tumor rather than hormonal status. In 1993, Driscoll and co-workers[20] reviewed the literature that examined the effect of pregnancy on the prognosis of melanoma and the effect on future pregnancies after diagnosis. Their review concluded that pregnancy after or at the time of diagnosis of stage I melanoma did not appear to alter the 5-year survival rate. However, there is little information about the prognosis of stage III and IV pregnancy-associated melanomas, as there have been no statistical trials for such cases.

Transplacental transmission of melanoma to the fetus is extremely rare, although placental metastases have been reported. Histological examination of the placenta is recommended, to look for metastatic disease in women presenting with melanomas during pregnancy. Metastases to the placenta are generally blood-borne and occur only in women with widely disseminated malignant disease[21].

DERMATOSES OCCURRING ONLY IN PREGNANCY

Obstetric cholestasis

Obstetric cholestasis is one of the few disorders that adversely affects both maternal well-being and fetal outcome. The condition was formerly known as pruritus gravidarum, although this term should be reserved for cases with pruritus and normal liver function. Obstetric cholestasis usually presents in the late second or third trimesters, whereas physiological pruritus is generally a characteristic feature of the first trimester. In obstetric cholestasis the pruritus is intense and generalized, often with nocturnal exacerbation and particularly targeting the palms and soles.

The pathogenesis of obstetric cholestasis is unclear, but multiple factors have been implicated. Reyes and Simon[22] suggested that affected patients might have a genetic predisposition that alters the membrane composition of bile ducts and hepatocytes, increasing their sensitivity to sex steroids, particularly estrogens. Often high levels of serum bile salts and serum aminotransferases are seen in this condition, and should alert one to the diagnosis. High serum levels of alkaline phosphatase are usually found in obstetric cholestasis, but these values tend to overlap with the increased levels often seen in the last few weeks of normal pregnancy, owing to the contribution of an isoenzyme of placental origin[23]. Recurrence of the condition is expected in at least 50% of cases[24], and there is also said to be a familial predisposition with a positive family history in up to 50% of cases in association with the HLA antigen haplotypes HLA-B8 and HLA-BW16[25]. Family studies suggest an autosomal dominant inheritance[26].

The management of obstetric cholestasis is overshadowed by the increased risks of fetal distress, spontaneous preterm delivery and fetal death, the causes of which remain unknown. The risk of stillbirth increases towards term and appears to be unrelated to maternal symptoms[27]. One group reported 56 pregnancies complicated by obstetric cholestasis in which there were five intrauterine deaths, one neonatal death, 18 spontaneous premature deliveries and five mothers who required blood transfusion for severe unexplained postpartum hemorrhage[28]. Treatment options available include cholestyramine, phenobarbitone, charcoal, ultraviolet light, evening primrose oil, intravenous S-adenosyl-L-methionine and epomediol, but most of these have proved disappointing[29]. Ursodeoxycholic acid (UDCA) is an endogenous bile acid that reduces serum bile acids. It is not yet licensed for use in pregnancy, although small studies have so far revealed impressive relief of pruritus and improvement in total bile acids and liver function[30]. Maternal morbidity in this condition is often underestimated. Nocturnal itching causes insomnia and fatigue, while anorexia, malaise, mild epigastric discomfort, steatorrhea and dark urine are also common. Malabsorption of fat can lead to weight loss and vitamin deficiency, particularly of vitamin K, which may account for some cases of uterine and intracranial hemorrhage[29]. Quoted risks of spontaneous preterm labor are between 12 and 44%, and of fetal distress and meconium staining about 30%[31]. Constant serum monitoring of liver function tests, bile acids and prothrombin time are now recommended, and fetal ultrasound and Doppler blood flow studies should be performed regularly. Early elective delivery at 38 weeks' gestation is now considered mandatory[29].

Impetigo herpetiformis

Impetigo herpetiformis is a rare acute form of pustular psoriasis that is precipitated by pregnancy[32]. It can occur without a prior history of psoriasis and generally presents in women in their third trimester, with symptoms often persisting until delivery and, in some cases, postpartum. It is reminiscent of pustular psoriasis and classically presents with erythematous patches and pustulation at the margins. These typically begin in flexural areas and spread centrifugally onto the trunk and around the umbilicus, but they usually spare the hands, feet and face. Mucosal sites such as the tongue, buccal mucosa and esophagus can also become affected. Lesions tend to heal with postinflammatory hyperpigmentation. There is often accompanying constitutional upset with fever, delirium, diarrhea and vomiting and tetany due to hypocalcemia.

Histopathology of a skin biopsy is identical to that of pustular psoriasis, with spongiform pustules of Kogoj and large collections of neutrophils within foci of spongiotic epidermis.

Laboratory investigations often reveal hypocalcemia (in some cases associated with hypoparathyroidism), an elevated leukocyte count and high erythrocyte sedimentation rate (ESR). One group recently showed extremely low levels of epidermal skin-derived antileukoproteinase/elafin in a single case of impetigo herpetiformis when compared with three cases of generalized pustular psoriasis and six with plaque psoriasis[33]. The authors speculated that this enzyme may be relevant in pustule formation.

Management is usually with systemic corticosteroids, with doses of prednisolone up to 30–40 mg daily. However, stillbirth and placental insufficiency are still seen frequently, even when disease activity appears to be controlled. Remission postpartum is common, but recurrence in successive pregnancies is typical, often with increased severity and at an earlier gestation, so that careful counseling is essential. Recurrence with the contraceptive pill has also been described[34].

SPECIFIC DERMATOSES OF PREGNANCY

The specific dermatoses of pregnancy have led to much confusion in the past, owing to the clinical overlap between the various conditions. A rationalized clinical classification is now widely recognized[35] (Table 3). Apart from pemphigoid gestationis, no reliable diagnostic criteria exist to differentiate between these conditions. It was hoped that this classification would facilitate clinical investigation

Table 3 Specific dermatoses of pregnancy

New classification	*Previous terminology*
Pemphigoid gestationis	herpes gestationis
Polymorphic eruption of pregnancy	toxemic eruption of pregnancy
	late-onset prurigo of pregnancy
	pruritic urticarial papules and plaques of pregnancy
	toxic erythema of pregnancy
	erythema multiforme of pregnancy
Prurigo of pregnancy	prurigo gestationis of Besnier
	early-onset prurigo of pregnancy
Pruritic folliculitis	unknown

and thereby improve our understanding of the etiology of these dermatoses. Papular dermatitis of pregnancy as described by Spangler and co-workers[36] is not included in this classification and is now thought to overlap with prurigo and polymorphic eruption of pregnancy (PEP) and not to be a separate clinical entity.

Only one recent prospective study, by Roger and colleagues[37], has been performed to examine the incidence of these disorders in a pregnant population. These authors published data on 51 women.

Pemphigoid gestationis

Over recent years, significant advances have been made in our understanding of this condition. It is a rare, organ-specific, autoimmune bullous disease previously named 'herpes gestationis' because of the morphological similarity of individual lesions to herpetic vesicles[38]. It has a consistent relationship to pregnancy, the puerperium and, rarely, hydatidiform mole[39] and choriocarcinoma[40]. Its incidence has been reported in the literature as between one in 10 000 and one in 60 000 pregnancies[41,42]. In a study by Zurn and colleagues[43], the incidence of pemphigoid gestationis was one in 7000 pregnancies. The onset of a rash varies from 9 weeks' gestation to 1 week postpartum, but presents most frequently in the second and third trimesters[44]. Characteristically it recurs with increased severity and at an earlier gestational age in subsequent pregnancies, although 'skipped' pregnancies can rarely occur. A patient is said to have a 'skipped pregnancy' when she presents with classical pemphigoid gestationis in one pregnancy, but in a subsequent pregnancy does not develop a cutaneous eruption; this is said to occur in approximately 5% of pemphigoid gestationis pregnancies. The reasons for this are not entirely understood, although some authors have hypothesized that this situation arises when the fetus

has the HLA-DR antigens possessed by the mother[45]. The proposed mechanism may be via the induction of an exaggerated supressor T-cell response in the presence of common HLA-DR antigen subtypes[45,46]. A change of partner may also influence disease activity or expression[47].

In pemphigoid gestationis, early lesions are pruritic, erythematous urticated plaques, which may become annular or polycyclic (Figure 6). Gradually, vesicles or bullae predominate, so that lesions can closely resemble bullous pemphigoid. Lesions are most marked in the periumbilical skin in 87% of cases[46] before spreading over the abdomen, thighs, palms and soles.

The histopathological features include marked edema with subepidermal separation and eosinophilic spongiosis (Figure 7). Basal cell necrosis may be a prominent feature; however, the diagnosis is confirmed by direct IMF that demonstrates linear C3 basement membrane zone deposition in all cases, and in addition IgG in 27% of cases[46]. Circulating antibodies are often detected by indirect IMF and are usually of the complement-binding IgG1 subclass. These antibodies classically bind to the epidermal side of saline-split normal human skin (Figure 8). Transplacental transfer of these antibodies can occur and may result in a neonatal blistering eruption that is milder and more transient than the maternal eruption[44]. The fetal prognosis in pemphigoid gestationis has been a controversial issue, with results from only a few studies available. Shornick and Black[47] compared fetal outcome in pregnancies from 74 women with pemphigoid gestationis with normal pregnancies from the same women. Their results clearly indicated a significant increase in premature deliveries in the pemphigoid gestationis pregnancies, as well as a tendency for small-for-dates babies. They concluded that these findings were compatible with low-grade placental dysfunction in pemphigoid gestationis.

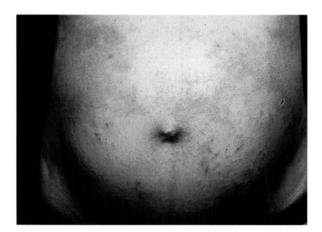

Figure 5   Dermatitis on the central abdomen in pregnancy with no previous history of atopic dermatitis. Note the absence of periumbilical sparing, which helps to distinguish this eruption from polymorphic eruption of pregnancy

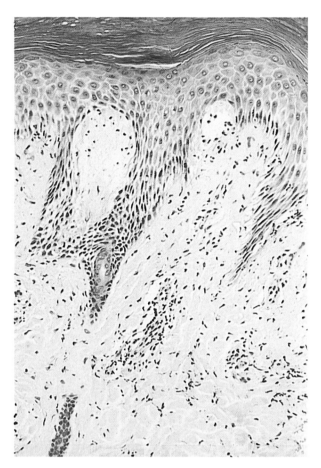

Figure 7   High-power histopathology of a skin biopsy in pemphigoid gestationis (× 90), demonstrating the severe papillary dermal edema leading to early subepidermal separation

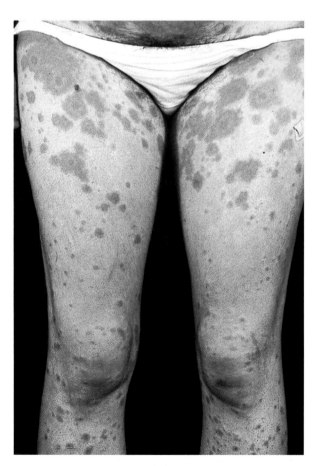

Figure 6   Pre-bullous stage of pemphigoid gestationis, showing the typical annular urticated plaques on the lower abdomen and upper thighs

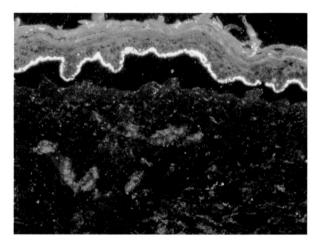

Figure 8   Indirect immunofluorescence using serum from a patient with pemphigoid gestationis applied to saline-split normal human skin (× 6.2). A bright linear basement membrane zone band of complement 3 deposition is seen only on the epidermal side of the split skin

The close similarities between pemphigoid gestationis and bullous pemphigoid have been noted, not only clinically and immunopathologically, but also in the response to systemic corticosteroids. Both are autoimmune bullous diseases characterized by subepidermal blisters, circulating and tissue-bound autoantibodies reacting against similar determinants; both immunoblotting and immunoprecipitation techniques demonstrate two major antigenic targets, termed BP1AG and BP2AG, with molecular weights of 230 and 180 kDa, respectively[48–51]. In addition, 100% of pemphigoid gestationis sera and over 50% of bullous pemphigoid sera contain IgG autoantibodies, which avidly fix complement *in vitro*[52,53]. The histopathological findings of subepidermal bullae with numerous eosinophils can be indistinguishable, and IMF and immunoelectron microscopy demonstrate deposition of C3 and IgG in the lamina lucida of the basement membrane zone in both conditions[54,55].

However, all the evidence suggests that pemphigoid gestationis and bullous pemphigoid are distinct conditions with divergent clinical features. The pattern of clinical involvement in pemphigoid gestationis, initially with distribution around the umbilicus, sparing of the face and mucosal surfaces, is very different from that of bullous pemphigoid, where lesions occur on the trunk and limbs, sometimes with involvement of mucosal surfaces. Pemphigoid gestationis typically occurs in the second and third trimesters of pregnancy, often with exacerbation postpartum, whilst bullous pemphigoid is described in patients usually older than 50 years of age with no evidence of direct hormonal modulation. In addition, there is no reported HLA antigen association in bullous pemphigoid, whereas pemphigoid gestationis is linked to HLA-DR3, -DR4[56] and a C4 null allele[57]. One group recently studied 39 cases of pemphigoid gestationis for the presence and specificity of anti-HLA antibodies, and found these in 100% of cases; almost all of them were cytotoxic. Specificity was against class I antigens in 98% and class II antigens in 25%[58].

We previously reported two cases, both initially presenting with a bullous disorder of pregnancy typical of pemphigoid gestationis but later progressing into bullous pemphigoid over a long period of time[59]. This indicates that the two conditions are part of the same continuum of disease, but with differing clinical patterns. One of these patients responded initially to treatment with a luteinizing hormone releasing hormone analog, inducing a reversible chemical oophorectomy[60], but relapsed and continues to have active disease, despite hysterectomy and bilateral oophorectomy. The other patient also developed ulcerative colitis and thyrotoxicosis due to underlying Graves' disease, again highlighting the overlap with other autoimmune diseases. A higher incidence of antithyroid autoantibodies in patients with a history of pemphigoid gestationis has already been established[61].

Although rare, pemphigoid gestationis is perhaps the most frequently studied and well understood of the specific pregnancy dermatoses. Its relationship to the pregnancy hormones, other autoimmune diseases and immunogenetics has been clearly established[61]. Pemphigoid gestationis is clearly a unique autoimmune disease that has profound potential implications for both mother and fetus. The primary event that triggers the pathogenesis is still unknown, and the exact molecular nature of the pemphigoid gestationis antigen also remains unclear. Its close relationship to bullous pemphigoid provides an area for future research, and further cases will need to be studied to examine the immunopathological overlap between these two conditions.

Our group has reported on a patient with pemphigoid gestationis who showed clinical features that were entirely typical, but whose immunopathological profile was extremely atypical, with both cell surface staining and linear basement membrane zone IgG staining on direct and indirect immunofluorescence[62]. Immunoelectron microscopy of the skin biopsy did show labelling of immunogold particles on the lamina lucida just below the hemidesmosomes, and immunoblotting of the serum confirmed the presence of antibodies directed against the 180-kDa bullous pemphigoid antigen-2 (BP-Ag 2), with no other antibodies detectable. Both these features were confirmatory for the diagnosis of pemphigoid gestationis, despite the unusual IMF findings. To our knowledge, this is the first report of these atypical features in pemphigoid gestationis.

Polymorphic eruption of pregnancy

PEP (previously named pruritic urticarial papules and plaques of pregnancy or PUPPP) was first described in 1979[63]. Although the latter term is still used to describe this condition, particularly in the USA, it is generally agreed that PEP and PUPPP are identical dermatoses[64,65]. PEP more accurately describes the variable morphology of individual lesions, which can be papular, plaque-like urticated wheals, vesicular and bullous. PEP is the commonest gestational dermatosis with an incidence of approximately 1 : 160 pregnancies. It is now regarded as a distinct clinical entity, although the clinical features can resemble other specific dermatoses of pregnancy[66]. The common clinical presentation of PEP in abdominal striae suggests that abdominal distension may be an important factor in the etiology (Figure 9). Indeed, there is a significant association with excess maternal weight gain[67,68] and increased fetal weight, while PEP in twin pregnancies tends to be more severe[69] (Figure 10). One group has postulated that increased maternal weight gain and abdominal girth due to rapid abdominal expansion may cause trauma to the overlying skin, triggering the inflammatory response of PEP[67]. We reported two severe cases of PEP, one the first report in a triplet pregnancy, of a woman who presented at 24 weeks' gestation, by which stage she already had marked abdominal distension. An elective Cesarean section was performed at 34 weeks' gestation, and the next day her eruption had begun to resolve[69]. An earlier study described 25 patients with PEP[70] and found four cases with twins (16%) compared with the national incidence of twins reported as 1 : 85 (1.2%) births[71], although the significance of this is unknown. Three-quarters of patients are primigravid and the eruption usually develops in the third trimester or the postpartum period. In contrast to pemphigoid gestationis, PEP is predominantly a disease of women in their first pregnancy[72], and when it recurs the second eruption is less severe than the first. Unlike pemphigoid gestationis, there is no association with autoimmune disease or HLA type, and the fetal prognosis is normal. A study of sex hormones in this condition (serum β-human chorionic gonadotropin (β-hCG), estradiol and cortisol) found no significant differences compared with controls[73]. So far no direct hormonal influence has been established, although this needs to be investigated further.

The eruption tends to be short-lived, with an average duration of 6 weeks. Lesions begin on the lower abdomen within striae, but spare the umbilicus. Urticarial papules develop which coalesce to produce plaques, vesicles, target lesions and polycyclic wheals, and subsequently spread to distal sites. Pruritus is a prominent symptom and, as the lesions resolve, fine scale and crusting appear, reminiscent of dermatitis. Clinically, the lesions can occasionally appear similar to pemphigoid gestationis and can also be confused with scabies and drug eruptions. In PEP the umbilicus is frequently spared, in marked contrast to pemphigoid gestationis, and this can be a helpful distinguishing feature between the two conditions.

The histopathology of PEP varies with the clinical stage of the eruption[72], but often demonstrates variable features including upper dermal edema, scanty eosinophils and a perivascular lymphohistiocytic infiltrate. Some of these histopathological features are also seen in the other specific dermatoses of pregnancy[74]. Direct and indirect IMF and immuno-electron microscopy are characteristically negative and are important investigations to distinguish this condition from pemphigoid gestationis, which can appear clinically similar[75]. Recently, several studies have demonstrated circulating antibasement membrane zone antibodies of IgM class raising the question of an immune pathogenesis[43,76]. A single case report of linear IgM dermatosis of pregnancy has also been described which the authors felt may represent a subtype of PEP with features of early pemphigoid gestationis[77]. However, this has not been fully substantiated. Immunohistochemical studies in PEP have been limited, but have so far suggested a predominantly T-helper lymphocytic response[78,79].

As PEP is self-limiting and often resolves after delivery without sequelae, symptomatic treatment alone is required. Moderately potent topical corticosteroids are usually more effective in relieving pruritus than antihistamines and, in addition, the new non-sedating antihistamines are not recommended during pregnancy[9]. The eruption can be severe for 1–2 weeks, when a short reducing course of oral prednisolone may be indicated[69]. A severe case of PEP unresponsive to therapy dramatically improved within 2 h of Cesarean section delivery[80].

Polymorphic eruption is a relatively common dermatosis of pregnancy, with an incidence of approximately 1 : 120[66]. Despite the frequency of this pregnancy dermatosis, little is known about the exact pathogenesis of this condition, although many theories exist. Several hypotheses have been put forward, including the association of increased maternal weight gain[67,68] with large infants and multiple pregnancy[69].

Direct IMF studies in PEP have occasionally been reported to show a linear or speckled band of fluorescence with IgM at the basement membrane zone. This has been labelled as 'linear IgM dermatosis of pregnancy', although this label has not gained universal acceptance[77]. The original description was based on a single case report of a pregnant woman in her third trimester with erythematous follicular papules on the forearms, abdomen and thighs[77]. Direct immunofluorescence of perilesional skin demonstrated a dense deposition of IgM at the basement membrane zone. Both the eruption and the immunopathological findings disappeared at the end of the puerperium, suggesting that it had been immune-mediated. However, it is likely that the eruption described was more suggestive of either PEP or prurigo of pregnancy. A further report of five pregnant women with a cutaneous eruption clinically distinct from PEP described erythematous papular and urticarial lesions on the trunk and limbs. Direct IMF findings were negative, but indirect IMF demonstrated circulating IgM class antibasement membrane zone antibodies[43]. Another group found 25 cases out of 2271 with linear deposits of IgM on direct immunofluorescence, but the authors made no comment on whether any of these had occurred in pregnant women[81].

Maternal morbidity is a significant consideration in this group of patients, as the eruption classically occurs late in pregnancy, when intense pruritus can cause loss of sleep, with severe depression in some cases. For some patients elective cesarean section is chosen as the best mode of delivery after liaison between the patient, the obstetricians and dermatologists.

In the remaining cases the most effective treatments used are antihistamines (chlorpheniramine), emollients (aqueous cream with 1–2% menthol) and topical corticosteroids (clobetasone butyrate 0.05% or betamethasone valerate 0.1%). Although the use of systemic corticosteroids has been reported in this condition[69], this is generally reserved for severe cases.

Prurigo of pregnancy

In 1904, the term 'prurigo gestationis' was introduced to refer to all patients with a pregnancy-related dermatosis other than herpes gestationis[82]. Some years later, in 1941, the prevalence of this condition was estimated at about 2% of all pregnancies[83]. Since then, prurigo of pregnancy has remained perhaps the least studied and least understood of all the pregnancy dermatoses.

A group of 40 pregnant patients was studied over a 3-year period[84] and grouped together under the diagnostic heading of 'prurigo of pregnancy'. However, within this group, two well-defined subgroups were recognized and defined as 'early' and 'late' type of prurigo of pregnancy, respectively, referring to the stage of pregnancy at which the eruption began. Thirty-one cases were found to have the so-called 'early' type, the eruption beginning between 25 and 29 weeks' gestation with resolution occurring within 3 months of delivery. Individual lesions were excoriated papules, sometimes accompanied by eczematous patches, distributed mainly on the extensor aspects of the limbs (Figure 11). Three of these patients gave a history of a similar rash occurring during a previous pregnancy. Nine patients were also described with the so-called 'late' type of prurigo, characterized by urticarial papules, plaques and occasionally target lesions on the lower abdomen, later spreading to the limbs[84]. In seven of these cases the lesions began within abdominal striae and often exhibited the Koebner phenomenon within excoriations. The eruption occurred within the last 2 weeks of pregnancy and had resolved in all cases within a month postpartum. These 'late-onset' cases are now considered in retrospect to be polymorphic eruption of pregnancy. This original study remains the only detailed clinical description of this disorder.

In both subtypes of prurigo described, both maternal and fetal prognosis were normal, apart from one stillbirth within the 'early' type. No data were given in this study for histopathological findings or hormonal investigations on either subtype of patients. The overall incidence of prurigo was estimated at between 0.3 and 0.5%.

On comparison of these patients with those from earlier studies, the 'early' subtype appeared clinically indistinguishable from prurigo gestationis[82], while the 'late' subtype corresponded to the disorder described as 'toxemic rash of pregnancy', which we would now regard as PEP[85].

Since the original description, there have been two further studies of patients with similar eruptions. One group discussed five patients with what they described as 'prurigo of late pregnancy'[86] and noted some additional features. Histopathological examination in four cases demonstrated a perivascular lymphohistiocytic infiltrate with occasional eosinophils, with both upper dermal edema and focal epidermal edema causing areas of vesicular spongiosis. IMF studies in all cases were negative.

A further seven patients with prurigo were described, some of whom had vesicular lesions[87]. In one of these cases, direct IMF demonstrated C3 deposition along the basement membrane zone, although the authors made no comment as to whether this was in a patchy, linear or continuous distribution. However, the authors did not feel that this meant that these patients had pemphigoid gestationis. Indeed, this finding is often seen in the IMF results of patients with chronic itching and excoriation, both of which are characteristic features of patients with prurigo. The nature of the infiltrate in frozen skin sections was also studied using pan-T-cell monoclonal antibodies, and the perivascular infiltrate was found to comprise mainly T lymphocytes[87]. In addition, intracutaneous endocrine skin tests using progesterone and estradiol revealed no abnormal immediate or delayed responses, thereby excluding an autoimmune response to progesterone, as has previously been described[88]. The authors[87] concluded that their

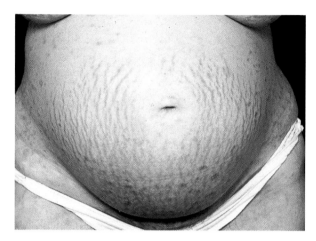

Figure 9   Early polymorphic eruption developing on abdominal striae in a primiparous woman in her third trimester. This case demonstrates typical periumbilical sparing

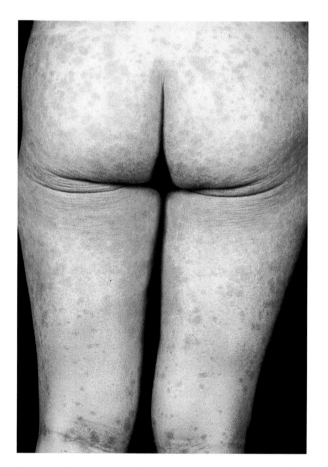

Figure 10   Urticated erythematous lesions becoming confluent on the buttocks and upper thighs in a woman with twins and early polymorphic eruption

patients had the same disorder as toxemic rash of pregnancy[85]. They felt that the possibility that this condition was an early form of pemphigoid gestationis was worthy of further investigation.

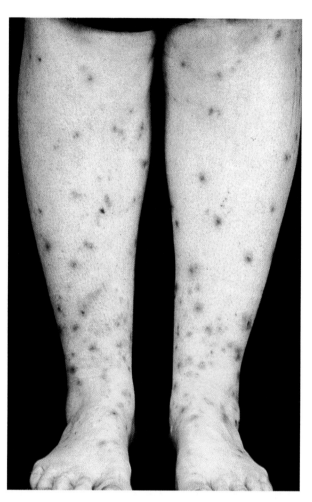

Figure 11   Prurigo of pregnancy, showing excoriated papules on the extensor aspect of the lower legs

A later study of eight patients with prurigo found that each patient had features of an underlying atopic diathesis, although none had typical eczematous lesions[46]. The authors therefore postulated that prurigo of pregnancy may arise as a result of pruritus gravidarum occurring in atopic women. They based this argument on the finding that 18% of pregnancies are complicated by pruritus[89] and that 10% of the population demonstrate atopy[90]. It would therefore be predicted that both conditions would coexist in approximately 2% of pregnancies.

Papular dermatitis of pregnancy

Papular dermatitis was first described by Spangler and colleagues[36] in a group of 12 patients among those with pruritic papular eruptions of pregnancy. They described an eruption with variable onset from the 1st to the 9th month of gestation and resolution within a week of delivery. Recurrence of the eruption occurred in all six patients who became pregnant again subsequently. The individual

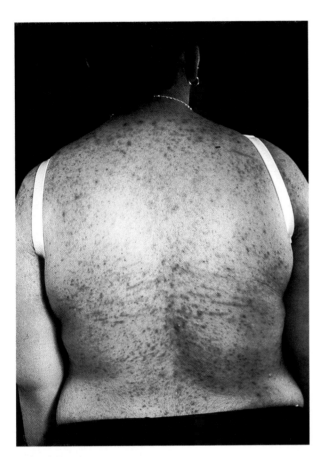

Figure 12 Pruritic folliculitis of pregnancy in an Afro-Caribbean mother showing an extensive eruption on the upper back with small erythematous papules and postinflammatory hyperpigmentation in a follicular distribution

lesions consisted of pruritic, erythematous, soft papules with secondary excoriations, widely distributed on the trunk, limbs, face and scalp. One of the major features described was the high fetal mortality of 27–37%, which they claimed could be considerably reduced by the administration of systemic corticosteroids. This has aroused much controversy, among both dermatologists and obstetricians, but there have been no subsequent studies that have objectively examined the evidence since the original description. Spangler and colleagues considered that papular dermatitis could be differentiated from prurigo of pregnancy both clinically and biochemically[36]. On clinical grounds the lesions were diffusely scattered and the pruritus was unresponsive to topical therapy, whereas in prurigo[82] the lesions were often clustered on the limbs and the pruritus invariably responded to topical therapy. However, the feature that Spangler and co-workers felt was of particular importance was the high level of urinary hCG during the last trimester which returned to normal following treatment with

systemic corticosteroids[36]. The authors also noted reduced plasma hydrocortisone and a shortened plasma hydrocortisone half-life in their group of patients. No histopathological data were recorded in the patients of Spangler and associates, so that no clinicopathological correlation is possible in retrospect. Unfortunately, no systematic study to date has compared these potentially important biochemical abnormalities of papular dermatitis of pregnancy (PDP) with the commoner and similar condition of prurigo of pregnancy, or with the other specific dermatoses of pregnancy. Indeed, considerable doubt exists as to whether papular dermatitis does exist as a separate entity or whether these cases represent more widespread cases of either prurigo or PEP, particularly as histopathological data are not available on the original 12 cases[36]. This important question about the validity of PDP cannot be resolved until biochemical data are available for the other specific dermatoses of pregnancy.

A further study of PDP was carried out[91] in which the role of urinary estriol levels and treatment with estrogen therapy was examined. In eight out of 14 of their cases the urinary estriol levels were low, although the significance of this finding is uncertain, as many of these patients were taking systemic prednisone at doses between 40 and 200 mg daily when the estriol assays were performed. One author has shown that this can be a cause of low urinary estriol itself[92]. Spangler and Emerson treated nine out of their 14 cases with diethylstilbestrol at doses ranging from 600 to 2500 mg daily, resulting in clearance of the skin lesions within 1 week. As there was no fetal mortality in this study, they concluded that estrogen therapy might be a useful alternative therapy to corticosteroids. However, the following year, the authors withdrew this statement[93] because of a newly recognized association between the administration of diethylstilbestrol during pregnancy and subsequent development of vaginal carcinoma during adolescence in the female offspring[94].

The histopathological features of PDP were not mentioned in either of the reports by Spangler and colleagues. A further 12 cases were then described and both the fetal prognosis and the histopathological features were studied[95]. In these cases, the epidermis showed mild acanthosis, focal parakeratosis and some crust formation, with upper dermal edema and a perivascular mixed inflammatory cell infiltrate. However, there was no evidence of high fetal mortality in contrast to the observations of Spangler and co-workers, and therefore conservative treatment was recommended.

Several case reports of PDP have been documented since then[96,97], in which the benefits of treatment with reducing courses of systemic prednisolone were found. No additional data on the biochemical or endocrine investigations in these patients have been reported.

In view of much of the controversy surrounding the diagnosis of PDP, the term has not gained universal acceptance as one of the specific dermatoses of pregnancy.

Pruritic folliculitis of pregnancy

The term 'pruritic folliculitis' of pregnancy was first introduced in 1981[98] to describe six patients with pruritic erythematous follicular papules (Figure 12), and urticarial lesions in addition in two cases. In one case the eruption was confined to the limbs and abdomen, but in all others it was widespread. Onset during pregnancy was variable with the majority between the 4th and 9th months of pregnancy, with resolution within 2–3 weeks of delivery. One patient experienced premenstrual recurrence of the rash, and two other patients gave a history of a similar eruption during a previous pregnancy. There were no other systemic features associated with this eruption, and both the maternal and the fetal prognosis were normal. Histopathological features of the papular lesions showed acute folliculitis in five of the six cases, with intrafollicular pustules comprising mixed inflammatory cells and some eosinophils. In some cases there was destruction of the follicular wall, and additional features included upper dermal edema and mild focal spongiosis. Direct immunofluorescence in four cases was negative, and bacteriological examination of the lesions with Gram staining revealed no significant organisms.

The incidence of this eruption is not known, but it is thought to be a hormonally induced acne[46]. The clinical appearances are of a papulopustular folliculitis similar to the monomorphic acne seen in patients taking corticosteroids or progestogenic steroids[66], but the appearances described suggest some clinical similarities to PDP. It classically occurs on acneiform sites, i.e. on the upper chest and upper back, but it is also frequently seen on the lower limbs. There are no specific immunopathological features, and the histopathology is that of an inflammatory folliculitis. Later, a single case report described a primigravid woman in her third trimester with pruritic folliculitis whose serum androgens were elevated[99]. However, the authors concluded that this may have been due to high levels of pregnancy-induced androgens or end-organ hypersensitivity to normal pregnancy levels of androgen. No subsequent studies have confirmed or refuted these findings.

REFERENCES

1. Siazinski L, Degefu S. Herpes gestationis associated with chorionocarcinoma. *Arch Dermatol* 1982;118: 425–8
2. Fitzpatrick TB, Eisen AZ, Wolff K, *et al. Dermatology in General Medicine.* New York: McGraw-Hill, 1979:1363–70
3. Sanchez NP, Pathak MA, Sato S, *et al.* Melasma: a clinical, light microscopic, ultrastructural and immunofluorescent study. *J Am Acad Dermatol* 1981;4:698–710
4. Chernosky ME, Knox JM. Atrophic striae after occlusive corticosteroid therapy. *Arch Dermatol* 1964;90:15
5. Zheng P, Lavker RM, Kligman AM. Anatomy of striae. *Br J Dermatol* 1985;112:185–93
6. Winton GB. Skin diseases aggravated by pregnancy. *J Am Acad Dermatol* 1989;20:1–13
7. Jenkins RE, Black MM. Effect of pregnancy on other skin disorders. In Black MM, McKay M, Braude P, eds. *Colour Atlas and Text of Obstetric and Gynaecologic Dermatology.* London: Mosby Wolfe, 1995:47–62
8. Kemmet D, Tidman MJ. The influence of the menstrual cycle and pregnancy on atopic dermatitis. *Br J Dermatol* 1991;125:59–61
9. Jurecka W, Gebhart W. Drug prescribing during pregnancy. *Semin Dermatol* 1989;8:30–9
10. Rayburn WF. Glucocorticoid therapy for rheumatic diseases: maternal, fetal and breast-feeding considerations. *Am J Reprod Immunol* 1992;28:138–40
11. Bartelsmeyer JA, Petrie RH. Erythema nodosum, estrogens and pregnancy. *Clin Obstet Gynecol* 1990;33:777–81
12. Urowitz MB, Gladman DD, Farewell VT, *et al.* Lupus and pregnancy studies. *Arthritis Rheum* 1993;10: 1392–7
13. Ruiz-Irastorza G, Lima F, Alves J, *et al.* Increased rate of lupus flare during pregnancy and the puerperium: a prospective study of 78 pregnancies. *Br J Rheumatol* 1996;35:133–8
14. Petri M. Systemic lupus erythematosus and pregnancy. *Rheum Dis Clin North Am* 1994;20:87–118
15. Formby B. Immunologic response in pregnancy. *Endocrinol Metab Clin North Am* 1995;24:187–205
16. Terpestra H, de Jong MCJM, Klokke AH. *In vivo* bound pemphigus antibodies in a stillborn infant. *Arch Dermatol* 1979;115:316–19
17. Yair D, Shenhav M, Botchan A, *et al.* Pregnancy associated with pemphigus. *Br J Obstet Gynaecol* 1995;102:667–9
18. Goldberg NS, DeFeo C, Kirshenbaum N. Pemphigus vulgaris and pregnancy: risk factors and recommendations. *J Am Acad Dermatol* 1993;28:877–9

19. Mackie RM, Bufalino R, Morabito A, *et al*. Lack of effect of pregnancy on outcome of melanoma. *Lancet* 1991;1:653–5

20. Driscoll MS, Grin-Jorgensen CM, Grant-Kels JM. Does pregnancy influence the prognosis of malignant melanoma? *J Am Acad Dermatol* 1993;29:619–30

21. Ferreira CMM, Maceira JMP, de Oliveira Coelho JMC. Melanoma and pregnancy with placental metastases. *Am J Dermatopathol* 1998;20:403–7

22. Reyes H, Simon FR. Intrahepatic cholestasis of pregnancy: an estrogen-related disease. *Semin Liver Dis* 1993;13:289–301

23. Girling JC, Dow E, Smith JH. Liver function tests in pre-eclampsia: importance of comparison with a reference range derived for normal pregnancy. *Br J Obstet Gynaecol* 1997;104:246–50

24. Holzbach RT, Sanders JH. Recurrent intrahepatic cholestasis of pregnancy – observations on pathogenesis. *JAMA* 1965;193:542–4

25. Fagan EA. Disorders of the liver, biliary system and pancreas. In: de Swiet M, ed. *Medical Disorders in Obstetric Practice*, 3rd edn. Oxford: Blackwell Science, 1995:332

26. Hirvioja ML, Kivinen S. Inheritance of intrahepatic cholestasis of pregnancy in one kindred. *Clin Genet* 1993;43:315–7

27. Davies MH, da Silva RCMA, Jones SR, *et al*. Fetal mortality associated with cholestasis of pregnancy and the potential benefit of ursodeoxycholic acid. *Gut* 1995;37:580–4

28. Reid R, Ivey KJ, Rencoret RH, Storey B. Fetal complications of obstetric cholestasis. *Br Med J* 1976;1:870–2

29. Fagan EA. Intrahepatic cholestasis of pregnancy. *Br Med J* 1994;309:1243–4

30. Nelson-Piercy C. Liver disease in pregnancy. *Curr Obstet Gynaecol* 1997;7:36–42

31. Floreani A, Paternoster D, Grella V, *et al*. Ursodeoxycholic acid in intrahepatic cholestasis of pregnancy. *Br J Obstet Gynaecol* 1994;101:64–5

32. Lotem M, Katzenelson V, Rotem A, *et al*. Impetigo herpetiformis: a variant of pustular psoriasis or a separate entity? *J Am Acad Dermatol* 1989;20:338–41

33. Kuijpers ALA, Schalkwijk J, Rulo HFC, *et al*. Extremely low levels of epidermal skin-derived antileucoproteinase/elafin in a patient with impetigo herpetiformis (IH). *Br J Dermatol* 1997;137:123–9

34. Oumeish OY, Farraj SE, Bataineh AS. Some aspects of impetigo herpetiformis. *Arch Dermatol* 1982;118:103–5

35. Holmes RC, Black MM. The specific dermatoses of pregnancy: a reappraisal with special emphasis on a proposed simplified clinical classification. *Clin Exp Dermatol* 1982;7:65–73

36. Spangler AS, Reddy W, Bardawil WA, *et al*. Papular dermatitis of pregnancy. *JAMA* 1962;181:577–81

37. Roger D, Vaillant L, Fignon A, *et al*. Specific pruritic diseases of pregnancy – a prospective study of 3192 pregnant women. *Arch Dermatol* 1994;130:734–9

38. Milton JL. *The Pathology and Treatment of Diseases of the Skin*. London: Robert Hardwick, 1872;205

39. Dupont C. Herpes gestationis with hydatidiform mole. *Trans St Johns Hosp Dermatol Soc* 1974;60:103

40. Tillman WG. Herpes gestationis with hydatidiform mole and chorion epithelioma. *Br Med J* 1950;1:1471

41. Sasseville D, Wilkinson RD, Schnader JY. Dermatoses of pregnancy. *Int J Dermatol* 1981;20:223–41

42. Shornick JK. Herpes gestationis. *J Am Acad Dermatol* 1987;17:539–56

43. Zurn A, Celebi CR, Bernard P, *et al*. A prospective immunofluorescence study of 111 cases of pruritic dermatoses of pregnancy: IgM anti-basement membrane zone antibodies as a novel finding. *Br J Dermatol* 1992;126:474–8

44. Black MM. New observations on pemphigoid gestationis. *Dermatology* 1994;189(suppl 1):50–1

45. Holmes RC, Black MM, Jurecka W, *et al*. Clues to the aetiology and pathogenesis of herpes gestationis. *Br J Dermatol* 1983;109:131–9

46. Holmes RC, Black MM. The specific dermatoses of pregnancy. *J Am Acad Dermatol* 1983;8:405–12

47. Shornick JK, Black MM. Fetal risks in herpes gestationis. *J Am Acad Dermatol* 1992;26:63–8

48. Stanley JR, Hawley-Nelson P, Yuspa SH, *et al*. Characterization of bullous pemphigoid antigen: a unique basement membrane protein of stratified squamous epithelia. *Cell* 1981;24:897–903

49. Labib RS, Anhalt GJ, Patel HP, *et al*. Molecular heterogeneity of the bullous pemphigoid antigens as detected by immunoblotting. *J Immunol* 1986;136:1231–5

50. Morrison LH, Labib RS, Zone JJ, *et al*. Herpes gestationis autoantibodies recognize a 180-kD human epidermal antigen. *J Clin Invest* 1988;81:2023–6

51. Kelly SE, Bhogal BS, Wojnarowska F, *et al*. Western blot analysis of the antigen in pemphigoid gestationis. *Br J Dermatol* 1990;122:445–9

52. Kelly SE, Cerio R, Bhogal BS, Black MM. The distribution of IgG subclasses in pemphigoid gestationis: PG factor is an IgG1 autoantibody. *J Invest Dermatol* 1989;92:695–8

53. Suzuki M, Harada S, Yaoita H. Purification of bullous pemphigoid IgG subclasses and their capability for complement fixation. *Acta Derm Venereol (Stockh)* 1992;72:245–9

54. Kaparti S, Stolz W, Meurer M, *et al*. Herpes gestationis: ultrastructural identification of the extracellular antigenic sites in diseased skin using immunogold techniques. *Br J Dermatol* 1991;125:317–24

55. Schaumberg-Lever G, Rule A, Schmidt-Ullrich B, Lever W. Ultrastructural localization of *in vivo*

bound immunoglobulins in bullous pemphigoid – a preliminary report. *J Invest Dermatol* 1975;64:47–9

56. Shornick JK, Stastny P, Gilliam JN. High frequency of histocompatability antigens HLA-DR3 and DR4 in herpes gestationis. *J Clin Invest* 1981; 68:553–5

57. Shornick JK, Artlett CM, Jenkins RE, *et al.* Complement polymorphism in herpes gestationis association with C4 null allele. *J Am Acad Dermatol* 1993;29:545–9

58. Shornick JK, Jenkins RE, Briggs DC, *et al.* Anti-HLA antibodies in pemphigoid gestationis. *Br J Dermatol* 1993;129:257–9

59. Jenkins RE, Vaughan Jones SA, Black MM. Conversion of pemphigoid gestationis to bullous pemphigoid – two refractory cases highlighting this association. *Br J Dermatol* 1996;135:595–8

60. Garvey MP, Handfield-Jones SE, Black MM. Pemphigoid gestationis response to chemical oophorectomy with goserelin. *Clin Exp Dermatol* 1992;17:443–5

61. Shornick JK, Black MM. Secondary autoimmune diseases in pemphigoid gestationis. *J Am Acad Dermatol* 1992;26:563–6

62. Vaughan Jones SA, Bhogal BS, Black MM, *et al.* A typical case of pemphigoid gestationis with a unique pattern of intercellular immunofluorescence. *Br J Dermatol* 1997;136:245–8

63. Lawley TJ, Hertz KC, Wade TR, *et al.* Pruritic urticarial papules and plaques of pregnancy. *JAMA* 1979;241:1696–9

64. Alcalay J, Wolf JE. Pruritic urticarial papules and plaques of pregnancy: the enigma and the confusion. *J Am Acad Dermatol* 1988;19:1115–16

65. Stoller HE. Pruritic urticarial papules and plaques of pregnancy. *JAMA* 1980;243:2156

66. Black MM, Stephens CJM. The specific dermatoses of pregnancy: the British perspective. *Adv Dermatol* 1991;7:105–26

67. Cohen LM, Capeless EL, Krusinski PA, *et al.* Pruritic urticarial papules and plaques of pregnancy and its relationship to maternal weight gain and twin pregnancy. *Arch Dermatol* 1989;125:1534–6

68. Bunker CB, Erskine K, Rustin MHA, *et al.* Severe polymorphic eruption of pregnancy occurring in twin pregnancies. *Clin Exp Dermatol* 1990;15:228–31

69. Vaughan Jones SA, Dunnill MGS, Black MM. Pruritic urticarial papules and plaques of pregnancy (polymorphic eruption of pregnancy): two unusual cases. *Br J Dermatol* 1996;135:102–5

70. Yancey K, Hall RP, Lawley TJ. Pruritic urticarial papules and plaques of pregnancy. *J Am Acad Dermatol* 1984;10:473–80

71. Greulich WW. The incidence of human multiple births. *Am Nature* 1930;64:142

72. Holmes RC, Black MM, Dann J, *et al.* A comparative study of toxic erythema of pregnancy and herpes gestationis. *Br J Dermatol* 1982;106:499–510

73. Alcalay J, Ingber A, David M, *et al.* Hormone evaluation and autoimmune background in pruritic urticarial papules and plaques of pregnancy. *Am J Obstet Gynecol* 1988;158:417–20

74. Black MM. Prurigo of pregnancy, papular dermatitis of pregnancy and pruritic folliculitis of pregnancy. *Semin Dermatol* 1989;8:23–5

75. Holmes RC, Jurecka W, Black MM. A comparative histopathological study of polymorphic eruption of pregnancy and herpes gestationis. *Clin Exp Dermatol* 1983;8:523–9

76. Borradori L, Didierjean L, Bernard P, *et al.* IgM autoantibodies to 180 and 230-kD human epidermal proteins in pregnancy. *Arch Dermatol* 1995; 131:43–7

77. Alcalay J, Ingber A, Hazaz B, *et al.* Linear IgM dermatosis of pregnancy. *J Am Acad Dermatol* 1988; 18:412–15

78. Carli P, Tarocchi S, Mello G, Fabbri P. Skin immune system activation in pruritic urticarial papules and plaques of pregnancy. *Int J Dermatol* 1994; 12:884–5

79. Tarocchi S, Carli P, Caproni M, Fabbri P. Polymorphic eruption of pregnancy. *Int J Dermatol* 1997;36:448–50

80. Beltrani VP, Beltrani VS. Pruritic urticarial papules and plaques of pregnancy: a severe case requiring early delivery for relief of symptoms. *J Am Acad Dermatol* 1992;26:266–7

81. Velthuis PJ, deJong MCJM, Kruis MH. Is there a linear IgM dermatosis? Significance of linear IgM junctional staining in cutaneous immunopathology. *Acta Dermatol Venereol (Stockh)* 1988;68:8–14

82. Besnier E, Brocq L, Jacquet L. *La Pratique Dermatologique*. Paris: Masson, 1904;1:75

83. Costello MJ. Eruptions of pregnancy. *N York St J Med* 1941;41:849–55

84. Nurse DS. Prurigo of pregnancy. *Australas J Dermatol* 1968;9:258–67

85. Bourne G. Toxaemic rash of pregnancy. *Proc R Soc Med* 1962;55:462–4

86. Cooper AJ, Fry JA. Prurigo of late pregnancy. *Australas J Dermatol* 1980;21:79–84

87. Faber WR, van Joost T, Hausman R, Weenik GH. Late prurigo of pregnancy. *Br J Dermatol* 1982; 106:511–16

88. Bierman SM. Autoimmune progesterone dermatitis of pregnancy. *Arch Dermatol* 1973;107:896–901

89. Kasdon SC. Abdominal pruritus in pregnancy. *Am J Obstet Gynecol* 1953;65:320–4

90. Rapaport HG, Appel SJ, Szanton VL. Incidence of allergy in a pediatric population. *Am J Allergy* 1960;18:45–9

91. Spangler AS, Emerson K. Estrogen levels and estrogen therapy in papular dermatitis of pregnancy. *Am J Obstet Gynecol* 1971;110:534–7

92. Ismail AAA. *Biochemical Investigations in Endocrinology*. London: Academic Press, 1981;126

93. Spangler AS, Emerson K. Diethylstilbestrol in the management of papular dermatitis of pregnancy. A reply to the editor. *Am J Obstet Gynecol* 1972; 113:571

94. Herbst AL, Ulfeder H, Poskanzer DC. Adenocarcinoma of the vagina: association of maternal stilbestrol therapy with tumor appearance in young women. *N Engl J Med* 1971;284:878–81

95. Rabhari H. Pruritic papules of pregnancy. *J Cut Pathol* 1978;5:347–52

96. Michaud RM, Jacobson D, Dahl MV. Papular dermatitis of pregnancy. *Arch Dermatol* 1982;118: 1003–5

97. Nguyen LQ, Sarmini OR. Papular dermatitis of pregnancy – a case report. *J Am Acad Dermatol* 1990;22:690–1

98. Zoberman E, Farmer ER. Pruritic folliculitis of pregnancy. *Arch Dermatol* 1981;117:20–2

99. Wilkinson SM, Buckler H, Wilkinson N, *et al.* Androgen levels in puritic folliculitis of pregnancy. *Clin Exp Dermatol* 1995;20:234–6

Drug use in pregnancy

Joseph A. Witkowski

34

The use of a medication in any patient requires acceptance of possible risks and benefits[1]. In the pregnant patient, pharmacotherapy requires consideration of an additional risk, the fetus who will also receive the drug. The benefit of the drug to the mother should outweigh the possible risks to the baby she is carrying.

Ideally a woman who is pregnant should not receive any drug. Once a decision is made to treat, however, it should be based on an accurate diagnosis with knowledge of the course of the disease. The stage of pregnancy at that time should be determined. The medication with the best benefit/risk ratio should be selected, and the therapy should contain as few active drugs as possible[2].

The therapeutic decision must be thoroughly discussed with the patient, her spouse or partner and the obstetrician with regard to benefit, risk and possible alternatives. Women who are pregnant and who have a chronic disease require additional counseling, as they may need intermittent or continuous therapy during pregnancy. They must be given information regarding the effect of the underlying disease on the pregnancy, its treatment during pregnancy and the effect of the pregnancy on the course of the pre-existing disease[2]. Informed consent must be obtained and the information documented.

MATERNAL PHYSIOLOGY

Fetal exposure to a drug depends on the rate of uptake by the mother, maternal excretion and metabolism. All of these processes are altered by the pregnant state and may require modification of the drug dose and its adminstration interval.

Absorption

Because of decreased acid production and increased mucus secretion[3], the absorption of weakly acidic and basic drugs may be decreased[4]. The rates of both gastric emptying and motility are decreased late in pregnancy[5]. The decreased motility of the small intestine may lead to increased absorption from this site in the gastrointestinal tract[4].

Elimination

Hepatic blood flow remains unchanged in pregnancy and first-pass metabolism of drugs by the portal circulation is not altered[6]. The activity of the hepatic microsomal enzyme system, however, is enhanced, thereby increasing the metabolism of certain drugs[7]. Cholestasis may occur during pregnancy, causing retention of drugs excreted in bile[8]. Renal blood flow and creatinine clearance increase in pregnancy, having the potential for increasing the clearance of drugs primarily excreted by the kidneys[9].

Distribution

During pregnancy there is a progressive expansion of both the intra- and the extravascular compartments. The maternal plasma volume increases by up to 50% late in pregnancy, causing a dilution of ingested drugs[4]. Drug binding capacity is decreased because of the decreased albumin concentration[10]. Protein binding is further reduced because of the high levels of steroid hormones in pregnancy[11]. This may result in higher levels of free drug when a drug is normally highly bound. The free fraction of drugs may require monitoring.

THE FETUS

The fertilized ovum and embryo receive a drug through the maternal circulation. Placental transport to the fetus of substances ingested by the mother begins about the 5th week of gestation[4]. Following placental transfer, 20–40% of umbilical blood bypasses the fetal liver by shunting directly to the inferior vena cava via the ductus venosus. This permits a significant portion of any drug direct access to the fetal heart and brain without hepatic modification[4].

Unbound drug or an active metabolite should cross the placenta easily unless it has a large molecular weight or a large spatial configuration[12]. While some drugs cross the placenta more easily than others, any drug, when given in large doses for a significant time, will cross the placenta and will have the potential for affecting fetal development[13].

Exposure to drugs occurs during three periods following conception:

(1) The preimplantation period from fertilization to implantation;

(2) The period of organogenesis, from the 2nd to the 8th week;

(3) The fetal period, from the beginning of the 9th week until term.

The effect of a teratogenic agent is related to a large extent to the period of development when the fetus is exposed[14]. During the preimplantation phase, exposure to a drug either kills the conceptus or produces no congenital malformation. The period of organogenesis is the most critical time with respect to malformations. The embryo is maximally susceptible to teratogenic effects on major organs. When more than one organ is developing simultaneously, the same agent can cause several malformations in the embryo[15]. Some drug effects on the fetus are limited to a narrow window of a few weeks of fetal development when a particular organ is differentiating[16]. Other drugs have less specific effects, exerted over a greater period of time.

Because of their mode of action, some drugs can cause adverse effects when taken after the 8th week. Organs that are still growing and developing can be affected. In this instance the malformations may be present at birth or become manifest some time later. Early manifestations include craniofacial abnormalities, intrauterine growth retardation, differentiation of the external genitalia, temporary hematological abnormalities and transient immunosuppression[17]. An example of a later-occurring abnormality is the staining and abnormalities of the diciduous teeth following tetracycline ingestion by the mother. Late manifestations include defective intellectual development and vaginal adenocarcinoma. The latter may appear as long as 20 years after *in utero* exposure to diethylstilbestrol[18]. Near term is another important time, when a drug given to the mother can adversely affect the neonate, which is less able than the adult to metabolize and excrete the drug[19].

TERATOGENS

A teratogen is defined as a drug, chemical, virus, physical agent or deficiency state that, by acting during the embryonic or fetal period, alters morphology or subsequent function in the postnatal period[13]. A pregnant woman has a 2–3% chance of giving birth to an infant with a major malformation[13]. This baseline risk of malformations without

discernible cause exists for every woman who becomes pregnant. Three to five per cent of these anomalies are the result of a known teratogen[13]. While most anomalies cannot be definitely linked to a known teratogen, there are some suggestive findings. A teratogenic effect is suspected when the range in the general population is exceeded[20]. Malformations occurring in aborted fetuses, stillborn and live infants of mothers who took the drug during pregnancy suggest a causal relationship[15]. A consistent pattern of malformations from similar drugs is also suggestive[21].

DRUG SELECTION

The choice of a medication for a pregnant woman should be based on the human data available; how long the drug has been in clinical use; and animal studies[22]. Human data are usually sparse, as information depends on voluntary reporting from occasional case reports of unintentional or accidental drug exposures. Since over 50% of all pregnancies are unplanned, documentation of pregnancy outcomes after exposure to drugs is a complex problem, because women may have been taking over-the-counter or prescribed medication before they knew they were pregnant[20]. Only reported pregnancies are available for review. Since the number of unreported medication-related adverse events and the number of pregnancies without adverse effects is not known, this source of information does not permit valid conclusions to be drawn regarding safety. While a double-blind placebo controlled study would provide the most information, it would be difficult to justify on ethical grounds[23]. Prospectively monitored cohort studies[24] and prospective controlled observational studies[20] have been performed to obtain information about the reproductive safety of drugs. In all these studies the sample size should be adequate, otherwise the statistical power will be limited[23].

The length of time a drug has been in clinical use can also provide useful information[1]. The longer the time interval the more likely it is that teratogenicity would surface. The safety profile of a new drug is generally not known for at least 2–3 years after its introduction[25].

Negative animal studies are considered reassuring[22]. However, they are not infallible. Interspecies variations may lead to false assumptions of human safety. This is best illustrated by the experience with thalidomide, where phocomelia was initially not demonstrated in rats. Malformations occurring in positive studies in animals should be regarded as

Table 1   Food and Drug Administration pregnancy categories

Pregnancy category	Definition
A	Adequate studies in pregnant women have not demonstrated a risk to the fetus in the first trimester of pregnancy and there is no evidence of risk in later trimesters.
B	Animal studies have not demonstrated a risk to the fetus, but there are no adequate studies in pregnant women. OR Animal studies have shown an adverse effect, but adequate studies in pregnant women have not demonstrated a risk to the fetus during the first trimester of pregnancy, and there is no evidence of risk in later trimesters.
C	Animal studies have shown an adverse effect on the fetus, but there are no adequate studies in humans; the benefit of the drug in pregnant women may be acceptable despite its potential risks. OR There are no animal reproduction studies and no adequate studies in humans.
D	There is evidence of human fetal risk, but the potential benefits from the use of the drug in pregnant women may be acceptable despite its potential risks.
X	Studies in animals or humans demonstrate fetal abnormalities, or adverse reaction reports indicate evidence of fetal risk. The risk of use in a pregnant woman clearly outweights any possible benefit.

evidence of potential risk[26]. Of interest is the observation that more than 600 drugs cause congenital abnormalities in animals, while fewer than 25 of these drugs are known teratogens in humans[13].

SOURCES OF INFORMATION

Because of a lack of published studies on reproductive safety in humans, manufacturers of drugs have not labelled their products as safe for use in pregnancy[27]. It is thought that, in some instances, such studies have been commissioned by the manufacturers but not published. This probably represents the defensive stance of the companies engendered by our legal system and litiginous society. Until 1993 women of childbearing potential were excluded from participating in investigational drug trials[28]. Including this segment of the population will permit discovery of medication efficacy and untoward effects resulting from female steroid hormones. Women have other unique biological features that may influence their response to drugs. An example of this was recently brought to light by a study on the cardiac effect of erythromycin[29]. Women have a longer QTc interval than men of the same age that may predispose them to torsades de pointes cardiac arrythmia. Pregnant and lactating women are still excluded from premarket testing of drugs, even those that might be used during gestation for obvious reasons.

In order to aid the clinician in drug prescribing decisions, the Food and Drug Administration mandated a risk classification for drugs introduced after 1980[30]. The categories (Table 1) are based on the available information concerning risk to the human fetus, animal studies and the drug's potential benefit to the mother. A drug that is not absorbed systemically and not known to have a potential for indirect harm to the fetus is not labelled. There are very few medications with a category A rating. Categories B and C include most medications that are assumed to be relatively safe, although not without possible risk[31]. Categories D and X include drugs that are teratogenic. Drugs for which there is no safer alternative are given a D rating, while those for which there is no justification for their use during pregnancy have an X rating. The categories may be found on the drug package insert, *The Physician's Desk Reference* and Mosby's *Gen Rx*, a complete reference for generic and brand drugs.

Regardless of the designated pregnancy category or presumed safety, no drug should be adminstered during pregnancy unless it is clearly needed and potential benefits outweigh potential risks.

Sources of information and the effects of particular drugs on pregnancy are listed in Appendix 1.

CONCLUSIONS

The pregnant woman should take as few medications as possible. Medical necessity should be the sole determining factor upon which the decision to treat is made. Selection of a drug should be determined by the known safety data. There are very few drugs with a listing of category A. It is essential that the patient, spouse or partner and obstetrician be a part of this decision-making process.

APPENDIX 1
Sources of information on the effect of drugs on pregnancy

Computer on-line service

Subscribing to Microdex Computerized Clinical Information Systems.

Teratogen information services

National Collaborative Perinatal Project, Washingtons DC; The Boston Collaborative Program, Boston MA; The Motherisk Program, The Hospital for Sick Children, Toronto, Ontario, Canada; The Pregnancy Healthline, Philadelphia PA; Reproductive Toxicology Service (REPROTOX), Columbia Hospital for Women, Washington DC; Teratogen Information Service (TERIS), University of Washington, Seattle WA; United States Pharmacopeial Dispensing Information.

Books

Drugs in Pregnancy and Lactation, Briggs *et al.*; *Catalogue of Teratogenic Agents*, Sheppard; *Physician's Desk Reference*.

Literature

Case reports on adverse effects of medications in pregnancy.

Untoward reactions to drugs can be reported to the Food and Drug Administration (FDA) Drug Bulletin and Dermatology Hotline.

Dermatological medications

The drugs listed have been rated on the basis of FDA categories, information from the Motherisk Program and the literature. Drugs introduced before 1982 do not have an FDA rating.

Acne medications

(1) Antibacterials – see Antibacterials;
(2) Benzoyl peroxide – category C.
    On the basis of available data the drug is safe for use in pregnancy[2];
(3) Resorcin – category unknown.
    Use should be limited to the late second and third trimesters[32];
(4) Salicylic acid – see Antivirals;
(5) Tretinoin – see Vitamins.

Analgesics

Acetaminophen – category B
    No adverse effects with short-term use[33]
Aspirin – category C
    Near term chronic high dose may cause prolonged gestation and fetal neonatal hemorrhage[33]
Codeine – category C
    No evidence of teratogenicity[34]
Ibuprofen – category B
    Late in pregnancy may close ductus arteriosus and prolong labor[35]
Indomethacin
    Not recommended during pregnancy because of cardiac, pulmonary and renal effects[36]
Ketoprofen – category B
    Same as ibuprofen
Naprosyn – category B
    Same as ibuprofen
Propoxyphene – no pregnancy category
    No clear link with teratogenicity[34]; may cause neonatal withdrawal symptoms[37]

Anesthetics

Lidocaine – category B
    No teratogenic risk when used for local anesthesia[34]
Lidocaine with epinephrine – category B
    Same as lidocaine

Antibacterials

Aminoglycosides
    Amikacin, gentamycin, kanamycin, neomycin, spectinomycin, streptomycin and tobramycin may cause nephrotoxicity, ototoxicity and neuromuscular paralysis.
    Kanamycin, streptomycin and tobramycin – category D
        Neonatal damage to eighth cranial nerve[38]
    Amikacin, gentamycin, neomycin and spectinomycin – category C
        Parenteral spectinomycin is safe for use in pregnancy[32]
        Topical use of gentamycin and neomycin is safe for use in pregnancy[32]
    Bacitracin topical – category C
        Topical use in pregnancy is safe[32]
β-lactam antibiotics
    Include the penicillins, semisynthetic penicillins, cephalosporins, carbapenems and monobactams – most are category B
        Semisynthetic penicillins are safe for use in pregnancy[32]
        Cephalosporins – category B
            Oral use in pregnancy is safe[32]

Clindamycin topical – category B
  Topical use in pregnancy is safe[32]
Co-trimoxazole – category C
  Potential cause of jaundice and kernicterus in fetus[38]
  Safe for use in pregnancy[32]
Fluoroquinolones
  Ciprofloxacin – category C
    Causes arthropathy in immature animals[39]
Macrolides
  Erythromycin – category B
    Topical use in pregnancy is safe[32]
    Erythromycin estolate may cause cholestatic hepatitis in pregnant women[40]
  Clarithromycin – category C
Azalide
  Azithromycin – category B
Metronidazole
  Oral – category B
    Contraindicated during the first trimester of pregnancy[41]
  Topical – category B
Rifampin – category C
  Induces cytochrome P450 enzymes, causing interferences and enhancement of the metabolism of other drugs that are metabolized in the same fashion[41]
Tetracyclines – category D
  Causes staining of the diciduous teeth if given after the 3rd month of pregnancy[42]
  Demeclocycline causes similar staining, while minocyline should cause the least discoloration[15]

Antifungals

Systemic
  Amphotericin B – IV category B, oral category C
    No adverse fetal effects when given to pregnant women[38]
  Clotrimazole – oral category C; vaginal category B; topical category B
    Topical safe for use in pregnancy[32]
  Fluconazole – category C
  Flucytosine – category C
    Not recommended for use in pregnant women[32]
  Griseofulvin – no category
    Use contraindicated in pregnancy[32]
  Itraconazole – category C
  Ketoconazole – oral category C; topical category C
    Not recommended for use in pregnancy[43]
  Miconazole – vaginal no category. Not recommended in first trimester

  Topical – no category. Safe for use in pregnancy[32]
  Nystatin – vaginal category C; topical no category
  Potassium iodide – category D
    Administration should be limited to the period before fetal thyroid development[32]
  Terbinafine – oral category B; topical category B
Topical
  Ciclopirox – category B
  Haloprogin – category B
  Naftifine – category B
  Oxiconazole – category B
  Econazole – category C
  Terbinafine – category B

Antihistamines

Astemizole – category C
  Use is safe during pregnancy[44]
Cetirizine – category B
  No increased risk for major malformations when used during organogenesis[45]
Cimetidine – category B
Cyproheptadine – category B
  No problems in animal studies[46]
Diphenhydramine – category B
  No evidence that exposure during pregnancy will elevate baseline risk for malformations[32]
Fexofenadine – category C
Hydroxyzine – category C
  Not associated with increased teratogenic risk[45]
Loratadine – category B
Terfenadine – category C
  Exposure during period of organogenesis should be avoided[47]

Antimalarials

Chloroquin and hydroxychloroquin
  Treatment of malaria – category unknown
    Risk of birth defects is unlikely to be increased above baseline[32]
  Treatment of collagen vascular disease – category unknown
    Use not recommended[32]

Antiparasitics

Systemic
  Ivermectin – category unknown
  Co-trimoxazole – category C
    May cause jaundice and kernicterus in fetus[41]
Topical
  Crotamiton – category C
    No unwanted systemic side-effects have been reported[2]

Lindane – category B
No evidence that it will elevate baseline risk for malformations[32]
Permethrin – category B
Pyrethrum with piperonyl butoxide – category unknown

Antiviral

Systemic
Acyclovir – category C
Exposure to oral and topical acyclovir will not affect the fetus[32]
Famciclovir – category B
Valacyclovir – category B
Zidovudine – category C
No adverse effects in children followed for 5.6 years after exposure[48]
Didanosine – category B
Zalcitabine – category C
Lamivudine – category C
Stavudine – category C
Nevirapine – category C
Delaviradine – category unknown
Saquinavir – category B
Ritonavir – category B
Indinavir – category C
Nelfinavir – category unknown
Topical
Cantharidin – category unknown
Will not elevate baseline risk for malformations[32]
Podophyllin – category C
Not recommended for use in pregnancy[32]
Salicylic acid – category unknown
Will not elevate baseline risk for malformations in early pregnancy, avoid in late pregnancy[32]
Imiquimod – category B

Chemotherapeutics

Azathioprine – category D
Bleomycin – category D
Carmustine – category D
Cyclophosphamide – category D
Cyclosporin – category C
Fluorouracil
Topical – category X
Parenteral – category D
Mechlorethamine – category D
Vinblastine – category D

Hormones

Adrenocorticosteroids
Systemic

Prednisone, prednisolone – category C
Neither drug has the potential to raise the risk for birth defects[32]. High doses may be associated with intrauterine growth restriction and adrenal suppression[49]
Topical
Betamethasone valerate and dexamethasone – category C
Not associated with congenital defects in humans[38]
No risk to developing fetus during any stage of pregnancy[32]
Betamethasone dipropionate – category C
Clobetasol propionate – category C
Diflorasone diacetate – category C
Fluocinonide – category C
Halobetasol propionate – category C
Triamcinolone acetonide – category C
Androgens
Danazol – category D
Spironolactone – category C
No known teratogenic effects[46]
Estrogens
Ethinyl estradiol – category X
Mestranol – category X
Progestogens
Norethindrone – category D
Norgestrel – category D
Norethynodrel – category D

Vitamins

Beta carotene – category C
Nicotinamide – category C
No fetal abnormalities reported[38,46]
Puridoxine – category A
Vitamin A and derivatives
Acitretin – category X
Not recommended during pregnancy
Etretinate – category X
Data on teratogenicity are inconclusive[32]
Isotretinoin – category X
Retinol – category X
Chronic ingestion of 20 000 IU per day should be discontinued[32]
Tretinoin – topical category C
Short-term use over a small area is safe during pregnancy[32]

Miscellaneous medications

Topical – anthralin – category C
Not recommended for use in pregnancy[32]
Systemic – cholestyramine – category C

Adverse effect could theoretically occur, owing to impaired absorption of fat-soluble vitamins[46]

Topical – coal tar – category C
  Use should be limited to the second and third trimesters[32]

Topical – hexachlorophene – category C
  Should not be used during pregnancy[32]

Topical – povidone iodine – no pregnancy category
  Use during pregnancy should be avoided[32]

Systemic – psoralens – category C

Topical – silver sulfadiazine – category B
  Application to large areas near term may cause jaundice, hemolytic anemia and kernicterus[50]

REFERENCES

1. Schatz M, Pettito D. Antihistamines and pregnancy. *Ann Allergy Asthma Immunol* 1977;78:157–9

2. Jurecka W, Gebhart W. Drug prescribing during pregnancy. *Semin Dermatol* 1989;8:30–9

3. Gryboski WA, Spiro HM. The effect of pregnancy on gastric secretion. *N Engl J Med* 1958;255:1131–7

4. Montella KR. Pulmonary pharmacology in pregnancy. *Clin Chest Med* 1992;13:587–95

5. Davison JM, Davis MC, Hay DM. Gastric emptying time in late pregnancy and labour. *J Obstet Gynaecol Br Commonw* 1970;77:37–41

6. Dvorchik BH. Drug disposition during pregnancy. *Biol Res Preg* 1982;3:129

7. Krauer B, Krauer F. Drug kinetics in pregnancy. *Clin Pharmacokinetics* 1977;2:167

8. Brooks PM, Needs CJ. Antirheumatic drugs in pregnancy. *Baillier's Clin Rheumatol* 1990;4:157–71

9. Krauer B, Krauer F. Drug kinetics in pregnancy. In Gilbaldi M, Prescott L, eds. *Handbook of Clinical Pharmacokinetics.* Sydney: Adis Press, 1983:1–17

10. Wood M, Wood ATJ. Changes in plasma drug binding and a1-acid glycoprotein in mother and newborn infant. *Clin Pharmacol Ther* 1981;29:522

11. Battino D, Granata T, Binelli S, *et al.* Intrauterine growth in the offspring of epileptic mothers. *Acta Neurol Scand* 1992;86:555–7

12. Rayburn WF. Connective tissue disorders and pregnancy: recommendations for prescribing. *J Reprod Med* 1998;43:341–9

13. Shepard TH. Teratogenicity of therapeutic agents. *Curr Probl Pediatr* 1979;10:1–43

14. Council on Scientific Affairs. Effect of toxic chemicals on the reproductive system. *JAMA* 1985;253:3431–7

15. Stockton DL, Paller AS. Drug administration to the pregnant or lactating woman: a reference guide for dermatologists. *J Am Acad Dermatol* 1990;23:87–103

16. Smith DW. Dysmorphology (teratology). *Med Prog* 1966;66:1150–69

17. Livesey G, Rayburn W. Principles of perinatal pharmacology. In Rayburn WF, Zuspan FP, eds. *Drug Therapy in Obstetrics and Gynecology*, 3rd edn. St Louis: Mosby-Year Book, 1992:5–7

18. Horbst AL, Ulfelder H, Poskanzer DC. Adenocarcinoma of the vagina; association of maternal stilbestrol therapy with tumor appearance in young women. *N Engl J Med* 1971;284:878–80

19. Mirkin BL, Singh S. Placental transfer of pharmacologically active molecules. In Mirkin BL, ed. *Perinatal Pharmacology and Therapeutics.* New York: Academic Press, 1976:1–69

20. Pastuszak A, Schick B, D'Alimente D, *et al.* The safety of astemizole in pregnancy. *J Allergy Clin Immunol* 1996;98:748–50

21. Lione A, Scialli AR. The developmental toxicity of the Hl histamine antagonists. *Reprod Toxicol* 1996;10:247–55

22. National Asthma Educational Program Report of the Working Group on Asthma and Pregnancy. *Management of Asthma during Pregnancy.* NIH Publication Number 93-3279. Bethesda, MD: National Institutes of Health, 1993

23. Kelso JM, Schatz M. Astemazole use in pregnancy. *J Allergy Clin Immunol* 1998;99:144

24. Schatz M, Zeiger RS, Harden K, *et al.* The safety of asthma and allergy medications during pregnancy. *J Allergy Clin Immunol* 1997;100:301–6

25. Hararmburu F, Lindoulsi T, Bavoux F, *et al.* Strategy of treatment of pruritus during pregnancy: the Drugs and Pregnancy Study Group. *Ann Pharmacother* 1994;28:17–20

26. Stern L. *In vivo* assessment of the teratogenic potential of drugs in humans. *Obstet Gynecol* 1981;58(suppl):3–8

27. Krogh C, ed. *Compendium of Pharmaceuticals and Specialties*, 29th edn. Ottawa: The Canadian Pharmaceutical Association, 1994;556

28. Morrell MJ. The new antiepileptic drugs and women: efficacy, reproductive health, pregnancy and fetal outcome. *Epilepsia* 1996;37(suppl 6):S34–44

29. Drici MD, Knollmann BC, Wang WX, *et al.* Cardiac actions of erythromycin: influence of female sex. *JAMA* 1998;280:1774–6

30. Code of Federal Regulations. Title 21, vol 4, Parts 200–99. US Government Printing Office via GPO access, April 1998. CITE 21 CFR 201, 57:19–20

31. Hornby PJ, Abraham TP. Pulmonary pharmacology. *Clin Obstet Gynecol* 1996;39:17–35

32. Bologa M, Pastuszak A, Shear NH, *et al.* Dermatologic drugs in pregnancy. *Clin Dermatol* 1992;9:435–51

33. Rudolph AM. Effects of aspirin and acetaminophen in pregnancy and in the newborn. *Arch Intern Med* 1981;141:358–63

34. Heinomen JP, Sloane D, Shapiro S. *Birth Defects in Pregnancy.* Littleton, MA: Publishing Science Group, 1977:286–95

35. Levin DL. Effects of inhibition of prostaglandin synthesis on fetal development, oxygenation and the fetal circulation. *Semin Perinatol* 1980;4:35–44

36. Sifton DW, ed. *Physicians Desk Reference*. Montvale NJ: Medical Economics Company, 1997:1723–7

37. Tyson HK. Neonatal withdrawal symptoms associated with maternal use of propoxyphone hydrochloride (Darvon). *J Pediatr* 1974;85:684–5

38. Briggs GG, Freeman RK, Yaffe SJ, eds. *Drugs in Pregnancy and Lactation*, 3rd edn. Baltimore: Williams and Wilkins, 1990

39. Maggiolo F, Caprioli S, Suter F. Risk/benefit analysis of quinolone use in children. The effect on diarthodial joints. *J Antimicrob Chemother* 1990;26:469–71

40. McCormack WM, George M, Danner A, *et al.* Hepatotoxicity of erythromycin estolate during pregnancy. *Antimicrob Agents Chemother* 1977;12:640–5

41. Stiefeld SM. Toxicities of antimicrobial agents used to treat osteomyelitis. *Orthop Clin North Am* 1991;22:439–65

42. Cohlan DS. Tetracycline staining of teeth. *Teratology* 1977;15:127–30

43. McGregor JA, Pont A. Contraindications of ketoconazole in pregnancy. *Am J Obstet Gynecol* 1984;150:793–4

44. Mazzotta P, Koren G. Nonsedating antihistamines in pregnancy: considering astemazole. *Can Fam Med* 1997;43:1509–11

45. Einarson A, Bailey B, Jung G, *et al.* Prospective controlled study of hydroxyzine and cetirizine in pregnancy. *Ann Allergy Asthma Immunol* 1997;78:183–6

46. *United States Pharmacopeia Dispensing Information*, 9th edn. Rockville, MD: The United States Pharmacopeial Convention, 1989

47. Schatz M, Pettiti D. Antihistamines and pregnancy. *Ann Allergy Asthma Immunol* 1997;78:157–9

48. Culnane M, Fowler M, Lee SS, *et al.* Lack of long-term effects of *in utero* exposure to zidovudine among uninfected children born to HIV infected women. *JAMA* 1999;281:151–7

49. Corticosteroids/corticotropin–glucocorticoid effects, systemic. In *United States Pharmacopeial Dispensing Information: Drug Information for the Health Care Professional*. Taunton MA: Rand McNally, 1995:878–906

50. Lucey JF, Driscoll TJ Jr. Hazard to newborn infants of administration of long-acting sulfonamides to pregnant women. *Pediatrics* 1959;24:498–9

Cultural attributes

African-American women   **35**

Amy J. McMichael

INTRODUCTION

Cultural attributes can help to define ethnic groups and can become shared traits that allow members of an ethnic group to converse and live together using a cultural shorthand. There is no ethnic group that can be stereotyped in the practice of cultural attributes, but enumerating some medical attributes can help to improve communication between healthcare providers and patients. In considering dermatological cultural attributes, one can discuss the attributes of the skin, hair and nails separately. In the case of African-American girls and women, there are several dermatological cultural attributes that can be examined. In this chapter, the attributes of skin, hair and nails are discussed for this group, as well as the role that they play in health and disease.

HAIR

With any characteristic such as hair, there is an unaltered state and, in many cases, a treated state. The unaltered clinical appearance of the hair shaft in African-Americans tends to be coarse and curly, or even frizzy. This appearance stems from the histological orientation of the hair in African-Americans which can be elliptical or flattened in cross-section and spiral or tightly curled in its tertiary structure. Variations may be seen in any race and African-Americans are no exception. In many members of this ethnic group, the follicle where the hair is formed is just as curved as the hair itself[1].

In women, there is a societal assumption that hair will be present covering the entire scalp. The popular media have superimposed the assumption of full, long, luxurious hair as the societal expectation. In African-American women, hair is of major importance. The amount spent on hair products by African-Americans is estimated at billions of dollars[2]. Secondary to personal style and acceptable societal style in the USA, there is pressure to have shiny, bouncy hair. The unaltered state of the hair in African-American women does not conform to many of the bouncing and shiny criteria. This sets up a contradiction in how to treat the hair to conform to societal norms while still maintaining personal and cultural preferences[3]. Often the only way to satisfy or bridge the gap between norm and cultural preference is significant chemical and heat use along with topical product use.

Heat and chemicals are common modalities utilized by African-American girls and women to straighten the hair. Heat was at one time the preferred modality of hair straightening with the use of a straightening comb heated to high temperatures and then passed through wavy or coarse hair (also referred to as pressing the hair). The final effect is a temporary straightening that lasts until the hair is washed. Hair pressing allows for more versatility in styling for those with coarse, wavy or curly hair that is often set as a general societal norm. Straightening the hair using this method is time consuming, as the hair must be divided into small sections and then combed thoroughly with the hot comb to assure an even straightening. In part, as a result of the time spent on the pressing process, other practical cultural attributes evolved such as washing the hair only once weekly or even every 2 weeks in order to preserve the hair in the straightened form for as long as possible. Patients may be alienated by physicians who do not understand that frequency of hair washing differs in different ethnic groups. Patients should not be told that they must wash their hair daily or even every other day. Although this may be the norm in some ethnic groups, it is usually not the case for African-American women. Often, washing the hair too frequently can cause dryness of the hair shaft in this group of patients that may already have dry hair secondary to chemical or heat manipulation.

With the advent of the chemical relaxer, African-American women had yet another means by which to straighten the hair[4]. These chemical relaxers quickly gained popularity over pressing with a hot comb, primarily because the re-formation of the hair bonds achieved by relaxers is permanent and allows for less time for care and treatment of the hair as compared to the pressing modality. In this form of straightening, chemicals are used to break

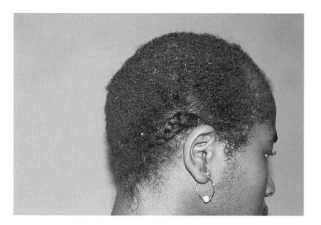

Figure 1 Young woman with severely damaged and broken scalp hair several days after use of a chemical relaxer

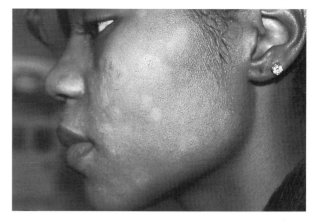

Figure 4 Dramatic hypopigmentation of the face in a young woman with sebopsoriasis

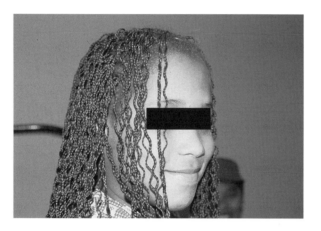

Figure 2 Braids with hair extensions in a teenager

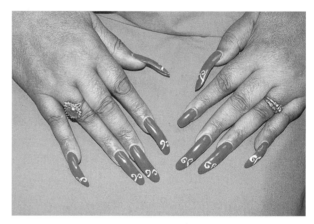

Figure 5 Long acrylic nails with intricate designs on the distal-most portion of the nail

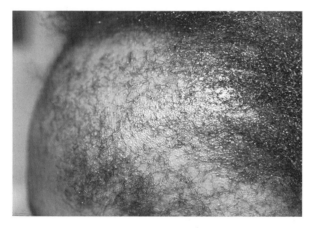

Figure 3 Traction alopecia in a middle-aged woman with a many-year history of loss of hair at the frontal hair line

and then reset the bonds of the hairs in a straighter configuration. The chemical is applied to hair in the native, unaltered state and must be repeated every 6–8 weeks to new growth of hair at the base of the scalp to maintain the straightened look. This has allowed African-American women more flexibility in washing, styling and time spent on the

hair, by freeing up the time that would normally be spent on pressing the hair.

The age at which chemical relaxers are first used by African-American women varies. There are a variety of chemical products that can relax the hair, offering something for every patron, including: children's chemical relaxers, relaxers with moisturizers, relaxers that are mild enough for home use and varying strengths from mild to strong[5]. Most often, chemical relaxers are not used in the hair until the child is old enough to sit still for application of this potentially irritating chemical.

There are many women of color who have become less enthusiastic about chemical and heat treatment of the hair, because of the damage that can occur, the time involved in performing these processes and the fluctuation in societal norms (Figure 1). In these women and girls, the hair is worn in a manner in which the natural curl of the hair is utilized in a style that is less straight. During certain periods of history, such as the late 1960s, the 1970s and in more current times, there has been less of a unifying idea of beauty; the natural curl of the hair is often displayed as a sign of personal style.

The natural curl of the hair in many African-American women and girls allows for unique and attractive styles that those with straight hair cannot achieve. There are short and long styles that may be worn with the hair in the natural state. Personal preference dictates the style and allows for considerable individualism, since there are so many variations on the native curl pattern in the hair of African-American women and girls. Often the natural styles will be achieved with the use of styling gels or mousse that can help to coat the hair and maintain the style without worry that the humidity or any mild water exposure might cause frizzing of the hair.

The use of greases and other emollient products in the hair is often observed in African-American girls and women. These products can serve a number of purposes and are often part of the daily personal care regimen. First, these products can control and lubricate the hair shafts. The hair can be combed and styled more easily with an increase in tensile strength, a function that the emollients may lend temporarily. Second, a lubricant of some kind must be used in the hot-comb straightening method to minimize overheating of the hair shafts and facilitate smooth combing through coarse or wavy sections of hair. Last, the weekly or less than weekly hair washing practice can make some dermatological scalp conditions more noticeable, such as seborrheic dermatitis or psoriasis of the scalp. Lubricants can be applied to the scalp to control flaking temporarily without treating the underlying problem and, in some cases, worsening the skin condition.

Girls and women often develop personal care regimens that save time and meet the style of the times. One of the time-saving methods is braiding of the hair. In young African-American girls, braiding of the hair is one of the almost universal attributes. Whether hair is long or short, wavy or straight, young African-American girls from the approximate age of 1 year to the prepubertal years typically wear braids of some kind. Braids may vary from a single braid to more than 50 ornate braids, some of which may be connected or corn-rowed along the scalp (Figure 2). The braided styles allow for ease of control without heat or chemical relaxation, and can often stay in place for longer than 24 h in the case of small, neat rows of braids.

Among adult African-American women, braided styles are an option to control the hair in a more natural style than a straightened look. It can be a method used to avoid the use of chemicals but still restrain very thick or coarse hair. The braids are often interwoven with hair pieces that allow for dramatic styling options. A variation on braids is the style of 'locking' the hair, in which the hair is twisted until the natural curl of the newly grown hair follows the locked hair twist and pattern. These locked styles are more recent attributes of African-American women than the straight and natural short styles, although these styles are historically a part of African and West Indian hair styling.

While the braiding technique of hair treatment is a long-practiced one, some problems may arise. Traction on the hair in an attempt to make braiding neat may cause significant traction-related alopecia, usually at the hairline but often at the bitemporal–preauricular site[6–8] (Figure 3). If traction is removed early in life, there are few sequelae of this practice. If the traction continues into the adult years, there can be permanent damage in the affected areas. It is important to note that not all braids cause traction and that a loosely braided style may give the wearer respite from other damaging hair-care practices, thereby encouraging a healthier scalp and healthier hair.

SKIN

Deeply pigmented skin commonly shows dryness with a very noticeable, whitish scaling. This inherited attribute of the deeply pigmented skin, along with tradition, leads many African-American girls and women to use emollients liberally on the skin. Daily emollients after showering or bathing are commonly used. Lotions and thicker emollients, such as petroleum jelly and/or products containing cocoa butter, are used to keep skin lubricated and to make it appear less scaly. Often, in childhood, these lubricants are used on the face. When these products are used on the adult face, they may exacerbate acne or mask seborrheic dermatitis[9]. It is important to understand what a patient may use in deciding treatment, since a patient with oily-appearing skin may not need drying agents to improve complexion, but may need only to minimize the use of emollients to the skin.

Skin color is determined by both genetic and environmental factors, such as exposure to sunlight, trauma, and/or chemical exposures. When the skin is deeply pigmented, even a slight color change can be easily noticed. Postinflammatory dyschromia is a common problem among African-Americans and, when this problem occurs on exposed areas in women, there is a tendency to use over-the-counter products to attempt to return the skin to its original color. Bleaching creams, α-hydroxyacids and other emollients with or without proven treatment value are often used to fade the dark spots that occur from acne, trauma, atopic dermatitis and other inflammatory conditions. Other deeper processes may cause hypopigmentation (Figure 4). Even treatments believed to be routine in those with light skin must be considered for the possibility of causing post-traumatic dyschromia in deeply pigmented patients. It is not uncommon for women to try many over-the-counter treatments prior to seeking the advice of a physician, and African-American women are no exception. Often, these products will cause further irritation or mask the original hyper- or hypopigmentation.

Once the patient does consult the dermatologist for treatment, a full questioning of product use is necessary. There has been some concern regarding misuse of potent hydroquinone-containing topical agents and the development of hydroquinone-caused pseudo-ochronosis[10]. Many products claim to 'fade blemishes' but may not actually contain chemicals that can lighten pigmentation. Patients may use these products with a false sense of security that there is an active ingredient at work in the product. In reality, few of these products contain chemical bleaching agents and patients should be apprised of this possibility. In many cases, women realize that time will fade postinflammatory hyper-pigmentation and do not seek medical help.

NAILS

The practice of wearing acrylic nails over the original nail has been in vogue for the past 10 years. This is a widespread phenomenon that crosses cultural barriers and affects African-American girls and women as well. Although no comparison studies have been carried out, African-Americans may be a large part of the consumer group for this practice. Certainly, many African-American girls and women wear intricate styles and designs on acrylic nails. These nail designs can range from conservative manicured styles to dramatic and colorful ones (Figure 5). A possible effect of wearing acrylic nails is the damage that can be done to the original nail, which can result in bacterial or fungal infection of the nail. Irritant or allergic contact dermatitis

can ensue on the nail fold and periungual skin from chemical exposure from the acrylics used[11]. For the number of consumers wearing these nails, there appear to be few who develop severe side-effects.

CONCLUSIONS

Stereotyping of cultural attributes must be avoided. Still, there is some value to examining attributes that may lead to better skin care by physicians. Understanding at least some of the practices that fit into the life style of the patient can improve compliance and outcome. Physicians must allow patients to participate in their care, especially if treatment is to be used for any long duration. The time that it takes to learn what may be helpful or detrimental in a patient's personal care regimen may save the dermatologist and the patient several unnecessary visits. African-American girls and women are a diverse and varied group and each patient encounter will show this diversity. A general understanding of cultural attributes in this population will improve treatment regimens and patient–doctor rapport.

REFERENCES

1. Lindelof B, Forslind B, Hedblad M, Kaveus U. Human hair form. *Arch Dermatol* 1988;124:1359–63
2. Khalil EN. Cosmetic and hair treatments for the black consumer. *Cosmet Toil* 1986;101:51–8
3. Draelos ZD. Black individuals require special products for hair care. *Cosmet Dermatol* 1993;6:19–20
4. Harris RT. Hair relaxing. *Cosmet Toil* 1979;94:51–6
5. Brooks GB, Lewis A. Treatment regimens for 'styled' black hair. *Cosmet Toil* 1983;98:59–68
6. Sleyan AH. Traction alopecia. *Arch Dermatol* 1958;78:395–8
7. Lipnik MJ. Traumatic alopecia from brush rollers. *Arch Dermatol* 1961;84:183–5
8. Rudolph RI, Klein AW, Decherd JW. Corn-row alopecia. *Arch Dermatol* 1973;108:134
9. Fulton JE, Pay SR, Fulton JE III. Comedogenicity of current therapeutic products, cosmetic and ingredients in the rabbit ear. *J Am Acad Dermatol* 1984;10:96–105
10. Grimes PE, Stockton T. Pigmentary disorders in blacks. *Dermatol Clin* 1988;6:271–8
11. Hemmer W, Fockes M, Wantke F, *et al.* Allergic contact dermatitis to artificial fingernails prepared from UV light-cured acrylates. *J Am Acad Dermatol* 1996;35:377–80

African women

E. Joy Schulz

36

OVERVIEW

Sub-Saharan Africa is beset with many problems that adversely affect health. These include heat, humidity, lack of infrastructure, poverty, illiteracy, shortage of medical personnel and drugs, and civil war. Social conditions vary greatly from country to country, depending on their degree of industrialization and political stability.

The dermatological priorities of the women of Africa vary considerably, depending on whether they live in an urban or a rural environment, and on their economic circumstances. The poor, whether in rural villages or urban slums, are mainly concerned with obtaining treatment for infections and serious disease. Affluent urban women, like their Western counterparts, are increasingly preoccupied with cosmetic problems and the pursuit of a perfect complexion. Cultural traditions continue to exert a strong influence on the lives of women throughout the social spectrum.

INTRODUCTION

The continent of Africa consists of three main regions: north, central and south. In the north are situated the mainly Muslim, Arab countries. Black or Negroid races predominate in sub-Saharan Africa, which stretches down from the Sahara desert, through central, equatorial Africa, southwards to the Republic of South Africa at the tip of the continent (Figure 1). Climatic conditions in sub-Saharan Africa vary greatly from the hot, humid jungles of the Congo to cool, dry mountainous regions in Kenya. Countries such as Zambia and Namibia are mainly hot and arid, and regularly threatened by drought. The heat and humidity in tropical Africa favor the spread of bacterial infections, and vectors of serious diseases such as malaria and onchocerciasis abound. Tropical diseases have played a major role in retarding development in Africa in the past[1]. At present, HIV infection and AIDS pose grave health and economic threats to the whole of sub-Saharan Africa.

Most African countries have multiethnic populations, with different languages and cultural practices. Some countries, notably Rwanda[2], are densely populated while others, such as Namibia, are sparsely populated. In Nigeria, the most populous country on the continent, polygamy and the uncontrolled birth rate are major problems[3]. The health of populations in many regions is adversely affected by poor socioeconomic conditions, lack of infrastructure, rapid urbanization, low levels of literacy and superstition. Most countries have a dearth of medical personnel, and drugs are costly and in short supply. Unfortunately, in some countries these problems are compounded by civil war and the influx of refugees.

In rural Africa, women traditionally till the fields, while men tend the cattle. The women often need to carry water over long distances from rivers or waterholes. The men may leave home for months, or even years, to earn a living in industrialized areas in their own or in other countries, while the women remain at home to provide for the children. In the large cities of industrialized countries, women may belong to affluent professional classes, or be domestic workers with a regular if modest income, while others may be poor slum dwellers without regular employment.

While skin diseases are among the commonest causes of morbidity in rural Africa, there are few dermatologists to attend to them[1]. This lack is being redressed by specialized training centers such as the Institut Marchoux in Bamako, Mali and the Regional Dermatology Training Centre in Moshi, Tanzania.

CULTURAL FACTORS
Traditional healers

The practice of traditional medicine is based on the belief that disease is a supernatural phenomenon in which ancestral spirits play a cardinal role[4]. In South Africa, traditional healers are of two main types: inyangas and isangomas[4]. The inyangas are almost exclusively men and are essentially herbalists. Isangomas, of whom 90% are women, are diviners who determine the cause of illness by consulting ancestral spirits. Isangomas are 'called' by their ancestors to take up the profession and undergo many years of training before they can practice[5]. Traditional healers play an important role in both urban and rural communities and are highly respected and often affluent members of society. They are known to be astute observers of human nature and are particularly successful in treating psychosomatic disorders that may be inexplicable to Western practitioners unfamiliar with native languages and cultures.

In Africa traditional healers vastly outnumber practitioners of Western medicine; in South Africa their number is estimated at up to 35 000[5]. The official status of traditional healers varies in different countries. They are officially recognized in Zimbabwe; in South Africa they are not, but are registered with many organizations[4]. Some patients use traditional healers exclusively, while others use them in addition to Western doctors[4]. In Tanzania traditional healers are not anxious to treat skin diseases, as they have no effective remedies for them[6]. In Rwanda most patients first consult traditional healers, who make use of charms and incantations as well as topical and oral medicines prepared from plants[2]; two of these, used to treat scabies and tinea versicolor, respectively, are marketed commercially[2]. In South Africa traditional healers are willing to tackle all skin ailments and are currently claiming success treating AIDS with an indiginous plant, the African potato.

Tribal scarifications

Tribal marks are commonly used in many parts of Africa for purposes of identification, healing and beauty[1] (Figure 2). The skin is scarified with a blade, after which materials made from burnt leaves or wood are rubbed into the wound. Traditional healers always administer scarifications used for healing purposes themselves, and their localization identifies the site of a medical problem. Marks used for identification and adornment are administered by 'lay' persons. Scarifications sometimes result in hypertrophic scars (Figure 3).

In some African tribes piercing of ears, nose and lips is used for purposes of identification and cosmesis[7]. The earlobes and lips may be progressively dilated to accommodate large ornamental plates.

Body image

Traditional African men prefer their women well endowed, as this indicates that they are providing well for them. In South Africa obesity in middle-aged and elderly women in urban areas is often severe and commonly associated with osteoarthritis, diabetes and hypertension. Obesity was found to be rare in a rural population in Tanzania, where women are active in tilling the fields and fetching water[8]. The younger generation of urban women is persuing a more slim figure and, at least in South Africa and Zambia, 'working out' is becoming increasingly popular among them.

Grooming

Skin

As elsewhere in the world, the woman in Africa desires a smooth skin without blemishes. Previously it was fashionable to have a light complexion and this was encouraged by the cosmetics industry, which promoted the use of bleaching creams. Today an artificially pale skin is no longer fashionable in upper-class women who are proud of their natural, dark complexions. In South Africa sunscreens are now widely advertised and increasingly used by women to prevent pigment darkening on sun-exposed areas, and to avoid premature aging. Photoaging occurs late in a dark skin, first becoming apparent in the fifth or sixth decade, but having become aware of it, modern women hope to retard the process.

It is a popular misconception among whites that Africans, particularly the women, desire a shiny skin, when what they really strive for is smoothness. Dryness of the skin causes scaling, which feels rough and appears ashy. The desire for a smooth skin has led to the universal use of petroleum jelly (Vaseline) in Africa, as it is cheap and readily available. On the face in young people, prolonged use of petroleum jelly invariably leads to acne. It is occasionally suspected of causing dermatitis, possibly due to impurities in inferior products. Commercially available moisturizers are widely used, although many women prefer glycerine, as this imparts a moist feel to the skin. Glycerine has the added advantages of being cheap and non-comedogenic. In upper- and middle-class South African women, a shiny facial skin is avoided and matt, tinted foundations, often incorporating sunscreens, have become increasingly popular.

Many people make use of a stone to achieve cleanliness and smoothness of the skin on the body and limbs. This may be a naturally occurring stone (Figure 4) or a commercially available pumice stone.

Hair

Negroid hair differs from other racial types of hair by being tightly coiled. Contrary to general belief,

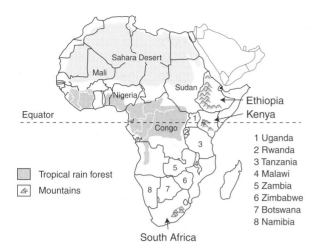

Figure 1   Map of Africa

1 Uganda
2 Rwanda
3 Tanzania
4 Malawi
5 Zambia
6 Zimbabwe
7 Botswana
8 Namibia

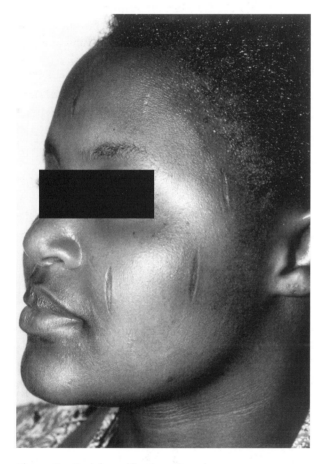

Figure 2   Facial scarifications for adornment

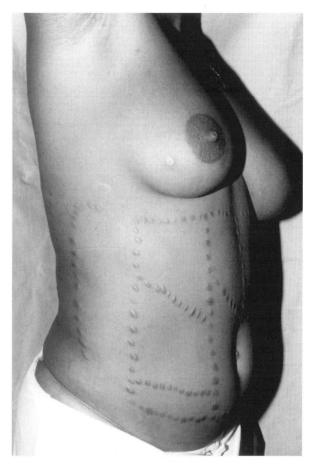

Figure 3   Hypertrophic scars following scarifications for adornment

the hair is dry and fragile and very susceptible to damage. The dryness may be due to the fact that the tight coils prevent the distribution of natural oils along the hair shaft[9]. The dryness explains why Africans need to shampoo infrequently, at intervals of 1–3 months or longer. Glycerine and commercially available creams and gels are used liberally to relieve dryness. If hair is left in its natural state, adjacent hairshafts become entangled; the hair needs to be combed daily to prevent matting, and

trimmed about once a month (Figure 5). Many urban women have their hair washed only in salons, where the hair is disentangled and conditioned.

African women seldom if ever leave their hair in a natural, uncovered state. In some regions it is customary for women to wear traditional headgear (Figure 6). Rural and more traditional older women cover their heads with a scarf or beret. Wigs were popular until about two decades ago. Plaiting or braiding of hair has long been customary, often starting very young and continued well into old age. Today, hair extensions are often incorporated into the braids (Figure 7). Braids may be left in place for periods varying from 3 weeks to 6 months, during which time the hair is shampooed at intervals. The natural African look is not popular at the moment and young women follow styling fashions such as perming and relaxing[9] (Figure 8). Most women enjoy varying their hair styles at frequent intervals.

DERMATOLOGICAL DISORDERS AFFECTING AFRICAN WOMEN

Publications concerning skin diseases in Africa are relatively few in number. Many observations date

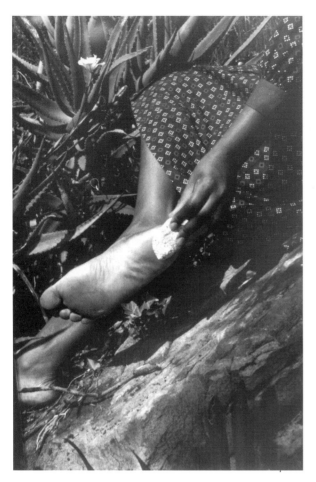

Figure 4   Scrubbing the soles with a natural stone

back to earlier times and may no longer be true for the present. In addition, studies done in different regions are not neccessarily comparable and results may not be relevant to other parts of Africa.

Many diseases that affect women in Africa need further investigation. Those skin disorders which form part of common experience, and those recorded in the literature from Africa, are reviewed below.

Postinflammatory pigmentary changes

Postinflammatory hypopigmentation

The commonest causes of postinflammatory hypopigmentation are eczema and tinea versicolor, but the genders are equally affected. Discoid lupus erythematosus is more prevalent in women than in men (see below); the permanent loss of pigment that may follow the acute inflammatory stage is a major cause of disfigurement in a black skin.

Postinflammatory hyperpigmentation

Postinflammatory hyperpigmentation is a cause of much distress to many people throughout sub-Saharan Africa. In 1991 Olumide and colleagues[10]

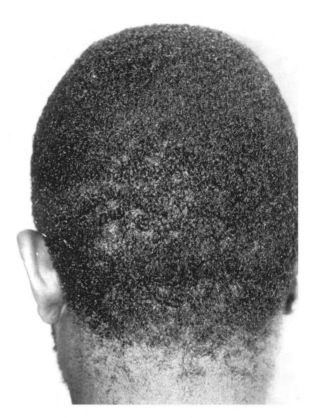

Figure 5   Natural hair – 1 month's growth, combed daily

reviewed the causes of facial hyperpigmentation in Nigeria. Topical applications included hydroquinone in bleaching creams and mercury in cosmetic creams and antiseptic soaps. Systemic causes included drugs such as antimalarials, thiazides and clofazimine. In Nigeria, herbal concoctions are bathed in or drunk to prevent or treat various diseases. These concoctions contain psoralens which cause photodermatitis and hyperpigmentation[10]. In South Africa, acne and exogenous ochronosis are by far the most important causes of distressing facial hyperpigmentation in black women.

Fixed drug eruptions may occasionally involve the face. In Nigeria the commonest causes are pyrazolone analgesics and sulfonamides[10]; in South Africa phenolphthalein is most often implicated.

In their search for remedies for postinflammatory hyperpigmentation, many African women self-medicate with topical steroids; continued use invariably leads to acne and further hyperpigmentation. Hydroquinone has received such adverse publicity in South Africa that women tend to avoid it. Commercially available creams containing α-hydroxy acids, kojic acid and liquorice are becoming increasingly popular as relatively safe alternatives with patients and doctors alike.

Dermatologists encourage patients to cover blemishes with tinted cosmetic foundations, but

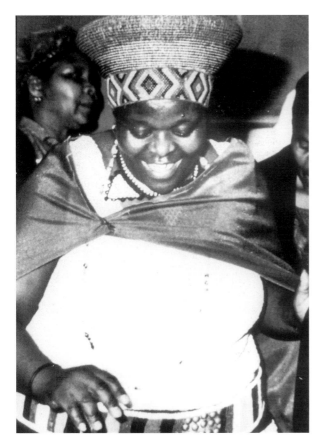

Figure 6   Traditional Zulu headdress

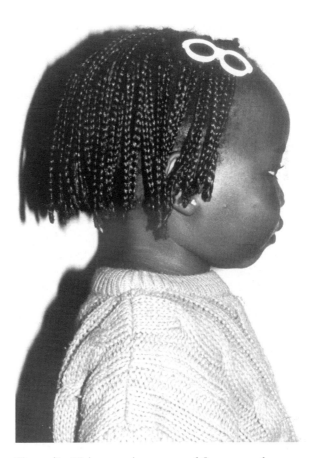

Figure 7   Hair extensions are used from an early age

their use is forbidden by some husbands who associate make-up with loose morals. Unsophisticated women often cover blemishes with light brown shoe polish, which is very effective but, being greasy, tends to cause acne.

Melasma (chloasma)

Melasma is common in African women, usually first noticed during pregnancy or following the use of oral contraceptives. Melasma is particularly noticeable on dark skins, and women demand some form of treatment. Some dermatologists prescribe the Kligman hydroquinone formula[11], which consists of retinoic acid 1%, hydroquinone 4% and a topical steroid, but it is less effective in dark skins than in white. Black patients do not like the irritant properties of the retinoic acid in the formula and they prefer to use a combination of 2% hydroquinone with glycolic acid. The mainstay of treatment recommended by dermatologists remains the regular use of sunscreens.

Acne

The incidence of acne vulgaris is similar in both sexes but women are more affected by the cosmetic disturbance and are also prone to develop cosmetic acne. Cosmetic acne is common, owing to the almost universal use of petroleum jelly and other emollients on the face. In addition, greasy applications used on the hair tend to spread down onto the forehead, causing so-called pomade acne.

In treating black patients with acne, the dermatologist often finds it difficult to persuade patients to stop using greasy creams. It is also difficult to persuade them to use topical retinoic acid because of its drying effect. The pigmentation resulting from deep acne lesions takes months to fade and women often request intralesional injections of corticosteroids to hasten resolution.

Dermatitis due to bleaching creams

Cosmetic disturbances due to the use of bleaching creams have plagued African populations for decades. The problem seems to have been greatest, or at least most documented, in South Africa. Although bleaching cream dermatitis is seen almost exclusively in women, men are occasionally affected.

History

In the earlier part of the twentieth century ammoniated mercury was widely used as a skin-lightening

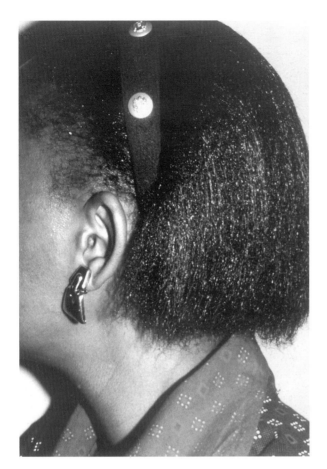

Figure 8   Straightened ('relaxed') hair – about 5 years' growth

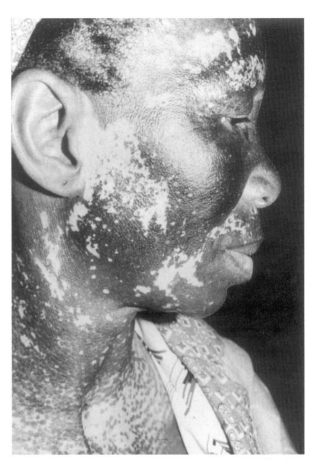

Figure 9   Leukomelanoderma from monobenzone in the 1970s

agent. In 1972, following reports of nephrotoxicity, all creams containing mercury were banned in South Africa. Unfortunately, as late as 1991, skin-lightening creams and antiseptic soaps containing mercury were still being imported into several African countries, including Nigeria[10].

In South Africa ammoniated mercury was replaced in some bleaching creams by the monobenzyl ether of hydroquinone (monobenzone) which, like mercury salts, could be dispensed in wide-mouthed jars that were popular at that time[12]. This resulted in an 'epidemic' of leukomelanoderma, which was reported by Dogliotti and co-workers in 1974[12]. In patients with leukomelanoderma, patches of depigmentation and mottled areas of hyperpigmentation affected the face, neck and upper chest (Figure 9). Monobenzone bleaching creams were consequently banned in 1975.

From 1966 certain bleaching creams containing 6–8% hydroquinone were marketed in South Africa and, from 1969 onwards, Findlay and co-workers observed the emergence of a new disease which they reported in 1975 as 'exogenous ochronosis and colloid milium from hydroquinone bleaching creams'[13]. Following prolonged and intense lobbying

by South African dermatologists, eventually in 1983 a limit of 2% was placed on hydroquinone in commercially available bleaching creams, which were further required to contain a sunscreen and carry a warning label. Since then, partly as a result of the legislation but perhaps mainly owing to the adverse publicity given to hydroquinone in the media, the number of cases of severe exogenous ochronosis has gradually declined.

Exogenous ochronosis

Changes affect sun-exposed skin on the malar areas, cheeks, and sides and back of the neck[13]. Early signs consist of erythema and mild, sooty pigmentation in the malar areas[14]. Soon small black micropapules may be detected within the area of hyperpigmentation, easily visible if the skin is stretched. White, confetti-like macules are usually seen within the hyperpigmented area (Figure 10). On histological examination thick, brown, banana-shaped ochronotic fibers are seen in the dermis (Figure 11). At a later stage collections of pigmented papules – the colloid milia – appear. On histological examination they are seen to consist of blocks of hyaline, lightly

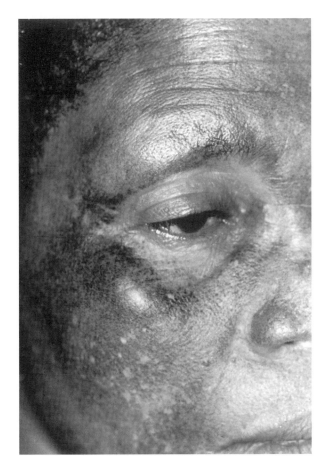

Figure 10   Exogenos ochronosis due to hydroquinone

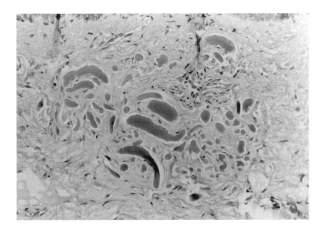

Figure 11   Ochronotic fibers in dermis (magnification × 47)

pigmented ochronotic material in the upper dermis[13]. At a later stage eruptive papulonodular lesions with a granulomatous histological picture may develop[14]. In some of these lesions transepidermal elimination of ochronotic fibers is seen on biopsy[15]. Annular lesions with the histological appearance of sarcoidosis occasionally appear within areas of ochronosis on the face (Figure 12). In some of these patients evidence of systemic sarcoidosis has been found[16].

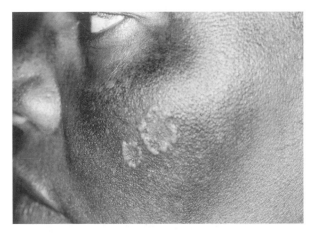

Figure 12   Annular sarcoidal lesions in ochronotic skin

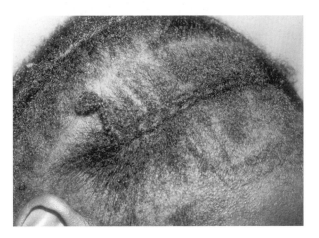

Figure 13   Advanced traction alopecia in an elderly woman

There is no effective treatment for exogenous ochronosis but lesions do slowly lighten and flatten after several years. Patients are advised to use sunscreens and to hide the pigmentation with colored cosmetic foundations. The observation by Fisher that oral tetracycline is effective for sarcoid-like ochronosis due to hydroquinone[17] was confirmed in a patient in Johannesburg who had widespread annular lesions on the face.

Alopecia

Traction alopecia

Traction alopecia due to tight plaiting or braiding is common, often causing severe permanant hair loss around the scalp margins (Figure 13). Hair extensions braided onto natural hair also result in traction alopecia if used for long periods (Figure 14).

Friction and pressure from heavy head ties worn as part of traditional costume are a cause of marginal alopecia in Nigeria[3].

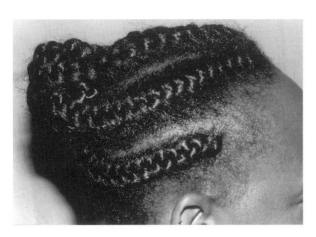

Figure 14   Artificial braids and traction alopecia in a young woman

Hot comb alopecia (follicular degeneration syndrome)

This type of scarring alopecia, which starts on the crown and spreads down laterally and frontally on the scalp, is found in African-American women in the USA[9]. It does not ever seem to have been a problem in Africa and has not been observed in South African women.

Androgenetic alopecia

Male-pattern hair loss is rarely, if ever, seen in black women, in South Africa at any rate.

Hirsutism

The prevalence of facial hirsutism in black women is unknown, but it appears to be far less than in whites. Black women in South Africa do not seek treatment for it, as they believe that any interference worsens the condition.

Contact dermatitis

The causes of contact dermatitis in Africa are likely to vary considerably in different countries according to climate and degrees of industrialization. Most information on the subject comes from Nigeria[3,18], but isolated observations have been recorded in the literature from other countries.

Nigeria

Olumide has reported on causes of contact dermatitis in Nigeria[3,18]. Nickel in jewelry, shoes and clothing is the most common cause of contact dermatitis in the general population[3]. On investigating hand dermatitis in women in Lagos, she found nickel to be the commonest sensitizer, with dressmaking as the single most important cause[18].

Dressmaking is a popular occupation in Nigeria and scissors, pins and needles are sources of nickel exposure, the dermatitis affecting mainly the finger tips. The next most common contact allergy on the hands of women was to the essential oil of orange peel. The women affected are fruit vendors who customarily peel the oranges for their customers[18].

Housewives' dermatitis as such is not common in Nigeria, presumably because the hands of women are 'hardened' by domestic chores from childhood[3]. Housewives' dermatitis was not diagnosed in Olumide's study of hand dermatitis in women in Lagos, as causes other than domestic work were identifiable in all the affected women[18]. Most women in Nigeria are self employed in various occupations, for example selling fruit or working as hairdressers from home[18].

South Africa

In South African women contact dermatitis due to nickel in jewelry and in belt and shoe buckles is common, but no incidence studies are available. Shoe dermatitis is seen regularly. Housewives' dermatitis is relatively uncommon in South Africa, although many women are employed as household helpers and do a lot of washing for their employers in addition to their own. In these women candidal or bacterial paronychia is the commonest disorder resulting from constant working in water.

Mali

In Bamako 2.2% of dermatological consultations were classified as contact dermatitis; irritant dermatitis consisted mainly of occupational dermatitis in housewives[19].

Rwanda

Contact dermatitis is very common in Rwanda, mainly in the urban population[2]. Common causes are application of traditional herbal medicines and topical antibiotics such as penicillin and neomycin.

Zambia and Malawi

Contact dermatitis was reported to be uncommon in Zambia in 1979[20] and in Malawi in 1994[21].

Sycosis cruris

Long-term use of petroleum jelly or other oily substances on the legs leads to an eczematous folliculitis on the shins; in longstanding cases the skin is shiny and atrophic and studded with small pustules[3]. The condition is well known in Nigeria, where it was initially called 'dermatitis cruris pustulosa et atrophicans'[3]. It is one of the most common eczematous eruptions in Malawi[21]. Sycosis cruris was previously seen regularly in South Africa, mainly in women, but seems to be on the decline. The eruption tends to be aggravated by topical treatment and responds best to systemic steroids and antibiotics.

Acquired keratodermas

Walking barefoot is still popular in rural areas and usually results in dry, cracked soles. Women working barefoot in the fields tend to develop plantar keratoderma consisting of hyperkeratosis and painful fissures[2]. This so-called African keratoderma is highly prevalent in Tanzania, where it is regarded as normal[6]. Most cases of keratoderma in Mali are acquired and involve the soles, being due to chronic trauma[19]. In Malawi it is customary to treat skin lesions by rubbing them with a stone. This results in a linear neurodermatitic thickening of the skin along the tendons on the backs of the hands and feet[21].

Podoconiosis (endemic non-filarial elephantiasis)

Podoconiosis is a disabling condition of socio-economic importance. It is endemic in humid regions of central Africa; countries affected include Ethiopia[22,23], Nigeria[22] and Tanzania[6]. Podoconiosis follows on long-term trauma to the feet in agricultural laborers who work barefoot in moist volcanic clays[22]. Microparticles of silica and aluminosilicates enter through the skin and accumulate in the lymphatics and lymph nodes of the legs. Clinical signs start in one limb with burning or pruritus and swelling of the forefoot; this is followed by thickening, hyperkeratosis and cracking of the skin[22,24]. Eventually both lower limbs are involved in an asymmetrical fashion[24]. Whether men or women are most affected in a particular region depends on their respective involvement in agricultural work[22,23].

Disorders associated with reproductive life

Puberty

In rural Tanzania the onset of puberty is late and the average age of acne patients is in the early twenties; this is ascribed to nutritional deficiency in childhood[8].

Marriage

Female circumcision is practiced in many African countries[1,7,25]. It is considered to be a prerequisite for marriage and in some tribes is performed as part of a premarriage ceremony; in other tribes young girls are circumcised in adolescence or childhood[7]. Female circumcision is widely practiced in Nigeria, where the great majority of women are in favor of the custom[25]. Resultant scars could be confused with lichen sclerosus et atrophicus[1], but complications are gynecological and urological rather than dermatological[25].

Customs regarding marriage may determine the occurrence of reccessive genetic disorders. In South Africa there are two main ethnic groups – the Zulu–Xhosa in whom intermarriage is taboo and the Sotho–Tswana in whom it is encouraged in order to keep wealth, that is cattle, in the family. Tyrosinase-positive oculocutaneous albinism is relatively common in the latter[26]. Similarly, a high prevalence of albinism due to intermarriage is found in southeastern Nigeria[1]. Although the sexes are equally affected, it is easier for albino men to be accepted by society; women suffer greater loss of marriage prospects.

Pregnancy

Little is known about the prevalence of skin diseases associated with pregnancy in Africa. In South Africa herpes gestationis and impetigo herpetiformis seem to be more common in blacks than in whites, but this is likely to be an erroneous impression, as blacks constitute 75% of the population. Papular pruritic eruptions of pregnancy appear to be rare.

Breast feeding

In rural areas breast feeding tends to continue for at least 2 years, or until the next pregnancy[1]. Prolonged lactation does not cause any dermatological problems, such as nipple eczema, in the mother. The child abruptly weaned because of a new pregnancy is in danger of developing the protein calorie deficiency disease kwashiorkor[1,7,25].

Vascular sequelae of pregnancy

Varicose veins and venous ulcers are far less common in African than in Western countries. Although women may have multiple pregnancies, early mobilization after delivery is the rule. Henderson noted the rarity of deep vein thrombosis and venous hypertension in rural Tanzania[8] and Lomholt the rarity of venous ulcers in Malawi[21].

Infections

Although skin infections occur mostly in children and do not affect women significantly more than men, the burden of combatting the causes and obtaining treatment for the family falls mainly on the women.

In Nigeria 30% of patients seeking medical help suffer from skin disease and 60–75% of these skin diseases are communicable[3]. In rural Tanzania, where 74% of skin disease is transmissable, household density was found to be the most significant associated factor[6]. Similarly, overcrowding was found to be the main predisposing factor for skin infection in Ethiopia[23].

Bacterial infections and infestations

Bacterial infections may be primary pyodermas such as impetigo or folliculitis, or secondary to eczematized dermatoses. Undoubtedly, the most important predisposing cause of bacterial skin infection is scabies, which is endemic in Africa[7]. At a skin clinic in Lilongwe, Malawi, 37% of patients were found to have scabies and 28% were suffering from skin infections[21]. In Bamako, Mali, scabies accounted for 16.6% of skin disease[19]; similar rates have been recorded in Rwanda[2].

Papular urticaria due to bites of insects such as mosquitoes, fleas and sandflies is common in Africa. The papules are intensely itchy, are scratched and usually become secondarily infected. Although papular urticaria is primarily a disease of children, in Nigeria it frequently occurs as persistent papules in adults, particularly young women[3]. Infected insect bites and minor injuries on the lower legs often result in ecthymatous ulcers, which are followed by scarring. Although probably more common in young men[8] the permanent atrophic scars cause most distress to young women who wish to wear short skirts.

Fungal infections

Fungal infections are highly prevalent in Africa, particularly in hot, humid regions[3]. Superficial fungal infections account for 13.6% of dermatoses in Mali[19] and 15–25% of dermatoses in Nigeria[3]. Although scalp ringworm is largely a disease of children, trichophytic tinea capitis has been found in adult women in Rwanda[2].

Sexually transmitted diseases and HIV infection

Sexually transmitted diseases are highly prevalent in Africa[2,21]. The genital ulceration resulting from early contagious syphilis, chancroid and lymphogranuloma venereum is an important risk factor for the transmission of HIV infection[27], which affects the sexes equally in Africa. The HIV epidemic in sub-Saharan Africa has spread downwards from the north, with South Africa lagging a decade behind its neighbors[28]. In South Africa the spread of HIV infection is monitored by anonymous testing of pregnant women attending antenatal clinics. HIV positivity in these women rose from 4.25% in 1993 to 10.44% in 1995. The highest rates were in women in their twenties and there was a high and rising prevalence rate in pregnant teenagers[28]. Since 1995 the rate of HIV infection has continued to increase, creating grave personal, social and economic problems.

Lupus erythematosus

Lupus erythematosus affects black races more than white, and women more than men. In 1966 Shrank and Harman showed that lupus erythematosus was twice as common in Nigerians as in Londoners[29]. In South Africa the ratio of blacks to whites with lupus erythematosus is about 3 : 2[30]. Most cases of lupus erythematosus are of the discoid type. In Kenya in 1968 the relative numbers were 40 discoid, five chronic disseminated and three systemic[31]. In black South Africans in 1982 the proportion was 55 cases of discoid to 6 of systemic[32].

The female preponderance in lupus erythematosus is confirmed by several studies undertaken in Africa. In 1962 Schaller found that 63.4% of cases of lupus erythematosus (type not specified) in Ethiopia were women[33]. Recent reports concerning relatively large numbers of patients with systemic lupus erythematosus show an even higher female preponderance. The percentage of women with systemic lupus erythematosus was 81 in Uganda[34], 97 in Kenya[35], 97 in Zimbabwe[36] and 85 in South Africa[37]. In two of these studies photosensitivity was found to be relatively infrequent[36,37], presumably because of the protective effect of melanin[36].

In South Africa, subacute lupus erythematosus, although not mentioned in previous surveys, is seen fairly regularly in black patients (Figure 15). Discoid lupus erythematosus is often difficult to manage successfully, because of the long-term treatment required and lack of regular follow-up, particularly in rural areas. The resultant atrophy and depigmentation are particularly disfiguring in a dark skin (Figure 16).

Pemphigus

The prevalence of pemphigus in sub-Saharan Africa is similar to that in Europe and North America, but

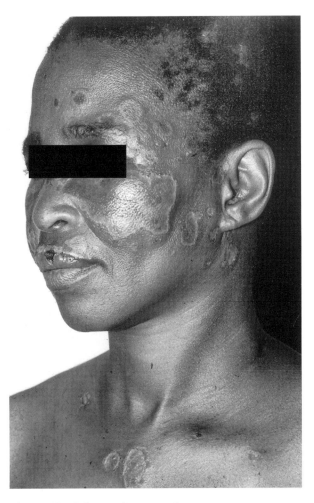

Figure 15   Subacute lupus erythematosus

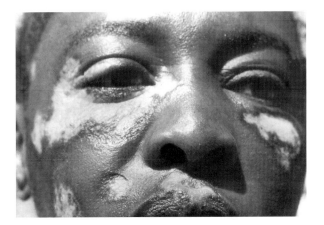

Figure 16   Depigmentation and atrophy in discoid lupus erythematosus

few individuals who do seek medical advice readily appreciate that any treatment is likely to cause more cosmetic disturbance than the lesions themselves.

Nevus of Ota

Nevus of Ota (oculodermal melanocytosis) is common in Orientals and blacks, affecting women significantly more than men[39]. The macular pigmentation is almost always unilateral, involving the upper part of the face, eye and mucous membranes. It is not uncommon in Nigeria[10] and is occasionally seen in South Africa.

Syringomas of the eyelids

In 1968 Verhagen and associates[31] stated that syringoma and adenoma sebaceum were the commonest tumors on the face in Kenya; the type of syringoma was not specified. Multiple syringomas of the eyelids occur fairly regularly in young black women in South Africa; white women and males seem to be rarely, if ever, affected. As the small tumors gradually increase in number and size, they become cosmetically disturbing. The easiest and safest form of treatment on a black skin is scissors excision of the larger, most troublesome lesions, without cauterization.

Malignant melanoma

South African studies have confirmed that in black patients most malignant melanomas occur on the soles of the feet or palms of the hands; women in the older age group are most affected[40]. In black South Africans the lifetime risk for melanoma is estimated to be 1 in 588 for women and 1 in 833 for men[41]. Survival rates are more favorable for women but unfortunately they often present at a late stage with disseminated disease[40].

the disease pattern is different[38]. The conclusion was reached by Mahé and co-workers from their recent study in Mali[38]. Of their 30 cases, 83% were pemphigus foliaceus, whereas in Europe and North America 80% of cases are due to pemphigus vulgaris. There was a female to male preponderance of 4 : 1, whereas the usual ratio is 1 : 1[38]. In 1968 Verhagen and co-workers reported from Kenya that pemphigus occurred almost exclusively as pemphigus foliaceus and erythematosus, but the sex ratio was not stated[31]. Among black patients with pemphigus in Johannesburg, South Africa, there is a female preponderance of 2.9 : 1 and 49% of cases are of the foliaceus type (E.C. Bue, unpublished data).

Nevoid conditions and skin tumors

Dermatosis papulosa nigra

This common, often familial, condition shows a slight preponderance for women[39]. The small dark papules which resemble sebborrheic keratoses, clinically and histologically, first appear in early adulthood and increase with age. The malar areas and sides of the face and neck are mainly affected. The

POSTSCRIPT AND ACKNOWLEDGEMENTS

Writing on tropical dermatology, Ryan stated in 1994: 'There is much evidence that skin disease occurring in women is diagnosed much later than in men. Many conditions of the skin also occur predominantly in women and have so far received little investigation into their pathogenesis'[42]. He added that the profession of dermatology was attracting women with talent, energy, intellect and empathy for the problems of their own sex.

The present South African government is committed to the empowerment of women, and women are playing an ever more important role in society. Black women physicians show great interest in dermatology and their ability to communicate with patients in their own languages, coupled with their understanding of the special problems of women, are proving to be of great benefit to the community.

I should like to thank two young African women, Dr Pholile Mpofu, dermatologist in private practice and part-time consultant, Johannesburg Hospital and University of the Witwatersrand, and Dr Ntebaleng Makhera, resident in dermatology at the same institutions, for their advice on aspects of African customs and culture.

REFERENCES

1. George AO. Africa. In Parish LC, Millikan LE, eds. *Global Dermatology. Diagnosis and Management According to Geography, Climate and Culture.* New York: Springer-Verlag, 1994:64–70
2. Van Hecke E. Rwanda. In Parish LC, Millikan LE, eds. *Global Dermatology. Diagnosis and Management According to Geography, Climate and Culture.* New York: Springer-Verlag, 1994:265–71
3. Olumide YM. Nigeria. In Parish LC, Millikan LE, eds. *Global Dermatology. Diagnosis and Management According to Geography, Climate and Culture.* New York: Springer-Verlag, 1994:242–62
4. Kale R. Traditional healers in South Africa: a parallel health care system. *Br Med J* 1995;310: 1182–5
5. Jones JS. Interview. A 'traditional' traditional healer: Philip Kubukeli. *S Afr Med J* 1997;87:917
6. Gibbs S. Skin disease and socioeconomic conditions in rural Africa: Tanzania. *Int J Dermatol* 1996;35: 633–9
7. Donofrio LM, Millikan LE. Dermatologic diseases of Eastern Africa. *Dermatol Clin* 1994;12:621–8
8. Henderson CA. Skin disease in rural Tanzania. *Int J Dermatol* 1996;35:640–2
9. Wilborn WS. Disorders of hair growth in African Americans. In Olsen EA, ed. *Disorders of Hair Growth. Diagnosis and Treatment.* New York: McGraw-Hill, 1994:389–407
10. Olumide YM, Odonowo BD, Odiase AO. Regional dermatoses in the African. Part I. Facial hypermelanosis. *Int J Dermatol* 1991;30:186–9
11. Kligman AM, Willis I. A new formula for depigmenting human skin. *Arch Dermatol* 1975;111:40–8
12. Dogliotti M, Caro I, Hartdegan RG, Whiting DA. Leukomelanoderma in blacks. A recent epidemic. *S Afr Med J* 1974;48:1555–8
13. Findlay GH, Morrison JGL, Simson IW. Exogenous ochronosis and pigmented colloid milium from hydroquinone bleaching creams. *Br J Dermatol* 1975;93:613–22
14. Dogliotti M, Leibowitz M. Granulomatous ochronosis – a cosmetic-induced skin disorder in blacks. *S Afr Med J* 1979;56:757–60
15. Jordaan HF, Van Niekerk DJT. Transepidermal elimination in exogenous ochronosis. A report of two cases. *Am J Dermatopathol* 1991;13:418–24
16. Jacyk WK. Annular granulomatous lesions in exogenous ochronosis are manifestations of sarcoidosis. *Am J Dermatopathol* 1995;17:18–22
17. Fisher A. Tetracycline treatment for sarcoid-like ochronosis due to hydroquinone. *Cutis* 1988;42: 19–20
18. Olumide Y. Contact dermatitis in Nigeria (1). Hand dermatitis in women. *Contact Dermatitis* 1987;17: 85–8
19. Mahé A, Cissé IA, Faye O, *et al.* Skin diseases in Bamako (Mali). *Int J Dermatol* 1998;37:673–6
20. Ratnam AV, Jayaraju K. Skin diseases in Zambia. *Br J Dermatol* 1979;101:409–53
21. Lomholt G. Malawi. In Parish LC, Millikan LE, eds. *Global Dermatology. Diagnosis and Management According to Geography, Climate and Culture.* New York: Springer-Verlag, 1994:236–41
22. Kloos H, Bedri Kello A, Addus A. Podoconiosis (endemic non-filarial elephantiasis) in two resettlement areas in western Ethiopia. *Trop Doct* 1992;22:109–12
23. Figueroa JI, Fuller LC, Abraha A, Hay RJ. Dermatology in southwestern Ethiopia: rationale for a community approach. *Int J Dermatol* 1998; 37:752–8
24. Price EW. Pre-elephantiasic stage of endemic non-filarial elephantiasis of lower legs: 'podoconiosis'. *Trop Doct* 1984;14:115–19
25. Onadeko MO, Adekunle LV. Female circumcision in Nigeria: a fact or a farce? *J Trop Ped* 1985;31: 180–4
26. Kromberg JGR, Jenkins T. Prevalence of albinism in the South African Negro. *S Afr Med J* 1982;61:383–6
27. Mroczkowski TF, Martin DH. Genital ulcer disease. *Dermatol Clin* 1994;12:753–64
28. Küstner HGV, Swanevelder JP, van Middelkoop A. National HIV surveillance in South Africa – 1993–1995. *S Afr Med J* 1998;88:1316–20

29. Shrank AB, Harman RM. The incidence of skin diseases in a Nigerian teaching hospital dermatological clinic. *Br J Dermatol* 1966;78:235–41

30. Schulz EJ. South Africa. In Parish LC, Millikan LE, eds. *Global Dermatology. Diagnosis and Management According to Geography, Climate and Culture.* New York: Springer-Verlag, 1994:272–83

31. Verhagen ARHB, Koten JW, Chaddah VK, Patel RI. Skin diseases in Kenya. A clinical and histopathological study of 3,168 patients. *Arch Dermatol* 1968;98:577–86

32. Schulz EJ. Skin disorders in black South Africans. A survey of 5000 patients seen at Ga-Rankuwa Hospital, Pretoria. *S Afr Med J* 1982;62:864–7

33. Schaller KF. Hautkrankheiten in Äthiopien. *Hautarzt* 1962;13:289–98

34. Kanyerezi BR, Lutalo SK, Kigonya E. Systemic lupus erythematosus: clinical presentation among Ugandan Africans. *East Afr Med J* 1980;57:274–9

35. Otieno LS, Wairagu SG, Waweru HW. Systemic lupus erythematosus at Kenyatta National Hospital 1972–1984. *East Afr Med J* 1985;62:391–6

36. Taylor HG, Stein CM. Systemic lupus erythematosus in Zimbabwe. *Ann Rheum Dis* 1986;45:645–8

37. Jacyk WK, Steenkamp KJ. Systemic lupus erythematosus in South African blacks: prospective study. *Int J Dermatol* 1996;35:707–10

38. Mahé A, Flageul B, Cissé IA, *et al.* Pemphigus in Mali: a study of 30 cases. *Br J Dermatol* 1996;134: 114–19

39. Rosen T. *Clinical Dermatology in Black Patients*. Bari: Grafica 080, 1995:80–81, 102–103

40. Rippey JJ, Rippey E. Epidemiology of malignant melanoma of the skin in South Africa. *S Afr Med J* 1984;65:595–8

41. Sitas F, Blaauw D, Terblanche M, *et al. Incidence of Histologically Diagnosed Cancers in South Africa, 1992. National Cancer Registry of South Africa.* Johannesburg: South African Institute for Medical Research, 1997:19

42. Ryan TJ. United Nations and nongovernmental organizations: healthy skin for all. *Dermatol Clin* 1994;12:611–20

Arab women

Oumeish Youssef Oumeish

37

At the close of the second millennium, the beauty of Arab women had its foundations in culture, traditions and folklore. The beauty of Arab women has not lost its vitality, its vigor, or its ability to reveal itself, captivate the attention, stir the imagination and arouse the desire, indignation, anger, compassion and pleasure of the Arab man. It has been the source of elation and jubilation, and an important factor in human attractiveness.

The standards of beauty for an Arab woman depend on biological inheritance, cultural standards and the natural interpersonal processes of identification, socialization and attraction.

Through many centuries, Arabs have promoted knightly virtues, equality, virility and a sense of honor, generosity and magnanimity. Men practiced swordsmanship to defend the honor of the tribe, and in particular that of women. At the same time, Arabs appreciated women's beauty in terms of philandering, dallying and the writing of love and erotic poetry[1]. Their love poetry was famous, especially that describing the beauty of women's eyes.

Arab women have used many available materials and invented many cosmetics to look beautiful in the eyes of men. They also embellished themselves, and tried always to be esthetically attractive to men, especially their lovers. They also meant to intimidate enemies, mask the effects of advancing age and compensate for defects, whether real or imagined. They used every possible way to excite the keenest of pleasure and stir the emotions of men through their senses. They also used all styles of traditional costume, folk jewelry and cosmetics that were part of Arab culture. This was also meant to show that some women were comely and simple, as a sign of purity, especially young and virgin women. Above all, Arab women are keen to get married and secure their future. Arab women, through the centuries, have been influenced by different ethnic traditions, such as those of the Arab Bedouin, Romans, Greeks and Turks.

The woman's skin has its effect on self image in many ways. Woman's beauty has been represented in different patterns through the fine arts of many civilizations. Woman's skin has been visualized on many statues and paintings through the centuries[2].

Since the invention of motion pictures and television, the depiction of women's skin features has been explored and used for different purposes, but mainly the expression of beauty[3].

ARAB WOMEN AND COSMETICS

For thousands of years, the Arabs as well as other nations have interacted with one another across the Arab land that extends from the north of Africa to south of Aden and from the east of the Arabian peninsula to the west of the African coast. They transmitted to us an enduring legacy of arts, crafts, architecture and shared values. The natural beauty of Arab women is enhanced by the use of cosmetics, jewelry and clothes. Cosmetics have a major purpose to accentuate overt signals of sexuality and social identity. Cosmetics are used mainly on the face, as the most exposed part in the majority of Arab women. The eyes are accentuated by lining and shadowing with kohl[4]. Eyebrows are usually accentuated by cosmetics, and the orbital ridges are emphasized. The eyes are clearly outlined, with the eyelashes thickened with kohl, or even long artificial eyelashes. The lips are usually reddened or darkened; lipstick is used to create a focus of attention. Arabic herbal perfumes are also used.

Creams

Arabs have been influenced by the Old Egyptian civilization, which goes back to 4500 BCE. The Pharaohs began aromatherapy, using oils of a sweet and delicate scent, extracted from flowers and pine trees. In addition, they used different types of salts and alabaster to improve the skin. They also produced creams that contained fruit acids (glycolic acid) from sugar cane, mangoes, apples and other fruits that were used by women of the royal family and the rich. They also used sour milk, which contains lactic acid, to smooth the skin.

Arab women used and still use extracts of roses and lemon flowers diluted with water or mixed with glycerine as cleansers and moisturizers for the face, neck and hands. They also use extracts or pieces of fruit such as avocados, lemons, oranges, apples and mangoes as masks for the face as they contain glycolic acid, in addition to pieces of cucumber applied directly on the face. They also use yogurt and sour milk (skimmed) as cleansers, and peels, to smooth the skin, as they contain lactic acid. Honey is also used on the belief that it enriches the skin and improves its quality. They use olive oil for the scalp both as a skin moisturizer and for styling and softening dry hair, and to prevent its splitting. Women in certain desert areas and villages also use the urine of pregnant cows and camels to wash their hair, because they believe that this will lengthen it.

Kohl

Arab women used the black powder 'kohl', one of the most famous cosmetics known until now. It is used as a powder or smear to darken the edges of the eyelids, similarly to eye-liner[5]. Kohl was introduced into Europe in the 13th century by the crusaders, and is still used today. Some men from certain Arab Bedouin tribes also traditionally use kohl as an eye-liner. It is also used as a treatment for blepharitis and is believed to lengthen the eyelashes and improve vision.

Hair cosmetics

Women and men have always been concerned about their hair and have sought to modify it by growing, coloring and cutting it, and by the use of wigs. Arab women's concern about their hair has a psychological as well as a sexual importance in addition to its esthetic base. They have used cosmetic hair coloring materials both to hide gray hair and for reasons of fashion and beauty. The most famous coloring material is henna.

Henna

Arabs were one of the first nations to use henna, a vegetable dye, the product of a tropical and subtropical shrub or small tree (*Lawsonia inermis*) of the loosestrife family with small opposite leaves and white flowers[6]. A reddish brown or blackish dye is obtained from the dried leaves of henna plants. The shrubs are found in North Africa and the Middle East, especially Saudi Arabia, Yemen and Oman. The active principle is an acidic naphthoquinone, which is used to give reddish auburn shades. It was used instead of metallic or synthetic organic dyes, partly on the basis of religion, and that is why some men use henna to dye the scalp, mustache and beard hair. Powdered henna is used by women to dye hair. It is made into a paste or pack by being mixed with tea or water, with a small amount of olive oil, and applied to the hair for 2 h, after which the paste is washed out and the hair is shampooed and dried. The effect lasts for 8–12 weeks. If it is mixed with powdered indigo leaves it will produce blue–black shades[7]. To hide gray hair the procedure is repeated every 2–3 weeks. It is also used in marriage ceremonies, by different shapes and figures being painted on the hands and feet of women and children. Intricate patterns are painted on the hands of young girls, especially in Morocco, Jordan, Yemen and Oman. Henna is also applied to the hands and feet to treat some skin diseases such as eczema, or as a camouflage for depigmented lesions such as vitiligo or skin scars. Poultices have also been used for skin infections, abscesses, skin burns and scabies. It is also useful for sciatica when applied to the back, and if mixed with vinegar and applied to the forehead it is thought to cure headache[8]. It is also useful in treating oral ulcers if it is chewed, and as a paint for brittle and dystrophic nails[9]. It is believed by some women to lengthen the hair and make it thick.

Tattooing

Tattooing has been known for several centuries. Originally it was associated with religious ceremonies and fertility and marriage rites. It is still commonly practiced by Arab women as a tribal custom and for decoration. The chin, lips, back of the hands and the feet are tattooed. The technique is painful and includes the use of needles to introduce the particles of pigment into the dermis. The pigments are chosen according to psychological, traditional and cultural factors[10]. Black–blue is produced by carbon, red by cinnabar, green by chromic oxide, yellow by cadmium sulfide and brown by iron oxide.

Tattoos can be in the form of lines, dots and figures, as a sign of one's career, especially in men, and for tribal identification or decoration, especially in women. People also believe that tattooing brings them happiness and protects them from illness.

Tattooing is commonly used by women of desert tribes, who are usually Arab Bedouin, in addition to villagers. The common pigment used is the blue–black carbon. Usually it is done in vertical lines or dots on the chin, or starts from the edge of the lower lip downwards. Sometimes a few dots are produced on the cheeks and forehead. Pigment is also applied in different shapes on the dorsum of the hands, fingers, feet and on the shins.

Tattooing is considered taboo in the Muslim faith due to the fact that the technique itself causes severe pain.

Micropigmentation

Modern tattooing for esthetic purposes is practiced by Arab women, especially Westernized women, and it is considered a semipermanent make-up. The pigment used is iron oxide, which usually does not cause allergic reactions. Micropigmentation is applied to eyebrows, eyelids and lips. A skin test is carried out for possible allergy to the pigment prior to the procedure. This is done by applying a small amount of pigment on one side of the ear, and waiting 48 h before the treatment is carried out.

A topical anesthetic cream, usually EMLA cream 5%, which contains lidocaine 25 mg and prilocaine 25 mg per gram of cream, is used. A special machine with a microneedle inserts the pigment into the surface of the skin. The skin become tight following the procedure, and the color will get darker for up to 5 days, when an exfoliation process will occur.

Lip liner or full lip color can be applied to change the size and shape of the lips as well as deepening their color. It also camouflages facial aging lines around the lips. Sometimes women use a more dramatic color, according to personal preference.

Eyebrow coloring aims to give the appearance of hair in the browline and more fullness for sparse eyebrows or for creating artificial brows when the hair is absent, as in alopecia. The pigment can be applied to eyelashes, giving the appearance of thicker lashes.

Micropigmentation can be used for areola restoration, and for the camouflage of scars, burns, cleft lip, vitiligo and alopecia areata anywhere on exposed skin. Minor side-effects in the form of erythema and swelling can occur.

Tattooing in general has many complications such as the introduction of pyogenic infection, tuberculosis, syphilis, infective hepatitis, or acquired immunodeficiency syndrome, through the use of unsterilized needles and poor technique[11]. Allergic reactions and hypersensitivity to the pigment and development of keloids or hypertrophic scars might also occur[12].

Hair removers

Many methods have been used to remove unwanted hair[13]. In the past, abrasives such as stones and sandpaper were used by women[14]. Bleaching is also used, especially on the upper lip, cheeks, neck, forearms and upper arms, in particular in women with blond hair. Hydrogen peroxide 6–9% in cream form is popular, and is applied on the hairy area for 15 min and then washed out. This is repeated every 2–3 weeks.

Hair plucking by forceps is widely performed. Threading is also practiced; this involves pulling a twisted loop of thread across the skin, catching hairs and either pulling them out or breaking them[15]. This procedure is commonly used to epilate the face, neck, shoulders, back and chest hair, especially 2–4 days before a woman's marriage. Shaving is used mainly for the legs, thighs, upper arms and forearms, but women often avoid it as they believe it leads to a masculine quality of hair. It has some side-effects, such as pseudofolliculitis and superficial irritation. Waxing is performed by the application of a warm molten sheet of wax with or without resins to the hair-bearing skin; as soon as it has hardened with the hair shafts embedded, it is abruptly peeled off the skin in the direction against which the hair lies on the skin[16]. The procedure is painful and is often complicated by contact dermatitis, postinflammatory pigmentation, folliculitis, pseudofolliculitis and sometimes scarring[17].

The most popular method of hair removal by Arab women is the use of a 'sugar pack'. This is more efficient, less traumatizing and can be used on any hairy area of the body. White sugar 0.25 kg is mixed with half a cup of water (125 ml) and the juice of one lemon. It is boiled until the color becomes light brown, and then poured on a wet piece of marble, where it cools. The pack is applied to the hairy area in sheet form, and then removed against the direction of the hair on the skin, when it pulls out the hair from its shaft. The sugar pack can be kept in a nylon bag in a freezer, to be thawed when used again. The procedure is repeated every 2 months. It is painful and can cause pseudofolliculitis, erythema and irritation.

Electropilation (electrolysis) has been introduced for hair removal and used for limited areas, especially the face[18,19]. Modern methods of hair removal by the use of lasers are now available, and are used by Arab women[20–22].

ARAB WOMEN AND FOLK JEWELRY

Folk jewelry for Arab women is used for adornment. It is similar throughout all Arab countries, with some variations in the shape, size and color of the jewelry. The basic common similarities are the use of geometric and floral designs and the use of semiprecious stones.

Jewelry is considered the personal and most valuable property of an Arab woman[23]. Many Arab women believe that certain types of jewelry have talismanic properties. They believe that jewelry protects the body and soul from injury and harm. They also believe that jewelry made of gold, silver and metal protects the woman who wears it from misfortune and drives away bad spirits and evil from the soul and body in states of illness or catastrophes, and brings luck. Many still believe in the *jinn* and the evil eye (*al'ayn*), a glance that is supposed to harm those on whom it falls, especially young and beautiful women, or prosperous, healthy and elegant ones. The *jinn* (plural, *jinni*) could bring good as well as bad luck, and so some jewelry, while protecting a woman from the evil eye, could also be a source of envy and one of the causes of *al'ayn*.

Jewelry is more often worn on major occasions such as weddings, parties and official or private family celebrations. Jewelry as a traditional custom is also considered a luxury if it is expensive, such as diamonds. They also give the impression that a woman who wears them is wealthy and cultured. All this will enhance her attention and attraction. Precious stones and metals are also criteria for social class identification. Folk jewelry has been influenced by tribal migrations, and has changed in style through many centuries. Modern jewelry has been imported to the Arab world from both east and west: India, Pakistan, Armenia, Turkey, Greece and Italy. In addition, the jewelry of pre-Islamic and Arab–Islamic civilizations is used or imitated nowadays. All kinds of jewelry, such as necklaces, rings, earrings, bracelets, chains, chokers and amulets, are hand made. Nose-rings are worn by many Arab Bedouin women, especially in Arab North African and Gulf countries, and anklets are worn by both Bedouin and rural women.

Coins or chains are also used or attached to a *hijab* (veil). Diamonds, crystals, precious and semi-precious stones in addition to their shape, color and quality, are valued for their influence on the beauty of Arab women. They are also valued for their healing influences, based on the belief that their energies can be used in the healing of a disease, trauma or injury. It is holistic healing, and many claim benefits from this kind of therapy.

The quality, shape and color of the gemstones are also important in their effect. Some women feel more self-confident when they wear certain stones such as amazonite. The wearing of a purple necklace is spiritual, and some believe that placing it on the abdomen might cure intestinal problems, and placing it on the pelvis will treat infertility. Rose quartz and aquamarine have much to do with the mood and love. Cape amethyst, for example, is believed to be useful for arthritis, when strands are wrapped around the joint. Carnelian is used to treat allergic reactions, hay fever and asthma. Coral,

diamond, emerald, and green and purple fluorite are used for emotional stress and hormonal imbalance, and jade for relaxation. Arab women also select precious stones according to their birth dates and they are classified according to their horoscopes.

Types of jewelry used by Arab women

(1) *El-orjeh*. This is more known in the north of Jordan and Syria. It is a wool band knitted by hand, containing colored, twined and interlaced threads. The main band, which is worn around the head and wrapped on the upper part of the forehead, is usually covered with two lines of coins made of gold and silver, and in between these are thin lines of colored beads. The coins and the beads are attached by fine chains made of silver.

(2) Earrings or eardrops. Earrings are used to illuminate both the ears and the neck. They are sometimes known as *al-khars*, and are also worn by a few men in one ear. In pre-Islamic and Islamic civilizations, earrings were made mainly from silver, and they used to be long, and fixed with small bells, leaves, or crescent-shaped silver pieces. The latter lunate-shaped earrings were believed to keep away *al'ayn*, or the evil eye, in addition to its suitability for the lower part of the ear. Earrings can cause contact dermatitis, and pyogenic infection.

(3) Funnel. This is made of pure silver, 10 cm in length, and decorated with silver coins (in quarters). It is attached to the head cover to be hung over the chest and shoulders, or it might reach the waist, or be attached to a pigtail or braid.

(4) *Al-shinaf* (*zamimah*). This is a small ring with a small bead attached to it, and it is used as a nose ring by Arab Bedouin women. It is also currently used as a fashion statement by teenagers. It can cause secondary infection to the nose and interfere with breathing.

(5) Necklaces, neck bands, collars, chockers and lavalieres[24]. They are round trinkets, that surround the neck. They can have a special meaning for an Arab woman. Some of them contain a piece of paper with a written verse of the Holy Koran to make the woman rich, to protect her from jealousy and to keep her from *al'ayn* or the evil eye. They also might cause contact dermatitis.

(6) Bracelets and bangles. The bracelet is a very ancient form of human adornment, like so many other kinds of jewelry. It was originally a

form of talisman or magic charm. In the past, bracelets were made of wood, stone and metals ranging from copper to silver and gold. Apart from their esthetic qualities, bracelets are believed to be useful as complementary medicine. Copper bracelets are still believed to relieve pains in the joints, and to reduce blood pressure if placed tight on the wrist. Bracelets containing agate were believed to protect the wearer against bites by snakes and scorpions.

(7) Amulets. Amulets are prescribed, prepared and advised by certain clergymen or magicians or sometimes ordinary people who claim to possess knowledge of the secrets of amulets. Amulets or periapts are usually made of different kinds of cloth, often silk or cotton, with different colors and in different shapes. They usually include a piece of paper with written incantations, either religious phrases or words that can work as an exorcism of evil. Some amulets also contain pieces of hair from a man. They might also contain nonsense words, or nothing. Arab women who carry amulets believe and are told to believe that amulets are useful to bring good luck and health to them. Sometimes they are meant also to intimidate an enemy or make sterile women conceive. Amulets are hung around the neck or placed near the chest, abdomen, umbilicus, or pubic region and genitalia. They are also placed under the main steps of the house or bedroom or under the pillow or bed.

(8) Anklets or *khilkhal*. These are bracelets worn around the ankles, and are called *Balbal*, an Arabic word meaning 'ankle'. They are made of pure silver, round in shape and opened from one side to be easy to wear on the ankle. Some of them are concave and hollow and contain a few pieces of metal or semiprecious stones that give a sound when the woman walks. Particular sounds of anklets are used by men to identify a woman. Some anklets contain semiprecious stones or colored beads, and some are made from a string of hollow spheres containing tiny metal beads, so that they make a pleasant tinkling sound.

Most jewelry can cause contact dermatitis when it contains metals such as nickel, chrome, cobalt and copper.

BODY PIERCING

Body piercing is used to pierce the earlobe with a needle or a special piercing instrument to apply ornaments such as earrings or eardrops. Nowadays, ear piercing has been modified to have more than one piercing and more than one earring. Body piercing is used as a tribal fashion in some Afro-Arabian countries and is used for the nose, lips and tongue. Today, some young people practice body piercing in unusual ways. In addition to the ears, piercing is also done to the nose, tongue, nipples, navel and vulva.

Body piercing has adverse effects such as secondary infection and abscess formation, and the risk of contracting diseases through unclean needles. It also causes contact dermatitis due to nickel and chrome materials incorporated in the ornament.

REFERENCES

1. Oumeish YO. Traditional Arabic medicine in dermatology. *Clin Dermatol* 1999;17:13–20
2. Marchionini A. The relationship of dermatology to the arts and sciences. *Arch Dermatol* 1961;83:15–25
3. Reese V. Dermatology in the cinema. *J Am Acad Dermatol* 1995;33:1030–4
4. Ebling FJG. The role of colour in cosmetics. In Counsell JN, ed. *Natural Colours for Food and Other Uses*. London: Applied Sciences Publishers, 1981:55–81
5. Oumeish YO. The philosophical, cultural, and historical aspects of complementary, alternative, unconventional, and integrative medicine in the old world. *Arch Dermatol* 1998;134:1380
6. Dawber RPR, Ebling FJG, Wojnarowska FT. Disorders of hair: cosmetic hair colouring. Vegetable dyes. In Rook, Wilkinson, Ebling, eds. *Textbook of Dermatology*, vol 4. Blackwell scientific publications, 1992;629
7. Natow AJ. Henna. *Cutis* 1986;38:21–5
8. Avicenna. *The Canon of Medicine*. Beirut, Lebanon: Izeldeen Publishing Foundation, 1993;1:510–11
9. Immam Shams Ibn Kaim Al-Jouzieh. *Medicine of the Prophet*. Beirut, Lebanon: Izeldeen Publishing Foundation, 1991:100–1
10. Rook AJ, Thomas PJB. Social and medical aspects of tattooing. *Practitioner* 1952;169:60–6
11. Biro L, Klein WP. Unusual complication of mercurial (cinnabar) tattoo. *Arch Dermatol* 1967;96:165–7
12. Taaffe A, Knight A, Marks R. Lichenoid tattoo hypersensitivity. *Br Med J* 1978;1:616–18
13. Olsen EA. Continuing medical education. Methods of hair removal. *J Am Acad Dermatol* 1999;40:146–7
14. Ridley CM. A critical evaluation of the procedures available for the treatment of hirsutism. *Br J Dermatol* 1969;81:146–53
15. Richards RN, Uy M, Meharg G. Temporary hair removal in patients with hirsutism: a clinical study. *Cutis* 1990;45:199–220

16. Rentoul JR. Aitken AB. The cosmetic treatment of hirsutism. *Practitioner* 1980;24:1171–84
17. Wright RC. Traumatic folliculitis of the legs: a persistent case associated with use of a home epilating device. *J Am Acad Dermatol* 1992;27:771–2
18. Wagner RF, Tomich JM, Ghande DJ. Electrolysis and other thermolysis for permanent hair removal. *J Am Acad Dermatol* 1985;12:441–9
19. Richards RN, McKenzie MA, Meharrg GE. Electroepilation (electrolysis) in hirsutism. *J Am Acad Dermatol* 1986;15:693–7
20. Wheelard RG. Laser assisted hair removal. *Dermatol Clin* 1997;15:459–77
21. Finkel B, Eliézri YD, Waldman A, Slatkine M. Pulsed alexandrite laser technology for noninvasive hair removal. *J Clin Laser Med Surg* 1997;15:225–9
22. Dierich CC, Grossman MC, Farinelli WA, Anderson RR. Permanent hair removal by normal-mode ruby laser. *Arch Dermatol* 1998;134:837–42
23. Bienkowski P. *The Art of Jordan*. Stroud, Gloucestershire: Alan Sutton Publishing, 1996: 162–3
24. Mershen B. Amulets and jewellery from Jordan. A study on the function and meaning of recent bead necklaces. *Tribus* 1989;38:43–58

Korean women

Hae-Shin Chung

38

The 20th century has brought many changes to the lives of Korean women, from the ever-changing environment exacerbated by longevity and the contact with the Western world. Before modern medicine was introduced into Korea, the Korean spa (i.e. hot-spring water therapy) was used successfully for treatment of most of the chronic skin diseases. For skin diseases such as psoriasis, the first treatment would be a spa, and atopic dermatitis has also responded well to this form of therapy. The sulfur-rich spa is known to be especially effective in the treatment of diseases such as psoriasis. The sulfur that penetrates the skin is oxidized and evokes various physiological responses, such as vasodilatation in the microcirculation, an analgesic influence on the pain receptors and inhibition of the immune response[1].

BATHING

Bathing for Korean women also involves scraping away a part of the stratum corneum (called *Tte*). Korean women routinely scrape away their *Tte* with

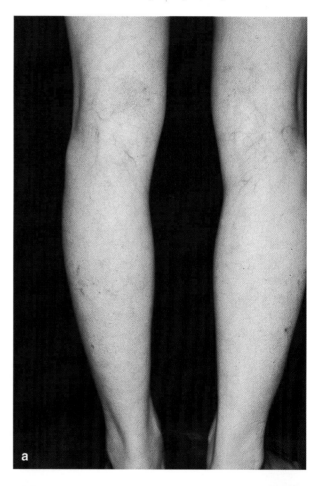

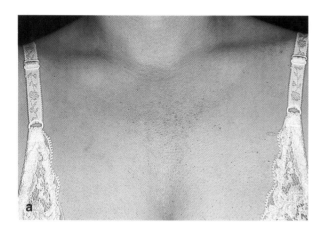

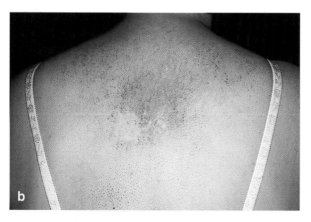

Figure 1 Lichen amyloidosis on the front (a) and back (b) of a woman

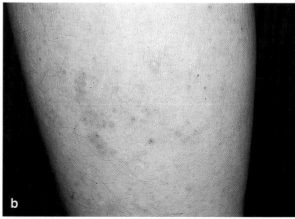

Figure 2 (a) and (b) Irritant dermatitis

stiff towels or a stone until their skin becomes red and then they will use soap and water again, to make sure all the *Ttes* are removed. In severe cases, this may cause injury to the skin and women will visit the hospital for severe pruritus, irritation dermatitis and lichen amyloidosis (Figures 1 and 2). This phenomenon more often occurs in women, because Korean women tend to scrape their skin for cleanliness more than do men.

TRADITIONAL KOREAN MEDICINE

Korean women still tend to depend for their treatment on traditional Korean medicine, which is heavily influenced by Chinese culture, which asserts that internal organs combine physiological, psychological and dermatological functions. The stomach and lungs are considered to be particularly susceptible to ill effects as a result of anxiety, worries and sadness. This is why Korean women always associate their skin problems with food. Patients will ask the dermatologist what kinds of foods they must take and what kinds of food to avoid[2].

Postmenopausal Korean women sometimes visit the dermatology clinic because of hot flushes. Although there may be many causes of flushing, Korean women call this *Hwabyung*. *Hwabyung* is a widely held Korean popular belief concerning suppressed anger as the cause of a variety of somatic illnesses. *Hwabyung* is associated with the Korean historical and socioeconomic environment, with Korean ways of thinking and perceiving and with Korean medical beliefs and practices. Suppression of emotions is taught in Korean society. This contributes to the development of *Hwabyung* through a process of internalization. Suppression of emotions such as anger, hatred, revengefulness, frustration, depression, anxiety and disappointment disturbs the physiological harmony from the perspective of Korean traditional medical principles. Emotional distress is manifested as somatic symptoms such as flushing.

In the past, Korean people were forbidden to cut any of their body hair. Even men grew their hair and twisted it up into a topknot. That is why Korean women are reluctant to shave their axillary hair.

IN RETROSPECT

Korean women have many different pigmentary diseases such as nevus of Ota, melasma, acquired bilateral nevus of Ota-like macule (ABNOM), lentigo and freckles. For these reasons, Korean women are attracted to any whitening products on the market. Korean women love the thought of pure white skin.

REFERENCES

1. Hann SK. Mineral water and spas in Korea. *Clin Dermatol* 1996;14:633–5
2. Hann SK. Traditional Korean medicine in dermatology. *Clin Dermatol* 1999;17:29–31

Caucasian women

39

Mary P. Lupo

Caucasian women, like women of other races, have physical features typically associated with their race. There is great heterogenicity within the Caucasian race, because Caucasians evolved in distinct genetic pools throughout Europe and the Mediterranean.

Owing to mixing of the gene pools in the USA, it is there that we see the most variety of physical attributes that constitute 'Caucasian' features. As a result of their phenotype, Caucasian or 'white' women have distinct dermatological features. Most significantly, their phenotype results in vulnerability to solar damage and subsequent skin problems.

WHO ARE CAUCASIANS?

The race of humans referred to as Caucasians is largely derived from peoples found all over the world who trace their ancestry to Europe, the Mediterranean and Western Asia. Their phenotype conforms to 'arbitrary criteria of skin color or facial shape'[1]. Although there is variability of skin color from Northern European Caucasians to Mediterranean Caucasians, this racial group is commonly also referred to as 'white'. Indeed, this color designation probably dates back to ancient Greek times when whiter, paler skin was the preferred beauty standard for women. Only in the later part of the 20th century did tanner, darker skin become an ideal for Caucasian women.

HAIR

When describing racial characteristics, it is often easier to cite differences and comparisons between different races. For example, the hair of Caucasians is narrower in diameter than that of Asians[2]. In cross-section, Caucasian hair is oval, and is flatter in blacks and rounder in Asians. As a result of these differences, Caucasians have less straight and less shiny hair than Asians, and it is less curly than the classic kinkiness of African (black) hair.

The hair of Caucasians is heterogeneous in its appearance. Hair color of whites varies from light blond to dark brown and, in some groups, it is red. It can also range in texture from straight to curly. There is follicular form variation among races, with Caucasian hair follicles being a variation between the more extreme helical form of blacks and the straight follicles of Asians[3]. Among Caucasians, the variation of curvature of the hair follicle determines the degree of curling of the hairs themselves.

FACIAL SHAPE

Compared to other races, Caucasians tend to have slimmer faces with more prominent cheek bones. The nose is high and slim and not flat in profile, and the lips are thinner. Asians, in comparison, have flat profiles, with eyelids in line with the brows, wider jawlines and less protruding chins than whites[4].

Extensive variability in facial size and proportion exists among this ethnic group[5]. Measurements of distances between various areas of the head and face were taken and averages obtained for comparison with similar measurements by scholars and artists of the Renaissance. The height from the top of the head to the frontal hairline (calva height), the forehead height and the nose length were always each smaller than the lower face height from beneath the nose to the chinline in modern American Caucasians.

In an elaborate study on Caucasian subjects' evaluation of attractiveness of photographs of Caucasian women, composites using exaggerated features were preferred over the average composites[6]. Most important were higher cheekbones, thinner jaw and larger eyes. In a different study, a survey that consisted of 92% of Euro-American Caucasians, anatomical traits that were derived as a result of evolutionary changes in humans (such as bipedal locomotion, omnivorous diets and an increased dependence on visual acuity over olfactory or gustatory senses) were overwhelmingly preferred[7]. These preferences are important to understand, because being deemed 'attractive' increases one's chances of procreation and thus the propagation of one's genes. As one author states: 'Our perceptions of facial beauty are based on a complex mix of evolutionary biological characteristics and the social environment'[8].

SKIN COLOR

Besides differences in facial features compared to other races, there is the obvious difference in skin color. These differences are due to real variations seen on histopathology. While there are the same number of melanocytes in the skin of all races, there are functional differences. In Caucasians of all skin colors, from darkly tanned Southern Europeans to fair untanned Northern Europeans, there are fewer and smaller melanosomes per cell and no central clumping of melanosomes in corneocytes, as seen in Africans and Asians, whether they are light or dark[9]. These melanosomes are also smaller in whites. Melanin in all layers of skin is variable within racial groups, depending on the level of natural fairness and derived tanning of the individual. Melanin is scant in the basal layer of Caucasian skin, and is rarely capped with melanosomes. Caucasian skin is more likely to have spotty islands of pigment, with melanosomes in the keratinocytes grouped and surrounded by a membrane. This is found in the skin layers from the basal cell layer up to the stratum granulosum[10]. After ultraviolet irradiation, melanosomes increase in keratinocytes of all races, but the clumpiness remains in Caucasians while Negro skin melanosomes remain individually dispersed.

AGING EFFECTS

Female Caucasian skin also exhibits differences after the menopause. In one study, postmenopausal white women were found to have a higher prevalence of skin atrophy, senile dry skin and skin wrinkling than in a similar group of African-American women[11]. Estrogen use reduced senile dry skin only in the white women exhibiting this finding. They also found a 'statistically significant protective effect of estrogen use on wrinkling' in the white women. This was not seen in the African-American women studied.

SKIN DISEASE

The most obvious Caucasian physical attribute, the fairer skin color, is responsible for most of the skin diseases that are more prevalent in whites. Compared to more darkly pigmented races, Caucasian patients with minor cosmetic skin problems may find these conditions more noticeable, owing to the fairness of their skin. Non-bulging telangiectatic vessels of the lower extremity are always more noticeable in lighter skin. This sometimes results in

the patient sunbathing to conceal this problem with a tan, but self-tanners with dihydroxyacetone would be a safer option. Tinea versicolor, in contrast, is usually more noticed by the Caucasian who tans. This condition is more common in tropical climates where Caucasians get more sun. The causative organism, *Pityrosporum orbiculare*, causes pigment disruption that is most noticeable as white skin tans.

Owing to the lack of those protective individually dispersed melanosomes seen in black skin, Caucasian skin is vulnerable to skin diseases from sunlight. The melanosome complexes of Caucasians poorly absorb and scatter ultraviolet radiation. This lack of protection results in the precancerous and malignant transformation seen more commonly in Caucasian skin. Indeed, even slight but regular lifetime ultraviolet exposure leads to many concerns of less medical, but often cosmetic, significance including senile lentigines, solar purpura, solar elastosis and rhytides. Poikiloderma of Civatte is a benign discoloration of the lateral neck and upper chest seen exclusively in Caucasians. The pattern spares the area under the chin, clearly delineating the photodistribution of this condition.

In a recent survey of female Caucasian patients seeing dermatologists, the top three complaints were all related to the vulnerability of Caucasian skin to solar damage[12]. Fine wrinkling, solar keratosis and hyperpigmentation were the most common chief complaints for the dermatology visits evaluated in this study.

Public education programs have only recently begun to educate the Caucasian population about the risks of ultraviolet exposure, the vulnerability of white skin and the need for a lifetime of protection and ultraviolet radiation avoidance. It will probably take a generation for this message to have an impact that decreases the incidence of sun-induced skin problems in Caucasians.

CONCLUSIONS

Caucasians constitute a heterogeneous group derived from peoples of Europe and the Mediterranean that now inhabit distant places around the world. Within this group there is variation in skin tone, hair color and texture, and facial proportions and shape. It is owing to recognizable contrasts to members of other races that the features of Caucasians are identified as their own. Basic functional differences in the skin of Caucasians result in an inability to protect itself from ultraviolet radiation. The result is that the most distinct attribute of Caucasians, lighter skin, is the very source of the most common and more noticeable skin diseases.

REFERENCES

1. Stowell H. The most beautiful people. *Nature Genet* 1996;12:361–2

2. Bertolino AP, Klein LM, Freedberg IM. Biology of hair follicles. In Fitzpatrick TB, Eises AZ, Wolff K, *et al.*, eds. *Dermatology in general Medicine*, 4th edn. New York: McGraw-Hill, 1993:289–93

3. Lindelof B, Forslind B, Hedblad M, Kaveus U. Human hair form. *Arch Dermatol* 1988;124:1359–63

4. Kouga F. Ochoboguchi. Facial beauty and the Japanese art of make-up. *Koku Eisei Gakkai Zasshi* 1978;28:116–24

5. Farkas LG, Hreczko TA, Kolor JC, Monro IR. Vertical and horizontal proportions of the face in young adult North American Caucasians: revision of neoclassical canons. *Plast Reconstr Surg* 1985;75:328–38

6. Perrett DI, May KA, Yoshikawa S. Facial shape and judgements of female attractiveness. *Nature (London)* 1994;368:239–42

7. Mangro AM. Why Barbie is perceived as beautiful. *Percept Mot Skills* 1997;85:363–74

8. Larrabee WF. Facial beauty: myth or reality? *Otolaryngol Head Neck Surg* 1997;123:571–2

9. Jimbow K, Quevedo WC, Fitzpatrick TB, Szabo G. Biology of melanocytes. In Fitzpatrick TB, Eisen AZ, Wolff K, *et al.*, eds. *Dermatology in General Medicine*, 4th edn. New York: McGraw-Hill, 1993:261–89

10. Szabo G, Gerald AB, Pathad MA, Fitzpatrick TB. Racial differences in the fate of melanosomes in human epidermis. *Nature (London)* 1969;i:1081–2

11. Dunn LB, Damesyn M, Moore AA, *et al*. Does estrogen prevent skin aging? *Arch Dermatol* 1997;133:339–42

12. Grimes PE. White, ethnic women differ on reasons for visiting Derm. *Skin/Allergy News* 1998;29:32

Expatriate women

40

Tanya O. Bleiker and Robin A. C. Graham-Brown

In this chapter we illustrate and discuss some of the dermatological problems encountered by women who are part of a migrant community and are living among what is usually called an 'ethnic minority'. The word 'ethnicity' is derived from the Greek word meaning people or tribe. Thus, 'ethnic minority' identifies people with a shared origin or social background, with distinctive traditions that are maintained between generations and often with a common religion and language[1].

Over the years there have been large influxes of immigrants into the United Kingdom, most recently from the Indian subcontinent and from the West Indies. The first significant movements occurred in the 1950s and 1960s, at a time when the prosperity and very low levels of unemployment in Europe and North America led to the migration, often by direct invitation, of Third World people in search of jobs and a higher standard of living. These were mainly men who were willing to take on unpopular, poorly paid jobs. Such individuals often came alone and supported their families from a distance. There then followed a second phase of migration of wives, fiancées and elderly relatives.

Because of the British role in the Indian subcontinent, many migrants have come to Britain from India and Pakistan (West and East – now Bangladesh). These have mainly been Bengalis and Pakistanis (almost all Muslim), Gujaratis (the majority of whom are Hindu) and Sikhs and other religious groups from the Punjab. The Immigration Act of 1962 effectively marked the end of large-scale immigration; however, a further influx occurred in the early 1970s, when many people of Indian (Gujarati) origin, who had lived for generations in East Africa, came to the UK as refugees from the racist policies of the then-President Idi Amin. These East African Indians were often of a higher social class than those directly from India[2]. Many were highly successful in business and the professions and had to start all over again in their new cultural surroundings.

Settlement within the UK was not uniform; immigrants headed for places where friends and relatives lived. Therefore, Jamaicans settled in South London and West Birmingham, Muslims in Bradford, Sikhs in Birmingham and Southall, London and Gujarati Hindus in Leicester and Wembley. These minority communities tend to function as a separate group keeping the same social, marital and dietary habits of their original home nation.

Our experience of dealing with an ethnic minority population is based on the fact that, in Leicester, where we work, there is an Asian community that comprises 18% of the city's population. Three-quarters are Gujarati[3]. It is important to stress that the term 'Asian' in Britain generally describes people originating from India, Pakistan or Sri Lanka. This is in comparison to the USA, where 'Asian' is used to describe people from Japan or South East Asia.

WOMEN IMMIGRANTS

Asian women are traditionally home-based and often treated, by Western standards, as inferior. They have always been the last to emigrate in any major population movement, following their husbands and fathers. The practice of arranged marriages has meant that there has been a continuing flow of small numbers of women (and also some men) in recent years. Women in such situations are often the most disadvantaged of all, having little or no English, no knowledge of how industrialized societies function and very limited opportunities for developing experiences outside the family home. Upon marriage, the wife normally moves in with her husband's family and is expected to look to her mother-in-law and sisters-in-law for advice and instruction. Children are the desired outcome of the union, with failure potentially resulting in disgrace or divorce[4]. In traditional families, adolescent girls, whether born in the UK or abroad, have a particularly restricted lifestyle, and finding a suitable husband is of critical importance to her parents; cosmetic abnormalities such as pigmentary disorders are therefore of great concern.

IMMIGRANTS' HEALTH

It is well recognized that ethnic minorities pose a number of special problems distinct to themselves[2]. Certain physical and psychiatric problems have long been associated with migration and adjustment to life in a different society. Important considerations in Asian women include language, religion, expectations of treatment and diet. For example, many Hindus are vegans and women frequently suffer from low-grade, or even quite pronounced, iron deficiency. The gender of any examining doctor is also an issue. Many Asian women refuse to be examined by men, particularly if the examination involves the genital area.

SKIN DISEASE IN ASIAN EXPATRIATE WOMEN

There are two main areas of difficulty with skin disease in this population: the fact that common diseases may be expressed or appreciated differently from the indigenous population, and that, in comparison to white women, a number of conditions are generally only seen in Asian women, recently arrived in the UK (Table 1).

Infections

Asian women are, of course, liable to present in the skin clinic with the effects of a number of the common cutaneous pathogens, such as warts, impetigo, erysipelas and cellulitis. There are, however, some infections that cause particular problems, because of their relative frequency as compared to the indigenous population, because of the ways in which they present or because of the stigma attached to them.

Cutaneous tuberculosis

The incidence of tuberculosis (TB)[5] in England and Wales in 1988 was 5 : 100 000 per year[6]. The annual incidence among Asian immigrants, however, is 120 : 100 000 overall and 500 : 100 000 in those described as 'recent' immigrants. TB is becoming more common, despite the availability of effective treatments. This is due to a number of factors, including the arrival of immigrants from countries with a high prevalence of TB, HIV infection, poverty and decline in good contact tracing. Cutaneous TB makes up only a small proportion of these; in USA cutaneous TB made up 1.5% of all cases in 1987[7]. Atypical forms[8,9] and even standard presentations may be overlooked through lack of familiarity.

Classification of cutaneous tuberculosis

Cutaneous TB can be classified into four groups: inoculation TB, secondary TB, hematogenous TB

Table 1 Disorders that may present differently or present special problems in Asian expatriate women in the UK

Exotic and tropical diseases
Unusual forms of tuberculosis
Leprosy
Madura foot
Disorders of pigmentation
Vitiligo
Macular amyloid
Dermatosis papulosa nigra
Postinflammatory hyper- or hypopigmentation
Mongolian blue spot
Other/miscellaneous
Common conditions
Acne
Allergic contact dermatitis
Atopic dermatitis

and eruptive TB (the tuberculides) (Table 2). A brief description of the different types follows, with a more complete discussion on lupus vulgaris and erythema induratum, which affect Asian women in particular.

Tuberculous chancre

This is rare outside Asia, where it most commonly presents as a nondescript brown nodule, papule or ulcerated lesion that heals slowly and rarely develops into lupus vulgaris. It is due to direct inoculation of the mycobacterium into the skin of a non-immune patient.

Warty tuberculosis (syn. tuberculosis verrucosa cutis)

The lesions present as chronic, indolent, warty plaques, which extend slowly and respond to antituberculous therapy. It is due to inoculation of the mycobacterium into the skin of an immune patient. Active disease elsewhere may coexist and should be investigated.

Scrofuloderma

This is a bluish-red nodule overlying a focus of TB infection, in particular in gland and joint disease.

Orificial tuberculosis (syn. tuberculosis cutis orificialis, acute tuberculosis ulcer)

This is TB infection of the mucosa or skin adjacent to an orifice in patients with advanced internal TB, particularly in intestinal, anogenital and pulmonary infection. It is probably due to autoinoculation.

Table 2 Classification of cutaneous tuberculosis (TB). Adapted from reference 5

	Classical terminology of TB
Inoculation TB (exogenous source)	TB chancre
	warty TB
	lupus vulgaris
Secondary TB (endogenous TB)	
contiguous spread	scrofuloderma
autoinoculation	orificial TB
Blood borne TB	acute miliary TB
	lupus vulgaris
	TB gumma
Eruptive TB (the tuberculides)	
micropapular	lichen scrofulosorum
papular	erythema induratum (Bazin's)
nodular	? nodular vasculitis

Miliary tuberculosis

This is as a result of acute hematogenous spread of TB, mainly in children. Cutaneous features include crops of bluish papules, vesicles, pustules or hemorrhagic lesions.

Tuberculosis gumma (syn. metastatic tuberculosis ulcer)

These develop owing to the hematogenous spread from a primary focus in patients with lowered resistance. Clinically, there is a firm subcutaneous nodule or an ill-defined fluctuant swelling on the extremeties, which ulcerates.

The tuberculides

These are a group of eruptions arising as a response to an internal focus of TB, probably secondary to hematogenous spread. They have a variable clinical appearance but similar histology, with features of caseation necrosis and giant cell formation. They all respond to antituberculous therapy.

Lupus vulgaris

Definition

Lupus vulgaris is a progressive cutaneous TB in immune patients[5]. It characteristically presents with reddish-brown nodular plaques and scaly surface which on diascopy are referred to as 'apple-jelly' nodules (Figure 1).

Incidence

Lupus vulgaris is now uncommon in Europe and the USA, but when it occurs, it most frequently involves the head, particularly the face (over 80% of European cases). Lupus vulgaris is the most common type of cutaneous TB in India[10]. In India it is more common in women than men and affects the buttocks and trunk more frequently than the face.

Pathogenesis

It is due to direct inoculation, extension from infected glands or joints or lymphatic spread; however, the origin is often obscure and culture of the organism is difficult.

Histopathology

Histology of the lesion is variable; in most cases there are tubercles in the upper part of the dermis. Bacilli are rarely seen.

Clinical features

Five patterns of disease have been described, depending on the local tissue response to infection: serpiginous plaques; ulcerative and scarring; vegetating; tumor-like; and papular/nodular forms. The nasal, buccal and conjunctival mucosa must be examined carefully for involvement. Active lupus vulgaris can be a destructive process to deep tissues and cartilage, with contractures and deformities developing, especially with the ulcerating and tumor-like forms. It has been found to be associated with an active focus elsewhere, mainly glandular, in 11% of cases[11].

Prognosis

Lupus vulgaris is a progressive disease, with more rapid spreading in older patients. Spontaneous resolution may occur, with scarring and tissue destruction, but active disease often recurs. Squamous cell and less commonly basal cell carcinomas may occur within the scar many years later.

Treatment

Standard antituberculous therapy should be given.

Erythema induratum

Definition

Erythema induratum[5] is a persistent or recurrent nodular eruption, usually on the legs, secondary to TB elsewhere in the body.

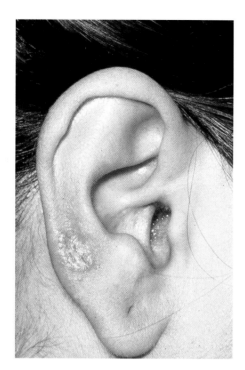

Figure 1 Lupus vulgaris of the outer helix of the right ear

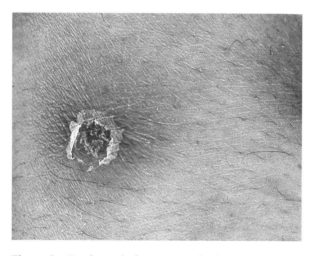

Figure 2 Erythema induratum on the leg

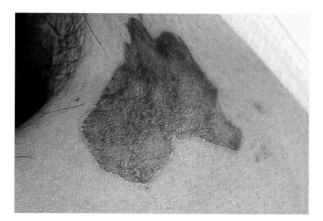

Figure 3 Pigmented lichen planus on the side of the neck

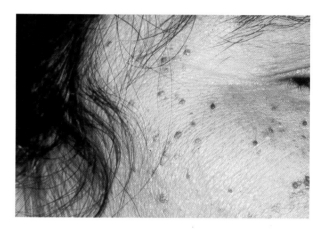

Figure 4 Dermatosis papulosa nigra on the right cheek of an Asian woman

Histopathology

Histology is non-specific, with features of nodular vasculitis and areas of tuberculoid granulomas, fat necrosis and foreign-body giant-cell reaction. Caseation is rarely seen.

Clinical features

There is an indolent eruption of nodules on the legs in young and middle-aged women, often with plump legs and an erythrocyanotic circulation. The nodules eventually ulcerate to form ragged, shallow ulcers with a bluish irregular edge (Figure 2).

Treatment

Resolution is slow, even with treatment.

Leprosy

Leprosy is endemic in India and the Far East and is regularly imported into Northern Europe and North America. It therefore remains a significant problem. The full clinical features may take years to

Incidence

It is extremely rare in Western countries today, but when it is seen in Britain it is almost always in an Asian woman.

Pathogenesis

Patients are tuberculin test-positive with a past or present history of active infection. Mycobacteria are rarely cultured. Erythema induratum is often found in association with nasopharyngeal, renal and endometrial infection.

Figure 5 Macular amyloidosis, with characteristic 'rippled' hyperpigmentation on the upper back

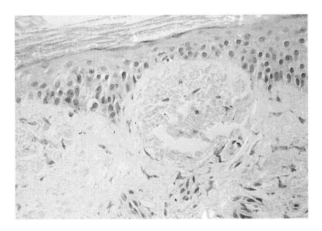

Figure 6 Histology of macular amyloid (hematoxylin and eosin section): amorphous eosinophilic mass in the upper dermis, with lateral displacement of the rete ridges and sparse lymphohistiocytic infiltrate

develop in immigrants who may have originated from the endemic areas many years previously, and the diagnosis is often delayed.

DISORDERS OF PIGMENTATION

In Leicester, some years ago, we looked at 1000 consecutive new referrals to our out-patient clinic[12]. Pigmentary conditions, as the main presenting condition, were far more common among Asians, whereas skin cancers were, as expected, almost exclusively seen in whites. The main conditions we see are discussed briefly below.

Postinflammatory pigmentary changes

Inflammation in pigmented skin may provoke hyperpigmentation or hypopigmentation that persists after the initial eruption has faded. These pigmentary changes are often of more concern to patients, particularly females, than the primary dermatosis, and are the reason for seeking medical advice.

Secondary hypopigmentation can result from many common conditions such as eczema, pityriasis alba, tinea versicolor, herpes zoster infection and less commonly sarcoid and leprosy. Iatrogenic causes include cryotherapy, topical or intralesional corticosteroids, in particular fluorinated corticosteroids, and the use of hydroquinone 'skin lightening' creams.

Secondary hyperpigmentation, similarly, is seen in a variety of skin conditions including acne, eczema, psoriasis, lichen planus, lichen simplex chronicus, mycosis fungoides and fixed drug eruptions.

Lichen planus in Asians is commonly associated with hyperpigmentation[13] and may present with nothing more than pigmented macules (Figure 3).

Vitiligo

Vitiligo has the same incidence in all races[14], but its manifestations have a greater social impact in people with pigmented skin. For example, facial vitiligo in a young, unmarried Asian female can have enormous implications for her 'marriageability'.

Dermatosis papulosa nigra

This is a condition in which there are hyperpigmented, smooth-surfaced, round or filiform papules usually occurring on the face, neck or upper trunk, and often causing cosmetic concern in Asian (and in Afro-Caribbean) women (Figure 4).

Amyloidosis
Definition

Amyloid[15,16] is a proteinaceous substance with abnormal extracellular deposition. It has characteristic staining properties with congo red, a distinctive fibrillar ultrastructure and cross β-pattern on X-ray diffraction.

Classification

Amyloid is divided into systemic and organ-limited disease and is classified according to the biochemical nature of the fibril proteins (Table 3). Systemic disease is further divided into primary and secondary amyloid. Primary localized cutaneous amyloid is divided into three groups: macular, papular (or lichen amyloidosis) and nodular or tumefactive forms in which there is amyloid deposition in previously normal skin with no internal involvement.

Table 3   Biochemical nature of amyloid fibril proteins associated with skin lesions. From references 15 and 16

Clinical type	Amyloid fibril protein	Precursor substance
Systemic		
Primary	AL	immunoglobulin light chains
myeloma associated	AL	immunoglobulin light chains
Secondary	AA	SAA
hemodialysis associated	β_2-microglobulin	
heredofamilial e.g. hereditary	AA	SAA
Mediterranean fever		
Organ-limited		
Primary localized cutaneous		
nodular	AL	immunoglobulin light chains
macular and lichen amyloidosis	? altered keratin	? keratin filaments

AL, amyloid light chain protein; SAA, serum amyloid A protein

Pathogenesis

Amyloid is composed of fibril proteins, glycosamino-glycans and a protein termed amyloid P (plasma) component. The biochemical composition of amyloid varies according to the clinicopathological type. Primary, myeloma-associated, systemic disease is derived from immunoglobulins and is termed AL amyloid. Secondary systemic disease is due to a variety of chronic diseases, e.g. rheumatoid arthritis, inflammatory bowel disease and chronic infection. Secondary amyloid can also be caused by a number of dermatoses, e.g. generalized psoriasis and hidradenitis suppurativa. Secondary disease is derived from serum amyloid A protein (SAA), an acute phase reactant, and is known as AA amyloidosis. Nodular cutaneous amyloid is derived from immunoglobulin light chains (AL type), and is thought to be due to aberrant light chain production by clonally expanded plasma cells. Fibrils in lichen and macular amyloid are probably keratin derived.

Histopathology

Examination with light microscopy shows amorphous, homogeneous, eosinophilic material. In cutaneous amyloid, deposits are often sparse and a number of stains can be used, including PAS, Congo red with green birefringence when viewed under polarized light, crystal violet metachromasia of amyloid deposits and thioflavine T fluorescence[16].

Cutaneous amyloidosis

Cutaneous involvement is seen in 40% of primary systemic disease. Cutaneous features include petechiae, purpura and ecchymoses after minor trauma, especially in flexural areas, owing to amyloid deposition in blood vessels. Waxy, translucent nodules, papules and plaques are also commonly seen. Rarer features include pigmentary changes, scleroderma-like infiltrates, bullous lesions, cord-like blood vessel thickening, amyloid elastosis, cutis laxa and nail dystrophy.

Clinically insignificant, microscopic deposits of amyloid are commonly seen in association with a variety of tumors, such as intradermal nevi, pilomatricoma, dermatofibroma, seborrheic keratoses and basal cell carcinomas.

Primary localized cutaneous amyloidosis

A brief description of the nodular and lichen forms is given below, with more emphasis on macular amyloid, which is more common in Asian women.

Nodular cutaneous amyloid presents as single or multiple lesions indistinguishable from primary systemic amyloid. It may follow a benign course or later develop a paraproteinemia and systemic amyloid.

Lichen amyloidosis is a persistent, pruritic eruption of multiple discrete hyperkeratotic papules mainly on the shins which coalesce to form plaques. It is particularly common in Chinese people. Lichen and macular amyloid may coexist[17].

Macular amyloidosis

This is a pruritic eruption often mistaken for postinflammatory pigmentation, resolving lichen planus or neurodermatitis. The etiology is unknown, although it has been reported following chronic friction[18]. It normally starts in early adulthood, with equal sex incidence, and tends to persist. It is common among Asians[19], and is normally confined to the interscapular regions or more extensively over the back, chest or extensor aspects of the limbs. A reticulate or 'rippled' pattern of pigmentation is characteristic (Figure 5). Histologically, amyloid deposits are confined to the papillary dermis and displace the rete ridges laterally with a sparse lymphohistiocytic infiltrate; there is no involvement of the blood vessels or adnexae (Figure 6). Treatment is disappointing.

COMMON CONDITIONS

Certain conditions that are commonly seen in dermatology clinics may present differently, may present more frequently, or may require a different treatment approach in the Asian community.

Atopic dermatitis

In Leicester, we found[12] that referral of Asian children with atopic dermatitis was three times more common than in white children. A subsequent cohort study in Leicester[20], however, found that the prevalence of atopic dermatitis was similar in both Asian and white European children. A family history of atopic disease was significantly less common in Asian families. Apart from the obvious implication that something in the 'new' environment in which Asian children were growing up must be responsible, we concluded that the increased referral pattern in Asians was probably due to a low level of familiarity of the disease within the community as a whole.

Acne

The incidence of acne is the same in the Asian as in other ethnic groups. However, because of the disfiguring, hyperpigmented scarring that may occur in young women, we believe that aggressive treatment should be considered earlier than in other skin types.

Contact dermatitis

There is no racial predisposition to allergic contact dermatitis. However, certain patterns of allergic contact dermatitis are recognized, owing to the use of traditional or ethnic preparations.

Bindi dermatitis

Bindi (also known as *kum kum* or *tilak*) is applied to the forehead by Hindu women for socioreligious reasons. *Bindi* is a vermilion powder containing carbon soot. Recently, artificial forms, particularly felt- or plastic-covered disks with adhesive backs, have been introduced. Lipstick is also used.

Various dermatoses have been associated with their use[21]. Contact dermatitis can develop to the vermilion powder, the azo-dyes or the artificial *bindi*, adhesive or lipstick. The incidence is unknown. Hyperpigmentation can occur after long use of vermilion powder. Depigmentation has also been described with the use of artificial *bindi*, probably due to the epoxyresin in the adhesive.

CONCLUSIONS

Asian women are a distinct group within the immigrant population of Britain. This is not merely because of the spectrum of disease, but is also because of the important cultural and religious traditions and communication difficulties. Many presentations in this population are due to pigmentary problems and the subsequent cosmetic disfigurement, which can have major implications for the future of women within their family environment. Such issues can be difficult to deal with and to treat. It is important, therefore, to look behind any presentation to the clinic by a woman from an ethnic minority and deal sympathetically with the problem, always bearing cultural differences in mind.

REFERENCES

1. Senior PA, Bhopal R. Ethnicity as a variable in epidemiological research. *Br Med J* 1994;309:327–30
2. Cruickshank JK, Beevers DG. *Ethnic Factors in Health and Disease*. London: Wright, 1989
3. Graham-Brown RAC, Neame RL. The United Kingdom. In Parish LC, Millikan LE, eds. *Global Dermatology*. Heidelberg: Springer-Verlag, 1994:56–61
4. Karseras P, Hopkins E. *British Asians: Health in the Community*. Topics in Health. Chichester, UK: John Wiley and Sons, 1987
5. Gawkrodger DJ. Mycobacterial infections. In Champion RH, Burton JL, Burns DA, Breathnach SM, eds. *Textbook of Dermatology*, 6th edn. Oxford: Blackwell Science, 1998:1181–214
6. MRC Cardiothoracic Epidemiology Group. National survey of notifications of tuberculosis in England and Wales in 1988. *Thorax* 1992;47:770–5
7. Block AB, Rieder HC, Kelly GD, *et al*. The epidemiology of tuberculosis in the United States. *Clin Chest Med* 1989;10:297–313
8. Graham-Brown RAC, Sarkany I. Lichen scrofulosum and tuberculosis dactylitis. *Br J Dermatol* 1980;103:561–4
9. Milligan A, Chen K, Graham-Brown RAC. Two tuberculides in one patient – a case report of papulonecrotic tuberculide and erythema induratum occurring together. *Clin Exp Dermatol* 1990;15:21–3
10. Ramesh V, Misra RS, Jain RK. Secondary tuberculosis of the skin: clinical features and problems in diagnosis. *Int J Dermatol* 1987;26:578–81

11. Kanon MW, Ryan TJ. Endonasal localization of blood borne viable and non-viable particulate matter. *Br J Dermatol* 1975;92:475–8

12. Sladden MJ, Dure-Smith B, Berth-Jones J, Graham-Brown RAC. Ethnic differences in the pattern of skin disease seen in a dermatology department – atopic dermatitis is more common among Asian referrals in Leicester. *Clin Exp Dermatol* 1991;16: 348–9

13. Fallowfield ME, Harwood C, Cook MG, Marsden RA. Lichen planus in Asians. *Br J Dermatol* 1993;129 (suppl 42):59

14. Kenney JA. Vitiligo. *Dermatol Clin* 1988;6:425–34

15. Breathnach SM. Amyloid and amyloidosis. *J Am Acad Dermatol* 1988;18:1–16

16. Black MM. Cutaneous amyloid. In Champion RH, Burton JL, Burns DA, Breathnach SM, eds. *Textbook of Dermatology*, 6th edn. Oxford: Blackwell Science, 1998:2626–37

17. Brownstein MH, Hashimoto K, Greenwald G. Biphasic amyloidosis: link between macular and amyloid forms. *Br J Dermatol* 1973;88:25–9

18. Wong CK, Lin CS. Friction amyloidosis. *Int J Dermatol* 1988;27:302–7

19. Black MM, Wilson Jones E. Macular amyloid. *Br J Dermatol* 1971;84:199–209

20. George S, Berth-Jones J, Graham-Brown RAC. A possible explanation for the increased referral of atopic dermatitis from the Asian community in Leicester. *Br J Dermatol* 1997;136:494–7

21. Kumar AS, Pandhi RK, Bhutani LK. Bindi dermatoses. *Int J Dermatol* 1986;25:434–5

Women in the Indian subcontinent 41

*Kazal Rekha Bhowmik, Hirak Behari Routh
and Narayan Krishna Bhowmik*

The Indian subcontinent – extending from Bangladesh in the east to Pakistan in the west and from the Himalayas in the north to the Bay of Bengal and the Arabian sea to the south – has a population of more than 1 300 000 000 or one-fourth of the world's population, nearly half of whom are women. The people of this region have varied social, environmental and cultural differences, but traditionally there is one thing in common: women are not treated equally. Their share of justifiable equal treatment in comparison with men has been, and still is, mostly denied or ignored.

Diseases of women are not the priority or of importance in this male-dominated society. Multiple factors play a role in the causation of this situation. Some of these rely on women, but most of them are due to the society's male domination and its outlook towards women. These factors are[1]:

(1) Poverty and backwardness;

(2) Ignorance;

(3) Illiteracy;

(4) Social injustice and inequalities;

(5) Dependency of women throughout life;

(6) Social stigmata;

(7) Rapid industrialization, leading to overcrowded cities;

(8) Natural calamities such as floods and cyclones, resulting in overcrowded temporary housing;

(9) Discriminatory government policies towards women.

With the vicious cycles of these multiple factors, combined with religious superstitions, there is little wonder that the rights of women are curtailed, and they have limited possibilities of taking advantage of modern medical treatment for their illnesses. Modern treatment of skin diseases is not a priority for most women.

Skin, ranging from skin color to cutaneous diseases, has a profound influence in society. In the Indian subcontinent, brighter skin color has become a measure of beauty and superiority, whereas darker color is regarded as inferior. The social impact of skin color affects every part of daily living, from marriage to employment.

The stigmata of leprosy and other disfiguring conditions have not changed for thousands of years. If these conditions occur in women, the entire family pays a heavy toll[2–4]. Women's dermatological diseases are rarely presented separately. This finding is based upon our own experience, working in medical college hospitals, in updated facilities with the standards of a developing country, or in rural health centers with the minimum resources of modern medicine. Reports of skin disorders of women and data of individual diseases are scanty, at best.

Dermatological disease profiles of women in this region are different from those in other developing countries, owing to differences in environmental conditions, social customs and life style[5]. Skin disorders of girls and women may vary from common dermatoses to specific dermatitides, ranging from cosmetic-related minor dermatitis to severe pigmentary changes, including vitiligo, which carries significant social impact. Bacterial, parasitic and fungal skin lesions are common in this region, owing to prolonged exposure to high temperatures and humidity, which contribute to the growth and survival of potential pathological organisms[6].

Scabies, pediculosis, pyoderma and dermatophytoses are more common than in other countries. When scabies occurs, it affects the whole family. Pediculosis capitis is a common condition among girls and women, as a result of unhygienic and overcrowded living conditions. Pediculosis is also prevalent. Smuggling and trading of young girls and women for sex from one region to another is a major tragedy. These frightened people often have no knowledge of sexually transmitted diseases, and usually have no opportunity for treatment. Even rescue from this situation is no salvation; their family and society no longer accept them[7]. Sexually transmitted diseases are occasionally reported when these occur in women, but far more young girls and women are affected.

The injuring and burning of girls and women for different social reasons is growing. Severe burning has been reported to lead to disfigurement, deformity, disability and sometimes death. In a 1998 report from Bangladesh, 164 cases of burns resulted from acids being thrown onto the face and body of young girls (Figures 1 and 2)[8]. Violence and rape are two other crimes where girls and women are easy victims. The social consequences are enormous and may lead to suicide. The victims often cannot marry. Most cases are not reported.

CULTURAL AND SOCIAL ASPECTS

In the Indian society gender plays a crucial role, where women are placed in a disadvantageous position and given lower status, owing to unique social factors. This leads to dependence on men[9]. Traditionally, boys and men, who are treated as superior and enjoy a better position in the family, are given more nutritious food. This leaves girls and women at risk for anemia, which leads to various infections, both bacterial and parasitic[10,11].

Women have less access to and utilization of treatment and other health-care services than do men. Women have minimum care during illnesses. There is a heavy burden on the family and an overall negative impact[12]. Little or no explanation is given to women about their condition, which is underestimated or attributed to psychosomatic reasons. The educational status of women is lower than that of men, and this may affect basic nutrition and sanitation. The perception of diseases in men and women differs, because skin conditions in women are seen as a curse or punishment by God for their wrongdoings. Such women are isolated and dishonored by society. Financial hardship also plays a role in the treatment of women.

Sometimes social customs such as the use of *kumkum*, a traditional vermilion colored mark, mainly worn by Hindu married women, leads to *kumkum* dermatitis, a type of contact dermatitis. The *burkha* worn by Muslim women as a veil or *purdah*, may also cause dermatitis (discussed below)[13]. Indiscriminate spitting, another common practice, may help transmit diseases. Early marriage and multiple pregnancies may also decrease the resistance of young mothers, in whom tuberculosis is common[14]. Ignorance and negligence combined with poverty add to the transmission of microbes and promote water-borne, feco-oral, vector-borne and environmental infectious diseases[5].

Lack of education and resources often leads to the seeking of help from so-called traditional health professionals including sorcerers and faith healers. Women in this region prefer to take advice for their conditions first from these traditional healers, because they are more approachable. The explanations seem understandable and are economical. Anxiety and confusion are increased by ignorance, illiteracy and lack of proper knowledge of the signs and symptoms of diseases, modes of transmission and preventive measures[15]. Finally, the decision for their therapy is greatly influenced by men and often by female relatives.

SPECIFIC DISEASE CONDITIONS
Leprosy

Leprosy is a chronic condition with global distribution, but most cases are in Asia and Africa. It is estimated that about half of the leprosy patients live in the Indian subcontinent, where there is a prevalence of 6 per 1000[16]. The stigmata of leprosy have been known since antiquity and have not changed for thousands of years. This condition has been attributed to a curse or punishment from God. It is also believed in Indian society that this incurable disease is caused by bad habits or deviant sexual behavior, and imbalance of hot and cold[2]. As in most other tropical countries, leprosy in men and women is at a ratio of 2 : 1. The greater resistance of women to leprosy has been postulated to be due to levels of estrogen and other female sex hormones. During pregnancy and lactation, there may be disastrous changes and exacerbation of a pre-existing condition due to a decrease in immunity[17]. Infants born to mothers with lepromatous leprosy usually have a lower weight.

Leprosy in the poorer section of society causes much more devastation in women. Twenty-five per cent of women have strained relationships with their husbands and another 25% with family members[18]. In the extended Indian family, 33% of these women were discriminated against by the members of the family. The attitude of the community towards these women are as follows: 31% are not allowed to use the popular community sites; 62% suffer disability; and 45% have to compromise their routine work. During pregnancy, drug therapy for women with leprosy is often discontinued, owing to the fear of adverse effects of the medication. Usually, treatment of leprosy in women is delayed, compared with that of men[19].

Most women in Indian society for cultural reasons do not allow male health workers for skin screening and especially areas such as the buttocks, trunk and proximal extremities. It takes a long time to diagnose skin conditions because women do not come forward, for many reasons. They tend to suffer silently so that the whole family will not

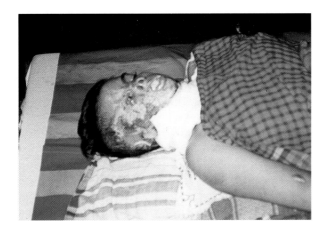

Figure 1 Facial disfigurement as a result of acid thrown on the face for revenge. Courtesy of Biswajit Bhowmik, MD, Dhaka, Bangladesh

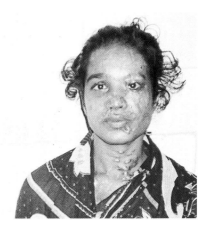

Figure 2 Disfigurement of the face, neck and arms from acid thrown for spite. Courtesy of Biswajit Bhowmik, MD, Dhaka, Bangladesh

bear the consequences. Women continue to work with infected hands and feet, putting themselves at greater risk of burns and ulcers, leading to disfigurement and deformity. Women face physical, mental and social problems irrespective of the family status. Drop-out rates of treatment among the 15–44 year age group of women are more common, owing to shyness[20]. Nutritional factors also play an important role in leprosy, as women traditionally have less food compared with men. The stigmata of leprosy mainly arise because it usually affects visible parts of the body[21]. Social rejection of the woman and her family forces her to hide her illness until obvious deformity is noted.

Vitiligo

Vitiligo presents in both men and women, but in women it has much more devastating cosmetic and social effects. In most Indian languages, vitiligo means white leprosy and causes an increase in social isolation and rejection. The society's attitude towards vitiligo is negative and its social consequences are serious, ranging from psychological upset to divorce, with discrimination in the community. In Indian society, the prevalence of vitiligo ranges from 2 to 4% with a male preponderance[22]. In one study, patients attributed their vitiligo to magicoreligious causes such as the evil eye, sorcery and possession by deities and demons[2]. The highly unpredictable course of the disease and the similarly unsatisfactory response to therapy cause many problems for women.

Filariasis

Lymphatic filariasis is an endemic condition on the Indian subcontinent. It usually affects poor people living in crowded or substandard conditions; many of these are women. Initial manifestations are acute filarial attacks with fever and lymphangitis. After 10–15 years of filarial infection, the chronic stage begins. In the sequence of events, the following occur: filarial fever, lymphangitis, lymphatic stagnation and, finally, elephantiasis[4]. The clinical and pathological changes induced in the skin lead to elephantiasis, a condition of great concern.

Massive swelling, especially of the legs, causes deformity and, ultimately, difficulty in normal movement and function, with disability in life style. In women the arm, vulva or breast may also be involved. The most dependent part of the breast thickens first, progressing upwards. Hypertrophy and fibrosis of the skin and subcutaneous tissue occur, but the glandular tissue of the breast remains unaffected. Picking the skin up from the underlying tissue is not possible. The skin does not pit under pressure.

The skin changes cause psychosocial problems and economic hardship for the family[23]. The deformity and discomfort along with other secondary changes of a swollen extremity ultimately lower the patient's self-esteem and confidence.

Kumkum dermatitis

Kumkum (*bindi* or *tilak*) is a traditional mark for Hindu married women, being compulsory and worn on the center of the forehead. Some men also use this mark for religious purposes. This vermilion colored substance may be in powder, liquid or paste form. In the past, it was made from turmeric powder mixed with lime juice, plus alum and dye. The commercially available *kumkum* contains either scarlet red or rhodamine B and red sulfide of mercury (*sindur*). Multicolored disks with an adhesive back and sometimes red lipstick are also used. Frequent sweating will cause the color to be leeched out of the *kumkum* and lead to contact dermatitis[24]. The dermatitis may be irritant or allergic in nature owing to either the alum or the alkalinity. It may appear within hours of application, followed by a burning sensation, leading to postinflammatory hyperpigmentation or depigmentation. Allergic contact dermatitis presenting with itching and oozing with crusting may also occur. Patients may react to different brands of *kumkum*.

CONCLUSIONS

Many of the dermatological conditions present in this region among girls and women remain a significant problem. Early diagnosis and recognition of the social and epidemiological factors are very important in the management of these conditions. This is a multifactorial problem and its solution will depend upon many social as well as health-care improvements. These may include public awareness of women's diseases, improvement of financial and living conditions, a direct approach, permitting women to come forward to seek medical help, a promotion of women's health services, a change in social customs and behavior and community's attitude towards women, an improvement of women's education, and the implementation of policies to improve the overall status of women.

Development of a safe and secure environment with privacy maintained for women to discuss and obtain help for skin disease is necessary, so that women can come forward without hesitation or social isolation. Lack of initiative and implementation of the existing resources for women's health care remains a huge hurdle. Appropriate therapy for both disability and deformity and the establishment of rehabilitation centers is a necessary step. Women dermatologists and dermatological health assistants may help, as many women will not visit a male physician or dermatologist.

REFERENCES

1. Khan A. Nari, nirapatta, hefazat and mananadhikar [Women, security, protection and human rights]. Bengali. *Probashi-Bengali News Weekly*, New York, 4 September 1998
2. Krause IB. The cultural construction of illness of the skin. In Parish LC, Millikan LE, eds. *Global Dermatology: Diagnosis and Management According to Geography, Climate, and Culture*. New York: Springer-Verlag, 1994:25–34
3. Finlay AY, Ryan TJ. Disability and handicap in dermatology. *Int J Dermatol* 1996;35:305–11
4. Routh HB, Bhowmik KR. Elephantiasis. *Dermatol Clin* 1994;12:719–27
5. John TJ. An Indian point of view. Tropical medicine. *Lancet* 1997;349(suppl III):S31–2
6. Routh HB, Parish LC. Tropical dermatology. In Goldstein BG, Goldstein AO, eds. *Practical Dermatology*. St Louis: Mosby, 1997:286–308
7. Homicide, rape and burning by throwing acids: 1998 report from Bangladesh. *Thikana-Bengali News Weekly*, New York, 8 January 1999
8. Begum N. Patitabritta kaj noy [Prostitution not a profession]. Bengali. *Parichoy*, New York, 30 September 1998
9. Rathgaber E, Vlassof C. Gender and tropical diseases: a new research focus. *Soc Sci Med* 1193;35:513
10. Khan ME, Tamang AK, Patel BC. Work pattern of women and its impact on health and nutrition – some observation from urban poor. *J Fam Welfare* 1990;36:3–5
11. Hossain MM, Glass RI. Parental son preference in seeking medical care for children less than five years of age in a rural community of Bangladesh. *Am J Pub Health* 1988;78:1349
12. Wyon JB, Gordon JE, eds. *The Khanna Study: Population Problems in the Punjab*. Cambridge: Harvard University Press, 1971:23–30
13. Sehgal VN. Cutaneous tuberculosis. Contemporary tropical dermatology. *Dermatol Clin* 1994;12:645–53
14. Park JE, Park K. *Textbook of Preventive and Social Medicine*. Jabalpur: Messers Banarsidas Bhanot, 1983:276–308
15. Kaur V. General consideration: tropical diseases and women. *Clin Dermatol* 1997;15:172–8
16. Sehgal VN. Leprosy. *Dermatol Clin* 1994;12:629–44
17. Duncan ME, Person JMH. The association of pregnancy and leprosy. *Lepr Rev* 1984;55:129–42
18. Kaur H, Ramesh V. Social problems of women leprosy patients: a study conducted at 2 urban centres in Delhi. *Lepr Rev* 1994;65:261–71
19. Krishnamurthi P, Subramaniam M, Reddy BN, *et al*. Time lag between case registration and commencement of treatment in leprosy control unit. *Indian J Lepr* 1992;64:8–13
20. Gopalakrishnan S. Drop outs during treatment for leprosy: a study in ELEP leprosy control project, Dharampuri district, Tamilnadu during 1975–77. *Indian J Lepr* 1986;58:431–40
21. Kumar JHR, Verghese A. Psychiatric disturbances among leprosy patients: an epidemiologic study. *Int J Lepr* 1980;48:431–4
22. Yesudian P. India. In Parish LC, Millikan LE, eds. *Global Dermatology. Diagnosis and Management of Illness According to Geography, Climate and Culture*. New York: Springer-Verlag, 1994:289–96
23. WHO division of Control of Tropical Diseases (CTD). UNDP/World Bank/WHO Special Programme for Research and Training in Tropical Diseases (TDR). *Tropical Diseases 1990: Filariasis*. Geneva: WHO, 1990:8–9
24. Kumar AS, Pandhi RK, Bhutani LK. Bindi dermatises. *Int J Dermatol* 1986;25:434–5

Native American women

*Maria-Teresa Hojyo-Tomoka, María-Elisa Vega-Memije
and Léon M. Waxtein*

42

Genetic factors and racial susceptibility may contribute to the higher prevalence of the following skin problems in native American women. Environmental factors, cultural customs and labor-related activities seem to play a very important role in their etiology.

OCCUPATIONAL LENTICULAR ACRAL KERATOSIS

This is also called lenticular acral keratosis in washerwomen.

Clinical description

In Latin American countries, especially in patients who belong to lower social strata, it is frequent to see lesions on the hands of working women that are clinically similar to those described by Costa as acrokeratoelastoidosis[1,2]: accentuation of the cutaneous folds on the knuckles, and numerous small, flat, flesh-colored hyperkeratotic papules and plaques in a cobblestone pattern at the transition between the dorsal and volar surfaces of the skin of the hands (Figures 1 and 2). The medial border of the palm and fifth fingers, the lateral border of the thumb and thenar eminence, and the volar surface of the wrist are the most affected areas.

Practically all of these patients are working-class women, with a mean age of 39 years, who spend many hours a day washing clothes on stone washboards. Therefore, chronic trauma might be the cause of these dermatoses. This type of dermatosis is virtually unheard of among men, possibly because, in Latin American society, the washing of clothes is performed by women[3].

Histologically, individual lesions are characterized by a lenticular area of hyperkeratosis overlying compressed epidermis (Figure 3). The epidermal rete pegs tend to coalesce and form thick epidermal processes. In the mid- and reticular dermis there is an increased amount of elastic fibers, which are coarse and tortuous (Figure 4)[3].

The differential diagnosis must include entities manifested by acral keratotic papules (Table 1)[4].

Acrokeratoelastoidosis, although clinically similar to lenticular acral keratosis, presents histologically as a decrease in the amount and fragmentation of elastic fibers. The incidence appears unaffected by sex and race, and most cases are sporadic, with some reports of familial transmission[5–12].

Focal acral hyperkeratosis corresponds to abnormalities of keratinization, with onset in childhood, differing from acrokeratoelastoidosis by the absence of elastic fiber alterations. Focal acral hyperkeratosis seems to be more common in black people, with a frequent familial incidence[13].

Marginal keratoelastoidosis is characterized by acral keratotic papules in manual laborers, and occupational trauma associated with actinic damage is suggested as a possible cause of these dermatoses in elderly men. Histologically, hyperkeratosis and acanthosis, elastic actinic degeneration and vasodilatation are seen[14–16].

Management

There is no specific treatment. Keratolytics and topical tretinoin have not shown any improvement. Avoiding the mechanical trauma during daily activities may be the best preventive[3].

FRICTION MELANOSIS

Synonyms are friction amyloidosis and nylon brush macular amyloidosis.

Clinical description

Friction melanosis is an acquired pigmentary disorder affecting bony prominences and first described by Japanese authors. It mainly affects young and thin women between 20 and 35 years of age[17–20]. It appears to be related to ethnic factors, since the majority of cases have been reported from Oriental and Latin American patients with skin types IV and V[17–20].

The lesions are characteristically located on bony prominences, predominating on the clavicular area, neck and upper trunk. They are hyperpigmented macules with a dark brown to a grayish-blue hue with a reticulated pattern and irregular shape, size

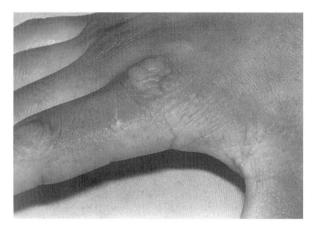

Figure 1   Accentuation of the cutaneous folds on the knuckles

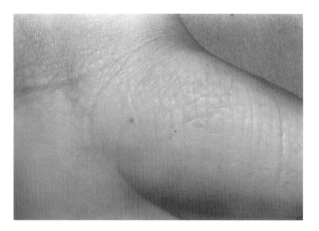

Figure 2   Small, flat, hyperkeratotic papules in a 'cobblestone' pattern at the transition of the dorsal and volar surfaces of the hand

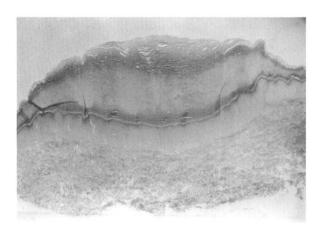

Figure 3   Lenticular area of hyperkeratosis overlying compressed epidermis (10 ×)

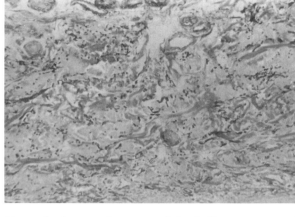

Figure 4   Increased amount of elastic fibers, coarse and tortuous (40 ×)

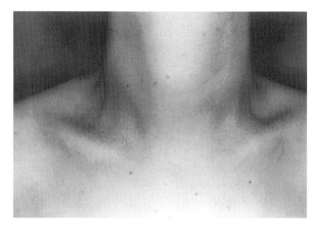

Figure 5   Hyperpigmented macules predominating on bony prominences

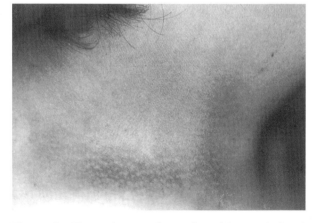

Figure 6   Hyperpigmented macules with a reticulated pattern

and undefined borders. They are usually asymptomatic and have a chronic course for many decades. The main cause of consultation is related to esthetic aspects[21-23] (Figures 5 and 6).

The histopathology shows a flattened or normal epidermis with increased melanin pigment and

vacuolar degeneration at the basal cell layer. In the dermis, a scarce perivascular lymphocytic infiltrate and melanophages can be seen (Figure 7). These findings correspond to a non-specific melanosis[20-22].

There are no specific studies to support the clinical diagnosis, but the history of having the habit of

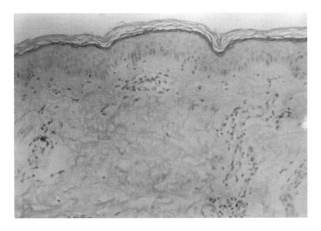

Figure 7 Increased melanin pigment at the basal cell layer and a scarce perivascular lymphocytic infiltrate in the dermis (non-specific melanosis) (20 ×)

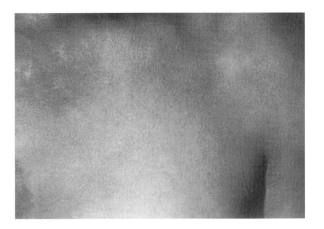

Figure 8   Hyperpigmented macules

scrubbing daily with rough nylon towels, vegetal fibers and brushes during bathing for long periods should be considered[20–23].

The most important differential clinical diagnosis is with macular amyloidosis, which affects the upper trunk in mainly older patients[22–25].

Friction melanosis has been considered by some authors to be an early stage of macular amyloidosis, owing to the basal cell layer damage. The damaged keratinocytes can potentially produce amyloid deposits (amyloid K)[25–27]. Some cases can be confused clinically with other acquired pigmentary disorders such as ashy dermatosis, confluent and reticulated papillomatosis, which are also of unknown etiology.

Management

There is no specific treatment. Avoiding scrubbing or rubbing habits during bathing is the main preventive in predisposed individuals. It is usually refractory to any measures of treatment.

ASHY DERMATOSIS

This is sometimes called erythema dyschromicum perstans.

Clinical description

Ashy dermatosis affects young women around 33 years of age. It predominates in skin types IV and V[28–32]. It is an uncommon disease. The lesions are located on the trunk and upper limbs in a bilateral and symmetric disposition. They consist of

Table 1   Lenticular acral keratosis: differential diagnosis (%). From reference 4

	Acrokerato-elastoidosis	Focal acral hyperkeratosis	Marginal keratoelastoidosis	Occupational lenticular acral keratosis*
Onset before age 20 years	57	87	0	40
Familial incidence	57	40	0	20
Caucasian	79	0	95	0
Black	7	100	5	0
Mestizo	11	0	?	100
Hand involvement	96	100	100	100
Feet involvement	61	100	0	0
Elastorrhexis	36	0	0	0
Actinic elastosis	4	0	100	0
Collagen densification	36	0	29	0

*Column not included in reference 4

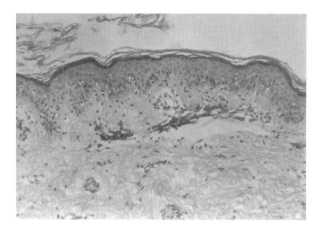

Figure 9 Hyperpigmentation and vacuolization of the basal cell layer. A slight perivascular lymphohistiocytic infiltrate in the dermis (20 ×)

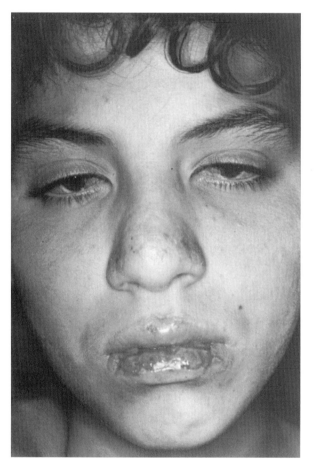

Figure 10 Polymorphic lesions on sun-exposed areas of the face. Note the involvement of the conjunctiva and lips

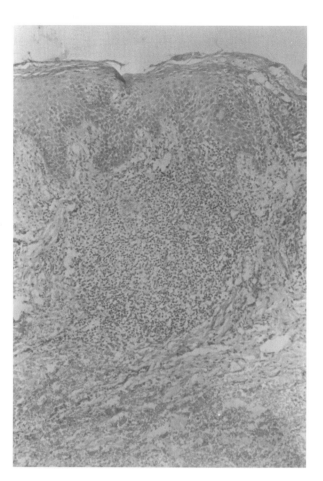

Figure 11 A dense lymphocytic infiltrate in a follicular pattern with germinal centers (lip biopsy, 10 ×)

hyperpigmented macules and patches with a grayish-blue (ashy) hue and variable shapes and sizes. At an early stage they can show an erythematous active border, sometimes elevated and polycyclic in configuration, that eventually disappears. The hyperpigmented macules are asymptomatic and have a chronic course (Figure 8)[28–32].

The histopathology is non-specific, showing hyperkeratosis, a slightly flattened and irregular epidermis, vacuolization and hyperpigmentation of the basal cell layer. A slight perivascular lymphohistiocytic infiltrate with melanophages can be seen in the dermis[28–30] (Figure 9).

There are no specific laboratory studies to confirm the diagnosis. Although the etiology is unknown, an immunological etiology is suspected. Immunohistochemical studies have shown an increased expression of ICAM-1 and HLA-DR in the basal keratinocytes of the erythematous active border of the lesions, while the keratinocytes of the upper epidermal layers expressed CD36 thrombopostin receptor, usually not present in normal skin. The dermal infiltrate showed mainly CD8 positive cells (90%), also expressing the activating molecule AIM/CD69 and the CD94 cytotoxic cell marker[33,34].

The keratinocytes from the inactive lesions did not show increased expression of ICAM-1, HLA-DR, CD36 or CD69, although an increased number of Langerhans cells was seen after treatment with clofazimine[33,34].

Management

There is no specific treatment. Keratolytics, topical steroids, oral antimalarials and sunscreens have been tried with variable results. Clofazimine in doses of 200 to 300 mg/week has been reported to be beneficial. The orange-brown pigmentation resulting from clofazimine use camouflages the lesions. The immunomodulatory and anti-inflammatory effects of clofazimine are suspected to be beneficial in ashy dermatosis[34].

ACTINIC PRURIGO

Synonyms are light-sensitive eruption in American Indians[35], solar prurigo[36], solar dermatitis[37], familial actinic prurigo[38], hereditary polymorphic light eruption of American Indians[39], polymorphous light eruption: prurigo type[40], solar prurigo of high plateau[41] and Guatemalan cutaneous syndrome[42].

Clinical description

The lesions are polymorphic and characterized by macules, papules, plaques, eczema and lichenification on sun-exposed areas of the face, neck and upper limbs; the lips and conjunctiva are frequently involved (Figure 10).

Pruritus is always present, and as a result patients present secondary lesions such as exulcerations, crusts, lichenification and residual hyperpigmentation.

It affects mestizo women (Amerindians) predominantly with skin types IV and V. The signs appear early in life between 6 and 8 years of age, and have a chronic course with partial or no remissions, especially in tropical countries where there is sun all year long[43]. The histopathology has been considered to be non-specific, but some reports have shown distinctive characteristics: epidermal hyperkeratosis, regular acanthosis and a dense lymphocytic infiltrate with a follicular pattern with germinal centers, although in some cases the infiltrate tends to be arranged in a 'band-like' disposition[44] (Figure 11).

The immunohistochemistry of the infiltrates has shown the presence of B and T lymphocytes. In the lymphoid follicles B cells are in the center and T cells in the periphery[45].

Tumor necrosis factor-α (TNF-α) immunoreactivity has been observed in keratinocytes in all suprabasal layers and in inflammatory cells (monocytes, macrophages, dendrocytes) in the superficial dermis and in the vicinity of the lymphoid follicles. Extracellular deposits of IgM, IgG and C3 were present in the papillary dermis[46]. The increase of total T cells, T helper and Ia antigen-marked cells in the infiltrates suggest an abnormal immune response in the skin[47].

The immunogenetic studies suggest a genetic predisposition influenced by ethnic ancestry. A high prevalence of HLA-A24 and HLA-C4 has been reported in Cree Indians in Canada[48], and HLA-C4 in Chimila Indians of Colombia[49], whereas in Mexican mestizos, HLA-28 and HLA-DR4 are most frequent[50].

The clinical lesions can be reproduced by repeated exposure of uninvolved skin to artificial UVA and/or UVB light[51].

Differential diagnoses include entities such as polymorphous light eruption, photosensitized atopic dermatitis and chronic photocontact dermatitis[52]. Most of the American and European authors consider actinic prurigo to be a variant of polymorphous light eruption[39,47]. Polymorphous light eruption has a worldwide distribution, affects all races and presents seasonal remissions and recurrences.

Photosensitized atopic dermatitis patients have a familial or personal atopic history and present other atopic skin signs such as xerosis and ichthyosis. They usually respond to antihistaminics and topical steroids, in contrast to patients with actinic prurigo who respond poorly to these agents.

Chronic photocontact dermatitis is very common in underdeveloped countries where self-medication with over-the-counter medicines and home remedies with photosensitizing potential such as vegetables and plants are a common practice, leading to chronic photosensitized dermatoses. The diagnosis can be supported by photopatch testing.

Management

Sun exposure avoidance and adequate clothing protection is crucial. This is especially difficult when the affected individuals have low socioeconomic status and have to work outdoors.

Antihistaminics, antimalarials[53,54], β-carotenes[55,56], PUVA[57–59] and systemic and topical steroids provide temporary relief[60]. The most effective drug for the treatment of actinic prurigo is thalidomide; its effect lasts while the patient is taking the drug, but relapses are frequent after discontinuation. The recommended dose is 100 mg/day. Adequate contraceptive measures are mandatory[61–63].

REFERENCES

1. Costa OG. Acrokeratoelastoidosis. Presented at the meeting of the *Minas Gerais Branch of the Brazilian Society of Dermatology*, September 1952, and at the *10th Brazilian Congress of Hygiene*, Belo Horizonte, Brazil, October 1953

2. Costa OG. Acrokeratoelastoidosis. *Arch Dermatol* 1954;70:228–31

3. Waxtein ML, Teixeira F, Cortes FR, *et al.* Lenticular acral keratosis in washerwomen. *Int J Dermatol* 1998;37:532–7

4. Zukervar P, Vigneaud H, Balme B, Perrot H. Acrokérato-élastoïdose. A propos dúne forme atypique. *Nouv Dermatol* 1990;9:544–5

5. Masse R, Quillard A, Hery B, *et al.* Acrokeratoelastoidose de Costa. *Ann Dermatol Venereol* 1977; 104:441–5

6. Civatte J, Hincky M, Barranger C, *et al.* Acrokéato-élastoïdose. *Ann Dermatol Venereol* 1977;104:877–8

7. Civatte J, Mousset S, Marinho E, Zeraffa J. Acrokéato-élastoïdose. *Ann Dermatol Venereol* 1982;109:757–8

8. Mathews CNA, Harman RRM. Acrokeratoelastoidosis in a Somerset mother and her two sons. *J Dermatol* 1977;42:42–3

9. Andersen BL, Bierring F. Acrokerato-elastoidosis: a case report. *Acta Derm Venereol (Stockh)* 1981;61: 79–82

10. Highet AS, Rook A, Anderson JR. Acrokeratoelastoidosis. *Br J Dermatol* 1982;106:337–44

11. Nelson-Adesokan P, Mallory SB, Lombardi C, Robert L. Acrokeratoelastoidosis of Costa. *Int J Dermatol* 1995;34:431–3

12. Redondo Mateo J, Niembro de Rasche E. Acrokeratoelastoidosis. *Med Cut Ilero Latino Am* 1990;18: 245–8

13. Dowd PM, Harman RRM, Black MM. Focal acral hyperkeratosis. *Br J Dermatol* 1983;109:97–103

14. Kocsard E. Keratoelastoidosis marginalis of the hands. *Dermatologica* 1965;131:169

15. Burks JW, Wise LJ, Clark WH. Degenerative collagenous plaques of the hands. *Arch Dermatol* 1960;82:362–6

16. Ritchie EB, Williams HM Jr. Degenerative collagenous plaques of the hands. *Arch Dermatol* 1966;93: 202–4

17. Asai Y, Hamada T, Suzuki N, *et al.* Acquired hyperpigmentation distributed on the skin over the bones. *Jpn J Dermatol* 1983;93:405–14

18. Hidano A, Mizuguchi M, Higaki Y. Mélanose de friction. *Ann Dermatol Venereol* 1984;111:1063–71

19. Tanigaki T, Hata S, Kitano Y, *et al.* Unusual pigmentation on the skin over trunk bones and extremities. *Dermatologica* 1985;170:235–9

20. Amador ME, Arenas R, Navarrete G, *et al.* Melanosis por fricción. Estudio clínico-patológico de 17 casos. *Dermatol Rev Mex* 1988;32:15–21

21. Magaña-García M, Carrasco E, Herrera-Goepfert R, *et al.* Hyperpigmentation of the clavicular zone: a variant of friction melanosis. *Int J Dermatol* 1989;28:119–22

22. Domínguez-Soto L, Hojyo Tomoka MT, Vega Memije ME, *et al.* Pigmentary problems in the tropics. *Dermatol Clin* 1994;12:777–84

23. Wong CK, Lin CS. Friction amyloidosis. *Int J Dermatol* 1988;27:302–7

24. Hashimoto K, Ito K. Nylon brush macular amyloidosis. *Arch Dermatol* 1987;123:633–7

25. Kobayashi H, Hashimoto K. Amyloidogenesis in organ-limited cutaneous amyloidosis: an antigenic identity between epidermal keratin and skin amyloid. *J Invest Dermatol* 1983;80:66–72

26. Iwasaki K, Mihara M, *et al.* Bifasic amyloidosis in frictional melanosis. *J Dermatol* 1991;18:86–91

27. Sumitra S, Yesudian P. Friction amyloidosis: a variant or an etiologic factor in amyloidosis? *Int J Dermatol* 1993;32:422–3

28. Ramírez O. The ashy dermatosis (erythema dyschromicum perstans). Epidemiological study and report of 139 cases. *Cutis* 1967;3:244–7

29. Vega-Memije ME, Waxtein ML, Arenas R, *et al.* Ashy dermatosis and lichen planus pigmentosus: a clinico-pathologic study of 31 cases. *Int J Dermatol* 1992;31:90–4

30. Convit J, Piquero-Martin J, Pérez RM. Erythema dyschromicum perstans. *Int J Dermatol* 1989;28: 168–9

31. Vega-Memije ME, Waxtein ML, Arenas R, *et al.* Ashy dermatosis vs lichen planus pigmentosus: a controversial matter. *Int J Dermatol* 1992;31:87–8

32. Domínguez-Soto L, Cortés-Franco R, Vega-Memije ME, *et al.* Dermatosis cenicienta. Experiencia del Departamento de Dermatología del Hospital 'Gea González' de la ciudad de México. *Arch Argent Dermatol* 1998;48:109–13

33. Baranda L, Torres-Alvarez B, Cortés-Franco R, *et al.* Involvement of cell adhesion and activation molecules in the pathogenesis of erythema dyschromicum perstans (ashy dermatitis). The effect of clofazimine therapy. *Arch Dermatol* 1997;133:325–9

34. Piquero-Martin J, Pérez-Alfonso R, Abrusci V, *et al.* Clinical trial with clofazimine for treating erythema dyschromicum perstans. Evaluation of cell mediated immunity. *Int J Dermatol* 1989;28:198–200

35. Everett MA, Crocket W, Lamb JH, *et al.* Light-sensitive eruption in American Indians. *Arch Dermatol* 1961;83:243–6

36. López-González G. Prúrigo solar. *Arch Argent Dermatol* 1961;11:301–18

37. Escalona E. *Dermatología. Lo esencial para el estudiante.* México: Impresiones Modernas SA, 1964;194

38. Londoño F, Murdi F, Giraldo F, *et al.* Familial actinic prurigo. *Dermatol Iber Lat Am* 1968;11:61–71

39. Birt AR, Davis RA. Hereditary polymorphic light eruption of American Indians. *Int J Dermatol* 1975;14:105–11

40. Hojyo-Tomoka MT, Domínguez-Soto L. Clinical and epidemiological characteristics of polymorphous light eruption. *Castellania* 1975;3:21–3

41. Flores O. Prúrigo solar de la altiplanicie. Resultados preliminares del tratamiento con talidomida en 25 casos. *Dermatol Rev Mex* 1975;19:26–39

42. Cordero CFA. Síndrome cutáneo Guatemalense en la dermatitis actínica. *Med Cut ILA* 1976;4:393–400

43. Hojyo-Tomoka MT, Vega-Memije E, Granados J, *et al*. Actinic prurigo: an update. *Int J Dermatol* 1995;34:380–4

44. Vega ME. Características histopatológicas del prúrigo actínico. *Dermatol Rev Mex* 1993;37 (suppl 1):295–7

45. Guevara E, Hojyo-Tomoka MT, Vega-Memije ME, *et al*. Estudio inmunohistoquímico para demostrar la presencia de linfocitos T y B en el infiltrado inflamatorio de las biopsias de piel, labio y conjuntiva de pacientes con prúrigo actínico. *Dermatol Rev Mex* 1997;41:223–6

46. Arrese JE, Vega Memije ME, Cortés-Franco R, *et al*. Effectors in inflammation in actinic prurigo. *J Am Acad Dermatol* 2000;in press

47. Moncada B, González-Amaro R, Baranda L, *et al*. Immunopathology of polymorphous light eruption. *J Am Acad Dermatol* 1984;10:970–3

48. Sheridan DP, Lane PR, Irvine J, *et al*. HLA typing in actinic prurigo. *J Am Acad Dermatol* 1990;22:1019–23

49. Bernal JE, Durán MM, Ordoñez CO, *et al*. Actinic prurigo among Chimila Indians in Colombia: HLA studies. *J Am Acad Dermatol* 1990;22:1049–51

50. Hojyo-Tomoka MT, Granados J, Vargas-Alarcon G, *et al*. Further evidence of the role of HLA-DR4 in the genetic susceptibility to actinic prurigo. *J Am Acad Dermatol* 1997;36:935–7

51. Hojyo-Tomoka MT. Pruebas fotobiológicas en prúrigo actínico. *Dermatol Rev Mex* 1993;37(suppl 1):295–7

52. Hojyo-Tomoka MT. Prúrigo actínico: diagnóstico diferencial. *Dermatol Rev Mex* 1993;37(suppl 1):303

53. Cahn MM, Levy EJ, Shaffer B. The use of chloroquine diphosphate (Aralen) and quinacrine (Atabrine) hydrochloride in the prevention of polymorphous light eruptions. *J Invest Dermatol* 1954;22:93–6

54. Knox JM. Use and abuse of antimalarials in the treatment of light induced diseases. In Pathak MA, Fitzpatrick TB, eds. *Sunlight and Man*. Tokyo: University of Tokyo, 1974;779

55. Swanbeck G, Wennersten G. Treatment of polymorphous light eruption with beta-carotene. *Acta Derm Venereol (Stockh)* 1972;52:462–4

56. Nordland JJ, Klaus SN, Mathews-Roth MM. A new therapy for polymorphous light eruption. *Arch Dermatol* 1973;108:710–13

57. Schenck RR. Controlled trial of methoxsalen in solar dermatitis in Chipewa Indians. *JAMA* 1960; 172:1134–5

58. Parrish JA, Levine MJ, Morrison Wl, *et al*. Comparison of PUVA and beta-carotene in the treatment of polymorphous light eruption. *Br J Dermatol* 1979;100:187–91

59. Gschnait G, Honigsman H, Brener W, *et al*. Induction of UV light tolerance by PUVA in patients with polymorphous light eruption. *Br J Dermatol* 1978;99:293–5

60. Lane PP, Moreland AA, Hogan DJ. Treatment of actinic prurigo with intermittent short course of topical 0.05% clobetasol 17-propionate. *Arch Dermatol* 1990;126:11–13

61. Londoño F. Thalidomide in the treatment of actinic prurigo. *Int J Dermatol* 1973;12:326–8

62. Saul A, Flores O, Novales J. Polymorphous light eruption: treatment with thalidomide. *Australas J Dermatol* 1976;17:17–21

63. Vega ME, Hojyo-Tomoka MT, Domínguez-Soto L. Tratamiento del prúrigo actínico con talidomida: estudio de 30 pacientes. *Dermatol Rev Mex* 1993;37(suppl 1):342–3

Miscellaneous topics

Battered women and children   43

Karolina M. Leonik and Tomasz F. Mroczkowski

Violence against women has been called a national epidemic in the USA. Political leaders and governments and medical authorities around the globe are searching for appropriate solutions to this problem[1,2]. Fifty per cent of all women in America have reported being battered at some point in time and one in five reports regular assaults[3]. It is estimated that domestic violence may occur in as many as one of every four American families[4]. By some estimates, 3–4 million women are assaulted by male partners each year in the USA, and in only approximately 10% of these cases is the assault followed by effective protection or permanent estrangement from the aggressor. A large majority of these beatings are reported to be part of an identifiable pattern of ongoing, systematic and usually escalating abuse that often extends over a long period of time[5,6].

Violence against women by their intimate partners is a leading cause of injury and death to women not only in the USA but worldwide[7]. Half of battered women suffer serious injuries at the hands of their husbands, boyfriends or former partners, and 2–4 thousand lose their lives each year as a result of battery[8]. Almost 30% of the women who are murdered are killed by their partners[9].

BATTERER AND BATTERED

Battering men and battered women occur in families of every racial and religious background and in all socioeconomic strata, although younger, lower income, less-educated men who have observed parental violence in their own homes, or were abused themselves as children, are at higher risk of abusing their spouses[8,10]. Other risk factors for men include antisocial personality disorder, depression, and/or alcohol and drug abuse[8]. Abusive husbands tend to be immature, dependent and non-assertive, and to suffer from a strong feeling of inadequacy. Their aggression is bullying behavior, designed to humiliate their spouses to improve their own low self-esteem, and the abuse is most likely to occur when the man feels threatened or frustrated at home, at work, or with peers. Frequently, abusive husbands physically displace aggression provoked by others onto their wives[8,10–13].

Battered women, on the other hand, show no consistent prebattering risk markers, other than a history of parental violence in their family of origin, psychiatric history, divorce, marriage counseling and a trait of strong dependency[10,11,13]. As with battering men, women of all social classes, educational levels and ethnic groups are battered. While younger women are more likely to be battered than older women[11], age is no protection, since the battering of wives accounts for a significant amount of elder abuse[14]. Pregnancy is also no protection against being battered; in fact, it appears to increase the risk of battering[15,16].

The act of battery itself is reinforcing. Once a man has beaten his wife, he is likely to do so again. When an abused wife tries to leave her oppressor, he often becomes doubly intimidating; however, some may feel remorse and guilt after an episode of violent behavior and become particularly loving. This frequently gives a battered wife false hope and she remains until the next cycle of violence, which inevitably occurs.

The most common myth about battered women is that they do not leave violent relationships and are being masochistic. The implications of this belief are that she asks for it; she enjoys being beaten; it is her own fault; she should control the batterer's behavior; and, finally, if she doesn't like being beaten why doesn't she leave? In fact, most battered women do eventually leave, and the reasons for procrastination are very prosaic. Some try desperately to preserve the family in order to provide a father for their children. Others lack economic resources and the independent ability to provide for themselves and their children. In some instances, a woman defers leaving because of the fear that her husband or partner will carry out his threats to kill her, or himself, or the children, or all of them, if she does leave. While any or all of these reasons may account for an individual decision to stay in a violent relationship, many battered women do make active and continued efforts to stop the violence, including, ultimately, leaving[8,17].

BATTERING INJURIES

Battered women are struck with fists, hands and tools. They are grabbed (Figure 1), choked, slammed against the walls, beaten in the head, the neck, the abdomen and breasts. When knocked down they are kicked or stepped upon. Some battered women are stabbed, shot or imprisoned. Many of them are sexually assaulted in various ways[18–23].

The most characteristic assault in woman-battering is punching of the head, face and arms (69%), followed by kicking (21%), knocking down (15%), choking (15%) and head-banging against the wall or floor (11%) (Table 1). High percentages of women are struck with weapons; this is far more common in the USA, where a firearm is a common feature of an American household. It should be emphasized that a typical assaultive episode involves a combination of assaultive acts combined with verbal abuse and threats.

Injury pattern

Violence against women usually results in multiple soft tissue injuries, which often appear to be of varying age, owing to the cyclic course of repeated periods of physical violence[24]. The scope of injuries ranges from minor cuts or bruises, black eyes (Figure 2), concussions, broken bones and miscarriages to permanent injuries such as damaged joints, decreased or loss of hearing or vision, and scars from burns or bites or knife wounds. Several studies have concluded that there are specific injury types that are more common in battered women than in those injured by other causes[19,23]. Table 2 lists the differences in injury location between battered women and other injured women for whom injury location and types were known[23]. The most common sites of injuries in battered women are the face and head, followed by injuries to the torso, spine and abdomen, whereas women injured by other mechanisms (usually accidents) are more likely to be injured in the spine and lower extremities[24].

The most common lesions encountered among battered women are bruises and abrasions (Figure 3), followed by fractures, concussion, eardrum perforation and thoracic and abdominal injuries (Table 3). These are also the injury types often found among emergency room patients but, when compared to location and lesion type found in women injured by other mechanisms, some specific injury types appear to be more frequent in the first group[24].

Because many physicians do not routinely screen for battering, and women frequently do not acknowledge the cause of their injuries voluntarily, the presence of specific injuries and their distribution should alert clinicians to probe more deeply

Table 1 Mechanism of battering injuries[*]. Data from reference 19

Mechanism	%
Punching	69
Kicking	21
Knocking down	15
Choking (strangle grip)	15
Head banging	11
Striking with weapon	11
Rape	3
Other	11
Unknown	3

[*]Some women were exposed to more than one mechanism of violence

into the cause of injuries in female patients which may reveal domestic violence.

Psychological and social impact

As with other types of violent assault, the primary focus of the victim during domestic violence is on self-protection and survival. Initial psychological reactions include shock, denial, confusion, numbing and fear. Usually, during and shortly after battery, women offer little or no resistance in an attempt to reduce the threat of injury and to prevent new aggression. Long-term reactions include fear, anxiety, fatigue, sleeping and eating problems, and physical complaints. Battered women frequently become dependent and suggestible, and may find it difficult to make decisions alone[18]. Psychological trauma is exacerbated by the fact that the assailant is someone they love, trust and are dependent on. It is further complicated by the numerous relationships they have with their assailants, such as financial, legal and the 'role' relationship, all confounding their decision on what to do about the violence. Many battered women have a profound perception of vulnerability, loss, betrayal and hopelessness. A high prevalence of depression and suicide attempts is common[25].

SEXUAL ABUSE
Marital rape

Sexual abuse is a very serious form of marital violence. Numerous studies have found that women in the USA are more likely to be assaulted and injured, raped or killed by a current or ex- male sexual partner than by all other types of assailants combined[26–28]. In severely abusive relationships, violent sexual assault may occur as often as several times a month[18]. The National Victims Center estimated

Table 2 Injury location among battered women and caused by other mechanisms*. Data from reference 23

Body region	Battered patients		Control group†	
	n	%	n	%
Face	121	51.1	233	10.5
Head	55	23.2	129	5.8
Thorax	48	20.3	97	4.4
Lower extremities	43	18.1	696	31.5
Spine	34	14.4	506	22.9
Abdomen	29	12.2	31	1.4
Neck	5	2.1	3	0.1
Total	237		2211	

*Some women had injuries in more than one body region
†Total number of women presented to the emergency room for any reason

Table 3 Characteristic injuries found in battered women*. Data from reference 19

Type of injury	%
Bruises	77
Abrasions	48
Fracture(s)	12
Concussion	11
Eardrum perforation	5
Thoracic injury	2
Abdominal injury	1

*Some women had multiple injuries

that 9% of women have been raped by their husbands and ex-husbands, while other studies have put the estimate even higher[29]. Marital rape has been reported in relationships in which no other forms of physical abuse occur, and empirical research has shown that marital rape is an integral part of marital violence[26,30]. Marital rape is often accompanied by beatings or other forms of violence[27,31]. In one report, out of 137 women beaten by their husbands, 34% were subsequently raped as part of their 'punishment'[32]. Marital rape seems to be motivated by the same factors as any other rape – power, anger and sadism, and marital rape is not less criminal than rape committed by a stranger. Sexual abuse is reported by over one-third of women victims who are being physically assaulted by their partners and yet, except for child sexual molestation, it is the type of violence least likely to be reported by victims[18].

Sexual abuse causes both physical and psychological injury. It is possible to inflict an intense level of physical pain over a long period and to cause numerous injuries, from superficial bruises or tearing, to serious internal injuries. The psychological impact of sexual assault, especially by an intimate, can also be extreme. Many victims of marital rape suffer the same reactions as other rape victims and exhibit both severe physical and emotional sequelae, including severe depression and a tendency to suicide[18].

Sexual assault in a dating relationship (date rape)

Violence in a dating relationship until recently has been considered relatively non-serious and negligible. However, recent evidence on the prevalence, morbidity and increasing number of male-perpetrated homicides in these relationships have shed new light on this phenomenon[18].

The term 'date rape' is used to describe sexual assault that takes place during a social encounter agreed to by the victim. In most instances it is committed by a person the victim has known and thus is frequently called acquaintance rape. The term itself is unfortunate, because it may imply that it is somehow different from rape by a stranger. Some people are less sympathetic and attribute some blame to the victims of acquaintance rape – more than they would to victims of rape by a stranger. This also holds true for police and medical personnel, which may influence the patient's treatment. It should be made very clear that rape by a date or an acquaintance is no less real than rape by a stranger[33–35].

Sexual assault among dating and cohabiting couples is more prevalent than has been previously thought[36]. A survey of several thousand college students revealed that 42% of women students reported some type of sexual assault, from forcible sexual contact or attempted rape to completed rape[37]. Interestingly, the rate of rape victimization was reported to be about the same, regardless of the size of the school or its location

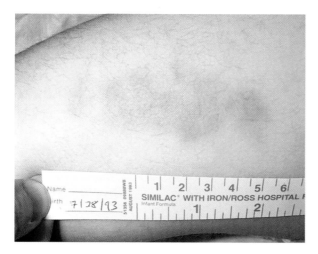

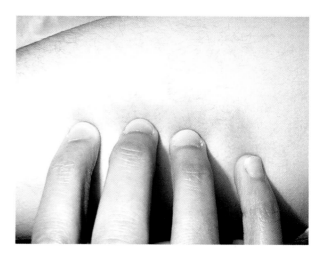

Figure 1 'Finger-tip' contusions consistent with a history of grabbing. Courtesy of Scott A. Benton, MD, New Orleans, LA

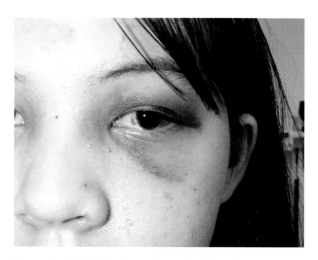

Figure 2 Periorbicular ecchymosis with subconjunctival hemorrhage after an assault. (Note the pupil dilated iatrogenically). Courtesy of Scott A. Benton, MD, New Orleans, LA

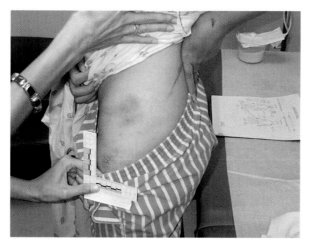

Figure 3 Multiple contusions to hip and thigh. Note the abrasion across the back. Acute sexual assault victim. Courtesy of Scott A. Benton, MD, New Orleans, LA

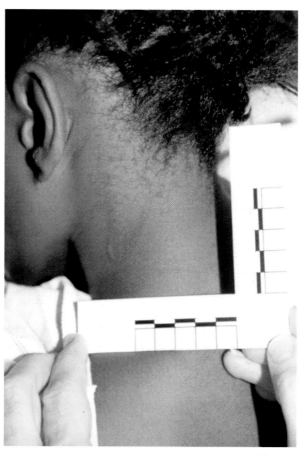

Figure 4 'Loop mark' to neck, indicative of whipping with a looped object. Courtesy of Scott A. Benton, MD, New Orleans, LA

(metropolitan, urban, or in rural areas). Rape victimization for females was highest in the 16–19-year-old age group, and the next highest was in the 20–24-year-old age group. Overall rates were approximately four times higher than the mean for all women[38]. Similarly to what has been reported for marital relationships, rapes and attempted rapes among dating couples involve greater levels of violence, resulting in more serious physical and psychological injuries than in non-sexual assault. Unfortunately, the rate of females killed by dating or cohabiting partners is quite substantial and still rising[18].

Rape

In the last two decades the legal definitions of rape have undergone numerous revisions and many statutes now define rape as the 'nonconsensual penetration of an adolescent or adult obtained by physical force, by threat of bodily harm, or when the victim is incapable of giving consent by virtue of mental illness or retardation or intoxication'[39]. FBI records show that there are over 100 000 reported cases of rape in the USA annually. Even though this is a large number, many researchers agree that the actual number of rapes committed each year is far higher. The Justice Department (Bureau of Justice Statistics, 1995) estimated that there are 170 000 rapes and 140 000 attempted rapes committed each year in the USA, while the National Victims Center estimates that there are over 600 000 rapes of adult women a year[33].

Although women between 16 and 24 years of age are the most frequently reported victims of rape (51% are under the age of 18), the record shows that anyone can be a victim of rape, including young girls, elderly women and even men[33]. Prevalence studies indicate that at least 20% of adult women, 15% of college women and 12% of adolescent girls have experienced sexual abuse and assault during their lifetime, with rates for African-American women even higher[40]. Some researchers estimate that a woman living in the USA has a one in four chance of being raped in her lifetime[41].

Psychological and medical impact of sexual abuse

Reactions to sexual abuse (rape) can be divided into two phases: the initial effect (an acute phase) which begins right after the rape and continues for several weeks, and the long-term effects. During the acute phase the victim's body has to recover from the physical damage that may have been caused by the rape and to begin to recover from the psychological damage that was done. The victim then enters a period of long-term reorganization (long-term effects) when the woman attempts to regain control of her life[18].

Initial effect

Initial reactions to sexual assault include shock, numbness, withdrawal and denial. Those raped by strangers typically fear their assailant(s) will return and harm them again. Victims of attacks by acquaintances or intimates are frequently stunned that someone known to them, whom they trusted, could attack them in this manner. In initial presentation to medical staff or police, victims often appear unnaturally calm and detached, or they may be crying or angry[18]. Many of them are shaking, and their skin temperature may be low. About one-fourth of rape victims suffer minor injuries, and about 4% are seriously injured[33]. Some victims become very expressive about their feelings while others experience severe depression, become fearful, or experience great anxiety. Some of the rape victims may demonstrate what is called a controlled reaction, as if they were trying to deny that the rapist had affected them in any way. Many women experience dissociative symptoms (detachment from other people, affect restriction, concentration problems), and the presence of these symptoms is associated with long-term post-traumatic stress syndrome[42]. Headaches, sleeplessness and/or restless behavior are not uncommon among rape victims. Typically there is a lessening of initial symptoms after the first 2 weeks, and the victim enters a denial phase in which there is an outward appearance of adjustment[18]. However, studies suggest a period, from 2 weeks to several months after the assault, in which symptoms return and may even intensify[43]. This may be the time when a raped woman begins a pattern of help-seeking for these symptoms, without informing those she contacts of the sexual assault that underlies them[18].

Long-term effects

Numerous studies document that the after-effects of sexual assault are persistent and can be long-lasting. Victims suffer from chronic anxiety and feelings of vulnerability, loss of control, and self-blame, even long after the incident has occurred[44]. Long-term reactions include anxiety, nightmares, catastrophic fantasies, feelings of alienation and isolation, and physical distress[18,37]. Many victims lose their desire for sex and have trouble becoming sexually aroused[45]. Some show a decreased frequency of sexual relations that lasts for years. Other long-term effects include mistrust of others, different phobias, depression, hostility and somatic symptoms[44]. Suicidal thoughts are common (33–50%)[18]. The psychological picture often meets criteria for the post-traumatic stress disorder (PTSD), the hall-marks of which include psychological numbing, intrusive re-experiencing of the trauma and psychological distress. Women with a history of prior victimization suffer especially severe after-effects[46].

Medical concerns

Immediate medical concerns include local and distant injuries, infections with sexually transmitted agents and possible impregnation. Physical injuries that result from sexual assault usually include soreness, bruises and vaginal and/or rectal and/or anal bleeding. Ongoing health concerns include gynecological trauma and hidden internal injuries.

While the risk of pregnancy resulting from rape is low (one pregnancy in 100 assaults of women of reproductive age), the risk of contracting one or more sexually transmitted diseases (STDs) is quite high[47]. Many studies have found that some rape victims are infected with sexually transmitted agents (2–13% have gonorrhea; 8–26% chlamydia; 5–22% trichomoniasis; 2% syphilis)[47–50]. Considering the high prevalence of these diseases among adolescents and young adults, it is obvious that not all of the infected victims who have been studied contracted the disease during rape. In some, the infection existed before the assault, whereas in others the infections were acquired from new partners in the interval between the assault and the time of testing. Nevertheless, some women do in fact contract STDs at the time of sexual assault[50,51].

Even though expert opinion is that the chance of being infected with the human immunodeficiency virus (HIV) during rape is very low[52], the risk of HIV infection is of increasing concern to rape victims. With the rising number of heterosexually transmitted cases of the acquired immunodeficiency syndrome (AIDS), one must take into account a possibility that the rape victims are at risk of being infected with all sexually transmitted agents, including HIV.

CHILD BATTERY

Children can be affected by home violence in two ways: first, by being witnesses to battery of their mothers (indirect assault); and second, by being directly assaulted.

Indirect assault

The effects of exposure to violence on children and teenagers can be enormous[53]. Children who witness violent assault on their mothers are at greater risk of cognitive and social problems as well as behavioral disorders, depression and aggression (predominantly boys) and a high likelihood of suffering assault themselves (predominantly girls)[54]. Those children who not only witness but are also attacked by their father's or their mother's lovers are at even higher risk of psychological, social and school problems[55]. Moreover, children who witness marital violence are more likely to consider violence as an appropriate means of solving conflicts in their future lives[56].

Exposure to violence affects children of all ages, including the very young. Many people erroneously assume that very young children are too young to know or remember what has happened. Recent research contradicts that belief and provides evidence that, even in the earliest phases of infant and toddler development, there is a clear association between exposure to violence and post-traumatic symptoms and disorders[57,58].

The first 3 years of life are characterized by very rapid and complex changes, in which developmental factors influence the young child's perception. Practically any traumatic experience at this age, such as exposure to violence, has a negative impact. Infants exposed to violence may demonstrate increased irritability, excessive screaming, sleep disturbances and fears of being alone. Exposure to trauma interferes with their normal development of trust and with the later emergence of autonomy through exploration[59]. Regression in developmental achievements such as toileting and language is common[57] as is evidence of PTSD symptoms[60].

Preschoolers often display hiding, shaking and stuttering, as well as excessive irritability and yelling. In this age group, somatic symptoms and behavioral regression are very common.

At school age, gender-related differences usually appear. Boys are more disruptive, are more aggressive and throw severe temper tantrums. Girls are more likely to become withdrawn, passive and clingy and/or to display a wide array of somatic symptoms. As they mature, they are more likely to be victims of physical violence from boys they date than are girls from non-violent homes. Similarly, the boys exposed to home violence are more likely to be physically violent to the girls they date and marry[8].

Children of school age often demonstrate anxiety and sleep disturbances after exposure to violence. Some of them have difficulty paying attention and concentrating, owing to frequently present intrusive thoughts. Both preschoolers and school-age children exposed to violence are less likely to explore their physical environment and play freely, showing less motivation to master their environment[53]. All children exposed to violence and who live in a violent environment generally show signs of PTSD that is often modified because of their age.

Direct assault

Direct assault on children includes physical abuse, neglect, and/or sexual exploitation. Unfortunately, all of these are far from rare, and every year more and more children suffer from abuse by their parents, close relatives and strangers.

The most conspicuous physical manifestations of direct child abuse are seen on the skin (Figure 4), although other organ injuries such as bone fractures, chest or abdominal injuries and ocular or intracranial hemorrhages are not uncommon[61]. As most of the injuries of child battery are visible on the skin, dermatologists should be particularly alerted, and should consider the possibility that they might have resulted from child abuse. This is very important, since children rarely volunteer information on abuse, being afraid of the consequences to themselves.

Suspicion that child abuse took place should be aroused by certain clinical features that are highly suggestive for battery. They are primarily related to the location and pattern of skin lesions. Other factors such as the presence of multiple lesions of different ages, or failure of new lesions to appear after child isolation, may suggest child abuse or neglect[62]. Lesions on the sides of the face, scalp, inner thighs, buttocks and genitals are more likely to be the result of battery than accidental[63]. The same can be said of some lesions on the ears, neck or extremities. Some lesions are considered pathognomonic for child battery, e.g. focal hair loss, which often results from jerking or dragging a child, lashes, cord or knife marks, rope burns or bruises. The latter often take the shape of recognizable objects (belt buckles, kitchen utensils, etc.)[64]. Moreover, bruises that include ecchymoses and hematomas that occur on the buttocks or in the genital area are rarely accidental and are most likely to be the result of an assault. Human bite marks are also pathognomonic for non-accidental trauma, and in most instances differ from dog bites or puncture wounds. The size and the shape of the mouth as well as the number of teeth allows one to distinguish between animal and human bites. All burns must also be assessed as to whether they were caused by accident or were intentional. Deep, crater-like changes are suggestive of

cigarette burns[65] (Figure 5); scald lesions caused by hot tap water could also be a sign of child abuse.

Many of the aforementioned skin lesions may not be individually pathognomonic of child battery; however, when viewed in the context of other injuries it may become obvious that physical assault is the only tenable diagnosis. It is also important to know that certain features of medical history may be very helpful in revealing child battery. Such elements as lack of concern by the person bringing the child to the medical facility, delay in seeking medical help, vague and inconsistent information about the cause of injuries, the account given not being compatible with the clinical picture, an abnormal reaction of a parent, e.g. hostility towards the medical staff, or abnormal demeanor of the child can be characteristic of child abuse. Occasionally, children themselves disclose the origin of an injury, making the process of establishing the diagnosis much easier.

SEXUAL ABUSE OF CHILDREN

Sexual abuse of children is more common than was previously thought, and recent data show that at least twice as many girls as boys are targeted as victims. Comprehensive reviews of many studies have estimated that sexual abuse of girls is 6–62% and of boys 3–31%[66,67]. The YWCA Rape Crises Program indicates that one out of every four girls and one out of every seven boys will be the victim of some form of sexual abuse before they reach the age of 18[68].

Many sexual contacts with children involve fondling of the genitals, and children, especially young ones, do not understand the sexual significance of these behaviors. However, recent studies have found that an increasingly greater proportion of child molestation cases involve vaginal, anal or oral sex[69,70].

Dermatological manifestations of sexual abuse in children

Intercrural intercourse with a young girl may produce no dermatological signs whatsoever. Occasionally swelling or patchy redness of the labia and perineum may occur; however, these signs are common in other conditions not related to sex, e.g. enuresis, poor hygiene, etc.[71] Sometimes the rounded labial contour may be flattened; again, this is not a reliable sign, since it can be caused by wearing tight clothing. A split of the posterior fourchette and subsequent scar can be the sign of molestation of a girl.

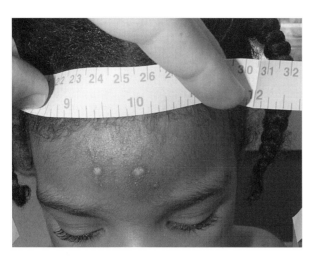

Figure 5   Healed cigarette burns on forehead of chronically abused and neglected child. Courtesy of Scott A. Benton, MD, New Orleans, LA

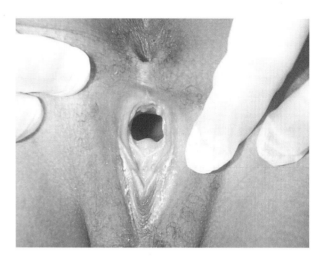

Figure 7   Knee chest view of introitus with posteriorly scarred hymen indicative of previous blunt penetrating trauma. Courtesy of Scott A. Benton, MD, New Orleans, LA

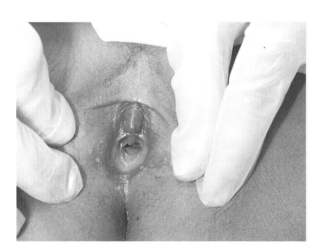

Figure 6   Supine view of introitus with posteriorly scarred hymen indicative of previous blunt penetrating trauma. Courtesy of Scott A. Benton, MD, New Orleans, LA

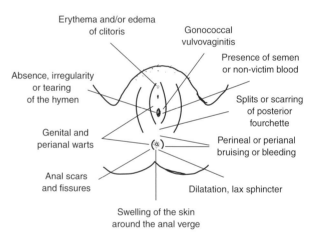

Figure 8   Dermatological findings in the genitoanal area that may indicate sexual child abuse

The pressure of a penis against the hymen may stretch it so the child may think that there has been penetration. Since the size of the erect penis is several times greater than the unstretched hymenal orifice, true vaginal penetration usually causes hymenal damage with significant bleeding and causing irregularity or tearing of the hymen[71] (Figures 6 and 7). Semen and blood of a group different from that of the child, if present within the vagina or rectum or on the perineum of a child, can be conclusive evidence of sexual abuse, but such cases are uncommon in forensic practice. Lubricants or hairs are of similar importance. Perineal bruising or bleeding without a credible explanation should be regarded as suspicious for sexual abuse.

In case of anal abuse multiple fissures due to overstretching of the sphincter may occur. Their extent is usually in proportion to the disparity in size between the assailant and the child, and the degree of force used. They may leave scars and skin tags[71], but it must be remembered that these should be distinguished from prominent folds in the anal canal. Swelling of the skin around and on the anal verge may be a sign of recent anal abuse, whereas thickening is seen after repeated abuse. The skin of the anal verge may become rounded and smooth. Veins in the skin may become dilated, giving a bruised appearance, but caution is needed in interpretation, since these may result from other disorders such as certain bowel diseases. However, if the bowel is normal and the child is free from any

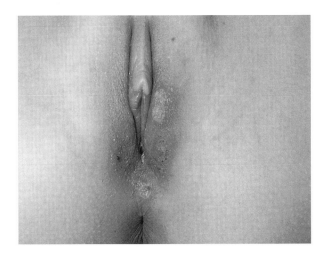

Figure 9 Herpes simplex infection in a prepubertal girl. Courtesy of Scott A. Benton, MD, New Orleans, LA

neurological diseases, abnormal anal dilatation may be indicative of anal abuse (penis penetration, use of foreign bodies, etc.)[71] (Figure 8).

The presence of sexually transmitted disease (STD) in children beyond the neonatal period is strongly suggestive of sexual abuse. Genital gonorrhea (in prepubertal girls, infection with *Neisseria gonorrhoeae* causes vulvovaginitis) is indicative of sexual contact with infected persons in 98% of instances. However, the presence of other STDs should be regarded with caution, as they can be transmitted in circumstances or conditions other than sexual intercourse[72]. Infection with *Chlamydia trachomatis* among children may be the result of perinatally acquired infection which can persist for as long as 3 years. Genital warts, bacterial vaginosis and genital mycoplasmas have been diagnosed in children who have been abused and in those not abused. Warts around the vaginal introitus or anus may be sexually transmitted, especially if caused by the human papilloma viruses (HPV) types 6 and 11. They usually produce condyloma acuminata which are different in appearance from common warts, and appear as multiple papules along the inner surface of the labia or circumferentially around the anus[72]. However, one must remember that parents or children who have common warts on their hands may infect the skin in the anogenital region by innocent handling or accidental autoinoculation, usually during toileting. In very young infants, the presence of genital warts can be explained as a result of infection acquired from infected mothers during passage through the birth canal.

Genital herpes in prepubertal children is relatively uncommon (Figure 9). Herpes simplex virus can be transmitted through sexual intercourse, but accidental inoculation into the skin of the anogenital region from lesions of other locations, e.g. the mouth or from a parent, cannot be ruled out.

As to the transmission of hepatitis B virus, there are several modes by which this is transmitted to children. The most common appears to be household exposure to persons who have chronic hepatitis B infection.

Psychological and social impact

The effects of sexual abuse in children include impact on emotions, on self-perception and on social functioning[73]. Approximately 20% of child molestation victims evidence serious long-term psychological effects[74]. These include disassociative responses and other PTSD indicators such as numbing of affect, chronic states of arousal, nightmares and flashbacks[74]. The prevalence of depression among adult survivors of child abuse is higher than among non-victims[18]. A high prevalence of suicide attempts and higher incidence of self-destructive behavior, both suicidal ideation and deliberate self-harm, has been found in adult survivors of child sexual abuse[18].

Those girls who have been sexually assaulted by their fathers or stepfathers appear to be at high risk for severe long-term sequelae[74]. The most troubling is the increased risk of these girls being re-victimized later in life (33–68%). Moreover, victims of child abuse are more likely to be physically abused by husbands and other adult partners[75].

Several somatic disorders, such as chronic abdominal pains, headaches and eating disorders, e.g. anorexia and bulimia, are more prevalent among victims of sexual child abuse, and female victims are also at higher risk for substance abuse and development of alcoholism than women without this childhood history[18,76].

MANAGEMENT OF BATTERED WOMEN AND CHILDREN

Management goals for battered women include the attainment of physical health, mental health and safety from further harm. Routine screening for domestic violence should be carried out at the entry point of contact between women and medical care, usually primary care, emergency services, obstetric/gynecological services, psychiatric services and pediatric care.

Women patients rarely volunteer a history of domestic violence when they see their physicians, and few primary care physicians question all female patients about the underlying causes of the injuries they treat. Treatment of symptoms alone may be ineffective for victims of violence, especially if assaults are ongoing and their sequelae continually recur. Failure to reveal domestic violence promptly may initiate a cyle of patient contacts with various doctors at various health service establishments, with the attendant risks of increasingly severe and debilitating sequelae for the patients.

The list of symptoms that have often been found in battered women is very long, and practically any complaint that women bring to a physician can be an indicator of abuse. Even though battered women experience certain injury types more frequently than women injured by other mechanisms (Table 3), the low positive predictive value of these injuries supports the use of universal screening for domestic violence in all injured women. Moreover, certain mental problems that are often the result of the battering of women such as affective and anxiety disorders, sleep disturbances, drug and alcohol abuse or chronic pains, justify inquiry about domestic violence as part of every routine clinical examination.

As a result of recommendations from the American Medical Association for routine inquiry about family violence, since January 1992 all emergency rooms have been required by the Joint Commission on Accreditation of Health Care Organizations (JCAHO) to have a protocol for inquiry about domestic violence.

After a disclosure of victimization, referral should be made as quickly as possible to specially trained staff within the setting, or to outside resources. Whenever possible, the resources should be 'trauma-specific', which means that rape victims should be referred to those with expertise in rape crisis and physically abused women and children should be referred to those with expertise in domestic violence. However, one should remember that referring a victim to counseling together with her assailant may be inappropriate, since the victim may resist discussing the issue, or may completely deny that a problem exists, in an attempt not to anger her batterer or endanger herself in the future. Interviews should be conducted in a safe environment, on a one-to-one basis, while encouraging the possibility of a follow-up visit.

The role of the dermatologist

The role of the dermatologist in the problem of battered women is usually secondary. Dermatologists are rarely primary-care or emergency-room physicians, but they may be asked for consultations in order to distinguish lesions caused by skin diseases and physical assault. Those dermatologists who specialize in cosmetic surgery may be asked to perform corrective surgery on the victims of domestic violence. In the USA, the UK and a few other countries, all dermatologists are trained in STDs. Therefore, they are frequently asked to evaluate and treat the victims of sexual assault for STDs.

EVALUATION FOR SEXUALLY TRANSMITTED INFECTION

Initial examination

According to the Centers for Disease Control and Prevention, an initial examination of sexual assault victims should include:

(1) Cultures for *Neisseria gonorrhoeae* and *Chlamydia trachomatis* from specimens collected from any sites of penetration or attempted penetration. If chlamydial culture is not available, non-culture tests can be performed, but a positive result should be verified with a second test based on a different diagnostic principle. Enzyme immunoassay and direct fluorescence antibody assay are not recommended in rape victims because of their lower reliability.

(2) Wet mount and culture for *Trichomonas vaginalis* and, in cases suggesting bacterial vaginosis (malodorous discharge), appropriate tests for bacterial vaginosis (clue cells, KOH test and others, if available).

(3) Collection of serum sample for evaluation for syphilis, HIV and hepatitis B.

Follow-up examination

Because of extended incubation periods for certain STDs, all tests performed during the initial visit, if negative, should be repeated 2 weeks after the assault, unless prophylactic treatment has already been provided.

Serological tests for syphilis and HIV infection should be repeated 6,12 and 24 weeks after the assault, if initial test results are negative.

Prophylaxis

Many experts recommend routine preventive therapy after a sexual assault. The following prophylactic regimen is recommended by the Centers for Disease Control[77].

(1) Post-exposure hepatitis B vaccination.
(2) An empirical antimicrobial treatment for gonorrhea, chlamydia, trichomoniasis and bacterial vaginosis:
   (a) ceftriaxone 125 mg intramuscularly in a single dose plus

(b) metronidazole 2 g orally in a single dose plus

(c) azithromycin 1 g orally in a single dose or

(d) doxycycline 100 mg orally twice a day for 7 days.

Other considerations

All victims of sexual assault should be counseled regarding symptoms of STDs and the need for immediate examination if symptoms occur. They should also be advised to refrain from any sexual activity until STD prophylactic treatment is completed.

Evaluation for STDs in children

The risk for a child's acquiring an STD as a result of sexual abuse has not been determined, but it is believed to be low. The decision to evaluate the child for STDs must be made on an individual basis. It should be considered if:

(1) A suspected offender is known to have an STD or be at high risk for STDs;

(2) The child has symptoms or signs of an STD;

(3) The prevalence of STDs in the community is high.

For more detailed information see reference 77.

REFERENCES

1. Jones RF. Domestic violence: let our voice be heard. *Obstet Gynecol* 1993;81:1–4
2. Marvick C. Health and justice professionals set goals to lessen domestic violence. *JAMA* 1994;271: 1147–8
3. Clarke PN, Pendry NC, Kim YS. Patterns of violence in homeless women. *West J Nurs Res* 1997;4:490–500
4. Novello AC, Rosenberg M, Saltzman L, Shosky J. From the Surgeon General, US Public Health Service. *JAMA* 1992;267:3132
5. Stark E, Flitcraft A. *Women at Risk. Domestic Violence and Women's Health.* Thousand Oaks, CA: Sage Publications, 1996;3
6. Dobash RE, Dobash R. Wives: the appropriate victims of marital violence. *Victimology* 1977/78;2: 426–42
7. Mills L. Empowering battered women transnationally: the case for postmodern interventions. *Soc Work* 1996;41:261–8
8. Keller LE. Invisible victims: battered women in psychiatric and medical emergency rooms. *Bull Menninger Clin* 1996;60:1–22
9. Margolin G, Sibner LG, Gleberman L. Wife battering. In Hasselt VB, Morrison RL, Black AS, *et al.*,

eds. *Handbook of Family Violence.* New York: Plenum Press, 1986
10. Burge SK. Violence against women as a health care issue. *Fam Med* 1989;21:368–73
11. Hotaling GT, Sugarman DB. An analysis of risk markers in husband to wife violence: the current state of knowledge. *Violence Victims* 1986;1:101–24
12. Dinwiddie SH. Psychiatric disorders among wife batters. *Compr Psychiatry* 1992;33:411–16
13. Appleton W. The battered women syndrome. *Ann Emerg Med* 1980;9:84–91
14. Arnold JF, Jeffries PF. Spouse abuse. In Taylor RB, ed. *Family Medicine. Principles and Practice.* New York: Springer-Verlag, 1983:202–6
15. McFarlane J, Parker B, Soeken K, Bullock L. Assessing for abuse during pregnancy. *JAMA* 1992;267:3176–8
16. Helton AS, McFarlane J, Anderson ET. Battered and pregnant: a prevalence study. *Am J Pub Health* 1987;77:1337–9
17. Pfouts JH. Violent families: coping responses of abused wives. *Child Welfare* 1978;57:101–11
18. Council on Scientific Affairs. Violence against women. Relevance for medical practitioner. *JAMA* 1992;263:3184–9
19. Bismar B, Bergman B, Larsson G, Strandberg A. Battered women: a diagnostic and therapeutic dilemma. *Act Chir Scand* 1987;153:1–5
20. Grisso JA, Wishner AR, Schwartz DF, *et al.* A population based study of injuries in inner-city women. *Am J Epidemiol* 1991;134:59–68
21. McLeer SV, Anwar R. A study of battered women presenting in an emergency department. *Am J Pub Health* 1989;79:65–6
22. Abbot J, Johnson R, Koziol-McLain J, *et al.* Domestic violence against women. Incidence and prevalence in an emergency department population. *JAMA* 1995;273:1763–7
23. Muelleman RL, Lenaghan PA, Pakieser RA. Battered women: injury locations and types. *Ann Emerg Med* 1996;28:486–92
24. Walker L. The battered woman. New York, NY: Harper and Row, 1979
25. Stark E, Flitcraft A. Violence against intimates: an epidemiological review. In Van Hasselt VB, Morrison RL, Bellack AS, Hersen M, eds. *Handbook of Family Violence.* New York, NY: Plenum Press, 1988:293–318
26. Russell DEH. *Rape in Marriage.* New York, NY: MacMillan Publishing, 1982
27. Finkelhorn D, Yllo K. *License to Rape: Sexual Abuse of Wives.* New York: Holt Rinehart & Winston, 1985
28. Browne A, Williams KR. Exploring the effect of resources availability and the likelihood of female-perpetrated homicides. *Law Soc Rev* 1989;23: 75–94
29. Russell DEH. *Rape in Marriage.* Bloomington, IN: Indiana University Press, 1990

30. Walker LE. *The Battered Woman Syndrome*. New York: Springer Publishing, 1984

31. Frieze IH, Browne A. Violence in marriage. In Ohlin L, Tonry M, eds. *Family Violence: Crime and Justice, A Review of Research*. Chicago: University of Chicago Press, 1989:163–218

32. Frieze IH. Investigating the causes and consequences of marital rape. *Signs* 1983;8:532–53

33. King BM. Sexual abuse. In *Human Sexuality Today*. Saddler River, NJ: Prentice Hall, 1996:343–77

34. Barnett MA. Factors affecting reactions to rape victim. *J Psychol* 1992;126:609–20

35. Bridges JS, McGrail CA. Attributions of responsibility for date and stranger rape. *Sex Roles* 1989; 21:273–86

36. Berkowitz A. College men as perpetrators of acquaintance rape and sexual assault: a review of recent research. *J Am Coll Health* 1992;40:175–81

37. Koss MP, Harvey M. *The Rape Victim: Clinical and Community Aproaches to Treatment*. Beverly Hills, CA: Sage Publications, 1991

38. Bureau of Justice Statistics. *Criminal Victimization in the United States. 1982*. Washington, DC: US Department of Justice, 1984

39. Searles P, Berger RJ. The current status of rape reform legislation: an examination of state statutes. *Wom Rights Law Reporter* 1987;9:25–43

40. Koss MP. Hidden rape: sexual aggression and victimization in a national sample of students in higher education. In Burgess AW, ed. *Rape and Sexual Assault*. New York: Gorland Publishing, 1988;2:3–25

41. Russell DEH, Howell N. The prevalence of rape in the United States revisited. *Signs* 1983;8:688–95

42. Foa EB, Riggs DS. Posttraumatic stress disorder following assault: theoretical considerations and empirical findings. *Curr Dir Psychol Sci* 1995;4: 61–5

43. Forman B. Psychotherapy with rape victims. *Psychother Theory Res Pract* 1980;17:304–11

44. Resick P, Calhoun K, Atkenson B, *et al.* Adjustment in victims of sexual assault. *J Consult Clin Psychol* 1981;49:705–12

45. Gilbert B, Cunningham J. Women's post rape sexual functioning: review and implications for counseling. *J Counsel Dev* 1987;65:71–3

46. Sorenson SB, Golding JM. Depressive sequelae of recent criminal victimization. *J Trauma Stress* 1990; 3:1154–64

47. Davis AG, Clay JC. Prevalence of sexually transmitted disease infection in women alleging rape. *Sex Transm Dis* 1992;19:298–300

48. Estreich S, Forster GE, Robinson A. Sexually transmitted diseases in rape victims. *Genitourin Med* 1990;66:433–8

49. Glaser JB, Hammerschlag MR, McCormack WM. Epidemiology of sexually transmitted diseases in rape victims. *Rev Infect Dis* 1989;11:246–54

50. Jenny C, Hooton TM, Bowers A, *et al.* Sexually transmitted diseases in victims of rape. *N Engl J Med* 1990;322:713–16

51. Glaser JB, Schachter J, Benes S, *et al.* Sexually transmitted diseases in postpubertal female rape victims. *J Infect Dis* 1991;164:726–30

52. Hearst N, Hulley SB. Preventing the heterosexual spread of AIDS: are we giving our patients the best advice? *JAMA* 1988;259:2428–32

53. Osofsky JD. The effects of exposure to violence on young children. *Am Psychol* 1995;9:782–8

54. Rosenbaum A, O'Leary D. Children: the unintended victims of marital violence. *Am J Orthopsych* 1981;51:692–699

55. Hughes H. Psychological and behavioral correlates of family violence in child witnesses and victims. *Am J Orthopsychiatry* 1988;58:77–90

56. Jaffe PG, Wilson SK, Wolfe D. Specific assessment and intervention strategies for children exposed to wife battering: preliminary empirical investigation. *Can J Community Ment Health* 1989;7:157–63

57. Drell M, Siegel C, Gaensbauer T. Post-traumatic stress disorder. In Zeanah C, ed. *Handbook of Infant Mental Health*. New York, NY: Guilford Press, 1993:291–304

58. Osofsky JD, Cohen G, Drell M. The effects of trauma on young children: a case of two-year-old twins. *Int J Psychoanal* 1995;76:595–607

59. Osofsky JD, Fenichel E. *Caring for Infants and Toddlers in Violent Environment: Hurt, Healing and Hope*. Arlington VA: Zero to three/National Center for Clinical Infant Programs, 1994

60. Scheeringa MS, Zeanah CH, Drell M, Larrieu JA. Two approaches to the diagnosis of posttraumatic stress disorder in infancy and early childhood. *J Am Acad Child Adolesc Psychiatry* 1995;34:191–200

61. Ellerstein NS. The cutaneous manifestations of child abuse and neglect. *Am J Dis Child* 1979;133:906

62. Reece RM, Grodin MA. Recognition of non-accidental injury. *Pediatr Clin North Am* 1985;32: 41–60

63. Pascoe JM, Hildebrandt HM, Tarrier A. Patterns of skin injury in non-accidental and accidental injury. *Pediatrics* 1979;64:245–7

64. Raimer BG, Raimer SS, Herbeler JR. Cutaneous signs of child abuse. *J Am Acad Dermatol* 1981; 5:203–12

65. Hobbs CJ. ABC of child abuse: burns and scalds. *Br Med J* 1989;298:1302–5

66. Peters SD, Wyatt GE, Finkelhorn D. Prevalence. In Finkelhorn D, ed. *A Source of Child Sexual Abuse*. Beverly Hills CA: Sage, 1986:15–59

67. Laumann E, Michael R, Gagnon J, Michaels S. *The Social Organization of Sexuality. Sexual Practice in the United States*. Chicago, IL: University of Chicago Press, 1994

68. Becker JV, Coleman EM. Incest. In Van Hasselt VB, Morrison L, Bellack AS, Hersen M, eds. New York: Plenum Press, 1988

69. Moore KA, Nord CW, Peterson JL. Nonvoluntary sexual activity among adolescents. *Fam Plann Perspect* 1989;21:110–14

70. Leventhal JM. Have there been changes in the epidemiology of sexual abuse in children during the 20th century? *Pediatrics* 1988;82:766–73

71. Bamford F, Roberts R. Child sexual abuse II. *Br Med J* 1989;299:377–82

72. Mroczkowski TF. *Sexually Transmitted Diseases.* New York, NY: Igaku-Shoin Medical Publisher, 1990

73. Gold E. Long-term effects of sexual victimization in childhood: an attributional approach. *J Consult Clin Psychol* 1986;54:471–5

74. Browne A, Finkelhorn D. The impact of child sexual abuse: a review of the research. *Psychol Bull* 1986; 99:66–77

75. Russell DEH. *The Secret Trauma: Incest in the Lives of Girls and Women.* New York, NY: Basic Book, 1986

76. Miller BA, Downs WR, Gondoli DM, Keil A. The role of childhood sexual assault in the development of alcoholism in women. *Violence Victims* 1987; 2:57–172

77. Sexual assault and STDs in 1998. Guidelines for treatment of sexually transmitted diseases. *Morbid Mortal Weekly Rep* 1998;47:108–16

Transsexuality

44

John A. Cotterill

---

*We live in kaleidoscopes of fragmented
and differing realities*[1]

INTRODUCTION

Skin is a major organ of communication and has been modified in three basic ways since time began: by scarification, by tattooing and by body painting. Indeed, these modifications can be regarded as a major feature distinguishing human beings from so-called lower animals[2]. Cutaneous communication is aided and abetted by modification of body hair, and scalp hair in particular, which can be easily utilized to irritate authority, whilst changes in shaving habits may be used in men to signal positive or negative changes in masculinity.

From the anthropological point of view, body painting becomes more widely practiced at times of love or during preparation for war. Modern cosmetics, as used in the developed world, could be regarded as an extension of body painting.

THE SKIN AND BODY IMAGE

Concepts about what is desirable in terms of body image vary, not only geographically, but also with time. For instance, the modern Miss World is taller and much slimmer, with smaller hips and smaller breasts, than her forerunner almost 90 years ago.

The skin of the ideal woman in the developed world must be odor-free, wrinkle-free, grease-free and spot-free. It should also be largely hair-free, apart from the scalp, eyebrows and eyelashes. Adipose tissue is definitely out, but large lips are now desirable. Whilst the cosmetic industry targets women in particular, there are also pressures on men to conform to accepted body image patterns, and so there is a definite market for calf expansion and penile augmentation.

The cosmetic industry encourages women to be infantile about their body image. The shelves in many supermarkets and pharmacies contain products labelled 'baby oil', 'baby talc' or 'baby shampoo'. These products are not intended primarily for babies, but are encouraging women to be infantile about their skin care.

As far as body image is concerned, therefore, the woman of today is expected to deny nearly all her secondary sex characteristics in a quest for youthful, 'perfect' and babylike skin. In the writer's opinion, these social pressures are likely to be, at least in part, important in the pathogenesis of anorexia nervosa.

The skin is a very important part of the perception of body image. The most important skin body areas involved in image include the face, eyes, mouth, nose, hair, scalp, breasts in women and genital area in men. Body odor is also important in body image and usually largely cutaneous in origin. Individuals with a strong, positive body image usually have high self-esteem and confidence. Society demands that one should look good to feel good, and this is reflected by success within a society which responds to and rewards individuals with a positive body image. It is known, for instance, that individuals without acne have a better chance of gaining employment than those with acne[3], so individuals perceived as more attractive have numerous advantages over those perceived as less attractive. More worrying for the aging writer of this chapter is that outwardly attractive geriatric patients are looked after far better than those perceived as unattractive by their carers[4].

To achieve these advantages cosmetics can be used to reinforce an individual's body image. It has been postulated that everyone is unconsciously or consciously seeking to attain the status of a Confident Nude, and cosmetics may have a place in this quest[5].

A standard range of cosmetics has been evaluated to see how attractive they are when used by women or men in both day-time and night-time social situations. The one cosmetic used by women that was rated as the most attractive by men was perfume, both for night-time and for day-time use, whilst mascara gained the highest rating by women when rated both for use at night and during the day.

VULNERABLE PERSONALITY

Some individuals have a very vulnerable personality as far as body image, perception, self-esteem and confidence are concerned. In this type of situation even the slightest blemish can produce disparate misery in these anxious, obsessional, ruminating, mirror-checking, dermatologist-shopping individuals with low self-esteem. It is no coincidence that women with such personality traits often become beauticians and attract other women with similar personality characteristics.

Kathryn Phillips has estimated that up to 1.5% of Americans see themselves as ugly, i.e. 1.5% of Americans have a significant body image problem which they have not been able to modify using convectional techniques such as cosmetics[6].

The ultimate rejection of body image occurs when a man wants to become a woman, or a woman wants to become a man.

TRANSVESTISM, TRANSSEXUALISM AND GENDER DYSPHORIA

Transvestism, transsexualism and gender dysphoria are not uncommon. Anatomy is the ultimate proof of being a man or a woman, whilst gender is a more complex social issue[1].

Sex reassignment can be regarded as a biological fix. Men may be asked to prove their ability to take on a female role in society by undergoing a 1-year real-life test before surgery is offered.

The dermatologist and the transsexual

The dermatologist is likely to be consulted by a transsexual or potentially transsexual patient from time to time. The frequency with which this occurs depends on the interest of the individual dermatologist and, in particular, on whether he/she is sympathetic to transsexuals or not. The frequency of consultation also depends on whether there are psychiatrists in the immediate area who are seeing transsexuals on a regular basis for counseling about sex change operations and are organizing grooming clinics.

It is very important that the dermatologist refrains from adopting a moralist stance when confronted with this clinical situation. Doctors are there to help their patients and not to moralize. Almost all the patients are men wanting to become women; so far, the writer has never encountered a woman wanting a sex change to a man.

Transsexual patients present with three main areas of dermatological concern. The main problems experienced evolve around concerns about male pattern alopecia; unwanted body hair, including the beard, limbs and truck; and tattoos.

Tattoos

In the writer's experience, there is a high incidence of both amateur and professional tattoos in transsexual individuals and, moreover, these tattoos are often in highly visible areas. Obviously, a highly masculine type of tattoo in visible areas, such as the face, hands and arms, is unacceptable for an individual wanting to undergo a sex change. Such patients are referred to a dermatologist with a request for the tattoos to be removed.

The optimum way of removing an amateur tattoo is with the Q-switched frequency-doubled Nd : YAG laser emitting at 1064 nm or with the Q-switched ruby laser or Q-switched alexandrite laser. Most amateur tattoos respond satisfactorily to treatment and the average number of treatments is two to eight to achieve clearance in most patients, although in some patients a little ghosting of pigment remains.

Professional tattoos are more difficult to remove, particularly those containing green pigment, which may require more than 20 treatments with either the Q-switched ruby laser or Q-switched alexandrite laser. Even then, not all the green pigment may totally disappear.

It is very important that the patient's expectations regarding the treatment and eradication of the tattoos are realistic. Extensive professional tattoos may take a long time to treat and the final results may be less than perfect, so other ways of management may have to be looked at, including cosmetic camouflage.

Most potential health-care purchasers are not prepared to pay for tattoo removal in transsexuals, so there may be considerable economic pressures on individual transsexuals undergoing repeated treatment for tattoo removal.

Male pattern alopecia

Male pattern alopecia is a problem in a significant proportion of men wanting to become women. This hair loss may be arrested or helped to some extent by treatment with cyproterone acetate, which has the added bonus of inducing some breast growth and inhibiting secondary sex hair growth to some extent. Topical minoxidil may also be helpful, especially in individuals with fairly recent male pattern hair loss; however, as a practical proposition, a significant proportion of male transsexuals require wigs. In the UK wigs are prescribable on a National Health Service basis, but many purchasing authorities are now unwilling to provide wigs for transsexual individuals, who then have to buy their own.

Unwanted facial and body hair

Large doses of cyproterone acetate help contain hair growth in secondary sexual body areas to some extent, but there are requests from transsexuals that dermatologists remove unwanted facial hair, particularly in the beard and on the trunk and limbs, using lasers. There are several different laser systems which can be used, including the free-running ruby laser, the long pulse Nd : YAG laser, the Q-switched frequency-doubled Nd : YAG laser, with or without endogenous pigment, and even photodynamic therapy.

There have been no good long-term studies on the effect of these lasers on hair removal in the male transsexual. It is known, however, that hair in the male beard area is particularly difficult to treat, and many treatments will be necessary to achieve perhaps only a 50% clearance. Electrolysis may also have a part to play in the management of this problem, but many transsexuals with thick, coarse, black terminal hair have to resort to shaving on a regular basis.

CONCLUSION

A well-motivated dermatologist may be able to give some assistance to the transsexual in helping to modify and, possibly, in some instances, eliminate masculine cutaneous messages from the skin. It remains to be seen whether more recent antiandrogens such as finasteride, a selective 5α-reductase inhibitor, will have a place in management.

REFERENCES

1. Moynihan C. Theories in health care and research. Theories of masculinity. *Br Med J* 1998;317:1072–5
2. Scutt R, Gotch C. *Skin Deep. The Mystery of Tattooing.* London: Peter Davies, 1974:21–37
3. Cunliffe WJ. Unemployment and acne. *Br J Dermatol* 1986;115:386
4. Kligman AL, Graham JA. The psychology of cutaneous ageing. In Balin AK, Kligman AM, eds. *Ageing and the Skin.* New York: Raven Press, 1989:347–55
5. Ryan TJ. The confident nude – or – whither dermatology? *Dermatol Pract* 1987;5:8–18
6. Phillips KA. Body dysmorphic disorder. Data presented at the *6th International Congress – a Meeting of the European Society for Dermatology and Psychiatry,* Amsterdam, 1995

Use and abuse of tobacco, alcohol and drugs

45

Ronni Wolf

Cigarette smoking, an uncommon habit in 1900, escalated to dizzying proportions in the 20th century, peaking in 1964, when more than 40% of all adult Americans were habitual smokers. Since that time, smoking has decreased at a slow but steady rate; however, 28% of all adults in the Western world are still following Mark Twain's rules of 'not to smoke more than one cigar at a time...never to smoke when asleep, and never to refrain when awake'. The rates of smoking are even higher in underdeveloped areas of the world and in the developing nations.

Cigarette smoking, the chief preventable cause of illness and death in the Western world, continues to exact an enormous health toll on our society, being directly responsible for one in every five deaths each year. It is incumbent upon all those directly or indirectly involved with smoking and disease to become more active in this vital and challenging aspect of health care.

Although the deleterious effects of smoking on the skin pale into insignificance compared to the effects it has on other body systems, the range of damage caused to the skin by smoking cannot and should not be ignored. The skin is directly and intensely exposed to cigarette smoke and its exhalation. It is also exposed to toxic substances reaching it via the bloodstream. It is not surprising, therefore, that smoking has manifold effects on the skin and is associated with significant morbidity of this organ.

In the Western world, alcohol consumption has doubled in the past 40 years, and this has been accompanied by a parallel rise in alcohol-related diseases, violence, accident rates and psychosocial problems. It is estimated that up to 40% of all current hospitalizations are related directly or indirectly to alcohol. Scientific advances over the past two decades have revolutionized our understanding of substance abuse and its determinants, sequelae and treatment.

Ethanol has many effects on the lipid and protein components of cell membranes and it affects almost every organ, including the skin and its vasculature. The increased alcohol consumption in the Western world has resulted in the recognition of numerous alcohol-related skin disorders. Furthermore, dermatological diseases are now emerging as an important marker of alcohol misuse at an early, and possibly reversible, stage in the disease, hence their importance to both general practitioners and dermatologists.

WHY A SPECIAL FOCUS ON WOMEN'S SMOKING- AND ALCOHOL-RELATED PROBLEMS?

Women smokers are numbered in the millions throughout the world. In the developed countries, smoking by women was socially unacceptable for many years but increased rapidly in most developed countries by the mid-20th century. Although the prevalence of smoking among American women declined from 34% in 1965 to 24% in 1991, the rate of cessation of smoking is lower among women than among men, and the prevalence of smoking women is expected to have surpassed that of men in the year 2000[1]. Over the next 30 years, tobacco-related deaths among women will more than double, so that by the year 2020 well over one million adult women will die every year from tobacco-related illnesses and millions will suffer from smoking-related diseases and disabilities.

The last half century has witnessed a rise in the prevalence of alcoholism and drug abuse among women in the Western world. The well-documented convergence of women's drinking patterns with men's has paralleled women's successful competition with men for equality in the workplace. There are an estimated six million women with alcohol-related problems in America today. More women consume alcohol than ever before, and alcohol dependence among women has grown steadily: about one-third of all persons with drinking problems are women[2,3].

There is no doubt that the extent of the problem of smoking and of substance abuse among women is considerable and is on the increase. Although there has been a broadening of interest in women's issues in relation to both smoking and substance abuse over the past 30 years, the gap between awareness and knowledge of men's problems versus those of women is still large and, to our regret, most research, policy and treatment initiatives still focus on men, with scant attention being paid to special features of women abusers.

The differences between men and women are not merely chromosomal, sexual, reproductive and hormonal. There are profound gender differences of skin anatomy, morphology and physiology, as well as of the metabolism of drugs and reaction to exogenous factors[4]. Beyond these physiological differences, there are major psychological, social and emotional differences. Over the past two decades, investigations have distinguished men and women on a number of differences in the characteristics, epidemiology, symptoms, clinical consequences, complications, associated problems, potential etiologies and treatments of cigarette smoking and of alcohol dependence.

WOMEN AND TOBACCO USE: EPIDEMIOLOGY AND TRENDS

Smoking has not always been socially acceptable for men and, during the 1800s and early 1900s, tobacco use by women was largely unacceptable. In most developed countries, smoking by women was considered to be vulgar, improper and even immoral, and the antismoking movements in several countries were often led by women or women's organizations. Such attitudes began to change with the coming of women's emancipation. Since the Baroness de Dudevant (Chopin's mistress, Paris, ca. 1840) purportedly became the first woman to don men's trousers and smoke in public, smoking by women became indelibly intertwined with images of independence, fashion, emancipation, equality and attractiveness. Smoking became fashionable in the 1930s, particularly among urban women. In real numbers, however, few women smoked at the turn of the 20th century. Female smoking prevalence did not exceed 25% until World War II, when it was still half that of men. As women contributed to the national war effort, smoking by women became associated with the pride of going out to work, and with independence, emancipation, defiance and patriotism. After the war, the prevalence of smoking among women was about 40% in the UK, 30% in Austria and 25% in the USA. In the UK, the prevalence rate of smoking among women was 38% in 1950 and reached

45% in 1966 before starting to fall as the risks of smoking became evident, but this occurred later than for men and in fewer countries.

The awareness of health hazards of tobacco also led to the decline in the prevalence of smoking among men in some developed countries. It went from 51.9% in 1965 to 28.1% in 1991, while women's prevalence had diminished by only about one-third, from 33.9% to 23.5%. In general, the countries in which smoking was first taken up were the first to show a decline in the prevalence of smoking among women. Initiation rates in young men also began to decrease in the mid-1960s, whereas for women they actually increased abruptly around 1967 (when tobacco advertising aimed at selling specific brands to women was introduced) and peaked at around 1973[5,6]. Currently, in some developed countries, the numbers of men and women who smoke are converging. In Sweden, smoking prevalence among men is 22% and that of women is 24%; in Denmark it is 37% for both sexes; and for men and women, respectively, in Norway it is 36.4% vs. 35.5%; in the UK 28% vs. 26%; in Ireland 29% vs. 28%; in the USA 27.7% vs. 22.5%; and in Canada 31% vs. 29% (these data were collected in 1991–94)[7]. With fewer men than women taking up smoking, more women than men may well become dependent on tobacco.

Smoking was first adopted by the more affluent and educated women, and these women were also the first to give it up. The female smoker is now more likely to have a limited education, have a job of lower status or be unemployed and have a low income, be single, separated or divorced, or be subject to various forms of deprivation. National trends in smoking prevalence by educational category from 1974 to 1985 show that education has replaced gender as the major sociodemographic predictor of smoking status. Although smoking prevalence has declined across all educational groups, the decline has occurred five times faster among the higher educated compared with the less educated segments of the population.

Poor families give priority to essential items such as housing, fuel and food and severely restrict spending on non-essential and personal items (such as clothes, hobbies and alcohol). Consequently, minimal spending by women might be anticipated, as they are usually responsible for making ends meet, particularly those in households with children where the needs of the youngsters place additional financial burdens on the adults[8]. An interesting study on the budgeting strategies of poor households in the UK showed that tobacco was an exception to the economic rules by which low-income families organize their finances. Unlike most categories of household expenditure, spending on tobacco is inversely related to income. Furthermore, spending on tobacco among low-income households with children is higher than among low-income households without children, the highest per capita expenditure on tobacco being among one-adult households with children.

Another study[9] investigated the smoking habits of 10 000 men and women who were both unemployed and of full-time workers throughout Scotland. For both sexes, the proportion of current smokers and ever smokers was found to be considerably higher among the unemployed. Interestingly, among current smokers, the unemployed men reported smoking fewer cigarettes a day, whereas unemployed women smoked more than did full-time working women.

In 1987 there was a sudden and large decline in initiation of smoking among less-educated women in the USA. The changes in initiation patterns by educational level suggest that the converging of smoking prevalence between the genders may not continue and that it may again become greater among men[10].

WHY DO WOMEN SMOKE?

Many factors affect the initiation and maintenance of tobacco use by girls and women. Both internal ones such as self-esteem and self image, as well as external influences such as social acceptability and tobacco advertising are important.

An overview of the estimated prevalence of smoking among women in various developing countries indicates that women are sensitive to social or religious acceptability, factors that contributed to keeping prevalence rates low among women in developed countries in the past and which are responsible for keeping rates low in most developing countries today.

In developed countries, girls in particular appear to be influenced by their parents' smoking behavior and attitudes, although this decreases as they become older. Mothers have a particularly strong impact on their daughters' smoking behavior whenever they are chosen as role models.

Smoking is portrayed in advertising as a means of attaining maturity, adulthood and popularity, and of being sophisticated, elegant, glamorous, sociable, feminine and sexually attractive. Studies have repeatedly found that girls who have low self-esteem are more likely to take up the habit. A study

in the UK showed that having positive beliefs about the advantages of smoking was an important predictor of starting smoking in girls but not boys. Girls who thought that smoking made people look more grown-up, helped calm nerves and control weight, gave confidence and was enjoyable were the most likely to start smoking. Girls' perceptions of their physical appearance and overall sense of self-worth are much lower than those of boys and fall with increasing age during early adolescence, and these perceptions are associated with regular smoking. Young women may be faced with gender role conflicts different from those of young men and may be more concerned about what is socially desirable. Social preoccupation with female thinness is another factor that affects adolescent girls' perceptions of the benefits of smoking.

In direct contradiction to all this, girls at the top of the social pecking order who projected an image of high self-esteem were identified as most likely to smoke, while only a small minority of girls fitted the stereotype of the young female smoker who has poor social skills and low self-esteem. Boys of high social status were less vulnerable, since interests in sports and a desire to be fit protected them to some extent[11].

Tobacco companies have identified women as a key target group, therefore particular attention is given to ways in which they have attempted to reach women through advertising and other marketing strategies. The fact that smoking became a symbol of emancipation and defiance was not lost on the tobacco industry, which captured the wide-open women's market with advertising campaigns. As early as 1919, Lorillard used images of women smoking to market its Murad and Helman brands. The links to fashion and slimness were not far behind; Marlboro unveiled its 'mild as May' campaign in the sophisticated fashion magazine *Le Bon Ton* in 1927, and a 1928 advertisement for Lucky Strike encouraged women to 'Reach for a Lucky Instead of a Sweet'[12]. Lucky Strike hired debutantes and models to smoke in public places and prevailed on the fashion industry to choose the color of the Lucky Strike package (green) as the fashion color of the year.

Advertising and sales promotion have an important influence on smoking initiation. Pierce and Gilpin[13] showed sex-specific temporal associations between major cigarette marketing campaigns and increases in youth smoking initiation. Analyzing data from National Health Interview Surveys on age of initiation of smoking for males and females aged 10 to 20 years, from 1944 to the middle of the 1980s, Pierce and colleagues[5] documented that tobacco advertising campaigns targeting women were associated with abrupt increases in smoking initiation by girls 11 to 17 years old – a finding unique to this gender and age group. In women younger than 18 years, smoking initiation increased abruptly around 1967, when tobacco advertising that was aimed at selling specific brands to women was introduced. This increase was particularly marked among those women who never attended college (1.7-fold higher). Initiation rates for women younger than 18 years peaked around 1973, at about the same time sales of these brands peaked. Initiation rates for boys younger than 16 years showed little change during the entire study period.

Fashion is a powerful route for reaching young women, who use fashion trends to enhance their image. The tobacco industry itself proclaims 'Brands can serve as strong fashion statements' and 'Brands are frequently a personal emblem, identifying to others a smoker's status and aspiration'[14]. For the young woman more prone to rebellion, there is the Virginia Slims biker ensemble promotional offer. The young women seeking enlightenment may choose Natural American Spirit, marketed by the Sante Fe Natural Tobacco Company with claims of 'pure, unadulterated leaves' (no chemical additives) and sold alongside tofu, whole-grain cereal and health books in 2000 specialty groceries throughout the USA[14].

It is noteworthy that many women in developed countries are very concerned that smoking cessation might lead to weight gain (and studies have indeed shown that, on average, sustained quitters do gain about 5–6 kg in weight[15]). The tobacco industry exploits and reinforces this vulnerability by linking smoking to fashion, where unnaturally slim models epitomize beauty and glorify images that most young girls cannot hope to attain.

CIGARETTE SMOKING AND FACIAL WRINKLING

We live in a youth-oriented culture, a culture geared to success and physical perfection, with large resources invested in holding back the ravages of time. Women, particularly, are motivated to avoid or eliminate facial wrinkles and/or other signs of age. Tens of thousands of facial cosmetic operations are performed yearly in the USA for the major purpose of removing facial wrinkles. American women spend more than 7 billion dollars per year on over 20 000 different cosmetic products promising youth and beauty. For many individuals, particularly

young women, evidence that smoking might affect their appearance and cause conditions such as wrinkles, bad breath, or yellow teeth is much more compelling than the evidence that smoking kills.

The relation between smoking and the complexion was suggested as early as 1856, when in a large series of British subjects undergoing insurance examinations, smokers were found to have a sallow complexion and markedly wrinkled skin[16]. One year later, a similar difference was noted among British Army officers stationed in India[17].

In 1965, Ippen and Ippen[18] first studied the association between complexion and smoking. They conducted their study on women only, because they did not believe that the same changes were found in men. Two hundred and twenty-four women, aged 35–84 years, were examined with no knowledge of their smoking habits. The authors found that 79% of female smokers had 'cigarette skin', compared with only 19% of the non-smokers. 'Cigarette skin', according to the authors, exhibited a loss of turgor, a pale color with a grayish hue without local variations of pigmentation, and prevalent wrinkles with thick skin between the wrinkles. Their description of 'cigarette skin' or 'smoker's face' is similar to that of Solly[16] some 100 years earlier. Although this investigation can be criticized for many reasons – in particular, the lack of control or adjustment for age, sun exposure and body mass index – its importance lies in the fact of its being a pioneer study in this field.

Four years after the study of Ippen and Ippen, Daniell, who has become the protagonist of the idea of using the smoking–wrinkle association for the antismoking campaign and education, published a Letter to the Editor stating that 'There must be a close relation between the presence of wrinkling of the facial skin and habitual cigarette smoking'[19]. Indeed, he later succeeded in proving his clinical observation in a large, well-controlled study[20]. He established a method of grading the severity of facial skin wrinkling that 'can be rapidly learned and easily used by untrained students'. In a study of 1104 subjects, he found that the association between cigarette smoking and wrinkling was striking in both sexes after the age of 30 years, that it was related to the duration and intensity of the smoking, and that it was more pronounced than was the association between wrinkling and outdoor exposure. He found that smokers in the 40–49-year-old age group were as likely to be prominently wrinkled as non-smokers who were 20 years older. A correlation between prolonged sun exposure and increased wrinkling was shown among smokers of both sexes: it was less striking among non-smoking men and was not found among non-smoking women. Although Daniell was convinced that 'there must be a close relation' between smoking and wrinkling before he proved it in his study, he succeeded in performing an objective, 'blind', well-controlled study.

The role of smoking in premature facial wrinkling was challenged two years later[21] when 650 patients were examined for wrinkling in the crow's foot area. Among the subjects, 137 blacks (91 smokers) showed minimal or no wrinkles whether or not they smoked and whether or not they had more than 2 hours of daily sun exposure. Smoking had no effect on the so-called facial smoker's wrinkles. Several authors believe that this conclusion is not supported by the data presented in the article. Although the results appeared to refute Daniell's findings, the data supported an association between smoking and skin wrinkling in whites (of 513 white subjects, data were given on only 15).

While Daniell's study[20] was mainly concerned with the grading of the degree of facial wrinkling and relating it to the number of cigarettes smoked in a day, other investigations[22,23] emphasized and defined the characteristics of 'smoker's face', which has features similar to those described by Ippen and Ippen[18] 20 years earlier. With no knowledge of smoking history, 116 white English patients, aged 35–69 years, attending a general medical clinic were examined. Smoker's face was present in 46% of current smokers, 8% of former smokers and none of the non-smokers. The relationship between smoking and smoker's face seemed to be independent of social class, duration of daily sun exposure or recent weight change. Further studies that used 'smoker's face' as a diagnostic sign confirmed the results[24,25].

The first study to indicate differences between the sexes concerning susceptibility to the wrinkling effect of smoking was a Danish one[26], probably the largest to date, involving 4485 women and 2485 men. In this study, the degree of wrinkling lateral to the canthus of the right eye was described without the investigator being aware of the smoking habits of the individual concerned. The results showed a significant association between the cumulative cigarette consumption and the amount of deep wrinkles in men, but not in women. The authors found no definite explanation for this difference between the sexes, but speculated that a difference in exposure to sunlight and/or use of face cream might have been the reasons.

Another study indicating a gender difference in the susceptibility to the wrinkling effects of smoking

appeared in 1995[27]. An analysis of the facial wrinkles of 911 men and women between 40 and 69 years of age who had completed a multiphasic health screening examination at a medical center was reported. Objective, blinded evaluations of wrinkling were performed, and potential confounding variables, including age, sex, sun exposure, alcohol consumption and body mass index were taken into account. The data on 227 individuals who had never smoked, 456 former smokers and 228 current smokers were analyzed. Although both male and female current smokers had elevated risks of moderate or severe facial wrinkling compared with never smokers, this was greater for women (the estimated risk for wrinkling in smokers compared to non-smokers was 3.1 in women vs. 2.3 for men). As for former smokers, for women, there was a marginally significant risk of wrinkling (odds ratio 1.8; 95% confidence interval (CI) 1.0–3.1), while this was not the case for men. These results are in sharp contradiction to those of the previous study[26], where the association between smoking and wrinkling was observed only in men. Among current and former smokers, individuals with more than 20 pack-years of exposure were more likely to be classified in the moderate or severe wrinkling category than those with ten or fewer pack-years of exposure. For both sexes, a significant risk of wrinkling was associated with more than 20 pack-years of smoking. However, age was the strongest independent predictor of facial wrinkle category. Average daily sun exposure of 2 h or more was also associated with an increased risk of wrinkling for both men and women, while higher body mass index categories were associated with a lower risk. Perhaps the most convincing and illustrative data were those of a multiple regression analysis of the relationship of pack-years of smoking to facial wrinkle score. This showed that ten pack-years of smoking was equivalent for both sexes to about 1.4 years of aging.

SMOKING AND HORMONAL CHANGES IN WOMEN

Several clinical and epidemiological observations have indicated a decreased incidence of estrogen-linked syndromes among women who smoke, such as a reduced incidence of carcinoma of the endometrium and endometriosis, but an increased incidence of conditions associated with estrogen deficiency, such as osteoporosis and earlier onset of menopause. In other words, women who smoke cigarettes display patterns as though they were relatively estrogen deficient.

Furthermore, there are convincing studies indicating that smoking might affect estrogen metabolism. A study on human granulosa cell aromatase *in vitro* has shown that aqueous extracts of cigarette smoke inhibited the conversion of androstenedione to estrone in a dose-dependent manner[28]. A similar effect was found on choriocarcinoma cell cultures and in preparations of term placental microsomes, where nicotine, cotinine and anabinase inhibited the conversion of testosterone to estradiol[29]. Women smokers excreted only one-third as much estrogen during the luteal phase of the ovulatory cycle than did either non-smokers or ex-smokers, suggesting an effect of smoking on the biosynthesis of estrogen[30]. Smoking-induced alteration in estrogen metabolism was suggested by the observation of lower serum estrogen levels in estrogen-treated women who smoke, compared with their non-smoking counterparts. Tobacco components were found to induce an increase in estradiol metabolism via the hepatic cytochrome P-450 enzyme system. A significant increase in 2-hydroxylation of estradiol (to its inactive product, 2-hydroxyestrone) was found in women who smoked at least 15 cigarettes per day. Women who smoke are usually thinner than non-smokers. Combining this with the fact that thin women produce less estradiol and more 2-hydroxyestrone than their overweight counterparts makes the association of slender women and smoking in terms of estrogen economy very sinister.

In conclusion, although clinical epidemiological studies have linked smoking to antiestrogenic effects, laboratory confirmation of these data is sometimes controversial or of borderline significance. A possible explanation for the discrepancy between the results of laboratory studies and epidemiological studies may be that the acute effect of cigarette smoking on endocrine metabolism (which is usually the effect studied in experimental studies) is less significant and notable than that of the cumulative effect (usually analyzed in epidemiological studies).

SMOKING, WOUND HEALING AND FACE-LIFT SURGERY

Smokers have worse cosmetic results after surgery and have a higher incidence of skin-flap necrosis and skin sloughs after face-lift surgery. Women are the principal candidates for face lifts, rhytidectomies and other types of elective cosmetic surgery. Dermatological surgeons should be aware of this effect of cigarette smoking and take it into account when selecting patients for cosmetic procedures, when advising them of their prognosis and when obtaining informed consent.

Surgeons have long noted a relationship between smoking and defective wound repair. Because of their clinical experience, many surgeons routinely asked their patients to abstain from smoking during the immediate preoperative period. Despite centuries of clinical experience and decades of scientific evidence, it was not until 1977 that it was declared that smoking is detrimental to the healing of wounds[31]. One year later, this group showed that systemic administration of nicotine impaired wound healing in an experimental animal model[32], further confirmed in 1984[33] and in 1985[34,35].

One of the few controlled studies on surgical wound healing focused on 120 women who had undergone laparotomic sterilization[36]. The method of skin suture was standardized and, using a uniform scoring system, the investigators determined that cosmetic scar results were significantly poorer in 69 smokers than in 51 non-smokers. Scarring was unsatisfactory in 25% of the smokers, compared with none of the non-smokers.

Compromised wound healing is a particular concern in smokers undergoing plastic or reconstructive surgery. Likewise, a face lift carries with it a high risk of skin slough, since in this procedure, as in skin grafting, the skin of the face is detached from the subcutaneous tissue and from most of its blood supply.

In a retrospective review of 1186 face-lift procedures, the investigators concluded that skin slough was significantly more likely to occur in smokers than in non-smokers[37]. The results showed that 74% of skin sloughs were due to smoking, independent of those associated with hematoma. The risk of skin slough was calculated as being 7.5% in smokers vs. 2.7% in non-smokers. In a subsequent prospective study[38], 83 patients who underwent face lift by the same surgeon were examined: there were nine skin sloughs. Five per cent of non-smokers, 8.3% of ex-smokers and 19.4% of current smokers had skin slough. Because of the risks of performing surgery on smokers, Webster and co-workers[39] devised a modification of the face lift in which they performed only limited undermining. They recorded no skin slough among 407 patients, including 32% who were smokers. Even with this limited procedure, however, there was a statistically significantly higher incidence of hair loss at the surgical sites in smokers compared to non-smokers.

Similar issues arise with regard to breast reduction and mastectomies. The incidence of wound healing complications was found to be an astounding 30–50% higher in smokers than non-smokers undergoing breast surgery[40].

There are many possible mechanisms by which smoking may affect wound healing. A common end feature of several mechanisms is apparently a decrease in tissue oxygen content or PO_2.

SMOKING AND SEXUAL BEHAVIOR

A considerable body of evidence, mainly from the USA, supports the view that a variety of 'problem behaviors' are related, and that individuals with such behaviors are more likely than others to take risks leading not only to physical illness, but also to accidental injury and death[41]. Another recent study[42] confirmed this position by questioning whether adolescent male involvement with pregnancy is associated with other risk behaviors. It showed that high school adolescents who had early experiences with cocaine and tobacco were more likely to indulge in sexual experimentation resulting in pregnancy. Also, these adolescents were more prone to engage in risky behaviors, such as driving while drinking alcohol, or having multiple concomitant sexual partners, thus increasing the risks of HIV infection.

Smoking is *per se* a 'risk behavior'. It is not unexpected that it would be associated with other problem behaviors, and public health researchers have found that smoking is associated with alcohol, caffeine and psychoactive drugs. In an interesting recent study using a large representative sample of the general American population[43], early-onset smoking was a significant predictor of lifetime drinking, and the subsequent development of DSM-IV alcohol abuse and dependence. The results also showed a relationship that generally remained consistent for males, females, whites and blacks. Early-onset smoking was significantly associated with more excessive alcohol consumption and more severe alcohol use disorders relative to late-onset smokers and non-smokers. Smokers were less likely to use seat belts, apply sunscreens or obtain necessary vaccinations. Female smokers have been noted to be more sexually active, with an earlier age at first intercourse and more lifetime sexual partners and to have had more pregnancies and more live births.

In a recent study[44] on contraceptive use among women, sexually active smokers were less likely than non-smokers to use contraceptives, especially oral contraceptives, while smokers over the age of 30 were more than twice as likely as non-smokers to

have been sterilized. The finding that women smokers were younger at first intercourse and had a higher number of lifetime sexual partners was confirmed repeatedly. The association between smoking and a risky sexual behavior, i.e. a behavior that increases risk for HIV and other sexually transmitted diseases, was also observed in numerous other studies on adolescents of both sexes.

Interestingly, even women exposed to passive smoke differed from those not exposed on several factors that would mark them as being more likely to be involved in risk-taking behavior[45]. It is not only personal smoking that was related to problem behavior: adolescent school truants were found to score higher on all negative social indices, including parents who smoked[46].

Until recently, the notion of a global healthy or unhealthy life style has been more an epidemiological concept. One of the new developments in epidemiology was the awareness of underlying global or generalizable factors that might predispose individuals to choose a risky life style, and the consequent elaboration of the subdiscipline of behavioral epidemiology[47]. The challenge for epidemiology has become to move beyond its usual biomedical scope and try to understand and explain the causes and circumstances that bring about risk-taking behavior.

SMOKING AND HUMAN PAPILLOMA VIRUS

The relationship between smoking and cervical cancer has been extensively studied. Since there is a strong link between cigarette smoking and sexual activity or, more specifically, high-risk sexual behavior, and an association between these factors and cervical cancer, several studies that dealt with risk factors for cervical cancer also examined the association between smoking and human papilloma virus (HPV) infection. However, most of the studies primarily addressed the association between HPV and cervical neoplasia and showed that it persisted after adjustment for smoking and other sexual risk factors.

Rohan and colleagues[48] studied student health clinic patients using the polymerase chain reaction (PCR) to establish the prevalence of cervical HPV infection and the association between this and known risk factors for cervical carcinoma. Overall, the prevalence of HPV infection was 18.1%, which is similar to previous estimates using the same methods. The authors found a statistically significant increase in risk of overall HPV infection with a history of having ever smoked cigarettes, but not for HPV-16 alone, or for usually having sexual intercourse during menstrual periods. These associations were independent of the effects of several other factors, including age at first sexual intercourse and number of sexual partners.

Another study showed an increase in the prevalence of HPV DNA with cigarette smoking and sexual activity, and a decrease in prevalence with age, in 1126 Alaskan native women seeking routine care and colposcopy or from population-based lists[49].

Other investigators examined 181 women with reported cervical cytological abnormality[50]. Oncogenic HPV was found in the cervix of 41% of women who did not smoke, 58% of those who smoked 1–10 cigarettes a day, 61% of those who smoked 11–20 cigarettes a day and 76% of those who smoked 20 or more cigarettes a day. The prevalence of the virus thus increased in parallel with the number of cigarettes smoked. This relationship persisted after adjustment for parameters of sexual activity. The authors concluded that 'the dose dependent effect of cigarette smoking on the occurrence of oncogenic HPV favors a causal relation between these risk factors for cervical neoplasia'. This conclusion on a direct causal relationship between smoking and HPV infection was severely criticized by Phillips and Smith[51]. They suggested that the cigarette smoking status is probably a better indicator of sexual activity than standard criteria, such as the lifetime number of sexual partners and age at first intercourse. This, they stated, explained why the association between smoking and oncogenic HPV was found even after adjustment for the usual parameters of sexual activity.

In a more recent study[52], a significant independent effect of smoking on the occurrence of HPV was demonstrated, and confirmed previous results.

Several experimental studies examined the interaction of smoking and HPV infection in an attempt to find a biological plausibility for the relationship. A significant finding is the reduced number of Langerhans cells in the cervical epithelium of smokers. Cigarette smoking was found to be associated with a reduction in the Langerhans cell count in both normal and diseased epithelium.

One must not neglect the male factor: Lovejoy[53] reviewed the literature on 'male factors' associated with precancerous and cancerous lesions of the cervix and found that, in a number of studies, smoking in the male partner was linked to an increased risk of development of cervical cancer.

Examination of the male factor in cervical carcinogenesis among Indian women with one lifetime partner indicated that *bidi* smoking for more than 20 years was a significant risk factor (RR = 2.4) whereas cigarette smoking was not. (*Bidi* is a cheap smoking stick consisting of a rolled piece of dried temburi leaf (*Diospyres melanoxylon*) containing 0.15–0.25 g of coarsely ground tobacco)[54].

In the debate on the role of smoking in the etiology of HPV infection, there is one central point of agreement: women who smoke are at increased risk of contracting HPV infection. Apart from the theoretical considerations of the question of predisposing factors and immunological status of the host, finding a satisfactory answer also has practical importance from the standpoint of public health and preventive medicine.

SMOKING AND HERPES SIMPLEX VIRUS

In 1976, Smith and co-workers[55] found that smokers had higher antibody titers to herpes simplex virus (HSV) than did non-smokers. IgA antibodies to HSV were detected six times more frequently in the sera of smokers than in non-smoking controls. IgG and IgM anti-HSV antibodies were detected with comparable frequencies in both groups, but the antibody titers were significantly higher in the smoking group. Only after 6 years had elapsed were these findings confirmed by another study[56]. This investigation demonstrated significantly higher antibody titers to HSV-1 in smokers compared with non-smokers. Since individuals with a history of recurrent herpetic infection were excluded from this study, the authors suggested that the HSV-1 antibody differences probably resulted from exposure to HSV antigens due to symptomless reactivation of a latent infection. They hypothesized that cigarette smoke reactivated a latent HSV-1 infection, leading to symptomless shedding of the virus into the mouth and consequently to boosting of the antibody titer. In an earlier experimental study, the same group had demonstrated that polycyclic aromatic hydrocarbons related to those of cigarette smoke can induce HSV-1 shedding in mice[57].

There have been only a few studies that have dealt with the relationship between smoking and recurrent herpetic lesions, all of them on herpes labialis. The frequency of recurrent herpes labialis was examined in 20 333 adult Swedish individuals[58]. Their results indicated that the prevalence of recurrent herpes labialis was influenced by some tobacco habits: it was significantly lower among smokers, and especially among pipe smokers, compared with non-smokers. Snuff dipping did not seem to influence the prevalence values. Young and Rimm[59] did not find a significant difference in the frequency of recurrent herpes labialis between smokers and non-smokers among 446 consecutive blood donors.

Interesting experimental investigations on the relationship between smoking, nicotine and HSV led to the formation of a hypothesis on the synergistic oncogenic action of tobacco products and HSV. Hirsch and associates[60] demonstrated that tobacco water extracts inhibited the replication of DNA virus in cultured monkey kidney cells in a dose-dependent manner. The tobacco-induced block of HSV replication was found to be at an early stage, i.e. before or at the level of viral DNA synthesis. Non-toxic concentrations of nicotine restricted HSV replication but not to the same extent as did the snuff extracts. These authors and others[61] suggested that nicotine was probably one, but not the only, substance contributing to the overall HSV inhibition observed with snuff extracts.

The oncogenic capacity of HSV-1 and HSV-2 has been well established in many epidemiological and molecular biology studies. However, a prerequisite for HSV to cause cell transformation and induce carcinomas is the prevention of virus-induced cell lysis. Several methods have been used to inactivate the virus and thus inhibit virus-induced cell lysis. In a series of animal studies, prolonged exposure to formalin-inactivated HSV-1 or HSV-2 (or to HSV-2 inactivated by ultraviolet light) produced premalignant and malignant cervical lesions similar to those occurring in women. Herpetic lesions of mouse lips could be transformed into malignant squamous cell carcinomas by the use of a tumor-promoting agent, provided that the virus was previously inactivated by ultraviolet irradiation. Experimentally, cellular transformation has been demonstrated with ultraviolet-irradiated HSV, fragments of viral DNA and photodynamically inactivated virus.

Although both viral genomic DNA and viral proteins are detected in transformed cells at early passages, the cells or tumors have no detectable viral information later on. This is different from transformation by other oncogenic DNA viruses such as SV-40 and adenoviruses, where viral DNA and proteins remain in the transformed cells. It has been postulated that malignant transformation by HSV occurs by a 'hit and run' mechanism, at a very early stage after infection. If virus-induced cell lysis is inhibited, the mutated cells could survive and later undergo malignant transformation.

Park and colleagues[62] examined the histopathological changes of hamster buccal pouches after repeated HSV inoculation and exposure to long-term simulated snuff dipping. Neither simulated snuff dipping nor HSV infection alone induced neoplastic changes in the hamster buccal pouches; however, herpetic infection in combination with simulated snuff dipping resulted in epithelial dysplasia and invasive squamous cell carcinoma in more than 50% of the animals. When simulated snuff dipping and HSV inoculation were combined, the development of clinical herpetic lesions was very mild compared to the clinical findings in the group inoculated with HSV without snuff dipping.

Taken together, these data suggest that when HSV is inactivated and has thus lost its cytolytic activity by exposure to certain chemicals or ultraviolet irradiation, it can be associated with neoplastic changes in mammalian cells. Therefore, substances that inhibit HSV replication for prolonged periods of time might be of potential danger for the development of cancer. This mechanism of oncogenesis has been proposed for smoking and tobacco in the presence of HSV infection.

SMOKING AND HUMAN IMMUNODEFICIENCY VIRUS

The first association between smoking and acquired immunodeficiency syndrome (AIDS) was observed in a study of homosexual men; 51.5% of patients with AIDS were smokers compared with 24.1% of control subjects[63]. Several additional studies confirmed the association between smoking and AIDS[64–66], although some did not[67]. In a multicenter AIDS cohort study of 2499 homosexual men, cigarette smoking did not have a major effect on the progression of HIV-1 infection to AIDS or death[68].

The reasons for hypothesizing that smoking might have an accelerating effect on the natural history of HIV infection and its progression to AIDS were its well-known effects on the immune system. Despite these logical theoretical considerations, results of the published investigations failed to show that cigarette smoking was associated with an altered rate of progression to AIDS.

SMOKING AND BACTERIAL VAGINOSIS

An association between cigarette smoking and bacterial vaginosis has been reported in several studies. In one of these, on 400 women with bacterial vaginosis and 400 women without it, it was noted that the former smoked or had smoked more often, and that they had a similar sexual behavior pattern to those at risk for sexually transmitted diseases (STDs)[69].

An assessment of the relationship between bacterial vaginosis and dyskaryotic cells in a group of 280 women revealed a significant association of bacterial vaginosis with the number of cigarettes smoked per day[70]. In a 7-year case–control study on the prevalence of genital *Chlamydia trachomatis* infection in pregnant adolescents in east Tennessee, smoking was not associated with the infection[71].

A positive correlation between smoking and bacterial vaginosis has been reported from Bulgaria[72]. The prevalence of bacterial vaginosis was evaluated and correlated with the history and clinical manifestations in 156 women attending an STD clinic.

SMOKING AND CERVICITIS AND PELVIC INFLAMMATORY DISEASE

Cervical ectopia has been implicated as a possible risk factor for the acquisition or shedding of certain sexually transmitted pathogens, although it remains uncertain which is the cause and which is the effect[73]. The principal aim of the study was to identify non-microbial determinants of cervical ectopia and cervicitis. These results showed that cervical ectopia was negatively associated with current smoking. Cervicitis was most prevalent among women with cervical infection, ectopia and the use of oral contraception. It was not related to current smoking. A link between cervical *Chlamydia trachomatis* and both the presence of ectopia and smoking had been demonstrated in a previous study[74].

The cervical mucus of smokers compared to non-smokers had a greater number (colony counts > 8500/ml) of micro-organisms, including yeast and non-pathogenic normal flora other than lactobacilli; this result was even more pronounced for heavy smokers and persisted after adjustment for number of sexual partners. Female smokers were significantly more likely to have had a greater number of lifetime sexual partners, to have been pregnant, and to have a history of chlamydia, gonorrhea and/or pelvic inflammatory disease (PID)[75].

Using univariate analysis, it was found that smoking was associated with current STDs, such as *Chlamydia trachomatis*, but such a link was no longer significant after adjustment for age and social class[76].

To examine the relationship between cigarette smoking and PID, data from a hospital-based, case–control study of PID were analyzed[77]. The case subjects were 197 women hospitalized with their first episode of PID and the control subjects were 667 women hospitalized with non-gynecological conditions. Compared with women who had never smoked, current cigarette smokers had a significantly elevated relative risk of PID of 1.7 (95% CI 1.1–2.5). Similarly, former cigarette smokers had a significantly elevated relative risk of PID, confirmed by another case–control study[78].

SMOKING AND ECTOPIC PREGNANCY

Cigarette smoking has been implicated as a risk factor for ectopic pregnancy. Increasing the risk of PID is one mechanism by which smoking might be implicated.

SMOKING AND PSORIASIS

In recent years, smoking has been repeatedly incriminated as a potential risk factor for psoriasis. The risk appeared to be modified by gender, and was found to be greater in women.

O'Doherty and McIntyre[79] were the first to draw attention to the strong link between smoking habits and palmoplantar pustulosis. Eighty per cent of patients with palmoplantar pustulosis were smokers at the time of onset of their disease, compared with only 36% of the controls; four out of five patients were women! Whether palmoplantar pustulosis is accepted as a variant of psoriasis or not, the strength of the relationship between smoking and this disease, according to this study, is of the order of magnitude of the well-known, and generally accepted, relationship of acute guttate psoriasis to streptococcal disease, especially in women.

Although the relationship between smoking and psoriasis is not nearly as strong, several studies have shown that there is a significant relationship.

The first epidemiologic study to draw attention to environmental factors in psoriasis vulgaris was conducted in Norway[80]. In this cross-sectional study based on data from a sample of 14 667 people, psoriasis was found to be directly associated with smoking and inversely associated with the intake of fruit and vegetables. Unfortunately, no evidence of an exposure–effect relationship was observed for smoking. Another cross-sectional population survey, also from Norway, confirmed these results[81]. Among psoriatic patients, 47.5% were daily smokers, whereas 35.5% of those without psoriasis smoked daily, the differences being greatest among females.

In an incidence study of psoriasis from Rochester, Minnesota, the overall crude incidence rate was 57 per 100 000 people per year[82]. Incident cases were defined as newly diagnosed at the Mayo

Clinic facilities, which cover the whole Rochester population. Interestingly, the smoking profile for male patients was similar to the profile from a random sample of the Minnesota population, whereas female patients smoked more than women in the general population (40.3% vs. 28.0%).

A group from Cardiff found a significant association betweeen psoriasis, current smoking status and smoking habits prior to the onset of disease, as well as a marked dose–response relationship[83]. A case–control study from Italy provides further evidence of a dose–response relationship for an association between smoking habits and psoriasis[84].

A case–control study limited to female psoriatic patients demonstrated its association with smoking before the onset of the disease[85]. In logistic regression analysis, the odds ratio for women smoking 20 cigarettes daily compared with non-smokers was 3.3. Interestingly, the same group had previously failed to document an association betweeen smoking and psoriasis in men[86]. Of further note is the finding that psoriasis changed women's attitude towards alcohol but not to smoking.

In conclusion, the available evidence suggests that smoking may be a risk factor for the onset of psoriasis, and that this was found to be greater in women than in men.

SMOKING, VULVAR AND ANOGENITAL CANCER

Cancer of the vulva is a rare malignancy whose incidence increases progressively with age. The age-standardized incidence averages between 1 and 2 per 100 000 women in Western countries[87]. The etiologies of vulvar intraepithelial neoplasia (VIN), *in situ* disease and invasive cancer appear to be different. VIN does not automatically progress to invasive cancer and is strongly associated with HPV infection and other risk factors including smoking. Vulvar cancer is common in older women who do not have evidence of HPV and who do not smoke[87,88].

In a study of 57 women with a new diagnosis of *in situ* or invasive vulvar carcinoma, the factors found to be associated with the disease were similar to those observed among women with cervical cancer, including smoking[89]. In a case–control study on 149 patients with histologically proven vulvar carcinoma and the same number of control subjects, a statistically significant risk for cancer of the vulva was found only in patients who smoked 10–20 cigarettes per day[90].

In another case–control study of 209 vulvar cancer patients, 49.3% of patients and 29.6% of control subjects were current smokers (relative risk, 2.03). There was a significant interaction between smoking and genital warts; women with both had 35 times the risk of vulvar cancer as those with neither factor[91].

Detailed information on smoking history was collected as part of population-based case–control studies of cancers from the anogenital region[92]. Although current smokers had an increased risk of cancer in all areas, vulvar, anal and penile cancers were more strongly associated with smoking than were vaginal and cervical cancer. Slightly over 40% of the cases of vaginal and cervical cancer to 60% of the cases of vulvar and anal cancers were current smokers, in contrast to only about 25% of the controls.

The association between cigarette smoking and vulvar carcinoma, and VIN has further been supported by other studies[88,93–96]. It is of note that smoking is also a risk factor for penile cancer in men[92,97,98].

WOMEN AND ALCOHOL CONSUMPTION: EPIDEMIOLOGY AND TRENDS

Although it is now clear that American women from all social classes have been consumers of a variety of drugs and alcohol for well over two centuries, this behavior has largely remained hidden from public scrutiny because of the social mores governing female behavior during the late 18th and early 19th centuries. Women learned to 'hide' their drug consumption by using patent medicines under the respectable cloak of treatment for 'female health conditions'. In fact, during the period from 1850 to 1880, women were twice as likely as men to be addicted to legal patent medicines. Patent medicine use became increasingly popular and flourished from the late 18th century until the early part of the 20th century, the majority of users being women. After the Harrison Act of 1914 in the USA outlawed non-prescription opiates, their use decreased considerably, and the majority of new addicts tended to be men.

Prevalence estimates of women alcoholics first appeared in the late 19th century; between 1884 and 1912, data on some 24 200 institutionalized alcoholics produced male/female patient ratios ranging from 3 : 1 to 9 : 1. These estimates, however, suffered from some of the same difficulties inherent in modern prevalence figures: 'hidden alcoholism' among women, a lack of treatment facilities and lower socioeconomic status of women, all leading to under-reporting of women[99].

Women's alcohol use has increased over the last half century, as have their alcohol problems. Although men still drink and use illicit drugs to a much greater extent than do women, young women are drinking in increasing numbers and are rapidly approaching males in numbers of new drinkers.

National surveys of quantity/frequency of drinking, conducted over the last half century, show that at least two-thirds of women over 18 years of age drank low to moderate levels of alcohol without personal, social, or environmental consequences. Women's drinking levels, however, are increasing and are approaching those observed in men. Assessment of drinking practices of women and men at a large urban university at two points in time, 1977 ($n = 1711$) and 1985 ($n = 1045$), showed that, although women's ethanol intake remained the same, significant changes in patterns of drinking were observed. The mean annual volume of beer consumed by females in 1985 showed a 33.9% increase over the mean annual volume in 1977. 'Binge' drinking increased for both sexes from 1977 to 1985. There was also a decrease in women's rate of abstention. Convergence with male drinking patterns was not just a trend, but had in fact occurred[100].

Alcohol is a complex subject to study, because it can be used both moderately, in a socially acceptable way, and in an excessive and destructive way. In most Western societies, the social use of alcohol by adults is commonplace and acceptable; however, the demarcation between what is regarded as social drinking and the use of alcohol that goes beyond this point produces problems of definition. Data on prevalence of female alcohol abuse, alcoholism or problem drinking are scarce, but with several surveys providing some useful information on the subject.

The results from a general population survey in the USA in 1987 showed a proportion of 5 to 6% of female drinkers from the ages of 18 to 49 years with dependence symptoms[101]. Surprisingly, the proportion was much higher for drinking-related problems (e.g. arrest, divorce, or traffic accidents). Twelve per cent of women in the 18–29 age range and 6% of women in the 30–40 age range reported having drinking-related problems.

Compared to white women, black women had higher rates of abstention and lower rates of heavy drinking[102]. Those black women who did drink heavily tended to become alcohol dependent and suffer alcohol-related biopsychosocial consequences more rapidly than did white women[103]. Asian[104] and Hispanic[105,106] American women also had high rates of abstention and lower rates of heavy drinking compared to white women. As younger Asian American women become increasingly integrated into American society, alcohol and other drug use may begin to reflect patterns similar to those in the dominant culture.

Based on an earlier general population survey and updated to account for population changes, it was estimated that there were 4 018 000 adult women (age > 18 years) in the USA who could be diagnosed as suffering from alcohol abuse or dependence according to the DSM-IV criteria. This compared with 11 167 000 adult affected men[107].

In the UK, the prevalence of alcohol dependence has been estimated to be 4.7% and drug dependence 2.2% in the general population. The male/female ratio was 2 : 1 for alcohol disorders and 4 : 1 for substance use disorders, close to that described in the USA[108]. A similar prevalence and male/female ratio was demonstrated in another American study, the Epidemiologic Catchment Area (ECA) Study[109], in which more than 20 000 respondents from five community sites were surveyed from 1980 to 1984 and found to have a lifetime prevalence of alcohol disorders of 13.5% and a current prevalence (active in the last 6 months) of 4.8%. These results were confirmed in a more recent study based on the National Institute on Alcohol Abuse and Alcoholism's National Longitudinal Alcohol Epidemiologic Survey (NLAES)[110].

An analysis of the files of all clients entering two private, non-profit in-patient substance abuse treatment facilities in Maryland during an 8-month period in 1989 showed a total of 181 men and 48 women. The women were similar to men with respect to sociodemographic characteristics, family history, alcohol/drug history and treatment completion[111].

Another study compared the prevalence of mental illness, including alcohol use disorders, of the ECA study with data obtained from Germany[112]. Alcohol use disorder was the most frequent category of mental disorder for men in both studies; for women, affective disorder and phobia were the most frequent categories.

The comparison of a 1974 study to data gathered in 1982 showed an increase both in heavy drinking (from 4.4 to 11.5%) and in various alcohol-related problems in college women[113]. An analysis of the drinking patterns of American and Polish university students in a cross-national study showed that significantly more drinks per week were consumed by both Polish male (24.9) and female (15.2) students compared to American male (15.0) and female (7.6) students, although American female students consumed more beer than their Polish counterparts[114].

In a study from Sweden, data from five cohorts of adult women ($n = 3130$) in mainly suburban areas were analyzed[115]. The lifetime prevalence of alcohol dependence and abuse was 3.27% and the 12-month prevalence was 1.49%.

Another study from Sweden focused on the question of to what extent female alcohol dependence and abuse is known in the health-care system. The results of this study revealed a lifetime prevalence of alcohol dependence and abuse of 3.3%. A total of 63.6% of the diagnosed women 45–65 years of age and 25.9% of the women 25–35 years of age were known in the health-care system[116].

A study from Scotland investigated the patterns of alcohol, tobacco and marijuana use in postsecondary helping-profession students (medical, nursing, education and psychology)[117]. The sample consisted of 717 male and 2537 female students. The results showed a slightly ($p < 0.05$) higher percentage of women (92.7%) who consumed alcohol compared to men (90%), but men consumed significantly ($p < 0.001$) more drinks per week (26.7) compared to women (17.3).

WHICH WOMEN DRINK AND WHY?

All drunks are not created equal, and the reasons for women to drink differ in many respects from those that lead men to drink. Several factors influence alcoholism and other drug dependence in women.

Genetic factors

Studies that have involved both men and women show differences in hereditary patterns between the sexes. An epidemiological sample of 1030 female–female twin pairs with known zygosity, retrieved from the Virginia Twin Registry, were evaluated for six major psychiatric disorders, including alcoholism[118]. The results demonstrated both specific genetic influences for alcoholism and interplay of genetic and environmental influences in the causation of both alcoholism and psychiatric co-morbidity in women. The same group also investigated the etiology of cannabis use and abuse in a population-based sample of female twins[119]. The results of this study showed that genetic risk factors in women had a moderate impact on the probability of ever using cannabis and a strong impact on the liability towards heavy use, abuse and, probably, dependence. In contrast, the family and social environment substantially influenced the risk of ever using cannabis, but played little role in the probability of developing heavy cannabis use or abuse.

Although it is difficult if not impossible to differentiate genetic influences from environmental influences, most studies estimated heritability at 50 to 60%. Genetic vulnerability to alcoholism was found to be equally transmitted from fathers and from mothers to their daughters[120,121].

Parental separation

In a study of female twin pairs, Kendler and colleagues[122] showed that childhood parental loss through separation, but not death, substantially increased the risk in adulthood for all definitions of alcoholism. Furthermore, both paternal and maternal alcoholism substantially increased the probability of parental separation from their children. When analyzing causality, the authors found that, while a significant proportion of the association was due to non-causal genetic mechanisms, childhood parental loss (or the familial discord that preceded or followed it) was probably a direct and significant environmental risk factor for the development of alcoholism in women. It is of note that this study was the first to investigate alcoholism and premature parental loss in women. In an investigation of predictors of problem drinking and alcohol dependence in female twins, personality characteristics and parental psychopathology were found to be important predictors of these behaviors, independent of their effect on risk for affective and anxiety disorders[123].

Traumatic events

There is general agreement in the literature that difficult life experience is a major cause of women turning to alcohol[2]. Childhood sexual abuse has been recognized as a common antecedent of problem drinking as well as of opiate and cocaine abuse. Past history of physical abuse or sexual victimization is not always confined to childhood and not necessarily done by parents. In one study, over half of the women alcoholics in the sample reported a history of at least one incident of rape[124]. Spouse-to-woman negative verbal interaction and violence are also strong predictors of alcoholism in women[125].

Victimization of women who drink is another aspect of the problem. In a study of social victimization related to drinking by another person, it was found that, unlike men, women who drink in bars are far more likely to be victimized, even if they were not themselves heavy or problem drinkers[126].

Self-esteem

The relationships between gender, self-esteem and DSM-III alcohol use disorder diagnoses were examined in a sample of 217 men and 240 women evaluated at four annual assessments over the college years[127]. The results indicated that low self-esteem played a particularly important etiological role in alcohol problems in women relative to men. Women who had an alcohol use disorder during those 4 years showed relatively low levels of self-esteem throughout the study period. Furthermore, the study provided clear evidence for prospective prediction from year 1 self-esteem to year 4 alcohol use disorder diagnosis for women, but not for men. There was minimal evidence that alcohol use predicts later self-esteem.

These findings supported those of previous studies which indicated that alcoholic women suffered from low self-esteem and feelings of inadequacy, incompetence and great anxiety[128]. These women felt chronically lonely, bored and depressed and had difficulty coping with marital conflict and life transitions[129,130].

Co-occurrence of other psychiatric disorders

All psychiatric diagnoses are more prevalent in female alcoholics than in female non-alcoholics[131]. The Epidemiologic Catchment Area sample found that 37% of women with alcohol disorders had comorbid mental illness, of which major depression was the most common[109]. This confirmed earlier results which found that 19% of the women who fulfilled diagnostic criteria for alcohol abuse also fulfilled criteria for a lifetime diagnosis of major depression, compared to 5% of men. The rate of lifetime diagnosis of major depression in alcoholic women was nearly three times the general population rate for women (7%)[131].

Alcoholic men outnumber alcoholic women in only two diagnostic categories: antisocial personality and pathological gambling.

Cohabiting with an alcohol-dependent partner may contribute to the development of addiction in women. The spouses of alcoholic women are three to five times more likely than non-alcoholic women's spouses to be alcoholic[132]. There is a strong positive correlation between a woman's level of drug or alcohol consumption and that of a partner or husband. Female drug addicts are usually initiated into use by men, yet women progress more quickly from initiation to addiction than do men. Women entering addiction treatment were more likely to be married to or living with an alcoholic or addicted sexual partner, or to be divorced or separated, while men entering treatment were more likely to be married to a non-addicted spouse.

GENDER DIFFERENCES IN ALCOHOL METABOLISM AND SUSCEPTIBILITY

Specific organ systems are differentially affected by alcohol in women compared to men. Dealing with all of them is beyond the scope of the present work, and we concentrate only on pharmacokinetic differences between the sexes.

Early studies of the pharmacology of alcohol and other psychoactive drugs were performed on male subjects, with the assumption that the findings would apply to women as well. Women achieve higher blood alcohol levels than men after equivalent dosing[133]. This was thought to be due to the higher average body water content in men than women. Because ethanol is distributed in total body water, a dose of ethanol will be distributed in a smaller volume of water in women than in men (a smaller volume of distribution), and so should be less diluted and produce higher concentrations in women's blood.

More recently, Frezza and co-workers found a substantial first-pass metabolism of ethanol in the human gastric mucosa, through oxidation by alcohol dehydrogenase[134]. They further proved that differences in this metabolism were the principal cause of the sex-related differences in blood alcohol concentration. In non-alcoholic subjects, the first-pass metabolism and gastric alcohol dehydrogenase activity of the women were 23% and 59%, respectively, of those in the men, and there was a significant correlation between first-pass metabolism and gastric mucosal alcohol dehydrogenase activity. The authors concluded that the increased bioavailability of ethanol resulting from decreased gastric oxidation of ethanol may contribute to the increased vulnerability of women to acute and chronic complications of alcoholism.

It is therefore understandable that the blood levels achieved for a given dose of alcohol are higher in women than in men. This effect is particularly striking in alcoholic women, but also has marked significance concerning social drinking in normal women. There are at least three reasons for these gender differences. First and most important of all is the first-pass metabolism by gastric alcohol dehydrogenase which is much lower in women, so that less of the ingested alcohol will be broken down in the stomach and more will reach the peripheral blood. Second, women are usually smaller than men, but the quantity of alcohol served to them in social settings does not take this gender difference into account. Finally, the alcohol consumed is distributed in a smaller water space (see above).

Women who drink amounts of alcohol comparable to those of men are more likely to be affected, both immediately and over time. Women have a greater vulnerability than men to the development of organ damage after chronic alcoholic abuse, in terms of both liver disease and brain damage. Medical complications occur sooner in women's drinking careers, and alcohol-related mortality is substantially higher in women than in men. There are probably important gender differences in the responses of other tissues to alcohol consumption as well. Further studies are needed to investigate such gender differences in tissue sensitivity to alcohol intake, and to unravel the mechanisms involved.

Women are commonly served amounts of alcohol comparable to those given to men in contemporary social settings. Making women aware of their increased vulnerability may strengthen their resolve to resist the social pressures that may lead to inappropriate levels of consumption, possibly resulting in impairment of the ability to drive an automobile and to perform other tasks requiring alertness. In addition, the increased bioavailability may influence the severity of medical problems related to drinking.

Women and men differ in other aspects of ethanol metabolism. Some studies have found that women eliminate ethanol more rapidly[135,136]. Furthermore, women have higher ethanol-induced acetaldehyde levels.

ALCOHOL INTAKE AND ENGAGEMENT IN 'UNSAFE SEX'

'A man hath no better thing under the sun, than to eat, and to drink, and to be merry' (Ecclesiastes 8 : 15). 'Soul, thou hast much goods laid up for many years; take thine ease, eat, drink, and be merry' (Luke 12 : 19).

Drinking and sex, two of life's greatest pleasures, have always been closely interrelated. In the present chapter, we critically evaluate and analyze the relationship between drinking, sex and STDs.

Although the relationship between alcohol and STDs has been investigated over many decades, the AIDS epidemic has brought in its wake a renewed interest in this topic. Indeed, since 1986, a vast number of interesting and informative papers have been published which examine the impact of alcohol consumption on numerous aspects of STDs, particularly on AIDS.

An evaluation of the impact of alcohol consumption on STDs must deal with two aspects of the problem:

(1) What, if any, is the circumstantial connection between drinking and STDs, i.e. the effects of alcohol consumption on the engagement in 'unsafe sex', thus increasing the risk of sexual transmission of diseases?

(2) Is there a causal relationship between alcohol and STDs, e.g. the influence of alcohol on the immune system and its ability to weaken individuals' physiological defenses against STDs and thereby increase the likelihood of contracting an STD?

Several alternative and contradictory theories have been proposed to explain the linkages between drinking and risky sexual behaviors:

(1) The disinhibition hypothesis, suggesting a causal link between alcohol and unsafe sex. Alcohol use lowers inhibition of sexual impulses, clouds judgment with regard to risky sex and consequently may predispose to the taking of risks. Furthermore, the culturally learned belief that alcohol impairs decision-making may in itself affect the dynamics of sexual encounters, and may provide individuals with a convenient self-justification for engaging in unsafe sex and allow them to abrogate responsibility for behaviors that they and their peers would otherwise find unacceptable.

(2) The association between alcohol and risky sexual behavior could stem from a third factor, one which could be correlated with both activities. The individual might have a personality disorder presenting as a 'risky personality' or a 'sensation-seeking personality' which may even be genetically determined, be based on some psychobiological defect, or may result from socioeconomic and/or sociocultural problems.

In 1993 Leigh and Stall[137] reviewed more than 50 published studies on the relationship between drinking and high-risk sexual behavior and divided them into three categories according to the research design: global association studies, situational association studies and event analysis. Together with other authors[138,139], they considered a causal association between alcohol and risky sexual behavior as being old-fashioned and based on poor-quality studies with many methodological shortcomings and limitations. We do not completely agree with this approach. Alcohol is an indisputable risk factor for many injuries including road accidents, homicides, suicides, falls, burns, drownings, overdoses, aviation accidents, child abuse, assaults and industrial accidents[140]. It seems to us to be highly unlikely that alcohol could be a proven major risk factor in so many and varied injuries and accidents and have a clear causal relationship between these accidents and other aggressive and unsafe behaviors, but that sexual behavior is the singular exception among these findings. In any event, as Leigh and Stall put it, 'there is one conclusion that can be drawn from the literature that will provoke little controversy: Both sex and substance use are complicated behaviors, and determining the nature of the relationship between them is not simple'[137]. There is also general agreement that, from a public health standpoint, an understanding of these behaviors is of the utmost importance and is essential for effective STD-preventive interventions.

An analysis of weekly and seasonal variation in sexual behaviors among adolescent women with STDs indicated that intercourse was least likely on Sunday (12.2%) and most common on Friday and Saturday (17.5%). Eight per cent of total coital events were associated with alcohol and drug use. Forty-six per cent of all substance-associated coital events occurred on Friday and Saturday. The proportion of coital events associated with drugs or alcohol increased from Sunday to Saturday, although the proportion of coital events in which a condom was used did not vary significantly. Intercourse was most common in spring and summer and least frequent in winter, and substance-associated intercourse occurred most frequently in spring and autumn[141].

In a study that comprised 83 HIV-positive single women, most of the subjects declared having only one partner who was aware of her serological status, and 26% of these partners were themselves HIV-positive. These women were using condoms when having sex with their main partner, but not with other partners. Factors found to be associated with not using condoms included young age, low educational level, HIV-positive partner, STD history, alcohol consumption and drug use when having sex[142].

In a study on the association between drug and alcohol use and sexual risk behaviors in 51 female prostitutes in south London, most of these women (76%) were found to be using condoms[143,144]. There was no overall association between any of the drug use variables and the likelihood of unprotected sex. A substantial minority (just under a quarter of the sample) reported that, for them, drug use did reduce the chance that they would use a condom. There was a link between willingness to have unprotected sex for more money and drinking larger amounts and drinking more often.

A completely different situation emerges from a community-based sample survey carried out among commercial sex workers in Calcutta[145]. Almost all of them (448 out of 450) were addicted to alcohol and 81% drank regularly. Only 1.1% reported that their clients used condoms regularly.

In a study that examined the prevalence and predictors of HIV risk behaviors among low-income, African-American women residents of inner-city housing developments, the women at high risk were younger, and reported higher rates of substance and alcohol use[146,147].

In a longitudinal study of 82 female adolescents (aged 16–19 years), the potential causal relationship between alcohol and drug use and behavior that increased the risk of STDs was examined[148]. Event-specific condom use was associated with a usual pattern of condom use, but not with event-specific variables of partner change or substance use before intercourse. Substance use did not cause an alteration of the adolescent women's behavior in a manner that increased the risk of STD.

In comparing women's beliefs regarding the effects of alcohol consumption on sexual behavior with its real effects, there was a contrast between the two variables[149]. While women believed that alcohol enhanced sexual desire, enjoyment and activity, results of the questionnaire showed the opposite. Female-initiated sexual activity was inversely related to alcohol use, with women initiating significantly fewer sexual activities following the consumption of alcohol. Alcohol consumption immediately prior to sexual intercourse did not significantly alter the use of contraceptives.

ALCOHOL INTAKE AND SEXUALLY TRANSMITTED DISEASES

In a recent study, the association between lifestyle and sexual behavior and HPV infection was analyzed in 608 college women who were followed at 6-month intervals for 3 years[150]. An increased risk was significantly associated with several factors, including alcohol consumption. This study confirmed the results of previous studies, which also showed a positive correlation between alcohol consumption and HPV infection[151–153]. All of these studies emphasized the point that this association is not causal, but that alcohol consumption is probably a surrogate for an unidentified life-style risk factor, i.e. that alcohol is a marker of 'risky' sexual behavior.

A study on vaginal pH among 273 healthy sexually active adolescents revealed that seven factors, alcohol consumption included, were significantly associated with a more alkaline vaginal pH, which might explain the associated decreased resistance to common vaginal infections[154]. Moreover, after step-wise multiple regression analysis, only three factors (black race, current alcohol use and parity) remained significantly related to vaginal pH.

The epidemiology of *Trichomonas vaginalis* infection was investigated in a large study from China[155]. A total of 1489 new cases of *T. vaginalis* infection were diagnosed with 132 946 person-years of observation. The study confirmed the relationship between *T. vaginalis* infection and multiple sexual partners and suggested that the risk for *T. vaginalis* infection may be related to life-style risk factors, alcohol and smoking included.

The relationship between alcohol consumption and AIDS is controversial. Dingle and Oei[156], who critically examined empirical research and reviewed the literature, came to the conclusion that it is premature to promote the role of alcohol as a co-factor in HIV and AIDS. *In vitro* immunological studies demonstrated that social drinking increased the susceptibility of human cells to HIV infection. Animal studies showed that acute and chronic alcohol ingestion increased the rate of progression from retrovirus to clinical illness. In humans with HIV, however, no experimental evidence showed that alcohol was a co-factor of AIDS.

In an interesting study from Spain, factors associated with rapid or slow progression of HIV infection were analyzed in a cohort of 1783 persons infected with HIV-1[157]. One hundred of the patients fulfilled the criteria of long-term non-progressors, i.e. patients with more than 8 years of confirmed HIV seropositivity and a CD4+ T-cell count above 500×10^6, in the absence of antiretroviral therapy or symptoms suggesting immunodeficiency. Surprisingly, alcohol intake was among the variables found to be associated with long-term non-progressors. This does not indicate that alcohol had any protective effect on the progression of HIV. Alcohol was probably associated with a third factor that influenced the progression of HIV, such as infection by intravenous drug abuse (as opposed to sexual infection) which was positively associated with slow progression of the infection.

ALCOHOL AND CANCER OF THE SKIN AND MUCOSA

A great amount of epidemiological data have identified chronic alcohol consumption as a significant risk factor for upper alimentary tract cancer, including the oropharynx, and for anorectal cancer. Although the exact mechanisms by which chronic alcohol ingestion stimulates carcinogenesis are not known, experimental studies in animals support the concept that ethanol is not a carcinogen, but rather a co-carcinogen and a tumor promoter under certain experimental conditions. The metabolism of ethanol leads to the generation of acetaldehyde and free radicals, both highly toxic compounds that bind to cellular protein and DNA if not further metabolized to acetate by acetaldehyde dehydrogenase. Other mechanisms that have been suggested include interference of alcohol with immune functions; suppression of antimicrobial activity; increase in lipid peroxidation; and increase in incidence of p53 mutation.

In a Swedish study, site-specific risks were evaluated in more than 15 000 alcoholic women[158]. An increased relative risk (RR) for any cancer was found (RR = 1.6). Site-specific risks were increased for the tongue (RR = 8.5), mouth (RR = 12), tonsil (RR = 11), hypopharynx (RR = 9.0), cervix uteri (RR = 3.9), vulva, vagina and unspecified female genital organs (RR = 4.0). In contrast, a decreased risk for malignant melanoma of the skin was calculated (RR = 0.5). Similarly, in another study of women, the association between alcohol consumption and the risk for melanoma was not statistically significant[159].

Other studies confirmed the association between alcohol consumption and the incidence of and mortality from malignant neoplasms of the female genital tract[160–162].

ALCOHOL INTAKE AND PSORIASIS

While early reports failed to find a correlation between alcohol intake and psoriasis, most of the studies conducted in the past decade do support a positive association between alcohol consumption and the disease.

Higgins and du Vivier[163,164], deeply involved with the effects of alcohol on skin diseases, suggested that the rising incidence of alcohol addiction and misuse in recent years had accentuated the association between alcohol consumption and other common diseases, which might explain the discrepancy between the results of earlier and recent reports.

Striking differences between the sexes were found in a study on the relationship between the severity of psoriasis and alcohol consumption in 100 consecutive, unselected patients with chronic plaque-type psoriasis of at least 1 year's duration who were attending an out-patient clinic. Only two of 45 women (4.4%) were heavy drinkers, compared to 14 of 55 men (25.5%). Alcohol-related medical problems were found in seven of the 32 men with severe psoriasis compared to only one woman with severe disease[165].

In another investigation, possible risk factors for psoriasis were studied among women[85]. This study consisted of 55 consecutive female psoriatic patients and 108 unmatched controls with other skin diseases, all from a department of dermatology in Helsinki. A questionnaire focused on two specified periods of time: 12 months before the onset of the skin disease and 12 months before the examination date. The results showed that, before the onset of the disease, psoriasis was associated significantly with smoking, but not with alcohol intake. After the onset of the disease, psoriasis was associated significantly with alcohol intake, smoking and the occurrence of negative life events. Among psoriatics, skin surface involvement was significantly associated with alcohol intake, but not with smoking or negative life events. These results indicate that smoking was a risk factor for psoriasis in women, and that alcohol intake worsened their psoriasis. In contrast, results of a similar study by the same researchers indicated that psoriasis was associated with alcohol intake, but not with smoking in young and middle-aged men[86]. Moreover, there was no significant correlation among men between the extent of body area affected and the average alcohol intake, in contrast to women.

In a study investigating the relationship between ethanol consumption and treatment outcome among 48 men and 46 women with moderate to severe psoriasis, a positive correlation was found in men, but not in women[166].

ALCOHOL INTAKE AND PORPHYRIA CUTANEA TARDA

The image of porphyria cutanea tarda (PCT) as a disease of hard-drinking, middle-aged men that emerged in the 1950s has become modified over the years, but still describes many patients. Regular ingestion of alcohol in moderate to large amounts over long periods of time is a common and consistent feature of all series[167–172].

The association of PCT with estrogen, the increasing use of estrogens (in oral contraceptives

and for hormonal replacement therapy), and changes in the social use of alcohol, may explain the changes in the traditional patient profile of PCT, with more women being affected[171–174].

Finally, there are over 50 reported cases of coexistent lupus erythematosus and PCT, most of them found among women[175].

ALCOHOL CONSUMPTION AND HORMONAL CHANGES IN WOMEN

There are a number of difficulties in assessing the effect of alcohol consumption on hormonal changes. First, there are significant individual variations in hormonal patterns during a normal menstrual cycle. Second, there are significant variations in individual responses to alcohol. Third, several other habits are correlated with alcohol consumption, e.g. cigarette smoking, predilection for certain foods and use of psychoactive drugs, and all of these may influence hormonal status. Finally, there are disagreements over the definition of alcoholism, and the methods for quantification of alcohol consumption.

Valimaki and associates[176] studied sex hormone levels and ultrasound findings of the ovaries and endometrium in premenopausal non-cirrhotic alcoholics during the menstrual cycle. Serum levels of follicle stimulating hormone (FSH), luteinizing hormone (LH) and prolactin were similar to those of the controls throughout the whole observation period, and their estrone and estradiol levels were normal as well.

At least two studies reported increased total estradiol levels in the periovulatory phase of alcoholic women. In one study, elevated estrone, estradiol and estriol levels were detected in the urine during the luteal phase; however, no changes were found in the bioavailable estradiol levels[177]. In the second study, the relationship between alcohol intake and serum total estradiol level was analyzed in premenopausal women[178]. In this study, blood was drawn from 60 premenopausal women twice, 1 year apart. Both blood samples were obtained on the same day of the luteal phase of the cycle, in the same month and in the same hour and minute of the day. A significant association between alcohol intake and estradiol was found when the estradiol levels were averaged across the two visits. The results of the study indicated that women showing consistently high estradiol levels at both visits were characterized by a significantly higher alcohol intake (92.8 g/week) in comparison with those showing consistently low estradiol levels at both visits (31.6 g/week). This finding may provide a possible explanation for a positive association between alcohol consumption and breast cancer.

Another interesting finding is the lower progesterone level and higher testosterone level during the luteal phase in drinkers compared to non-drinkers.

A number of studies in the past decade attempted to assess the effect of moderate alcoholic beverage consumption on endogenous sex hormones in postmenopausal women. Examining postmenopausal women has an advantage in that menstrual cycle variations in hormones no longer occur, and it is easier to optimize detection of differences in levels of hormones and hormone interrelationships in such a study population.

A strong and significant trend for increasing levels of estradiol with increasing alcohol consumption was demonstrated in 61 Japanese postmenopausal women. This association persisted after adjusting for age, height and body mass index[179]. A recent study on 125 postmenopausal women in five geographic regions of the USA confirmed these results[180].

The major source of endogenous estrogens in postmenopausal women is the aromatization of androgens to estrogens. Because alcohol is known to increase aromatization, the relationship between moderate alcoholic beverage consumption and serum estradiol levels was evaluated in postmenopausal women. In evaluating 128 of these women, a significant correlation was found between total weekly drinks and both the estradiol levels and the estradiol/testosterone ratio (a crude estimator of aromatization)[181]. The authors suggested that moderate alcohol use is an important factor for postmenopausal estrogen status and may offer a partial explanation for the reported protective effect of moderate alcohol consumption with respect to postmenopausal cardiovascular disease risk. Certainly, such a correlation would also have implications on the skin of postmenopausal women.

At least two papers have dealt with the impact of alcohol on estrogen metabolism in postmenopausal women who were on hormone replacement therapy[182,183]. In the first study[182], the effect of alcohol on hormone levels in postmenopausal women using transdermal estradiol patches (0.15 mg) was evaluated. Estradiol levels rose significantly above the mean baseline of 675 pmol/l after ethanol ingestion with a mean peak of 804 pmol/l 35 min after the onset of drinking, and were significantly greater than the estradiol levels that followed a carbohydrate drink. In another study by the same group[183],

healthy postmenopausal women receiving oral estrogen and progestin replacement therapy were compared with women who were not on this therapy. Each group drank alcohol (0.7 g/kg) and an isoenergetic placebo on consecutive days. Alcohol ingestion led to a three-fold increase in circulating estradiol in women on estrogen replacement therapy, but did not change estradiol significantly in the control women who were not on the therapy. No significant increase in circulating estrone was detected in either group. Blood alcohol levels did not differ in women who used replacement therapy and those who did not. In conclusion, acute alcohol ingestion may lead to significant and sustained elevations in circulating estradiol to levels 300% higher than those targeted in clinical use of estrogen replacement therapy. Such an effect on circulating hormones might have an impact on many end organs, including the skin.

REFERENCES

1. Anonymous. Surveillance for selected tobacco-use behaviors – United States, 1900–1994. *MMWR* 1994;43(SS-3):1–43

2. Cirillo J. Differential treatment: considerations for the female alcoholic. *Ann NY Acad Sci* 1996;789:83–99

3. North C. Alcoholism in women. More common – and serious – than you might think. *JAMA* 1996;100:221–33

4. Tur E. Physiology of the skin – differences between women and men. *Clin Dermatol* 1997;15:5–16

5. Pierce J, Lee L, Gilpin E. Smoking initiation by adolescent girls, 1944 through 1988. An association with targeted advertising. *JAMA* 1994;271:608–11

6. Gilpin E, Lee L, Evans N, Pierce J. Smoking initiation rates in adults and minors: United States 1944–1988. *Am J Epidemiol* 1994;140:535–43

7. World Health Organization (WHO). *Tobacco or Health. A Global Status Report.* Geneva: WHO, 1997

8. Graham H. The changing patterns of women's smoking. *Health Visit* 1989;62:22–4

9. Lee A, Crombie I, Smith W, Tunstall-Pedoe H. Cigarette smoking and employment status. *Soc Sci Med* 1991;33:1309–12

10. Pierce J, Fiore M, Novotny T, *et al.* Trends in cigarette smoking in the United States. Educational differences are increasing. *JAMA* 1989;261:56–60

11. Michell L, Amos A. Girls, pecking order and smoking. *Soc Sci Med* 1997;44:1861–9

12. Ernster V. Mixed messages for women: a social history of cigarette smoking and advertising. *NY State J Med* 1985;85:353–40

13. Pierce J, Gilpin E. A historical analysis of tobacco marketing and the uptake of smoking by youth in

the United States: 1890–1977. *Health Psychol* 1995;14:500–8

14. Kaufman N. Smoking and young women. The physician's role in stopping an equal opportunity killer. *JAMA* 1994;271:630

15. Froom P, Melamed S, Blair V. Smoking cessation and weight gain. *J Fam Pract* 1998;46:460–4

16. Solly S. Clinical lectures on paralysis. *Lancet* 1856;ii:641–3

17. Martin J. Effects of tobacco in Europeans in India. *Lancet* 1857;i:226

18. Ippen M, Ippen H. Approaches to a prophylaxis of skin aging. *J Soc Cosmet Chem* 1965;16:305–8

19. Daniell H. Smooth tobacco and wrinkled skin. *N Engl J Med* 1969;280:58

20. Daniell H. Smoker's wrinkles. A study in the epidemiology of 'crow's feet'. *Ann Intern Med* 1971;75: 873–80

21. Allen H, Johnson B. Smoker's wrinkles? *JAMA* 1973;225:1067–9

22. Model D. Smokers' face: an underrated clinical sign? *Br Med J* 1985;291:1760–2

23. Model D. Smokers' faces: who are the smokers? *Br Med J* 1985;291:1755

24. Soffer A. Smoker's faces: who are the smokers? *Chest* 1986;89:622

25. Kadunce D, Burr R, Gress R, *et al.* Cigarette smoking: risk factor for premature facial wrinkling. *Ann Intern Med* 1991;114:840–4

26. Schnohr P, Lange P, Nyboe J, *et al.* Does smoking increase the degree of wrinkles on the face? The Copenhagen City Heart Study. *Ugeskr Laeger* 1991;153:660–3

27. Ernster V, Grady D, Miike R, *et al.* Facial wrinkling in men and women by smoking status. *Am J Public Health* 1995;85:78–82

28. Barbieri L, McShane M, Ryan J. Constituents of cigarette smoke inhibit human granulosa cell aromatase. *Fertil Steril* 1986;46:232

29. Barbieri L, Goldberg J, Ryan J. Nicotine, cotinine and anabinase inhibit aromatase in human trophoblast *in vitro*. *J Clin Invest* 1986;77:1727–33

30. MacMahon B, Trichopulos D, Cole P, Brown J. Cigarette smoking and urinary estrogens. *N Engl J Med* 1982;307:1062–5

31. Mosley L, Finseth F. Cigarette smoking: impairment of digital blood flow and wound healing in the hand. *Hand* 1977;9:97–101

32. Mosley L, Finseth F, Goody M. Nicotine and its effects on wound healing. *Plast Reconstr Surg* 1978;61:570–5

33. Lawrence W, Murphy R, Robson M, *et al.* The detrimental effect of cigarette smoking on flap survival: and experimental study in the rat. *Br J Plast Surg* 1984;37:216–19

34. Craig S, Rees T. The effects of smoking on experimental skin flaps in hamsters. *Plast Reconstr Surg* 1985;75:842–6

35. Nolan J, Jenking R, Kurihara K, *et al.* The acute effects of cigarette smoke exposure on experimental skin flaps. *Plast Reconstr Surg* 1985;75:544–9

36. Siana J, Rex S, Gottrup F. The effect of cigarette smoking on wound healing. *Scand J Plast Reconstr Surg Hand Surg* 1989;23:207–9

37. Rees T, Liverett D, Guy C. The effect of cigarette smoking on skin-flap survival in the face lift patient. *Plast Reconstr Surg* 1984;73:911–15

38. Riefkohl R, Wolfe J, Cox E, McCarty KS Jr. Association between cutaneous occlusive vascular disease, cigarette smoking, and skin slough after rhytidectomy. *Plast Reconstr Surg* 1986;77:592–5

39. Webster R, Kazda G, Hamdan U, *et al.* Cigarette smoking and face lift: conservative versus wide undermining. *Plast Reconstr Surg* 1986;77:596–604

40. Silverstein P. Smoking and wound healing. *Am J Med* 1992;93(suppl):S22–4

41. Miller P, Plant M, Plant M, Duffy J. Alcohol, tobacco, illicit drugs, and sex: an analysis of risky behaviors among young adults. *Int J Addict* 1995;30:239–58

42. Spingarn R, DuRant R. Male adolescents involved in pregnancy: associated health risk and problem behaviors. *Pediatrics* 1996;98:262–8

43. Grant B. Age at smoking onset and its association with alcohol consumption and DSM-IV alcohol abuse and dependence: results from the National Longitudinal Alcohol Epidemiologic Survey. *J Subst Abuse* 1998;10:59–73

44. Cress R, Holly E, Ahn D, *et al.* Contraceptive use among women smokers and nonsmokers in the San Francisco Bay area. *Prev Med* 1994;23:181–9

45. Cress R, Holly E, Aston D, *et al.* Characteristics of women non-smokers exposed to passive smoke. *Prev Med* 1994;23:14–17

46. Ward R. Truancy and illegal drug use, and knowledge of HIV infection in 932 14–16 year old adolescents. *Mich Med* 1992;91:7

47. Jessor R. Risk behavior in adolescence: a psychosocial framework for understanding and action. *J Adolesc Health* 1991;12:597–605

48. Rohan T, Mann V, McLaughlin J, *et al.* PCR-detected genital papillomavirus infection: prevalence and association with risk factors for cervical cancer. *Int J Cancer* 1991;49:856–60

49. Davidson M, Schnitzer P, Bulkow L, *et al.* The prevalence of cervical infection with human papillomaviruses and cervical dysplasia in Alaska native women. *J Infect Dis* 1994;169:792–800

50. Burger M, Hollema H, Bouw A, *et al.* Cigarette smoking and human papillomavirus in patients with reported cervical cytological abnormality. *Br Med J* 1993;306:749–52

51. Phillips A, Smith G. Smoking and human papillomavirus infection. Causal link not proved. *Br Med J* 1993;306:1268–9

52. Burger M, Hollema H, Pieters W, *et al.* Epidemiological evidence of cervical intraepithelial

neoplasia without the presence of human papillomavirus. *Br J Cancer* 1996;73:831–6

53. Lovejoy N. The multi-cultural 'Male Risk' factor. *Oncol Nurs Forum* 1994;21:497–504

54. Agarwal S, Sehgal A, Sardana S, *et al*. Role of male behaviour in cervical carcinogenesis among women with one lifetime sexual partner. *Cancer* 1993;72:1666–9

55. Smith H, Horowitz N, Silverman N, *et al*. Humoral immunity to herpes simplex viral-induced antigens in smokers. *Cancer* 1976;38:1155–62

56. Shillitoe E, Greenspan D, Greenspan JS, *et al*. Neutralizing antibody to herpes simplex virus type 1 in patients with oral cancer. *Cancer* 1982;49:2315–20

57. Kao R, Shillitoe E. Interaction between herpes simplex virus and DMBA in epithelial tumorigenesis (abstr). *J Dent Res* 1980;59:332

58. Axell T, Liedholm R. Occurrence of recurrent herpes labialis in an adult Swedish population. *Acta Odontol Scand* 1990;48:119–23

59. Young T, Rimm EDD. Cross-sectional study of recurrent herpes labialis. *Am J Epidemiol* 1988;127:612–25

60. Hirsch J, Svennerholm B, Vahlne A. Inhibition of herpes simplex virus replication by tobacco extracts. *Cancer Res* 1984;44:1991–7

61. Park N, Weiss R, Sapp J. *In vitro* and *in vivo* effect of smokeless tobacco on the replication of herpes simplex virus (abstr 826). *J Dent Res* 1985;64:266

62. Park N, Sapp J, Herbosa E. Oral cancer induced in hamsters with herpes simplex infection and simulated snuff dipping. *Oral Surg Oral Med Oral Pathol* 1986;62:164–8

63. Newell G, Mansell P, Wilson MLH, *et al*. Risk factors analysis among men referred for possible acquired immune deficiency syndrome. *Prev Med* 1985;14:81–91

64. Royce R, Winkelstein W Jr. HIV infection, cigarette smoking and CD4+ T-lymphocytes count: preliminary results from the San Francisco Men's Health Study. *AIDS* 1990;4:327–33

65. Boulos R, Halsey N, Holt E, *et al*. HIV-1 in Haitian women 1982–1988. *J Acquir Immun Defic Syndr* 1990;3:721–8

66. Halsey N, Coberly J, Jolt E, *et al*. Sexual behavior, smoking, and HIV-1 infection in Haitian women. *JAMA* 1992;267:2062–6

67. Hardell L, Moss AOD, Voberding P. Exposure to hair dyes and polychlorinated dibenso-*p*-dioxins in AIDS patients with Kaposi sarcoma: an epidemiological investigation. *Cancer Detect Prev* 1987;1(suppl):567–70

68. Galai N, Park L, Wesch J, *et al*. Effect of smoking on clinical progression of HIV-1 infection. *J Acquir Immun Defic Syndr* 1997;14:451–8

69. Larsson P, Platz-Christensen J, Sundstrom E. Is bacterial vaginosis a sexually transmitted disease? *Int J STD AIDS* 1991;2:362–4

70. Peters N, Van Leuwer A, Pietens W, *et al*. Bacterial vaginosis is not important in the aetiology of cervical neoplasia: a survey on women with dyskaryotic smears. *Sex Transm Dis* 1995;22:296–302

71. Chokephaibulkit K, Patamasucon P, List M, *et al*. Genital *Chlamydia trachomatis* infection in pregnant adolescents in east Tennessee: a 7-year case–control study. *J Pediatr Adolesc Gynecol* 1997;10:95–100

72. Tchoudomirova K, Stanilova M, Garov V. Clinical manifestations and diagnosis of bacterial vaginosis in a clinic of sexually transmitted diseases. *Folia Med (Plovdiv)* 1998;40:34–40

73. Critchlow C, Woelner-Hanssen P, Eschenback DKNKL, *et al*. Determinants of cervical ectopia and cervicitis: age, oral contraception, specific cervical infection, smoking and douching. *Am J Obstet Gynecol* 1995;173:534–43

74. Shafer M, Pessione F, Schieux C, *et al*. *Chlamydia trachomatis*: facteurs de risque chez less femmes de la region Parisienne. *J Gynecol Obstet Biol Reprod Paris* 1993;22:163–8

75. Holly E, Cress R, Ahn D, *et al*. Characteristics of women by smoking status in the San Francisco Bay Area. *Cancer Epidemiol Biomarkers Prev* 1992;1:491–7

76. Willmott F. Current smoking habits and genital infections in women. *Int J STD AIDS* 1992;3:329–31

77. Marchbanks P, Lee N, Peterson H. Cigarette smoking as a risk factor for pelvic inflammatory disease. *Am J Obstet Gynecol* 1990;162:639–44

78. Scholes D, Daling J, Stergachis A. Current cigarette smoking and risk of acute pelvic inflammatory disease. *Am J Public Health* 1992;82:1352–5

79. O'Doherty C, McIntyre C. Palmoplantar pustulosis and smoking. *Br Med J* 1985;291:861–4

80. Kavli G, Forde OAE, Stenvold S. Psoriasis: familial predisposition and environmental factors. *Br Med J* 1985;291:999–1000

81. Braathen L, Botten G, Bjerkedal T. Psoriasis in Norway. A questionnaire study of health status, contact with paramedical professions and alcohol and tobacco. *Acta Derm Venereol (Stockh)* 1989;142(suppl):9–12

82. Bell L, Sedlack R, Beard M, *et al*. Incidence of psoriasis in Rochester, Minn 1980–1983. *Arch Dermatol* 1991;127:1184–7

83. Mills C, Srivastava E, Harvey M, *et al*. Smoking habits in psoriasis: a case control study. *Br J Dermatol* 1992;127:18–21

84. Naldi L, Parazzini F, Brevi A, *et al*. Family history, smoking habits, alcohol consumption and risk of psoriasis. *Br J Dermatol* 1992;127:212–17

85. Poikolainen K, Reunala T, Karvonen J. Smoking, alcohol and life events related to psoriasis among women. *Br J Dermatol* 1994;130:473–7

86. Poikolainen K, Reunala T, Karvonen J, *et al*. Alcohol intake: a risk factor for psoriasis in young and middle aged men? *Br Med J* 1990;300:780–3

87. Giles G, Kneale B. Vulvar cancer: the Cinderella of gynaecological oncology. *Aust NZ J Obstet Gynaecol* 1995;35:71–5

88. Andersen W, Franquemont DW, Williams J, *et al.* Vulvar squamous cell carcinoma and papillomaviruses: two separate entities? *Am J Obstet Gynecol* 1991;165:329–35

89. Newcomb P, Weiss N, Daling J. Incidence of vulvar carcinoma in relation to menstrual, reproductive and medical factors. *J Natl Cancer Inst* 1984;73: 391–6

90. Mabuchi K, Bross D, Kessler I. Epidemiology of cancer of the vulva. *Cancer* 1985;55:1843–8

91. Brinton L, Nasca P, Mallin K, *et al.* Case–control study of cancer of the vulva. *Obstet Gynecol* 1990;75:859–66

92. Daling J, Sherman K, Hislop T, *et al.* Cigarette smoking and the risk of anogenital cancer. *Am J Epidemiol* 1992;135:180–9

93. Kirschner C, Yordan E, De Geest K, Wilbanks G. Smoking, obesity, and survival in squamous cell carcinoma of the vulva. *Gynecol Oncol* 1995;56: 79–84

94. Ansink A, Heintz AP. Epidemiology and etiology of squamous cell carcinoma of the vulva. *Eur J Obstet Gynecol Reprod Biol* 1993;48:111–15

95. Jones R, Baranyai J, Stables S. Trends in squamous cell carcinoma of the vulva: the influence of vulvar intraepithelial neoplasia. *Obstet Gynecol* 1997;90: 448–52

96. Trimble C, Hildesheim A, Brinton L, *et al.* Heterogenous etiology of squamous cell carcinoma of the vulva. *Obstet Gynecol* 1996;87:59–64

97. Hellberg D, Valentin J, Eklund T, *et al.* Penile cancer: is there an epidemiological role for smoking and sexual behavior? *Br Med J* 1987;295:1306–8

98. Maden C, Sherman K, Beckmann A. History of circumcision, medical conditions, and sexual activity and risk of penile cancer. *J Natl Cancer Inst* 1985; 85:19–24

99. Lender M. Women alcoholics: prevalence estimates and their problems reflected in turn-of-the-century institutional data. *Int J Addict* 1981;16:443–8

100. Mercer P, Khavari K. Are women drinking more like men? An empirical examination of the convergence hypothesis. *Alcohol Clin Exp Res* 1990;14:461–6

101. Hilton M. Drinking patterns and drinking in 1984; results from a general population survey. *Alcoholism* 1987;11:167–75

102. Herd D. Drinking by black and white women: results from a national survey. *Soc Probl* 1988;35: 493–505

103. Amaro H, Beckman L, Mays V. A comparison of black and white women entering alcohol treatment. *J Stud Alcohol* 1987;48:220–8

104. Kitano H, Chi I, Rhee S, *et al.* Norms and alcohol consumption: Japanese in Japan, Hawaii and California. *J Stud Alcohol* 1992;53:33–9

105. Caetano R, Hines A. Alcohol, sexual practices, and risk of AIDS among blacks, Hispanics, and whites. *J Acquir Immun Defic Syndr Hum Retrovirol* 1995;10: 554–61

106. Wechsler H, Demone H, Gottlieb N. Drinking patterns of Greater Boston adults: subgroup differences on the QFU Index. *J Stud Alcohol* 1980; 41:672–81

107. Grant B. Alcohol consumption, alcohol abuse and alcohol dependence. The United States as an example. *Addiction* 1994;89:1357–65

108. Mason P, Wilkinson G. The prevalence of psychiatric, morbidity OPCS survey of psychiatric morbidity in Great Britain. *Br J Psychiatry* 1996;168:1–3

109. Regier D, Farmer M, Rae D, *et al.* Comorbidity of mental disorders with alcohol and other drug abuse. Results from the Epidemiologic Catchment Area (ECA) Study. *JAMA* 1990;264:2511–18

110. Grant B. Prevalence and correlates of alcohol use and DSM-IV alcohol dependence in the United States: results of the National Longitudinal Alcohol Epidemiologic Survey. *J Stud Alcohol* 1997;58:464–73

111. Wallen J. A comparison of male and female clients in substance abuse treatment. *J Subst Abuse Treat* 1992;9:243–8

112. Fichter M, Narrow W, Roper M, *et al.* Prevalence of mental illness in Germany and the United States. Comparison of the Upper Bavarian Study and the Epidemiologic Catchment Area Program. *J Nerv Ment Dis* 1996;184:598–606

113. Engs R, Hanson D. Drinking patterns and problems of college students. *J Alcohol Drug Educ* 1985;31:65–83

114. Engs R, Slawinska J, Hanson D. The drinking patterns of American and Polish university students: a cross-national study. *Drug Alcohol Depend* 1991;27:167–75

115. Spak F, Hallstrom T. Prevalence of female alcohol dependence and abuse in Sweden. *Addiction* 1995; 90:1077–88

116. Spak F. To what extent is female alcohol dependence and abuse known in the health care system? The use of multi-source information in a Swedish population survey. *Acta Psychiatr Scand* 1996;93:87–91

117. Engs R, Van Teijlingen E. Correlates of alcohol, tobacco and marijuana use among Scottish post secondary helping-profession students. *J Stud Alcohol* 1997;58:435–44

118. Kendler K, Walters E, Neale M, *et al.* The structure of the genetic and environmental risk factors for six major psychiatric disorders in women. Phobia, generalized anxiety disorders, panic disorders, bulimia, major depression, and alcoholism. *Arch Gen Psychiatry* 1995;52:374–83

119. Kendler K, Prescott C. Cannabis use, abuse, and dependence in a population-based sample of female twins. *Am J Psychiatry* 1998;155:1016–22

120. Kendler K, Neale M, Heath A, *et al*. A twin-family study of alcoholism in women. *Am J Psychiatry* 1994;151:707–15

121. Yates W, Cadoret R, Troughton E, Stewart M. An adoption study of DSM-IIIR alcohol and drug dependence severity. *Drug Alcohol Depend* 1996;41:9–15

122. Kendler K, Naele M, Prescott C, *et al*. Childhood parental loss and alcoholism in women: a causal analysis using a twin-family design. *Psychol Med* 1996;26:659–66

123. Prescott C, Naele M, Corey L, Kendler K. Predictors of problem drinking and alcohol dependence in a population-based sample of female twins. *J Stud Alcohol* 1997;58:167–81

124. Murphy W, Coleman E, Hoon E, Scott C. Sexual dysfunction and treatment in alcoholic women. *Sex Disabil* 1980;3:240–55

125. Miller B, Downs W, Gondoli D. Spousal violence among alcoholic women as compared to a random household sample of women. *J Stud Alcohol* 1989;50:533–40

126. Fillmore K. The social victims of drinking. *Br J Addict* 1985;80:307–14

127. Walitzer K, Sher K. A prospective study of self-esteem and alcohol use disorders in early adulthood: evidence for gender differences. *Alcohol Clin Exp Res* 1996;20:1118–24

128. McLachlan J, Walderman R, Birchmore D, Marsden L. Self-evaluation, role satisfaction and anxiety in the women alcoholic. *Int J Addict* 1979;14:809–32

129. Marsh J, Colten M, Tucker M. Women's use of drugs and alcohol: new perspectives. *J Soc Issues* 1982;38:1–8

130. Marsh J, Miller N. Female clients in substance abuse treatment. *Int J Addict* 1985;20:995–1019

131. Helzer J, Pryzbeck T. The co-occurrence of alcoholism with other psychiatric disorders in the general population and its impact on treatment. *J Stud Alcohol* 1988;49:219–24

132. Gomberg E. Women and alcohol: use and abuse. *J Nerv Ment Dis* 1993;181:211–19

133. Jones B, Jones M. Male and female intoxication levels for three alcohol doses or do women really get higher than men? *Alcohol Tech Rep* 1976;5:11–14

134. Frezza M, DiPadova C, Pozzato G, *et al*. High blood alcohol levels in women: the role of decreased gastric alcohol dehydrogenase activity and first-pass metabolism. *N Engl J Med* 1990;322:95–9

135. Cole-Harding S, Wilson J. Ethanol metabolism in men and women. *J Stud Alcohol* 1987;48:380–7

136. Mishra L, Sharma S, Potter J, Mezey E. More rapid elimination of alcohol in women as compared to their male siblings. *Alcohol Clin Exp Res* 1989;13:754

137. Leigh B, Stall R. Substance use and risky sexual behavior for exposure to HIV. Issues in methodology, interpretation, and prevention. *Am Psychol* 1993;48:1035–45

138. Weatherburn P, Cavies P, Hickson F, *et al*. No connection between alcohol use and unsafe sex among gay and bisexual men. *AIDS* 1993;7:115–19

139. McManur T, Weatherburn P. Alcohol, AIDS and immunity. *Br Med Bull* 1994;50:115–23

140. Glucksman E. Alcohol and accidents. *Br Med Bull* 1994;50:76–84

141. Fortenberry J, Orr D, Zimet G, Blythe M. Weekly and seasonal variation in sexual behaviors among adolescent women with sexually transmitted diseases. *J Adolesc Health* 1997;20:420–5

142. Clark R, Kissinger P, Bedimo A, *et al*. Determination of factors associated with condom use among women infected with human immunodeficiency virus. *Int J STD AIDS* 1997;8:229–33

143. Gossop M, Powis B, Griffiths P, Strang J. Female prostitutes in south London: use of heroin, cocaine and alcohol, and their relationship to health risk behaviours. *AIDS Care* 1995;7:253–60

144. Gossop M, Powis B, Griffiths P, Strang J. Sexual behaviour and its relationship to drug-taking among prostitutes in south London. *Addiction* 1994;89:961–70

145. Chakraborty A, Jana S, Das A, *et al*. Community based survey of STD/HIV infection among commercial sexworkers in Calcutta (India). Part I. Some social features of commercial sexworkers. *J Commun Dis* 1994;26:161–7

146. Sikkema K, Heckman T, Kelly J. HIV risk behaviors among inner-city African American women. The community Housing AIDS Prevention Study Group. *Wom Health* 1997;3:349–66

147. Sikkema K, Heckman T, Kelly J, *et al*. HIV risk behaviors among women living in low-income, inner-city housing developments. *Am J Public Health* 1996;86:1123–8

148. Fortenberry J, Orr D, Katz B, *et al*. Sex under the influence. A diary self-report study of substance use and sexual behavior among adolescent women. *Sex Transm Dis* 1997;24:313–19

149. Harvey S, Beckman L. Alcohol consumption, female sexual behavior and contraceptive use. *J Stud Alcohol* 1986;47:327–33

150. Ho G, Bierman R, Beardsley L, *et al*. Natural history of cervicovaginal papillomavirus infection in young women. *N Engl J Med* 1998;338:423–8

151. Sikstrom B, Hellberg D, Nilsson S, Mardh P. Smoking, alcohol, sexual behaviour and drug use in women with cervical human papillomavirus infection. *Arch Gynecol Obstet* 1995;256:131–7

152. Burkett B, Peterson C, Birch L, *et al*. The relationship between contraceptives, sexual practices, and

cervical human papillomavirus infection among a college population. *J Clin Epidemiol* 1992;45: 1295–302

153. Herrero R, Reeves W, Brenes M, *et al*. Invasive cervical cancer and smoking in Latin America. *J Natl Cancer Inst* 1989;81:205–11

154. Stevens Simon C, Jamison J, McGregor J, Douglas J. Racial variation in vaginal pH among healthy sexually active adolescents. *Sex Transm Dis* 1994;21:168–72

155. Zhang Z. Epidemiology of *Trichomonas vaginalis*. A prospective study in China. *Sex Transm Dis* 1996;23:415–24

156. Dingle G, Oei T. Is alcohol a cofactor of HIV and AIDS? Evidence from immunological and behavioral studies. *Psychol Bull* 1997;122:56–71

157. Soriano V, Martin R, Del-Romero J, *et al*. Rapid and slow progression of the infection by the type 1 immunodeficiency virus in a population of seropositive subjects in Madrid. *Med Clin Barc* 1996;107:761–6

158. Sigvardsson S, Hardell L, Pryzbeck T, Cloninger R. Increased cancer risk among Swedish female alcoholics. *Epidemiology* 1996;7:140–3

159. Holly E, Aston D, Cress R, Ahn D. Cutaneous melanoma in women. II. Phenotypic characteristics and other host-related factors. *Am J Epidemiol* 1995;141:934–42

160. Guo W, Chow W, Li J, *et al*. Correlations of choriocarcinoma mortality with alcohol drinking and reproductive factors in China. *Eur J Cancer Prev* 1994;3:223–6

161. Serur E, Fruchter R, Maiman M, *et al*. Age, substance abuse, and survival of patients with cervical carcinoma. *Cancer* 1995;75:2530–8

162. Grundmann E. Cancer morbidity and mortality in USA Mormons and Seventh-day Adventists. *Arch Anat Cytol Pathol* 1992;40:73–8

163. Higgins E, du Vivier A. Alcohol and the skin. *Alcohol* 1992;27:595–602

164. Higgins E, du Vivier A. Cutaneous disease and alcohol misuse. *Br Med Bull* 1994;50:85–98

165. Monk B, Neill S. Alcohol consumption and psoriasis. *Dermatologica* 1986;173:57–60

166. Gupta M, Schork N, Gupta A, Ellis C. Alcohol intake and treatment responsiveness of psoriasis: a prospective study. *J Am Acad Dermatol* 1993;28: 730–2

167. Brunsting L. Observations in porphyria cutanea tarda. *Arch Dermatol Syph* 1954;70:551–64

168. Grossman M, Bickers D, Poh-Fitzpatrick M, *et al*. Porphyria cutanea tarda. Clinical features and laboratory findings in 40 patients. *Am J Med* 1979;67:335–6

169. Herrero C, Vicente A, Bruguera M, *et al*. Is hepatitis C virus infection a trigger of porphyria cutanea tarda? *Lancet* 1993;341:788–9

170. Stolzel U, Kostler E, Koszka C, *et al*. Low prevalence of hepatitis C virus infection in Germany. *Hepatology* 1995;21:1500–3

171. Elder G. Porphyria cutanea tarda. *Semin Liver Dis* 1998;18:67–75

172. Elder G. Update on enzyme and molecular defects in porphyria. *Photodermatol Photoimmunol Photomed* 1998;14:66–9

173. Mor Z, Caspi E. Cutaneous complications of hormonal replacement therapy. *Clin Dermatol* 1997;15:147–54

174. Koszo F, Morvay M, Dobozy A, *et al*. Erythrocyte uroporphyrinogen decarboxylase activity in 80 unrelated patients with porphyria cutanea tarda. *Br J Dermatol* 1992;126:446–9

175. Gibson G, McEvoy M. Coexistence of lupus erythematosus and porphyria cutanea tarda in fifteen patients. *J Am Acad Dermatol* 1998;38:569–73

176. Valimaki M, Laitenen K, Tiitinen A, *et al*. Gonadal function and morphology in non-cirrhotic female alcoholics: a controlled study with hormone measurements and ultrasonography. *Acta Obstet Gynecol Scand* 1995;74:462–6

177. Reichman M, Judd J, Longscope C, *et al*. Effects of alcohol consumption on plasma and urinary hormone concentrations in premenopausal women. *J Natl Cancer Inst* 1993;85:722–7

178. Muti P, Trevisan M, Micheli A, *et al*. Alcohol consumption and total estradiol in premenopausal women. *Cancer Epidemiol Biomarkers Prev* 1998;7: 189–93

179. Nagata C, Kabuto M, Takatsuka N, Shimizu H. Association of alcohol, height, and reproductive factors in serum hormone concentration in postmenopausal Japanese women. *Breast Cancer Res Treat* 1997;44:235–41

180. Madigan M, Troisi R, Potischman N, *et al*. Serum hormone levels in relation to reproductive and lifestyle factors in postmenopausal women (United States). *Cancer Causes Contr* 1998;9:199–207

181. Gavaler J, Thiel D. The association between moderate alcoholic beverage consumption and serum estradiol and testosterone levels in normal postmenopausal women: relationship to the literature. *Alcohol Clin Exp Res* 1992;16:87–92

182. Ginsburg E, Walsh B, Gao X, *et al*. The effect of acute ethanol ingestion on estrogen levels in postmenopausal women using transdermal estradiol. *J Soc Gynecol Invest* 1995;2:26–9

183. Ginsburg E, Mello N, Mendelson J, *et al*. Effects of alcohol ingestion on estrogens in postmenopausal women. *JAMA* 1996;276:1747–51

Therapeutic considerations

46

Marianne N. O'Donoghue

Many women make appointments to see their dermatologists to inquire about skin care. The following recommendations are particularly helpful for girls and women.

CLEANSING

Skin

The skin-care market is heavily aimed at women and girls. This has both advantages and disadvantages. There are new products being developed by the day, with constant improvement of old products. Unfortunately, these often contain increased fragrance, preservatives and photosensitizers. These ingredients have often been proven to cause trouble[1]. The soap gels that are appropriate for the European market may be too drying for Midwestern American women, or women in other countries that are largely desert areas. Safe recommendations are as follows:

(1) Selection of a cleanser should be based on the type of skin and the ambient humidity where the patient lives. If the humidity is high, soap gels, liquid cleansers and perhaps even deodorant soaps may be appropriate. If the humidity is low, such as in the autumn and winter seasons, or climates such as the American Southwest or the Middle East, gentle face soaps may be the only cleansing products required for the body as well as the face.

(2) Many of the liquid cleansers contain more surfactants, which can interact at the dermal–epidermal junction, causing an irritant dermatitis. These may be tolerated by people with normal skin but not tolerated by people with asteatotic or atopic dermatitis. Some of the soaps and synthetic detergents that are recommended are Dove, Neutrogena, Aveeno, Basis, or Cetaphil liquid or bar soap. When women consult the dermatologist about skin care, all of these considerations should be considered.

Hair

If girls or women are prone to mild acne rosacea, seborrheic dermatitis of the face, or very oily skin in general, it may be necessary to adjust their shampoo regimen. The use of a zinc pyrithione shampoo two times weekly may decrease the amount of sebum in these oleaginous areas. The zinc pyrithione shampoos are cosmetically elegant and will not disturb hair color or texture.

For African-American women, and women with permanents or straightened or bleached hair, care must be used in the selection of shampoos. For example, although tar is an excellent ingredient for the treatment of scalp psoriasis, the use of tar in the special hair being discussed will be tolerated only about twice weekly. The special needs of these hair textures must be met. The addition of conditioners to any therapy will not undo the therapeutic effect. If the dermatologist in charge works with the patient's hairdresser, much can be accomplished. Selenium sulfide may also be hard on Negroid hair[2].

SHAVING IN WOMEN

Two areas of concern for women in skin care are hair removal from the legs, and hair removal from the axillae and bikini areas. The first concern on the legs is the development of irritant dermatitis and tiny cuts from shaving. The second is folliculitis which can occur in the axillae and the bikini area.

Legs

For women with very dry skin, it is important to apply a heavy emollient to the skin, such as petrolatum, 6–8 h before shaving. This will make the skin smooth, so that the hyperkeratotic surface projections will not be shaved off.

Bikini area and axillae

It is important to let the hair grow long enough for the patient to assess the direction of hair growth. She must then shave in the direction of hair growth using one of the non-allergic shaving gels or a gentle facial cleanser. Sometimes a single-edged razor may cause less folliculitis than a more efficient double-edged razor in the individual patient.

SKIN CARE FOR WOMEN WHO WORK OUT/EXERCISE

Many patients who initiate an exercise program develop intertrigo, body acne and facial acne. Recommendations for these patients are as follows:

(1) Always wear the highest percentage of cotton apparel as possible. Lycra may be more slenderizing, but it does not absorb as much perspiration as cotton.

(2) Dust the body folds with corn starch (cornflour) before the exercise. This will absorb perspiration and oils before they cause trouble.

(3) For facial acne – especially the tiny prickly-heat type of acne – the use of oil-free foundations is helpful. Some of the work-out make-up stays on longer, because it is occlusive. This type of product should be avoided. It is helpful to recommend astringent pads or astringent-soaked cotton balls to be applied to the face every 30 min while exercising.

ACNE

When treating acne in women, special considerations must be met. A woman's self-image is often based on her physical appearance. Occasionally the existence of one pimple may send her into the physician's office requesting isotretinoin. It is highly important to discuss realistic therapy and results with such a patient.

The first approach to these patients should be to exercise good health habits. It is important to sleep at least 7–8 h per day to have healthy skin. The intake of a moderate amount of water, fruits and vegetables may also contribute to good skin. While undergoing treatment for acne, the patient does not have to stop her cover-up or camouflage while at work or school. There are many color cosmetics available that are oil-free. Some dermatologists give their patients a list of locally available cosmetics that are effective for cover-up and may not aggravate the condition. These are perfectly acceptable to use during this time. It is important to use non-comedogenic hair conditioners, such as propylene glycol, to avoid pomade acne.

The choice of an acne lotion is made on the basis of skin type. If the patient has sensitive skin, gentle sulfur products may be the treatment of choice. If the patient has severe cystic acne, 5% benzoyl peroxide with or without the combination of topical clindamycin or erythromycin may be needed. It is advisable to start with 5% benzoyl peroxide and increase it to 10% if the area of the body (back vs. face) can tolerate a higher strength. If the patient has comedones, closed comedones, pustules, photoaging, or irregular pigmentation, topical tretinoin or adapaline cream or gel may be the treatment of choice. Combinations of a topical antibiotic such as clindamycin lotion 1% or erythromycin 2% may be used in the morning, and a tretinoin-type product applied at bedtime.

For more severe acne, oral antibiotics are very effective[3]. Tetracycline was reported many years ago to interfere with the absorption of oral contraceptives. This has not been substantiated; however, with the pharmacist's warning labels about this concern, it is often too complicated to prescribe these two drugs together. The other antibiotics – erythromycin, minocycline and doxycycline – have not been labeled with such a concern. If a patient's menstrual cycle is irregular, erythromycin may be the safest antibiotic to prescribe[4-6].

For the very severe cases of acne, isotretinoin at a dosage of 1 mg/kg for 20 weeks is the treatment of choice. This should not be prescribed for a patient unless there is absolutely no chance of pregnancy. The Guidelines of Care from the American Academy of Dermatology recommend two forms of contraception. A pregnancy test should be performed before the administration of this medication.

HANDS AND NAILS

Women are especially prone to housewives' dermatitis. This can be prevented by following several precautions:

(1) Purchase several pairs of cotton-lined rubber gloves to be left at the kitchen sink, bathroom and laundry room. These should be used for dishes, peeling fresh vegetables, and rinsing out clothes. If the patient's hands are very sore, using gloves while in the bathroom, then washing and drying the gloves similarly to bare hands may prevent severe hand dermatitis.

(2) Heavy emollients should be used on the hands. Lotion vehicles may be too thin and not occlusive enough to prevent the loss of moisture. Recommending only those moisturizers that are found in a jar or tube may be helpful. Fragrance should also be avoided.

(3) Liquid cleansers in attractive dispensers have become very popular recently. It is important to stress that antibacterial liquid cleansers and other strong products may actually cause more infection by causing dermatitic skin. Liquid facial cleansers may be more appropriate.

Many women complain of brittle nails. Several recommendations can help this problem:

(1) Use gloves for all housework.

(2) Use the same heavy emollient on the nails as on the hands.

(3) Never use nails as a tool.

(4) Never change nail polish more than once weekly. The nail polish remover dries out the nail plate too much.

(5) If a patient has onychoschizia (horizontal splitting), file the nails to prevent splitting them vertically. Avoid nail polish until the ends are all even. Moisturize the nail plates with petrolatum or another heavy emollient three or four times daily.

MELASMA

There is less melasma occurring in women today than previously because the anovulatory drugs have been improved. Occasionally hyperpigmentation is still present, however, from pregnancy, postmenopausal hormones, birth control pills and other medications.

There are many products available to bleach out the hyperpigmentation. All of these contain hydroquinone. The over-the-counter products contain 2% concentration, and the prescription products contain 3% in a highly penetrating solution, or 4% in several different bases. These are all quite effective.

For women with this problem, the most important recommendation is the avoidance of UVA exposure. This wavelength penetrates through window glass, so an effective sunblock must be used daily, even inside an automobile. The best ingredients against UVA are Parsol 1789, titanium dioxide, and zinc oxide. Ordinary SPF 15 sunblocks will not prevent this problem.

It is also important to stress to patients with this condition that, once the melanocytes are triggered to acquire melasma, they are rarely turned off. This is especially true if the cause is exogenous estrogen and not just pregnancy. Sunblocks against UVA will need to be used forever. Hyperpigmentation secondary to UVA is the same, whether the patient is outdoors at the equator or in the temperate zones.

SELF-TANNERS

The final advice to be given to girls and women about skin care concerns self-tanners. Because we desire the skin to stay healthy and avoid sun damage, those products containing dihydroxyacetone are appropriate for use. With the addition of silicone to these products for easy application and dispersion, they have become cosmetically much more appealing.

(1) If a patient has many seborrheic keratoses or lentigines, these may be accentuated.

(2) Washing the skin with a loofah-type sponge will allow a more even pigmentation.

(3) Patients should be aware that they must use sunscreen on top of the artificially tanned skin.

REFERENCES

1. deGroot AC, Frosch PJ. Adverse reactions to fragrances. A clinical review. *Contact Dermatitis* 1997;36:57–86

2. Wilborn WS. Disorders of hair growth in African Americans. In Olsen EA, ed. *Disorders of Hair Growth Diagnosis and Treatment.* New York: McGraw-Hill, 1994:389–406

3. Leyden JJ. Therapy for acne vulgaris. *N Engl J Med* 1997;336:16, 1157–62

4. Helms SE, Bredle DL, Zajic BS, *et al.* Oral contraceptive failure rates and oral antibiotics. *J Am Acad Dermatol* 1997;36:705–10

5. London BM, Lookingbill DP. Frequency of pregnancy in acne patients taking oral antibiotics and oral contraceptives. *Arch Dermatol* 1994;130:392–3

6. Back DJ, Grimmer SFM, Orme ML'E, *et al.* Evaluation of Committee on Safety of Medicines yellow card reports on oral contraceptive–drug interactions with anticonvulsants and antibiotics. *J Clin Pharmacol* 1988;25:527–32

Prevention and rejuvenation

Aging and sun damage

47

Susan Boiko

OVERVIEW

The 20th century saw girls and women shed long-sleeved, floor-length dresses, bonnets, parasols and gloves in favor of the 'New Look'. Popularized in the 1920s by French clothing designer Coco Chanel, abbreviated clothing and tanned skin replaced sun avoidance and pallid complexions for European and American women. With increased leisure time, more enthusiasm for outdoor pursuits and a longer lifespan, today's woman has turned the 'New Look' into the 'latest wrinkle'.

Awareness of sun-associated cutaneous damage is the first step in the prevention of deadly or disfiguring skin cancers, as well as undesired wrinkling. A newborn girl's 'place in the sun' will affect her mature skin's resistance to the ravages of ultraviolet (UV) radiation.

The 'New Look' tanning fad has begun to fade. George and colleagues posed the question, 'Will fashion make you look old and ugly?'[1] They reviewed the June issues of North American fashion magazines from 1983 to 1993. The overwhelming majority of the models pictured were Caucasian adult women. Photographs of men in editorial content and advertising showed darker tans than women. Adults had darker tans than children. Trends included lighter tans, more women wearing hats, more sunscreen advertisements and more sun awareness articles in the most recent issues.

'No tan is a healthy tan' for anyone under the sun, regardless of skin color[2]. This chapter will explore the major factors affecting cutaneous aging, and suggest specific ways girls and women can maintain healthy skin through a lifetime awareness of the hazards of sun overexposure.

FACTORS AFFECTING CUTANEOUS AGING

Genetic

Cutaneous aging may be defined as the changes in the skin's ability over time to function as an environmental barrier, sensory organ and immune system defense outpost. Intrinsic ('natural') aging is the genetically determined, chronological rate of decrease in cutaneous function. Skin of both genders shows the first signs of intrinsic aging after the age of 30 years[3].

The best place to observe intrinsic aging is in skin that is not normally sun exposed. Buttocks fold skin is a standard comparison site to sun-exposed areas for microscopic studies of aging skin[4]. Skin appears thinner, pale, dry and flaky, with fine wrinkling and decreased elasticity. Decreased sweat production contributes to dryness. Body and scalp hair is more sparse. Microscopically, intrinsically aged skin shows epidermal and dermal atrophy and loss of appendages[3].

For women, loss of ovarian estrogen production causes skin collagen content to decrease. Hormone replacement therapy may improve cutaneous thickness, and decrease laxity and fine wrinkling. Postmenopausal women on hormone replacement therapy have fewer facial wrinkles[5].

Environmental

Intrinsic aging is the background upon which sunlight and smoke leave their indelible marks on a woman's skin. These external factors, termed 'extrinsic aging', cause the majority of age-related cutaneous changes. Synonyms for UV light-induced extrinsic damage include photoaging, photodermatitis, dermatoheliosis and heliodermatitis.

Extrinsic cutaneous damage from sunlight has been described by Bergfeld as a 'state of chronic inflammation'[3]. Chronic UV light exposure causes cutaneous roughness, a leathery texture, scaling, xerosis, sallowness, fine and coarse wrinkling, laxity, mottled pigmentation, telangiectasia, open and closed comedones, neoplasms and, most severely, atrophy, purpura and stellate pseudoscars. The intensity of these changes depends on sun and/or tanning bed exposure, cigarette smoking, ethnicity, eye and hair color and tendency to form nevi and freckles. Extrinsic UV skin damage is independent of chronological age[3,6].

The key microscopic finding is solar elastosis. Solar elastosis consists of amorphous, basophilic-staining degenerated collagen and elastic fibers and increased glycosaminoglycans in the papillary and reticular dermis[2]. A thickened, disorganized epidermis, with parakeratosis and acanthosis contributes to the dry, rough sensation. The dermo-epidermal junction loses rete ridges and the flattened interface leaves the dermis more subject to shearing forces, producing hemorrhage and purpura with minimal trauma. Enlargement of melanocytes with a higher level of epidermal integration produces mottled pigment, and focal decreases in melanocytes yield hypo- and depigmentation[7].

UV light: sun

Most people know that a tan is a sign of sun damage, yet few realize that everyday sun exposure not intended to produce tanning accounts for 80% of a person's lifetime sun exposure[2]. UV light is the skin-damaging component of sunlight[7].

Whether as a consequence of sunbathing or during more casual exposure, UV radiation, even at suberythemogenic doses, damages keratinocytes by directly altering DNA, which leads to abnormal tumor growth. UV exposure to skin also causes suppression of the immune responses controlling the growth of abnormal cells, with resulting inability to suppress abnormal tumor growth[7]. UV light also affects cutaneous resilience. Pierard and co-workers studied the facial skin of Caucasian women with types II and III skin (always burns, sometimes tans). All women had indoor occupations and none were sun worshipers. On sun-exposed skin near the lateral angle of the eye, they found a significant decrease in elasticity with age in a time-related, logarithmic manner[8].

UV light: tanning beds

Most tanning beds have light bulbs that give off predominantly UVA with enough UVB to speed up the tanning process. UVA provided by tanning bed bulbs produces greater photodamage than 'solar simulator' bulbs with a more sunlight-like balance between UVB and UVA[9]. Beginning in adolescence, women use tanning beds at double the rate of men (see Primary prevention, below).

Cigarette smoke

Although cigarette smoking is responsible for three million deaths a year worldwide, the threat of wrinkles may be more powerful in convincing some smokers to quit than the threat of death[10]. Cigarette smoke contributes to wrinkling by decreasing hyaluronic acid and glycosaminoglycan synthesis and decreasing capillary blood flow in skin[5].

In one study, female smokers had a relative risk for facial wrinkling three times that of lifelong non-smokers and two times that of former smokers[5]. In a comparison of Caucasian male and female smokers with a blended standardized visual assessment, the estimated relative risk of moderate to severe wrinkling was significantly higher for women. For both genders, increasing number of pack-years correlated with increasing facial wrinkle scores[11].

PRIMARY PREVENTION OF UV-ASSOCIATED CUTANEOUS AGING

It is easy to practice sun safety if the 'sun ABCs' are remembered. This mnemonic was part of a sun-safety educational program prepared for elementary school students by the American Academy of Dermatology and the American Cancer Society in 1991, but its basic tenets apply to all ages and both genders:

A – stay away from the sun;

B – block the sun;

C – cover up;

S – speak out to teach others about sun safety.

Table 1 provides detailed recommendations on protecting skin from UV damage.

For infants, children and adolescents

The largest portion of lifetime exposure to sun occurs before the age of 20 years. Fifty per cent of lifetime UV exposure occurs before the age of 18 years[3]. Eighty per cent of non-melanoma skin cancers may be prevented in adulthood, and extrinsic cutaneous damage would be greatly decreased, if children less than 10 years old were adequately protected from the sun[2,14].

Sun protection begins at birth. An interventional program for mothers of healthy newborns began in a Connecticut, USA, hospital shortly after the mothers gave birth. Intervention, whether with basic written sun safety guidelines alone or with more elaborate written materials and free sunscreen, baby hats and umbrellas, was effective in decreasing the amount of time both newborns and their mothers spent in direct sunlight, compared to a control group that received nothing. Interestingly, the free hats and umbrellas were not used by mothers who received them[15].

Table 1 Primary prevention of ultraviolet (UV)-associated cutaneous aging. Suggestions for all age groups

A: stay away from the sun

Avoid tanning beds

Avoid sun exposure when your shadow is shorter than you are, or, if it is overcast, between 10.00 and 15.00

Indoors away from the window is best

Outdoors in the shade is next best

Avoid highly reflective surfaces including sand, snow, water and light-colored building walls

Avoidance plus sunscreen and protective clothing are especially recommended for photosensitive patients with:

    lupus erythematosus

    keratinizing disorders

    fair skin

    drugs: non-steroidal anti-inflammatory drugs, thiazides, tetracycline and (unique to women) oral contraceptives[2]

B: block the sun

Apply sunscreen, which blocks mostly UVB, some UVA, 30 min before outdoor activities

For an adult in a bathing suit, use one ounce (2 tablespoons) of sunscreen to coat all sun-exposed skin

Do not forget lips, hair parting, toes, ears (women are less likely to apply sunscreen to their ears[12])

Reapply sunscreen after exercise, swimming and sweating

Do not use sunscreen as a reason to stay in the sun longer

C: cover up

Choose a hair style that covers the forehead, ears and neck

Wear a hat with a 6-inch (15-cm) brim all the way around, made of tightly woven cloth

Wear wrap-around style sunglasses with wide templed earpieces that block 100% of UVA and UVB

Select clothing that is tightly woven and covers most skin (long sleeves, long trousers); repeated washing will shrink fabric weave and increase the UV protective factor[13]

Gloves are recommended for chronic sun exposure, especially if there is severe atrophy of the dorsal hand skin

Stand under a dark-colored umbrella, which will absorb, rather than reflect, UV light

S: speak out

Use your role as health professional, parent, teacher, friend, community leader, or outdoor hobbyist to spread the ABC message

Mothers' influence over their young children's sun protection habits continues from infancy to preadolescence. In Greece, mothers of children aged 1–12 years were randomly selected at a hospital out-patient department and questioned about sun safety practices. More than 97% of mothers knew that excessive sun exposure is harmful to the skin, and mothers who used sun protection for themselves also used it for their children[16].

Adolescent girls are still influenced by their parents to protect their skin from the sun, and this influence is stronger for girls than boys (press release, American Academy of Dermatology 30 April 1997, *Seventeen* magazine: Nivea Sun Skin Protection Survey, Elizabeth Brous, Beauty Director, *Seventeen*).

From Norway to Australia, there are striking gender differences in childhood and adolescence regarding sun safety practices. Girls usually spend less time in the sun than boys, but when they go outdoors girls deliberately seek a tan. Girls shun hats. Adolescent girls are twice as likely as boys to use tanning beds (press release[17–23]). Table 2 summarizes these differences.

Climate does not always determine the likelihood of harmful sun exposure. Even in the relatively cloudy climate of Sunderland, Great Britain, 38% of children up to the age of 20 years had been sunburned in the previous year[19]. Norway is a European country with a latitude higher than that of Juneau, Alaska, yet girls spent 22 days a year, boys 16 days a year, sunbathing[23].

Sunbathing may be perceived by physicians as a health risk, but adolescents also consider it a social event and a means of increasing attractiveness[23]. In Southern California during the 1950s to the 1970s, a concoction of iodine and baby oil was applied to the skin while sunbathing at the beach by adolescent sunbathers, especially girls with types I and II skin, in an effort to increase the darkness of a tan. Girls would sit at the beach, or in high school, and peel the sun-blistered skin off each other's arms and backs (S. Boiko, personal observation).

The role of parents, child-care workers, teachers, camp directors, sports coaches and other influential adults is essential in providing the sun protection message to girls and young women. This message needs to be specifically targeted to girls[20–22].

For young women

A telephone survey in Australia of men and women with a mean age of 19.7 years showed three significant variables related to gender: more women sought a tan, women spent more time deliberately seeking a tan and women rated their personal risk of skin cancer higher than did men[24]. Of women 20 years and older from rural North Carolina, more

Table 2 Gender differences in sun-associated behavior in childhood and adolescence

---

Safe attitudes and behaviors

Girls are more likely to use sunscreen regularly (press release[17,22,23])

Girls are more likely to have a friend who practices sun-safe behaviors[20]

Girls are more likely to have parents who influence healthy sun-safety behaviors (press release)

Girls are more likely correctly to estimate the amount of time one can safely stay in the sun[17]

Girls are more likely to wear clothing outdoors that covers at least part of the upper torso[19]

Girls are less likely to say that a tan protects against skin cancer[20]

Girls are less likely to feel that a tan makes a person look more athletic (press release)

Girls are less likely to spend time outdoors[18,22]

Girls are less likely to have occupational sun exposure[22]

Hazardous attitudes and behaviors

Girls are more likely to sunbathe[21–23]

Girls are more likely to say their friends think they look better with a tan[20]

Girls are more likely to use tanning beds[17,22]

Girls are less likely to wear hats[18,20–22]

---

than 40% regularly sunbathed to get a tan, and less than half regularly used a sunscreen[25].

Mawn and Fleischer surveyed North Americans aged 16–90 years in a shopping mall, at a social gathering and on a cruise ship. Women were three times as likely to sunbathe and/or use a tanning bed as men, but were also three times as likely to use sunscreen. Surprisingly, tanning bed users were better informed about UV damage than non-users[26].

In Israel, an educational program attempted, through a health education program of leaflets and newspaper advertising, to influence women clinic patients' behavior regarding several kinds of cancer prevention and early detection. The educators were unable to detect a change in suntanning behavior, showing the lack of success of a carefully planned educational endeavor[27]. For young women, a tan is still sought after. Additional work needs to be done to find an effective means of changing both attitudes and behavior in this age group.

For postmenopausal women

Some patients in Mawn and Fleischer's study fell in the over 50 age range. In New York, a survey of Caucasian persons between the ages of 17 and 74 years showed that 21% had used sun lamps, but

Table 3 Therapeutic options for women with cutaneous sun damage

---

Avoid the sun as much as possible (Table 1)

Quit smoking; avoid secondhand smoke

If postmenopausal, consider hormone replacement therapy

Use cosmetics as sun protection and camouflage

Work with a knowledgeable physician to use topical and systemic therapies on an individualized basis[2,3]

---

only 2.3% used them on at least a monthly basis. Women in the age range 16–24 years were much more likely to have used a sun lamp. No breakdown was given for older women[28].

SECONDARY PREVENTION OF SUN-ASSOCIATED CUTANEOUS AGING

Primary prevention of cutaneous aging can be accomplished by practicing the sun ABCs (Table 1). Secondary prevention of sun damage, in the form of skin cancer, means participating in a skin cancer screening program, to attempt to find a skin cancer, especially melanoma, at an early stage, so that it can be cured.

Australian researchers were able to find a link between sun-safe behaviors and early detection of skin cancer. They found that if a person had had a personal experience of skin cancer in relatives or friends, they were more likely to check their own skin for skin cancer[29]. In North Carolina, women were more likely than men to attend skin cancer screenings[24].

In my practice experience, many women have exclaimed as I entered the examination room, 'Oh thank goodness you're a woman!' Many confessed that they had been too embarrassed to have a complete skin examination done by male dermatologists, despite the fact that they were otherwise satisfied with their care. On the other hand, I have only had one male patient in 20 years of medical practice who refused to disrobe because I was female (S. Boiko, personal observation).

TREATMENT OF EXTRINSICALLY AGED SKIN

This subject is discussed in detail in Chapters 50 and 51. Table 3 offers a general therapeutic approach.

CONCLUSIONS

In the 21st century, skin cancer prevention, through the avoidance of excessive UV exposure, will begin at birth. A longer human lifespan will add to the current challenges women face: to change the attitude that a tan is desirable and worth the accompanying skin damage; to provide shelter from the sun at all opportunities; to replace hormone loss during menopause; and to end cigarette smoking and tobacco use. Successful achievement of these goals will mean that tomorrow's sunny-faced little girl will retain her youthful glow and a new, wrinkle-free look throughout her long and healthy life.

REFERENCES

1. George PM, Kuskowski M, Schmidt C. Trends in photoprotection in American fashion magazines 1983–1993. *J Am Acad Dermatol* 1996;34:424–8

2. Fenske NA. How to discuss photodamage with your patients. *Skin Aging* 1998;January:44–50

3. Bergfeld WF. The aging skin. *Int J Fertil* 1997;42:57–66

4. Bernstein EF, Chen YQ, Kopp JB, *et al.* Long term sun exposure alters the collagen of the papillary dermis. *J Am Acad Dermatol* 1996;34:209–18

5. Castelo-Branco C, Figueras F, Martinez de Osaba MJ, Vanrell JA. Facial wrinkling in postmenopausal women. Effects of smoking status and hormone replacement therapy. *Maturitas* 1998;29:75–86

6. Drake LA, Dinehart SM, Farmer ER, *et al.* Guidelines of care for photoaging/photodamage. *J Am Acad Dermatol* 1996;35:462–4

7. Coldiron BM. The UV index. A weather report for skin. *Clin Dermatol* 1998;16:441–6

8. Pierard GE, Henry F, Castelli D, Ries G. Aging and rheological properties of facial skin in women. *Gerontology* 1998;44:159–61

9. Spencer JM, Amonette R. Tanning beds and skin cancer. Artificial sun + old sol = real risk. *Clin Dermatol* 1998;16:487–501

10. Smith JB, Fenske NA. Cutaneous manifestations and consequences of smoking. *J Am Acad Dermatol* 1996;34:717–32

11. Ernster VL, Grady D, Miike R, *et al.* Facial wrinkling in men and women, by smoking status. *Am J Public Health* 1995;85:78–82

12. Loesch H, Kaplan DH. Pitfalls in sunscreen application [letter]. *Arch Dermatol* 1994;130:665–6

13. Stanford DG, Georgouras KE, Pailthorpe MT. Sun protection by a summer-weight garment. The effect of washing and wearing. *Med J Aust* 1995;162:422–5

14. Stern RS, Weinstein MC, Baker SG. Risk reduction for nonmelanoma skin cancer with childhood sunscreen use. *Arch Dermatol* 1986;122:537–45

15. Bologna JL, Berwick M, Fine JA, *et al.* Sun protection in newborns. A comparison of educational methods. *Am J Dis Children* 1991;145:1125–9

16. Kakourou T, Bakoula C, Kavadias G, *et al.* Mothers' knowledge and practices related to sun protection in Greece. *Pediatr Dermatol* 1995;12:207–10

17. Banks BA, Silverman WA, Schwartz RH, Tunnessen WW. Attitudes of teenagers toward sun exposure and sunscreen use. *Pediatrics* 1992;89:40–2

18. Fritschi L, Green A, Solomon PJ. Sun exposure in Australian adolescents. *J Am Acad Dermatol* 1992;27:25–8

19. Jarrett P, Sharp C, McLelland J. Protection of children by their mothers against sunburn. *Br Med J* 1993;306:1448

20. Lowe JB, Balanda KP, Gillespie AM, *et al.* Sun-related attitudes and beliefs among Queensland school children. The role of gender and age. *Aust J Public Health* 1993;17:202–8

21. McGee R, Wiliams S. Adolescence and sun protection. *N Z Med J* 1992;105:401–3

22. Robinson JK, Rademaker AW, Sylvester JA, Cook B. Summer sun exposure. Knowledge, attitudes and behavior of midwest adolescents. *Prev Med* 1997;26:364–72

23. Wichstrom L. Predictors of Norwegian adolescents' sunbathing and use of sunscreen. *Health Psychol* 1994;13:412–20

24. Clarke VA, Williams T, Arthey S. Skin type and optimistic bias in relation to the sun protection and suntanning behaviors of young adults. *J Behav Med* 1997;20:207–22

25. Michielutte R, Dinan MB, Sharp PC, *et al.* Skin cancer prevention and early detection practice in a sample of rural women. *Prev Med* 1996;25:673–83

26. Mawn VB, Fleischer AB. A survey of attitudes, beliefs and behavior regarding tanning bed use, sunbathing, and sunscreen use. *J Am Acad Dermatol* 1993;29:959–62

27. Biger C, Epstein LM, Hagoel L, *et al.* An evaluation of an educational programme, of prevention and early detection of malignancy in Israel. *Eur J Cancer Prev* 1994;3:305–12

28. Lillquist PP, Baptiste MS, Witzigman MA, Nasca PC. A population-based survey of sun lamp and tanning parlor use in New York state, 1990. *J Am Acad Dermatol* 1994;31:510–12

29. Anderson PJ, Lowe JB, Stanton WR, Balanda KB. Skin cancer prevention. A link between primary prevention and early detection? *Aust J Public Health* 1994;18:417–20

The use and role of cosmetics

48

Zoe Diana Draelos

OVERVIEW

Cosmetics are used to adorn, camouflage, highlight, color and dramatize the appearance of the face. The use of cosmetics is particularly important to dermatologists, because these products can cause acneiform eruptions, and create contact dermatitis, both irritant and allergic. Additionally, cosmetics impact the skin either alleviating or magnifying underlying dermatoses. This chapter presents the use and role of cosmetics for the face, eyes and lips, paying particular attention to pertinent dermatological aspects.

FACIAL FOUNDATIONS

Facial foundations are the most important class of colored facial cosmetics, from a dermatological standpoint, because the cosmetic is applied to the entire face, used on a daily basis and worn for an extended period of time. The foundation can be used to augment facial color, cover pigmentation irregularities, deliver treatment benefits and provide a vehicle for the application of sunscreen, moisturizers, or astringents.

The first facial foundations were developed for the theater in the form of a white powder incorporated into a liquid vehicle[1]. Later, pigments and fillers were added to oily vehicles to create a product known as 'grease paint'. The first major breakthrough in facial foundations outside the theater occurred when Max Factor developed cake makeup, a product patented in 1936[2]. This facial foundation provided excellent coverage, gave a velvety look and added facial color.

Formulation

There are four basic facial foundation formulations: oil-based, water-based, oil-free and water-free. Oil-based foundations are water-in-oil emulsions containing pigments suspended in oil, such as mineral oil or lanolin alcohol. Vegetable oils (coconut, sesame, safflower) and synthetic esters (isopropyl myristate, octyl palmitate, isopropyl palmitate) may also be incorporated. The water evaporates from the foundation following application, leaving the pigment in oil on the face. This provides facial skin with a moist feeling, especially desirable in women with a dry complexion.

Water-based facial foundations are oil-in-water emulsions containing a small amount of oil in which the pigment is emulsified with a relatively large quantity of water. The primary emulsifier is usually a soap, such as triethanolamine or a non-ionic surfactant. The secondary emulsifier, present in smaller quantity, is usually glyceryl stearate or propylene glycol stearate. These popular foundations are appropriate for minimally dry to normal skin.

Oil-free facial foundations contain no animal, vegetable or mineral oils. They may, however, contain other oily substances, such as the silicones dimethicone or cyclomethicone. These foundations are usually designed for individuals with an oily complexion. The pigment is dissolved in water and other solvents, leaving the skin with a non-greasy feel. This formulation is the most rapidly expanding area in facial foundation development. The silicone oils are non-acnegenic, non-comedogenic and hypoallergenic. These products can be adapted for a variety of skin types, depending on the amount of silicone incorporated into the formulation.

Anhydrous facial foundations are formulated without water and are therefore waterproof. Vegetable oil, mineral oil, lanolin alcohol and synthetic esters form the oil phase, which may be mixed with waxes to form a cream[3]. These products can be dipped from a jar, squeezed from a tube, wiped from a compact, or stroked from a stick. They have a slow drying time, no color drift and extended wear. They may be opaque, making them valuable for patients with facial scarring. Special removal products are required, however, since soap and water are inadequate for removal.

Therapeutic value

Facial foundations can provide the skin with therapeutic benefits, in addition to adding color or covering blemishes. For example, the coloring agents in facial foundations are based on titanium dioxide with iron oxides, occasionally in combination with ultramarine blue. Titanium dioxide acts both as a facial concealing or covering agent and as a physical sunscreen. Thus, most facial foundations provide broad-spectrum sun protection at a sun protection factor of approximately 5.

Facial foundations can also aid in oil control on the face. Most products contain varying concentrations of talc and kaolin, which function as fillers and blotters. A filler gives substance to the foundation while a blotter absorbs facial secretions. Oil-control foundations contain increased concentrations of talc, kaolin, starch, or other synthetic polymers to absorb facial sebum, thus preventing the development of facial shine. Oil-control foundations are not necessarily oil-free, however. The oil content of a foundation can be assessed by placing a drop of the product on a sheet of 25% cotton bond paper. Oil-containing foundations will leave an oil ring on the paper, while oil-free foundations will not. The size of the oil ring is proportionally related to the foundation's oil concentration[4].

Facial foundations can also be formulated to provide all-day moisturization for dry skin. Creamier, thicker foundations with a higher oil and/or wax content can successfully occlude a damaged skin barrier, decreasing transepidermal water loss and allowing the stratum corneum to repair.

Application

Application techniques for facial foundations vary depending on the intent of the product. Foundations used purely for adding color or blending uneven facial tone should be selected to match the natural facial color as closely as possible. This can be difficult, however, because the nose and cheeks have redder tones than the forehead and chin. The foundation is matched to the skin along the jawline, as this is where the color is carefully blended beneath the chin. A foundation color should also be selected in natural sunlight: the bright, artificial fluorescent lights used in most stores will distort color perception. This may result in selection of a dark foundation that will appear unnatural under more conventional lighting. The customer should be urged to apply a sample of foundation to the jawline in the store and then walk outside to examine the color match with a compact mirror.

In general, facial foundation should be applied with the fingertips. A dab of foundation should be placed on the forehead, nose, cheeks and chin and then blended with a light circular motion until it is evenly spread over all the facial skin, including the lips. Finally, a puff or sponge should be used, stroking in a downward direction, to remove any streaks and to flatten vellus facial hair. Special care should be taken to rub the foundation into the hairline, over the tragus and beneath the chin. Foundation should also be blended around the eyes and may even be applied to the entire upper eyelid if desired. The foundation should be allowed to set or dry until it can no longer be removed with light touch.

If the foundation is used to cover scarring and additional coverage is desired, a second layer of foundation can be applied after the first application has dried. Patients with severe color abnormalities may find that even two applications of a conventional facial foundation are inadequate; in this case a surgical camouflage product should be selected.

Surgical camouflage facial foundations are usually thick creams stroked from a jar or squeezed from a tube or stroked from a stick. They sometimes benefit from being warmed in the palm of the hand to become softened prior to application. These foundations must be pressed into scarred tissue, since rubbing will produce an uneven application. Care should be taken to press the cosmetic into all pores and depressed facial scars. Most surgical products require finishing of the application with a loose powder that must be pressed into the foundation. This sets the cosmetic and enhances its waterproof characteristics.

Adverse reactions

Facial foundations are a possible source of allergic and irritant contact dermatitis. Allergic contact dermatitis is rare, most commonly encountered in a preservative-sensitive individual. Irritant contact dermatitis is common, as the facial foundation is generally the first cosmetic applied to the face and the product is worn all day. Irritant reactions generally take the form of acneiform eruptions consisting of perifollicular papules and pustules. This reaction is due to the tendency of facial foundations to migrate towards the follicular ostia with wearing. Migration is more rapid in individuals with copious sebum production. Substances in the foundation formulation that could cause this reaction include vehicles and emulsifiers.

Facial foundations are best use-tested, rather than patch-tested. The product can be applied nightly for five nights to the skin beside the lateral canthus of the eye. This is some of the most sensitive skin on the face, providing an excellent site for evaluation.

FACIAL POWDERS

Facial powders are designed to augment the underlying skin tone, add shine to the face, absorb oil, increase the wear of the facial foundation and blend facial foundation tones. They are usually removed from a compact, an item with an interesting history. The modern compact is a descendant of the patch box, shallow metal boxes with a mirror in the cover. This box contained small silk pieces shaped as moons, stars, etc. that were applied to the face to cover smallpox scars. The box was carried everywhere to keep replacements handy should a patch fall off in public. With the development of the smallpox vaccine, the patch box evolved into the compact used today for the application of facial powder[5].

Formulation

Facial powders consist of talc, also known as hydrated magnesium silicate, and covering pigments, such as titanium dioxide, kaolin, magnesium carbonate, magnesium stearate, zinc stearate, prepared chalk, zinc oxide, rice starch and precipitated chalk. Most products contain magnesium carbonate to absorb oil, keep the powder fluffy and absorb any added perfume. Facial powder usually incorporates iron oxides as the main brownish pigment, but other inorganic pigments such as ultramarine, chrome oxide and chrome hydrate may also be used.

Other ingredients may be added to alter the surface characteristics of the powder. For example, some powders impart a light shine to the face produced by nacreous pigments, such as bismuth oxychloride, mica, titanium dioxide-coated mica, or crystalline calcium carbonate[6].

Application

Facial powders are removed from a compact with a puff or dusted loosely from a container with a brush. They impart a matte finish to the face. Women with dry complexions may wish to avoid facial powder, since it can further dry the skin. However, women with oily complexions will find powder an excellent method of absorbing excess facial oil. Rubbing powder into the forehead, nose and central chin will prevent an oily shine from developing and increase the wear of other facial cosmetics.

Adverse reactions

The most common problem encountered with facial powder is irritation of the lungs due to inhalation, especially in women with asthma or vasomotor rhinitis. The incidence of allergic contact dermatitis

to facial powder itself is low; however, added fragrances may pose a problem. Irritant contact dermatitis due to coarse particulate matter, such as nacreous pigments, in the formulation may contribute to perifollicular papules and pustules, as well as milia. Facial powder is best use-tested, in the same manner as facial foundation, by applying a small amount lateral to the eye for five consecutive nights.

FACIAL BLUSHES

Facial blushes, also known as rouges, are designed to enhance rosy cheek color. They are particularly valuable in mature women to add color to an otherwise pale face, imparting the appearance of health.

Formulation

Blush and rouge are synonyms for a cosmetic designed to add color to the cheeks, but to many consumers blush connotes a powdered product while rouge connotes a cream product. Powdered blushes are more popular and are formulated identically to compact face powder, except more vivid pigments are added. Because color rather than coverage is desired, powdered blushes do not contain much zinc oxide. Cream rouges are formulated like anhydrous foundations which contain light esters, waxes, mineral oil, titanium dioxide and pigments[7].

Application

For a natural appearance, cheek color should be applied beginning at a point directly beneath the pupil on the fleshy part of the cheek, sweeping upward beyond the lateral eye[8]. This placement is designed to create or accentuate high cheek bones, which are a desired quality among women[9]. Powdered blushes are stroked from a compact with a brush and brushed on the cheeks, while cream rouges are removed from the compact with a sponge and rubbed on the cheeks.

Adverse reactions

The adverse reactions with blushes and rouges are identical to those for facial powders, previously discussed.

SELF-TANNING CREAMS

Self-tanning creams are the safest method of obtaining the illusion of tanned skin, without sun exposure. The brownish color produced by these products offers minimal sun protection. Thus, they represent colored cosmetics.

Formulation

The active ingredient in self-tanning creams is 3–5% dihydroxyacetone incorporated into a glycerin and mineral oil base to form a white cream, which dyes the stratum corneum brown[10]. The brown color is the byproduct of a chemical reaction where dihydroxyacetone acts as a sugar to interact with amino acids in the stratum corneum to produce melanoidins[11–14]. The reaction occurs overnight, but the color is not permanent. It is sloughed as the stratum corneum desquamates; therefore, continued application is required.

Formulations are available for the face and body with varying viscosity to aid in application. Higher concentrations of dihydroxyacetone are used to produce darker coloring of the stratum corneum. Some products even incorporate protein to enhance the darkening of the stratum corneum.

Application

Self-tanning creams will tan any skin surface they contact, even the palms of the hands. The cream should therefore be washed from the hands immediately after application. The cream must also be applied evenly, or streaking will occur. Deeper staining of the follicular ostia, seborrheic keratosis, actinic keratosis, porokeratosis and icthyotic skin also occurs, owing to the increased amount of skin keratin. Many women are not aware that they have these skin conditions until the self-tanning cream highlights the irregularity.

Successful application depends on applying a constant amount of the self-tanning cream to smooth skin. The smoothness of the skin can be improved by shaving, using an exfoliant cream, or rubbing with a mild abrasive sponge. α-Hydroxyacid creams can also aid in removal of excess desquamating corneocytes.

The brown color achieved with self-tanning creams is quite acceptable on persons with blonde or light brown hair, who tend to have golden hues to their skin. The color appears somewhat artificial on Mediterranean individuals with an olive complexion or extremely fair persons with pink skin tones.

Adverse reactions

Allergic contact dermatitis from use of the product is infrequent, but several cases of dihydroxyacetone allergy have been reported[15]. Self-tanning creams can be open or closed patch-tested 'as is'.

EYE SHADOWS

Eye shadows are used to add interest to the eyes in a manner that is currently fashionable. Eyelid cosmetics were first used in 4000 BC and consisted of a green powder made from ground malachite. Eyelid glitter composed of ground beetle shells was also popular[5]. Modern colored eyelid cosmetics, consisting of a compact containing a pigmented powder, became popular between 1959 and 1962[16].

Formulation

Eye shadows are currently available as pressed powders, anhydrous creams, emulsions, sticks and pencils. The color variety is extensive, but no coal tar derivatives can be used in the eye area. Only purified natural colors or inorganic pigments can be used in the USA as a result of the Food, Drug and Cosmetic Act of 1938[7].

The surface characteristics of the eye shadow are just as important as the color. The texture can range from dull to a pearled shine to an iridescent finish (Figure 1). Bismuth oxychloride, mica and fish scale essence are the standard materials used to produce a pearly shine. A metallic texture can be created by adding copper, brass, aluminum, gold, or silver powders.

Pressed powder eye shadows are the most popular formulation and are applied to the eyelid by lightly stroking a soft sponge-tipped applicator across the skin. They are predominantly talc with pigments and zinc or magnesium stearate used as a binder. Kaolin or chalk may be added to improve oil absorption and increase wearability.

Anhydrous cream eye shadows contain pigments in petrolatum, cocoa butter, or lanolin. These formulations are waterproof, but have a tendency to migrate into the eyelid folds, especially in women with oily complexions or redundant eyelid skin. The product is applied with the finger and gently rubbed across the eyelid skin.

Anhydrous cream eye shadows have also been formulated as an emulsion applied with a sponge-tipped applicator or wand withdrawn from a cylindrical tube and stroked across the eyelid. These products, known as automatic eye shadows, are also waterproof, with increased wear duration over the creams. They contain beeswax, cyclomethicone and pigments in a volatile petroleum distillate vehicle.

Application

Eye shadows are stroked or rubbed across the eyelid, depending on the formulation. Selection of eye shadow color is a matter of personal preference and fashion, although colors complementary to the natural color of the iris are most attractive. Care should be taken not to allow the eye shadow to enter the eye.

Adverse reactions

The eyelid skin is the thinnest on the body and is frequently affected by both irritant and allergic contact dermatitis[17,18]. The North American Contact Dermatitis Group has determined that 12% of cosmetic reactions occur on the eyelid, but only 4% could be linked to eye make-up use[19]. Furthermore, it may be difficult to determine the etiology of the eyelid dermatitis with routine patch testing[20]. Many substances, such as nail polish, can be transferred to the eye area by the hands, complicating dermatological evaluation[21].

Open- or closed-patch testing can be performed with eye shadows, but automatic emulsions should be allowed to dry thoroughly prior to occlusion[22]. Use-testing is recommended, however, for eye cosmetics in the same manner as previously discussed.

MASCARA

Mascara, the most commonly used eyelash cosmetic, is intended to darken, thicken and lengthen the eyelashes. Because the eyelashes form a frame for the eye, luxuriant eyelashes are considered a prerequisite to facial attractiveness. The original mascara, worn by women of many ancient civilizations, was kohl, based on antimony trisulfide. The first modern mascara was a cake composed of sodium stearate soaps and lampblack, however, the product was very irritating to the eyes[23]. New formulations, developed by cosmetic chemists, are now safe to use around the eyes.

Formulation

Mascaras must be carefully formulated to allow easy and even application without smudging, irritancy or toxicity. Coal tar colors are prohibited by the US Food, Drug and Cosmetic Act for use on the eyelashes; therefore, mascara colorants must be selected from vegetable colors or inorganic pigments and lakes. Colors employed include iron oxide to produce black, ultramarine blue to create navy and umber or burnt sienna or synthetic brown oxide to create brown[24].

Liquid mascara has largely replaced cake and thicker cream mascara since development of the automatic mascara tube. This invention consists of a tube into which a round brush is inserted through a small aperture to remove a metered amount of product (Figure 2)[7].

Several formulations of liquid mascara are available: water-based, solvent-based and hybrid. Water-based mascara is formulated from waxes (beeswax, carnauba wax, synthetic waxes), in addition to pigments (iron oxides, chrome oxides, ultramarine blue, carmine, titanium dioxide) and resins dissolved in water. There are classified as oil-in-water emulsions. The water evaporates readily, creating a fast-drying product that thickens and darkens the lashes. The product is water-soluble, allowing for easy removal, but unfortunately smudges with perspiration and tears.

Some water-based mascaras are labeled 'water-resistant', if they contain an increased amount of wax or a polymer to improve adherence of pigment to the lashes. Specialty additives can be incorporated into the formulation to enhance the cosmetic appearance of the lashes. These substances include hydrolyzed animal protein to condition lashes, and nylon or rayon fibers to elongate lashes.

Solvent-based mascaras are formulated with petroleum distillates, to which pigments (iron oxides, chrome oxides, ultramarine blue, carmine, titanium dioxide) and waxes (candelilla wax, carnauba wax, ozokerite, hydrogenated castor oil) are added, thus making them waterproof. As a result, the product performs well with perspiration and tears, but removal is difficult and requires an oil-based lotion or cream. Deposits may form on the lashes if the product is incompletely removed. Care must be taken to avoid smudging immediately after application, as solvent-based mascaras have a prolonged drying time.

Some hybrid mascaras combine both solvent-based and water-based systems to form either a water-in-oil or an oil-in-water emulsion. The aim is to create an optimal product that thickens with a short drying time like the water-based mascaras, but provides waterproof lash separation like a solvent-based mascara. The water in the formulation requires incorporation of a good preservative system.

Application

Modern liquid mascaras utilize a multitufted applicator that is stroked across the eyelashes and inserted into the tube between uses, providing

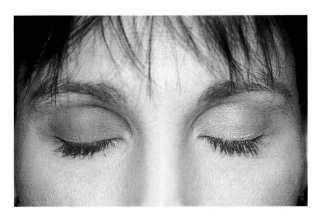

Figure 1 A shiny light-reflective eyeshadow is shown on the left eyelid compared to a matte-finish eyeshadow on the right eyelid

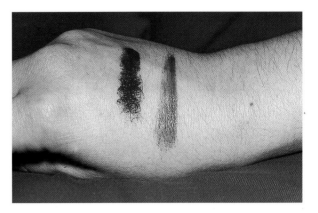

Figure 3 Transparent lipsticks, such as the product on the right, allow the underlying skin to be seen, while opaque lipsticks, such as the product on the left, cover the color of the vermilion

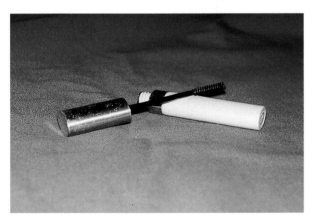

Figure 2 The modern mascara tube creates an environment for bacterial growth since the tufted brush is inserted and withdrawn from the tube multiple times

numerous opportunities to inoculate bacteria into the mascara. The most dangerous of these bacteria is *Pseudomonas aeruginosa*. Even though mascaras contain antibacterials, it is still wise to discard all mascara tubes after 3 months and not to allow more than one person to use the same mascara tube[25].

Mascara styles, dictated by fashion, are based on the type of applicator brush employed. If thick eyelashes are fashionable, lash-thickening mascaras are used with a larger, longer bristle brush applicator to apply mascara generously. If long eyelashes are fashionable, lash-lengthening mascaras with a short bristle brush are used to apply successive thin mascara coats and increase lash separation.

Adverse reactions

The most feared adverse reaction to mascaras is that of infection, particularly *Pseudomonas aeruginosa* corneal infections, which can permanently destroy visual acuity[26,27]. *Staphylococcus epidermidis* and *Staphylococcus aureus* may also proliferate in contaminated mascaras[28]. Infections are more

common if the eyeball is traumatized with the infected mascara.

Water-based mascaras are easily contaminated with bacteria, which readily grow in water, and must include preservatives, usually parabens. Thus, these products may potentially cause an allergic reaction in paraben-sensitive individuals; however, water-based mascaras are generally the least sensitizing of the mascara types. Some women may experience a contact irritancy from the emulsifiers required to maintain the pigment in solution.

Microbial contamination is not a great problem with solvent-based mascaras since the petroleum distillate is antibacterial. Individuals with recurrent bacterial infections, due to bacterial colonization, should probably select solvent-based mascaras[29]. Solvent-based mascaras can be a source of eye irritation.

Fungal organisms can also contaminate mascaras and result in eye infection[30]. This is rarer and usually only found in patients who are immunocompromised or wear contact lenses.

The pigment contained within mascaras can result in conjunctival pigmentation, if the mascara is washed into the conjunctival sac by lacrimal fluid[31]. This colored particulate matter can be observed on the upper margin of the tarsal conjunctiva. Histologically, the pigment is seen within macrophages and extracellularly with varying degrees of lymphocytic infiltrate. Electron microscopy suggests that ferritin, carbon and iron oxides are present within the tissues[32]. Unfortunately, there is no treatment for the condition, which is usually asymptomatic.

Allergic contact dermatitis has been reported to rosin (colophony)[33] and dihydroabietyl alcohol (Abitol)[34,35] contained in some mascaras. Mascaras can be open or closed patch-tested 'as is', but should be allowed to dry thoroughly prior to closed patch-testing to avoid an irritant reaction from the volatile vehicle.

EYELINER

Eyeliner defines the margins of the eye. It is placed immediately outside and sometimes inside the lash line, depending on current fashion. The first eyeliner was a dark kohl paste composed of powdered antimony, burnt almonds, black copper oxide and brown clay ocher. The eyeliner paste was stored in a pot and moistened with saliva, not a particularly hygienic practice.

Formulation

Eyeliner can be purchased as a cake, liquid, or pencil. Cake eyeliner has the same composition as eye shadow, except for the addition of surfactants promoting formation of a paste when the powder is mixed with water. Liquid eyeliner requires no mixing and contains the same pigments in a water-soluble latex base. It may be packaged as a marking pen or in a mascara-type tube with a unitufted applicator brush[7].

Pencil-type eyeliners are the easiest to apply and contain natural or synthetic waxes combined with pigments, mineral or vegetable oils and lanolin derivatives. The paste is extruded into rods and encased in wood. The pencil is then sharpened to the desired tip, which can be thin or broad, depending on the woman's preference. Resharpening removes exposed eyeliner, thus decreasing contamination.

Application

The eyeliner pigment is stroked across the upper and/or lower eyelid in the amount and position desired, dictated by current fashion. Eyeliner can be valuable in patients with absent eyelashes due to alopecia areata or scarring, since the line can simulate the appearance of eyelashes.

Adverse reactions

Eyeliners are subject to the same bacterial and fungal contamination seen with mascaras, especially if the liquid form is chosen, but the main adverse reaction is the possibility of conjunctival pigmentation, also seen with mascaras[36]. This problem is more commonly associated with eyeliner when it is applied within the lower lid margin. This practice is unsafe.

Allergic reactions to eyeliner are more common than with other facial cosmetics. Usually, the liquid latex-based eyeliners are the most problematic, with the cake eyeliners offering the least opportunity for allergic and irritant contact dermatitis. Open and closed patch-testing can be performed 'as is', but liquid eyeliner should be allowed to dry prior to occlusion. Use-testing is also recommended.

LIPSTICK

Lip cosmetics are valuable not only for accentuating the lips, but also for providing lip lubrication, camouflaging lip imperfections and acting as a sunscreen. Lip color has been used since the time of the Sumerians, dating back to 7000 BC. The practice has been handed down through many generations from the Egyptians to the Syrians to the Babylonians to the Persians to the Greeks to the Romans to present-day civilizations. The earliest lipsticks consisted of beeswax, tallow and red botanical pigments[37]. Modern lipstick formulations were introduced around 1920, when the 'push-up' holder, still used today, was invented[38].

Formulation

Lipsticks are mixtures of waxes, oils and pigments in varying concentration to yield the characteristics of the final product. For example, a lipstick designed to remain on the lips for a prolonged period of time is composed of high wax, low oil and high pigment concentrations. On the other hand, a product designed for a smooth creamy feel on the lips is composed of low wax and high oil concentrations (Figure 3)[38].

The waxes commonly incorporated into lipstick formulations are white beeswax, candelilla wax, carnauba wax, ozokerite wax, lanolin wax, ceresin wax and other synthetic waxes. Usually, lipsticks contain a combination of these waxes carefully selected and blended to achieve the desired melting point. Oils are then selected, such as castor oil, white mineral oil, lanolin oil, hydrogenated vegetable oils, or oleyl alcohol, to form a film suitable for application to the lips. The oils are also necessary for dispersion of the pigments. Preservatives, antioxidants, perfumes and surface characteristic additives complete the formulation[39].

Several types of coloring agents are used in lipsticks[40]. Indelible coloring, or lip staining, is achieved through the use of bromo acids, consisting of fluoresceins, halogenated fluoresceins and related water-insoluble dyes. Other pigments consist of insoluble dyestuffs and lake colors. Metallic lakes are insoluble dyes precipitated or 'laked' on a metallic substrate such as aluminum.

Application

Lipstick is applied by stroking the pigmented rod across the lips. The product must be artistically applied to color the entire vermilion, yet create a smooth, even, pleasant lip outline. The outline of the lips can be drawn in any fashion desired, making lipstick a useful camouflage cosmetic in patients with lip deformity.

Adverse reactions

Several ingredients unique to lipstick formulation can cause difficulty in the sensitized patient[41]. Castor oil, found in almost all lipsticks, owing to its excellent ability to dissolve bromo acid dyes, can rarely cause allergic contact dermatitis[42–44]. More common lipstick sensitizers in the mid 1920s were the bromo acid dyes, one of which is eosin (D&C Red No. 21)[45]. Eosin was commonly used in the indelible red lipsticks popular at that time. These indelible lipsticks are now making a comeback as active professional women want a long-wearing lip product. Other reports of lipstick dermatitis include ricinoleic acid[46], benzoic acid[47], lithol rubine BCA (Pigment Red 57-1)[48], microcrystalline wax[49], oxybenzone[50], propyl gallate[51] and C18 aliphatic compounds[52].

Lip cosmetics can be open or closed patch-tested 'as is', because their irritating potential is low; however, such cosmetics known as lip creams or gloss pots may be a source of perioral dermatitis and vermilion border comedones. The use of vegetable oils and other comedogenic substances in these products designed for adolescents may cause difficulty.

LIP LINERS

Lip liners are thin extruded rods encased in wood or placed in an automatic pencil-type holder. Their formulation is similar to that of lipsticks, except that stiffer waxes with higher melting points are used with minimal oil. This creates an extremely hard rod that applies a thick layer of pigment to the lips. Lip liners are used to define the outer edge of the lips and are valuable in reconstructing a normal lip contour. The thick wax layer applied around the lips also prevents creamier lip products from bleeding. Lip liner is usually selected one to two shades darker than the lipstick.

CONCLUSIONS

Cosmetics are an important aspect of self-image in women and girls. Part of the transformation from a girl to a woman involves the initial application of color to the face, eyes and lips. It is a ritual of adornment important to presenting an attractive appearance in modern society. Dermatologists should understand the formulation, application and possible adverse reactions to colored cosmetics so as to provide better care for their female patients.

REFERENCES

1. Schlossman ML, Feldman AJ. Fluid foundations and blush make-up. In de Navarre MG, ed. *The Chemistry and Manufacture of Cosmetics*, 2nd edn. Wheaton, IL: Allured Publishing Corporation, 1988:741–65
2. Wells FV, Lubowe II. *Cosmetics and the Skin*. New York: Reinhold Publishing Corporation, 1964: 141–9
3. Flick EW. *Cosmetic and Toiletry Formulations*, 2nd edn. Park Ridge, NJ: Noyes Publications, 1989:124–5
4. Fulton JE, Bradley S, Aqundez A, Black T. Noncomedogenic cosmetics. *Cutis* 1976;17:344–51
5. Panati C. *Extraordinary Origins of Everyday Things*. New York: Harper & Row, 1987:225–6
6. Wetterhahn J. Loose and compact face powder. In de Navarre MG, ed. *The Chemistry and Manufacture of Cosmetics*, vol 4, 2nd edn. Wheaton, IL: Allured Publishing Corporation, 1988:921–46
7. Lanzet M. Modern formulations of coloring agents: facial and eye. In Frost P, Horwitz SN, eds. *Cosmetics for the Dermatologist*. St Louis: CV Mosby, 1982: 133–51
8. Begoun P. *Blue Eyeshadow Should Be Illegal*. Seattle, WA: Beginning Press, 1986:62–4
9. Soldo BL, Drahos M. *The Inside-Out Beauty Book*. Old Tappan, NJ: Revell Company, 1978:78–9
10. Levy SB. Dihydroxyacetone-containing sunless or self-tanning lotions. *J Am Acad Dermatol* 1992;27: 989–93
11. Maibach HI, Kligman AM. Dihydroxyacetone: a suntan-simulating agent. *Arch Dermatol* 1960;35: 161–4
12. Goldman L, Barkoff J, Blaney D, *et al.* The skin coloring agent dihydroxyacetone. *GP* 1960;12:96–8
13. Wittgenstein E, Berry HK. Reactions of dihydroxyacetone (DHA) with human skin callus and amino compounds. *J Invest Dermatol* 1961;36:283–6
14. Wittgenstein E, Berry HK. Staining of skin with dihydroxyacetone. *Science* 1960;132:894–5
15. Morren M, Dooms-Goossens A, Heidbuchel M, *et al.* Contact allergy to dihydroxyacetone. *Contact Dermatitis* 1991;25:326–7
16. Wells FV, Lubowe II. Rouge and eye make-up. In Wells FV, Lubowe II, eds. *Cosmetics and the Skin*. New York: Reinhold Publishing Corporation, 1964:173–4

17. Fisher AA. Cosmetic dermatitis of the eyelids. *Cutis* 1984;34:216–21

18. Valsecchi R, Imberti G, Martino D, Cainelli T. Eyelid dermatitis: an evaluation of 150 patients. *Contact Dermatol* 1992;27:143–7

19. Adams RM, Maibach HI. A five-year study of cosmetic reactions. *J Am Acad Dermatol* 1985;13:1062–9

20. Wolf R, Perluk H. Failure of routine patch test results to detect eyelid dermatitis. *Cutis* 1992; 49:133–4

21. Nethercott JR, Nield G, Linn Holness D. A review of 79 cases of eyelid dermatitis. *J Am Acad Dermatol* 1989;21:223–30

22. Van Ketel WG. Patch testing with eye cosmetics. *Contact Dermatitis* 1979;5:402

23. Rutkin P. Eye make-up. In de Navarre MG, ed. *The Chemistry and Manufacture of Cosmetics*. Wheaton, IL: Allured Publishing, 1988:712–17

24. Wilkinson JB, Moore RJ. *Harry's Cosmeticology*, 7th edn. New York: Chemical Publishing, 1982:341–7

25. Bhadauria B, Ahearn DG. Loss of effectiveness of preservative systems of mascaras with age. *Appl Environ Microbiol* 1980;39:665–7

26. Wilson LA, Ahern DG. Pseudomonas-induced corneal ulcer associated with contaminated eye mascaras. *Am J Ophthalmol* 1977;84:112–19

27. MMWR Reports. *Pseudomonas aeruginosa* corneal infection related to mascara applicator trauma. *Arch Dermatol* 1990;126:734

28. Ahearn DG, Wilson LA. Microflora of the outer eye and eye area cosmetics. *Dev Ind Microbiol* 1976;17: 23–8

29. Ahern DG, Wilson LA, Julian AJ, *et al.* Microbial growth in eye cosmetics: contamination during use. *Dev Ind Microbiol* 1974;15:211–16

30. Kuehne JW, Ahearn DG. Incidence and characterization of fungi in eye cosmetics. *Dev Ind Microbiol* 1971;12:1973–7

31. Jervey JH. Mascara pigmentation of the conjunctiva. *Arch Ophthalmol* 1969;81:124–5

32. Platia EV, Michaels RG, Green WR. Eye cosmetic-induced conjunctival pigmentation. *Ann Ophthalmol* 1978;10:501–4

33. Fisher AA. Allergic contact dermatitis due to rosin (colophony) in eyeshadow and mascara. *Cutis* 1988;42:507–8

34. Rapaport MJ. Sensitization to abitol. *Contact Dermatitis* 1980;6:137–8

35. Dooms-Goossens A, Degreef J, Luytens E. Dihydroabietyl alcohol (Abitol), a sensitizer in mascara. *Contact Dermatitis* 1979;5:350–3

36. Stewart CR. Conjunctival absorption of pigment from eye make-up. *Am J Optom* 1973;50:571–4

37. deNavarre MG. Lipstick. In *The Chemistry and Manufacture of Cosmetics*, vol 4, 2nd edn. Wheaton, IL: Allured Publishing Company, 1975:767–9

38. Cunningham J. Color cosmetics. In Williams DF, Schmitt WH, eds. *Chemistry and Technology of the Cosmetics and Toiletries Industry*. London: Blackie Academic & Professional, 1992:143–9

39. Poucher WA. *Perfumes, Cosmetics and Soaps*, 8th edn. London: Chapman & Hall, 1984:196–207

40. Boelcke U. Requirements for lipstick colors. *J Soc Cosmet Chem* 1961;12:468

41. Sulzgerger MD, Boodman J, Byrne LA, Mallozzi ED. Acquired specific hypersensitivity to simple chemicals. Cheilitis with special reference to sensitivity to lipsticks. *Arch Dermatol* 1938;37: 597–615

42. Sai S. Lipstick dermatitis caused by castor oil. *Contact Dermatitis* 1983;9:75

43. Brandle I, Boujnah-Khouadja A, Foussereau J. Allergy to castor oil. *Contact Dermatitis* 1983;9:424–5

44. Andersen KE, Neilsen R. Lipstick dermatitis related to castor oil. *Contact Dermatitis* 1984;11:253–4

45. Calan CD. Allergic sensitivity to eosin. *Acta Allergol* 1959;13:493–9

46. Sai S. Lipstick dermatitis caused by ricinoleic acid. *Contact Dermatitis* 1983;9:524

47. Calnan CD. Amyldimethylamino benzoic acid causing lipstick dermatitis. *Contact Dermatitis* 1980;6:233

48. Hayakawa R, Fujimoto Y, Kaniwa M. Allergic pigmented lip dermatitis from lithol rubine BCA. *Am J Contact Dermatitis* 1994;5:34–7

49. Darko E, Osmundsen PE. Allergic contact dermatitis to Lipcare lipstick. *Contact Dermatitis* 1984;11:46

50. Aguirre A, Izu R, Gardeazabal J, *et al.* Allergic contact cheilitis from a lipstick containing oxybenzone. *Contact Dermatitis* 1992;27:267–8

51. Cronin E. Lipstick dermatitis due to propyl gallate. *Contact Dermatitis* 1980;6:213–14

52. Hayakawa R, Matsunaga K, Suzuki M, *et al.* Lipstick dermatitis due to C18 aliphatic compounds. *Contact Dermatitis* 1987;16:215–19

Adding and subtracting hair   **49**

Walter P. Unger and Paul C. Cotterill

Social image and acceptance is, for better or worse, very much tied to a person's physical appearance. How one sees oneself and how others see one therefore influences the way one acts, and is received. Women have always been viewed as the 'beautiful' gender, and hair is an important component of their beauty. Too little hair or too much hair in certain areas often leads to a poor body image and is socially unattractive. For unknown reasons, our modern society prefers women to have luxurious heads of hair with a totally hairless body. The aim of this chapter is to describe treatments that can help women enhance their physical appearance by adding or subtracting hair in the appropriate areas. The pathophysiology of excess hair growth and loss and the medical treatments for those conditions that cause them will not be discussed at length here, as they have been dealt with elsewhere in this text.

TOO MUCH HAIR
Physiology

Two factors – the rise of circulating androgens at puberty and the peripheral response of hair follicles to this increase – are responsible for the transition of fine-textured vellous hair into the coarser, longer terminal hair seen at puberty in both men and women.

When the amount of terminal hair in certain areas of a woman's body is enough to be socially unacceptable, it is referred to as hypertrichosis or hirsutism. As noted earlier, the causes and medical treatment of such excess hair are dealt with fully in this text. The type of hair, from fine vellous to coarse terminal hair, and in some cases its color, determine how well individual non-medicinal treatments for removing this hair will work. Common techniques such as plucking, shaving, waxing and chemical depilatories have all been employed by women seeking to reduce body hair[1,2]. Unfortunately, truly permanent hair removal is difficult to achieve.

Shaving is only temporary, with hair returning at the normal rate of hair growth, and with the same texture[3]. Waxing and plucking can, with time and numerous treatments, achieve total hair removal once enough traumatically induced inflammation has destroyed the follicle, but until such a time most patients will experience rapid hair regrowth.

Utilizing electricity for permanent removal of unwanted hair is one of the most time-proven and accepted techniques available[4]. Epilation using electricity was traditionally performed through electrochemical applications (electrolysis) and more recently via electrothermal treatments (electrothermolysis)[5–7]. In electrolysis a low level of direct or galvanic electric current passes between two electrodes. A chemical reaction occurs at the negative electrode, and adjacent tissue containing the hair follicle is destroyed. Unfortunately, electrolysis requires great skill and multiple treatments. It is also time consuming and uncomfortable. On the other hand, it has a low risk of producing scarring. Electrothermolysis is accomplished with needles that deliver a high-frequency current that produces thermolysis of the hair papilla without damaging the skin. It is growing in popularity as it is a faster process than electrolysis. Both techniques – electrochemical (electrolysis) and electrothermal (high-frequency electroepilation) – are common; the former is usually performed by non-medical practitioners and the latter by medical professionals.

Current epilation techniques employ fine tapered or untapered needles that have rounded or bulbous tips, and are insulated in order to limit heat generation to the base of the follicle with less disruption of the upper perifollicular dermis. This in turn reduces the chance of scarring. Electroepilation utilizes a needle that is 0.002–0.007 mm in diameter. The needle is inserted through the follicular ostium and follows the hair follicle usually to a depth of 3–4 mm. The epilating needle is attached either to a negative electrode for electrolysis or to the active electrode for thermolysis. Galvanic electrolysis units are usually set at 0.5–1.0 mA and activated for 15–20 s. Coarse hair generally requires a longer exposure time and higher power for removal than finer hair. An indication that the desired chemical destruction of the base of the follicles is occurring is the appearance of small bubbles of hydrogen gas at the follicular orifice.

Hair destruction via electrothermolysis is much faster than electrolysis, but is associated with a somewhat higher risk of scarring and pain. The current is applied either as a single application or as intermittent bursts to minimize pain. Vellous hairs may require a single very short (e.g. 0.125 s) application, whereas thick curly terminal hairs may require multiple applications of, for example, 5–8 0.125-s bursts. Sessions are usually spread a minimum of 7 days apart to allow any edema or erythema to dissipate. Additionally, it is usually preferable to refrain from treating hair follicles within 3–4 mm of each other in order to reduce thermal build-up. Treatments to the face can require multiple sessions spread over 1–2 years. Thereafter, occasional follow-up treatments are required for any vellous hairs that have transformed into terminal hairs. Axillary, mammary, forearm, leg and bikini hair can be permanently removed. The rate of permanent follicle destruction with thermolysis is 70–80%, compared with 80–90% with the slower galvanic electrolysis technique[8]. The patient should also be aware of the need for more treatments and a higher risk of scarring and infection[9] than are associated with electrolysis.

Laser hair removal

Laser hair removal requires a light source and an absorbing target or chromophore. The original concept of selective photothermolysis[10], currently called selective phototricholysis, operates on the principle that thermal injury will be restricted to a given target if that target is capable of absorbing light of a particular wavelength in a time period that is equal to or less than the thermal relaxation time (TRT) of the target[11]. This target, or chromophore, may be either endogenous melanin or exogenous carbon particles. The success of laser hair removal is based on two main theories: selective photothermolysis[10,12] and thermokinetic selectivity[13]. Both theories are based on the premise of melanin being the dominant absorbing chromophore in a hair shaft and follicle, and that the TRT for the target determines the optimal pulse duration for treatment. The ideal laser pulse duration should lie between the TRT for epidermis, which is approximately 3–10 ms, and the TRT for hair follicles. Wavelengths in a range from 600 to 1100 nm penetrate deeply enough into the dermal layers of the skin to reach both the follicular bulge and the papillae. These are the areas of the hair follicle that must be disabled or destroyed in order to achieve long-lasting or permanent hair removal.

Several different systems of laser hair removal have been developed. There have been marked inconsistencies amongst investigators in defining achievable goals, and in particular in their definition of 'permanent' hair removal. For some, 'permanent' is defined as complete loss of terminal hairs without any apparent clinical regrowth, while for others, 'permanent' means the induction of complete and permanent phototricholytic alopecia. Additionally, there is great variation in defining the success of hair removal because different anatomical sites have different anagen and telogen phase durations. A commonly used definition of 'permanent', as put forth by Rox Anderson, is 'significant and stable loss of hair for a period longer than the complete natural hair growth cycle'[14]. There are three distinct responses that can account for 'permanent' reduction of pigmented coarse hair[14]:

(1) Miniaturization of hair follicles and hair;
(2) Decreased pigmentation of regrowing hair;
(3) Degeneration of hair follicles with replacement by fibrosis.

Success may be gauged in terms of permanent hair loss – as defined above – or an increased percentage of vellous hairs (that are less cosmetically noticeable) over coarse terminal hairs. It should be emphasized, however, that permanent life-long and total hair removal has yet to be achieved.

Table 1 itemizes the current laser/light hair-removal systems available and the suggested wavelength, pulse length, fluence, spot size and repetition rate[15]. Thermolase was the first laser hair removal system to receive clearance by the United States Food and Drug Administration (FDA) (in April 1995) for its Soft Light Laser System. After wax epilation, microparticulate carbon is massaged into the follicles. This is followed by irradiation with a single pass of Q-switched Nd : YAG laser energy. It is in essence based on exogenous carbon particles that are forced into the hair follicle and act as the chromophore. Other systems, such as the pulse ruby laser light system, rely on endogenous melanin as the chromophore. A third type of system, nonselective phototricholysis, employs a non-laser broad-band light source (Epilight, ESC Medical Systems, Needham, MA). Figure 1 is an example of two laser/light hair removal systems in current use.

The success of each system depends on a variety of variables:

(1) The specific laser or light source employed;
(2) The area of the body treated;
(3) The color and caliber of hair;
(4) The color of the surrounding skin.

Table 1 Hair removal lasers. From reference 15

Laser type	Product name	Manufacturer	Wavelength	Pulse length	Fluence (J/cm^2)	Spot size	Repetition rate
Nd : YAG	Softlight	Thermolase	1064 nm	5 ns	3	6–7 mm	1,2,5 and 10 Hz
	Medlite	Continuum Biomedical	1064/532 nm	7.7 ns	2–8	2, 4, 6, 8 mm	1,2,5 and 10 Hz
Ruby	Epitouch Ruby	ESC/Sharplan	694 nm	1.2 ns	15–40	3–6 mm	1.2 Hz
	Chromos 694	Mehl Group	694 nm	2 ms	5–20	4 × 6-cm hexagon scanner	1 Hz
	Epilaser	Coherent	694 nm	3 ms	10–40	7 and 10 mm	0.5 Hz
Alexandrite	Epitouch/Alex	ESC/Sharplan	755 nm	2 ms	10–50	5–7 mm	5 Hz
	Apogee LPIR	Cynosure	755 nm	5–10 ms	25	7–10 mm	1 Hz
	GentleLASE	Candela	755 nm	3 ms	10–100	8, 10, 12 mm	1 Hz
Diode	Light Sheer	Coherent	800 nm	5–30 ms	10–40	9 mm^2	1 Hz
	LaserLite	Diomed	810 nm	50–250 ms	450	1 and 2 mm	10 Hz
Xenon flashlamp device	Epilight	ESC	590–1200 mm	2.5–5 ms	30–65	8 × 35 mm 10 × 45 mm	2–5 pulses per sequence with 1–300 ms delay

Generally, the darker the hair color and the greater the contrast between the hair and skin color, the better the results will be. Patients with fine-textured lighter-colored hair have less melanin and fewer chromophores to act as targets. Patients with darker skin have a greater chance of scarring and hypopigmentation than faired-skin people, because of the greater amount of melanin in their skin. For example, a recent study examining the benefits of the diode laser[14] on the back or thigh of 58 patients with skin type I–V and any hair color revealed: a 70% hair loss 1 month after one treatment; a 28% hair loss 12 months after one treatment; a 45% hair loss 12 months after two treatments, given 2 months apart; 70% of patients with black, brown, auburn or red hair having 'long-term' reduction of hair; and 10% of patients with blonde hair having long-term reduction.

Conclusions

Since the first laser for hair removal was introduced in 1995, there has been a tremendous influx of techniques available. More clinical research is necessary to clarify optimal systems for different patients. The current literature suffers not only from differing definitions of 'permanent', but also from the pooling of data from multiple anatomical sites with disparate hair cycles, from a plethora of inadequate hair-growth evaluation methods, from the absence of histopathological data, from little statistical analysis and from too brief a follow-up[16]. Nonetheless, current laser light hair-removal systems do provide a range of prolonged if not truly permanent and total elimination of hair, and patients seem to be happy enough with this effect.

TOO LITTLE HAIR
Non-surgical options

Because women tend to maintain their frontal hairline and have a generalized thinning without total alopecia, they continue to have some hair that can be cosmetically treated to appear denser than it really is. Generally, a woman with darker hair and pale skin can make the existing hair look thicker if the hair color is lightened, as there will be less contrast between the lighter hair and the pale scalp. Hair dyes are grouped into four types: gradual, temporary, semipermanent and 'permanent'. Alternatively, there are various products available that will color the scalp and that also adhere to the thinning hair. The purpose is to camouflage the paleness of the scalp by changing the color of the scalp to a color similar to that of the thinning hair. Two examples of

this are Couvre alopecia masking lotion, and GLH Formula no. 9. Couvre is an emulsion with iron oxide pigment similar to a liquid make-up product and is available in most hair colors. GLH Formula no. 9 is an aerosol-delivered hair thickener and is available in numerous colors with a finishing shield aerosol spray that helps to hold the color fast.

'Streaking' the hair can also produce the appearance of increased thickness, not only because it reduces hair/scalp color contrast but also because it thickens the individual hair shafts. Certain shampoos or conditioners will form a thin layer or polymer, such as polyvinylpyrrolidone (pvp), over the hair shaft[17]. Examples include: Big Hair by Optaderm (active ingredients include pvp, hydrolyzed keratin protein and chitin from cactus extracts); and Hair Volume Tonic by J.F. Lazartique (active ingredients include pvp, vinylco prolactam and chitin from seashells; Courtesy of Delineation Hair & Skin Essentials, Toronto, Canada). Chemical hair procedures, such as permanent waving, alter the structure and color of the hair. Permanent waving, for example, consists of three components: chemical softening, rearranging and fixing. A permanent wave is designed to last 3–4 months and will make straight hair, when waved, appear thicker, as it gives more 'body' to the hair, which then covers the thinning scalp better.

Non-surgical hair replacement additions have been available for thousands of years. They can be appropriate for patients with female-pattern thinning, whose hair is too thin to benefit enough from the agents described above, who are unsuitable for hair transplantation or who have expectations that are greater than hair transplantation can satisfy. Individuals who have alopecia areata, totalis or universalis, and those undergoing chemotherapy can also benefit from external hair-bearing devices. These can be called a hair addition, hair weave, hair extension, hairpiece, toupee, wig, hair fusion, hair integration, prosthesis, or simply a non-surgical hair replacement. They can be ready made or custom made and are constructed of human hair, synthetic hair, or a combination of both. Because women generally tend to look for more volume and fullness than men, women are more amenable to a hair addition that is a full wig that covers the entire scalp.

Hair additions can be affixed either to the scalp or to the existing hair. Scalp attachment involves adhesives (glues or double-sided tape), vacuum-fitted prosthetic hair additions, or surgical attachment of the prosthesis to the scalp[18]. Complications secondary to surgical attachment, however, include ripping of a surgical attachment 'tunnel', or

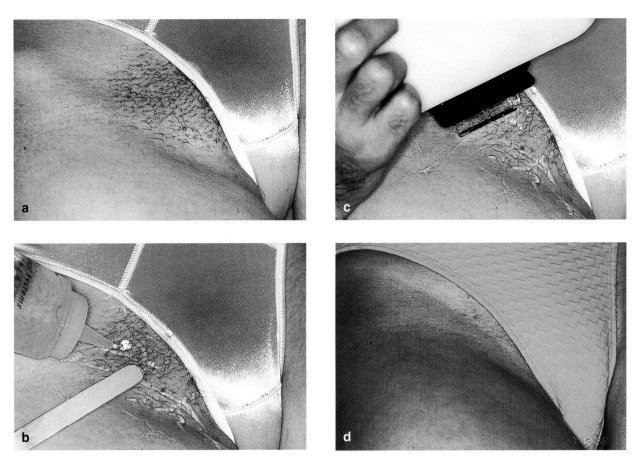

Figure 1   (a) Bikini area before treatment. (b) Skin with cold gel. (c) Application of the pulsed light. Fast Epilight (ESC Medical Systems) was used (filter 645, two pulses, 31 J, 5-ms duration, 20-ms delay). (d) Three months later, some hairs starting to grow. Typically 4–5 sessions will be needed. Courtesy of Dr Tykocinski, Sao Paulo, Brazil

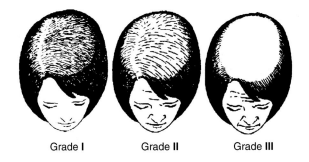

Grade I   Grade II   Grade III

Figure 2   Ludwig classification, illustrating typical female thinning patterns of increasing severity, with maintenance of the frontal hairline. Courtesy of reference 22

infection and discomfort associated with suture attachments. Hair additions can be attached to existing hair with clips, weaves or bonding. Bonding entails shaving the hair to approximately 2 cm in length at the area of attachment. The hair addition is applied to the matching area of the already cut hair that has had a sealant applied. The patient returns every 4–6 weeks for reapplication. Problems encountered with attachments to existing hair include traction alopecia, discomfort and seborrheic dermatitis.

Hair transplantation

Despite advances in the non-surgical methods of dealing with too little scalp hair in women described above, hair transplantation remains one of the best options for treatment of this problem. It can be utilized not only for androgenetic alopecia but also for scarring alopecias secondary to cutaneous disease, cosmetic surgery, trauma and burns, for adding hair to eyelashes, eyebrows and the pubic area, and even for enhancing the appearance of male to female transsexuals.

Androgenetic alopecia of course is the most frequent indication for hair transplantation. Its incidence in women seems to be increasing and may be as high as 20%. Its cause and medical treatment have already been dealt with in a previous chapter. As in men, it is very important to obtain a thorough family history. Often a similar problem has affected the patient's mother, sister(s), aunt(s), or grandmother(s), and they can provide some indication of the prognosis. The progression of androgenetic alopecia can be altered by factors such as stress, diet and general health. In particular, a low serum iron level, more commonly seen in women than in

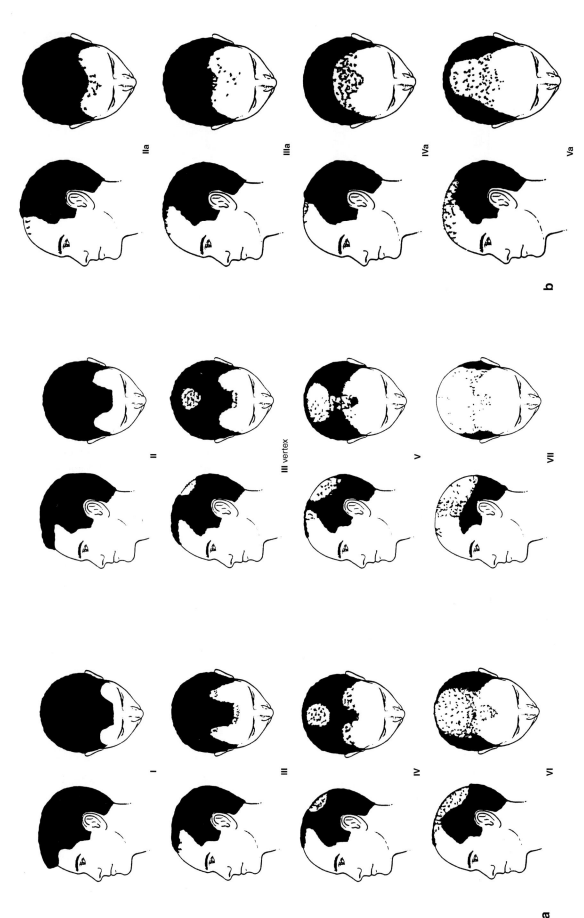

Figure 3 (a) Norwood classification of male-pattern baldness. (b) Type A variant male-pattern baldness. Courtesy of reference 23

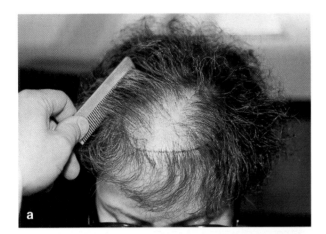

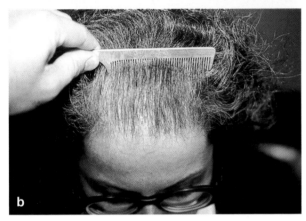

Figure 4 (a) Before first session, illustrating typical female pattern thinning with maintenance of the frontal hairline. Black grease pencil line demarcates the anterior limit of proposed grafting. (b) Eight months after a single session using a combination of 1–3-hair micrografts and 4–6-hair slit grafts. With the use of slit grafts to augment existing density without removing any previous hair, the result is very natural even on close inspection

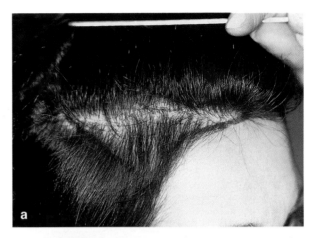

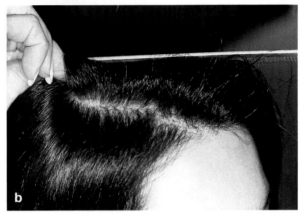

Figure 5 (a) Before transplantation. This woman had thinning of the fronto-temporal triangles and wanted a more feminine, denser hairline zone. (b) Five months after a single transplant session; 240 micrografts, 448 mini-slit grafts and 82 small slit grafts were used

men, may accelerate the disorder. If there is any suspicion of a testosterone excess syndrome (hirsutism, acne, lowering of voice, change in menses, rapid onset of male recessions), appropriate blood tests should be carried out, but they are not routinely performed in the absence of such clinical symptoms or signs. These tests include a complete blood count and measurement of thyroid stimulating hormone, testosterone, free testosterone, testosterone binding globulin, androstenedione, dehydroepiandrosterone sulfate, prolactin, serum vitamin B_{12} and serum ferritin. If the results are abnormal, the patient should be referred to an endocrinologist for full assessment and treatment.

The idea of a beautiful woman in society today includes a thick luxurious head of hair, regardless of age. Thinning hair anywhere on the scalp is seen not only as a component of decreased beauty, but also as a sign of age. Men are more willing to accept

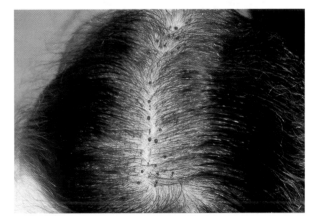

Figure 6 Slit grafts are used in areas with diffuse but low-density hair in combination with small round grafts that fill more or less round sites that are devoid of hair, and that are 'punched out' with a trephine

an area of thinning hair or are satisfied with transplantation of the front half of the scalp only – leaving the bald vertex untreated. This difference between men and women is referred to as gender

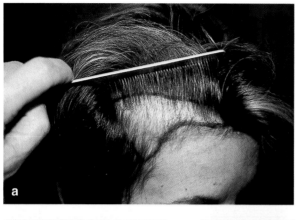

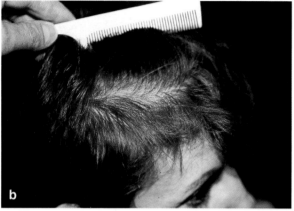

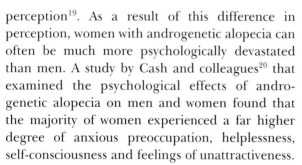

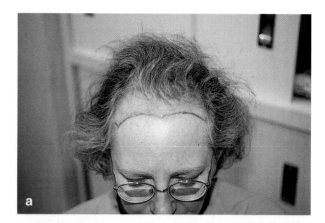

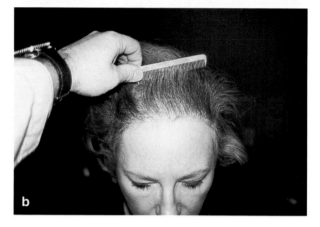

Figure 7 (a) Before hair transplantation, a black crayon line delineating the area to be transplanted. This woman wanted her male-type recessions thickened. (b) Five months after a single transplant session utilizing 200 micrografts and 268 mini-slit grafts

Figure 8 (a) Before first transplant. The black line denotes the anterior margins of a more feminine hairline. (b) Six months after the second transplant session with the hair pulled back for critical evaluation. Note the more rounded feminine hairline

perception[19]. As a result of this difference in perception, women with androgenetic alopecia can often be much more psychologically devastated than men. A study by Cash and colleagues[20] that examined the psychological effects of androgenetic alopecia on men and women found that the majority of women experienced a far higher degree of anxious preoccupation, helplessness, self-consciousness and feelings of unattractiveness.

Before a woman decides to undergo hair transplantation for androgenetic alopecia, other causes of diffuse loss of scalp hair must be ruled out[21]. Acute telogen effluvium, for example, presents as a rapid sudden increase in scalp hair shedding and is due to specific factors such as childbirth, febrile illness, stress, general anesthetic, certain drugs and crash dieting. Most importantly, it is self-limiting. Chronic telogen effluvium, in which there is a diffuse shedding of scalp hair of unknown origin, is common in middle age and can often mimic androgenetic alopecia. Androgenetic alopecia often begins sooner than chronic telogen effluvium (age 20–40), is more

gradual and typically is accompanied by a family history. A biopsy to distinguish between the two may be necessary. Once again, the course is self-limiting, so hair transplantation is not indicated.

Women tend to have hair that thins in different patterns from that of men. Ludwig divided the former pattern into three grades of increasing severity of thinning with preservation of the frontal hairline[22] (Figure 2). On the other hand, male-pattern baldness (MPB) as described by Norwood[23] typically is associated with total alopecia of portions of the top portion of the scalp and a fringe of persisting hair (Figure 3). As women tend to have a more generalized, gradual thinning pattern, many different scalp disorders can mimic female-pattern androgenetic alopecia[21]. Additionally, 13% of premenopausal and 37% of postmenopausal women exhibit some hair loss in the frontotemporal areas, creating some degree of the recessions that are more typical of MPB in men[24]. The following summarizes the differences between men and women as candidates for surgical hair restoration.

Women

Factors against:

(1) There are greater social expectations for a full head of dense hair. Therefore, women may be harder to please.

(2) The pattern of hair loss is often more diffuse, and frequently also affects the temporal, parietal and occipital potential donor areas, rendering them unusable or smaller than in their male counterparts.

(3) Women are not as amenable to alopecia reduction, owing to their general thinning pattern.

Factors in favor:

(1) There is maintenance of the frontal hairline. Therefore, one can use existing hair to provide better density and postoperative camouflage. The hairline itself, even if it is thickened by some transplanting, can look natural on even the closest examination (Figure 4).

(2) Usually fewer sessions are required to produce good hair density. With the use of micrografts and slit grafts, less or no existing hair is destroyed or removed, as occurred in the past with circular punch grafts.

Men

Factors in favor:

(1) Men can be happy with frontal coverage only and with a thinning look.

(2) Hair loss is more confined to the top of the scalp with maintenance of density in the temporal–parietal–occipital fringe regions.

(3) Men are more amenable to alopecia reduction, owing to their pattern of balding.

Factors against:

(1) Often there is total loss of the hairline with little or no hair to use for postoperative camouflage.

(2) Men generally require more grafting to achieve a natural-appearing hairline.

(3) Any pre-existing hair in the recipient region may eventually fall out, requiring further sessions.

In order to be a candidate for surgical hair restoration, two clinical criteria need to be satisfied[25]. First, a satisfactory donor/recipient 'area' ratio is required. If the intended recipient area is too large to be dealt with by the limited donor region, hair transplants should be avoided. Second, a satisfactory donor/recipient 'hair density' ratio is required. A positive exchange ratio is needed when transferring hair from the donor to the recipient area. This ratio is

not as crucial as it was before the advent of slit grafting and micrografting – which as noted earlier are used to augment the density of the recipient area without the removal of existing hair – but, if the density is the same in both recipient and donor areas, the value of hair transplantation is questionable. An argument might be made that, even if the density is the same in the donor and recipient areas, with the addition of more hair to the recipient area there will be improved density. The cosmetic change may not be enough to warrant transfer. One must keep in mind that women usually expect to see a substantial cosmetic change and are therefore unlikely to be happy with simply knowing that there is more hair in the recipient area. Hair color and quality can also affect a patient's candidacy for treatment. The patient may be a better candidate if, for example, they have lighter hair colour or coarser hair in the donor region. When hair with these characteristics is placed into the recipient area, it will give the appearance of more density than will darker or finer-textured hair.

Transplanted hair is initially shed 2–3 weeks after the surgery and regrows approximately 3 months after treatment. Sessions are performed no sooner than 6 months apart and patients are encouraged to wait 9–12 months before deciding on the need for another. Since the new hair is initially tapered, fine and short, it is not until 9–12 months after surgery that the full cosmetic benefit occurs. Women's hair may also look somewhat thinner for the first 3–6 months after a surgical procedure, owing to telogen and/or anagen effluvium affecting the transplanted hair and partial telogen effluvium of some of the surrounding pre-existing hair. They should always be forewarned of this possibility, but also reassured that all hair lost in this way will come back at the same time or slightly earlier than the transplanted hair regrows. We suggest 3% minoxidil applied twice daily for 1 month following the procedure, to decrease the likelihood of telogen and/or anagen effluvium of existing hair and to speed up regrowth of hair.

When transplanting women's hair – in comparison to men's – sessions are usually shorter, with a longer interval between them. This slower approach in women allows for:

(1) Easier postoperative camouflage of the recipient site with combed over non-treated adjacent-area hair (something that is often not possible for males with MPB);

(2) Untreated areas to be used as a 'control' with which to compare treated areas. This is

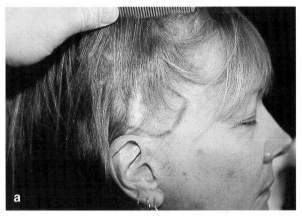

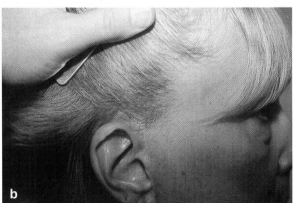

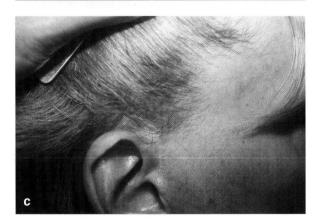

Figure 9   (a) Before transplantation, showing a white linear scar and thinning of the sideburn region after rhytidectomy. The black line delineates the area to be transplanted. (b) Nine months after one session using micrografts and minigrafts to thicken the scar and sideburn region. (c) Close-up of the area shown in (b)

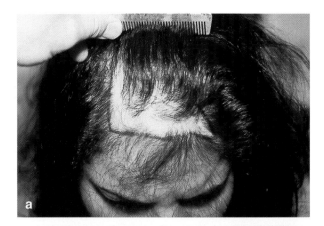

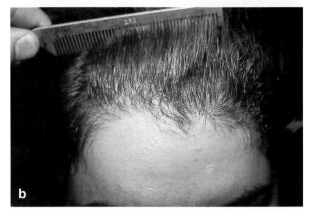

Figure 10   (a) Before transplantation. This woman was involved in a car accident and sustained scarring and hair loss. The black crayon line circumscribes the area to be transplanted. (b) Eight months after the third session of micrografts and minigrafts to the scarred region. The hair has been pulled back for critical evaluation

anesthetic solutions are used and there is less likelihood of temporary postoperative hair loss;

(5) Less postoperative discomfort. The use of nitrous oxide gas (Entonox) for minimizing pain at the time of the initial administration of local anesthetics should be avoided in pregnant women, owing to the possibility of inducing a miscarriage[26]. This concern applies to female surgical staff as well. A scavenging system is mandatory.

Graft selection

With the advent of mini/micrografting and improvements in donor harvesting techniques, more women are acceptable candidates and better candidates for transplantation today than they were when only large circular punch grafts were employed. The traditional 3–4-mm circular punch graft, while affording considerable hair density with each graft, had the disadvantage of removing hair in the recipient area in order to make room for the circular donor 'plug'. Since women generally maintain

important, as patients are better able to assess on the basis of one session whether or not to proceed with further treatment;

(3) Previously transplanted hair, when fully grown, to provide more camouflage for subsequent sessions;

(4) Somewhat smaller sessions, so that the procedure takes less time, smaller amounts of

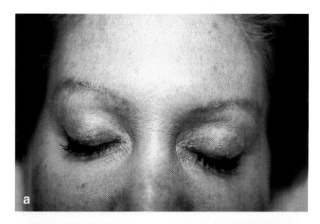

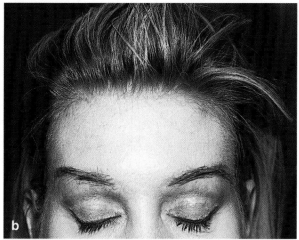

Figure 11   (a) Before hair transplantation. This woman over-plucked her eyebrows when she was younger and sustained permanent hair loss. Eyebrow pencil is in place for camouflage. (b) After three sessions of micrografts

some hair in the thinning area (compared to the potential for total loss in men), the removal of any hair in the recipient area constitutes the removal of at least some hair that is not destined to be lost. In addition, patients treated with 3–4-mm punch grafts would always initially have less hair than before surgery, and the improvement would be equal only to the difference between the number of hairs punched out and the number transplanted. Micrografts with 1–2 hairs and slit grafts with 3–5 hairs are inserted into sites that are made, respectively, with a small-bore needle or scalpel blade between existing hairs. They therefore allow for the addition of new hair without the removal of existing hair (Figure 5). Micrografts and minigrafts also minimize the possibility of a 'pluggy' look. In areas of the scalp that have diffuse thinning with discrete small areas devoid of hair, a combination of micrografts, slit grafts and small circular grafts can be employed. The round grafts are used in the small alopecic areas that are punched out in their entirety (Figure 6).

In the donor area, multiple strips or ellipses are harvested using multibladed scalpels or a no. 15 blade scalpel, respectively. The wound is sutured and produces a single fine scar line[27]. Subsequent donor area harvesting is designed to include the previous scar, so that no matter how many sessions are carried out, only a single scar line is left. This compares favorably to the old punch harvesting technique that left multiple rows of wider scars. The less scar produced, the more hair can be removed from the donor area without any thinning of that area being noticed. When selecting the donor area, it is important to remember that women often like to have a variety of hairstyles that may or may not expose a donor area scar. For example, women sometimes pull their hair up into a bun, so a scar in the inferior occipital area should be avoided.

The hairline in women normally lacks the alopecic frontotemporal recessions that are typically seen in men. Female hair transplanting therefore should include these areas if they are thinning or alopecic, and the anterior hairline should have a rounder, more concave configuration (Figures 7 and 8). Hair direction in the hairline zone can change dramatically as one goes from left to right. The use of fine-textured 1–2 hair micrografts to reconstitute a feathered feminine hairline is essential. Behind the hairline zone, the use of slightly larger 3–5 hair slit grafts and round minigrafts becomes more important for producing greater density. The authors' typical session will result in the transfer of between 2500 and 5000 hairs in the form of 500–1000 grafts of varying sizes.

The patient is presedated with 15–20 mg of diazepam and the procedure generally takes 3–4 h. A turban-like bandage is commonly applied at the conclusion of surgery and is removed the next day. At that time the scalp is also cleansed of any clotted blood and the hair is washed, blown dry and styled. Sutures are removed 1 week later. Patients are instructed to take 1 week off work, as there may be forehead edema as a result of the procedure. In rare cases, edema can be severe enough to cause ecchymosis around the eyes. This resolves in 7–10 days.

Non-androgenetic alopecia

The second most common reason for hair transplantation in women is scarring and hair loss after rhytidectomy[28]. Typically a coronal scar extends from ear to ear approximately 2.5–7.5 cm posterior to the anterior hairline (Figure 9). Scarring may also extend into the occipital region posteriorly and the sideburn area at the level of the ear anteriorly.

Endoscopic rhytidectomy can instead cause 2–4 scars, 1–2 cm in diameter, posterior to the hairline, while a brow lift can result in a noticeable hairline scar. All of these scars can be treated in 1–3 sessions utilizing micrografts and various sizes and types of minigrafts.

Finally, cicatricial alopecia secondary to burns and trauma (Figure 10) occurring anywhere on the body can be treated with hair transplantation. Eyelash and eyebrow hair loss in particular are amenable to grafting (Figure 11).

CONCLUSIONS

The role of hair as a component of female beauty has always been important. Too much hair in certain places or too little hair in others can be significantly detrimental to the aura of a woman's beauty and can affect the quality of life of that individual. New products and surgical techniques available today allow many more women to conform to their own and society's expectations. As a result, more women can now feel better about themselves and enjoy a better quality of life. Cosmetic surgery does more than simply improve appearance. Nowhere is this more true than in dealing with problems of too much or too little hair.

ACKNOWLEDGEMENT

The authors wish to thank Dr Harvey Jay for his assistance in writing the section on laser hair removal.

REFERENCES

1. Richards RN, Uy M, Meharg G. Temporary hair removal in patients with hirsutism: a clinical study. *Cutis* 1990;45:199–202
2. Olsen EA. Methods of hair removal. *J Am Acad Dermatol* 1999;40:143–55
3. Trotter M. The resistance of hair to certain supposed growth stimulants. *Arch Dermatol Syph* 1923;7:93–8
4. Sebenje JE. Cutaneous electrosurgery. In *Yearbook Medical*. Chicago: Yearbook Medical Publishers, 1989:57–60
5. Kalkworf KL, Hrejci RF, Edison AR, *et al*. Subjacent heat production during tissue excision with electrosurgery. *J Oral Maxillo Fac Surg* 1983;41:653–8
6. Wagner RF. Medical and technical issues in office electrolysis and thermolysis. *J Dermatol Surg Oncol* 1993;19:575–7
7. Wagner RF, Tomich JM, Grande DJ. Electrolysis and thermolysis for permanent hair removal. *J Am Acad Dermatol* 1985;12:441–9
8. Wheeland RG. Laser assisted hair removal. *Dermatol Clin* 1997;15:469–77
9. Wagner RF. Physical methods for the management of hirsutism. *Cutis* 1990;45:319–22
10. Anderson RR, Parrish JA. Selective photothermolysis: precise microsurgery by selective absorption of pulsed radiation. *Science* 1983;220:524–7
11. Van Scott EJ, Ekel TM, Auerback R. Determinance of rate and kinetics of cell division in scalp hair. *J Invest Dermatol* 1963;41:269–74
12. Clement M, Kiernan M, Bjerring P. *Depilation by Pulsed Ruby Laser: A Review.* UK; 1998:1–12
13. Fuchs M. Thermokinetic selectivity – a new highly effective method for permanent hair removal: experience with the LPIR alexandrite laser. *Derm Prakt Dermatol* 1997;5:1–7
14. Anderson RR. Clinical use of the light sheer diode laser system. *Coher Med* 1998:1–7
15. Ziering CL. Laser assisted hair removal: a review of current technology. *Int J Cosmet Surg* 1998;6:71–5
16. Tope WD, Hordinisky MK. A hair's breadth closer? *Arch Dermatol* 1998;134:867–9
17. Finkelstein P. Hair conditioners. *Cutis* 1970;6:542–5
18. Mahoney MJ. Non-surgical hair replacement. In Stough DB, Haber RS, eds. *Hair Replacement*. St Louis: Mosby, 1996:399–411
19. Friedman DO. Hair transplantation for female androgenetic alopecia. *Hair Loss J* 1992;7:1–7
20. Cash TF, Price VH, Savin RC. Psychological effects of androgenetic alopecia: comparisons with balding men and with female control subjects. *J Am Acad Dermatol* 1993;29:568–75
21. Orfanos CE, Happle R, eds. *Hair and Hair Diseases*. Berlin: Springer-Verlag, 1990:509–10
22. Ludwig E. Classification of the types of androgenetic alopecia (common baldness) arising in the female sex. *Br J Dermatol* 1977;97:247–54
23. Norwood O, Shiell R. *Hair Transplant Surgery*, 2nd edn. Springfield, IL: Charles C Thomas, 1984
24. Venning VA, Dawber RPR. Pattern androgenetic alopecia in women. *J Am Acad Dermatol* 1988;18:1073–77
25. Cotterill PC. Hair transplantation in females. In Unger WP, ed. *Hair Transplantation*, 3rd edn. New York: Marcel Dekker, 1995:287–92
26. Crawford J, Lewis M. Nitrous oxide in early human pregnancy. *Anaesthesia* 1986;41:900–5
27. Unger W. The donor site. In Unger W, ed. *Hair Transplantation*, 3rd edn. New York: Marcel Dekker, 1995:183–214
28. Cotterill PC. Application and approach to hair transplantation in females. *Am J Cosmet Surg* 1997;14:137–41

Facial rejuvenation

50

Anthony V. Benedetto and Paula Karam

Earth's noblest thing, A Woman perfected.
'Irene', James Russel Lowell

INTRODUCTION

The perception of beauty is certainly in the eyes of the beholder. From time immemorial the opposite sex has gazed upon girls and women, cherishing their beauty and immortalizing them in cave drawings and on wall mosaics, in epic poems and in love stories, in paintings on canvas and in film on the big screen. Women, like Hatchetsup of Egypt and Victoria of England have ruled nations, while others, like Helen of Troy and Cleopatra of Alexandria have precipitated international intrigue and wars of mass destruction all in the name of love and beauty. But beauty is evanescent and beautiful girls become 'older' women. How can a woman capture and retain the ephemeral beauty of youth? The early conquistadors of the Americas failed to do so in their futile search for the 'Fountain of Youth'; however, modern-day medicine and surgical techniques have attempted to bring a woman's desire for a perpetually youthful appearance closer to reality.

PATHOPHYSIOLOGY OF AGING

The relentless aging process can be caused by a variety of factors. Intrinsic or biological aging is a chronological phenomenon that interfaces with a woman's immune status, hormonal cycles and genetic profile. In biological aging, all the cutaneous anatomical infrastructures and their physiological functions inevitably and continuously regress with time[1]. This progressive deterioration of the integument and its supporting structures is enhanced by extrinsic aging[2]. Extrinsic aging is attributed to the skin's exposure to the environment, where the cumulative insults of chemical, physical and mechanical trauma from the elements can prematurely damage the skin, unless precautionary steps are taken[3].

Solar irradiation, including ultraviolet (UV) and infrared (IR) radiation, is the foremost environmental element that damages the skin[4]. The damage caused by UV and IR radiation is realized many years later, after its immediate consequences have long been forgotten. The changes of the cumulative effects of environmental exposure can be observed in later years as what are perceived as the clinical stigmata of old age[5]. Among the many different clinical and subclinical changes associated with photoaging are those that predominantly ravage a women's youthful appearance and mar her facial beauty. These include superficial and deep rhytides, as well as the dyspigmentary changes of lentigines, macular seborrheic and actinic keratoses. Solar elastotic changes can result in atrophic, inelastic, saggy, telangiectatic, yellow-colored, sallow facial skin that is fragile, redundant and coarse. Sometimes, photodamaged skin appears hypertrophic and dry, with cysts and comedones[6–8]. Moreover, those who experience repeated and severe episodes of sunburning also increase their probability of developing the more dangerous changes of premalignant and malignant skin lesions[9–12].

There are other factors that can contribute to aging and the wrinkling of a woman's face. Some are subtle. For example, tobacco smoking has recently been identified as causing facial wrinkles[13,14]. Occupational, geographical, cultural, or socioeconomic factors also will dictate to what extent and how rapidly a woman's skin ages and wrinkles[3].

What is a woman to do when she realizes her youthful appearance is waning? By the end of the 19th century, distinguished surgeons in Europe and the USA were trying to forestall the inevitable by developing surgical procedures that focused attention not only on the correction of inherited and acquired deformities, but also on esthetics and surgery that attempted to re-establish youthful beauty.

Dermatologists, by the very nature of their specialty, have always concerned themselves with the care and cosmesis of facial skin. Along with actively treating diseased and photodamaged skin, as well as helping patients prevent further changes of photoaging, dermatologists also possess a variety of medicosurgical techniques that can be used to rejuvenate the face. The range of interventional procedures of facial rejuvenation performed by dermatologists includes skin resurfacing techniques, intentional chemodenervation of facial mimetic muscles by injection and the implantation of soft tissue fillers. Many of these procedures have been developed or refined by dermatologists. The following sections discuss the many different options that are used by the dermatologist to rejuvenate the face of women.

FACIAL SKIN RESURFACING
Chemical peeling

From early recorded history, women have applied various potions and lotions to their faces to reduce wrinkling and other signs of photoaging. Cleopatra was known to bathe in sour milk, while French women coated their skin with wine, unaware that both sour milk and wine contain α-hydroxy acids[15].

In 1903, the New York dermatologist George M. MacKee was one of the first to use a solution of phenol or carbolic acid for chemical exfoliation of acne pits and scars. Many of his patients were followed for up to 30 years and no serious side-effects were ever encountered[16]. In the early 1960s Thomas J. Baker and Howard L. Gordon established the modern procedure of cosmetic phenol peeling with their formula, some form of which is still widely used today[17,18] (Table 1). The work of Baker and Gordon removed chemical peeling and facial rejuvenation from the depths of what previously was considered chicanery and a questionable procedure practiced by lay beauticians, elevating it to a loftier position of legitimacy and an ethical medicosurgical procedure practiced by reputable physicians. Baker and Gordon established that phenol is the most penetrating of all the known chemexfoliants, and that it is more penetrating at an aqueous concentration of 50% than it is at the higher concentration of 88%. By adding other epidermal irritants, such as croton oil, the penetration of phenol was enhanced. With the resurgence in popularity of chemical peelings in the 1960s and 1970s, came reports of experimentation with different formulas of phenol and various other chemexfoliants. Ayres[19], a dermatologist, used equal mixtures of phenol, trichloroacetic acid and alcohol. Aronsohn[20] used phenol with saponated cresol (Lysol®) and croton oil. Litton preferred 50% phenol with glycerol, water and croton oil, because it remained stable for 3–4 months[21].

Trichloroacetic acid, resorcinol, salicylic acid and many other exfoliants, irritants, enzymes, as well as solid carbon dioxide (CO_2) have been used alone and in combination to reduce wrinkling and to rejuvenate facial skin. Recently, newer and more

Table 1 Baker/Gordon formula of 50% phenol (carbolic acid)

Phenol 88%	3 ml
Distilled water	2 ml
Croton oil	3 drops
Septisol	8 drops

Table 2 Skin types classified according to pigmentation ability: the ability to tan after sun exposure. From reference 22

I	Burns easily and severely; never tans
II	Burns easily; tans minimally with difficulty
III	Burns moderately; tans moderately and uniformly
IV	Burns minimally; tans easily and moderately
V	Rarely burns; tans darkly and profusely
VI	Never burns; tans a deep brown or black

effective and, perhaps, less painful modalities other than chemicals to produce skin peeling and facial skin resurfacing have been developed. In certain situations, these newer modalities (e.g. dermabrasion and laser resurfacing) have replaced the use of chemical peeling.

Histopathological studies done on facial skin before and after different resurfacing procedures have revealed similarly beneficial changes in photodamaged skin, whether the resurfacing was done by chemical peeling, physical sanding (dermabrasion) or by laser ablation. The goal of facial skin resurfacing is the removal of aged and actinically damaged skin, replacing it with new epithelium and dermal connective tissue. With any resurfacing technique, the epidermis, papillary dermis and the upper to midportions of the reticular dermis can be removed without causing clinical scarring, provided that the supporting soft tissue has a sufficient amount of adnexal structures. The risk of dyspigmentation increases with a patient's increased ability to tan[22] (Table 2). The more darkly pigmented a patient is, the more likely it is for that patient to develop hyperpigmentation early in the postoperative period (i.e. 1–2 months after the peel) and hypopigmentation 1 year or longer after chemical peeling or any other resurfacing procedure.

The art of chemical peeling was transformed into a true science when, in the 1980s, Samuel J. Stegman, a dermatologist, published his seminal work comparing the histological changes produced by 50% trichloroacetic acid (TCA), full-strength phenol, Baker/Gordon formula phenol and dermabrasion in both animals and humans[23,24]. He found that the depth of wounding was related to the strength of the chemical agent used; i.e. Baker/Gordon formula was stronger than full-strength phenol, which was stronger than 50% TCA. Tape occlusion increased the depth of wounding after the application of phenol but not after TCA. Solar elastosis had no effect on the depth of wounding. The clinical signs of wounding and healing correlated with the depth of penetration of the dermabrasion or of the chemical exfoliant used.

Since Stegman's studies, our knowledge and the science of facial rejuvenation using chemical exfoliants alone or in combination with other chemical or physical agents has expanded. In the past two decades, the practice of chemical peeling has become more sophisticated, with dozens of new techniques described. The following is an overview of the different chemical peeling agents currently in use by dermatologists.

Classification of peeling agents

Peeling agents are classified as superficial[25–27], medium[28–32] and deep[33–35], depending on the depth of the wound they produce (Table 3).

Superficial peels

Superficial peels are produced by agents that wound the epidermis and part of the papillary dermis (Table 3). They can be repeated weekly, biweekly or monthly to obtain the desired effect. The main indications for superficial peels are melasma, photodamaged skin, acne, fine wrinkles, freckles, superficial scars and postinflammatory dyspigmentation secondary to acne or other skin conditions.

Medium-depth peels

Medium-depth peels are produced by agents that wound the epidermis and the dermis as deep as the reticular dermis (Table 3). They can be repeated every 3 months. The main indications for a medium-depth peel are depressed scars, melasma, photodamaged elastotic skin, fine wrinkles and actinic keratoses.

Deep peels

Deep peels are produced by agents that wound the epidermis and the dermis up to the mid-reticular dermis (Table 3). Deep peels should not be repeated sooner than 1 year after a previous peeling. The main indications for deep chemical peeling are photodamaged skin, rhytides and deep scars.

Factors affecting the absorption of a peeling agent

Besides the type of agent used, many factors play a role in the absorption of the peel and therefore in the depth of wounding. The use of medications prior to peeling, e.g. topical tretinoin or α-hydroxy acids or both, can also increase the absorption of the peeling agent[30–32].

The concentration of the different peeling agents will determine how deeply they are absorbed. For example, higher concentrations of TCA produce deeper wounds[28], while more concentrated phenol (carbolic acid) paradoxically produces more superficial wounds[32]. Degreasing the skin prior to a peel removes excess sebum and keratin, thereby promoting the absorption of the peel. It has been found that 70% glycolic acid is more effective after the skin has been rubbed with acetone for 2 min, than when the same skin has been rubbed with milk cleanser. The longer a peeling agent is kept on the skin, the deeper the penetration and wounding. This is seen with α-hydroxy acids[24] and resorcin peels[26], but it does not affect the peels done with TCA if it is kept on the skin for more than 2 min[29].

The mode of application of the peeling agent is also important. When using a liquid, rubbing with a cotton-tipped applicator or a gauze pad will promote its absorption. Reapplication of the peeling agent can enhance absorption. This has been documented with TCA and Baker's formula when the reapplication of either of these agents 10 min after an initial frost caused an increase in the wounding depth[33]. Occlusion increases the wounding depth of a phenol peel, but it does not affect a TCA peel[23,35]. Photodamaged skin can react more than normal skin when the dermis is thinner, and the peeling agents are metabolized less rapidly. When adnexal structures are fewer in number, re-epithelialization can be slower. There is an inverse relationship of wounding depth to epidermal thickness. For example, on the eyelids, where both the epidermis and the dermis are very thin, the absorption of any chemical occurs more rapidly. Therefore, lower concentrations and less time of application or both are necessary to prevent complications. Included in Table 4 are many of the relative contraindications for performing chemical peeling[36,37].

Complications of chemical peels

In general, the incidence of complications increases directly with the depth of tissue wounding[34,36,37]. Superficial chemical peels are the safest, while deep

Table 3 Types of chemical peels

Superficial	Medium depth	Deep
50–70% glycolic acid	50% TCA	50% phenol occluded
10–30% TCA	CO_2 slush + 35% TCA	
50% resorcin	Jessner's solution + 35% TCA	
Jessner's solution:	70% glycolic acid + 35% TCA	
resorcinol 14 g	50% phenol unoccluded	
salicylic acid 14 g	50% resorcin	
lactic acid (85%) 14 g		
ethanol (95%) qs ad 100 ml		

TCA, trichloroacetic acid; qs ad, sufficient quantity to make

Table 4 Relative contraindications for performing chemical peeling

Patients	Risk
Of skin types IV–VI	dyspigmentation
On oral contraceptives	
On postmenopausal hormonal therapy	
With active or past history of infection	disseminated infection with *Herpes simplex*, verrucae planae, bacteria or yeast
With diabetes mellitus	
With an immune compromising process	
Within 1 year of isotretinoin therapy	abnormal wound healing and scarring, especially after deeper peelings
On anticoagulation therapy	
With connective tissue disease	
After recent surgery involving extensive tissue undermining	
Pregnant or lactating	potential injury to fetus or infant

peels carry the highest risk for complications. The more significant adverse sequelae are seen after medium-depth to deep chemical peelings, and include dyspigmentary changes, scarring, infection, prolonged erythema, pruritus, skin atrophy and milia. Cardiac arrhythmias and laryngeal edema can be seen with peels done with phenol[38,39] (Table 5).

Dermabrasion

Background

Dermabrasion is the surgical removal of the epidermis and upper to mid-dermis by either a diamond fraise or wire brush which is attached to a motorized instrument that rotates it at high speeds parallel to the surface of the skin. This form of facial skin resurfacing was first used in Germany in 1905 by Ernst Kromayer, a dermatologist, who removed acne and smallpox scars, benign skin lesions and abnormal pigmentation[40,41]. He developed a variety of cylindrical steel burrs, knives, augers, bores and rasps, which he attached to a motor-driven rotary device commonly used by dentists. He observed that abrasions and lacerations confined to the epidermis and papillary dermis often healed without scarring; however, deeper injuries to the level of the reticular dermis tended to heal with scarring. In 1933, Kromayer advocated freezing of the skin by applying CO_2 snow or spraying ether or ethyl chloride onto the face to anesthetize the skin surface and to make it rigid before dermabrading it[42].

Dermabrasion was essentially ignored during the late 1930s and 1940s. In the early 1950s, a dermatologist, Abner Kurtin, and an instrument maker, Noel Robbins, promoted their method for mechanically resurfacing facial skin, which now has become the basis for the modern-day technique of dermabrasion[43]. Robbins manufactured the sterilizable wire brush bits that Kurtin placed at the end of a high-speed rotary motor so that he could dermabrade skin. Over the patient's face, Kurtin sprayed ethyl chloride, which was then blown away by a fan. The ethyl chloride provided a semianesthetized, rigid skin surface and near-bloodless field necessary for wire-brush dermabrasion. The fan provided a means of removing the toxic vapors of ethyl chloride away from the immediate surgical field, so as not to intoxicate the patient or the surgical team[44]. Not only is ethyl chloride flammable, but it is also hepatotoxic and a potent general anesthetic. In 1955, Wilson and co-workers reported how they substituted dichlorotetrafluoroethane (Freon 114) for ethyl chloride in their technique, thereby eliminating the fan and the other potential hazards[45,46]. In 1956, Burks popularized dermabrasion with the publication of his text entitled *Wire Brush*

Table 5 Complications of chemical peels

Adverse sequelae	Reason
Dyspigmentation (hypo- or hyperpigmentation; demarcation lines between peeled and non-peeled areas)	occurs more frequently in patients with skin types IV–VI who have deeper peels done
Scarring	occurs more frequently with medium-depth to deep peelings done on thinned, aged skin; on non-facial skin; after recent undermining or resurfacing surgery or in patients while on or within 6–12 months of taking isotretinoin
Disseminated infections	occurs with medium-depth to deep peelings in predisposed patients (i.e. those with diabetes mellitus, or other immune compromising process). Prophylaxis is needed against Gram-positive or -negative bacteria, *Herpes simplex* or candidal contamination during the post-peel healing period
Erythema	regularly occurs with medium-depth to deep peels, lasts 1–3 months and is prolonged by alcoholic beverages and isotretinoin
Pruritus	usually occurs 2–4 weeks post-peeling, but if it persists or intensifies, rule out contact or irritant dermatitis
Atrophy	can occur in aged skin with or without photodamage
Milia	can occur within 1–2 months after peeling, especially when thick occlusive ointments are used in the post-peeling period
Cardiotoxicity	can occur during a phenol peel, and is avoided by applying phenol slowly to small segments of the face
Laryngeal edema	occurs in 1.2% of phenol peelings, and resolves within 48 h

Surgery[47]. Since then, refinements to the technique of dermabrasion have been numerous. Developed as a procedure for the revision of scars due to acne and other conditions, dermabrasion soon evolved into a resurfacing technique for the treatment and prophylaxis of the photoaged face[48]. A long-term study of the clinical and histological changes found after dermabrasion revealed that there was a new and orderly epidermis overlying a band of new collagen or 'scar' in the upper papillary dermis that developed and matured in time to resemble normal, non-photodamaged skin (Figure 1). Dermabrasion was found to eliminate wrinkles and photodamaged tissue, resulting in a rejuvenation of facial skin that persisted for as long as 8 years (Figure 2). It also prevented for as many years the additional development of premalignant and malignant skin lesions.

Technique

There are a few items of surgical equipment that are required in order to perform a dermabrasion. The most significant advancement in the technique was the development of the motorized rotary dermabrader in 1978 called the Hand Engine® by the Bell International Machine Company. These instruments have miniaturized motors encased in their hand piece. Only a thin electrical cord is attached to the motorized handpiece, making it light in weight, while providing unrestricted maneuverability. The handpiece of the Hand Engine turns between 15 000 and 35 000 rpm and maintains a constant rotational speed in either direction with a substantial amount of torque (Figure 3). With the success and popularity of the Bell Hand Engine®, similar hand-held machines for dermabrasion were subsequently manufactured by Osada, Mill-Bilt Equipment Company and Robbins Instrument Company.

Bits and fraises for dermabrasion

There are two types of dermabrasion cutting tips currently in use: the wire brush and the diamond fraise (Figure 4). The wire brush bit is a wheel made of multiple stainless steel wires arranged on a stainless steel hub. The ends are beveled and trimmed to create a wheel that has a flat or tapered cutting surface. The wire brush comes in different widths and degrees of coarseness. The wire brush is a more efficient cutting tool than the diamond fraise, especially when abrading thick sun-damaged skin[49].

The diamond fraise is a stainless steel wheel with diamond chips bonded onto its surface. The chips come in various degrees of coarseness or roughness. Diamond fraises also come in different shapes. One can choose various types of wheels, cylinders, or cones. Each physician dermabrader

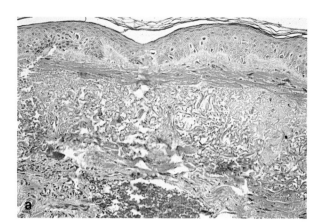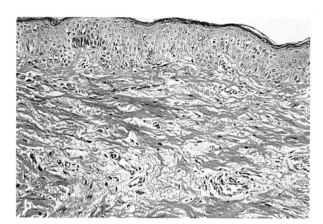

Figure 1   (a) Photomicrograph of sun-damaged facial skin showing evidence of solar elastotic amorphous material evident after Trichrome staining. Note the narrow Grenz area immediately beneath the epidermis. (b) A biopsy of the skin of the face of the same patient 5 years after a full face dermabrasion. Note the lack of amorphous, solar elastosis and the wide Grenz area with normal-appearing papillary dermis

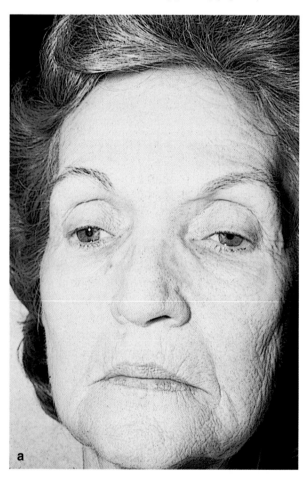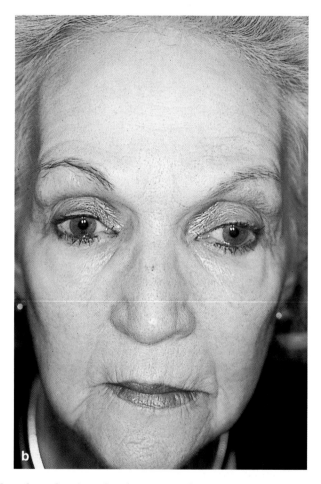

Figure 2   (a) Patient with signs of photoaging before total face dermabrasion. (b) The same patient 8 years after a full face dermabrasion. Figure reproduced with permission from Benedetto AV, Griffin TD, Benedetto EA, *et al.* Dermabrasion: therapy and prophylaxis of the photoaged face. *J Am Acad Dermatol* 1992;27:439–47

has his or her favorite shape for a given function and anatomical site.

Refrigerants

The function of a refrigerant is to anesthetize the surface of the skin as well as make the skin rigid so that the diamond fraise or wire brush can glide over the skin surface. Since the mid 1950s, Frigiderm® or Freon 114 (dichlorotetrafluoroethane) has been the most popular refrigerant for dermabrasion[50]. FluroEthyl®, which consists of 75% Freon 114 and 25% ethyl chloride, also can be used.

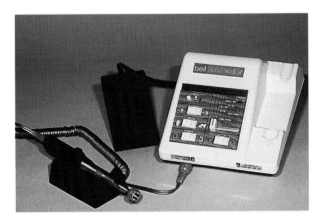

Figure 3 Bell Hand Engine®

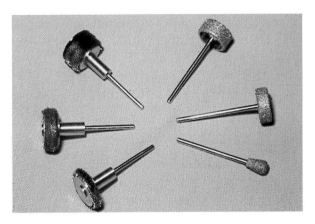

Figure 4 Wire brush bits on the left; diamond fraises on the right

Additional equipment and precautions

Surgical face masks, caps, gowns, gloves and face shields must be worn by the surgeon, surgical assistants and all those present at the operation during a dermabrasion procedure. This is to protect all those present from the aerosolized tissue and blood products that are produced during a dermabrasion[51,52]. The patient is draped, and the eyes are shielded and protected. The patient's face is painted with gentian violet prior to the procedure to mark the depths of the scars and areas of the face to be treated. Additionally, a benzodiazepine is administered preoperatively to induce postoperative amnesia, and an analgesic or a non-steroidal anti-inflammatory drug (NSAID) is administered to produce sufficient analgesia to make the surgical experience more tolerable for the patient. Postoperative wound care is similar to that given to anyone following a facial resurfacing procedure, including keeping the resurfaced areas moist with occlusive dressings with or without topical antibiotics[53]. Because of the recent emergence of an increased incidence of bacitracin contact allergy and irritation or both, a topical antibiotic free of bacitracin should be used[54]. Prophylaxis with oral antibiotics and antiviral medications is required during the postoperative period. A short course of analgesics and somnifacients can also be prescribed.

At about the same time that dermabrasion was becoming a popular technique for facial rejuvenation, David and colleagues, in 1989, reported their experience with 23 patients who had actinically damaged facial skin and were treated for cosmetic and medical purposes with CO_2 laser abrasion[55]. Since then, further refinements in the use of this new type of skin-resurfacing procedure have been developed and currently CO_2 laser resurfacing has become the preferred procedure of all the resurfacing techniques[56,57].

Lasers

Background

Einstein's quantum theory predicted the feasibility of the existence of laser light in 1917, long before the invention of the laser[58]. In 1959–60, Maiman was able to stimulate a synthetic ruby crystal by a helical flashlamp and he produced the first ruby laser[59]. Much of the interest in applying laser technology in medicine can be attributed to Leon Goldman, a dermatologist from Cincinnati, Ohio, who is considered the 'godfather' of laser medicine. He was the first to adapt laser light sources in the treatment of different vascular and cutaneous disorders, using the ruby, argon and neodymium : yttrium–aluminum–garnet (Nd : YAG) lasers[60,61].

The word laser is an acronym for *l*ight *a*mplification by the *s*timulated *e*mission of *r*adiation[61]. A laser is a device that generates an intense beam of light. Laser light is produced by the medium contained within a laser's resonating chamber or optical cavity. The medium can be a gas, a liquid, a solid crystal or a semiconductor diode. A laser is usually identified and named according to the active medium that is the source of its light. Examples of gas lasers are the CO_2 and argon lasers. The liquid lasers use liquid rhodamine dye as the active medium and are called dye lasers. The solid crystal lasers include the ruby, Nd : YAG, alexandrite and erbium : YAG lasers.

The medium is stimulated by the 'pump' of an external energy source, which can be a radiofrequency (as in the case of the newer high-energy pulsed CO_2 lasers), or an electrical, chemical, thermal or optical source. The external energy source excites the molecules and atoms of the laser medium inside the optical cavity, causing electrons orbiting around the nucleus of an atom to jump to an outer, unstable, higher-energy orbit. Because of the instability of this excited state, the electron soon returns to its normal, lower-energy more stable orbit, releasing the acquired excess energy in the form of a photon. This process is called the spontaneous emission of radiation. When most of the atoms in the laser medium are stimulated and the majority of their electrons are in their higher energy metastable state, population inversion occurs. Once population inversion is established, photons are randomly striking other atoms, stimulating them to emit additional photons of light energy. Because this light energy is being produced by the molecules of the single element in the laser medium, the photons emerge or radiate from their atoms in a single or narrow band of wavelengths (i.e. monochromatic), in phase with one another (i.e. coherent) and traveling in the same direction (i.e. collimated). This process is called the stimulated emission of radiation.

Mirrors at either end of the resonating chamber reflect the emitted photons, causing them to bounce back and forth within the resonating chamber. This amplifes the light created, and stimulates the creation of additional photons of light energy with each ricochet. At the front end of the laser tube, the mirror is only partially reflective, allowing for the passage of a small amount of the laser light to beam out of the optical cavity and into the laser's delivery system. The delivery system of a laser can consist of either flexible fiberoptics or an articulating hollow tube with mirrors on the inside of each articulating joint, directing the flow of the exiting laser light.

Laser–tissue interaction

The three unique properties of monochromation, coherence and collimation make the laser a very powerful and precise tool, and its light brighter than that from any other natural light source. The effects of laser light on tissue depend upon several attributes of the laser light beam. The wavelength of a laser determines its absorption characteristics, i.e. different wavelengths are absorbed by different types of tissue and at different depths. The intensity of the effects of laser light on tissue depend on the diameter of the laser beam, the power at which it is discharged, the frequency of each discharged exposure and the length of time the laser beam irradiates the targeted tissue; these are expressed in terms of energy, power, irradiance and fluence[62]. Energy is work expended and is measured in joules (J). The amount of energy delivered per unit area of skin surface is the dose or fluence, sometimes

called energy density, and is measured in joules per square centimeter. Power is the rate at which the energy is delivered (i.e. the flow of energy), and is measured in watts. A watt is the rate of energy per time of its application (J/s). Power density, also called irradiance, refers to the intensity or rate of energy of a continuous wave laser beam delivered per unit area of skin surface and is measured in watts per square centimeter. In conventional laser terminology, the joule is used to measure the energy of a single pulse of a pulsed laser. The watt, on the other hand, is used to measure the power of a continuous wave laser. The intensity or brightness of either energy density (i.e. fluence) or power density (i.e. irradiance) is predicated upon the spot size or the diameter of the beam of laser light. The smaller the diameter of the spot of the laser light, the more concentrated and intense the energy or power of that laser beam. The frequency of each discharged laser pulse is measured in hertz (Hz) or pulses per second.

Facial resurfacing with the carbon dioxide laser

The technique of CO_2 laser resurfacing is still in its developmental stages. Developed in 1964 by Patel[62], the CO_2 laser emits light energy in the invisible mid-infrared range of the electromagnetic spectrum at a wavelength of 10 600 nm. The laser medium is a mixture of CO_2, nitrogen and helium gasses. The newer generation of high-energy, pulsed CO_2 lasers of the 1990s are excited by the discharge of a radiofrequency. The light of the CO_2 laser is not tissue color selective, but is efficiently absorbed by water to a depth of only 20–30 μm[62]. Since skin is composed of mostly water, when CO_2 laser light reaches the skin surface, most of the laser light energy is instantaneously absorbed by the water in the epidermis and dermis and converted into heat. This raises the temperature of the tissue to above the boiling point of 100°C, causing instantaneous water vaporization and the release of steam and remnants of ablated skin in the plume of laser smoke. Although vaporization is limited to those cells immediately in the path of the laser beam, there is a narrow band of thermally damaged cutaneous tissue adjacent to the center of the treatment site that is exposed to conducted heat below the vaporization temperature. The depth and width of this zone of charred (burnt) skin depends upon the pulse width or the length of time that the target tissue is irradiated and the energy density or fluence used to irradiate it[63,64]. Higher fluences and shorter pulse widths conduct a minimal amount of

Table 6 Comparison of carbon dioxide lasers for skin resurfacing

	ESC Sharplan's SilkTouch/FeatherTouch™	Coherent's UltraPulse® 5000C
Delivery method	spiral scan	individual pulses
Beam configuration	non-Gaussian	Gaussian
Power	low average power (20, 30, 40 W); continuous-wave; non-collimated	high peak power (500 W); pulsed; collimated
Power source	direct current excited tube	radio frequency excited gas-slab
Irradiance	high	high
Energy fluence	$\geq$ 5–15 J/cm²/ms; 1400 mJ/pulse	5–7 J/cm²/ms; 500 mJ/pulse
Effect of increasing power setting	↑ thickness of tissue removed with each scanned pulse	↑ rate of pulsing only and no change in thickness of tissue removed by each pulse
Spot size	2-mm focused non-collimated spot; 1–9 mm scan pattern size with 0.1–0.25 mm focused beam; repeat mode of 0.2 s on and 0.3 or 0.4 s off	3-mm collimated spot for resurfacing
Ablation depth	$\approx$ 150 µm	$\approx$ 75 µm
Pulse duration	0.2 s scan duration; tissue-dwell time of a spot of scanned pulse < 1 ms	< 1 ms
Beam delivery method	SilkTouch 'scanning' (optomechanical flashscanner)	'Ultrapulsed' computer pattern generator (CPG)
Hand-held robotic device	SilkTouch: computer-driven mirrors to focus and manipulate round, square, elliptical doughnut-shaped scanned beam	CPG: parallel preprogrammed patterns; 2.25-mm spots: 9 different pattern shapes, 7 different pattern sizes and 9 different pattern densities

lowered temperature (i.e. less than 100°C) laser energy peripheral to a treatment site.

The newer generation of high-energy, ultra-pulsed CO_2 lasers used for skin resurfacing conform to the three principles of selective photothermolysis that require irradiation of laser energy of a specific wavelength precisely at a particular tissue chromophore or target without producing any additional change in adjacent tissue[65]. This is accomplished by irradiating skin with high enough energy to cause instantaneous vaporization of tissue in a single, very short pulse. This rapidly discharged single-pulse vaporization minimizes charring, producing only a very narrow band of burnt tissue adjacent to the target zone.

There are two CO_2 laser systems that are currently used to resurface facial skin[66] (Table 6). The first CO_2 laser system designed for skin resurfacing was the UltraPulse® 5000C laser (Coherent Medical Group, Palo Alto, CA) (Figure 5). It is a high-energy, pulsed CO_2 laser that can accomplish single pulse vaporization. Each individual pulse of the laser beam is discharged with a pulse energy of up to 500 mJ at a spot size of 3 mm of collimated light with a repetition rate of 6–10 Hz in less than 1 ms. Since 1995, a computer pattern generator (CPG) (Figure 6) using a 2.25-mm beam at 300 mJ per

pulse and a power of 60 W was incorporated into the delivery system of the UltraPulse® laser[67]. With the CPG, larger areas of skin surface can be treated in a shorter amount of time. The other type of CO_2 laser system used for facial skin resurfacing is the Silk-Touch/FeatherTouch® laser (ESC/Sharplan Laser Company, Allendale, NJ). This laser rapidly scans a high-power non-collimated continuous wave CO_2 laser beam, highly focused to a 0.2-mm spot. The laser beam is pulsed and rotated by mirrors revolving within the flash-scanner handpiece fast enough for the beam of laser light to sweep across the skin surface so quickly that the laser light's dwell time inany given spot on the skin's surface is less than 1 ms[68] (Table 6). Both the UltraPulse and the Silk-Touch/Feather Touch lasers irradiate the skin so rapidly and with such intense energy that the conduction of heat into adjacent tissue is negligible, minimizing thermal damage and tissue charring.

Each pass of the laser light over facial skin produces grayish-white, desiccated debris composed of necrotic proteinaceous epidermal and dermal tissue that accumulates on the surface of the skin. This debris should be wiped away with saline-soaked gauze prior to exposure of this treated area to another pass of the laser light. Depending on which proprietary CO_2 laser is used, the first pass is usually

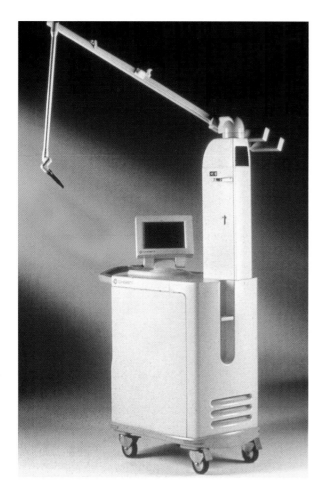

Figure 5   UltraPulse® 5000C CO$_2$ laser. Figure reproduced by permission of Coherent

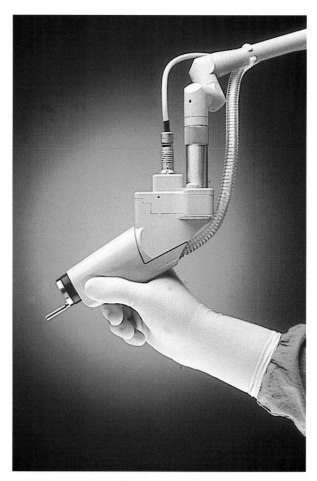

Figure 6   Computer pattern generator (CPG) for the UltraPulse® 5000C CO$_2$ laser. Figure reproduced by permission of Coherent

strong enough to remove the epidermis and some dermis to an overall depth of at least 20–50 µm, leaving a minimum of residual thermally damaged skin of about 10–40 µm in depth[64,66]. Additional passes over the surface of the skin will remove less tissue, because more and more desiccated, thermally denatured collagen is produced. This tissue with a reduced amount of water is less of a target for the CO$_2$ laser light. This results in a decrease in the tissue vaporization depth, and more of the energy is diffused into the surrounding tissue, causing additional thermal necrosis[63]. The endpoint of treatment is reached when either a wrinkle or a scar is eliminated, or when no additional skin tightening is observed, or when a yellow/brown or chamois discoloration of the remaining surface tissue is observed (Figure 7). In the recent past there have been a number of newer lasers released on the market, but they all still function using either the pulsed or the scanning type of laser light delivery system.

Laser safety

The wavelength of the CO$_2$ laser is invisible to the human eye. Consequently, a low power, visible red helium neon (He Ne) laser beam, which is coaxial with the invisible CO$_2$ laser beam, is used for aiming the light of the CO$_2$ laser. The CO$_2$ laser light is instantaneously absorbed by the first absorbent material it contacts. It can also reflect off smooth metallic surfaces, even though they may be blackened[69]. A CO$_2$ laser beam can ignite most non-metallic materials. Fire retardant drapes and gowns must be used at all times during a CO$_2$ laser procedure.

Because there is the potential for irreversible damage and scarring of a person's cornea and sclera, appropriate protective eyewear with side shields should be worn at all times by everyone in the vicinity of an actively operating CO$_2$ laser. The protective eyewear should have an optical density (OD) specific for the wavelength of the CO$_2$ laser. Because prescription spectacles made of glass can be shattered by a high-energy density laser light beam, spectacles or clear plastic wrap-around goggles made of polycarbonate can be used as an alternative. Dulled, metallic corneal eye shields must be inserted in the patient's eyes during laser resurfacing[70]. In addition, saline-soaked gauze should be placed over the patient's teeth to prevent laser beam pitting of tooth enamel. Also, the treatment room door must remain shut with a sign posted on the outside of the door, warning anyone attempting to enter that protective eyewear and barrier clothing must be donned prior to entering.

The plume of smoke generated by the CO_2 laser contains blood and soft tissue debris that may be contaminated with various biological agents, including pathogenic bacteria, viral DNA or other viable cells of infectious potential that can cause hepatitis, AIDS and other dangerous diseases[71–73]. Also, the particulate matter in the smoke plume can act as an irritant to the respiratory mucosa. Vacuum smoke evacuators with filters that are rated for ultra-low penetration of air (ULPA) have been designed for use during laser surgery to rid the operating room environment of most, if not all, of the laser plume as it is being generated. The smoke evacuator tip must remain no farther than 1 cm away from the target zone during a resurfacing procedure in order to remove the bulk of the laser plume effectively. In addition, all members of the laser surgical team must wear specially designed micropore laser plume barrier face masks during a laser procedure. These laser plume barrier face masks must have a particulate filtration efficiency (PFE) rating of at least 95% for filtering particulate matter 0.1 µm or larger in size, since human papilloma viruses can be as small as 0.45 µm and HIV 0.18 µm in diameter. However, hepatitis viruses can be as small as 0.042 µm, i.e. less than 0.1 µm in diameter, and therefore can conceivably pass through the special micropore laser plume barrier face masks.

All essential flammable materials at the perioperative site must be protected with wet towels or gauze sponges. A CO_2 laser must never be operated in the presence of flammable anesthetics, solutions used for preoperative disinfection of the patient's skin (e.g. iodoform-based solutions or 4% chlorhexidine gluconate (Hibiclens)) or other materials containing flammable volatile solvents, e.g. alcohol, acetone, etc. A fire or an explosion could occur. Fire extinguishers and an abundant supply of water should be readily available. Plastic devices such as specula or eye shields may melt when impacted by the CO_2 laser beam[74]. More importantly, the operation of a CO_2 laser in the vicinity of an endotracheal tube and oxygen can increase the risk of fire unless proper precautions are taken[75]. The endotracheal tube must be made of red rubber, silicone, or flexible stainless steel, and approved by the United States Food and Drug Administration (FDA) for use

during CO_2 laser procedures. Otherwise, not only can the anesthetic gases be ignited at the perioperative site, but they can also be flash ignited down the endotracheal tube and melt it.

Erbium : YAG laser resurfacing

The erbium : yttrium–aluminum–garnet (Er : YAG) laser emits a beam of light whose wavelength is 2940 nm, which is absorbed by water approximately ten times more strongly than the light of a CO_2 laser[76]. Consequently, the Er : YAG laser ablates an even thinner layer of skin (4 µm per 1 J/cm^2) per laser pass, leaving behind an even narrower zone of thermally damaged tissue[77]. Because Er : YAG laser light is absorbed so strongly, there is less scattering of the laser light in tissue, and thermal necrosis is limited to 5–20 µm. This is much less than the 20–50 µm of thermally damaged skin seen with each pass of the high-energy, pulsed CO_2 lasers. Unlike the CO_2 laser, the Er : YAG laser induces much less tissue desiccation and the depth of tissue vaporization remains the same. Because there is a narrow zone of thermal damage produced with each pass of the laser, coagulation of deeper dermal vessels is not complete and bleeding can be bothersome with successive passes during a resurfacing procedure. In general, Er : YAG lasers are being used for more superficial resurfacing procedures in younger patients with much less photodamage[78]. The Er : YAG laser is to the CO_2 laser much like 70% glycolic acid or 20% TCA is to a phenol peel or a dermabrasion (Table 7). As with the CO_2 lasers, computerized scanners are available for a variety of Er : YAG lasers.

Postoperative erythema in most clinical studies has lasted noticeably shorter with the Er : YAG laser than with the CO_2 laser, as has the overall healing time. Re-epithelialization can occur almost 30% more rapidly with the Er : YAG laser than with the CO_2 laser. It is probably the deeper thermal damage produced by the CO_2 laser that results in more prolonged wound healing after CO_2 laser surgery. However, even with more aggressive Er : YAG laser resurfacing, the overall cosmetic result as assessed by overall wrinkle reduction was found to be better with the CO_2 laser in most cases[79]. Consequently, the combined use of a CO_2 laser with an Er : YAG laser has recently been advocated. The purpose of this technique is for the CO_2 laser to ablate the skin and coagulate the microvasculature as far down as the papillary dermis, and then the Er : YAG laser ablates the residual layer of charred and desiccated tissue. This hypothetically leads to a reduction in

Table 7 Depth of UltraPulse® CO_2 and Er : YAG resurfacing compared with other resurfacing techniques

Number of laser passes	Ablation depth (μm)		Residual thermal damage (μm)		Level of damage	Other resurfacing procedures
	CO_2	Er : YAG	CO_2	Er : YAG		
1	50–100	10–20	50–100	5–20	epidermis/superficial papillary dermis	medium depth peel (TCA)
2	35–50	10–20	50–100	5–20	papillary dermis	medium depth peel (TCA) and DA
3	25–40	10–20	50–100	5–20	superficial reticular dermis	DA and phenol peel

TCA, trichloroacetic acid; DA, dermabrasion

the intensity and duration of postoperative erythema, because, by removing the charred tissue, less of an inflammatory response is needed during wound repair. As a result, re-epithelialization occurs sooner. The Er : YAG laser also heats the dermal collagen to about 60–65°C, producing additional skin tightening and stimulating the formation of new collagen[80]. Because the Er : YAG laser ablates tissue more superficially than does the CO_2 laser, it has been used to resurface areas that ordinarily could not be done safely with the CO_2 laser, e.g. the neck, chest, hands and arms[81]. Further studies are needed to verify the safety and efficacy of both CO_2 and Er : YAG lasers in resurfacing facial and non-facial skin[82].

Because there are many different reasons for the aging face to develop wrinkles, there are also many different ways to rejuvenate it. Facial skin resurfacing is only one of those ways. Another is the injection of botulinum toxin type A (BTX-A) into certain mimetic muscles of the face. Only since the late 1980s and early 1990s has BTX-A become a popular alternative used to relax some of the mimetic muscles of facial expression, thereby eliminating some of the inadvertent and dynamic wrinkling so often seen in the aging face.

WRINKLE REDUCTION
Botulinum toxin type A
Background

Excessively prominent facial lines are the result of many factors including age, photodamage and the pull of the underlying mimetic facial musculature, causing creases and furrows of the overlying skin. When the cause of excessive facial wrinkling, especially of the upper third of the face, is due mainly to hyperfunctional mimetic facial musculature, then chemodenervation by injections of BTX-A may be beneficial. BTX-A, also identified commercially as BOTOX®, is derived from the

neuroexotoxin produced by the Gram-positive spore-forming, obligate anaerobic bacillus *Clostridium botulinum*. This neurotoxin has been purified since the 1920s and is now commercially manufactured in crystalline form for use as a therapeutic agent in humans. Vacuum-dried BOTOX is distributed in over 60 countries worldwide and shipped frozen at −5°C. It should remain frozen at this temperature until it is ready to be injected[83].

BOTOX has been approved by the FDA for use in various dystonias of striated muscles including strabismus, blepharospasm and other types of focal muscle spasms. BOTOX is commercially available in vials containing 100 units of purified, crystalline botulinum exotoxin serotype A. A unit of BOTOX is a measurement of the bioactivity or potency of the neurotoxin. It is not a measurement of weight or volume. In the 20 years that it has been available for human use, there have never been any reported cases of systemic toxicity resulting from accidental injection or overdose of BOTOX. An intramuscular injection of BOTOX typically results in a dose-dependent reduction of hyperactive muscle contraction that lasts anywhere from 3 to 6 months and sometimes even longer, but ultimately is reversible. BOTOX is thought to produce its therapeutic effect of chemodenervation by acting selectively on peripheral cholinergic motor nerve endings to inhibit the release of the neurotransmitter acetylcholine at the neuromuscular junction[84]. The onset of striated muscle weakness occurs anywhere between 48 and 72 h after an injection of BOTOX and is dose dependent. It takes at least 1–2 weeks for the total effect to occur which means that retreatment with BOTOX should take place only 3–4 weeks after an initial treatment session.

When reconstituting the vial of 100 units of purified crystalline BOTOX, sterile normal saline without preservative must be used; otherwise, the potency of the neurotoxin can be compromised[85]. There are many different dilutions by which

Table 8 Acceptable dilutions of BOTOX®

Diluent added (ml) (0.9% NaCl without preservative)	Resulting dose	
	Units per 0.1 ml	Units per 0.01 ml
1.0	10.0	1.0
2.0	5.0	0.5
4.0	2.5	0.25
8.0	1.25	0.125
10.0	1.0	0.1

Table 9 Prevention of adverse side-effects after BOTOX® injections

Physician

Inject minimal and concentrated volumes

Use precise reconstitution and dose-measuring techniques

Place the needle accurately into the muscles being treated and at least 1 cm above, below or lateral to the bony orbital rim

Patient

Must not manipulate injected areas for 2–3 h after treatment

Must remain vertical 3–4 h after treatment

Must contract treated muscles for 2–3 h after injection, because the toxin selectively seeks and adheres to actively moving muscles

BOTOX can be reconstituted (Table 8). The preferred dilution amount is 1 ml or 2 ml of preservative-free normal saline. One milliliter of diluent in a vial of 100 units of crystalline BOTOX produces 10 units of BOTOX in 0.1 ml of solution or 1 unit of BOTOX in 0.01 ml of solution. The reconstituted solution of BOTOX can then be injected using a 0.5-ml U100 insulin syringe with an attached 28G needle that is either 13 mm or 25 mm long. BOTOX can be denatured by bubbling or similar violent agitation, so care must be taken when handling and reconstituting the product[83,85]. After reconstitution, BOTOX must be kept refrigerated at all times at 2–8°C and should be used within 4 h after it has been reconstituted. There have been a few studies that have disputed this[86,87]. One must keep in mind, however, that when using normal saline without preservative, there is an increased risk of bacterial contamination and colonization of the solution the longer it remains unused. On the other hand, diluting BOTOX with saline containing preservative can diminish its potency. Most importantly, injecting higher volumes of a more diluted solution causes diffusion of the diluent and toxin

Table 10 Muscles of facial expression of the upper third of the face and the direction of the wrinkle lines they produce

Muscles	Location and function	Direction of facial lines
Frontalis	Forehead (elevator)	horizontal
Corrugator supercilii	Glabella (depressors)	vertical
Orbicularis oculi, medial orbital portion		vertical
Depressor supercilii		vertical
Procerus		horizontal
Orbicularis oculi, lateral orbital portion	Lateral canthus (crow's feet)	horizontal

well beyond the area injected. This can lead to ptosis of the eyelids and even diplopia when injecting BOTOX in the periorbital area. Higher dilutions have been found to cause a decrease in the potency and in the duration of action of BOTOX. Table 9 identifies some of the ways physicians and patients can prevent ptosis and other side-effects when BOTOX is injected.

BOTOX is contraindicated in anyone who might be allergic to any one of its components (botulinum toxin, human albumin or saline). Certain medications that interfere with neuromuscular impulse transmission (e.g. aminoglycosides, penicillamine, quinine and calcium channel blockers) can theoretically potentiate and intensify the effects of the botulinum neurotoxin[88]. BOTOX is classified as a pregnancy category C drug and should not be deliberately injected into women who are known to be pregnant or actively nursing.

Technique of injecting BOTOX

In order to use BOTOX effectively when treating creases and furrows of the upper third of the face, one needs to be thoroughly familiar with the anatomy and function of the muscles of facial expression[89]. The directions of facial lines and wrinkles of the skin usually appear perpendicular to the direction of the muscle fibers creating them (Table 10). For example, the horizontal lines of the forehead are created by the frontalis, whose muscle fibers are vertically oriented and perpendicular to the forehead wrinkle lines. The frontalis is the only levator muscle of the forehead that elevates the eyebrows and the skin of the forehead. The action of the frontalis opposes the depressor action of the

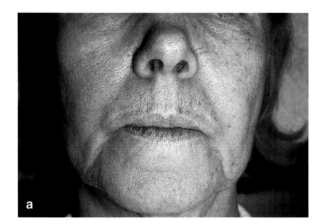

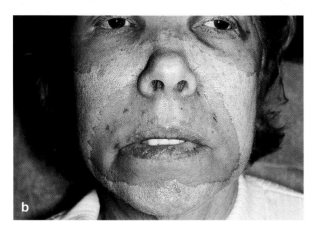

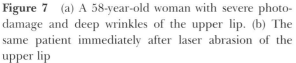

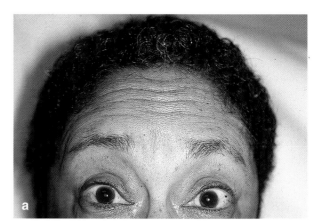

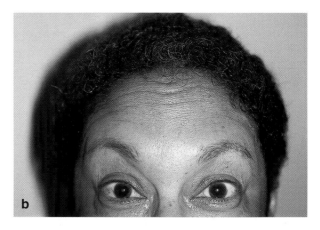

Figure 7 (a) A 58-year-old woman with severe photo-damage and deep wrinkles of the upper lip. (b) The same patient immediately after laser abrasion of the upper lip

Figure 8 (a) Patient with deep wrinkles of the forehead and glabella produced by elevating the brow. (b) The same patient 2 weeks after injections of BOTOX® into the forehead

muscles of the glabella and brow. Multiple injections of small amounts of BOTOX are used in the forehead to create only a weakening of the muscle instead of a total paralysis, so that the patient does not remain expressionless. Injections in three or four sites on either side of the midline are all that is necessary to reduce or eliminate all the horizontal forehead lines (Figure 8). Weakness of the frontalis should last approximately 4–6 months.

The most popular area of the face to treat with BOTOX is the glabella and its frown lines. The horizontal and vertical creases of the glabella are caused by four depressor muscles[89] (Table 10). These muscles help one to squint by lowering the eyebrows and adducting them medially. The muscles that produce the vertical lines of the glabella are the corrugator supercilii, the medial orbital portion of the orbicularis oculi and the depressor supercilii. The horizontal lines of the glabella and nasal root are produced by the procerus. In order to elimate glabellar vertical lines, BOTOX is injected into the belly of the corrugator, orbicularis oculi and depressor supercilii into two sites at the medial end

of the eyebrow on either side of the midline. In order to eliminate glabellar horizontal lines, BOTOX is injected into the belly of the procerus, at a point in the center of the nasal root. Weakness of the glabellar depressors should last approximately 4–6 months.

To eliminate the wrinkles of the lateral ocular canthus or crow's feet, BOTOX is injected into the lateral orbital portion of the orbicularis oculi (Table 10). Much of the wrinkling of this area is caused by aging and photodamage, but there is a component of hyperactivity of the lateral aspect of the orbicularis oculi that can be reduced by injections of small amounts of BOTOX. The injection of small quantities of concentrated BOTOX will prevent the migration of the toxin medially, which, if it occurs, can result in ectropion of the lower eyelid and even lead to corneal exposure. Weakness of the lateral aspect of the orbicularis oculi should last approximately 4–6 months.

BOTOX is always injected with the patient sitting up[90]. It is important that the injections be done symmetrically in all the areas treated in order to maintain a certain natural balance in the resultant facial expressions, and to avoid any unevenness of facial movement after BOTOX injections.

Injections of BOTOX, as we have seen, are most useful in treating the upper third of the face. The lower third of the face can also appear aged, especially in someone with a long history of chronic sun exposure. However, BOTOX should not be used in this area, because of the grouping and overlapping of muscles of facial expression and mastication. Injections of BOTOX in this area can cause eklabion, drooling, difficulty with lip pursing and temporary disfigurement. Instead, facial fillers and implants take a prominent role for the rejuvenation of the lower face. Because of the diminution in soft tissue support from chronic sun exposure and aging, the lower face takes on a sunken-in, wasted appearance and the melolabial sulci and folds become more prominent; women appear gaunt and haggard. The chin becomes more prominent and the upper and lower lips become thinned and studded with fine and deep rhytids and furrows, a hallmark of the senescent woman. For these changes, various types of facial fillers and implants are the treatment of choice.

FACIAL FILLERS AND IMPLANTS

Background

The challenge of augmenting the skin of the face to bolster sunken, sagging, wrinkled skin has been the objective of many a cosmetic surgeon since the end of the 19th century. Gersuny was one of the first to use injections of a low-melting petroleum jelly or paraffin to augment facial and nasal contour deformities, which eventually was found to cause local diffuse infiltrative deformities, ulcerations, scarring, foreign-body granulomas (paraffinomas), and even migration of the paraffin to distant sites and pulmonary embolism[91,92]. Consequently, the practice of paraffin injections was abandoned in the USA around the second decade of the 20th century. Up until the 1940s in the USA for a variety of reasons and defects, other questionable substances such as linseed and flax oils and fatty acids were injected into human skin to bolster different defects, furrows and wrinkles.

Silicone

The next promising injectable implant to be used as a tissue filler was liquid silicone. Silicone is the generic term for a family of synthetic compounds that are colorless, odorless and tasteless. Their viscosities vary according to the extent of their polymerization and cross-linkage, which determines whether they exist as a liquid, gel, foam or solid (elastomer)[93]. The name 'silicone' was coined in the early 1900s by F.S. Kipping, an English chemist, who created a number of silicon–carbon compounds that turned out to be mostly synthetic adhesives. He used the term 'silicone' to describe this family of polymers that contained the element silicon and appeared to be chemical analogs of organic ketones. Silicone polymers are contaminated easily by heavy metals, low chain-length polymers and other impurities during their manufacturing process. Medical-grade silicones require specialized filtration of these impurities and sterilization before they are deemed suitable for implantation into the human body.

When liquid silicone was first used for soft tissue augmentation in the 1940s, adulterants or irritants were added to the silicone in order to create a more vigorous fibroblastic tissue response. The first injections of liquid silicone were probably performed in Japan, where much of the injected silicone was adulterated with 1% olive oil, croton oil, talc and paraffins[94]. This 'Sakurai' formula was injected in large volumes into the face and breasts for tissue augmentation. Silicones adulterated with sesame oil or 1% oleic acid were subsequently used in the USA. In 1962, the Medical Products Division of Dow Corning was established in order to manufacture and distribute pure medical-grade silicone. In 1964 the FDA declared that injectable silicone used clinically was to be regulated as a 'new drug', and only designated investigators were authorized to conduct controlled investigations of the injectable medical-grade liquid silicone. A highly purified medical-grade silicone MDX4-4011® was produced in 1965 for this purpose, and was to be used to correct major bodily defects. During the 20 years of this controlled therapeutic trial, it was soon observed that silicone MDX4-4011 also successfully corrected minor cosmetic defects of the face, which included facial rhytids, melolabial creases and other small facial depressions[95]. The rate of complications and adverse reactions reported during the FDA-supported trial with MDX4-4011 silicone was low. However, in the USA and elsewhere, non-FDA-sanctioned clinicians were treating patients with other non-FDA-approved silicones of unknown quality and purity and by questionable techniques. Foreign-body granulomas at silicone injection sites in the face, breasts and genitalia were subsequently reported[96–99]. Over the years, disfiguring silicone-induced inflammatory reactions often requiring surgical intervention have been reported as long as 20 years after silicones of questionable sources and grade were injected into various parts of the body. Silicone has been found to migrate to distant sites, cause granulomatous hepatitis, acute silicone-induced pneumonitis and late-onset leg ulceration, as well as posterior ciliary artery occlusion resulting in blindness, and fatal intravascular silicone embolization[98]. However, there are as many, if not more, reports by physicians who have treated large numbers of patients with injectable medical-grade liquid silicone of known purity for facial soft tissue augmentation and who have observed no adverse complications[99]. Because of all this confounding intrigue with the sanctioned and the non-sanctioned use of injectable medical-grade and possibly even industrial-grade silicones, the FDA has yet to approve injectable liquid silicone for tissue augmentation.

Injectable collagens

Background

The search for the ideal cutaneous tissue filler continues to challenge the imagination and resourcefulness of clinicians and scientists alike. At the very least, the implant should be physiologically inert, biocompatible, safe, long-lasting, easily administered and stored with a long shelf life, giving predictable and reproducible results. The early 1980s witnessed a resurgence of interest in implantable soft tissue fillers mainly because of the release and FDA approval of injectable Zyderm® bovine collagen, followed shortly thereafter by the approval and release of the degraded porcine collagen gelatin powder Fibrel®[100]. In addition, techniques for the reinjection of autologous fat soon became popular. Even more recently, there has been a plethora of different types of implantable soft tissue fillers that are now being tested for future approval and release in the USA.

Zyderm/Zyplast® collagen

The most widely used implantable material for tissue augmentation is injectable reconstituted xenogeneic bovine collagen. In 1979, solubilized collagen was developed by the Collagen Corporation and, by July 1981, injectable Zyderm collagen implant for soft tissue augmentation was the first product of its kind to receive FDA approval for the production, distribution and use in tissue augmentation in the USA. Subsequently, Zyderm II was approved and released in 1983, and then Zyplast in 1985.

The normal human dermis is composed mostly of collagen, which is one of the body's most abundant proteins. Approximately 80% of dermal collagen is composed of type I collagen and 20% of type III collagen. Collagen proteins are trimers of a relatively rigid triple helix made up of three individual polypeptide chains called alpha chains. About 96% of the collagen molecule is helical, flanked by non-helical 'telopeptides' at the amino and carboxy terminals on the surface of the molecule. Different collagens are composed of distinct combinations of alpha chains, which aggregate to form rigid cross-linked collagen fibrils and fibers. Selective pepsin hydrolysis separates the antigenic non-helical telopeptides from a collagen molecule, thereby reducing the antigenicity of the solubilized collagen[101]. In the preparation of Zyderm collagen (ZC), the undisturbed, rigid, cross-linked, helical collagen fibrils are harvested by centrifugation and resuspended in phosphate-buffered physiological saline with 0.3% lidocaine. Injectable ZC contains 95–98% type I collagen and the remaining is type III collagen. Injectable ZC is distributed in prefilled syringes that should be refrigerated at about 4°C so that the dispersed fibrils remain fluid and small. This allows for passage of the implant material through 30G needles. Once injected into the skin, body temperature (37°C) causes the intermolecular cross-linking of the implant to occur, and its suspension consolidates into a gel as it forms larger fibrils. Injectable ZC is a sterile purified fibrillar suspension of dermal collagen derived from the cowhide of ranch-bred American cattle, free of infection with bovine viral spongiform encephalitic disease.

Injectable liquid ZC is currently available in three forms. Two forms of ZC differ only in the concentration of the suspended material: Zyderm I (Z-I), the original implant, contains 35 mg/ml bovine collagen, and Zyderm II (Z-II) contains 65 mg/ml bovine collagen. The third form of ZC, identified as Zyplast collagen (ZP), is the same 35 mg/ml of bovine collagen that is cross-linked by the addition of 0.0075% glutaraldehyde, producing a covalently bonded latticework between the collagen fibrils, which creates a thicker, longer-lasting product that is more resistant to proteolytic degradation and tissue mobilization[102]. Injectable ZP has been found to be less immunogenic than Z-I or Z-II[103]. Clinical use has revealed ZP to persist for up to 12 months and, as it is resorbed, the implant is replaced by new host collagen[103].

It has been estimated that, by the year 2000, more than 1 500 000 patients will have been treated successfully with some form of ZC, and all without significant adverse side-effects, improving superficial acne scars, steroid-induced atrophy, glabellar furrows, crow's feet, fine to medium depth wrinkling and depressed scars that can be distended.

The safety of injectable liquid collagen has been extensively studied in animals and in humans[104]. In contrast to the development of injectable liquid silicone, the development of these three collagen implants was carefully monitored by the Collagen Corporation and no material was released for sale until full studies had been completed and FDA approval had been secured.

Injectable collagen is one of the safest materials that is implanted for facial rejuvenation. However, local test site reactions occur in 1–5% of patients who are skin tested prior to treatment with Zyderm I skin test[105]. This is usually done in the volar surface of a forearm. A positive reaction at this test site is characterized by erythema, induration, pruritus or pruritic papules occurring within 72 h of the test[106]. Most positive skin tests are transient and resolve within days to several weeks or even months. Persistent nodular positive test site reactions can occur, lasting for more than 1 year, occasionally leaving permanent scars. These positive skin test reactions represent a type II hypersensitivity response and biopsy specimens of the test site reactions have shown foreign body granuloma formation[107]. Approximately 1–4% of patients with a negative pretreatment skin test have developed allergic reactions at the treatment site[108]. For this reason, a series of two collagen skin tests are performed 2–4 weeks apart before initiating treatment with collagen implantation[109]. Other reactions to collagen implantation include local abscess formation, bruising, infection, localized necrosis and granulomas[105–108]. Permanent unilateral blindness has resulted from an embolus occluding a branch of the ophthalmic artery when collagen was injected into a glabellar frown line. Injectable collagen is not known to induce any type of permanent systemic reaction or autoimmunity.

Currently, injectable bovine collagen remains the most popular injectable implant for facial rejuvenation and soft tissue augmentation. With careful patient selection, appropriate pretreatment evaluation and proper injection technique, injectable bovine collagen can be safely and effectively used in women who have a wide range of facial contour changes. The beneficial results from collagen implants are another adjunctive procedure in the rejuvenation of the aging face, albeit transient.

Implantation techniques

Any patient who has a known allergy to either lidocaine or bovine collagen should not be tested with ZC. If there is no positive reaction after two test doses applied to the volar forearm of the patient 2–4 weeks apart, then treatment with injectable Z-I or Z-II or ZP can commence.

The patient should be treated in the sitting position and the area to be treated should be well lit. While still cold from storage, Z-I can be injected using either a 30G needle or the 32G metal hub needle specially supplied in the package with the product. Z-I is then injected in a continuous flow of serially repeated injections until the area to be treated is completely filled. Because about 30% of the Z-I implant remains in place after product condensation and resorption of the saline and lidocaine, many physicians deliberately overcorrect the area, whereas others avoid this, because signs of overcorrection can often persist. Lesions most amenable to Z-I correction are soft, distensible, superficial defects and lines. Shallow acne scars, horizontal forehead lines, crow's feet, glabellar lines and furrows, nasolabial, accessory nasolabial and perioral lines, lateral commissure drool grooves and marionette lines respond well to Z-I. Injectable Z-II is a more concentrated form of Z-I. It requires greater force to inject it, and Z-II undergoes less condensation, leaving behind approximately 60% of the material at the implantation site. Therefore, overcorrection is not advisable. Because of its increased viscosity, Z-II can be injected only with a 30G needle. The technique for injecting Z-II is identical to that of Z-I. Z-II is useful for injecting deep acne scars, deep glabellar furrows and certain defects that do not respond to Z-I.

ZP is a longer-lasting form of injectable bovine collagen. The rigid cross-linked lattice network and the absence of microfibrils results in little condensation of ZP after implantation, so overcorrection should be avoided. ZP works best when placed in the mid-dermis using a 30G needle. As with Z-I and Z-II, ZP is deposited serially in small volumes. ZP should be injected at such a depth that minimal blanching and no beading should be seen at the completion of the injections. The skin should rise to the desired level of correction as the material is being implanted (Figure 9). Some clinicians massage or mold the ZP after injection. Others prefer to layer Z-I over the injected ZP. This has been found to improve both the esthetic result and the longevity of the treatment. Defects most amenable to ZP include deep nasolabial folds, deep distensible acne scars and deep lateral commissure drool grooves. ZP is not recommended for crow's feet or use in the glabellar frown lines.

Two to three treatment sessions are usually necessary to achieve optimal correction. Approximately 30% of individuals have reported the duration of their correction to be as long as 18 months, while

70% have required touch-up treatments at intervals of 3–12 months. Glabellar frown lines and distensible acne scars appear to retain correction the longest. The variability in longevity in different patients treated could be explained by the continued mechanical stress at the treatment sites, and the patient's individual response to ZC.

Fibrel

Fibrel was approved by the FDA for use in the USA in 1985. It was first manufactured and distributed by Serono Laboratories of Italy, and then marketed and distributed in the USA by the Mentor Corporation (Goleta, CA, USA). Fibrel is composed of a lyophilized mixture of 100 mg of absorbable degraded porcine gelatin powder and 125 mg of ε-aminocaproic acid (EACA)[110]. Fibrel is distributed in a sterile treatment kit complete with everything needed to reconstitute the gelatin powder and to inject the final product. The kit, stored at room temperature, has a long shelf life. The absorbable Fibrel gelatin powder provides a matrix framework in which a clot can form and remain stable under a scar or depressed area on the face. The enzyme EACA is added to the product to inhibit fibrinolysin. By preventing fibrinolysin production, host fibrin can form within the Fibrel matrix framework, allowing collagen to be produced within the clot matrix, permanently filling in the soft tissue defect.

To reconstitute the lyophilized Fibrel, approximately 10 ml of the patient's blood is drawn and then centrifuged for 10–15 min, so that 0.5 ml of clear plasma can be obtained. This 0.5 ml of the patient's plasma and the 0.5 ml of sterile 0.9% normal saline supplied with the Fibrel kit are then added to the syringe containing the gelatin powder. The kit also comes with a syringe adaptor so that the gelatin powder/EACA mixture can be easily reconstituted by having it and the plasma/saline diluent passed back and forth from one syringe to another. Unlike silicone and Zyderm collagen, that remain as foreign body implants within the dermis, the clot matrix of Fibrel is re-absorbed as the host's new collagen is gradually incorporated into the gel matrix.

Fibrel is indicated for the correction of depressed scars that are distensible and easily effaced by stretching of the skin. Fibrotic or ice-pick types of scars that do not elevate well with stretching are not satisfactorily treated with Fibrel. However, deeper creases, furrows and grooves may be amenable to injections of Fibrel. The fine creases on the eyelids and lips as well as facial wrinkling due to photoaging do not respond well to Fibrel injections,

because of its viscosity and the attendant inflammatory response experienced after implantation. In order for Fibrel to work, an inflammatory reaction to stimulate wound healing and collagen overgrowth is a necessary component of the treatment. Patients should expect to develop erythema, induration and edema at the treated sites that may last as long as 5 days. Collagen synthesis and rebuilding may take 6–12 weeks. Fibrel is injected from a syringe equipped with a 30G needle. Before injecting Fibrel, the technique of subcision (i.e. dissection and undermining with the needle) should be attempted, so as to release the scar from the tether of the surrounding tissue and to create a void or pocket into which Fibrel is subsequently injected. Intentional overcorrection to about 150% should be achieved, causing blanching and creating a *peau d'orange* effect on the surface of the skin.

Just like silicone and ZC, Fibrel must be used as an intradermal implant. Interestingly, there seems to be no cross-reactivity with autoantibodies to ZC and Fibrel, and patients who are allergic to ZC have been successfully treated with Fibrel without any adverse side-effects. There has been no association of Fibrel with any systemic adverse reaction, disease or autoimmune process.

Unfortunately, Fibrel is more cumbersome to use than ZC, because Fibrel requires the acquisition and addition of the patient's serum to reconstitute the product before it can be injected. Moreover, there is an increase in morbidity associated with post-treatment inflammation. Although clinical experience has indicated that the effect of Fibrel may last longer than ZC, the handling and use of Fibrel proved to be too cumbersome for the majority of the practicing physicians in the USA. Consequently, since 1998, Fibrel has no longer been available for use in the USA.

Since the development of ZC and Fibrel as soft tissue fillers, additional alternative forms of injectable tissue fillers and implantable materials, either synthetic or biological, have appeared both in the USA and in other countries around the world (Table 11). Alternative forms of injectable bovine collagen produced outside the USA are Koken Atelocollagen™ and Resoplast®.

Koken Atelocollagen

Koken Atelocollagen implant is a 2% monomolecular non-fibrillar aqueous solution of bovine collagen manufactured by the Koken Company of Japan. It is not approved for use in the USA. Koken Atelocollagen contains only collagen molecules, unlike ZC, which is a 3.5% dispersion of collagen

Table 11   Injectable soft tissue fillers

Product name	Product compostion	Implant placement	Manufacturer
Silicone	silicone	mid-dermis	Dow-Corning, USA
Zyderm® collagen	bovine collagen and lidocaine	upper and mid-dermis	Inamed Corporation
Zyplast® collagen	bovine collagen and lidocaine	mid- to lower dermis	through McGhan Medical Corporation, Santa Barbara, CA, USA
Fibrel®	porcine collagen	mid- to lower dermis	Serono Labs, Italy
Koken Atelocollagen®	2% monomolecular bovine collagen solution	mid-dermis	Koken Co, KTD Tokyo, Japan
Resoplast®	3.5% or 6.5% monomolecular bovine collagen solution	mid-dermis	Rofil Medical Int'l NV, Breda, the Netherlands
Artecoll®	PMMA in 3.5% collagen solution	subdermis	Rofil Medical Inc., USA Oakdale, MN, USA
Hylaform®	cross-linked hyaluronic acid gel	superficial and deep dermis	Biomatrix, Inc., Ridgefield, NJ, USA
Restylane™	cross-linked hyaluronic acid gel	mid-dermis	Q-Med, Uppsala, Sweden
Autologen®	4% processed autologous donor collagen solution	mid- to deep dermis and subcutaneous junction	Collagenesis, Inc., Beverly, MA, USA
Autologen® XL	6% processed autologous donor cross-linked collagen solution	mid- to deep dermis and subcutaneous junction	Collagenesis, Inc., Beverly, MA, USA
Isolagen®	cultured autologous live fibroblasts and collagen matrix solution	superficial, mid- and deep dermis and subcutaneous plane	Isolagen Technologies, Inc., Paramus, NJ, USA
Dermalogen™	injectable human collagen from US tissue banks	mid-dermis	Collagenesis, Inc., Beverly, MA, USA
Fascian™	injectable fragmented human fascia lata	subdermis and mid-dermis	Fascia Biosystems, LLC, Beverly Hills, CA, USA
AlloDerm®	acellular dermal allograft sheets from cadveric skin	subdermis	Life Cell Corporation, The Woodlands, TX, USA

PMMA, polymethylmethacrylate

molecules, fibrils and fibers. Indications for Koken Atelocollagen are the same as those for ZC. Users of Koken Atelocollagen hypothesize that the monomolecular solution forms a collagen matrix with a finer structure capable of retaining more water and glycosaminoglycans, therefore achieving a better correction than that seen with ZC.

Resoplast

Resoplast is the first European-produced injectable liquid collagen implant. It is a bovine monomolecular collagen in solution available in either 3.5% or 6.5% concentrations. The calfskins used to produce Resoplast come from healthy calves raised in Germany, and they are free of bovine spongiform encephalopathy virus. Indications for the use of Resoplast injections are the same as those for ZC. It is manufactured and distributed by Rofil Medical International NV in the Netherlands and it is currently not available for use in the USA.

Some of the other alloplastic injectable and surgically implantable materials that have been developed and are in use in different parts of the world are polymethylmethacrylate microspheres (Artecoll®); injectable hyaluronic acid; cross-linked polydimethylsiloxane (Bioplastique®); teflon paste; porous mesh-form polyethylene (Marlex®); hydroxyapatite; different proprietary forms of expanded poly-tetrafluoroethylene (ePTFE); and surgically implantable autologous dermal tissue (Autologen® and Isolagen®) or homologous, dermal tissue (Dermalogen™, Fascian® and AlloDerm®) (Table 11).

Artecoll

Artecoll is a suspension of polymethylmethacrylate (PMMA) microspheres that are 32–40 μm in diameter, have a smooth round surface and are suspended in a solution of partially denatured 3.5% bovine collagen and 0.3% lidocaine hydrochloride[111]. It is the successor to Arteplast which consisted of the PMMA microspheres in a medium of Tween 80. Arteplast is no longer available. Artecoll was developed using collagen as the carrier for the microspheres and it is manufactured and distributed by Rofil International NV in the Netherlands. Artecoll is an injectable implant used in Europe.

Developed by the German chemist Rohm in 1902, PMMA was patented in 1928 as Plexiglas® and has been used in industry, dentistry (Paladon), and medicine (bone cement) since that time. There have been no proven immunological reactions with its use. However, since bovine collagen can elicit an immunological response, it is recommended that a test injection be done in the volar aspect of the forearm 4 weeks prior to treatment. Artecoll is stable at room temperature, but should be stored refrigerated. Because of its consistency, Artecoll is more difficult to implant. Artecoll is less forgiving, because it is long-lasting, so good or poor results will persist. Artecoll is supplied in 1.0-ml or 0.5-ml syringes with an attached 27G needle that is 0.5 inch long. It should be injected subdermally between the dermis and the subcutaneous fat, and should not be implanted intradermally. A slight or minimal overcorrection should be created by serially injecting Artecoll in multiple adjacent sites, but in a continuous fashion similarly to the implantation of ZC. Common reactions to Artecoll implantation are edema, erythema, moderate pain and pruritus, lasting for a few days. Pruritus can last even longer. Hypertrophic scarring and an acute allergic reaction have been reported. There have been no reports of microsphere migration or carcinogenesis associated with the implantation of Artecoll. The main areas for treatment with Artecoll are glabellar, nasolabial and perioral lines and furows. Augmentation of other facial soft tissue areas include the lips, horizontal chin and forehead furrows. Artecoll has been used for therapeutic reasons in a variety of dermatological, ophthalmic, urological and orthopedic conditions.

Hyaluronic acid-derived products

Hyaluronan or hyaluronic acid is one of the naturally occurring glycosaminoglycans (GAGs) in the skin, and is a major component of the intercellular connective tissue matrix, in which collagen and elastic fibers are embedded. The natural depletion of hyaluronic acid over time causes a decrease in dermal hydration and the increased wrinkling often seen with aging. Since hyaluronan has the same chemical composition and molecular structure in all species and tissues, it displays no species or tissue specificity and consequently is not perceived as foreign by the human body when it is used as a soft tissue filler[112]. However, its half-life is only 1–2 days long in all connective tissues in the body (except in the vitreous of the eye), making it inadequate for long-lasting implantation in its natural form. Consequently, three generations of hyaluronan gels currently exist. The first-generation hyaluronan gel is not cross-linked, but is hyperpolymerized at a molecular weight of 10–20 mg/ml, which forms a viscoelastic gel. It is used clinically in ophthalmic and orthopedic surgery. Second-generation hyaluronan gels (e.g. Hylaform®) are cross-linked at a molecular weight of 5 mg/ml and are used in ophthalmic surgery and for dermal implantation. The third generation hyaluronan gels (e.g. Restylane™) are cross-linked and stabilized with a higher molecular weight of 20 mg/ml and are used for dermal implantation.

Hylaform™ Hylan B gel (Hylaform™) is a second-generation cross-linked derivative of natural hyaluronan developed in the mid-1980s. Hylan B gel is water insoluble, and has greater elasticity and viscosity than the water-soluble unmodified native polymer[113]. Highly elastic hylan B gel, when implanted in skin, resists degradation and does not migrate. Its high water content parallels the natural dermal hydrating properties of native hyaluronic acid.

Hylaform is the tradename of the viscoelastic hylan B gel developed, manufactured and marketed for use in Europe by the Biomatrix Corporation, Inc., Ridgefield, NJ, USA. It is indicated for the treatment and correction of facial soft tissue defects including depressed cutaneous scars and wrinkles. It is distributed by the Inamed Corporation through McGhan Medical Corporation, Santa Barbara, CA, for use in North America, but it is still not available for use in the USA.

Injections of Hylaform are placed in both the superficial and the deep dermis, and work best in areas known to respond to other types of soluble soft tissue fillers, such as ZC or Fibrel, e.g. glabellar frown lines, melolabial folds and distensible scars. Two to four touch-up injections 2–4 weeks apart are usually required, before the correction of a facial defect is stabilized. Traumatic and surgical scars seem to respond better and last longer (24 weeks) than facial wrinkles and furrows (18 weeks). Skin testing prior to treatment with Hylaform is not required.

After injections with Hylaform, transient and mild erythema, pruritus, edema and pain can be experienced by the patient. Approximately 2% of all patients treated experienced persistent erythema, ecchymosis and acneiform eruptions, but all resolved without sequelae. No known antigenic or immunogenic responses have been observed.

Restylane This is a third-generation, cross-linked, stabilized, non-animal, high molecular weight hyaluronan gel that retains the biological compatibility of native hyaluronic acid. It dissolves more slowly and lasts longer after implantation. It is not water soluble, but retains its hydrophilic properties, forming hydrated co-polymers. Restylane is transparent, and is distributed in sterile syringes containing 0.7 ml of gel product with no local anesthetic additive. Restylane is injected into the mid-dermis with a 27- or 30-G needle, and is indicated for the correction of glabellar and melolabial folds, oral commissures, furrows and depressed, distensible acne scars and hypoplastic lips. Touch-up injections can be given 1–2 weeks after an initial treatment session. About 75% of patients treated have experienced marked or moderate improvement 8 months after the initial treatment. Adverse side-effects have been localized and transient. They included erythema, edema, pain and tenderness, which all resolved spontaneously. There have been no systemic or hypersensitivity reactions observed. Restylane is manufactured by Q-Med, Uppsala, Sweden, and is not approved for use in the USA.

Autologous collagen implants

Autologous collagen soft tissue fillers include Autologen and Isolagen.

Autologen This is processed collagen removed from cutaneous tissue obtained from biopsies of the patient's own skin and prepared by proprietary purification and extraction processes by Collagenesis, Inc., Beverly, MA. Autologen is composed of intact autologous naturally cross-linked collagen fibers dispersed in an injectable neutral pH phosphate-buffered suspension. It is offered in a standard 4% concentration or a cross-linked 6% concentration, or it can be custom made to suit the individual patient's needs (e.g. in concentrations as low as 25 mg/ml or 2.5%, or as high as 100 mg/ml or 10%). After a specimen of skin is excised, it must be promptly wrapped in sterile saline-soaked gauze and placed in a special express mailer container kit supplied with dry ice packs by Collagenesis Inc. The excised skin can be refrigerated for several days or stored frozen for up to 2 weeks before being mailed. Individual specimens are carefully processed in an aseptic environment by a single, highly-trained technician. The preparation from start to finish usually requires 3 to 4 weeks. This includes tissue processing, sterility testing and delivery to the treating physician. Autologen can be stored for at least 5 years in the BioBank™, which is a highly sophisticated and safe storage system. The usual yield of injectable 4% Autologen (40 mg/ml) is approximately 1.0 ml per 125 cm² of donor skin, excluding eyelid or foreskin tissue. After it has been processed, the final product is then placed into sterile, 1.0-ml Luer-Lok syringes and hand-labeled with the donor/recipient's identification codes. When received by the treating physician, Autologen must be stored refrigerated, and not frozen. It should be removed from the refrigerator at least 30 min prior to injection. Autologen should be injected deep into the lower dermis, but not into the subcutaneous space. Multiple injections of small volumes are given into a particular defect, whose correction must be appreciated immediately, otherwise the injection was given too deeply. Indications for the use of Autologen are the same as for those of any other injectable soft tissue implantable filler including glabellar frown lines, horizontal forehead furrows, lateral canthal rhytides, nasolabial folds, marionette lines and perioral vertical rhytides. Small to medium rhytides and furrows are best overcorrected by 20% and treated with the standard 4% Autologen, which can be injected through a 30G needle. Deeper defects requiring a significant volume of implant are best treated with the cross- linked 6% Autologen XL injected through a 27G needle. Autologen is best injected in 2–4 sessions given at intervals of 2–4 weeks each, before complete correction is accomplished, because only a small residue of the autologous collagen implant will remain after the phosphate-buffered saline is resorbed. Fewer booster injections are required when injecting the 6% Autologen XL. Local or regional anesthesia is required prior to treatment, since an injection of Autologen can be very painful, especially when using the 6% concentration. Histopathological studies of implanted Autologen revealed a complete absence of inflammatory changes, which confirms Autologen's lack of a reactive host immunological response after implantation. Heterogeneic implantable soft tissue fillers such as ZC usually demonstrate a brisk reactive host immunological response with a series of inflammatory changes.

Isolagen This is an injectable solution of living, cultured and expanded fibroblasts in an extracellular matrix prepared by Isolagen Technologies, Inc., Paramus, NJ. Fibroblasts extracted from biopsy

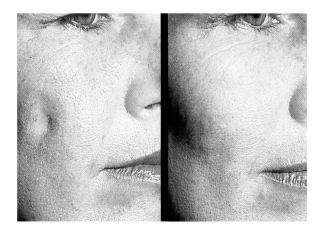

Figure 9 Patient before (left) and after (right) an injection of Zyplast collagen. Copyright McGhan Medical Corporation

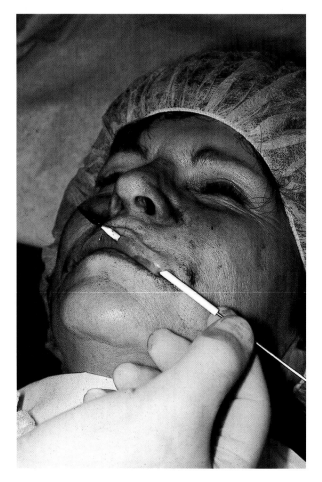

Figure 10 Trocar and Soft Form™ implant just released from the cannula and just prior to the removal of the trocar

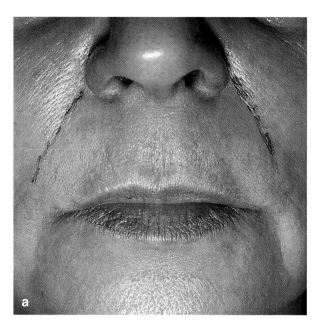

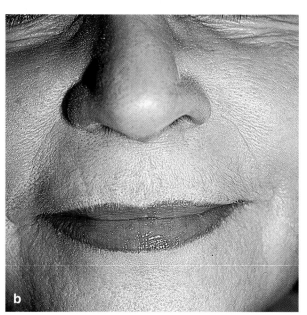

Figure 11 (a) Patient before Soft Form™ implantation. (b) The same patient 2 years after the implantation

specimens of the patient's skin and mucosa are expanded by a proprietary tissue-culture technique. Similar to the tissue-processing procedure of Autologen, donor skin biopsy specimens are placed in designated holding tubes containing special transport media, which are then placed on ice in a thermos flask and shipped overnight to the laboratories at Isolagen Technologies. Six weeks following donor skin harvesting, the patient is given a test injection in the volar surface of the forearm. Eight weeks from the acquisition of the biopsy, a 1.2-ml sterile vial containing Isolagen is shipped back to the treating physician in a thermos flask packed in ice. Injections must be administered within 24 h after shipping, to ensure that 95% of the cultured fibroblasts are alive and viable, because 48 h after shipping, the viability of the product

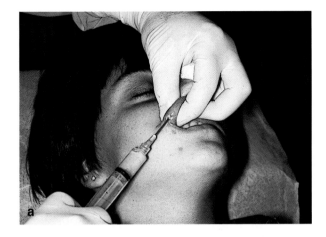

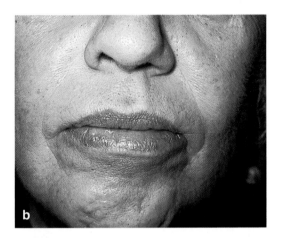

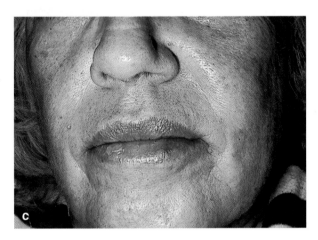

Figure 12 (a) Patient during autologous fat injection of the upper lip. (b) A patient's lips before autologous fat implantation. Note the thinness of the upper lip. (c) The same patient 1 month after autologous fat re-implantation

drops to 85%, and at 72 h it drops to 65%. Once the initial skin biopsy has been obtained, the fibroblasts can be expanded repeatedly without the need for additional biopsy specimens. Isolagen can be stored indefinitely in liquid nitrogen and can be renewed at any time.

Isolagen is injected with a 30G needle into the superficial, mid- and deep dermis and subcutaneous plane. Multiple passes with a 30G needle are made, to create pockets within the dermis (i.e. the subcision technique) before the Isolagen is injected. This is similar to the technique of Fibrel injections. Theoretically, injections of Isolagen provide a gradual and continual correction of dermal defects and facial wrinkles, restoring dermal collagen and fibroblasts lost as a result of aging, photodamage and scarring. Injections of Isolagen have maintained their correction up to 2.5 years after implantation[114]. Since there are no exogenous proteins added to Isolagen, there have been no reports of an allergic response to the implant.

Homologous collagen implants

Homologous soft tissue fillers include Dermalogen, Fascian and AlloDerm.

Dermalogen This is a suspension of injectable acellular homologous human collagen fibers prepared from live, human donor skin obtained from a tissue bank in New Jersey accredited by the American Association of Tissue Banks (AATB). A patented process renders the suspension essentially acellular without altering the collagen fibrils and matrix. The advantages of Dermalogen over Autologen or Isolagen is that Dermalogen is immediately available for use, whereas the injectable autologous collagens must first be harvested from the patient's own skin and then sent to a processing laboratory where the tissue is prepared and rendered into injectable autologous collagen before it can be returned at a later date to the treating physician.

The human tissue that is procured from the tissue bank in preparation for the processing of Dermalogen has been screened and cleared of all potentially infectious diseases, according to the AATB guidelines that are regulated by the FDA. The tissue is then processed in an aseptic environment and rendered acellular. Indications for the use of Dermalogen are the same as those for other soft tissue fillers. Typically, two or three treatments over a 3-month period are necessary to correct most dermal defects. There have been no reports of any adverse reactions to Dermalogen, and clinical trials are currently in progress.

Fascian™ This is a suspension of injectable collagen derived from preserved human fascia lata or gastrocnemius that is freeze-dried, irradiated, fragmented and vacuum sealed. It is prepared from AATB human tissue bank material, and thoroughly tested and certified to be free of any infectious material. Fascian is supplied in particle sizes of 0.10 mm, 0.25 mm, 0.50 mm, 1.0 mm, and 2.0 mm in ready-to-inject sterile 3 ml Luer-Lock syringes with an appropriate size needle, and it can be stored at room temperature. Syringes are available containing either 50 or 80 mg of the suspended collagen particles. The 0.1 mm particle size of Fascian can be injected through a 27G needle and placed intradermally or subdermally, which can be used to correct superficial and distensible scars. The 0.25 mm particle size of Fascian is injected from a sterile 3 ml syringe supplied with a needle as small as 22G, and placed intradermally or subdermally. The larger particle sizes of Fascian need to be injected subdermally with large-bore needles as large as 20–16G (e.g. 0.50 mm Fascian is injected with a 20G or 18G needle preferably only subdermally; 1.0 mm Fascian is injected with an 18G needle only subdermally; and 2 mm Fascian is injected with a 18G or 16G needle only subdermally). The larger particle sizes of Fascian are ideal in the treatment of deeper facial defects, scars, depressions and wrinkles of the lips, cheeks and melolabial folds. Prior to injection, the product has to be rehydrated with 2–4 ml of normal saline solution or lidocaine, and agitated for 5–10 min in order to soften and separate the particles thoroughly, so that they can form a homogeneous, crystalline slurry prior to injection. If normal saline is used to rehydrate the product, then the treatment site needs to be anesthetized prior to implantation, especially when injecting larger particle sizes (0.5 mm–2.0 mm). The preserved fascia has been shown to induce the deposition of the patient's own native collagen (i.e. recollagenation) and can be long lasting. There have been to date no cases of cross-contamination or allergic reactions, and skin testing is not required.

AlloDerm   This is an acellular non-immunogenic human dermal allograft that is distributed as implantable sheets, processed from the skin of human cadavers. It is prepared by the patented AlloDerm Process, in which antigenic tissue components (i.e. epidermis and collagen fibers) are removed from the dermis without damaging the matrix. It is then rendered acellular, freeze-dried and commercially distributed. Grafts should be refrigerated until implanted, and can be stored for at least 2 years. Prior to implantation, the graft is rehydrated in sterile normal saline. These sheets of dermal grafts are inserted under the area to be treated through small incisions in the skin. AlloDerm can be used as grafts for full-thickness tissue loss (e.g. burns and surgery), in nasolabial folds and lip augmentation, in the revision of depressed scars and rhinoplasties and for glabellar contouring. There have been no reports of prolonged edema, erythema or discomfort. There have been no reports of infection, rejection, resorption or extrusion of the graft when implanted under strict sterile technique.

Because of the inability of Zyderm collagen or other injectable soft tissue fillers to last for more than 1 year before additional filler needs to be reimplanted, a new more permanent type of facial soft tissue filler has been developed. This new implant can be used to restore the fullness of the lips and to augment and soften the deep folds of the melolabial area. This new implant is permanent, but reversible, soft and supple, safe and biocompatible, and it is made of the inert material expanded polytetrafluoroethylene (ePTFE).

ePTFE   This is a type of synthetic microporous polymer that has been expanded and extruded to form interconnecting fibrils and nodes; it is generally referred to as expanded polytetrafluoroethylene (ePTFE). It is highly biocompatible and has been used extensively since the 1970s in vascular, dental and general surgical procedures. Recently, it has been adapted for facial soft tissue augmentation[115–117]. A proprietary form of ePTFE called Soft Form™ facial implant is manufactured and distributed by the Inamed Corporation through McGhan Medical Corporation (Santa Barbara, CA) as a hollow tube 5, 7 and 9 cm long with a large lumen, whose outer dimensions measure 2.4, 3.2 or 4.0 mm. Soft Form has a soft and natural feel to it and is chemically stable and biologically inert. Soft Form is distributed in a closed delivery system that is sterile, fully assembled and ready to implant. The method of its implantation is a simple office procedure that has been standardized. The Soft Form hollow tubular configuration is designed to promote connective tissue ingrowth into the central lumen of the implant, resulting in enhanced stability[118]. It can be used in conjunction with other facial fillers; however, it is made of permanent, inert material that is the longest lasting of all the facial fillers. Soft Form can be used to enhance the vermilion border of the lips, giving them definition. It can also be used to fill in soft tissue deficiencies around the mouth and nasolabial areas.

Implanting Soft Form is a surgical procedure and should be done under sterile conditions. The area to be implanted with Soft Form is first marked with gentian violet, with the patient in the upright position. The area is anesthetized by regional and nerve blocks. The entrance and exit sites are created with the stab of a no. 11 surgical blade. The handling of the prepackaged delivery system of the Soft Form implant must be done in the prescribed manner, so that distortion of the implant can be avoided. The Soft Form delivery system is composed of a cannula and a small cutting trocar and shaft, which has been passed through the lumen of the Soft Form implant material. After the implant is inserted in the natural subcutaneous plane immediately beneath the dermis under the area to be augmented, the trocar is released from the cannula. With the implant still in place around the trocar (Figure 10), it is checked for proper positioning and, if necessary, it is readjusted so that it is placed under the skin smoothly and without crimping. The trocar is advanced and removed, leaving the implant in place under the area to be corrected. The exposed ends of the implant are then cut and trimmed, with care taken to ensure that its lumen is patent. The skin entry and exit incisional wounds are approximated with fine monofilament suture, and are virtually invisible within a few weeks' time. At the completion of the procedure, the implant can be felt when the surface of the skin is palpated, but it becomes less detectable in time (Figure 11). Because of the natural asymmetry of the body, precise symmetry may not be attainable, even after implanting different sizes of the Soft Form implants. However, revisions and adjustments can eventually be performed. Even additional fillers such as collagen or even autologous fat can be used at a later date, to enhance the final results. Postoperatively, patients should be given prophylactic antibiotics to avoid infection. The implant should not be visible at any time postoperatively if it is placed correctly. There can be pain in the immediate postoperative period as well as ecchymosis and edema. However, within less than 1 week, the soft tissue alterations should revert to normal. Soft Form has a low rate of postoperative infection if strict sterile technique is used during its implantation. Extrusion rates are negligible when compared to other forms of implantable ePTFE.

Autologous fat transplantation

The modern era of autologous free fat transplantation began in the late 1970s with the development of the technique of fat extraction by liposuction surgery first reported by Fischer and Fischer[119]. The mounting general frustration with the available injectable agents for soft tissue augmentation at that time eventually led to a renewed interest in using autologous fat for implantation, especially since now there was an easier way to harvest the fat by liposuction. Illouz extracted fat using the blunt cannula technique and reinjected it with a large-bore needle[120]. Initially, Fournier harvested fat by attaching a syringe with a large-bore needle to the distal end of the suction tubing during liposuction. Subsequently, he pioneered using only a syringe and needle to create the necessary suction to harvest fat. This occurs when, after inserting a 14G needle into subcutaneous fat, the plunger of the syringe is withdrawn. This created enough vacuum to harvest fat. Asken further modified the syringe technique by using blunt-tipped needles to extract the fat[121].

Dermatologists have played a very active role in the evolving technique of liposuction and autologous fat reimplantation. The most significant contribution was the development of tumescent anesthesia for liposuction surgery[122]. The pharmacokinetics for tumescent anesthesia was conceived and defined by a dermatologist, Jeff Klein, and its use in liposuction surgery was promoted by many other dermatologists.

The literature is replete with studies advocating different anatomical sites as the ideal one for harvesting longer-lasting fat. Different harvesting techniques are promoted one over another, as are whether and how to freeze the harvested fat for future touch-up procedures. The areas of the face that are best augmented with autologous fat and the appropriate defects are still questions that need to be answered.

Donor site harvesting

Whether it is because of ease of extraction or the quality and quantity of fat, the thighs, hips, abdomen and buttocks seem to be the preferred sites for donor fat harvesting. Very little equipment is necessary. To extract the fat, specially made resterilizable stainless steel blunt-tipped 16G and 18G needles are attached to 10 ml Luer-Lok disposable syringes. After the usual surgical preparation of the skin surface and the demarcation of the donor area is completed, the donor tissue is anesthetized. Depending on the size of the donor site, 1% lidocaine with epinephrine (adrenaline) 1 : 100 000 can be used for limited areas. Otherwise a reduced volume of Klein's tumescent anesthetic can be used for larger, more extensive donor sites. Klein's tumescent anesthetic modified for a reduced volume of solution is as follows: 250 ml normal saline 0.09%; 25 ml xylocaine 1%; 0.25 ml epinephrine 1:1000; 4 ml sodium bicarbonate 8.4%; to give a total of 250 mg xylocaine 0.1% in 1:1 000 000 epinephrine.

Once the donor site blanches and the tissue is totally anesthetized, fat extraction can commence. A blunt-tipped 14G or 16G fat-harvesting needle attached to a 10 ml Luer-Lok syringe is inserted through the skin and into the subcutaneous fat. Negative pressure is created in the syringe by withdrawing its plunger and keeping it in the fully retracted position either by hand or with the different types of devices made especially for this purpose (e.g. Tulip lipoextraction lock). With a back-and-forth motion, it is easy to draw fat into the syringe, because of the negative pressure maintained. Once the 10-ml syringes are full, they are placed tip down in a sterile holder of choice (e.g. stainless steel cup or test tube rack). After a few minutes, the fat rises as the supranatant and serum and blood drop down at the distal end of the syringe as the infranatant. The infranatant can now be expressed out of the syringe, leaving only fat behind. If the extraction of fat was somewhat traumatic and consequently tinged with blood, a few gentle washings with normal saline or lactated Ringer's solution will cleanse the fat, making it ready for implantation.

Recipient site treatment

The donor fat can be injected from the same syringe used to harvest it. Once the fat is cleansed and all the infranatant is ejected out of the syringe, a 16G or 18G disposable Luer-Lok needle is placed onto the syringe (Figure 12).

After selecting the area to be treated, one can begin injecting fat subcutaneously. Usually the pressure of the fat being injected causes immediate numbness in the area, so anesthesia of the recipient site is not necessary. Intentional overcorrection to about 150% is advisable. Massaging and molding the fat into the desired position in the subcutaneous strata is acceptable.

Postoperative care

Topical antibiotics are placed over all the skin puncture sites. Occasionally systemic oral antibiotics for approximately 7–10 days postoperatively can be administered. Analgesics can be prescribed, but most patients have no additional pain once the procedure is completed. Ice packs during the first 24 h will help reduce edema and inflammation. There have been cases of blindness following injection of autologous fat in the glabellar area, similar to that occurring with other tissue fillers[123]. With recent reports of successful long-term fat transplantation of scars and atrophies of the face, it seems that the best results are obtained when autologous fat is used to augment facial soft tissue defects that have dermal and subdermal components[124].

CONCLUSION

The new millennium will witness the 'graying' of the baby-boomers, many of whom possess an insatiable desire for a way to perpetuate youth, if not of bodily function at least of facial appearance. The average life span worldwide has jumped from 49.5 years in 1972 to more than 63 years in the 1990s[125]. This chapter on facial rejuvenation has attempted to touch upon the innumerable possibilities available to those who want to maintain a youthful appearance. Limiting one's exposure to intense solar radiation and environmental pollutants (e.g. tobacco smoke) is one way to forestall the obvious appearance of aging of exposed areas of the body, especially of the face. We have investigated some of the consequences of intrinsic and extrinsic aging and how to correct them, using techniques such as facial skin resurfacing, mimetic muscle denervation and soft tissue filling. Will many of our established techniques of the 20th century appear only as feeble attempts at facial rejuvenation in the 21st century? One can only hope that medical science will forge ahead and present us with even more ingenious ways to remain healthy and youthful. To be able to live longer and to maintain a youthful appearance is certainly an exciting prospect for the new millennium.

REFERENCES

1. Montagna W. Morphology of aging skin. In Montagna W, ed. *Advances in the Biology of Skin*. Oxford: Pergamon Press, 1965:1–16
2. Kligman AM, Lavker RM. Cutaneous aging: the differences between intrinsic and extrinsic aging and photoaging. *J Cutan Ageing Cosmetol Dermatol* 1988;1:5–12
3. Benedetto AV. Environment and skin aging. *Clin Dermatol* 1998;16:129–39
4. Kligman AM. Early destructive effect of sunlight in human skin. *JAMA* 1969;10:2377–80
5. Leyden JJ. Clinical features of aging skin. *Br J Dermatol* 1990;122(suppl 35):1–3

6. Sams WM. Sun-induced aging: clinical and laboratory observations in man. *Dermatol Clin* 1986;4:509–16

7. Kligman LH. Photoaging: manifestations, prevention and treatment. *Dermatol Clin* 1986;4:517–28

8. Gilchrest BA. Skin aging and photoaging: an overview. *J Am Acad Dermatol* 1989;21:610–13

9. Brownstein MH, Rabinowitz AD. The precursors of cutaneous squamous cell carcinoma. *Int J Dermatol* 1979;18:1–16

10. Freeman R. Carcinogenic effects of solar radiation and prevention measures. *Cancer* 1968;21:1114–20

11. Gellin GA, Kopf AW, Garfinkel L. Basal cell epithelioma: a controlled study of associated factors. *Arch Dermatol* 1965;91:38–45

12. Elmwood JM, Gallagher RP, Davison J, *et al.* Sunburn, suntan and the risk of cutaneous malignant melanoma. The Western Canada melanoma study. *Br J Cancer* 1985;51:543–9

13. Daniel HW. Smoker's wrinkles. *Ann Intern Med* 1971;75:873–80

14. Kanduce DP, Burr R, Gress R, *et al.* Cigarette smoking: risk factor for premature facial wrinkling. *Ann Intern Med* 1991;114:840–4

15. Marmelzat WL. Bits of history, bits of mystery – a historical review of chemical rejuvenation of the face. In Kotler R, ed. *Chemical Rejuvenation of the Face*. St Louis: Mosby-Year Book, 1992:1–39

16. MacKee GM, Karp FL. The treatment of post acne scars with phenol. *Br J Dermatol* 1952;64:456–9

17. Baker TJ, Jordan HL. The ablation of rhytides by chemical means: A preliminary report. *J Fla Med Assoc* 1961;48:451–4

18. Baker TJ, Gordon HL, Seckinger DL. A second look at chemical face peeling. *Plast Reconstr Surg* 1966;37:487

19. Ayers S III. Dermal changes following application of chemical cauterants to aging skin. *Arch Dermatol* 1960;82:578–85

20. Aronsohn RB. Facial chemosurgery. *Eye Ear Nose Throat* 1971;50:128–33

21. Litton C. Chemical face lifting. *Plast Reconstr Surg* 1962;29:371–9

22. Fitzpatrick TB. The validity and practicality of sun reactive skin type I through VI. *Arch Dermatol* 1988;124:869–73

23. Stegman SJ. A study of dermabrasion and chemical peels in an animal model. *J Dermatol Surg Oncol* 1980;6:490–7

24. Stegman SJ. A comparative histologic study of the effects of three peeling agents and dermabrasion on normal and sundamaged skin. *Aesth Plast Surg* 1982;6:123–35

25. Moy L, Murad H, Moy R. Glycolic acid for the treatment of wrinkles and photoaging. *J Dermatol Surg Oncol* 1993;19:243–6

26. Stagnone JJ. Superficial peeling. *J Dermatol Surg Oncol* 1989;15:924–30

27. Karam P. 50% Resorcin peel. *Int J Dermatol* 1993;32:569–74

28. Resnik SS. Chemical peeling with trichloroacetic acid. *J Dermatol Surg Oncol* 1984;10:549–50

29. Brody HJ. Medium depth chemical peeling of the skin: a variation of superficial chemosurgery. *Adv Dermatol* 1988;3:205–20

30. Monheit GD. The Jessner's + TCA peel: a medium depth chemical peel. *J Dermatol Surg Oncol* 1989;15:945–50

31. Coleman W III, Futrell J. The glycolic acid trichloroacetic acid peel. *J Dermatol Surg Oncol* 1994;20:76–80

32. Brody HJ. Variations and comparisons in medium-depth chemical peeling. *J Dermatol Surg Oncol* 1989;15:953–63

33. Brody HJ. Update on chemical peeling. *Adv Dermatol* 1992;7:275–89

34. Kligman AM, Baker TJ, Jordan HL. Long-term histologic follow-up of phenol face peels. *Plast Reconstr Surg* 1985;75:652–9

35. Peikert JM, Kaye VN, Zachary CB. A reevaluation of the effect of occlusion on the trichloroacetic acid peel. *J Dermatol Surg Oncol* 1994;20:660–5

36. Collins PS. Trichloroacetic acid peels revisited. *J Dermatol Surg Oncol* 1989;15:933–40

37. Brody HJ. Complications of chemical peeling. *J Dermatol Surg Oncol* 1989;15:1010–19

38. Beeson WH. The importance of cardiac monitoring in superficial and deep chemical peeling. *J Dermatol Surg Oncol* 1987;13:949–50

39. Klein DR, Little JH. Laryngeal edema as a complication of chemical peel. *Plast Reconstr Surg* 1983;71:419–20

40. Kromayer E. Rotationsinstrumente: ein neues technisches Verfahren in der dermatologischen Kleinchirurgie. *Derm Z* 1905;12:26–36

41. Kromayer E. *Cosmetic Treatment of Skin Complaints* [English translation of the 2nd German (1929) edition]. New York: Oxford University Press, 1930;9

42. Kromayer E. Das Frasen in der Kosmetik. *Kosmetol Rundschau* 1933;4:61–74

43. Kurtin A. Corrective surgical planing of skin. *Arch Dermatol Syphilol* 1953;68:389–97

44. Robbins N. Dr Abner Kurtin, father of ambulatory dermabrasion. *J Dermatol Surg Oncol* 1988;14:425–31

45. Wilson JW. Dichlorofluoroethane for surgical planing. *Am Med Assoc Arch Dermatol* 1955;71:523–5

46. Wilson JW, Ayres S III, Luikart R. Mixtures of fluorinated hydrocarbons as refrigerant anesthetic: a hazard in use in surgical skin planing. *Arch Dermatol* 1956;74:310–11

47. Burks JW. *Wire Brush Surgery*. Springfield, IL: Charles C Thomas, 1956

48. Benedetto AV, Griffin TD, Benedetto EA. Dermabrasion: therapy and prophylaxis of the

photoaged face. *J Am Acad Dermatol* 1992;27: 439–47

49. Yarborough JM. Dermabrasion by wire brush. *J Dermatol Surg Oncol* 1987;13:610–15

50. Strick RA, Moy R. Low skin temperatures produced by new skin refrigerants. *J Dermatol Surg Oncol* 1985;11:1196–8

51. Kemsley GM. Transmission of hepatitis B in dermabrasion. *Plast Reconstr Surg* 1975;56:440

52. Vaugh RY, Lesher JL, Chalker DK, *et al*. HIV and the dermatologic surgeon. *J Dermatol Surg Oncol* 1990;16:1107–10

53. Branham GH, Thomas JR. Rejuvenation of the skin surface: chemical peel and dermabrasion. *Facial Plast Surg* 1996;12:125–33

54. Smack DP, Harrington AC, Dunn C, *et al*. Infection and allergy incidence in ambulatory surgery patients using white petrolatum versus bacitracin ointment. *JAMA* 1996;276:972

55. David LM, Lask GP, Glassberg E, *et al*. Laser ablation for cosmetic and medical treatment of facial actinic damage. *Cutis* 1989;43:583–7

56. Dover JS. CO_2 laser resurfacing – why all the fuss? *Plast Reconstr Surg* 1996;98:506–11

57. Roenigk HH Jr. The place of laser resurfacing within the range of medical and surgical skin resurfacing techniques. *Semin Cutan Med Surg* 1996; 15:208–13

58. Einstein A. Zur Quantentheorie der Strahlung. *Physiol Z* 1917;18:121–8

59. Maiman TH. Stimulated optical radiation in ruby. *Nature (London)* 1960;187:493–4

60. Goldman L. Pathology of the effect of the laser beam on the skin. *Nature (London)* 1963;197: 912–15

61. Wheeland RG, Walker NPJ. Lasers – Twenty five years later. *Int J Dermatol* 1986;25:209–16

62. Herd RM, Dover JS, Arndt KA. Basic laser principles. *Dermatol Clin* 1997;15:355–72

63. Fitzpatrick RE, Smith SR, Sriprachya-Anunt S. Depth of vaporization and effect of pulse stacking with a high-energy, pulsed carbon dioxide laser. *J Am Acad Dermatol* 1999;40:615–22

64. Kauvar AN, Geronemus RG. Histology of laser resurfacing. *Dermatol Clin* 1997;15:459–67

65. Anderson RR, Parish JA. Selective photothermolysis: precise microsurgery by selective absorption of pulsed radiation. *Science* 1983;220:524–7

66. Alster TS, Nanni CA, Williams CM. Comparison of four carbon dioxide resurfacing lasers: a clinical and histopathologic evaluation. *Dermatol Surg* 1999;25:153–9

67. David LM, Sarne AJ, Unger WP. Rapid laser scanning for facial resurfacing. *Dermatol Surg* 1995;21: 1031–3

68. Lask G, Keller G, Lowe N, *et al*. Laser skin resurfacing with the Silk Touch flashscanner for facial rhytides. *Dermatol Surg* 1995;21:1021–4

69. Wood RL, Sliney DH, Basye RA. Laser reflections from surgical instruments. *Laser Surg Med* 1992; 12:675

70. Ries WR, Clipner MA, Reinisch L. Laser safety features of eye shields. *Lasers Surg Med* 1996;18: 309–15

71. Baggish EA. Presence of human immunodeficiency virus DNA in laser smoke. *Lasers Surg Med* 1991;11: 197–200

72. Research confirms earlier study on plume hazard: viral contaminates. *Clin Laser Monthly* 1989;7:43–4

73. Mullarky MB, Norris CW, Goldberg ID. The efficacy of the carbon dioxide laser in the sterilization of skin seeded with bacteria: survival at the skin surface and in the plume emissions. *Laryngoscope* 1985;95:186–7

74. Rohrich RJ, Gyimesi IM, Clark P, Burns AJ. CO_2 laser safety considerations in facial skin resurfacing. *Plast Reconstr Surg* 1997;100:1285–90

75. Wald D, Michelow BJ, Guyuron B, Gibb AA. Fire hazards and CO_2 laser resurfacing. *Plast Reconstr Surg* 1998;101:185–8

76. Kaufman R, Hibst R. Erbium : YAG laser ablation in cutaneous surgery. *Lasers Surg Med* 1996;19:324–8

77. Kauvar ANB, Grossman MC, Bernstein LJ, *et al*. Erbium YAG laser resurfacing. A clinical histopathological evaluation. *Lasers Surg Med* 1998; (suppl 10):33

78. Hohenleutner U, Hohenleutner S, Baeumler M, *et al*. Fast and effective skin ablation with an Er : YAG laser: determination of ablation rates and thermal damage zones. *Lasers Surg Med* 1997;20: 242–9

79. Teikemeier G, Goldberg DJ. Skin resurfacing with the erbium : YAG laser. *Dermatol Surg* 1997;23: 685–9

80. Goldman MP, Manuskiatti W. Combined laser resurfacing with the 950 μsec pulsed CO_2 + Er : YAG lasers. *Dermatol Surg* 1999;25:160–3

81. McDaniel DH, Ash K, Lord J, *et al*. The erbium YAG laser: a review and preliminary report on resurfacing of the face, neck and hands. *Aesthetic Surg J* 1997;17:157–64

82. Goldman MP, Fitzpatrick RE, Manuskiatti W. Laser resurfacing of the neck with the erbium YAG laser. *Dermatol Surg* 1999;25:164–8

83. Schantz EJ, Johnson EA. Preparation and characterization of botulinum toxin type A for human treatment. In Jankovic J, Hallet M, eds. *Therapy with Botulinum Toxin*. New York: Marcel Dekker, 1994: 41–9

84. Coffield JA, Considine RV, Simpson LL. The site and mechanism of action of botulinum neurotoxin. In Jankovic J, Hallet M, eds. *Therapy with Botulinum Toxin*. New York, NY: Marcel Dekker, 1994: 3–13

85. Klein AW. Dilution and storage of botulinum toxin. *Dermatol Surg* 1998;24:1179–80

86. Garcia A, Fulton JE. Cosmetic denervation of the muscles of facial expression with botulinum toxin. *Dermatol Surg* 1996;22:39–43

87. Gartland MG, Hoffman HT. Crystalline preparation of botulinum toxin type A (BOTOX): degradation impotency with storage. *Otolaryngol Head Neck Surg* 1993;108:135–40

88. Argov Z, Mastaglia FL. Disorders of neuromuscular transmission caused by drugs. *N Engl J Med* 1979;301:409–13

89. Wieder JM, Moy RL. Understanding botulinum toxin: surgical anatomy of the frown, forehead and periocular region. *Dermatol Surg* 1998;24:1172–4

90. Carruthers A, Kiene K, Carruthers J. Botulinum A exotoxin use in clinical dermatology. *J Am Acad Dermatol* 1996;34:788–97

91. Gersuny R, Ueber eine subcutane prosthese. *Z Heilkd* 1900;1:199–204

92. Khoo Boo-Chai MB. Paraffinoma. *Plast Reconstr Surg* 1965;36:101–10

93. Duffy DM. Silicone: a critical review. *Adv Dermatol* 1990;5:93–110

94. Rapaport MJ. Injectable silicone: cause of facial nodules, cellulitis, ulcerations and migration. *Aesth Plast Surg* 1996;20:267–76

95. Ashley FL, Thompson DP, Henderson TH. Augmentation of surface contour by subcutaneous injections of silicone fluid. *Plast Reconstr Surg* 1973;51:8–13

96. Wilkie TF. Late development of granuloma after liquid silicone injections. *Plast Reconstr Surg* 1977;60:179–88

97. Milojevic B. Complications after silicone injection therapy in aesthetic plastic surgery. *Aesth Plast Surg* 1982;6:203–6

98. Ellenbogen R, Rubin L. Injectable silicone therapy: human morbidity and mortality. *JAMA* 1974;229:1581

99. Orentreich DS, Orentreich NO. *Injectable Fluid Silicone: Principles of Dermatologic Surgery*. New York: Marcel Dekker, 1988

100. Pollack SV. Silicone, fibrel and collagen implantation for facial lines and wrinkles. *J Dermatol Surg Oncol* 1990;16:957–61

101. McPherson JM, Wallace DG, Piez KA. Development and biochemical characterization of injectable collagen. *J Dermatol Surg Oncol* 1988;14:13–20

102. Elson M. Clinical assessment of Zyplast implant: a year of experience for soft tissue contour correction. *J Am Acad Dermatol* 1988;16:707–13

103. Kligman AM. Histologic responses to collagen implants in human volunteers: comparison of Zyderm collagen with Zyplast implant. *J Dermatol Surg Oncol* 1988;14:35–8

104. DeLustro F, Smith ST, Sundsmo J, *et al*. Reaction to injectable collagen: results in animal models and clinical use. *Plast Reconstr Surg* 1987;79:581–92

105. Siegle RJ, McCoy JP, Schade W, *et al*. Intradermal implantation of bovine collagen: humoral immune responses associated with clinical reactions. *Arch Dermatol* 1984;120:183–7

106. Barr RJ, Stegman SJ. Delayed skin test reaction to injectable collagen implant (Zyderm): the histopathologic comparative study. *J Am Acad Dermatol* 1984;10:652–8

107. Brooks N. A foreign body granuloma produced by an injectable collagen implant at a test site. *J Dermatol Surg Oncol* 1982;8:111–14

108. Stegman SJ, Chu S, Armstrong RC. Adverse reactions to bovine collagen implant: clinical and histologic features. *J Dermatol Surg Oncol* 1988;14:39–48

109. Elson ML. The role of skin testing in the use of collagen injectable materials. *J Dermatol Surg Oncol* 1989;15:301–3

110. Millikan L, Rosen T, Monheit G. Treatment of depressed cutaneous scars with gelatin matrix implant: a multicenter study. *J Am Acad Dermatol* 1987;16:1155–62

111. Lemperle G. PMMA microspheres (Artecoll) for skin and soft tissue augmentation. Part II. Clinical investigations. *Plast Reconst Surg* 1995;96:627–34

112. Richter W, Ryde E, Zetterstroem EO. Non-immunogenicity of purified sodium hyaluronate preparations in man. *Int Arch Allergy Appl Immunol* 1979;59:45–8

113. Larsen NE, Pollack CT, Reiner K, *et al*. Hylan gel biomaterial: dermal and immunological compatiblity. *J Biomed Mat Res* 1993;27:1129–34

114. Boss WK, Marks O. Isolagen. In Klein AW, ed. *Tissue Augmentation in Clinical Practice: Procedures and Techniques*. New York: Marcel Dekker, 1998:335–47

115. Lassus C. Expanded PTFE in the treatment of facial wrinkles. *Aesth Plast Surg* 1991;15:167

116. Cisneros JL, Singla R. Intradermal augmentation with expanded polytetrafluoroethylene (Gore-Tex) for facial lines and wrinkles. *J Dermatol Surg Oncol* 1993;19:539–42

117. Artz JS, Dinner MI. The use of expanded polytetrafluoroethylene as a permanent filler and enhancer of experience: an early report of experience. *Ann Plastic Surg* 1994;32:457–62

118. Greene D, Pruitt L, Maas CS. Biochemical effects of e-PTFE implant structure on soft tissue implantation stability: a study in the porcine model. *Laryngoscope* 1997;107:957–62

119. Fischer A, Fischer GM. Revised technique for cellulitis fat. Reduction in riding breeches deformity. *Bull Int Acad Cosmet Surg* 1977;2:40–5

120. Illouz YG. The fat cell 'graft': a new technique to fill depressions. *Plast Reconstr Surg* 1986;78:172

121. Asken S. *Liposuction Surgery and Autologous Fat Transplantation*. East Norwalk, CT: Appleton & Lange, 1988

122. Klein JA. The tumescent technique for liposuction. *Am J Cosmet Surg* 1987;4:263–7

123. Feinendegen DL, Baumgartner RW, Vuadens P, *et al*. Autologous fat injection for soft tissue augmentation in the face: a safe procedure? *Aesth Plast Surg* 1998;22:163–7

124. Schuller-Petrovic S. Improving the aesthetic aspect of soft tissue defects on the face using autologous fat transplantation. *Facial Plast Surg* 1997;13:119–24

125. Longman PJ. The world turns gray. *US News World Rep* 1999;March 1:30–9

Body rejuvenation

51

Timothy Corcoran Flynn and W. Patrick Coleman IV

A wish for body rejuvenation is common for women of all ages. Dermatological science and surgery have brought about great advances in body improvements. Minor problems such as leg telangiectasias and major afflictions such as hyperhidrosis can be treated with simple techniques. Advanced dermatological surgical procedures, such as tumescent liposuction, are now available for the body with excellent, safe, long-lasting results.

BODY REJUVENATION WITH SOFT TISSUE AUGMENTATION

Depressed scars, acne scars, and distended or spread scars in women can be lessened with filler substances. Injectable bovine collagen (Zyderm and Zyplast) may be used to augment depressed scars and some body wrinkles. Zyderm I is useful for fine wrinkles and superficial scars, whereas Zyderm II is useful for moderately deep creases and scars. Zyplast, a form of bovine collagen cross-linked with glutaraldehyde, is helpful for improving deeper wrinkles and scars. It is important to remember that injectable bovine collagen is a dermal filler and should be placed in the dermis, directly underneath the depressed scar. Pretreatment skin testing is done before use of bovine collagen, as a 1–8% rate of antibodies to bovine collagen has been documented[1].

Newer filler substances include injectable hyaluronic acid derivatives such as Hylaform Gel and Restylane, which may be used for wrinkle and scar rejuvenation on the body. The materials are hyaluronic acid derivatives that are capable of binding multiple molecules of water, plumping up the dermal tissue.

Acne scars are frequently rejuvenated by first lysing the underlying collagen fibers that tether the skin to deeper subcutaneous tissue. This is often done with the use of a cutting needle, which serves to break the fibrous bands. Filler substances may then be injected in order to elevate these scars.

BODY REJUVENATION WITH FAT TRANSPLANTATION

Fat transplantation, or microlipoinjection, has been shown to be effective and safe for body rejuvenation.

This technique has been used for soft tissue contour defects for over a century. Fat transplantation involves injecting autologous adipose tissue as a filler substance. An area of donor fat is identified and instilled with tumescent anesthesia. A standard solution used for liposuction (0.05% lidocaine with 1 : 1 000 000 epinephrine in normal saline) is employed. After obtaining the maximal epinephrine vasoconstrictive effect, a 14G aspiration minicannula is connected to a 3-ml Luer-Lock syringe. With the plunger drawn back, donor fat is aspirated through a small cutaneous incision. The filled syringe is placed plunger-up in a laboratory test tube holder. After approximately 20 min, natural separation occurs and the extra saline and liquefied adipose tissue is expelled from the syringe. The remaining fat is then implanted into the recipient area using a 16 or 18G needle. It is important to remember that fat is not a dermal filler. Placement of the fat graft should occur into a space that contains some fat. Some molding of the injected fat can be done.

Fat transplantation is helpful for areas of localized fat loss or atrophy, such as contour defects following tumescent liposuction or as soft tissue augmentation to the back of aging hands[2] (Figure 1). Between 30 and 40% of the graft is retained after 1 year. Multiple fat transfers to the same area have filled out areas of fat atrophy with long-lasting results[3,4].

LIPOSUCTION

Liposuction is a vacuum-assisted removal of fat. Subcutaneous fat is often unequally distributed and often has a familial pattern. This is illustrated in families having a tendency towards excessive adiposity in the lateral thighs with mothers and daughters all having 'saddle bags'. In aging, there is natural loss of lean body mass and accumulation of excess fat.

Not all fat is the same throughout the body. There are site-specific differences in adipose tissue. Variable fatty acid composition occurs in fat in different areas, and not all areas of adiposity respond the same to weight gain or loss. Indeed, many individuals who have attempted to shrink a certain body area by excess exercise or caloric restriction have found that, while fat seems to be lost from some areas, there are certain trouble areas that appear to be resistant to shrinkage. Liposuction is necessary to remove the adipocytes storing fat in these resistant areas (Figure 2).

Liposuction is not a treatment for generalized obesity. The ideal liposuction patient is one who is of relatively normal body weight for height, with localized areas of adipose excess[5]. Tumescent liposuction is designed to remove these areas of localized adiposity by instilling a dilute solution of lidocaine and epinephrine followed by gently aspirating the excess adipose tissue. Fat does not appear to be regained in these areas as many of the offending fat cells have been removed. Liposuction, when performed under tumescent local anesthesia, is a safe procedure that has been performed in thousands of individuals without complications.

The patient should be in general good health and should have good skin elasticity over the areas being treated with tumescent liposuction. Poor candidates include those individuals who are excessively overweight and who, upon examination, show decreased skin elasticity with poor turgor and irregular waviness[5]. Caution must be exercised in a site with numerous surgical scars, especially in the abdomen, where weakness in the underlying muscle structure or hernias may be present.

Common areas for performing liposuction include the lateral thighs and the lower part of the abdomen[5]. The upper part of the abdomen is an area that often contains excess subcutaneous fat, and liposuction in the area is probably best performed in combination with aspiration of the lower aspect of the abdomen. Fat can accumulate in the neck, arms[6], upper and lateral parts of the back, and the posterior axillary fold. The flanks are a common area of excess fat. These areas, commonly called 'love handles', are a frequent site of fatty accumulation in men, and sometimes in women. Fat may accumulate in the buttocks and inner portion of the thighs, as well as in a crescent-shaped area of fat adiposity below the intergluteal fold. Women often complain about this 'banana' fold which responds well to liposuction[7]. Liposuction may be successfully used on the knees and lower leg around the calves or ankles, but caution and experience is required in these areas.

Tumescent liposuction has few complications. The normal sequelae include skin bruising and edema, hyperpigmentation and small scars. Asymmetry may occur. Rare complications include hematomas, seromas, infection, pulmonary embolism, tissue necrosis, nerve injury and fluid and electrolyte imbalances. Most complications from liposuction, including rare deaths, have been reported in patients who have undergone liposuction with large volumes of fat being removed at any one time and/or in combination with other procedures, often under general anesthesia. Tumescent liposuction, when performed correctly, is used for one or two anatomic sites at a time, does not use an excess of lidocaine, is not done under general anesthesia and does not require intravenous fluid replacement.

The procedure is sterile and the patient is draped and prepped appropriately. A dilute solution of lidocaine with epinephrine (0.05% lidocaine, 1 : 1 000 000 epinephrine in normal saline) is instilled into the fat through a small anesthetized wheal in the skin using an infiltration cannula. The solution is slowly infused, assisted by a peristolic pump. Enough tumescent anesthesia is instilled to firm the area of adiposity to the point of overriding dimpling and blanching of the skin. The maximal safe lidocaine dosage using the tumescent technique is 45–55 mg/kg of body weight[8,9]. Overweight patients should have less than 55 mg/kg lidocaine used.

Once maximum vasoconstriction has been achieved, after 15–25 min, liposuction may begin. The most common method of removing fat uses suction aspiration machines, which produce a vacuum of approximately 29 mmHg. A clear, sterile tubing is connected to a blunt tipped liposuction cannula. This is inserted through the skin and, using a gentle back-and-forth motion, the excess adipose cells are gently aspirated into the reservoir of the aspiration unit. Alternatively, a few liposuction surgeons prefer the manual syringe technique.

Liposuction cannulas are manufactured in a variety of shapes, diameters and lengths. Over time it has become apparent that small-gauge (< 4 mm) blunt-tipped cannulas provide the most finesse. These cannulas create a series of tunnels in the underlying fat through several entry sites in the skin. The tunnels are laid one on top of the other in a criss-cross fashion. Over time, these small tunnels collapse upon themselves, further reducing the volume of excess fat and allowing for even skin retraction.

Upon completion of the liposuction, the small incision sites may be closed with suture or allowed to heal by secondary intention. Leaving entry sites open has the advantage of allowing excess tumescent anesthetic solution to drain out of these entry sites. These sites should be covered by an antibiotic ointment and absorbent materials placed over the areas to absorb the draining tumescent anesthetic solution.

Compression garments assist in the drainage of extra tumescent anesthetic solution and give patients a feeling of security following liposuction. They may also decrease hematoma and seroma formation. Many patients use ready-to-wear elastic garments. Following a brief period of recuperation, patients are allowed to resume their normal activities. Light exercise is encouraged within a few days.

The results of liposuction are not often appreciable for at least 3 months after surgery and the final results may not be seen before 6 months. Patients must be apprised that this recontouring of fat and collapse of the subcutaneous tunnels takes time. Patients can become discouraged over this initial recuperative phase and should be encouraged and reassured during this period.

Liposuction can be used for non-cosmetic applications[5]. Among them, lipomas can be safely aspirated using liposuction techniques. Small, soft lipomas are more amenable to liposuction extraction than large, fibrous lipomas. Axillary hyperhidrosis can be lessened by liposuction. A technique is used in which the cannula's open port is directed towards the subcutaneous dermis, designed to remove the excessively functioning sweat glands. Excessive fat can cause problems with skin maceration and hygiene. Liposuction can be used to improve skin folding.

MASSAGE AND ENDERMOLOGIE

Therapeutic benefits of massage have been widely touted in the lay medical literature. A variety of massage techniques exist and patients attest to the pleasurable aspect and temporary increase in a feeling of well-being. Massage is indicated for the treatment of chronic edema[10-12], traumatic and surgical scars[13], muscular tenderness and soreness, and sports-related injuries. Endermologie is a proprietary term which describes massage of skin and underlying subcutaneous fat with the use of an instrument that moves the skin between a series of motorized rollers. These vacuum-assisted massage systems have been claimed to improve body contour and skin texture, lessen cellulite and develop over-all body shape. Results of studies using these machines have shown slight improvements after completing 7 to 14 sessions. The long-lasting effectiveness of these instruments is unknown[14]. A 1-year clinical outcome study update[15] showed little improvement.

CHEMICAL PEELING FOR THE BODY

Many benefits can be obtained by chemical peeling of the face; however, less data are available on chemical peels for the body. α-Hydroxy acids and topical tretinoin are the mainstays of photodamage treatment and can be used on a daily basis as a mild chemical peel to improve body skin. Various α-hydroxy acids including glycolic, lactic, tartaric and citric acids have been promoted as skin rejuvenation compounds. β-Hydroxy acids and salicylic acid[16] have been used for this purpose as well. All have keratolytic effects and act as moisturizers. Glycolic acid is by far the most extensively studied of these acids. It appears to increase dermal glycosoaminoglycans and increase elastic fibers and collagen, especially when used for long periods of time in higher concentrations. Patients should gradually work up to higher concentrations of glycolic acid to avoid irritation. Salicylic acid, a β-hydroxy acid, has shown improvement in resurfacing the skin of the body, particularly the back of the hands[17,18]. Caution must be used when non-facial skin is chemically peeled. A medium-depth or deep chemical peel should not be used on the body as body skin[19] has less adnexae essential for healing. Complications from chemical peeling on the body include scarring, persistent erythema, hyper- and hypopigmentation, and irregular results.

HYPERHIDROSIS

Excessive sweating is a troublesome condition for some women. The most troubling areas include the palms, axillae, soles and forehead. Liposuction techniques and cold steel surgical excision of axillary skin have been used successfully for hyperhidrosis in the past[20]; however, the use of botulinum A toxin (Botox) has been a recent development[21-24]. Botox is injected subcutaneously in the areas of increased sweating such as axillae, palms or soles. Botox is carefully placed in the dermis, at 1-cm intervals with 2 units of Botox used with every intradermal injection. Approximately 50 units per axillary vault is required for the initial treatment, and palms may require up to 100 units each. This procedure is highly effective, and if missed or unresponsive areas are encountered, it may be necessary to retreat at 1 month. The Minor starch test should be used prior to Botox treatment and following the initial treatment, to document areas of unresponsiveness. Botox treatment of hyperhidrosis usually lasts 3–6 months. It is hoped that multiple treatments over a 1-year period may

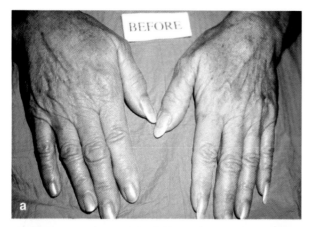

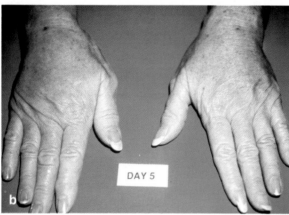

Figure 1 (a) Patient's dorsum of the hand before fat transplantation. Note the irregular texture on the dorsum of the hands and the prominence of dermal veins. (b) Fat transplantation to the back of the hand, showing an improvement in appearance with less noticeable skin irregularities and decreased prominence of veins. Photographs courtesy of W.P. Coleman III

result in a long-lasting decrease in excessive sweating. Expertise in Botox injections should be obtained before practitioners begin this therapy. Patients must be well apprised of the risk of temporary muscular weakness, particularly of the intrinsic muscles of the hand, and antibody formation against the botulinum A exotoxin protein, which may make treatments ineffective.

SCLEROTHERAPY

Prominent telangiectasias of the legs and excessive varicosities of the lower leg veins cause patients great concern. 'Spider veins' cause women embarrassment, and protuberant veins may be uncomfortable and painful. The incidence of telangiectatic leg veins in America is 29–41%, with varicose veins estimated at 10–20%[25]. Destruction can be accomplished by electricity, laser surgery and lesional injections.

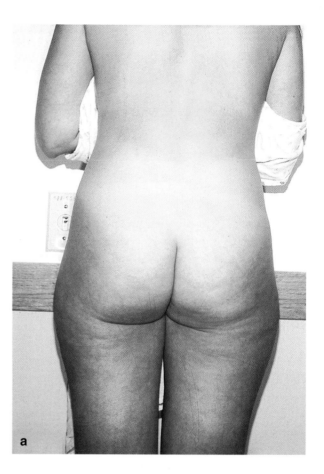

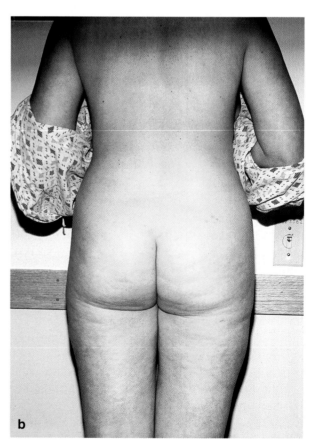

Figure 2 (a) Preoperative adiposity. (b) Improvement following tumescent liposuction

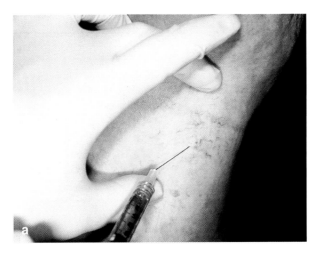

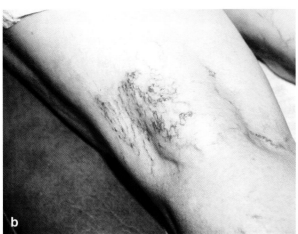

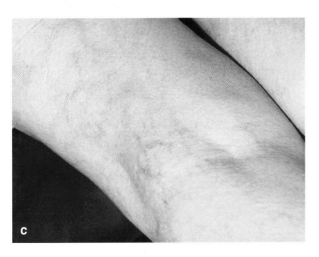

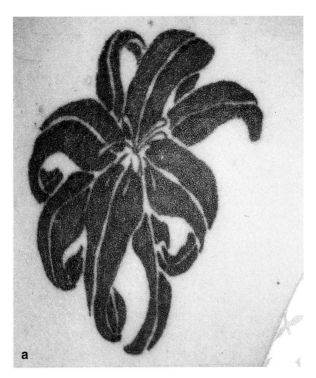

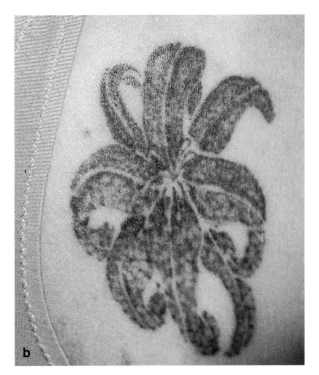

Figure 3 (a) Injection of hypertonic saline sclerosant solution into 'spider veins'. (b) Lower-extremity telangiectasias amenable to sclerotherapy. (c) Improvement of telangiectasias following sclerotherapy

Figure 4 (a) Preoperative view of a tattoo. (b) Lightening following one Nd : YAG laser treatment session

Sclerotherapy utilizes a sclerosing solution injected into the telangiectatic or varicose vein, followed by compression. This sclerosant solution causes necrosis and collapse of the vein with subsequent fibrosis. Typically, multiple treatments are necessary.

Sclerotherapy techniques can be used for both superficial and deep veins[26]. Patients with varicose veins need careful preoperative evaluation and may include a Doppler examination[27], photoplethysmography[28], or a duplex ultrasound examination. Advanced phlebologists can assist patients in the

Table 1   Sclerosant solutions

Sclerosant	Type	Advantages	Disadvantages	Treatment concentrations
Hypertonic saline	osmotic agent	non-allergic, commonly employed	painful upon injection, cutaneous necrosis	12–23.4% telangiectatic veins 20–23.4% reticular veins 23.4% varicose veins
Polidocanol (Aethoxyskerol)	urethane detergent	not painful, little risk of cutaneous ulceration	not approved for use in the USA	0.25–0.75% telangiectatic veins 0.5–1% reticular veins 1–3% varicose veins
Sodium tetradecyl sulfate (Sotraderol)	long-chain fatty acid	approved for use in the USA, less painful than hypertonic saline	skin necrosis, hyperpigmentation, rare anaphylactic reactions	0.1–0.3% telangiectatic veins 0.1–0.5% reticular veins 0.5–3% varicose veins

treatment of varicose veins by using a variety of sclerotherapy or ambulatory phlebectomy methods[29]. Superficial telangiectasias can be improved by the injection of a variety of sclerosing solutions (Table 1). Each sclerosing solution has its own advantages and disadvantages associated with side-effects[30]. Post-sclerotic pigmentation, pain with injection and intertelangiectatic matting following treatment are frequently seen. Less common side-effects include bruising around the injection site or contact dermatitis and blistering due to tape adhesions used in compression. Rare complications are intravascular hematoma and superficial thrombophlebitis. Extremely rare (but major) complications include inadvertent arterial injection, systemic allergic reaction and pulmonary embolism following deep vein thrombosis.

When beginning sclerotherapy, the degree of discomfort should be ascertained from injections by injecting one or two small sites. It is advisable to inject patients lying down to minimize vasovagal reactions. Successful treatment of leg veins is dependent on assessment for deeper valve incompetence or deeper varicosities. Optimal correction of superficial telangiectasia cannot occur without treatment of deeper varicose veins. Patients should return in 4–6 weeks to compare the test site with pretreatment photographs and pretreatment documentation.

Sclerotherapy should begin with treatment of larger phlebectasias proceeding to the smaller branching sites. With the patient in a supine position, a 1- or 3-ml syringe filled with sclerosing solution and a 30G needle is inserted bevel-up at a 30° angle (Figure 3). Helpful aids include the use of a magnifying lens and stretching the patient's skin between fingers of the non-dominant hand. Great care is needed to master the precise skill and touch required to place the 30G needle within the vessel.

A subtle sensation of the needle entering the telangiectasia can be felt. A helpful tip to ensure that the needle is present well within the telangiectasia is to inject a burst of air into the vein prior to administration of the sclerosant. This is accomplished by filling just the tip of the needle with a tiny amount of air so that, when the needle penetrates into the telangiectasia, air is initially injected which results in a clearing of blood from the vessel, demonstrating that the needle is within the telangiectasia. When certain that the needle is well within the telangiectasia, small amounts of the sclerosing solution are gently passed. Care must be taken not to extravasate the sclerosant. The key to non-extravasation is a very slow injection of the sclerosant and minimal volume and duration of the injection.

Immediately following injection, the treated area is gently massaged. This massage helps to distribute the sclerosing solution and is the first step in compression. Following massage, cotton balls or 5 × 5 cm gauzes are taped onto the injection sites using elastic surgical tape. Patients are encouraged to wear compression hose (30–40 mmHg) for 2–4 weeks following sclerotherapy. Treatment intervals for sclerotherapy are generally at 1–2 months.

AMBULATORY PHLEBECTOMY

Ambulatory phlebectomy treats varicose veins by extracting them through small incisions in the skin[31]. The technique uses specialized hooks, clamps and probes and is minimally invasive[32]. The technique extracts the varicosities segmentally through small openings. Multiple surgical sites are needed, owing to the fibrous tethers holding the veins to their surrounding adventitia. Although the technique has historical roots in ancient

Rome, the Swiss dermatologist Robert Muller developed the modern technique in 1966[31].

Preoperative evaluation involves a complete physical examination of the venous system of the lower extremity. Knowledge of venous anatomy is essential. Duplex ultrasound scanning of the varicose veins assists in proper patient assesment[33], and transillumination has significantly enhanced the success and ease of the procedure[34]. Local (1% xylocaine with epinephrine) or tumescent anesthesia[35] is used prior to puncturing the skin with a blood lancet or number 11 scalpel blade. Phlebectomy hooks and forceps are used to grasp the vein and exteriorize it. A probe may help to trace the vein's course. The vein is segmentally removed by cutting, tearing or dissection. Following the segmental 'harvesting', the patient wears compression bandages and elastic compression hose, usually for a period of less than 10 days[36]. The technique affords excellent cosmesis and is safe and effective.

LASER SURGERY

Vascular lesions in women can respond very well to laser surgery. Ample literature documents the excellent treatment of port-wine stains with the flash lamp-pumped pulsed dye laser (FLPPDL). This laser produces laser light with a 585 nm wavelength and a pulse duration of 450 ns. Selective photocoagulation of the vessels occurs, owing to the short pulse width, which allows destruction of the blood vessel without thermal damage to the surrounding tissue. Treatment of port-wine stains with the pulse style laser is associated with post-treatment purpura. The purple to gray discoloration, which commonly lasts 1–2 weeks on the face, often lasts longer when treatment is confined to the body. Four to five treatment sessions are frequently needed in order to achieve maximal response. Women with darker skin types are not as effectively treated with the FLPPDL, as melanin competes for the wavelength of the laser light. Other vascular lesions amenable to laser surgery include cherry angiomas, striae rubra, poikiloderma of Civatte and erythematous hypertrophic scars.

Newer developments in the treatment of vascular lesions include pulsed dye lasers which have longer pulse durations. These may be used to treat larger vessels including fine telangiectasias on the lower extremity not amenable to sclerotherapy, owing to their small size[37]. Lasers of 532 nm are also helpful for treatment of small telangiectasias (most commonly on the face) and have the benefit of producing no postoperative purpura. Instead,

an initial blanching of the lesion is seen. The use of other 532 nm wavelength lasers equipped with cooling devices and longer pulse durations has been found to be of benefit on selective lower extremity telangiectasias, provided they are small enough[38]. The long pulse alexandrite laser (755 nm) has been reported to improve leg veins[39]. Several treatment sessions may be necessary.

Laser therapy of tattoos has been found to be safe and effective (Figure 4). The most well-documented improvements have occurred with the use of the Q-switched neodymium: yttrium–aluminum–garnet Nd : YAG or Q-switched ruby laser in the treatment of homemade India-ink tattoos. These lasers produce high-intensity light, which is well absorbed by carbon particles with some absorption by melanin and minimal absorption by oxyhemoglobin. In this manner, selective treatment of the tattoo pigment occurs with these intense lasers. Several treatment sessions are often necessary for maximal lightening of the tattoo. Lasers of differing wavelengths may be necessary to treat women's tattoos that contain different colored pigments. Studies show that the alexandrite laser (with a wavelength of 755 nm) may be used to treat black or deep blue tattoos, is moderately effective for green and blue pigment, and minimally effective for red pigments[40–42].

Certain benign pigmented lesions respond well to laser therapy. Pigmented lesions commonly treated with visible light lasers include nevus of Ito[43], solar lentigines and flat seborrheic keratoses. A variety of lasers are used for treating benign pigmented lesions with the most common being the Q-switched Nd : YAG laser (frequency doubled at 532 nm) or the Q-switched ruby laser. The alexandrite laser and the copper vapor laser have also been used to treat benign pigmented lesions.

Cutaneous laser resurfacing using newer carbon dioxide lasers on the body has been associated with poor outcomes and irregular results[44]. Scarring, hypo- and hyperpigmentation, persistent erythema and other undesirable side-effects have been seen when the carbon dioxide laser is used on non-facial sites. The erbium laser[45–49] has shown some improvement when used on the skin of the neck in females in an attempt to improve wrinkling and dyschromia. The use of the erbium laser on non-facial skin may be helpful in improving actinic keratoses and seborrheic keratoses.

Good scientific data are now available to document the effectiveness of lasers in producing a long-lasting reduction in hair growth on face and body sites. The use of these lasers is reviewed in Chapter 49.

CONCLUSIONS

Several dermatological therapies and dermatological surgery procedures are available to assist the patient in body rejuvenation. Soft tissue augmentation and fat transplantation can assist with body rejuvenation. Liposuction can effectively remove areas of localized adiposity and is also indicated for non-cosmetic indications. Sclerotherapy is an elegant procedure commonly used to improve lower-extremity telangiectasia and varicosity. Cutaneous laser surgery can treat vascular and pigmented lesions as well as tattoos and unwanted hair. Body rejuvenation is possible through modern dermatological surgical techniques.

REFERENCES

1. DeLustro F. Immunology of injectable collagen in human subjects. *J Dermatol Surg* 1988;14 (suppl 1):49
2. Abrams HL, Lauber JS. Hand rejuvenation: state of the art. *Dermatol Clin* 1990;8:553–61
3. Peer LA. Loss of weight and volume in fat grafts with postulation of 'cell survival theory.' *Plast Reconstr Surg* 1950;5:217
4. Coleman SR. Long-term survival of fat transplants: controlled demonstrations. *Aesthetic Plast Surg* 1995;19:421–5
5. Flynn TC, Narins RS. Pre-operative evaluation of the liposuction patient. *Dermatol Clin* 1999;17: 729–34
6. Lillis PJ. Liposuction of the arms. *Dermatol Clin* 1999;17:783–97
7. Lack EB. Contouring the female buttocks. *Dermatol Clin* 1999;17:815–22
8. Klein JA. Anesthesia formulation of tumescent solutions. *Dermatol Clin* 1999;17:751–9
9. Ostad A, Kazeyama N, Moy RL. Tumescent anesthesia with a lidocaine dose of 55 mg/kg is safe for liposuction. *Dermatol Surg* 1996;22:921–7
10. Ko DS, Lerner R, Klose G, Cosim B. Effective treatment of lymphoedema of the extremities. *Arch Surg* 1998;133:452–8
11. Williams A. Lymphoedema. *Prof Nurse* 1997;12: 645–8
12. Ryan TJ, Mortimer PS, Jones RL. Lymphatics of the skin. Neglected but important. *Int J Dermatol* 1986;25:411–19
13. Beatty RC, Hestal BM. Guidelines in the management of traumatic scars and surgical incisions. *Semin Ophthalmol* 1998;13:171–6
14. Chang P, Wiseman J, Jacob T, *et al.* Non-invasive mechanical body contouring (Endermologie). A one year clinical outcome study update. *Aesthetic Plast Surg* 1998;22:145–53
15. Ersek RA, Mann EE II, Salisbury S, Salisbury AV. Non-invasive mechanical body contouring: a preliminary clinical outcome study. *Aesthetic Plast Surg* 1997;21:61–7
16. Vide DG, Bergfeld WF. Cosmetic use of alpha-hydroxy acids. *Cleve Clin J Med* 1997;64:327–9
17. Swinehart JM. Salicylic acid ointment peeling of the hands and forearms. Effective non-surgical removal of pigmented lesions and actinic damage. *J Dermatol Surg Oncol* 1992;18:495–8
18. Matarasso SL, Hanke CW, Alster TS, *et al.* Cutaneous resurfacing. *Dermatol Clin* 1997;15:569–82
19. Matarasso SL, Salman SM, Glogan RG, *et al.* The role of chemical peeling in the treatment of photo damaged skin. *J Dermatol Surg Oncol* 1990;16: 945–54
20. Stolman LP. Treatment of hyperhidrosis. *Dermatol Clin* 1998;16:863–9
21. Schnider P, Binder M, Kittler H, *et al.* A randomized, double-blind, placebo-controlled trial of botulinum A toxin for severe axillary hyperhidrosis. *Br J Dermatol* 1999;140:677–80
22. Glogau RG. Botulinum A neurotoxin for axillary hyperhidrosis. No sweat Botox. *Dermatol Surg* 1998;24:817–19
23. Odderson IR. Hyperhidrosis treated by botulinum A exotoxin. *Dermatol Surg* 1998;24:1237–41
24. Shelley WB, Talkanin NY, Shelley ED. Botulinum toxin therapy for palmar hyperhidrosis. *J Am Acad Dermatol* 1998;38:227–9
25. Engel A, Johnson ML, Hayes SG. Health effects of sunlight exposure in the United States: results from the first national health and nutrition examination survey 1971–74. *Arch Dermatol* 1988;124:72–9
26. Weiss RA, Weiss MA. Sclerotherapy in Wheeland RG, ed. *Cutaneous Surgery.* Philadelphia: WB Saunders, 1994:951–81
27. Weiss RA, Weiss MA. Doppler ultrasound findings in reticular veins of the thigh subdermic lateral venous system and implications for sclerotherapy. *Dermatol Surg Oncol* 1993;19:947–51
28. Weiss RA. Evaluation of the venous system by Doppler ultrasound and photoplethysmography or light reflection rheography before sclerotherapy. *Semin Dermatol* 1993;12:78–87
29. Guidelines of care for sclerotherapy treatment of varicose and telangiectatic leg veins. American Academy of Dermatology. *J Am Acad Dermatol* 1996;34:523–8
30. Weiss RA, Weiss MA. Incidence of side effects in the treatment of telangiectasias by compression sclerotherapy: hypertonic saline vs. polidocanol. *J Dermatol Surg Oncol* 1990;16:800–4
31. Ricci S. Ambulatory phlebectomy. Principles and evolution of the method. *Dermatol Surg* 1998;24: 459–64
32. Weiss RA, Weiss MA. Ambulatory phlebectomy compared to sclerotherapy for varicose and telangiectatic veins: indications and complications. *Adv Dermatol* 1996;11:3–16

33. Georgiev M. The pre-operative duplex examination. *Dermatol Surg* 1998;24:433–40

34. Weiss RA, Goldman MP. Transillumination mapping prior to ambulatory phlebectomy. *Dermatol Surg* 1998;24:447–50

35. Cohn MS, Sieger E, Goldman S. Ambulatory phlebectomy using the tumescent technique for local anesthesia. *Dermatol Surg* 1995;21:315–18

36. Neumann MA, DeRoos KP, Veraart JCJM. Muller's ambulatory phlebectomy and compression. *Dermatol Surg* 1998;24:471–4

37. Dover JS, Sadick NS, Goldman MP. The role of lasers and light sources in the treatment of leg veins. *Dermatol Surg* 1999;25:328–36

38. Massey RA, Katz BE. Successful treatment of spider leg veins with a high-energy, long-pulse, frequency-doubled neodymium : YAG laser (HELP-G). *Dermatol Surg* 1999;25:677–80

39. McDaniel DH, Ash K, Lord J, *et al*. Laser therapy of spider leg veins: clinical evaluation of a new long pulsed Alexandrite laser. *Dermatol Surg* 1999;25:52–8

40. Fitzpatrick RE, Goldman MP, Ruiz-Esparza J. Use of the alexandrite laser (755 nm, 100 nsec) for tattoo pigment removal in an animal model. *J Am Acad Dermatol* 1993;28:745–50

41. Dozier SE, Diven DG, Jones D, *et al*. The Q-switched Alexandrite laser's effects on tattoos in guinea pigs and harvested human skin. *Dermatol Surg* 1995;21:237–40

42. Alster TS. Q-switched alexandrite laser treatment (755 nm) of professional and amateur tattoos. *J Am Acad Dermatol* 1995;33:69–73

43. Michel S, Hohenleutner U, Baumler W, Landthaler M. (Q-switched ruby laser in dermatologic therapy. Use and indications). *Hautarzzi* 1997;48:462–70

44. Rather D, Tse Y, Marchell N, *et al*. Cutaneous laser resurfacing. *J Am Acad Dermatol* 1999;41:365–89

45. Goldberg DJ, Meine JG. Treatment of photoaged neck skin with the pulsed erbium : YAG laser. *Dermatol Surg* 1998;24:619–21

46. Alster TS. Clinical and histologic evaluation of six erbium : YAG lasers for cutaneous resurfacing. *Lasers Surg Med* 1999;24:87–92

47. Adrian RM. The erbium : YAG laser: facts and fiction. *Dermatol Surg* 1998;24:296

48. Goldman MP, Fitzpatrick RE, Manuskiatti W. Laser resurfacing of the neck with the erbium : YAG laser. *Dermatol Surg* 1999;25:164–7; discussion 167–8

49. Goldman MP, Fitzpatrick RE, Manuskiatti W. Laser resurfacing of the neck with the erbium : YAG laser. *Dermatol Surg* 1999;25:164–7

Body repair

Doris Maria Hexsel

52

Cellulite, stretch marks, telangiectasia and scars are common clinical esthetic conditions that can affect the bodies of girls and women, causing significant distress. The demand for consultation and effective therapeutic treatments for these conditions is increasing.

CELLULITE

The term cellulite originated in the French literature and has the following synonyms: *cellulalgie*[1,2], *infiltrat cellulalgiques*, fibrositis, *weichteilrheumatismus*, *pannikulose*, panniculitis and gynoid lipodystrophy[3]. Nürnberger and Müller[4] find the term 'dermopanniculosis' the most appropriate, from the histopathological point of view.

Clinical description

Known and used by physicians and lay people, the term cellulite is used to characterize unsightly lesions or alterations in the skin surface that tend to be chronic and give the skin an 'orange peel', 'quilted' or 'mattress' appearance[1,2]. The orange peel phenomenon is caused by pronounced follicular openings, sometimes with follicular keratosis[5]. The quilted phenomenon is due to the fibrous retinacula that connect the skin and fascia between the fat lobes[5–7]. It affects the thighs and buttocks as well as the abdomen and arms, the areas where, coincidentally, adiposities occur in women and an increase in subcutaneous fat may be found[1]. Cellulite can be found in all age groups and in both sexes (Figure 1). It is more frequently found in women, particularly in obese women, and is considered a normal manifestation of obesity[6]. The fat is divided into lobes[8] by a true connective structure. The fat lobes of women are larger and more rectangular than those of men[1,4,6,7]. These anatomic differences in this structure between men and women explain the quilted appearance characteristic of cellulite and help to account for the greater incidence in women[4].

The skin surface alterations that characterize the clinical state of cellulite are predominantly depressed compared with the normal skin surface of the affected area, but may also be raised. These alterations are rounded, oval, linear or varied in form, and the number varies from one to multiple (Figure 2). They have the same coloration and consistency as normal skin. Usually there are no symptoms. However, some patients complain of a feeling of heaviness and aching in the areas affected by cellulite.

Cellulite may be classified into four stages[4]:

(1) *Stage 0* is the situation in which the skin on the thighs and buttocks is smooth while a subject is standing or lying. The pinch test throws the skin into folds and furrows, but not into the quilt appearance. This stage is common in slim, heavy-armed women and in men who do not have a deficiency in androgens.

(2) *Stage I* is the condition in which the skin surface is smooth while a subject stands or lies, but in which the pinch test is positive for the quilt phenomenon. This is normal and typical for women, but in men is a sign of deficiency of androgens.

(3) *Stage II* is the condition in which the skin surface is smooth while a subject is lying, but shows the quilt phenomenon (dermopanniculosis deformans) spontaneously when standing. It is common in obese women over 35–40 years of age. It is seldom seen in men deficient in androgens.

(4) *Stage III* is the condition in which the quilt phenomenon (dermopanniculosis deformans) is spontaneously positive in both lying and standing positions. It is very common after the menopause and in obesity. Seldom is it seen in men deficient in androgens.

The standing position, muscle contraction, skin folding, or pinching of the affected area along with moderate lighting by dicroic lamps focused from above to below ease the visualization of the lesions. The prone position, muscle relaxation and intense environmental light directed at the affected region hinder visualization.

The patient should be examined in the standing position with relaxed muscles. From the clinical point of view, cellulite may be objectively classified as follows:

(1) *Degree 0* There are no alterations to the skin surface.

(2) *Degree 1*   There are no alterations to the skin surface; the quilted or orange peel appearance of the skin becomes visible by the pinch test or muscular contraction.

(3) *Degree 2*   The quilted or orange peel appearance of the skin is evident to the naked eye, without the help of any manipulation.

(4) *Degree 3*   The same alterations are present as are described in degree 2, with raised areas and nodules.

Two clinical conditions that frequently accompany and exacerbate cellulite are localized adiposities and flaccidity. The areas most affected by cellulite, the thighs and buttocks, are also areas where there is an increase in localized fat[6]. The clinical manifestation of localized adiposities is an increase in the ill-defined diffuse volume, symmetrical and bilateral, due to an increase in the adipose tissue. It is a widespread physiological condition in women, and is frequently aggravated by weight gain. Obesity promotes weight increase and, when a return to the original baseline weight is achieved, an increased accumulation of fat is observable[9]. This suggests the existence of fat deposit areas or areas predisposed to fatty accumulation[10]. Greater thickness in the subcutaneous fat may be seen by histopathological examination and measured by special instruments or by the pinch test (Figure 3)[9].

The increase of adipose tissue within the fat lobes imposes tension and traction forces on the upper adjacent skin, causing an effect similar to that of a stuffed quilt. The fibrous septa ascend vertically through the upper layer of the fat to become attached to the underside of the dermis of the skin[8]. The tension resulting from the increased volume of fat in the lobes causes the raising of the skin surface, by the projection of the subcutaneous fat into the reticular and papillary dermis[11]. The traction exercised by the tangential connective septa on the skin is responsible for the depressed skin alteration. Flaccidity is caused by a block ptosis of the skin and the subcutaneous structures, which become permanently hyperdistended and loose.

The affected area has a draped appearance (Figure 4). It is frequently located in the lower front and inner parts of the thighs and the inner surface of the arms, regions where the skin probably has less retentive capacity and suffers the mechanical action of weight exerted by the adipose tissue and by the other subcutaneous structures. The weight of these structures increases the effect of the force of gravity, working on progressively less elastic skin, causing alterations to the skin surface in these areas

seen as laxity and looseness, visible to the naked eye. The clinical manifestations of flaccidity clearly diminish without the action of the force of gravity, for example, when the block of skin and subcutaneous tissue is stretched in the direction toe to head or when the subject lies down (Figure 5).

It is more frequently found in patients over 30 years old or after sudden weight loss. Skin is elastic and the dermis is mainly responsible for its mechanical properties[12]. Excessive skin redundancy may be observed in cases of significant weight fluctuations or weight loss[13,14]. This may be related to the regional characteristics of the skin and to phenomena related to aging, such as decrease in skin elasticity[14], with a subsequent decrease in contraction after distension, a decrease in the retentive capacity of the skin and an increase in the cutaneous area.

Histopathology

Reports of the following histopathological findings are common[5,7,15]. The epidermis is essentially normal. In the dermis, the thickness is normal, with a slight perivascular lymphocytic infiltrate; there is slight edema in the superficial dermis; elastic fibers are mainly normal with a very slight focal reduction; there is vacuolization of the cells of piloerector muscles; and there is dilatation of superficial lymphatic vessels. In the subcutis, there are larger fat cells. No fibrosis, no sclerosis, no granuloma formation and no inflammation have been found. The fibrous septa may be involved[3]. The present author has found the same involvement in the few deep biopsies performed to study the depressed lesions of cellulite. The fibrous septa found were rigid and difficult to stretch (Figure 6).

Differential diagnosis

Differential diagnoses are localized adiposities[5] or alterations in the surface after liposuction and other traumas. Linear scleroderma may also be considered in unilateral cases.

Treatment

The discrete alterations in the surface of the quilted appearance corresponding to degree-I cellulite should be treated by hygienic–dietary measures, with special emphasis on weight loss[11] and the treatment of the clinical conditions that may be the cause of weight gain and fluid retention, although excess fat in this area is often difficult to eradicate by dieting[6]. Physical exercise and massage for

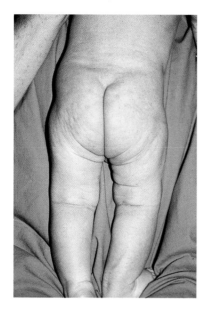

Figure 1 Two-month-old infant, presenting the 'quilt' appearance on the buttock

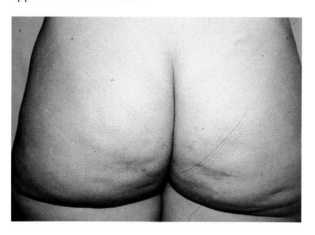

Figure 2 Clinical aspect of cellulite located in buttock area

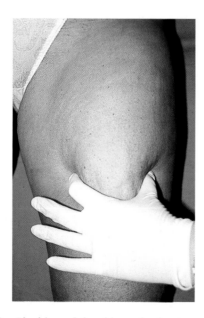

Figure 3 Pinching of the skin and subcutaneous tissue (pinch test)

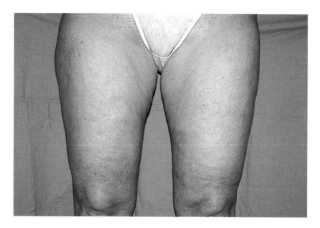

Figure 4 Clinical aspect of flaccidity

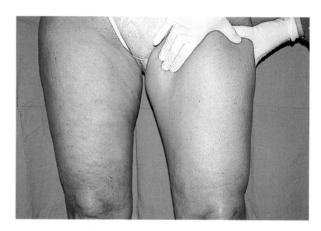

Figure 5 Stretching of a block of skin and subcutaneous tissue, diminishing the clinical aspect of flaccidity

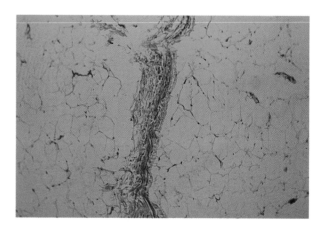

Figure 6 Thickened fibrous septa between the fat lobes. The fat cells are normal

lymphatic drainage[11], either manual or mechanical, may be equally useful. There is no proven evidence that either local or systemic medication or skin kneading (*endermologie*)[11] can directly affect the cellulite.

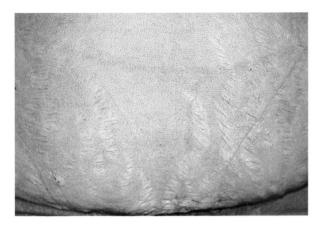

Figure 7   Old stretch mark shows the depressed, atrophic, stretched and wrinkled skin

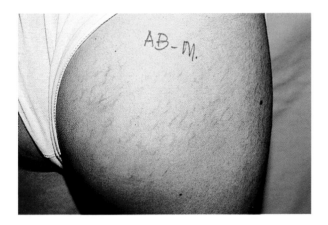

Figure 8   Recent stretch marks before treatment with superficial dermabrasions

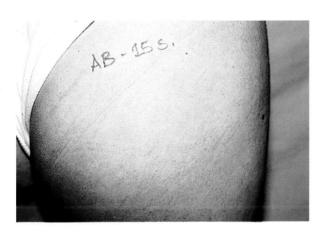

Figure 9   The same patient as in Figure 8, after 15 superficial dermabrasions

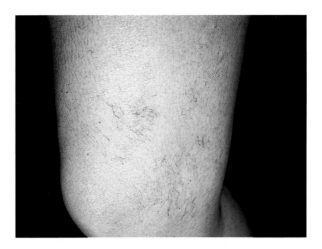

Figure 10   Telangectasia on the leg

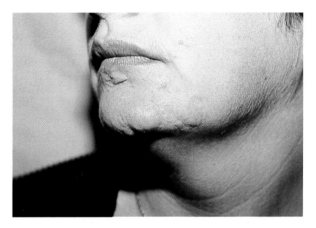

Figure 11   Scar resulting from car accident showing areas that are raised, depressed and retracted

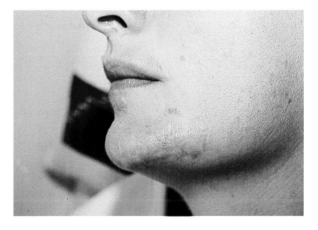

Figure 12   The same patient as in Figure 11, after treatment with synergic surgical techniques (subcision, soft tissue augmentation and intralesional corticoid administration)

Subcision is a simple surgical technique, originally described by Orentreich and Orentreich[16] in 1995, performed under local anesthesia, where subcutaneous fibrous septa are sectioned. The bruise formed by the procedure is desirable, to promote formation of new connective tissue. In 1997, Hexsel and Mazzuco[17] published the findings obtained from a study involving 46 patients, with moderate to severe alterations on thigh and buttock surfaces, treated as out-patients. The authors used the subcision technique at the level of the deep subcutaneous fat; they concluded that this was an efficacious technique for the treatment of these alterations. Inspection of the area with contracted gluteal muscles showed a worsening of many of these depressions, indicating the involvement of the fibrous septa of the superficial musculoaponeurotic system (SMAS)[17]. These data therefore indicate that subcision may be useful in the correction of such defects, since it sections the fibrous subcutaneous septa present in the anatomical basis of cellulite and those resulting from traumas such as liposuction[17].

Associated and exacerbating conditions, such as localized fat and flaccidity, may be treated surgically. Localized fat is effectively treated by liposuction[9,10]. Flaccidity may be treated by dermatolipectomy; however, the scars are large[9] and unsightly.

STRETCH MARKS

Synonyms are striae distensae and striae atrophicans.

Clinical description

Stretch marks are commonly found atrophic lesions that develop because of the rupture of the connective tissue due to mechanical structural stress[14,18]. In the initial phases, the epidermis has to accommodate and adapt to these alterations in spite of maintaining its normal histological structure. Its histogenesis is related to various factors[18–23], and is associated with an increased production of glucocorticoids by the adrenal[18,20].

Women are most commonly affected and the progressive stretch provoked by spurts of growth during adolescence, pregnancy[18,23], obesity or weight gain predisposes the skin to the development of stretch marks[22]. They occur in 90% of pregnant women on the abdomen and/or breasts[19]. Pregnancy has been reported as the only physiological condition in which they can occur[19].

From a clinical and histological point of view, there are no significant differences between stretch marks of different etiology or localization, or between stretch marks of patients of different sex or age group. Basically they differ with time of evolution and are classified as recent or old[18,21,22]. They are similar to early and old scars, respectively[22–24]. Therefore, for clinical, histological and therapeutic purposes, the very simple classification in Table 1 is suggested. Stretch marks are considered narrow if up to 5 mm in width.

Table 1 Simple classification of stretch marks

Recent stretch marks
Narrow
Wide

Old stretch marks
Narrow
Wide

The skin is pink in recent stretch marks. They may be raised or irritable, with burning or itching, but soon become flat, smooth and reddish[18], without significant alterations in the skin surface[23]. Skin in an old stretch mark is atrophic[18–21] and has a depression on the surface, with the outbreak of fine wrinkles. Cutaneous atrophy is clinically characterized by paleness, loss of normal texture and absence of cutaneous adnexae, mainly hair follicles[21]. These characteristics of atrophy are permanent in stretch marks (Figure 7).

Histopathology

Histopathological findings suggest that stretch marks are scars. The epidermis may be normal in recent, and atrophic in old, stretch marks[18]. In the dermis the inflammatory process causes destruction of the collagen and elastic fibers characterized by the fragmentation of these fibers, with perivascular lymphohistiocyte infiltration and telangiectatic vessels[20–22]. There is regeneration of the destroyed dermic elements as a result of the tissue repair process. In this stage collagen bands lie parallel to the surface, intertwined with similarly arranged elastic fibers[20–22]. The elastic fibers may be either absent in the stretch mark, or in increased number, forming an extensive network of fibers parallel to the collagen bands[18,21,22].

The histological aspect of the old stretch mark is that of a scar. The epidermis is atrophied, with rectification of the dermis–epidermis junction[18–22], but it may be structurally preserved. The atrophy of the epidermis may be found in diffuse areas of old stretch marks or in focal areas.

Treatment

Abrasive epidermic methods, whether mechanical, chemical, electrosurgical or laser, improve atrophied, distended and wrinkled epidermis and also act on the dermis. They improve the common aspects between photodamaged skin and stretch marks. We believe that recent and old stretch marks require different treatment.

It is very important to identify and treat the etiological factors involved when treating recent stretch marks. Early therapeutic interventions may guarantee better results by preventing or at least minimizing the structural alterations in the epidermis that follow this stage, altering and hindering its complete evolution. However, interventions that may cause untreatable side-effects or complications are neither recommended nor justifiable at this stage, when the epidermis, in general, is still preserved. Recent stretch marks behave dynamically. Thus the therapeutic procedures suggested should preferably be repeated until their stabilization, which coincides with the disappearance of the pinkish-violet coloring. The skin is very fragile in recent wide stretch marks, and subject to laceration. Skin moisturizing is useful and the patient should be directed to avoid friction or trauma. Tretinoin and/or other retinoids are useful for recent narrow stretch marks[24]. Dermabrasion, performed very superficially and repeatedly, gives good results on recent narrow stretch marks (Figures 8 and 9).

Old stretch marks, narrow or wide, when small in number, may be treated with surgical methods that cause epidermic contraction, besides dermic alterations. Trichloroacetic acid (TCA) and phenol both with or without occlusion, electrosurgery and laser are efficacious methods for the treatment of the atrophic and wrinkled aging skin[25–30]. These treatments within the lesion limits may produce improvements at this stage. However, these methods are not recommended in cases where the lesions are numerous, because of the risks of unsightly complications that may appear in the postoperative period.

Subcision may be useful when the stretch mark surface is very depressed, because it favors the formation of neocollagen, when performed in the dermis. Subcision is not very effective as an isolated method, because it is a procedure that does not structurally alter the epidermis[16] responsible for the unsightly appearance of the stretch marks.

Better therapeutic results are obtained at the recent stage of narrow stretch marks and at the late stage of wide stretch marks, when they are few in number.

The possibility of test sites should also be considered, as it allows the patient and the physician to assess beforehand the results that may be obtained with these techniques.

TELANGIECTASIA

A synonym is varix (plural varices).

Clinical description

The term telangiectasia was suggested by Von Graf in 1807 to describe a superficial vessel of the skin visible to the human eye[31,32], represented mainly by abnormal permanent dilatation of venules, but also, at times, of capillaries and arterioles[33]. The diameter of telangiectases is 0.1–1.0 mm[31,32]. Varicose veins measure more than 1 mm in diameter[31]. Both may arise from larger vessels (Figure 10)[34].

Regarding its clinical appearance and morphology telangiectasia may be classified into four types: sinus or simple (linear); arborizing; spider or star; and punctiform (papular)[31,32] or into three types: nodular; spider; and linear[35].

Acquired telangiectasia is generally an important diagnostic sign seen in many conditions. In collagenosis it is associated with other signs of inflammation. It is also prominent in acquired peripheral vascular disease. Generalized essential telangiectasia is most frequent in women in middle age[35]. On the body, telangiectases on the legs are a frequently cited motive for medical consultation. They are different from those on the face in both pathogenesis and vessel type[31]. They are widespread and directly associated with underlying varicose veins. Women between the ages of 30 and 50 are most commonly affected[31,35]. Pregnancy, the use of birth control pills, long hours of standing or sitting required for the patient's occupation and the incidence of the condition within the patient's family are commonly found in the personal history of patients[34]. Interestingly, pregnant women often develop telangiectases on the legs within a few weeks of conception. Pregnant women and those taking birth control pills have been shown to have an increase in the distensibility of vein walls.

The most common symptoms are aching and a sensation of fatigue of affected legs[34]. They worsen with prolonged standing[34].

Histopathology

Dilated blood channels are found in the upper part of a normal dermal stroma with a single endothelial cell lining, no muscularis and no adventitia[31,33].

Treatment

Many methods for treating all types of telangiectasia are described: electrosurgery, lasers, dermabrasion, medical treatments and sclerotherapy[31]. All these treatments are available and useful in the treatment of telangiectasia on particular areas of the body.

Treatment for telangiectases is most often sought when these occur on the legs, and sclerotherapy is the most frequent choice of treatment. A wide variety of substances have been used to obliterate both varicose veins and telangiectases. These foreign substances, injected into the lumen of vessels, cause thrombosis and subsequent fibrosis[31]. The best results are obtained on superficial linear or radiating vessels of the lower extremities. Currently, numerous sclerosing agents are used. These are hypertonic, detergent or chemical irritants: hypertonic saline 23.4%; combination dextrose (250 mg/ml) and NaCl (100 mg/ml) (Sclerodex); polidocanol (POL) (Aethoxysklerol) 0.5%, 1%, 2% or 3%; sotradecol (STS) 1% or 3%; sodium morrhuate; polyiodinated iodine (Varigloban) 2–12%, 72%; and glycerol with chromium salt (Scleremo)[34]. The most frequent side-effect reported with sclerosing agents is postsclerosing hyperpigmentation, which is temporary. This subject has been previously studied and many side-effects and complications, both common and rare, have been described[34,36,37]. Lasers can be used in one to four treatments. Good results are reported with long-pulsed dye and Photoderm lasers[38,39].

Telangiectases occurring on the neck and face are treated by different methods[32]. Lasers produce a high rate of clearance. Many lasers have been used; the Cooper vapor laser is reported as a good choice in cases of simple and arborizing facial telangiectasia[40].

SCARS

A synonym is cicatrix.

Clinical description and treatment

Scar formation is an attempt by an organism to restore its architecture. It is a lasting mark testifying to the healing of a wound or other morbid process. Although the psychological repercussion is comparable in scar carriers of both sexes, female patients more frequently seek therapeutic help to improve the appearance of the scar.

The clinical examination of a scar[41,42] involves the following: general appearance (perfect or imperfect), location, etiology, occurrences in the healing period, duration of evolution (which will determine whether it is old or recent), size, width, direction, shape and contours, level (atrophied, normotrophied, hypertrophied or keloid) and whether it is retractile or not. These are the outstanding

Table 2 The therapeutic techniques most frequently used in the treatment of the main features of scars

Large size, width and length
Serial excision
Z- or W-plasty
Skin grafts
Localization/direction contrary to force lines
Redirecting to a force line or natural furrow
Raised surface
Establish a waiting period
Intralesional infiltration with corticoid (triamcinolone)
Pressure therapy
Covering with silicone gel
Radiation therapy
Excision techniques
Depressed surface
Soft tissue augmentation techniques
Dermabrasion
Lasers
Subcision
Classical surgical treatments (excision, punch grafts, etc.)
Atrophy
Serial superficial dermabrasions
Cutaneous grafts of different thicknesses
Excision and/or Z- or W-plasty
Retraction
Subcision
Excision
Flap rotation
Grafting
Z- or W-plasty
Alopecia (baldness)
Transplantation with punch or micrografts
Serial or total surgical reduction
Flap rotation
Hyperchromia
Establish a waiting period
Topical depigmentation medications
Broad-spectrum sunscreen
Short-pulsed lasers
Hypo- or achromy
Establish a waiting period
Localized dermabrasion
Grafting with melanocyte transplant
Dermopigmentation
Multiple alterations
Diverse synergic techniques used in conjunction

characteristics. The skin that covers the scar should also be assessed. It may be normal or atrophied, with or without annexae. Regarding coloration, it may be achromatic, hypo- or hyperchromatic[41,42]. The skin surface of the scar may show a wide number of cutaneous lesions (telangiectases, tumors, ulcers, etc.). It is very important to feel and recognize the outstanding characteristics of a scar: those of which the patient complains as well as those most evident upon clinical examination[41].

Ideally, the opinion of the physician and the patient regarding these characteristics will coincide. These characteristics will guide the choice of treatment (Table 2)[41]. Scars may be corrected in order to improve their appearance and/or the function of the affected area[42]. In other cases, intervention is justified by the presence of marks or symptoms that disturb the patient. Each scar, like each patient, is unique and deserves individualized assessment and treatment[41]. Understanding the patient's dissatisfaction with a scar will help in the selection of the most adequate treatment[42]. In scar correction, invasive and non-invasive methods are described and may be useful[42].

Generally, scar intervention should take place after a stabilization period of 6 months to 1 year[41]. An exception should be made in cases of keloids and hypertrophic scars[43], where early intervention can guarantee better therapeutic success[41].

Hyperpigmentation in scars may be transitory but may be treated by using depigmentation substances, associated with sunblocks. Traumatic scars may sometimes show abnormal colorations due to the presence of the foreign materials that were not removed during the initial treatment. These foreign materials can be removed by dermabrasions or lasers[44–46]. Usually hypopigmentation is temporary, and thus does not require treatment. The following are regarded as permanent complications in scars: depigmentation, alopecia, retraction and atrophy.

The surgical techniques of grafting with melanocyte transplantation may be indicated to treat hypo- or achromic scars. Fallabela and other authors have published successful results with small, thin skin grafts in vitiligo and other hypochromic diseases[47–49]. Skin grafts with melanocyte transplantation may be successfully used in the treatment of scars. Dermopigmentation is an alternative that may be proposed in the correction of dyschromic scars.

Definitive alopecia occurs in hair-covered areas when the inflammatory process and/or necrosis had been produced at the follicle matrix level, thus sacrificing the hair follicles. Numerous modifications and refinements in hair transplantation have been reported and many surgical procedures may be useful: micrografts, minigrafts, square grafts, strip grafts, incisional slit grafting and minireductions[50].

The choice of surgical technique will depend especially on the sizes of donor and of recipient sites. Hair or single hair transplant by punch or micrografts may be carried out to restore hair to the bald area, if the patient has a donor area available[51]. Surgical reduction of the affected area may also be recommended. The scalp is not very elastic and this is a limiting factor if large bald areas need to be treated. In this case, serial surgical reductions may be chosen or even expanders used to ease the lifting of the scalp. Bald scar areas may be treated by rotation of flaps from an adjacent area[41].

Retraction in scars may be efficiently treated by subcision, a method that cuts subcutaneous fibrous septa using tribevelled or BD NoKor needles[14,15]. Subcision may be useful, either in isolation or in association with other procedures. Retraction may also be treated by conventional surgery.

Cutaneous atrophy is inevitable if the lesion that causes the scar extends beyond the subcutaneous tissue, because epithelium healing is difficult in deep tissues. An atrophic scar is thin and wrinkled[52]. Occasionally, or when in a small area, cutaneous atrophy may be treated with superficial and serial dermabrasion to induce new epithelium healing[45]. After a suitable healing period, the method can be repeated and additional dermabrasions can produce further improvement[45]. However, skin grafts of different thicknesses may be preferable.

The alterations of a depressed scar surface may be treated with filling techniques. Several filling materials – endogens or exogens, biological or non-biological – may be used, according to the recommendation and experience of the physician. Excision surgery, punch excision and grafts, dermabrasion[45] and lasers are also helpful.

Hypertrophic scars and keloids can appear early and may heal spontaneously in a few months. They are elevated, with excessive growth of fibrous tissue[52]. Some patients refer to symptoms such as pain and itching, both of which justify treatment. Triamcinolone is the preferred corticosteroid for intralesional treatment. Other treatments have been reported[43] and the most common are listed in Table 2. If the patient shows many outstanding features, synergic techniques can be used (Figures 11 and 12)[41].

Histopathology

Scars can be atrophic as well as hypertophic and both are histologically similar[21]. The main difference between them is the thickness of the scar[21].

Every recent scar is a new growth of connective tissue and has some characteristics seen in neoplasms: atypical proliferation of epithelium, fibrocytes and blood vessels[53]. The common histopathological findings in keloids and hypertrophic scars are fibroplasia, telangiectasia, inflammatory-cell infiltrate and mucin.

The three major features of scar tissue are as follows: collagen bundles run a fairly straight course parallel to the skin surface; small blood vessels extend perpendicularly between the epidermis and the subcutis; and elastic fibers either are absent or are thin and run parallel to the collagen bundles[53]. The hair follicles and sweat glands, the papillae and rete ridges may be absent.

CONCLUSION

Cellulite, stretch marks, telangiectasia and scars cause psychological and social discomfort, sometimes accompanied by other symptoms, especially in female patients. Although they are esthetic problems, they deserve careful medical assessment and suitable treatment.

REFERENCES

1. Scherwitz C, Braum-Falco O. So-called cellulite. *J Dermatol Surg Oncol* 1978;4:230–4
2. Segers AM, Abulafia J, Kriner J, Cortondo O. Celulitis. Estudio histopatológico e histoquímico de 100 casos. *Med Cut ILA* 1984;12:167–72
3. Ciporkin H, Paschoal LHC. Clínica da LDG. In Ciporkin H, Paschoal LHC, eds. *Atualização Terapêutica e Fisiopatogênica da Lipodistrofia Ginóide (LDG) 'Celulite'*. São Paulo: Santos, 1992:141–54
4. Nürnberger F, Müller G. So-called cellulite: an invented disease. *J Dermatol Surg Oncol* 1978;4:221–9
5. Braun-Falco O, Buddecke E, Karl HJ, *et al*. Zellulitis. Round-Table-Gespräch. *Med Klin* 1971;66:827–32
6. Burton JL, Cunliffe WJ. Subcutaneous fat. In Champion RH, Burton JL, Ebling FJG, eds. *Textbook of Dermatology*. Oxford: Blackwell, 1992;2140
7. Braun-Falco O, Scherwitz C. Zur histopathologie der sogenannten cellulitis. *Hautarzt* 1972;23:71–5
8. Salasche SJ, Bernstein G, Senkarik M. Superficial musculoaponeurotic system. In Salasche SJ, Bernstein G, Senkarik M, eds. *Surgical Anatomy of the Skin*. Norwalk: Appleton & Lange, 1988: 89–97
9. Coleman WP III. Liposuction. In Wheeland RG, ed. *Cutaneous Surgery*. Philadelphia: WB Saunders Company, 1994:549–67
10. Field LM, Narins RS. Liposuction surgery. In Epstein E, Epstein E Jr, eds. *Skin Surgery*. Philadelphia: WB Saunders Company, 1987:370–8
11. Draelos ZD, Marenus KD. Cellulite etiology and purported treatments. *Dermatol Surg* 1997;23: 1177–81
12. Archer CB. Functions of the skin. In Champion RH, Burton JL, Burns DA, Breathnach SM, eds. *Textbook of Dermatology*. Oxford: Blackwell, 1998;118
13. Matarasso A, Matarasso SL. When does your liposuction patient require an abdominoplasty? *Dermatol Surg* 1997;23:1151–60
14. Burton JL. Disorders of connective tissue. In Champion RH, Burton JL, Ebling FJG, eds. *Textbook of Dermatology*. Oxford: Blackwell, 1992: 1763–825
15. Braun-Falco O, Scherwitz C. Zur histopathologie der sogenannten cellulitis. *Hautarzt* 1972;23: 71–5
16. Orentreich DS, Orentreich N. Subcutaneous incisionless (subcision) surgery for the correction of depressed scars and wrinkles. *Dermatol Surg* 1995;21:543–9
17. Hexsel DM, Mazzuco R. Subcision: uma alternativa cirúrgica para a lipodistrofia ginóide ('celulite') e outras alterações do relevo corporal. *An bras Dermatol* 1997;72:27–32
18. Bittencourt-Sampaio S. *Striae atrophicae*. Thesis. Federal University of Rio de Janeiro, 1995
19. Pribanich S, Simpson FG, Held B, *et al*. Low-dose tretinoin does not improve striae distensae: a double-blind, placebo-controlled study. *Cutis* 1994; 54:121–4
20. Lever WF, Schaumburg-Lever G. Degenerative diseases. In Lever WF, Schaumburg-Lever G, eds. *Histopathology of the Skin*. Philadelphia: JB Lippincott, 1975:577–8
21. Ackerman BA. Fibrosing dermatitis. In Ackerman BA, ed. *Histologic Diagnosis of Inflammatory Skin Diseases*. Philadelphia: Lea & Febiger, 1978:748–55
22. Zheng P, Lavker RM, Kligman AM. Anatomy of striae. *Br J Dermatol* 1985;112:185–93
23. Alster TS. Laser treatment of scars and striae. In Alster TS, ed. *Manual of Cutaneous Laser Techniques*. Philadelphia: Lippincott-Raven, 1997:81–103
24. Kang S, Kim KJ, Griffiths CEM. Topical tretinoin (retinoic acid) improves early stretch marks. *Arch Dermatol* 1996;132:519–26
25. Gilchrest BA. A review of skin ageing and its medical therapy. *Br J Dermatol* 1996;135:867–75
26. Stuzin JM, Baker TJ, Gordon HL. Treatment of photoaging: facial chemical peeling (phenol and trichloroacetic acid) and dermabrasion. In McGrath MH, Turner ML, eds. *Clinics in Plastic Surgery – An International Quarterly – Dermatology for Plastic Surgeons*. Philadelphia: WB Saunders Company, 1993;20:9–25
27. Kligman AM, Baker TJ, Gordon HL. Long-term histologic follow-up of phenol face peels. *Plast Reconstr Surg* 1985;75:652–9

28. Roenigk RK, Brodland DG. Facial chemical peel. In Baran R, Maibach HI, eds. *Cosmetic Dermatology*. Baltimore: Williams & Wilkins, 1994:279–80

29. Glogau RG, Matarasso SL. Chemical peels (trichloroacetic acid and phenol). *Cosmetic Dermatol* 1995;13:263–76

30. Humphreys TR, Werth V, Dzubow L, Kligman A. Treatment of photodamaged skin with trichloroacetic acid and topical tretinoin. *J Am Acad Dermatol* 1996;34:638–44

31. Goldman MP, Bennett RG. Treatment of telangiectasia: a review. *J Am Acad Dermatol* 1987;17:167–82

32. Goldman MP, Weiss RA, Brody HJ, et al. Treatment of facial telangiectasia with sclerotherapy, laser surgery, and/or electrodesiccation: a review. *J Dermatol Surg Oncol* 1993;19:899–906

33. Ackerman AB. *Histologic Diagnosis of Inflammatory Skin Diseases: an Algorithmic Method Based on Pattern Analysis*. Baltimore: Williams & Wilkins, 1997;96

34. Weiss RA, Weiss MA. Sclerotherapy. In Wheeland RG, ed. *Cutaneous Surgery*. Philadelphia: WB Saunders Company, 1994:951–81

35. From L. Vascular neoplasms, pseudoneoplasms and hyperplasias. In Fitzpatrick TB, Eizen AZ, Wolff K, et al., eds. *Dermatology in General Medicine*. New York: McGraw-Hill, 1979;732

36. Scott C, Seiger E. Postsclerotherapy pigmentation. Is serum ferritin level an accurate indicator? *Dermatol Surg* 1997;23:281–3

37. Goldman MP, Sadick NS, Weiss RA. Cutaneous necrosis, telangiectactic matting and hyperpigmentation following sclerotherapy. Etiology, prevention and treatment. *Dermatol Surg* 1995;21:19–29

38. Alster TS. Laser treatment of vascular lesions. In Alster TS, ed. *Manual of Cutaneous Laser Techniques*. Philadelphia: Lippincott-Raven, 1997;27

39. Raulin C, Weiss RA, Schönermark MP. Treatment of essential telangiectasias with an intense pulsed light source. *Dermatol Surg* 1997;23:941–6

40. Waner M, Dinehart SM, Wilson MB, et al. A comparison of Cooper Vapor and Flashlamp Pumped Dye Lasers in the treatment of facial telangiectasia. *J Dermatol Surg Oncol* 1993;19:992–8

41. Hexsel DM. Manejo de cicatrizes pos-criocirurgia. In Stolar E, Turjansky E, eds. *Cryomedicine Argentina 1996*. Buenos Aires: Sociedad Argentina de Criocirugia, 1996:79–86

42. Rosio TJ. Revision of acne, traumatic, and surgical scars. In Wheeland RG, ed. *Cutaneous Surgery*. Philadelphia: WB Saunders Company, 1994:426–45

43. Ceilley RI. The treatment of hypertrophic scars and keloids. In Epstein E, Epstein E Jr, eds. *Skin Surgery*. Philadelphia: WB Saunders Company, 1987:580–9

44. Alster TS. Laser treatment of tattoos. In Alster TS, ed. *Manual of Cutaneous Laser Techniques*. Philadelphia: Lippincott-Raven, 1997:63–80

45. Orentreich D, Orentreich N. Acne scar revision update. *Dermatol Clin* 1987;5:359–68

46. Orentreich N, Durr NP. The four R's of skin rehabilitation. In Graham JAG, Kligman AM, eds. *The Psychology of Cosmetics Treatments*. New York: Praeger Scientific, 1985:227–37

47. Falabella R, Barona MI, Escobar C, et al. Surgical combination therapy for vitiligo and piebaldism. *Dermatol Surg* 1995;21:852–7

48. Suvanprakorn P, Dee-Ananlap S, Pongsomboon C, Klaus SN. Melanocyte autologous grafting for treatment of leucoderma. *J Am Acad Dermatol* 1985;13:968–74

49. Hann SK, Im S, Bong HW, Park YK. Treatment of stable vitiligo with autologous epidermal grafting and PUVA. *J Am Acad Dermatol* 1995;32:943–8

50. McGillis ST. Indications for and techniques of hair transplantation. In Wheeland RG, ed. *Cutaneous Surgery*. Philadelphia: WB Saunders Company, 1994:509–26

51. Brandy DA, Brandy KL. Hair replacement surgery. In Robinson JK, Kenneth AA, LeBoit PE, Wintroub BU, eds. *Atlas of Cutaneous Surgery*. Philadelphia: WB Saunders Company, 1996:281–93

52. Champion RH, Burton JL. Diagnosis of skin diseases. In Champion RH, Burton JL, Ebling FJG, eds. *Textbook of Dermatology*. Oxford: Blackwell Science, 1992:157–70

53. Pinkus H, Mehregan AH. Malformation and neoplasia. In Mehregan AH, ed. *A Guide to Dermatohistopathology*. New York: Appleton-Century-Crofts, 1976:590–621

Index

scalp biopsy 127–8
scarlet fever 269–72
    differential diagnosis, toxic shock syndrome 274
scarring, NICUs 54
scars 592–4
    stretch marks 589–90
    therapeutic techniques 592
SCC see carcinoma, squamous cell
Schistosoma spp. 299–300
    S. haematobium 299
        genital tract involvement 300
    S. japonicum 299
    S. mansoni 299
schistosomiasis 299–301
    perianal manifestation 370
Schnitzler's syndrome 218
SCLE see lupus erythematosus, subacute cutaneous
scleroderma
    en coup de sabre 209
    localized 209
    PBC association 244
    systemic (SSc) 206–8
        of childhood 207–9
        immunological markers 208
scleromyositis 212–13
    PM-Scl antibody association 214
sclerosing epithelial hamartoma see
        trichoepithelioma, desmoplastic
sclerosing periphlebitis of the chest wall
        see Mondor's disease
sclerosis
    systemic see systemic scleroderma
    tuberous, differential diagnosis, idiopathic
        guttate hypomelanosis 179
sclerotherapy 580–2
    sclerosant solutions 582
    telangiectasis 591, 593
    varicose veins 251
scoliosis, chondrodysplasia punctata 83, 90
Scopulariopsis brevicaulis infection,
        differential diagnosis, tinea unguium 286
scrofuloderma 454
scrub typhus diseases 275–6
sebaceous glands
    disorders 110–15
    ectopic 115
    hyperplasia 54, 76, 115
    structure and function, gender differences 109–10
seborrheic dermatitis see dermatitis
self-esteem 11–13
    alcoholism 504
    psychocutaneous diseases 14
    see also body image
Sennetsu fever 275
serotonin, selective serotonin reuptake
        inhibitors (SSRI) 15–16, 18, 21, 23
Sevestre and Jacquet syphiloid
        erythema 380, 383

sex hormone binding globulin (SHBG),
        hirsuties investigation 130
sexual abuse
    battered women 476
    children
        dermatological manifestations 481–3
        genitoanal lesions 482–3
        psychological and social impact 483
        vulvovaginal lesions 37
    date rape 477–9
    hymen examination 35
    prophylaxis 484–5
    psychological and medical impact 479–80
    PTSD 479–80
    rape 479
        marital 476–7
    STDs evaluation 484–5
sexually transmitted diseases (STDs) 303–16, 308–16
    African women 438
    alcohol consumption association 505–7
    bacterial infections 367
    children 483
    HIV 320–30
    Indian subcontinent 461
    oro-genital sexual tests 309–10
    rape 480
    screening questions 304
    serological testing 308
SHBG see sex hormone binding globulin
shoe fitting, onychodystrophy 122–3
sicca complex 354
    PBC association 244
sickle cell disease, parvovirus B19 278
silicone implants
    breasts 347
    facial 561–2
Simpson–Golabi–Bechmel syndrome,
        supernumerary nipple association 338
Sjögren's syndrome 354, 355
skeletal anomalies, supernumerary nipple
        association 338
skin
    African women 430
    African-American women 427–8
    appearance, birth 52
    appendages 76
    biopsy, drug eruptions 264
    Caucasian women 451
    cleansing 515
    color 75–6
        neonates 56
    grafts 593
    picking, BDD 17
    structure
        diseases, non-hereditary 109–59
        and function 49–51
    tags, pregnancy 65
    thickness